W9-ARC-798

The National Medical Series for Independent Study

3rd edition
medicine

Allen R. Myers, M.D.

Professor of Medicine
Temple University School of Medicine
Attending Physician
Temple University Hospital
Philadelphia, Pennsylvania

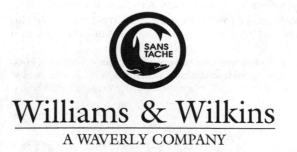

Williams & Wilkins
A WAVERLY COMPANY

BALTIMORE • PHILADELPHIA • LONDON • PARIS • BANGKOK
BUENOS AIRES • HONG KONG • MUNICH • SYDNEY • TOKYO • WROCLAW

Editor: Elizabeth A. Nieginski
Managing Editor: Amy G. Dinkel
Development Editor: Melanie Cann
Production Coordinator: Felecia R. Weber
Copy Editor: Patricia Nale
Cover Designer: Cathy Cotter
Typesetter: Maryland Composition
Printer: Port City Press
Binder: Port City Press

Copyright © 1997 Williams & Wilkins

351 West Camden Street
Baltimore, Maryland 21201-2436 USA

Rose Tree Corporate Center
1400 North Providence Road
Building II, Suite 5025
Media, Pennsylvania 19063-2043 USA

All rights reserved. This book is protected by copyright. No part of this book may be reproduced in any form or by any means, including photocopying, or utilized by any information storage and retrieval system without written permission from the copyright owner.

Accurate indications, adverse reactions and dosage schedules for drugs are provided in this book, but it is possible that they may change. The reader is urged to review the package information data of the manufacturers of the medications mentioned.

Printed in the United States of America

Third Edition.

Library of Congress Cataloging-in-Publication Data

Medicine / [edited by] Allen R. Myers. — 3rd ed.
     p.   cm. — (National medical series)
  Includes index.
  ISBN 0-683-18105-X
  1. Internal medicine—Outlines, syllabi, etc. 2. Internal medicine—Examinations, questions, etc. I. Myers, Allen R.
II. Series: National medical series for independent study.
  [DNLM: 1. Internal Medicine—examination questions. 2. Internal Medicine—outlines. WB 18.2 M489 1997]
RC59.M44 1997
616'.0076—dc20
DNLM/DLC   96-13091
for Library of Congress   CIP

The publishers have made every effort to trace the copyright holders for borrowed material. If they have inadvertently overlooked any, they will be pleased to make the necessary arrangements at the first opportunity.

To purchase additional copies of this book, call our customer service department at **(800) 638-0672** or fax orders to **(800) 447-8438.** For other book services, including chapter reprints and large-quantity sales, ask for the Special Sales department.

Canadian customers should call **(800) 268-4178,** or fax **(905) 470-6780.** For all other calls originating outside of the United States, please call **(410) 528-4223** or fax us at **(410) 528-8550.**

Visit Williams & Wilkins on the Internet: http://www.wwilkins.com or contact our customer service department at **custserv@wwilkins.com.** Williams & Wilkins customer service representatives are available from 8:30 am to 6:00 pm, EST, Monday through Friday, for telephone access.

97 98 99
1 2 3 4 5 6 7 8 9 10

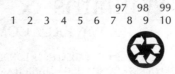

28⁹⁵

3rd edition
medicine

Dedication

To Rosina and Ellis Myers, for having the foresight to point me in the right direction, one of lasting interest and absolute joy.

To Ellen Myers, for journeying with me and being a superb partner.

To David, Rob, and Scott, for their inspiration.

To my teachers, for stimulating my interest, sharing their knowledge, and being excellent role models.

To Bobby Clarke, Brooks Robinson, and Johnny Unitas, for demonstrating that indomitable spirit and commitment that made them the winners they are.

To the legions of hardworking and inquisitive medical students and residents who constantly seek knowledge in their quest for clinical excellence.

Contents

11   Neurologic Disorders   595

Comprehensive Exam   661

Case Studies in Clinical Decision Making   693

Index   719

Contributors

E. Victor Adlin, M.D.
Associate Professor of Medicine
Endocrinology and Metabolism Section
Department of Medicine
Temple University School of Medicine
Attending Physician
Temple University Hospital
Philadelphia, Pennsylvania

Blase A. Carabello, M.D.
Charles Ezra Daniel Professor of Cardiology
Cardiology Division, Department of Medicine
Medical University of South Carolina School of
    Medicine
Attending Physician
Ralph Johnson Veterans Administration Medical
    Center
Charleston, South Carolina

Douglas C. Conaway, M.D.
Associate Professor of Medicine
Section of Rheumatology
Department of Medicine
Temple University School of Medicine
Attending Physician
Temple University Hospital
Philadelphia, Pennsylvania

Anthony J. DiMarino, Jr., M.D.
Professor of Medicine
Thomas Jefferson Medical College
Chief, Division of Gastroenterology
Thomas Jefferson University Hospital
Philadelphia, Pennsylvania

Thomas Fekete, M.D.
Associate Professor of Medicine
Infectious Diseases Section
Department of Medicine
Temple University School of Medicine
Attending Physician
Temple University Hospital
Philadelphia, Pennsylvania

Stanley B. Fiel, M.D.
Chief, Pulmonary and Critical Care Medicine
Department of Medicine
Medical College of Pennsylvania and
    Hahnemann University
Attending Physician
Medical College Hospital and
    Hahnemann University Hospital
Philadelphia, Pennsylvania

Stanley Goldfarb, M.D.
Clinical Professor of Medicine
University of Pennsylvania School of Medicine
Vice President for Patient Care, Education, and
    Research
Graduate Health System
Philadelphia, Pennsylvania

Donald P. Goldsmith, M.D.
Professor of Pediatrics
Temple University School of Medicine
Chief, Section of Rheumatology and Allergy
St. Christopher's Hospital for Children
Philadelphia, Pennsylvania

Donna Glover, M.D.
Associate Clinical Professor of Medicine
University of Pennsylvania School of Medicine
Chief, Division of Hematology and Oncology
Presbyterian University of Pennsylvania Medical
    Center
Philadelphia, Pennsylvania

Allen R. Myers, M.D.
Professor of Medicine
Temple University School of Medicine
Attending Physician
Temple University Hospital
Philadelphia, Pennsylvania

Ronald N. Rubin, M.D.
Professor of Medicine
Hematology Section
Department of Medicine
Temple University School of Medicine
Chief, Clinical Hematology
Temple University Hospital
Philadelphia, Pennsylvania

Barney J. Stern, M.D.
Professor of Neurology
Emory University School of Medicine
Chief of Clinical Services
Section of Neurology
The Emory Clinic
Atlanta, Georgia

Fuad N. Ziyadeh, M.D.
Associate Professor of Medicine
Renal Electrolyte and Hypertension Division
University of Pennsylvania School of Medicine
Attending Physician
Hospital of the University of Pennsylvania
VA Medical Center
Philadelphia, Pennsylvania

Preface

The easiest and surest way of acquiring facts is to learn them in groups, in systems, and systematized knowledge is science. You can very often carry two facts fastened together more easily than one by itself. . . .
—Oliver Wendell Holmes, "Scholastic and Bedside Teaching" from *Medical Essays*

In the natural method of teaching, the student begins with the patient, continues with the patient, and ends his studies with the patient, using books and lectures as tools, as means to an end.
—William Osler, 1901

Internal medicine is a vast and complicated field that is based upon strong scientific and clinical foundations. While certain pedagogical learning is unavoidable, an understanding of basic sciences, particularly pathophysiology, allows some meaning to be made of seemingly unrelated facts.

Any effort to provide a comprehensive review of internal medicine is destined to fall short of its goal. Despite this limitation, the authors have provided a framework for a working knowledge of internal medicine. It is not all-inclusive but nonetheless provides the essentials of the subject in an easily read and well-organized format. By necessity, NMS *Medicine* must be used as a companion to more extensive texts and monographs, but it can be considered a starting point. Internal medicine cannot be fully learned in a year or two, or in a lifetime, but its essence can be appreciated by students and house officers.

Medicine has been written primarily for students and residents. However, the authors believe it also can be used by all others who deal with patients who have medical illnesses.

This third edition has been extensively updated. The study questions with explanations are maintained as an aid to learning. The section on problem-solving exercises has been expanded in order to help the student develop clinical reasoning skills. The result of our efforts is a "user-friendly" review of internal medicine that enhances the educational process.

Allen R. Myers

Acknowledgments

The editor and contributing authors are grateful to Williams & Wilkins, particularly to Melanie Cann for her guidance and outstanding editorial contributions. The editor is also indebted to Anne Lewis and Betty Berdel for the invaluable, multidimensional assistance they provide, and for their enduring support.

Chapter 1

Cardiovascular Diseases

Blase A. Carabello

I. **CONGESTIVE HEART FAILURE**

A. **Definition.** Congestive heart failure is the inability of the heart, working at normal or elevated filling pressure, to pump enough blood to meet the oxygen requirements of the body tissues. Congestive heart failure should never be considered a diagnosis. Rather, it is a syndrome resulting from many diseases that interfere with cardiac function. In acting as a muscular pump the heart does only two things: it contracts (systole) and it relaxes (diastole). Therefore, heart failure can result from only two broad abnormalities—systolic dysfunction and diastolic dysfunction.

B. **Etiology**

1. **Systolic dysfunction.** Systole is governed by two cardiac properties, **contractility**—the ability of myocardium to generate force, and **afterload**—the force against which the heart must contract.
   a. **Decreased contractility.** Most cases of congestive heart failure occur when an insult to the myocardium reduces its ability to generate force, thus reducing its contractility.
      (1) **Myocardial infarction.** In myocardial infarction, a portion of the myocardium undergoes necrosis and can no longer generate force, resulting in weakening of the ventricle. If extensive areas of the myocardium are infarcted, congestive heart failure results.
      (2) **Valvular heart disease** results in stenosis or regurgitation of the cardiac valves, which places a **pressure** or **volume overload,** respectively, on the ventricles. Initially, compensatory mechanisms [see I B 1 c] accommodate these overloads and maintain normal cardiac output at acceptable filling pressure. However, eventually these mechanisms fail and heart failure ensues.
      (3) **Hypertension.** Many patients who develop congestive heart failure have had systemic hypertension at some time in the clinical course of their illness. **Persistent severe hypertension** is associated with a **contractile deficit** that leads to congestive heart failure.
      (4) **Cardiomyopathies** are diseases that directly injure the myocardium.
         (a) **Toxic.** Substances directly toxic to the myocardium (e.g., ethanol, cobalt, catecholamines) may damage its force-generating ability. Prolonged exposure to these agents may lead to the development of congestive heart failure.
         (b) **Idiopathic.** When the contractile function of the myocardium fails in the absence of a known etiology, a viral cause often is implied but frequently cannot be proven.
         (c) **Infiltrative diseases.** Infiltration of the myocardium by a variety of substances (e.g., amyloid) may reduce contractility.
   b. **Increased afterload.** Increasing the afterload makes it harder for the ventricular muscle fibers to shorten, reducing cardiac output. Afterload can be quantified by calculating the systolic force on the myocardium using the Laplace equation for stress:

$$\text{Stress} = (\text{pressure} \times \text{radius})/(2 \times \text{thickness})$$

Thus, disease states that increase either the systolic pressure (hypertension, aortic stenosis) or chamber radius (dilated cardiomyopathy, valvular regurgitation) increase afterload unless the wall thickness increases proportionately.

    c. **Compensatory mechanisms** develop in response to the ventricular pressure and volume overload that accompany decreased contractility.

      (1) The **Frank-Starling mechanism** is activated when reduced ventricular emptying results in more volume retained in the ventricles at the end of systole, which leads to a greater volume at the end of diastole. Increased end-diastolic volume increases sarcomere stretch, which increases the number of systolic actin–myosin crossbridges that develop. The increased number of crossbridges increases the strength of contraction.

      (2) **Cardiac hypertrophy** provides additional muscle mass to bear the burden of various overloads.

      (3) **Adrenergic stimulation** by endogenous catecholamines increases the inotropic state.

2. Diastolic dysfunction. Diastole is governed by **active** and **passive** properties. Active relaxation occurs early in diastole as calcium is pumped out of the myocardium, resulting in the near cessation of actin–myosin crossbridge interaction. Passive relaxation occurs as the mitral valve opens, allowing the blood stored in the atria to fill the ventricles.

    a. **Abnormalities in active relaxation.** Active relaxation is impaired when there is delay in calcium reuptake at the beginning of diastole. Myocardial ischemia and ventricular hypertrophy are two common causes of impaired active relaxation.

    b. **Abnormalities of passive relaxation.** Passive relaxation is impaired when the myocardium is stiffer than normal. Stiffness is defined as a change in pressure (ΔP) per unit change in volume (ΔV), or $\Delta P/\Delta V$. When stiffness is increased, any change in volume requires or causes a greater increase in pressure. Thus, in order to fill the heart to an adequate volume, high filling pressure occurs, which in turn leads to pulmonary and systemic congestion. Increased passive stiffness of the ventricles occurs when concentric hypertrophy causes the chamber wall to be thicker than normal as might occur in hypertension or when the myocardium is infiltrated by abnormal substances such as amyloid.

C. **Descriptive terminology**

1. High-output failure is characterized by cardiac output that may be several times higher than normal but still is not adequate to maintain tissue perfusion needs or, if adequate, is maintained with a higher than normal filling pressure. A classic example of high-output failure is **chronic severe anemia,** which causes a reduced oxygen-carrying capacity. In chronic severe anemia, the following occurs:

    a. Compensation is provided by increased forward cardiac output, which is facilitated by cardiac enlargement, decreased total peripheral resistance, and increased venous return to the heart.

    b. This causes a volume overload of ventricles.

    c. Eventually, the demands on the heart lead to cardiac failure; cardiac output, although high, still is not adequate to meet the circulatory demands placed on the heart by the anemia. Some other causes of high output failure include arteriovenous fistula, beriberi, and thyrotoxicosis.

2. Left-sided failure indicates that the left ventricle is the failing chamber. A disease that primarily affects the left ventricle (e.g., myocardial infarction) may reduce its contractile force, while the right ventricle continues to pump normally. Thus, left ventricular failure can occur without right ventricular failure.

3. Right-sided failure indicates that the right ventricle has failed, either as a result of left ventricular failure, or in isolation from the left ventricle.

    a. The **most common cause** of right ventricular failure **is left ventricular failure.** When left ventricular failure occurs, the filling pressure in the left ventricle becomes elevated, increasing the work load of the right ventricle (the chamber responsible for filling the left ventricle). Thus overtaxed, the right ventricle eventually fails also.

    b. The right ventricle also may fail in isolation from the left ventricle. In the presence of **chronic obstructive pulmonary disease (COPD),** increased pulmonary vascular resistance develops as a result of architectural changes in the lungs. The increased pulmonary vascular resistance, in turn, produces a pressure overload on the right ventricle, which leads to increased right ventricular work and eventual failure. Pulmonary embolism and primary pulmonary hypertension are some other causes of right-sided failure.

D. **Clinical features**

1. **Symptoms**
   a. **Dyspnea** is the most frequently encountered symptom of congestive heart failure.
      (1) The feeling of breathlessness is caused by **vascular congestion,** which reduces pulmonary oxygenation. In addition, the vascular congestion diminishes lung compliance, increasing the work of breathing, thus adding to the feeling of breathlessness.
      (2) Dyspnea also results from **reduced cardiac output to the periphery,** which triggers the symptom through neurohumoral mechanisms. In the early stages of congestive heart failure, dyspnea occurs only with exertion. As heart failure progresses, the amount of exertion required to produce dyspnea becomes progressively less until dyspnea may occur at rest.
   b. **Orthopnea** refers to dyspnea that occurs in the recumbent position and is relieved by elevation of the head. Orthopnea results from volume pooling in the central vasculature during recumbency, which leads to increased cardiac volume and, in turn, to increased left ventricular filling pressure, pulmonary congestion, and the feeling of dyspnea. The physician may gauge the degree of orthopnea by noting the number of pillows the patient uses to sleep. However, it should be recognized that many patients chronically sleep on more than one pillow out of habit, not because of breathlessness. **Nocturnal cough,** which has the same pathophysiology as orthopnea, may occur together with, or instead of, nocturnal dyspnea.
   c. **Paroxysmal nocturnal dyspnea** is the occurrence of sudden dyspnea that awakens the patient from sleep. Like orthopnea, it occurs during recumbency as a result of pooling in the central vasculature, which increases left ventricular filling pressure. Paroxysmal nocturnal dyspnea may occur in the orthopneic patient who inadvertently slips off the pillows used to elevate the upper body. Usually, the patient awakens from sleep and feels the need to sit upright or to go to an open window for increased ventilation. The symptom usually subsides after the patient has been in the upright position for 5–20 minutes.
   d. **Nocturia** develops in congestive heart failure as a result of increased renal blood flow when the patient is recumbent and asleep.
      (1) **During the day,** when the skeletal muscles are active, limited cardiac output is shifted away from the kidney toward the skeletal musculature. The kidney interprets this reduction in blood flow as **hypovolemia** and becomes sodium avid via activation of the **renin–angiotensin system.**
      (2) **At night,** when the patient is at rest, cardiac output is shifted toward the kidney and diuresis ensues.
   e. **Edema.** There are many causes of peripheral edema, several of which are noncardiac. **Cardiac edema** occurs when the systemic hydrostatic venous pressure is greater than the systemic oncotic venous pressure. Thus, cardiac edema is a sign of **right-sided failure;** it occurs because of the increased systemic venous pressure that results from right ventricular dysfunction.
   f. **Anorexia** may occur as a late manifestation of congestive heart failure. The exact mechanism leading to anorexia is unknown, but the occurrence of anorexia seems to correlate with hepatic congestion and right-sided failure.

2. **Physical signs**
   a. **Tachycardia** occurs in heart failure due to increased release of catecholamines as a compensatory mechanism for maintaining cardiac output in the presence

of decreased stroke volume. Catecholamines increase both the force and the rate of cardiac contraction.

b. Pulmonary rales. The increased left ventricular filling pressure associated with congestive heart failure is referred to the left atrium and pulmonary veins. The increased hydrostatic pressure produces transudation of fluid into the alveoli. As air circulates through the alveoli, crackling sounds (rales) are produced. It is important to note that there are multiple causes of pulmonary rales; the mere presence of rales does not necessarily indicate congestive heart failure.

c. Cardiac enlargement. As the failing heart relies more and more on the Frank-Starling mechanism, it dilates and may develop eccentric hypertrophy. In the presence of cardiac enlargement, the left ventricle's point of maximal impulse (PMI) is shifted downward and to the left. This shift is detected during a physical examination of the patient. Although much of the cardiac examination should be performed in the left lateral decubitus position, this position may artifactually shift the PMI. Thus, the PMI should be established with the patient lying supine.

d. Fourth heart sound (S_4). Patients in sinus rhythm and heart failure often have an S_4 (atrial gallop). The S_4 is produced as left atrial systole propels volume into the left ventricle just prior to ventricular systole. In congestive heart failure, the left ventricle is noncompliant and the S_4 probably results from the reverberation of the blood ejected from the left atrium into the left ventricle. In elderly patients, however, an S_4 may indicate reduced compliance of the stiff left ventricle as a result of aging rather than heart failure. The S_4 also may be heard over the right ventricle in right ventricular failure.

e. Third heart sound (S_3). An S_3 **(ventricular gallop),** which occurs early in diastole, probably is the single most **reliable sign of left heart failure** revealed during physical examination. The S_3 occurs during rapid filling of the left ventricle. Increased left atrial pressure (which propels the blood forward with increased force) and noncompliance of the left ventricle are two important factors in the production of this extra sound. While an S_3 is a reliable sign of heart failure in individuals over the age of 40, a similar sound may be heard in young, healthy athletes as a normal finding.

f. Neck vein distention. The neck veins can be considered manometers attached to the right atrium and, as such, reflect right atrial pressure.

(1) When the right ventricle fails, it relies increasingly on the Frank-Starling mechanism for compensation. This results in increased right ventricular volume and pressure, which is referred back to the right atrium.

(2) To estimate central venous pressure in cm H_2O, the patient's back is elevated or lowered so the point demarcating the distended from the nondistended portion of the neck vein can be discerned clearly. The vertical height is measured from this point to the manubrium. The average depth of the right atrium inside the chest cavity (5 cm) is added to the height of the neck vein. This sum approximates the right atrial pressure.

g. Edema. Lower extremity and presacral edema occur in right-sided failure as increased venous pressure results in transudation of fluid into these areas. For edema to be attributable to congestive heart failure, distended neck veins indicative of elevated right-sided filling pressure also should be present.

h. Ascites. Transudation of fluid into the **peritoneal space** also may occur as a result of increased systemic venous pressure. When ascites is caused by congestive heart failure, the neck veins typically are elevated, and the liver is distended from passive congestion.

E. **Diagnosis**

1. Etiologic approach. Because congestive heart failure is a syndrome that results from a disease, the management of congestive heart failure must focus on the cause of the heart failure, not simply on relieving the symptoms. Although a careful history and physical examination of the patient are the most important tools available in arriving at a diagnosis, in many cases a diagnosis may not be reached. In these instances, the following studies often are helpful.

a. The **electrocardiogram (ECG)** frequently is nonspecific. However, the presence of Q waves helps to confirm that myocardial infarction has been the cause of the patient's congestive heart failure.

b. The **chest radiograph** is useful in demonstrating cardiac chamber enlargement and in documenting congestion in the lungs. It provides objective evidence that heart failure is present.

c. The **echocardiogram** is useful in identifying chamber enlargement and in quantifying left ventricular function and valvular function. The most commonly employed descriptor of ventricular function is the **ejection fraction,** which is the percentage of the end-diastolic volume expelled during systole. For example, if a patient's end-diastolic volume is 150 ml and the stroke volume is 100 ml, then 67% (100/150) of the diastolic contents was ejected.

   (1) The end-diastolic and stroke volumes can be estimated from the echocardiogram.

   (2) Ejection fractions between 55% and 76% are normal.

d. **Doppler interrogation** measures the direction and acceleration of blood flow through the cardiac chambers and great vessels. This technique is useful for detecting blood flow moving in an abnormal direction, which is characteristic of valvular regurgitation and intracardiac shunts. In addition, Doppler interrogation can detect and quantify valvular stenoses by measuring how much acceleration is necessary to maintain constant blood flow through a stenotic valve.

e. **Radionuclide ventriculography** is used to measure right and left ventricular ejection fraction. It is an excellent noninvasive procedure to use when it is necessary to quantify precisely the degree of cardiac dysfunction present.

f. During **cardiac catheterization,** intracardiac pressures, chamber size, valvular stenosis, valvular regurgitation, and coronary anatomy can be evaluated. Often this is the **most accurate method for determining a specific cardiac diagnosis.** However, unlike the noninvasive tests mentioned above, catheterization has a small but finite risk. Therefore, cardiac catheterization is performed in congestive heart failure patients when the additional information the procedure provides is necessary for proper patient management. For example, cardiac catheterization is often necessary to help determine whether valve replacement will correct heart failure in a patient with valvular heart disease.

2. **Symptomatic approach.** In cases in which the definitive etiology is not thought to be important in the management of congestive heart failure (e.g., a patient with terminal cancer), some objective evidence of cardiac dysfunction is still advisable prior to therapy. Frequently, a patient with dyspnea on exertion and orthopnea is treated for congestive heart failure, but the symptoms have another cause. The chest x-ray and echocardiogram are useful adjuncts to the physical examination in providing objective evidence of cardiac dysfunction prior to therapy and also for gauging the effects of therapy.

F. Therapy

1. **Etiologic therapy.** It is important, when possible, to direct therapy at the etiologic agent responsible for the congestive heart failure. For example, if aortic stenosis is the cause of congestive heart failure, aortic valve replacement is the most effective therapy.

2. **Symptomatic therapy.** If the etiologic agent cannot be found, if the patient's condition does not permit direct intervention, or if the patient refuses to consider corrective surgery even if indicated, the physician must resort to therapy aimed at relieving the symptoms of heart failure.

   a. **Increasing the contractile state.** Contractile dysfunction is the most common mechanism producing heart failure; therefore, increasing the contractile state may result in symptomatic improvement. These therapies are not indicated in the treatment of pure diastolic dysfunction where contractile function is normal.

(1) Cardiac glycosides (e.g., **digoxin**) increase the contractile state by impeding the Na^+-K^+-ATPase–controlled intracellular pump. This results in the net influx of calcium into the myocardium, which increases contractile strength. The efficacy of cardiac glycosides in the chronic treatment of congestive heart failure is controversial. Although digoxin is used frequently in the United States, it does not form the mainstay of therapy in other countries, such as Great Britain. However, recent studies have found that heart failure worsens when the drug is discontinued, evidence that supports its efficacy.

(2) β-Adrenergic agonists (e.g., **catecholamines**) increase contractile function by increasing the production of cyclic adenosine monophosphate (cAMP), which results in increased myocardial calcium release. In end-stage heart failure, intravenous infusion of dobutamine for several days may help to restore and maintain pump performance even after the infusion is discontinued. The mechanism of this therapy's effectiveness is not well understood.

(3) Phosphodiesterase inhibitors increase contractile function by inhibiting the breakdown of cAMP. Cardiac-specific phosphodiesterase inhibitors include **amrinone** and **milrinone.** These agents act to enhance the inotropic state and reduce afterload by causing vasodilation. Currently, they are administered by intravenous infusion and are for short-term use only.

b. Reducing afterload. Agents that cause arteriolar dilatation reduce impedance of the outflow of blood from the left ventricle. By diminishing total peripheral resistance, cardiac output rises because the left ventricle can eject more completely against a lower afterload. The net effect is increased cardiac output without a serious fall in blood pressure, leading to symptomatic improvement.

(1) Currently, several **vasodilators** are used in the treatment of congestive heart failure to reduce afterload, including **angiotensin-converting enzyme (ACE) inhibitors** (e.g., **captopril, enalapril, lisinopril**), **nitrates,** and **hydralazine.**

(2) The combination of an ACE inhibitor, diuretic, and digoxin has been shown to reduce mortality associated with congestive heart failure and to extend the life span by 6 months to 1 year.

c. Reducing preload and left ventricular filling pressure. The increased preload resulting from volume retention in the ventricles is a compensatory mechanism that helps increase forward cardiac output by use of the Frank-Starling mechanism; however, an excessive increase in preload is associated with an increase in left ventricular and right ventricular filling pressures, which is responsible for symptoms of pulmonary and systemic congestion. Judicious reduction in filling pressures without excessive reduction in preload is indicated in the therapy of congestive heart failure.

(1) Diuretics reduce renal tubular absorption of sodium and water and increase the clearance of these substances from the body. The result is a reduction in central volume and in cardiac filling pressure.

(2) Vasodilators, which increase the capacity of the systemic venous system, transfer central volume to the periphery, thus reducing central preload and filling pressure. The nitrates and ACE inhibitors are effective as preload-reducing vasodilators.

d. Use of β-blocking agents. Because stimulation of the β receptor increases the force of cardiac contraction, β agonists have been used in the therapy of congestive heart failure [see I F 2 a (2)]. Paradoxically, cautious use of β-receptor antagonists has also been effective in reversing the same syndrome. The mechanism of action for this class of agents in the treatment of heart failure probably stems from protection of the heart from the toxic effects of prolonged exposure to the high levels of circulating catecholamines present in congestive heart failure.

e. Physical conditioning is an important adjunct to the medical treatment of congestive heart failure. Physical conditioning permits the peripheral tissues to use cardiac output more efficiently. Thus, the patient experiences an increase in tolerance to physical activity without an increase in cardiac output.

f. Cardiac transplantation may offer an improved quality of life to selected patients in whom control of congestive heart failure is not possible and prognosis is poor. The increasingly effective use of the immunosuppressive agent cyclosporine has greatly increased the success of this avenue of therapy. Currently, approximately 75% of patients undergoing cardiac transplantation achieve a 5-year survival rate. The paucity of cardiac donors is the primary factor limiting the use of this therapy.

3. **Therapy for cases involving pulmonary edema.** Pulmonary edema is the most extreme example of congestive heart failure, in which profound transudation of fluid into the pulmonary alveoli occurs because of a high left ventricular filling pressure. The result is impaired oxygenation and, if untreated, death. The goal of therapy is to improve oxygenation, to reduce left ventricular filling pressure, and to increase forward cardiac output.

   a. Oxygen therapy is a mainstay in the treatment of acute pulmonary edema. Oxygen should be administered by face mask, because patients in pulmonary edema are so dyspneic that they breathe primarily through their mouths.

   b. Diuretics. Furosemide probably is the single most commonly used medication in the treatment of acute pulmonary edema. This rapid-acting loop diuretic promotes an immediate diuresis in most cases.

   c. Morphine sulfate reduces patient anxiety, which may help to relieve the arterial vasoconstriction often present in acute pulmonary edema. This, in turn, helps to increase forward cardiac output. Morphine also is a venodilator and, therefore, acts to reduce central volume and left ventricular filling pressure.

   d. Other vasodilators. Nitroglycerine (administered sublingually or intravenously) or **nitroprusside** (administered intravenously) often is effective in treating pulmonary edema when other therapies fail. These drugs reduce central volume by venodilation and also increase cardiac output secondary to arteriolar vasodilation. However, the potent vasodilating ability of these drugs requires that blood pressure be monitored constantly during their administration in order to avoid hypotension.

   e. Intubation and positive-pressure ventilation. If the patient's oxygenation does not improve rapidly with the above therapies, intubation may be necessary to provide mechanical ventilation and to improve oxygenation.

   f. Cardiac glycosides are effective in increasing cardiac contractile function, which is beneficial in the treatment of heart failure. In the setting of acute pulmonary edema, however, these drugs provide only adjunctive therapy because symptomatic improvement usually occurs before the digitalis glycosides have a chance to take effect.

   g. Invasive hemodynamic monitoring. Most cases of pulmonary edema resolve quickly, making invasive hemodynamic unnecessary. However, in cases of recalcitrant pulmonary edema with severe cardiac compromise, exact knowledge of intracardiac filling pressure may be useful in guiding therapy. Hemodynamic monitoring (via Swan-Ganz catheterization) provides this information so that optimal filling pressure and cardiac output may be obtained.

II. CARDIAC ARRHYTHMIAS

A. Introduction. Bradyarrhythmias result from inadequate sinus nodal impulse production or from blocked impulse propagation and usually are not cause for concern unless the patient develops syncope or presyncope. Sustained atrial tachyarrhythmias usually permit adequate cardiac output and are less dangerous than sustained ventricular arrhythmias, which often cause collapse or death.

B. Atrial tachyarrhythmias. The atrial tachyarrhythmias can be classified into two subcategories, those that produce a regular cardiac rhythm and those that produce an irregular cardiac rhythm. In general, atrial tachyarrhythmias do not interfere with inter- or in-

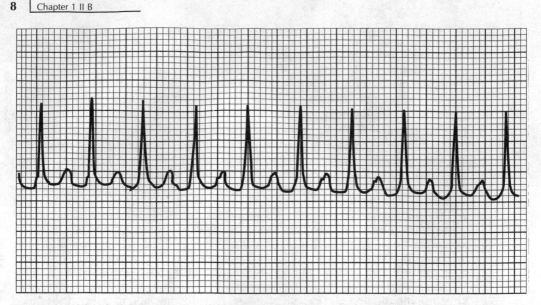

FIGURE 1-1. This rhythm strip demonstrates an episode of paroxysmal atrial tachycardia. The QRS complexes are narrow, and the heart rate is 165 bpm. The P waves are hidden in the T waves.

traventricular conduction of the cardiac impulse and therefore, the QRS complex (which is generated from the ventricles) remains narrow in form. Occasionally, however, atrial arrhythmias cause aberrant ventricular conduction with a wide QRS complex, which may mimic arrhythmias of ventricular origin.

1. Regular atrial tachycardias
   a. Sinus tachycardia. Sinus tachycardia represents a physiologic or pathophysiologic increase in the sinus rate ($\geq$ 100 bpm) and is often secondary to some other disease process. In general, the physician should treat the condition that is causing the sinus tachycardia, not the tachycardia itself. However, in some patients, such as those suffering from coronary artery disease, sinus tachycardia must be controlled to prevent myocardial ischemia. In this instance, β-blocking agents or calcium antagonists (either verapamil or diltiazem) may be effective in controlling heart rate.
   b. Paroxysmal atrial tachycardia. As the name implies, this arrhythmia is of sudden onset. This condition often exists in patients with otherwise normal hearts and is characterized by a heart rate of 150–250 bpm.
      (1) ECG identification. As demonstrated in the rhythm strip shown in Figure 1-1, the P waves are often not visible because they are buried in the QRS complex or the T wave.
      (2) Therapy
         (a) Therapies should be administered in a **quiet setting,** and the patient should be made as comfortable as possible, to reduce sympathetic discharge. As in the therapy of all arrhythmias, countershock may be necessary if the patient is hemodynamically unstable or if the arrhythmia has caused worsening of angina or congestive heart failure.
         (b) Because **most episodes** of paroxysmal atrial tachycardia are **secondary to electrical reentry around the atrioventricular (AV) node,** therapies that increase vagal tone usually succeed in halting the arrhythmia.
            (i) Mechanical maneuvers such as **carotid sinus massage,** the **Valsalva maneuver,** and **head immersion in cold water** are often effective in terminating the arrhythmia.
            (ii) Medical therapy includes the intravenous administration of **verapamil, esmolol, digoxin,** or **adenosine.**

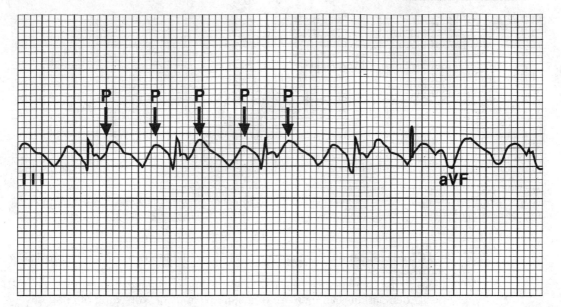

FIGURE 1-2. An episode of atrial flutter with 2:1 AV block is demonstrated. Note the frequency of the P waves, which represent the depolarization of the atria.

    c. Atrial flutter with constant conduction usually occurs in patients with anteced-ent heart disease, including coronary artery disease, pericarditis, valvular heart disease, and cardiomyopathy. Atrial flutter is characterized by an atrial rate of 240–400 bpm and is usually conducted to the ventricle with block so that the ventricular rate is a fraction of the atrial rate.

      (1) ECG identification. As shown in Figure 1-2, this arrhythmia produces a clas-sic sawtooth pattern on the ECG. In this example, there is 2:1 AV block with an atrial rate of 240 bpm and a ventricular rate of 120 bpm.

      (2) Therapy

        (a) Although intravenous administration of **digoxin, esmolol,** or **verapamil** may be effective in converting the arrhythmia to normal sinus rhythm, conversion is less likely than in paroxysmal atrial tachycardia. Usually these medications serve to control the ventricular response, which, in turn, helps to maintain hemodynamic stability. Once the ventricular rate has slowed as a result of increased AV block (3:1 or 4:1 conduc-tion), **quinidine** or other antiarrhythmic agents can be administered to restore sinus rhythm.

        (b) If medical therapy does not convert the patient to normal sinus rhythm, atrial flutter will usually convert itself over time, either to atrial fibrilla-tion or normal sinus rhythm.

        (c) As in all arrhythmias, **direct current (DC) cardioversion** is necessary if the arrhythmia has already produced hemodynamic instability.

  2. Irregular atrial tachycardias

    a. Atrial fibrillation. Atrial fibrillation is an **irregularly irregular** arrhythmia in which there is no ordered contraction of the atria but rather, multiple discoordi-nate wave fronts of depolarization that send a large number of irregular impul-ses to depolarize the AV node. The irregular impulses produce an irregular ven-tricular response, the rate of which depends on the number of impulses that are conducted through the AV node. Selected causes of atrial fibrillation include stress, fever, excessive alcohol intake, volume depletion, pericarditis, coronary artery disease, myocardial infarction, pulmonary embolism, mitral valve dis-ease, thyrotoxicosis, and idiopathic (lone) atrial fibrillation.

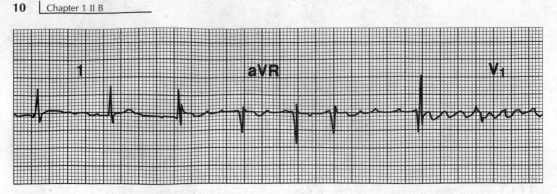

FIGURE 1-3. The irregularly irregular pattern of atrial fibrillation is demonstrated on this strip. Note the coarse fibrillatory waves in lead V_1. Although these could be confused with flutter waves, they are too irregular to be atrial flutter.

(1) ECG identification. An example of atrial fibrillation is shown in Figure 1-3.
(2) Therapy
    (a) If the patient with atrial fibrillation is hemodynamically unstable or demonstrates an increase in angina pectoris or worsening of congestive heart failure, immediate DC synchronous cardioversion is indicated.
    (b) If the patient is hemodynamically stable, the physician should first focus on controlling the ventricular response to the atrial fibrillation while simultaneously treating the cause of the arrhythmia. The ventricular response may be controlled by the intravenous administration of digoxin, verapamil, diltiazem, or esmolol.
    (c) Once the ventricular response has been controlled, cardioversion to sinus rhythm may be spontaneous or it may be induced by the oral administration of quinidine or by DC synchronous cardioversion.
    (d) If the atrial fibrillation has been present for more than 1 week prior to cardioversion, the risk of intra-atrial thrombus, and therefore, embolization, increases.
        (i) Many authorities advocate anticoagulation therapy for 10 days or longer prior to either pharmacologic or electrical cardioversion.
        (ii) An alternative strategy undergoing intensive investigation is the use of transesophageal echocardiography to image the left atrium and its appendage. If no thrombus is present, anticoagulation with heparin is begun and cardioversion is performed 24–48 hours later. Anticoagulation is then continued for up to 4 weeks. Post-cardioversion anticoagulation is advantageous because atrial mechanical activity often lags behind restoration of normal electrical activity, potentiating thrombus formation. Post-cardioversion anticoagulation is required whether or not pre-cardioversion anticoagulation is employed.
  b. Multifocal atrial tachycardia. In this arrhythmia, there is synchronous atrial contraction, but the contraction arises from many sites in the atria, not from the sinus node. In the majority of cases of multifocal atrial tachycardia, the patient has severe antecedent pulmonary disease.
    (1) ECG identification. The multiple sites of origin of the atrial contraction produce many different P wave configurations and different R-R intervals. At least three different P wave morphologies are required to make this diagnosis.
    (2) Therapy for multifocal atrial tachycardia is directed primarily at improving the patient's oxygenation, ventilation, and airway mechanics. If these measures fail, **verapamil** may be useful in controlling the heart rate.
  c. Atrial flutter with irregular conduction. If atrial flutter is conducted with varying block, the rhythm will be irregular. This arrhythmia is treated identically to atrial flutter with constant block [see II B 1 c (2) (a)–(c)].

C. **Bradyarrhythmias.** Bradyarrhythmias occur when sinus node impulse generation is slowed or when normal sinus node impulses cannot be conducted to the ventricles because of AV nodal block or ventricular conducting system disease. In general, bradyarrhythmias are only a cause for concern when the patient has become symptomatic with presyncope or syncope from the reduced cardiac output that the low heart rate produces [see IX C 1 a (1)–(2)].

1. **Sinus bradycardia**
   a. Sinus bradycardia may be a physiologic and normal response to cardiovascular conditioning, as is seen in trained athletes. In such cases, the arrhythmia is obviously a normal finding and requires no therapy. However, extreme sinus bradycardia (< 35 bpm) as a result of sinus node dysfunction may cause symptoms.
   b. **Therapy. Atropine** may be useful in temporarily increasing the sinus rate; the definitive therapy for symptomatic bradycardia is **pacemaker implantation.**

2. **Sinus pause** is an arrhythmia caused by the failure of the sinus node to generate an impulse on time. Such pauses may last for several seconds and induce syncope. Definitive therapy requires pacemaker implantation.

3. **AV block.** In AV block, all of the impulses generated from the sinus node are not conducted to the ventricles.
   a. **Types of AV block**
      (1) In **Mobitz type I (Wenckebach) block** there is a progressive prolongation in the P-R interval until a generated P wave is not conducted. This type of block usually occurs at the level of the AV node and is demonstrated in Figure 1-4. This type of block rarely produces symptoms.
      (2) In **Mobitz type II block** there is no prolongation of the P-R interval before the dropped beat. Often conduction in a 2:1 ratio is prolonged, leading to symptomatic bradycardia. This type of block can occur at the AV node or in the His–Purkinje system.
      (3) **Complete heart block.** In complete heart block, no impulses are conducted (Figure 1-5) and the ventricular rate becomes dependent on spontaneous ventricular depolarizations. Severe symptomatic bradycardia characterized by a heart rate of 25–40 bpm is the rule for complete heart block.

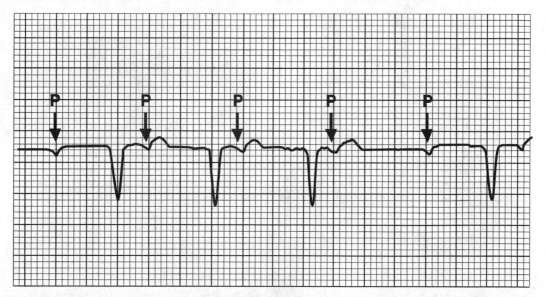

FIGURE 1-4. Electrocardiogram (ECG) rhythm strip produced by Mobitz type I second-degree atrioventricular (AV) nodal block. There is progressive prolongation of the P-R interval until finally a P wave is not conducted. In this example, there are four P waves for every three QRS complexes, resulting in a 4:3 Wenckebach block.

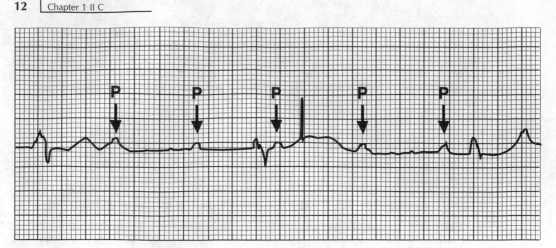

FIGURE 1-5. Complete heart block. In this strip, the P waves are regular and the atrial rate is 85. However, no relationship between the P waves and QRS complexes is present, indicating the presence of complete heart block.

    b. Therapy. Atropine and **isoproterenol** are often effective in temporarily increasing the ventricular response. If this therapy fails, transcutaneous pacing will temporarily increase heart rate. However, most forms of symptomatic AV block require the implantation of either a temporary (in the case of inferior myocardial infarction) or a permanent **cardiac pacemaker.**

D. **Ventricular tachyarrhythmias**

  1. Types of ventricular arrhythmias
    a. Premature ventricular contraction (PVC). In this arrhythmia, heart beats arise directly from the ventricles, bypassing the specialized cardiac His–Purkinje conduction system.
      (1) ECG identification
        (a) Because the His–Purkinje system is bypassed, the **QRS configuration** is typically **widened and bizarre** in appearance.
        (b) PVCs usually do not affect atrial depolarization, which proceeds normally and in dissociation with the PVC. Thus, the next sinus beat occurs at the same time it would have occurred if no PVC had been present. Accordingly, a PVC is usually followed by a **full compensatory pause** (Figure 1-6). The normally occurring P wave is usually buried in the PVC QRS complex.
      (2) Therapy. Most isolated PVCs are benign and should not be treated.
    b. Ventricular tachycardia is a regular rhythm that occurs paroxysmally and exceeds 120 bpm. **AV dissociation,** which causes the ventricular arrhythmia to proceed independently of the normal atrial rhythm, is the hallmark of the arrhythmia. During ventricular tachycardia, cardiac relaxation is impaired. This factor, together with loss of AV synchrony (i.e., loss of the atrial kick) and loss of the electrical coordination of the contraction by the His–Purkinje system, usu-

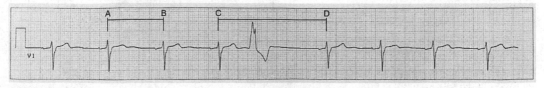

FIGURE 1-6. Premature ventricular contraction. The QRS is widened and bizarre in appearance and is followed by a compensatory pause—the R-R interval *C–D* is exactly twice the R-R interval *A–B*.

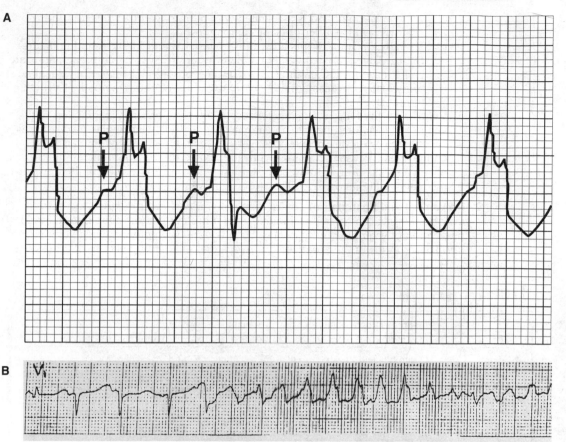

FIGURE 1-7. (*A*) Monomorphic ventricular tachycardia. There is a widened bizarre QRS complex, which has an inconsistent relationship to the preceding P wave. (*B*) Polymorphic ventricular tachycardia in a patient with a prolonged Q-T interval (torsades de pointes).

ally leads to severely reduced cardiac output, producing hypotension. **Sustained ventricular tachycardia is usually a life-threatening arrhythmia that degenerates into ventricular fibrillation and death if untreated.**

(1) **Physical examination.** In many cases of ventricular tachycardia, performance of a detailed physical examination is precluded by severe decompensation.

   (a) If the patient is relatively stable, physical diagnosis will reveal AV dissociation, manifested by the appearance of **cannon a waves** in the neck veins. Cannon a waves occur intermittently when the tricuspid valve is closed when right atrial contraction occurs during ventricular contraction. Because the atrial blood cannot go forward against the closed tricuspid valve, backward flow produces a large bulge in the neck veins.

   (b) **Variability in intensity of the S₁,** caused by variable positioning of atrial and ventricular contraction, can be auscultated.

(2) **ECG identification** (Figure 1-7)

   (a) The **QRS complex is widened and bizarre in appearance** because the arrhythmia does not use the specialized conducting system of the heart. Because the ventricles are operating independently of the atria, there is **no constant relationship between the P wave and the QRS complex.**

   (b) The QRS complex may be **monomorphic** (i.e., of one shape) as shown in Figure 1-7A, or it may be **polymorphic** as shown in Figure 1-7B. When the axis of a polymorphic arrhythmia appears to revolve about a central point and is associated with a prolonged Q-T interval, the arrhythmia is termed **torsades de pointes.**

(3) **Therapy.** Because of this arrhythmia's unstable and life-threatening nature, **DC cardioversion** is urgently required in most cases. While preparations are being made for DC cardioversion, intravenous administration of **lidocaine, bretylium,** or **procainamide** may be useful in returning the patient's rhythm to normal.

c. **Ventricular fibrillation** is characterized by a lack of ordered contraction of the ventricles; therefore, there is no cardiac output. Thus, **ventricular fibrillation is synonymous with death unless conversion to an effective rhythm can be accomplished.** The physician should begin cardiac resuscitation, including mechanical ventilation, cardiac compression, and drug and electrical therapy, immediately upon recognizing the presence of ventricular fibrillation.

2. **Prevention and treatment of ventricular arrhythmias.** Table 1-1 lists the current classification and some of the side effects of drugs currently available for chronic prevention of ventricular arrhythmias. Such therapy is employed when ventricular fibrillation occurs in the absence of a myocardial infarction (because of a high like-

TABLE 1-1. Antiarrhythmic Agents

Class	Major Electrophysiologic Properties	Specific Agents	Major Side Effects
Sodium channel blockers	Ia Inhibit rapid inward current Prolong repolarization	Quinidine	Proarrhythmia Diarrhea
		Procainamide	Proarrhythmia
		Disopyramide	Lupus-like syndrome Proarrhythmia Congestive heart failure Anticholinergic effects
	Ib Inhibit rapid inward current Accelerate repolarization	Lidocaine	CNS effects
		Tocainide	Proarrhythmia CNS effects
		Mexiletine	Neutropenia CNS effects
		Phenytoin	CNS effects
	Ic Inhibit rapid inward current Little effect on repolarization	Flecainide	Congestive heart failure
		Encainide	Proarrhythmia Proarrhythmia
Beta-blockers	II Accelerate repolarization Reduce ischemia Reduce sympathetic arrythmogenicity	Propranolol	Bradycardia Bronchospasm Congestive heart failure
		Acebutolol	Congestive heart failure
Potassium channel blockers	III Prolong action potential duration	Amiodarone	Pulmonary fibrosis Hypo- and hyperthyroidism
		Bretylium Sotalol	Orthostatic hypotension Proarrhythmia
Calcium channel blockers	IV Depress slow inward current	Verapamil (atrial arrhythmias)	Bradycardia

CNS = central nervous system.

lihood of recurrent arrhythmia) or with the occurrence of symptomatic or sustained ventricular tachycardia.

III. ISCHEMIC HEART DISEASE

A. Atherosclerotic coronary artery disease (ASCAD)

1. **Definition.** ASCAD is the focal narrowing of the coronary arteries as a result of intimal proliferation of smooth muscle cells and the deposition of lipids. The basic lesion is called a **plaque,** the chief components of which are diagrammed in Figure 1-8 and include:
   a. **Intimal smooth muscle cells,** which proliferate, probably as a result of endothelial damage
   b. **Lipids** (cholesterol esters and crystals), which are deposited at the center of the plaque and also accumulate within smooth muscle cells
   c. A **fibrous cap** made of connective tissue

2. **Incidence and risk factors.** Currently in the United States, the overall incidence of death as a result of ASCAD is 0.5 in 1000 and decreasing. However, ASCAD differs in frequency in subpopulations with the following risk factors:
   a. **Age.** The incidence of ASCAD increases progressively with age. The risk of death is 1.5 in 1000 individuals at age 50.
   b. **Gender.** ASCAD is more prevalent in men than in women. This difference is most marked in premenopausal women compared with men of similar age; 50-year-old men are affected five times more often than women of the same age.
   c. **Serum cholesterol.** The incidence of ASCAD increases with increasing total serum cholesterol levels, as shown in Figure 1-9.
      (1) Total serum cholesterol is carried in the blood by **low-density lipoprotein (LDL), very low-density lipoprotein (VLDL),** and **high-density lipoprotein (HDL).**
         (a) The higher the percentage of total cholesterol carried by LDL in relation to HDL, the higher the risk of ASCAD. Patients with LDL-to-HDL ratios of greater than 4:1 are particularly prone to ASCAD. Conversely, high levels of HDL seem to be protective. One theory is that HDL may allow for elution of cholesterol out of the coronary vessel.

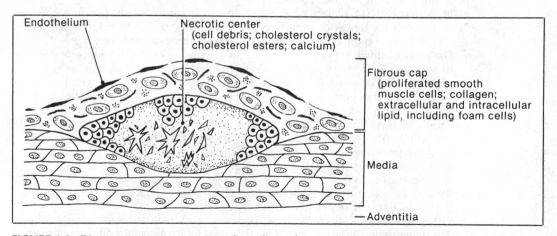

FIGURE 1-8. Diagrammatic representation of an atherosclerotic plaque, showing its composition. The *fibrous cap* of the plaque is linked to clinical events due to its tendency to fracture and ulcerate. The *necrotic core* of the plaque has clinical consequence as a result of its size, consistency, and thromboplastic components. (Adapted from Braunwald E: *Heart Disease,* 2nd edition. Philadelphia, WB Saunders, 1984, p 1186.)

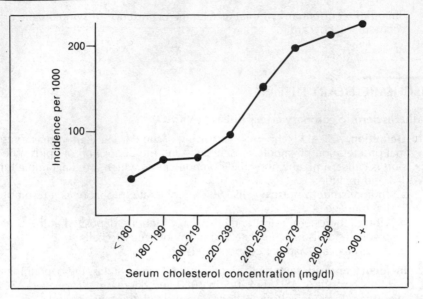

FIGURE 1-9. Graph showing the effect of increasing serum cholesterol concentration on the incidence of atherosclerotic coronary artery disease in men age 30–49 years. (Adapted from Cohn PF: *Diagnosis and Therapy of Coronary Artery Disease.* Boston, Little, Brown, 1979, p 27.)

      (b) It is desirable for the total cholesterol level to be less than 200 mg/dl.
          (i) The LDL cholesterol level should be less than 130 mg/dl; in pa-tients with known coronary disease, it should be less than 100 mg/dl.
          (ii) The HDL cholesterol level should exceed 40 mg/dl.
    (2) Several types of hyperlipidemia exist, and many are associated with an in-creased incidence of coronary artery disease. Table 1-2 presents an over-view of the hyperlipidemias.
  d. Smoking. Cigarette smokers are 60% more likely to develop ASCAD than non-smokers when other risk factors are controlled. Smoking increases carbon mon-oxide levels in the blood, which may, in turn, damage the coronary endothe-lium. Smoking also increases platelet adhesiveness and thus the likelihood of thrombotic coronary occlusion.
  e. Hypertension. The higher either the systolic or diastolic blood pressure, the more likely the development of ASCAD. This likelihood is noted in both men and women and becomes more pronounced with advancing age.
  f. Diabetes mellitus is associated with a 50% increase in the incidence of ASCAD in men and a 100% increase in women, explained in part by the increased platelet adhesiveness and increased serum cholesterol levels associated with dia-betes. In general, however, there is a poor correlation between the severity of the diabetes and the severity of ASCAD.
  g. Family history. A familial predisposition to coronary artery disease exists in part due to inheritance of the above risk factors (except smoking).
  h. Oral contraceptives are associated with an increased incidence of myocardial infarction, a clinical consequence of ASCAD. The incidence of myocardial in-farction rises from 0.01% to 0.04% in nonsmoking women between the ages of 30 and 40 who use oral contraceptives and, more dramatically, from 0.06% to 0.25% in similar women who also smoke.
  i. Other risk factors. Gout, "type A" personality, premature arcus corneae, obe-sity, hypertriglyceridemia, and a diagonal ear lobe crease are other conditions associated with an increased risk of ASCAD.

3. Pathogenesis. The previously mentioned risk factors do not constitute a known mechanism for ASCAD; however, two major theories of atherogenesis exist to ex-plain its origin.

TABLE 1-2. The Hyperlipidemias

Type of Hyperlipidemia	Lipid Abnormality	Lipoprotein Abnormality	Clinical Manifestations	Therapy
I Lipoprotein lipase deficiency	↑ Triglycerides	↑ Chylomicrons	Pancreatitis	Fat-free diet
			Eruptive xanthomas	
			Lipemia retinalis	
IIa LDL receptor deficiency	↑ Cholesterol	↑ LDL	Coronary disease	Restricted diet
			Tendon xanthomas	Bile acid–binding resins
			Xanthelasma	Nicotinic acid
				HMG-CoA reductase inhibitors
IIb	↑ Cholesterol	↑ LDL	Coronary disease	Restricted diet
	↑ Triglycerides	↑ VLDL		Bile acid–binding resins
				Nicotinic acid
				Gemfibrozil
				HMG-CoA reductase inhibitors
III Dysbetalipoproteinemia	↑ Triglycerides	↑ VLDL Remnants	Palmar fatty streaks	Gemfibrozil
	↑ Cholesterol		Tuberous xanthomas	
			Coronary disease	
			Peripheral vascular disease	
			Hypothyroidism	
IV	↑ Triglycerides	↑ VLDL	Eruptive xanthomas	Restricted diet
			Pancreatitis	Gemfibrozil
			Diabetes	
			± Coronary artery disease	
V	↑ Triglycerides	↑ VLDL	Eruptive xanthomas	Restricted diet
		↑ Chylomicrons	Pancreatitis	Gemfibrozil
			Diabetes	
			± Coronary artery disease	

HMG-CoA = β-hydroxy-β-methylglutaryl coenzyme A; LDL = low density lipoproteins; VLDL = very low-density lipoproteins.

    a. Response to injury theory. This theory states that some injurious stimulus (e.g., hypertension or hypercholesterolemia) causes endothelial damage, resulting in the release of various growth factors. These growth factors cause smooth cell proliferation and migration of macrophages into the vessel wall. At the same time, the now injured endothelium becomes more permeable, admitting lipid and cholesterol into the intima. These changes result in plaque formation, which may eventually compromise the vessel lumen enough to impede blood flow. If the plaque is disrupted, platelets are activated, leading to thrombus formation and worsening obstruction.

    b. Neoplasia theory. In women, smooth muscle cells in atherosclerotic plaques have the same glucose-6-phosphate dehydrogenase (G6PD) isoenzyme, suggesting a monoclonal origin of these cells. This theory postulates that a stimulus—perhaps vessel wall injury—leads to cell proliferation stemming from a single cell.

  4. Pathophysiology

    a. Supply–demand relationship. The oxygen needs of the myocardium can be roughly approximated by the product of heart rate and left ventricular systolic pressure or wall stress (see I B 1 b). As stress and heart rate increase (e.g., with exercise), myocardial oxygen consumption rises. This increased demand is normally met by autoregulated increases in coronary blood flow. If demand exceeds supply, ischemia results.

(1) **Increased demand.** In patients with ASCAD, stenosis of the coronary artery prevents the increase in coronary blood flow needed to compensate for an increased demand, resulting in oxygen demand exceeding oxygen supply. **Myocardial ischemia** is the result of this imbalance.

(2) **Reduced supply.** The atherosclerotic stenosis was once viewed as a fixed obstruction to coronary blood flow. In fact, the diseased area of the coronary artery often remains dynamic, and the effective lumen of the artery undergoes constant change. Changes are produced by vasoconstriction of the coronary artery, by production and degradation of local thrombi at the site of stenosis, and by progressive enlargement of the atherosclerotic plaque. Acute changes in lumen diameter may reduce the supply of coronary blood flow and, thus, produce ischemia without an increase in demand.

b. **Myocardial infarction** is the necrosis of myocardial tissue as a result of prolonged ischemia. The rapidity and extent of the infarction process are determined by the extent of reduction of blood flow to the area. In some cases, **collateral flow** may supply enough blood flow to prevent infarction despite a total coronary occlusion.

(1) Although the cause of **transmural (Q-wave) infarction** has been debated for much of the last century, it is now clear that most transmural myocardial infarctions are associated with early occlusion of a coronary artery by a **thrombus.**

(a) Usually, the thrombus is located adjacent to an atherosclerotic coronary stenosis, but the initial events causing the thrombus remain unclear.

(b) Aggressive lysis of the thrombus with agents such as **streptokinase** and **tissue plasminogen activator (t-PA)** reestablishes coronary blood flow, relieves pain, reestablishes contractile function of the segment of myocardium supplied by the thrombosed artery, and reduces myocardial damage [see III A 5 b (5) (b)]. These observations indicate that the thrombus is not merely a coincident event in myocardial infarction; rather, it is central to the infarction's pathogenesis.

(2) The pathogenesis of **nontransmural (non–Q-wave) infarction** is less clear, but the presence of total coronary occlusion is significantly less common, occurring in less than 50% of cases.

5. **Clinical consequences**

a. **Angina pectoris** is chest pain or pressure produced by myocardial ischemia.

(1) **Characteristic features**

(a) **Relation to exertion.** The single most important feature of angina pectoris is its precipitation by exertion. Exertion increases myocardial oxygen demand beyond the supply capabilities of diseased coronary arteries, producing ischemia. Other factors that increase myocardial oxygen demand (e.g., emotional upset, eating a meal, or the peripheral vasoconstriction caused by walking in cold weather) may also precipitate angina. In some patients, angina occurs predominantly at rest, but this is unusual. When rest pain does occur, it probably is produced by a reduction in coronary blood flow or by spontaneous increases in blood pressure, heart rate, or both.

(b) **Quality of pain.** Although many patients perceive angina as **chest pain,** others report a feeling of **pressure** in the chest area or complain of a **burning** sensation. In some patients, **exertional dyspnea** may represent an anginal equivalent.

(c) **Radiation of pain.** Radiation of anginal pain to the left arm is well-known. Pain also may radiate to the right arm, jaw, teeth, or throat. Occasionally, these radiation sites may be the only sites of pain, and the chest is free of discomfort; or the chest discomfort, when present, may not radiate at all.

(d) Progression of ischemia and duration of symptoms. Whatever the anginal symptom quality for a given patient, it usually will be reproduced upon repeated episodes of ischemia. The symptom complex usually begins at a low intensity, increases over 2–3 minutes, and lasts a total of less than 15 minutes. Episodes longer than 30 minutes suggest that myocardial infarction may have occurred. **Sudden onset of severe chest pain does not suggest ischemic pain.**

(2) Types of angina

(a) Chronic stable angina is angina that recurs under similar circumstances and with a similar frequency over time.

(b) Silent ischemia. For every episode of symptomatic ischemia that the patient suffers, there are usually four to five episodes of silent (asymptomatic) ischemia. These episodes can be detected by ECG monitoring but are less severe in nature and shorter in duration than the episodes that the patient perceives as angina. In some patients, especially diabetics, documentable ischemia occurs without the patient ever perceiving ischemic symptoms.

(c) Unstable angina is a term applied to angina when a change in status occurs (e.g., new-onset angina; angina of increasing severity, duration, or frequency; or angina occurring at rest for the first time). It is the progressive nature of unstable angina that is ominous, and the physician and the patient should be aware that close observation and intensive therapy are required. Unstable angina represents a more serious clinical situation than chronic stable angina because unstable angina may be an immediate precursor of myocardial infarction.

(i) Rest angina. Angina at rest is particularly worrisome because it implies that decreased supply, rather than increased demand, is causing the angina. This concept in turn suggests that arterial occlusion and possible infarction may be imminent.

(ii) New onset angina. In cases of new-onset angina, it is difficult to generalize about clinical outcome. New-onset angina that progresses in frequency, severity, or duration over 1 or 2 months is worrisome. Conversely, some cases of new-onset angina may simply be the first episode in what becomes a chronic stable anginal pattern.

(d) Variant (Prinzmetal's) angina

(i) The **hallmark** of variant angina is the appearance of transient **S-T segment elevation** on the ECG during the angina attack. The S-T segment elevation represents **transmural ischemia** produced by a sudden reduction in coronary blood flow.

(ii) The reduction in flow results from **transient coronary spasm,** which usually, but not always, is associated with a fixed atherosclerotic lesion. The spasm produces total, but transient, coronary occlusion. The cause of the spasm and its release are unknown.

(iii) Variant angina usually occurs at rest (often at night), and episodes frequently are complicated by complex ventricular arrhythmias.

(3) Diagnosis. When the patient exhibits chest pain characteristic of angina, the diagnosis can be suspected strongly by patient history alone. The suspicion that coronary disease is present is heightened by the presence of one or more coronary risk factors. However, the following procedures are useful in confirming the diagnosis.

(a) Physical examination. Patients experiencing an episode of angina are usually uncomfortable and anxious. Blood pressure and pulse rate are increased in most cases. Palpation of the precordium may reveal a **dyskinetic impulse** over the apex of the left ventricle. A new S_4 may appear, and **transient mitral regurgitation** as a result of ischemically produced papillary muscle dysfunction may produce a **holosystolic murmur.**

(b) Resting electrocardiography. The ECG taken in the absence of pain in patients with angina pectoris with no history of myocardial infarction is normal in 50% of cases. However, in many cases, efforts to obtain an ECG while the patient is experiencing chest pain are more rewarding.

  (i) The presence of **new horizontal** or **down-sloping S-T segments** on the ECG is highly suggestive of myocardial ischemia. **New T-wave inversion** also may occur, but this finding alone without S-T segment depression is less specific.

  (ii) In the presence of variant angina, the diagnostic finding is an acute current of injury indicated by transient S-T segment elevation. The S-T segment elevation normalizes as the pain wanes and no Q waves appear.

(c) Stress electrocardiography. Recording the ECG during exercise substantially increases the sensitivity and specificity of electrocardiography. In addition, a formal exercise test permits quantification of the patient's exercise tolerance and observation of the effects of exercise on the patient's symptoms, heart rate, and blood pressure.

  (i) The appearance of horizontal or down-sloping S-T segment depression of 1 mm or more during exercise has a sensitivity of approximately 70% and a specificity of 90% for the detection of coronary disease.

  (ii) The S-T criteria for positivity are less accurate in women than in men. The presence of **bundle branch block** or **left ventricular hypertrophy** or the use of **digitalis** by the patient **all reduce the accuracy of this test.**

(d) Stress scintigraphy, when used in combination with the stress ECG, has yielded increased sensitivity (80%) and specificity (92%) over the standard stress ECG alone. Therefore, it is a particularly useful diagnostic tool when the standard stress ECG is expected to be of low yield (e.g., in women and in patients with bundle branch block) and in patients in whom a previous stress ECG has produced equivocal results.

  (i) Method. When the radioactive isotope **thallium 201 (^{201}Tl)** or the technetium-based isonitrile **sestamibi** is injected into the peripheral venous blood, a portion of the substance will be taken up by the myocardium. The myocardial distribution of the substance is affected by blood flow and ischemia, with areas of less blood flow and ischemia taking up less ^{201}Tl or sestamibi than areas of normal blood flow. Normally, blood flow and, thus, the isotope, are distributed equally throughout the myocardium. With exercise, blood flow increases, but in patients with coronary artery disease, those parts of the myocardium supplied by diseased coronary arteries and areas of myocardial infarction take up less ^{201}Tl or sestamibi than normal areas, as shown in the scintigram in Figure 1-10. In patients unable to exercise, infusion of dobutamine (to increase oxygen demand) or dipyridamole (to cause coronary vasodilatation) are used to alter coronary flow in place of exercise.

  (ii) Enhancements. Thallium and sestamibi imaging can be further enhanced using **single-photon emission computed tomography (SPECT).** This technique uses a rotating gamma camera to acquire data at 32 to 64 stops in a 180°- or 360°- arc around the patient. A computer reconstructs the data into a two-dimensional image and assigns different colors to different levels of ^{201}Tl uptake. The sensitivity for detecting coronary disease with SPECT imaging is as high as 90%.

(e) Stress radionuclide ventriculography

  (i) Method. Pyrophosphate, injected peripherally, binds the radionuclide **technetium** to red blood cells. Radionuclide-tagged red

A. Normal myocardium

Initial   Delayed

B. Coronary artery disease

Initial   Delayed

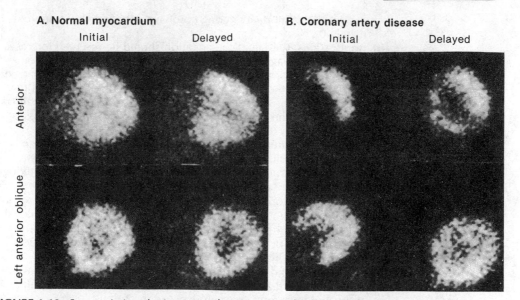

FIGURE 1-10. Stress scintigraphy in a normal patient (*A*) and in a patient with coronary artery disease (*B*). (A) Normal thallium study shows initial (i.e., immediately after exercise) and delayed thallium 201 (^{201}Tl) images in the anterior and left anterior oblique views. ^{201}Tl is taken up and released homogeneously throughout the myocardium, indicating equal coronary blood flow to all portions of the left ventricle. (*B*) A large defect (*black area from 5 o'clock to 11 o'clock*) is seen in the initial scintiscan in the anterior view. This area corresponds to the inferoapical area of the left ventricle. A defect also is seen in the left anterior oblique view (*black area from 6 o'clock to 9 o'clock*), which corresponds to the inferior portion of the left ventricular septum. Areas of decreased perfusion eventually demonstrate ^{201}Tl uptake, as seen in the delayed scintiscan. This study is consistent with exercise-induced hypoperfusion of the inferolateral and septal areas of the left ventricle and with obstructive disease of the right coronary artery. (Reprinted with permission from Johnson R, et al: *The Practice of Cardiology.* Boston, Little, Brown, 1980, p 1046.)

blood cells in the blood pool of the left ventricle can be used to produce a scintigraphic image of the left ventricle. By gating the fluctuations in tagged red blood cell count that occur within the ventricles over a number of cardiac cycles, a radionuclide ventriculogram can be produced.

   (ii) Interpretation. Coronary disease produces regional dysfunction by ischemia or infarction of those areas of the left ventricle not receiving an adequate blood supply. Exercise-induced ischemia produces transient regional dysfunction, which can be detected by radionuclide angiography. For example, in a patient with disease in the left anterior descending coronary artery, the anterior left ventricular wall may move normally at rest but become dyskinetic with exercise as a result of ischemia.

   (iii) Sensitivity. This test is sensitive (90%) for the detection of coronary artery disease but is not as specific because heart disease other than coronary artery disease may produce exercise-induced regional dysfunction.

 (f) Stress echocardiography. This technique is based on the same principles of ischemia as stress radionuclide ventriculography, but an echocardiograph, rather than a radioactive blood pool, is used to produce the images of wall motion abnormalities.

 (g) Cardiac catheterization with coronary arteriography allows for direct visualization of the coronary arteries by selective injection of radiographic contrast material and is the **most sensitive and specific test commonly employed for coronary artery disease.**

   (i) Risk. Unlike the previously mentioned tests, cardiac catheterization is an invasive procedure that carries a small but finite risk. The overall risk of mortality during coronary arteriography is approximately 0.2%.

    (ii) Applications. Cardiac catheterization should be reserved for cases in which the diagnosis is uncertain after noninvasive testing or when more information is needed to help determine whether medical or surgical therapy is most appropriate for the patient's coronary disease. If surgery is contemplated, the arteriograms obtained at catheterization guide the surgeon's placement of the bypass grafts.

  (h) Intravascular ultrasound using an echo transducer attached to a coronary catheter is an ultrasensitive experimental technique currently under investigation for the diagnosis of ASCAD. However, like arteriography, this procedure carries a risk.

(4) Therapy for angina pectoris is directed either at reducing myocardial oxygen demand to compensate for impaired flow through diseased coronary arteries or at increasing myocardial oxygen supply (i.e., blood flow).

  (a) Nitrates. This class of drugs produces venodilation and, to a lesser extent, arteriolar vasodilatation.

    (i) Venodilation and arteriolar vasodilatation decrease blood pressure and reduce cardiac size, thereby reducing left ventricular wall stress and myocardial oxygen demand.

    (ii) Direct coronary arterial vasodilation also may increase coronary blood flow, because even diseased portions of the coronary artery have been shown to dilate.

    (iii) Sublingual, oral, dermal, and intravenous nitrate preparations are available and effective.

  (b) β-Adrenergic blocking agents. β-Adrenergic receptor stimulation results in an increase in heart rate and in the force of myocardial contraction. Both events increase myocardial oxygen demand. β-Adrenergic blocking agents counteract these effects and act to **limit myocardial oxygen demand.**

    (i) Recent evidence suggests that β blockers also may diminish platelet activation, which could be important in stabilizing the coronary plaque and in preventing reduction in coronary blood flow.

    (ii) Currently, the **five β blockers approved for use in treating angina are propranolol, metoprolol, atenolol, nadolol,** and **timolol.**

    (iii) These drugs may precipitate congestive heart failure in some patients with severe systolic dysfunction. In addition, β blockers may precipitate bronchospasm in asthmatics and in patients with obstructive lung disease. They may also cause severe bradycardia in patients with SA node or AV node disease.

  (c) Calcium antagonists. Calcium regulates the contraction of smooth muscle, which is present in the walls of the coronary and peripheral arteries.

    (i) Calcium antagonists are particularly **effective in preventing the coronary spasm that causes variant angina.** They are also useful in treating cases of typical angina, in which they **act as coronary and peripheral arterial vasodilators.** Diltiazem and verapamil also reduce heart rate.

    (ii) Nifedipine, verapamil, diltiazem, amlodipine, and **nicardipine** are the calcium antagonists currently approved for the treatment of both typical and variant angina.

    (iii) All calcium blockers may cause hypotension. Verapamil and, more rarely, diltiazem may precipitate congestive heart failure or severe bradycardia.

  (d) Percutaneous transluminal angioplasty (PCTA). Angina can be alleviated by removing or reducing the obstructive coronary atherosclerotic lesion. Studies are currently underway to define the exact role of PCTA in the treatment of coronary disease.

(i) During angioplasty, a small balloon is inserted into a femoral or brachial artery and guided to the obstruction of the affected coronary artery. The balloon is inflated, dilating the stenosis and reducing the obstruction.

(ii) The initial success rate of PCTA approaches 90%, although there is a 33% restenosis rate after 6 months, making it necessary to repeat the procedure in some patients. The mortality rate is 1%, and 5% of the patients undergoing PCTA will require immediate surgery as a result of PCTA-related occlusions.

(e) **Atherectomy.** In some patients in whom PTCA is ineffective, atherectomy can be performed. **Directional atherectomy** involves removal of the lesion by cutting it away from the vessel wall. **Rotational atherectomy** involves the use of a high speed drill to remove the plaque.

(f) **Coronary artery bypass surgery.** Surgery offers a high incidence of symptomatic improvement (85%) at a 2%–5% operative risk and, thus, is indicated for patients whose lifestyles are seriously compromised by angina despite medical therapy. Additionally, coronary bypass surgery increases longevity in most patients with severe disease of the main left coronary artery and some anatomic distributions of triple-vessel coronary disease (see III A 6).

(g) **Therapy for unstable angina at rest.** Unstable angina occurring at rest is ominous because it is caused by a sudden decrease in blood supply, suggesting plaque instability. Bed rest, aspirin, intravenous heparin, and nitroglycerin are the mainstays of initial therapy. Cardiac catheterization is then performed to gauge the potential for revascularization.

b. **Myocardial infarction** occurs when the myocardium is deprived of its blood supply (and therefore, oxygen) for a significant amount of time. **Transmural myocardial infarction** results from the obstruction of the coronary arteries by **thrombi** or **coronary spasm.** Spasm is especially common in cocaine abusers. The cause of nontransmural (**subendocardial**) myocardial infarction remains uncertain.

(1) **Pathogenesis.** An abrupt change in the atherosclerotic plaque seems to be one of the events precipitating a myocardial infarction. At least in some instances, hemorrhage into the plaque disrupts it, leading to a break in the fibrous cap. The roughened surface attracts platelets that trigger thrombus formation, leading to total occlusion of the vessel. Antecedent endothelial dysfunction enhances potential for both vasospasm and thrombus formation.

(2) **Symptoms.** The patient usually experiences **severe, oppressive chest pain** or **pressure** that persists for more than 30 minutes and is unrelieved by nitroglycerin. The pain radiates in a pattern similar to that of angina pectoris.

(a) Frequently, **nausea, vomiting, diaphoresis,** and **shortness of breath** accompany the pain.

(b) The pain usually occurs when the patient is **at rest** or involved in minimal activity. However, recent studies show that myocardial infarction can be triggered by discrete events (e.g., **shoveling snow),** and an unusually large number of infarctions occur **between 6 A.M. and 10 A.M.,** when catecholamine levels increase upon awakening.

(3) **Diagnosis**

(a) **Physical examination.** The patient experiencing myocardial infarction is in obvious pain, is quite apprehensive, and often appears ashen. If the infarction is extensive, hypotension and tachycardia may be present. There also may be signs of congestive heart failure (e.g., elevation of the neck veins, pulmonary rales, and a cardiac gallop rhythm). The new murmur of mitral regurgitation may be present.

(b) **Electrocardiography.** The ECG is diagnostic in approximately 85% of cases. The remaining 15% of patients may experience myocardial infarction without manifesting clear-cut evidence on the ECG.

      (i) When **transmural myocardial infarction** is present, an injury current usually is demonstrated by S-T segment elevation in those leads reflecting the area of the myocardial infarction. As the S-T segments fall, Q waves appear and the T waves become inverted.

     (ii) In the presence of **subendocardial infarction,** the electrocardiographic diagnosis is less certain, and S-T segment depression may be the only finding.

   (iii) Because the presence or absence of Q waves on the ECG does not correlate well with transmural versus subendocardial infarction at autopsy, the current practice is to classify myocardial infarctions as either **Q wave or non–Q wave,** as opposed to transmural or subendocardial.

  (c) Cardiac enzyme studies

      (i) As myocardial necrosis occurs, the myocardium releases **creatine kinase (CK), aspartate aminotransferase** (AST or **SGOT),** and **lactic acid dehydrogenase (LDH),** thereby increasing serum concentrations of these enzymes.

     (ii) CK elevation appears 6 hours after infarction, AST elevation appears 12 hours after infarction, and LDH elevation appears 24 hours after infarction.

   (iii) Although these enzymes may be elevated in other disease states, isoenzyme studies can determine with a high probability whether or not the enzymes are cardiac in origin. It is the **MB isoenzyme** (i.e., the CK isoenzyme found primarily in the myocardium) that increases in the presence of myocardial infarction. In addition, LDH_1 **isoenzyme** levels are elevated so that they exceed LDH_2 isoenzyme levels.

(4) Complications. A myocardial infarction can occur with little clinical consequence; indeed, many are silent. The complications of myocardial infarction, however, produce clinically significant events.

  (a) Arrhythmias. A patient having an acute myocardial infarction is subject to acute, **lethal ventricular arrhythmias** (i.e., ventricular tachycardia or ventricular fibrillation), as well as **less serious atrial arrhythmias** (e.g., atrial fibrillation, atrial flutter).

      (i) Lethal arrhythmias often occur without warning, often within 24 hours of the infarction. Although many patients experience frequent premature ventricular contractions as a harbinger of lethal ventricular arrhythmias, other patients have sudden arrhythmias without lesser, premonitory rhythm disturbances.

     (ii) The need for detection of cardiac arrhythmias fostered the concept of the **coronary care unit.** By closely monitoring the patient with myocardial infarction, it is possible to detect and prevent severe cardiac arrhythmias before they become fatal.

  (b) Acute conduction system abnormalities. The specialized conducting system of the heart is itself myocardium, which may become ischemic or infarcted during a myocardial infarction. This may lead to bradyarrhythmias, heart block, or both.

      (i) Inferior-wall myocardial infarction usually occurs when the right coronary artery is diseased. Because this artery supplies the sinoatrial (SA) node in 55% of patients and the AV node in 85% of patients, it is not surprising that **sinus bradycardia** and varying degrees of **AV nodal block** occur during inferior myocardial infarctions.

     (ii) On the other hand, **anterior myocardial infarction** usually occurs from occlusion of the anterior descending coronary artery, which supplies the interventricular septum. Because the bundle branches course through the septum, acute **right** or **left bundle branch block** may occur during anterior myocardial infarctions. **Complete heart**

block also may occur due to dysfunction of both bundle branches or the bundle of His.

(c) Pump failure

  (i) When 30% of the myocardium is infarcted from one or more myocardial infarctions, **congestive heart failure** is likely to ensue.

  (ii) If more than 40% of the myocardium becomes infarcted, **cardiogenic shock** is likely to develop. In true cardiogenic shock, there is not enough myocardium to generate enough cardiac output to sustain bodily function. One definition of cardiogenic shock is a systolic blood pressure of less than 90 mm Hg together with a urinary output of less than 20 ml/hr in the presence of adequate left ventricular filling pressure. When cardiogenic shock occurs, the mortality rate is 50%–75%.

(d) Mitral regurgitation. The mitral valve is tethered by the **papillary muscles,** which are projections of the myocardium. Dysfunction or infarction of the papillary muscles together with ventricular dilatation may lead to systolic prolapsing of the mitral valve into the left atrium, causing varying degrees of mitral regurgitation. If the mitral regurgitation is severe, the cardiac output is decreased profoundly because a large part of the left ventricular stroke volume is ejected backward. At the same time, there is a precipitous rise in the left ventricular filling pressure that is transmitted to the lungs, resulting in pulmonary edema.

(e) Ventricular septal defect. The left ventricular septum may become infarcted in either anterior or inferior myocardial infarction, leading to rupture of the septum. Thus, a free communication between left and right ventricles (an acute ventricular septal defect) is formed. This defect diverts a significant percentage of the left ventricular stroke volume into the right ventricle, compromising forward cardiac output. Rupture of the septum occurs in approximately 2% of patients, usually 2–5 days after infarction.

(f) Cardiac rupture. Myocardial infarction of the free wall may lead to eventual perforation of the heart. This complication, which results in overwhelming **cardiac tamponade,** is nearly always fatal.

(g) Left ventricular aneurysm. The infarcted zone of the myocardium may evaginate and heal with fibrous connective tissue, forming a "fifth chamber" attached to the left ventricle. This useless chamber saps a portion of the left ventricular stroke volume. Left ventricular aneurysms may produce cardiac failure and angina, and they also may be the source of severe left ventricular arrhythmias and systemic emboli.

(5) Therapy. When a patient enters the hospital with a myocardial infarction, an intravenous cannula is placed percutaneously for use in administering medications. Intramuscular injections should be avoided because they may confuse interpretation of the cardiac enzymes. Oxygen is traditionally delivered via a nasal cannula.

(a) Treatment of pain

  (i) Nitroglycerin. Because approximately 4% of all acute myocardial infarctions are thought to be caused by **coronary spasm** (as opposed to thrombotic occlusive disease), sublingual nitroglycerin should be administered in case the patient is suffering from coronary spasm.

  (ii) Morphine sulfate. If nitroglycerin is not effective in relieving pain, enough morphine sulfate should be given intravenously to relieve the patient's pain and anxiety.

(b) Thrombolysis

  (i) The use of **thrombolytic agents** (e.g., streptokinase, t-PA, urokinase, anistreplase) to dissolve the occlusive thrombus and promote reperfusion of the infarct-related artery significantly reduces the mortality from myocardial infarction when administered within 6 hours of the onset of chest pain. Substantial evidence exists that if reperfusion can be accomplished within 3 hours of the onset of chest pain, a significant amount of myocardium can be salvaged, leading to lower acute mortality and, often, better left ventricular function. Concomitant administration of aspirin enhances the effectiveness of streptokinase, whereas coadministration of heparin, and perhaps aspirin, enhances the effectiveness of t-PA.

(ii) In some centers, **direct PTCA** of the occluded vessel is preferred over thrombolytic agents.

(c) **Treatment of arrhythmias**

(i) **Prophylactic lidocaine.** Lidocaine given intravenously reduces the number of episodes of serious ventricular arrhythmias during the early phases of myocardial infarction. However, lidocaine therapy may also increase the risk of asystole, especially in patients with inferior myocardial infarction. Therefore, lidocaine's prophylactic use has become controversial. When used, a loading dose is given, often followed by a second loading dose and then constant intravenous infusion.

(ii) **Additional antiarrhythmic therapy.** If serious ventricular arrhythmias occur despite lidocaine infusion, additional drugs may be necessary to control them. **Bretylium tosylate** and **procainamide** may be useful in controlling acute recalcitrant arrhythmias and are given intravenously with caution.

(d) **Treatment of serious conduction disturbances.** As noted, high-degree AV nodal block may occur during acute myocardial infarction, producing significant bradycardia and hypotension. Therapies for restoring heart rate include:

(i) **Atropine** (1 mg intravenously) may restore conduction and increase heart rate, especially in inferior infarctions. If this fails, an infusion of a positive chronotropic agent such as **isoproterenol** (or use of a **transcutaneous electronic pacemaker**) increases heart rate. These therapies are directed at maintaining heart rate until **temporary transvenous pacemaking** can be performed.

(ii) In cases of severe left ventricular dysfunction, atrial systole must be preserved to maintain cardiac output, and **AV sequential pacemaking** is the preferred treatment.

(iii) The occurrence of new **bundle branch block**—particularly the combination of right bundle branch block and left anterior hemiblock—may be an indication for **temporary prophylactic pacemaking** because these disturbances may presage the occurrence of complete heart block; however, this tactic is controversial and obviated by the availability of transcutaneous pacing.

(e) **Treatment of heart failure**

(i) Mild congestive heart failure in patients with myocardial infarction can be treated with **diuretics.**

(ii) The use of **digitalis** during acute myocardial infarction remains controversial; however, fears that digitalis may increase oxygen consumption and extend myocardial infarction do not appear justified if the patient is in congestive heart failure. In such cases, digitalis actually may reduce both cardiac size and myocardial oxygen consumption.

(iii) In more advanced cases of congestive heart failure, **vasodilators** may be useful in reducing cardiac afterload, allowing increased cardiac output.

(f) **Treatment of cardiogenic shock.** Shock in the presence of myocardial infarction usually is attributable to inadequate left ventricular filling, severe muscle damage, or a mechanical complication of the myocardial infarction. When shock ensues, an **echocardiogram** is performed to assess ventricular function, and a **Swan-Ganz catheter** should be placed to measure left ventricular filling pressure.

(i) If the pulmonary capillary wedge pressure is less than 18 mm Hg, **volume is infused to maximize left ventricular filling** and cardiac output. Additionally, if a new cardiac murmur is detected, the echocardiogram and the Swan-Ganz catheter are useful in making the diagnosis of acute mitral regurgitation or acute ventricular septal defect.

(ii) Alternatively, if cardiogenic shock is caused by severe muscle damage, **pressor agents** (e.g., dobutamine, dopamine) and **intra-aortic balloon pumping** may be used to stabilize the patient until coronary arteriography and reestablishment of coronary blood flow by **PCTA** are carried out. However, the prognosis for such patients remains very poor despite therapy.

(g) Treatment of mitral regurgitation and acute ventricular septal defect

(i) Arteriolar vasodilator therapy to lower systemic vascular resistance is the mainstay of medical therapy for these complications. Reduction of systemic vascular resistance preferentially increases forward cardiac output and reduces nonproductive cardiac output, either into the left atrium (in the case of mitral regurgitation) or through the ventricular septal defect.

(ii) Intra-aortic balloon pumping, which also increases forward cardiac output and reduces nonproductive cardiac output, is useful in stabilizing patients with mitral regurgitation or acute ventricular septal defect, especially in hypotensive patients where the use of vasodilators is contraindicated.

(iii) Surgical correction of mechanical complications often is required.

(h) Adjunctive therapy

(i) β **Blockers** administered hours to days after myocardial infarction reduce early mortality by reducing ventricular arrhythmias and the risk of reinfarction. Generally, however, these agents are avoided in patients with severe congestive heart failure, antecedent cardiac bradyarrhythmias, or bronchospasm.

(ii) ACE inhibitors. Changes in the infarct zone and forces placed on the noninfarcted portion of the ventricle lead to ventricular dilatation, which reduces ventricular efficiency. **Captopril** (and possibly all ACE-inhibitors) reduces the extent of remodeling and the incidence of late mortality.

(iii) Anticoagulants. In anterior infarction, especially an infarct involving the apex of the heart, there is a high risk of developing a mural thrombus, which can become a systemic embolus. Echocardiography should be performed during the first few days following anterior infarction. If a thrombus is detected, anticoagulation with heparin followed by oral administration of warfarin is indicated.

(iv) Aspirin. Administration of aspirin following acute myocardial infarction reduces subsequent mortality. The dose is controversial, but one baby aspirin per day is recommended.

(v) Diltiazem. Post-infarction administration of diltiazem in patients with non–Q wave infarcts reduces mortality.

(vi) Prevention. In patients who have survived a myocardial infarction, it is important to prevent subsequent infarctions. As mentioned in III A 5 b (5) (h), administration of aspirin, ACE inhibitors, and β blockers can reduce the risk of reinfarction. In addition, modification of major risk factors (e.g., hypercholesterolemia, hypertension, and smoking) reduces the risk of a second myocardial infarction.

c. Sudden death in patients with coronary artery disease is common; in fact, approximately one-third of patients with coronary disease experience sudden death without antecedent angina or myocardial infarction.

(1) Precipitating causes. It is believed that most patients die of **acute ventricular arrhythmias** precipitated by ischemia. Although sudden death may be the result of a myocardial infarction secondary to coronary artery disease, most patients who die suddenly and are resuscitated do not have an acute myocardial infarction documented. It is likely that in these patients, ischemia produces heterogeneous depolarization of the ventricle, which leads to ventricular tachycardia and ventricular fibrillation.

(2) Acute therapy

(a) Cardiopulmonary resuscitation (i.e., mouth-to-mouth resuscitation and external chest compression) must be initiated in the euthermic patient within 4 minutes of the cessation of effective ventricular contraction in order to preserve neurologic and myocardial function. Current evidence suggests that closed-chest compression does not produce cardiac output by external cardiac compression as was previously thought. Rather, the valves in the systemic veins allow chest compression to produce a pressure gradient between the relatively low pressure in the extrathoracic veins and the relatively high pressure in the intrathoracic cavity, thereby creating forward cardiac flow.

(b) Electrical defibrillation and **drug support** should be provided as soon as possible.

(3) Preventive therapy. It is estimated that cardiac resuscitation of patients experiencing out-of-hospital cardiac arrest is fully successful in only 10%–20% of cases. The goal of preventive therapy, then, is to identify high-risk patients and prevent sudden death from occurring. Patients with the following conditions are recognized as being at high risk for an episode of sudden death.

(a) Previous sudden death. Patients who have experienced one episode of sudden death and have been successfully resuscitated have a 30%–50% chance of a second episode if the first episode occurred in the absence of a myocardial infarction.

(i) In such patients, intensive diagnostic work-up is indicated and should include **invasive electrophysiologic testing** and **intensive antiarrhythmic therapy** (see Table 1-1).

(ii) If medical antiarrhythmic therapy fails to control the arrhythmia, **surgical or catheter ablation of the arrhythmogenic area** of the myocardium may be effective.

(iii) Another alternative to failed medical therapy is insertion of an **implantable defibrillator.** Electrode patches connect this device (usually implanted in the abdominal wall) with the heart. When a lethal arrhythmia is detected by the defibrillator, it automatically discharges a defibrillating electrical shock to the myocardium, thereby restoring effective cardiac contraction.

(b) High-grade ventricular ectopy (e.g., **coupled ventricular extrasystoles, short runs of ventricular tachycardia,** or **R on T phenomenon**) **following myocardial infarction.** Patients in whom electrocardiographic monitoring reveals high-grade ventricular ectopy have approximately a four times greater risk for sudden death than patients without these abnormalities.

(i) This risk factor applies to patients in whom these abnormalities are found in the late period (i.e., 2 weeks or more) following the myocardial infarction but does not extend to those experiencing severe ventricular arrhythmias during the acute phase.

(ii) Many authorities believe that these patients should undergo intensive antiarrhythmic therapy, although conclusive evidence that this therapy prolongs life or prevents sudden death is not available. In fact, some antiarrhythmic agents may actually worsen arrhythmias in this setting.

(c) Prolonged Q-T intervals. Patients demonstrating prolonged Q-T intervals on the ECG are also at risk for sudden death. Prolonged Q-T syndromes can be congenital or acquired.

6. Prognosis. The prognosis of patients with coronary artery disease is determined primarily by two variables: the extent of coronary disease in terms of the **number of**

vessels affected by the disease and the **extent of left ventricular damage** present as a result of previous myocardial infarctions.

    a. Patients with uncorrected **main left coronary artery disease** have approximately a 20% mortality rate in the first year after its discovery.

    b. Patients with **single-vessel coronary artery disease** have approximately a 2% annual mortality rate, those with **double-vessel disease** have approximately a 3%–4% annual mortality rate, and those with **triple-vessel disease** have approximately a 5%–8% annual mortality rate.

    c. The presence of significant **left ventricular dysfunction** (as identified by an ejection fraction of less than 40%) approximately doubles the yearly mortality rate at each level of extent of coronary disease.

    d. Revascularization improves the prognosis for patients with main left coronary disease and for those with triple-vessel disease associated with left ventricular dysfunction.

B. **Nonatherosclerotic coronary artery disease.** Although the majority of cardiac ischemic events are caused by atherosclerotic coronary disease, nonatherosclerotic disease also may produce clinical ischemia.

    1. **Coronary embolism** occurs in infective endocarditis, from mural thrombus formation following myocardial infarction, and in the presence of atrial fibrillation. Coronary embolism frequently produces myocardial infarction.

    2. **Collagen vascular disease.** The collagen vascular diseases that affect medium-sized arteries, including the coronary arteries, are: **polyarteritis nodosa, Wegener's granulomatosis, systemic lupus erythematosus (SLE),** and, occasionally, **rheumatoid arthritis.**

    3. **Radiation therapy.** Tumor irradiation, in which the field of radiation includes the heart, damages the coronary arteries and leads to nonatherosclerotic coronary artery disease.

    4. **Transplantation.** The development of coronary disease following cardiac transplantation is a major factor in limiting the success of this therapy. Post-transplant coronary disease tends to be distal in location and diffuse in nature. It is probably partially attributable to chronic rejection of the organ and is not closely related to the presence of the standard coronary disease risk factors.

IV. VALVULAR HEART DISEASE

A. **Aortic stenosis**

    1. **Etiology**

        a. **Congenital aortic stenosis** usually is detected in pediatric patients but occasionally becomes apparent in early adulthood.

        b. **Senile calcific aortic stenosis** is a degenerative condition of the aortic valve, in which scarring and calcification of a tricuspid aortic valve lead to stenosis in the sixth, seventh, and eighth decades of life.

        c. **Bicuspid aortic stenosis** is a common congenital cardiac abnormality. The flow characteristics of the bicuspid valve are more turbulent than those of the normal valve, leading to valve degeneration, calcification, and stenosis in the fourth and fifth decades of life.

        d. **Rheumatic aortic stenosis** never occurs alone and always is associated with mitral valve disease.

    2. **Pathophysiology.** Aortic valve stenosis produces a pressure overload on the left ventricle due to the greater pressure that must be generated to force blood past the stenotic valve.

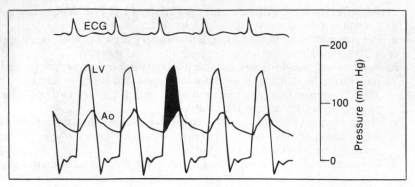

FIGURE 1-11. Diagram showing simultaneous recording of the electrocardiogram (*ECG*), left ventricular pressure tracing (*LV*), and aortic pressure tracing (*Ao*) in a patient with aortic stenosis. A large pressure gradient (*black area*) is evident. (Reprinted with permission from Grossman W: *Cardiac Catheterization and Angiography*, 2nd edition. Philadelphia, Lea & Febiger, 1980, p 128.)

    a. As shown in Figure 1-11, the systolic pressure inside the left ventricle is greater than in the aorta, producing a pressure gradient across the aortic valve. The pressure overload produced by the disease leads to the development of concentric left ventricular hypertrophy.

    b. Hypertrophy is a compensatory mechanism that reduces wall stress (afterload) on the left ventricle during systole. Thus, increased thickness of the ventricular wall as a result of concentric hypertrophy helps offset the increased pressure, which, in turn, reduces wall stress (the force each unit of myocardium must generate in order to shorten).

3. Clinical features

    a. Symptoms. Asymptomatic patients with aortic stenosis are at little risk for sudden death. However, this risk increases dramatically when symptoms develop.

        (1) Angina occurs in 35%–50% of patients with aortic stenosis.

            (a) Fifty percent of patients who develop this symptom die within 5 years of its onset unless aortic valve replacement is performed.

            (b) Although the exact mechanism of angina is unknown, current data suggest that coronary blood flow reserve is impaired in the severely hypertrophied left ventricle. Impairment of the coronary blood flow reserve limits oxygen delivery to the myocardium and produces angina during exercise.

        (2) Syncope occurs during exercise when total peripheral resistance falls due to local autoregulatory mechanisms [see IX B, C 1 b (2) (b)]. When aortic stenosis is present, cardiac output across the stenotic aortic valve cannot increase during exercise. Because total peripheral resistance falls, blood pressure must also fall and syncope occurs.

            (a) Other causes of syncope in aortic stenosis include **atrial** or **ventricular arrhythmias** and **heart block** as a result of conduction system calcification.

            (b) After syncope occurs in patients with aortic stenosis, expected survival is 2–3 years without valve replacement.

        (3) Heart failure. Fifty percent of patients who develop heart failure die within 1–2 years of presentation if the stenosis is not corrected. Heart failure occurs because the afterload placed on the myocardium becomes excessive and also because both contractile dysfunction and diastolic muscle dysfunction occur when the myocardium is exposed to a prolonged, severe pressure overload.

    b. Physical signs

        (1) Delayed carotid upstroke. In the presence of aortic stenosis, the carotid upstroke typically is delayed in its timing and reduced in volume. This finding is the most reliable physical sign in gauging the severity of the disease.

    (2) Systolic ejection murmur. A harsh, late-peaking systolic ejection murmur is heard in the aortic area and is transmitted to the carotid arteries. The murmur also may be reflected to the mitral area, producing the false impression that mitral regurgitation also is present **(Gallavardin's phenomenon).**

    (3) Soft, single S$_2$. Because the aortic valve is stenotic, its motion is severely impaired. The reduction in motion of the valve causes the **aortic component (A$_2$)** of the S$_2$ to be absent. Thus, the only component of the S$_2$ that is heard is the **pulmonic component (P$_2$),** which is normally soft.

    (4) An S$_4$ **usually is heard** as a result of the reduced left ventricular compliance that occurs in left ventricular hypertrophy.

    (5) Sustained, forceful apex beat. The point of maximal cardiac impulse usually is not displaced unless heart failure has occurred; however, the impulse is sustained and forceful throughout systole.

4. Laboratory diagnosis

    a. Electrocardiography. The ECG usually shows evidence of left ventricular hypertrophy.

    b. Fluoroscopy. Calcium is present in the aortic valve in most cases of aortic stenosis and can be demonstrated by fluoroscopy. The absence of calcium suggests that the stenosis is not severe.

    c. Echocardiography can rule out significant aortic stenosis if valve motion is shown to be normal, but the standard echocardiogram generally cannot prove that severe aortic stenosis definitely is present. However, Doppler examination of the aortic outflow tract during echocardiography can accurately measure the pressure gradient across the aortic valve, more precisely defining the severity of the pressure overload produced by the stenotic valve.

    d. Cardiac catheterization. Diagnosis and evaluation of the severity of aortic stenosis may be confirmed by cardiac catheterization, during which the pressure gradient across the valve is measured and the degree of stenosis is calculated.

5. Therapy

    a. Palliative therapy

        (1) Medical therapy has no definitive role in the treatment of aortic stenosis, but **digitalis** and **diuretics** may temporarily improve heart failure until mechanical relief of the obstruction is performed.

        (2) Insertion and inflation of a large balloon in the aortic valve orifice **(balloon valvuloplasty)** may also produce a moderate improvement in the amount of obstruction and in the patient's symptoms, but relief using this technique is usually only temporary. It does not reduce the mortality expected if the disease is left untreated.

    b. Curative therapy requires **aortic valve replacement.** Aortic valve replacement can be performed using a preserved human homograft valve, a porcine biprosthetic heterograft valve, or a mechanical valve.

        (1) Homograft valves have an excellent hemodynamic flow pattern and patients with homograft valves do not require anticoagulation therapy. Availability of these valves is limited because most suitable donors are also acceptable for whole heart donation in cardiac transplantation.

        (2) Heterograft valves. Patients with heterograft valves do not require anticoagulation therapy, but the durability of the valve is limited and deterioration after 10 years is common.

        (3) Mechanical valves are more durable than bioprostheses; however, patients do require anticoagulation therapy.

B. **Mitral stenosis**

1. Etiology. Almost all cases of mitral stenosis in adults are **secondary to rheumatic heart disease.** Most cases of mitral stenosis occur in women.

2. Pathophysiology

    a. Mitral valve stenosis impedes left ventricular filling, thereby increasing left atrial pressure as a pressure gradient develops across the mitral valve. Elevated left atrial pressure is referred to the lungs, where it produces **pulmonary congestion.** As the stenosis becomes more severe, it may significantly reduce forward cardiac output.

   b. Because the right ventricle is responsible for filling the left ventricle, the burden of propelling blood across the stenotic mitral valve is borne by the right ventricle. The overload on the right ventricle may be increased further when secondary pulmonary vasoconstriction occurs. Thus, the right ventricle must generate enough force both to overcome the resistance offered by the stenotic valve and to propel blood through constricted pulmonary arteries. Consequently, pulmonary arterial pressure may increase to three to five times normal, eventually resulting in **right ventricular failure.**

3. **Clinical features**
   a. **Symptoms**
      (1) **Left-sided failure. Dyspnea on exertion, orthopnea,** and **paroxysmal nocturnal dyspnea** occur as a result of reduced left ventricular output and increased left atrial pressure. In mitral stenosis, the symptoms of left ventricular failure usually are not attributable to left ventricular dysfunction but, rather, to the mitral stenosis itself.
      (2) **Right-sided failure.** When pulmonary hypertension occurs, the right ventricle may fail, producing **edema, ascites, anorexia,** and **fatigue.**
      (3) **Hemoptysis.** The high left atrial pressure produced in mitral stenosis may lead to rupture of small bronchial veins, producing hemoptysis.
      (4) **Systemic embolism.** Stagnation of blood in the enlarged left atrium and left atrial appendage occurs in mitral stenosis, particularly if atrial fibrillation is present. Under these circumstances, a thrombus may form in the left atrium and can become a source of systemic embolism.
      (5) **Hoarseness** may occur in mitral stenosis as the enlarged left atrium impinges on the left recurrent laryngeal nerve.
   b. **Physical signs**
      (1) **Atrial fibrillation.** Frequently, an irregularly irregular cardiac rhythm indicative of atrial fibrillation is present.
      (2) **Carotid pulse.** The carotid pulse is brisk in upstroke but diminished in volume as a result of reduced cardiac output.
      (3) **Pulmonary rales.** Bilateral pulmonary rales occur secondary to elevated left atrial and pulmonary venous pressures.
      (4) **Increased intensity of the S_1.** The S_1 usually increases in intensity because stenosis limits spontaneous diastolic mitral valve closure. Thus, the mitral valve remains open until ventricular systole closes it forcibly, resulting in an increase in S_1 intensity. Late in the course of the disease, the valve may become so stenotic that it no longer opens or closes, reducing the intensity of S_1.
      (5) **Increased intensity of the P_2 component of the S_2.** The P_2 component of the S_2 is usually increased in intensity if pulmonary hypertension has developed.
      (6) An **opening snap is heard following the S_2** as the stenotic valve is forced open in diastole by the high left atrial filling pressure. The higher the pressure, the sooner the mitral valve opens. Thus, a short S_2-opening snap interval (less than 0.10 second in duration) indicates relatively high left atrial pressure and severe stenosis.
      (7) **Diastolic rumble.** The murmur of mitral stenosis is a low-pitched apical rumble, which begins after the opening snap. If the patient is in sinus rhythm, atrial systole produces a presystolic accentuation of this murmur.
      (8) **Sternal lift.** Enlargement of the right ventricle as a result of pulmonary hypertension produces a systolic lift of the sternum.
      (9) **Neck vein distention, edema, hepatic enlargement,** and **ascites** may be present if right ventricular failure occurs.

4. **Laboratory diagnosis**
   a. **Electrocardiography.** The ECG may show atrial fibrillation and signs of left atrial enlargement and right ventricular hypertrophy.

   b. Chest radiography
      (1) Straightening of the left heart border and a double density along the right
      heart border (formed by the right and left atria) occur as a result of left
      atrial enlargement.
      (2) Signs of pulmonary venous hypertension, including an increase in pulmo-
      nary vascular markings and **Kerley's lines,** are likely to be present.
      (3) When **pulmonary hypertension** leads to right ventricular enlargement, the
      lateral view shows a **loss of the retrosternal airspace.**
   c. Echocardiography usually provides excellent images of the mitral valve.
      (1) The echocardiogram shows reduction in the excursion of the valve leaflets
      and thickening of the valve. Two-dimensional echocardiography can be
      used to visualize and measure the residual mitral valve orifice. Invariably,
      left atrial enlargement is present.
      (2) Doppler examination of the mitral valve can also help to quantify the sever-
      ity of the stenosis.
   d. Cardiac catheterization. Although the echocardiogram often can precisely and
      noninvasively quantify the severity of mitral stenosis, cardiac catheterization is
      still used frequently to perform coronary arteriography in coronary disease-
      prone patients.

5. Therapy
   a. Medical therapy is reserved for patients with mild to moderate symptoms of
      left-sided failure.
      (1) Diuretics are the mainstay of treatment. Diuretics are used to **control pul-
      monary congestion** and to **limit dyspnea and orthopnea.**
      (2) Digitalis. Because left ventricular muscle function usually is normal in mi-
      tral stenosis, the use of digitalis is of little benefit to patients in sinus
      rhythm. In patients in **atrial fibrillation,** however, digitalis is used to slow
      ventricular rate. A rapid ventricular rate in mitral stenosis shortens diastole,
      thereby reducing left ventricular filling, which, in turn, further increases left
      atrial pressure and reduces cardiac output.
      (3) Anticoagulants. Patients with mitral stenosis and coexistent atrial fibrillation
      have a **high incidence of systemic embolism.** In such patients, anticoagula-
      tion therapy (e.g., with **warfarin**) usually is indicated.
   b. Balloon valvuloplasty. Unlike balloon valvuloplasty for aortic stenosis, balloon
      valvuloplasty for mitral stenosis can offer effective long-term improvement. The
      best candidates for balloon mitral valvuloplasty are those in sinus rhythm with
      relatively mild mitral regurgitation and mild to moderate thickening of the mi-
      tral valve leaflets.
      (1) Valvuloplasty for mitral stenosis produces a commissurotomy similar to that
      produced by open heart surgery. During balloon mitral valvuloplasty,
      transseptal catheterization of the interatrial septum is performed, allowing
      passage of the balloon catheter from right atrium to left atrium. From the
      left atrium, the balloon catheter is advanced to the mitral valve and in-
      flated.
      (2) Although long-term follow-up data are not yet available, it is likely that this
      technique will be as effective as surgery in reducing symptoms and prolong-
      ing life.
   c. Surgical therapy is effective in relieving the symptoms of mitral stenosis and in
      prolonging life in symptomatic patients. Surgery should be performed prior to
      the development of pulmonary hypertension, which increases surgical risk.
      However, if pulmonary hypertension is present and surgery is successful, pulmo-
      nary hypertension usually regresses postoperatively.
      (1) Mitral commissurotomy. In young patients without significant valvular calci-
      fication or mitral regurgitation, commissurotomy allows relief of the stenosis
      without valve replacement.
      (2) Mitral valve replacement. If commissurotomy cannot be performed, valve
      replacement relieves the stenosis and the patient's symptoms.

C. **Aortic regurgitation**

1. Etiology

    a. Idiopathic aortic root dilatation. Aortic root dilatation is a frequent cause of aortic regurgitation. It is more frequent in patients with hypertension but correlates best with increasing age.

    b. Rheumatic heart disease. Aortic insufficiency usually is present to some degree in most cases of rheumatic heart disease. While mitral stenosis usually predominates, aortic insufficiency occasionally is the most severe manifestation of rheumatic heart disease.

    c. Infective endocarditis. Infection of the aortic valve may lead to **perforation or partial destruction of one or more aortic leaflets,** producing aortic insufficiency.

    d. Marfan syndrome may produce aortic insufficiency in two ways.

        (1) Proximal root dilatation. The extreme expansion of the proximal aortic root seen in Marfan syndrome may produce aortic insufficiency.

        (2) Aortic root dissection. The advanced cystic medial necrosis present in Marfan syndrome may lead to an intimal tear and dissection of the aorta. If the dissection involves the proximal aortic root, the supporting structures of the aortic valve are disrupted, and the valve is rendered incompetent.

    e. Aortic dissection. Any cause of aortic dissection other than Marfan syndrome may lead to aortic insufficiency.

    f. Syphilis may produce **aortitis,** which may extend to the aortic valve and produce aortic incompetence.

    g. Collagen vascular disease. SLE and ankylosing spondylitis may cause aortic insufficiency.

2. Pathophysiology

    a. A portion of the left ventricular stroke volume ejected during systole regurgitates into the left ventricle during diastole. If no compensation occurs, left ventricular forward output decreases. However, chronic regurgitation of blood into the left ventricle stimulates sarcomere replication in series, producing eccentric cardiac hypertrophy and an increase in end-diastolic volume. Because the stroke volume equals the end-diastolic volume minus the end-systolic volume, the total stroke volume increases, helping to compensate for the volume that is regurgitated. The increase in total stroke volume leads to an increase in pulse pressure and increased systolic pressure. This second type of overload is compensated by the additional development of concentric hypertrophy. **The additional volume and pressure that the left ventricle must generate eventually lead to left ventricular dysfunction and congestive heart failure.**

    b. An additional pathophysiologic consequence of aortic insufficiency is a **reduction in systemic diastolic blood pressure.**

3. Clinical features

    a. Symptoms

        (1) Left ventricular failure

            (a) Chronic aortic insufficiency may cause left ventricular dysfunction, leading to symptoms of **dyspnea, orthopnea,** and **paroxysmal nocturnal dyspnea.**

            (b) In **acute aortic insufficiency,** normal muscle function may coexist with heart failure. In this circumstance, reduced forward output and elevated left ventricular filling pressure occur prior to **compensatory left ventricular enlargement.**

        (2) Syncope. Reduction in diastolic systemic arterial pressure produces a reduction in mean arterial pressure. If the mean arterial pressure is reduced significantly, cerebral perfusion is compromised and syncope may occur.

        (3) Angina occurs less commonly in aortic insufficiency than in aortic stenosis. Angina in aortic insufficiency is caused by **reduced coronary blood flow.** Coronary blood flow occurs primarily in diastole and is driven by the aortic diastolic blood pressure. This driving pressure is reduced in aortic insufficiency, in turn reducing coronary blood flow.

b. Physical signs

(1) **Left ventricular impulse.** The PMI is **hyperdynamic** and is **displaced downward and to the left** as a result of left ventricular enlargement.

(2) **Diastolic murmur.** The murmur of aortic insufficiency is a **high-pitched, diastolic blowing murmur** heard along the left sternal border. Often the murmur is heard best when the patient is sitting up and leaning forward.

(3) **Austin Flint murmur.** A **low-pitched diastolic rumble** similar to that heard in mitral stenosis may be present in patients with aortic insufficiency. The Austin Flint murmur **usually indicates moderate to severe insufficiency.** The murmur is believed to be caused by reverberation of the regurgitant flow against the mitral valve, although the exact mechanism is unclear.

(4) **Total stroke volume** and consequently, **pulse pressure, increases** in chronic aortic insufficiency, because

$$\text{pulse pressure} = \frac{\text{stroke volume}}{\text{aortic elasticity}}.$$

The increased stroke volume and pulse pressure lead to many physical signs, some of which are listed below. These signs may be absent in acute aortic insufficiency because compensatory increases in end-diastolic volume and stroke volume have not yet occurred.

(a) **Corrigan's pulse.** The carotid pulse has a rapid rise and full upstroke with a rapid fall in diastole.

(b) **Hill's sign** refers to a disproportionate increase of systolic blood pressure (i.e., greater than 20 mm Hg) when measured in the leg, as compared with the systolic blood pressure measured in the arm. Hill's sign suggests severe aortic insufficiency.

(c) **Pistol-shot femoral pulses.** Auscultation over the femoral arteries reveals a pulse that sounds like a pistol shot.

(d) **Duroziez's sign.** A stethoscope is placed over the femoral artery with enough pressure to produce a systolic bruit. The concomitant occurrence of a diastolic bruit constitutes Duroziez's sign.

(e) **de Musset's sign** refers to a bobbing movement of the head caused by the increased stroke volume and pulse pressure.

(f) **Quincke's pulse** is systolic blushing and diastolic blanching of the nail bed when gentle pressure is placed on the nail.

4. Diagnosis

a. **Electrocardiography.** The ECG usually shows left ventricular hypertrophy.

b. **Chest radiography.** Unless the aortic insufficiency is mild or acute, **cardiac enlargement** is usually present, and often, the proximal aorta is dilated. The absence of cardiac enlargement militates against the diagnosis of severe chronic aortic insufficiency.

c. **Echocardiography.** Evidence of an enlarged left ventricular cavity is usually present in aortic insufficiency. Frequently, diastolic vibration of the mitral valve, produced by the regurgitant flow striking the valve, is present. Doppler examination of the aortic outflow tract will reveal abnormal diastolic flow from aorta to left ventricle.

d. **Cardiac catheterization.** Aortography is performed during cardiac catheterization. Contrast material is injected into the aorta, and the amount that regurgitates into the left ventricle is analyzed qualitatively. The regurgitant volume also can be calculated.

5. Therapy. If aortic insufficiency is severe, **aortic valve replacement** eventually is necessary.

a. Timing of surgery is difficult, however, because the lesion may be tolerated for several years. Careful follow-up is required to detect early signs of decompensation, at which time, valve replacement is advisable. In most cases, valve replacement should be performed before the left ventricular echocardiographic end-systolic dimension exceeds 55 mm and the ejection fraction falls below 55%.

    b. If surgery is not possible, therapy with **digitalis, diuretics,** and **vasodilators may afford symptomatic relief.**

D. **Mitral regurgitation**

    1. Etiology

      a. Rheumatic heart disease. Scarring and retraction of the mitral leaflets as a result of rheumatic heart disease causes mitral regurgitation.

      b. Ruptured chordae tendineae. Spontaneous rupture of the chordae tendineae may occur in otherwise healthy individuals. Chordal rupture permits prolapse of a portion of a mitral valve leaflet into the left atrium, rendering the valve incompetent.

      c. Coronary artery disease may lead to ischemia or infarction of the papillary muscles to which the mitral valve is tethered, thereby producing mitral incompetence.

      d. Infective endocarditis. Infection of the mitral valve may cause its destruction with subsequent regurgitation.

      e. Mitral valve prolapse and click-murmur syndrome are terms that describe a group of diseases in which the mitral valve or chordae are redundant, permitting systolic prolapse of the mitral valve into the left atrium with resultant mitral regurgitation.

        (1) This syndrome usually is benign but in some cases may be associated with significant mitral regurgitation. Additional complications include atypical chest pain, cardiac arrhythmias, and an increased risk of embolic stroke. Most clinically important sequelae occur in those patients whose mitral valves are clearly thickened and echocardiographically abnormal.

        (2) A midsystolic click and a late systolic murmur typically are heard on physical examination.

    2. Pathophysiology. Mitral regurgitation permits a portion of the left ventricular stroke volume to be pumped backward into the left atrium instead of forward into the aorta, resulting in **increased left atrial pressure and decreased forward cardiac output.** Preload is increased by the volume overload, and afterload is initially decreased as the left ventricle empties a portion of its contents into the relatively (i.e., compared to the aorta) low-pressure left atrium. This augments ejection performance and helps to compensate for the regurgitation.

      a. Initially, compliance of the left atrium is low, and the regurgitant volume produces high left atrial pressure with resultant congestive symptoms.

      b. With time, the left atrial compliance and volume increase, allowing accommodation of the regurgitant volume at more physiologic filling pressures.

      c. The development of left ventricular eccentric cardiac hypertrophy restores forward stroke volume.

      d. After a prolonged period of compensation, left ventricular muscle dysfunction eventually occurs, resulting in a fall in ejection fraction from supranormal to normal or even subnormal values.

    3. Clinical features

      a. Symptoms of mitral regurgitation are those of left ventricular failure (i.e., **dyspnea, orthopnea,** and **paroxysmal nocturnal dyspnea**).

        (1) If mitral regurgitation is severe and chronic, **pulmonary hypertension** and **symptoms of right-sided failure** also may occur.

        (2) Patients in atrial fibrillation may experience **symptoms of systemic embolization.** The risk of embolization appears to be less in patients with mitral regurgitation than in those with mitral stenosis, although this is debatable.

      b. Physical signs

        (1) Left ventricular impulse. As with aortic regurgitation, the PMI is hyperdynamic and displaced downward and to the left.

        (2) Carotid upstroke. The upstrokes are brisk but diminished in volume as a result of reduced stroke volume.

        (3) Murmur. The murmur of mitral regurgitation is a holosystolic apical murmur that radiates to the axilla and frequently is **accompanied by a thrill.**

(4) An S_3 **usually is heard** in mitral regurgitation and may occur even in the absence of overt heart failure. The S_3 is caused by the rapid filling of the left ventricle by the large volume of blood accumulated in the left atrium during systole.

4. Diagnosis

  a. Electrocardiography. The ECG shows signs of left ventricular hypertrophy and left atrial enlargement.

  b. Chest radiography shows cardiac enlargement. Vascular congestion indicates heart failure.

  c. Echocardiography

  (1) In cases of a **ruptured chorda** or **mitral valve prolapse,** the mitral valve can be seen extending into the left atrium during systole.

  (2) When the mitral valve has been damaged by **endocarditis,** vegetations on the cardiac leaflets frequently are demonstrated. Transesophageal echocardiography is better than transthoracic echocardiography for detecting vegetations.

  (3) Regardless of the cause of the mitral regurgitation, **left atrial** and **left ventricular enlargement occur** if the condition is chronic.

  (4) Doppler examination reveals abnormal systolic flow from the left ventricle into the left atrium.

  d. Cardiac catheterization. Right-heart catheterization yields a **pulmonary capillary wedge tracing** that often displays a **large v wave** representative of the systolic volume overload on the left atrium. **Left ventriculography** demonstrates systolic regurgitation of contrast material into the left atrium.

5. Therapy

  a. Medical therapy. The goal of medical therapy is to relieve symptoms by increasing forward cardiac output and reducing pulmonary venous hypertension.

  (1) **Digitalis** is useful in controlling heart rate when atrial fibrillation occurs. In chronic mitral regurgitation with muscle dysfunction, digitalis may be useful in increasing the inotropic state. Digitalis is not indicated in cases of acute mitral regurgitation when no inotropic deficit exists.

  (2) **Diuretics** are used to reduce central volume overload, which in turn reduces pulmonary venous hypertension and congestion.

  (3) **Vasodilators.** Arteriolar vasodilators are **particularly useful** in managing acute mitral regurgitation. These agents **reduce resistance to aortic outflow,** thereby preferentially increasing forward output while reducing the amount of regurgitation. Vasodilators also **reduce left ventricular size,** which helps to reestablish mitral competence.

  (4) **Anticoagulants.** Patients with mitral regurgitation and atrial fibrillation are at some risk for systemic embolism; thus, anticoagulants usually are indicated.

  b. Surgery. Mitral valve replacement or repair is indicated for chronic mitral regurgitation, even if symptoms are mild, if there is evidence of ventricular dysfunction.

  (1) **Valve replacement** must be performed prior to the onset of significant muscle dysfunction, which limits the success of operative intervention. To help ensure preservation of ventricular function, surgery should occur before the ejection fraction falls below 60%.

  (2) **Valve repair** offers several advantages over replacement, including eliminating the introduction of a prosthesis and decreasing the need for anticoagulation therapy. Furthermore, repairing, rather than replacing, the valve helps preserve left ventricular function because the mitral valve apparatus, which plays an important role in ventricular contraction, is preserved.

E. **Tricuspid regurgitation**

1. Etiology

  a. Infective endocarditis is a common cause of tricuspid regurgitation in drug abusers who inject drugs under septic conditions.

    b. **Right ventricular failure.** Sustained pressure or volume overload on the right ventricle leads to right ventricular dilatation and improper alignment of the papillary muscles, which produces tricuspid regurgitation.

    c. **Rheumatic heart disease.** In rheumatic heart disease, tricuspid regurgitation may occur, secondary to right ventricular pressure overload from left-sided valvular lesions. Tricuspid regurgitation also may occur as a result of primary rheumatic involvement of the tricuspid valve.

    d. **Right ventricular infarction.** Right coronary artery occlusion with subsequent right ventricular infarction may lead to papillary muscle dysfunction and ventricular dilatation, which in turn may produce tricuspid regurgitation.

2. **Pathophysiology.** During systole, the dysfunctioning tricuspid valve allows blood to flow backward into the right atrium, leading to systemic venous congestion and venous hypertension.

3. **Clinical features**
    a. **Symptoms** of tricuspid regurgitation include those of right-sided failure (i.e., **edema, ascites**). In severe and acute cases, **hepatic congestion** may be extensive enough to produce **right upper quadrant pain.** Passive hepatic congestion also may lead to hepatocellular damage and **jaundice.**
    b. **Physical signs**
      (1) **Right ventricular lift.** The enlarged right ventricle may be palpated as a systolic lift of the sternum.
      (2) **Murmur.** A holosystolic murmur that increases with inspiration is heard along the left sternal border.
      (3) **Jugular venous pulsation.** A large **v wave** is seen in jugular veins during systole.
      (4) **Pulsatile liver.** Systolic expansion of the liver frequently is present.

4. **Diagnosis**
    a. **Electrocardiography** reveals signs of right ventricular and right atrial enlargement.
    b. **Chest radiography.** Right ventricular enlargement is seen as an obliteration of the retrosternal airspace on the lateral view.
    c. **Echocardiography** demonstrates enlargement of the right atrium and right ventricle. Doppler examination is highly effective in demonstrating tricuspid regurgitation.

5. **Therapy.** Left-sided failure frequently is the cause of right-sided failure and tricuspid regurgitation. Effective treatment of left-sided failure reduces right ventricular pressure overload, which may decrease right ventricular size, thus restoring valvular competence. If tricuspid regurgitation is caused by organic valvular disease, surgical repair or replacement of the tricuspid valve may be necessary.

V. CARDIOMYOPATHIES

B. **Dilated (congestive) cardiomyopathy**

1. **Definition.** Dilated cardiomyopathy is defined as a diminution in the contractile function of the left, right, or both ventricles in the absence of pressure overload, volume overload, or coronary artery disease. The loss of cardiac muscle function results in congestive heart failure.

2. **Etiology.** The cause of most cases of dilated cardiomyopathy is unknown. Viral infection has been implicated in the pathogenesis of this disease, but proof of cause generally is lacking. The following other conditions have been linked to cardiomyopathy.
    a. **Prolonged ethanol abuse** is the most common reversible cause of cardiomyopathy.

    b. Doxorubicin therapy. High doses of doxorubicin, a commonly used antitumor drug, may result in irreversible dilated cardiomyopathy.

    c. Exposure to cobalt, mercury, lead, and or **high-dose catecholamines** may cause myocardial damage and dilated cardiomyopathy.

    d. Endocrinopathies, including **thyrotoxicosis, hypothyroidism,** and **acromegaly,** have been reported to cause dilated cardiomyopathy. In thyrotoxicosis and in hypothyroidism, the myopathy usually is reversed when the endocrinopathy is corrected.

    e. Metabolic disorders (e.g., **hypophosphatemia, hypocalcemia, thiamine deficiency**) may produce reversible cardiomyopathy.

    f. Hemoglobinopathies (e.g., **sickle cell anemia, thalassemia**) are associated with myocardial dysfunction.

    g. Genetic abnormalities. In some families, the development of dilated cardiomyopathy is linked to specific genetic abnormalities.

3. Clinical features

    a. Symptoms of dilated cardiomyopathy are those of both left- and right-sided congestive heart failure as described in I D 1.

        (1) Generally, the symptoms of left-sided failure (i.e., **orthopnea, paroxysmal nocturnal dyspnea,** and **dyspnea on exertion**) precede those of right-sided failure.

        (2) Chest pain may occur in the absence of obstructive coronary disease. The cause of the chest pain may be the excessive oxygen demands of an enlarged, thin-walled ventricle.

    b. Physical signs in dilated cardiomyopathy are those of congestive heart failure. A gallop rhythm is usually present. The murmur of mitral regurgitation also may be present. Mitral regurgitation occurs due to ventricular dilatation and improper alignment of the papillary muscles.

4. Diagnosis

    a. Electrocardiography. Left ventricular hypertrophy and nonspecific S-T– and T-wave abnormalities are seen frequently. Left bundle branch block is common.

    b. Chest radiography. The heart is enlarged in dilated cardiomyopathy and there is evidence of pulmonary vascular congestion.

    c. Echocardiography reveals dilated and poorly contracting left and right ventricles. In addition, secondary left and right atrial enlargement usually is seen.

    d. Gated blood pool scanning in dilated cardiomyopathy reveals reduction of the ejection fraction of both ventricles. There usually is global dysfunction, but regional contractile abnormalities also may exist.

    e. Cardiac catheterization usually is not necessary to make the diagnosis of dilated cardiomyopathy. However, because surgical correction of ischemic heart disease can occasionally improve left ventricular function, ischemic heart disease should be excluded prior to making the diagnosis of cardiomyopathy. In such cases, cardiac catheterization may be indicated.

5. Therapy

    a. Removal of an offending agent. The most hopeful situation is one in which a known toxin has caused ventricular dysfunction. Removal of the toxin from the patient's environment may lead to significant improvement in ventricular function.

    b. Supportive therapy. When dilated cardiomyopathy is idiopathic, the symptoms of congestive heart failure can be improved by such measures as **salt restriction** and **administration of cardiac glycosides, diuretics,** and **vasodilators.** Recent evidence shows that the addition of vasodilators (e.g., nitroglycerin and hydralazine or ACE inhibitors) to a standard regimen of digoxin and diuretics increases longevity.

    c. Cardiac transplantation. Cardiac transplantation may offer an improved quality of life to selected patients when control of congestive heart failure is not possible and prognosis is poor.

B. **Hypertrophic obstructive cardiomyopathy**

1. **Definition.** Hypertrophic obstructive cardiomyopathy, which previously was referred to as **idiopathic hypertrophic subaortic stenosis** or **asymmetric septal hypertrophy,** is a disorder in which the interventricular septum hypertrophies excessively. The hypertrophied septum and the anterior leaflet of the mitral valve produce left ventricular outflow obstruction.

2. **Etiology.** Most cases are inherited through an autosomal dominant mode of transmission, but sporadic cases also occur. Specific abnormalities in cardiac myosin resulting from several abnormal genes have been identified.

3. **Pathophysiology**
   a. **Method of obstruction**
      (1) As shown in Figure 1-12, the hypertrophied septum encroaches on the left ventricular outflow tract and comes into close approximation with the anterior leaflet of the mitral valve.
      (2) During systole, a low-pressure zone may develop as blood flow accelerates through the narrowed area between the septum and the anterior leaflet, generating a **Bernoulli effect.** Thus, the anterior leaflet of the mitral valve is drawn into the septum (systolic anterior motion), leading to outflow obstruction.
      (3) The septum itself shortens very little during systole because of its catenoid shape. Because the septum does not shorten, it cannot thicken. Therefore, it is the anterior leaflet of the mitral valve that plays the active role in creating the obstruction.

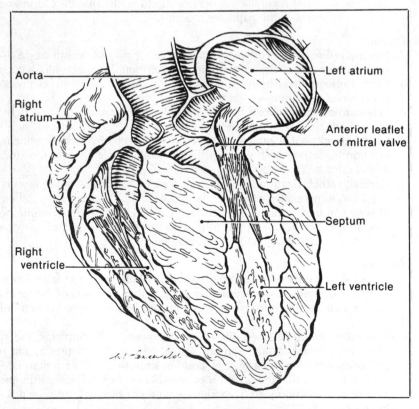

FIGURE 1-12. Cardiac cross-section cut from the apex to the base in a patient with hypertrophic obstructive cardiomyopathy. The upper portion of the septum is thickened and comes into close proximity with the anterior leaflet of the mitral valve. (Adapted from Johnson R, et al: *The Practice of Cardiology.* Boston, Little, Brown, 1980, p 648.)

b. The **degree of outflow obstruction** varies from patient to patient and from time to time in the same patient.

(1) Physiologic conditions that enlarge the left ventricle (e.g., increases in pre-load and afterload) separate the septum and anterior leaflet of the mitral valve and reduce the obstruction.

(2) Physiologic conditions that make the ventricle smaller or that increase the velocity of blood flow (e.g., dehydration, positive inotropic drugs) increase the degree of obstruction.

c. The obstruction to outflow may cause secondary cardiac hypertrophy of the nonseptal portions of the ventricle, but septal thickness generally remains greater than that of the free wall of the ventricle.

4. Clinical features

a. Symptoms

(1) **Angina.** Patients with obstructive cardiomyopathy frequently complain of chest pain.

(a) The pain usually has **atypical features;** that is, the pain may occur at rest and is not always related to exercise.

(b) The pathophysiology of angina in hypertrophic obstructive cardiomyopathy is unclear, but coronary blood flow is subnormal, potentially causing ischemia.

(2) **Syncope**

(a) Syncope usually occurs after exercise in patients with obstructive cardiomyopathy as a result of reduced left ventricular size and the consequent increased obstruction to outflow.

(i) After exercise, **afterload is reduced** because of peripheral vasodilatation.

(ii) **Preload is reduced** because of the decreased activity of the contractions of the leg muscles, which help to return blood to the heart.

(iii) The **inotropic state remains elevated** because of the increased catecholamine level after exercise.

(b) **Arrhythmias,** which are common in this disorder, also may precipitate syncope.

(3) **Congestive heart failure.** Dyspnea on exertion, orthopnea, and paroxysmal nocturnal dyspnea occur in patients with obstructive cardiomyopathy. Systolic function usually is normal or supranormal and the ejection fraction often exceeds 80%.

(a) The symptoms of heart failure usually are not caused by systolic malfunction, but rather, occur as a result of increased diastolic stiffness.

(b) The thickened myocardium requires an increased filling pressure for adequate diastolic distention. The increased filling pressure is reflected to the lungs and produces pulmonary congestive symptoms.

(c) In the later stages of the disease, however, systolic dysfunction also may occur, contributing to the symptoms of congestive heart failure.

b. Physical signs

(1) **Carotid upstroke.** In patients with the obstructive form of the disease, the carotid upstrokes have a **spike and dome character** (Figure 1-13). This configuration indicates early systolic outflow followed by a period of obstruction, during which flow falls. The dome portion of the curve reflects the period near the end of systole when obstruction diminishes and aortic outflow again commences.

(2) **Murmur.** The murmur is a systolic ejection murmur, heard along the left sternal border. Unlike the murmur in valvular aortic stenosis, it does not usually radiate to the neck.

(a) **Increasing the intensity of the murmur**

(i) Maneuvers that diminish left ventricular size (e.g., the **Valsalva maneuver**) cause an increase in both the obstruction to outflow and the intensity of the cardiac murmur. Thus, the Valsalva maneuver,

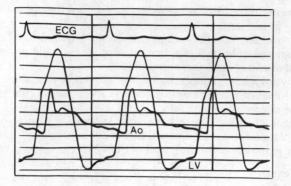

FIGURE 1-13. Diagram showing simultaneous recording of the electrocardiogram (*ECG*), left ventricular pressure tracing (*LV*), and aortic pressure tracing (*Ao*) in a patient with hypertrophic obstructive cardiomyopathy. A large pressure gradient exists between the left ventricle and aorta. The aortic pressure tracing (similar to the carotid pulse) demonstrates a spike and dome configuration. (Reprinted with permission from Cohn PF, Wynne J: *Diagnostic Methods in Clinical Cardiology.* Boston, Little, Brown, 1982, p 147.)

which diminishes the murmur in valvular aortic stenosis by diminishing flow, increases the murmur in obstructive cardiomyopathy by increasing obstruction.

 (ii) Having the patient stand or inhale amyl nitrite also diminishes left ventricular size and, therefore, increases the intensity of the murmur.

 (b) Diminishing the intensity of the murmur. Squatting, which increases myocardial afterload and venous return to the heart, increases cardiac size and, therefore, diminishes the murmur.

 5. Diagnosis

  a. Electrocardiography. The ECG almost always is abnormal, usually showing evidence of left ventricular hypertrophy, nonspecific S-T– and T-wave abnormalities, and left atrial enlargement.

  b. Echocardiography establishes the diagnosis in most patients.

   (1) In patients with **asymmetric septal hypertrophy without obstruction,** increased septal thickness results in a **septum-to-free wall thickness ratio of 1.3:1** or greater.

   (2) Findings in the obstructive form of the disease include **systolic anterior motion of the mitral valve, systolic fluttering of the aortic valve leaflets,** and **early closure of the aortic valve,** corresponding to the spike and dome seen in the carotid pulse.

  c. Cardiac catheterization is performed in patients with obstructive cardiomyopathy to quantify the degree of obstruction prior to surgery.

 6. Therapy. Unlike aortic stenosis, in which relief of valvular obstruction relieves symptoms and prolongs life, there is no conclusive evidence that surgical relief of obstruction in obstructive cardiomyopathy prolongs life. Therefore, medical therapy is employed first in an attempt to improve symptoms.

  a. Medical therapy

   (1) β-Adrenergic blocking agents (e.g., **propranolol**) are effective in relieving symptoms in this disease.

    (a) β blockade **slows the heart rate,** which increases left ventricular filling and size, diminishing obstruction.

    (b) β blockade also reduces the vigor of left ventricular contraction and, thus, **decreases the velocity of blood flow,** which also reduces the degree of obstruction.

   (2) Calcium channel blocking agents. Although currently not approved for treatment of obstructive myopathy, calcium channel blockers have been shown to **diminish the left ventricular outflow gradient. Verapamil** is the calcium channel blocker most widely used in the treatment of this disease. Caution must be exercised in congestive heart failure patients because verapamil may worsen failure and precipitate acute pulmonary edema.

(3) **Digitalis** is **contraindicated in the hyperdynamic phase** of the disease when obstruction is present and the left ventricular cavity is small, because digitalis increases the vigor of left ventricular contraction and, thus, increases the outflow obstruction. In the end stages of the disease **when ventricular dilatation has occurred,** standard therapy for congestive heart failure (i.e., **digitalis** and **diuretics) may be beneficial.**

b. **Surgical therapy**

(1) **Myomectomy.** Surgical reduction of the thickness of the left ventricular septum relieves the outflow gradient and symptoms in those patients who have not responded to medical therapy.

(2) **Mitral valve replacement.** Because it is the anterior leaflet of the mitral valve that produces the obstruction, mitral valve replacement is also effective in relieving obstruction.

(3) **Pacemaker implantation.** Recent studies have shown that implantation of an AV sequential pacemaker can dramatically reduce outflow obstruction probably by altering the sequence of septal contraction in relation to the rest of the ventricle. Trials are underway to study the long-term efficacy of this therapy.

C. **Restrictive cardiomyopathy**

1. **Definition.** The restrictive cardiomyopathies are a group of diseases in which the composition of the myocardium has changed so that it becomes stiffer. The **increased stiffness of the myocardium** restricts left ventricular filling, reducing stroke output and increasing left ventricular filling pressure.

2. **Etiology. Infiltrative diseases** of the myocardium, which produce restrictive cardiomyopathy, include **amyloidosis, hemochromatosis, idiopathic eosinophilia, carcinoid syndrome, sarcoidosis,** and **endomyocardial fibroelastosis.**

3. **Pathophysiology.** Systolic function usually is normal in the early stages of the disease, but the altered properties of the myocardium increase diastolic stiffness. Thus, the left ventricular pressure is above normal at any diastolic left ventricular volume. Increased filling pressure produces pulmonary congestion. As the infiltrative process progresses, systolic function also is compromised.

4. **Clinical features**
   a. **Symptoms of both left-sided and right-sided congestive heart failure** usually are present; the symptoms of right-sided failure are usually more prominent.
   b. **Physical signs** include those present in left-sided and right-sided congestive heart failure.

5. **Diagnosis**
   a. **Electrocardiography.** The ECG frequently shows low QRS voltages and nonspecific S-T– and T-wave abnormalities. Conduction abnormalities are common.
   b. **Radiographs.** Signs of pulmonary vascular congestion may coexist with normal heart size because, even when left ventricular systolic function fails in the later stages of the disease, the restriction to cardiac filling prevents cardiac dilatation.
   c. **Echocardiography**
      (1) The echocardiogram demonstrates thickening of the left and right ventricles. The combination of increased left ventricular thickness on the echocardiogram and decreased left ventricular voltage on the ECG is highly suggestive of restrictive cardiomyopathy.
      (2) Left and right ventricular chamber sizes usually are normal, while the left and right atria are increased in size.
      (3) In amyloidosis, the myocardium may appear brighter than normal.
   d. **Cardiac catheterization.** Often it is difficult to distinguish restrictive cardiomyopathy from constrictive pericarditis using cardiac catheterization.

      (1) A **dip** and **plateau** in the left and right ventricular filling pressures may be seen in both diseases.

      (2) In restrictive cardiomyopathy, **left and right atrial pressures and left and right ventricular filling pressures** usually are **not identical,** as they are in constrictive pericarditis.

      (3) **Endomyocardial biopsy** during cardiac catheterization may help to establish the diagnosis.

  6. Therapy for this group of diseases is limited.

    a. In cases with a **reversible etiology** (e.g., hemochromatosis), **direct therapy** such as iron chelation may result in improvement.

    b. When the cause of the disease cannot be treated, **symptomatic therapy with diuretics** to reduce the symptoms of congestion is indicated. **Vasodilators** must be used with caution because a reduction in preload causes a reduction in both left ventricular filling and cardiac output.

VI. PERICARDIAL DISEASE

A. Acute pericarditis

  1. Etiology

    a. Myocardial infarction. Pericarditis may occur in the first 24 hours following transmural myocardial infarction, because the inflamed surface of the infarcted area of myocardium produces **pericardial irritation.** A second type of pericarditis, called **Dressler's syndrome,** also may be seen from 1 week to several months after myocardial infarction and may occur as the result of an autoimmune reaction to the damaged heart muscle.

    b. Viral infection. Many cases of acute pericarditis have no known etiology. However, because **pericarditis frequently follows upper respiratory tract viral infections,** a viral etiology has been implicated.

    c. Collagen vascular disease. Acute pericarditis may be a clinical manifestation of SLE, or, less commonly, scleroderma.

    d. Infectious pericarditis. Tuberculosis, streptococcal infection, staphylococcal infection, and the sequelae of infective endocarditis all may produce pericarditis.

    e. Drugs. Commonly used drugs that may cause acute pericarditis include **procainamide, hydralazine,** and **isoniazid.**

    f. Malignancy. Pericarditis may occur secondary to metastatic involvement of the pericardium. **Pulmonary and breast carcinomas** are the most **common primary sites.**

    g. Uremia. Pericarditis is common in untreated or undertreated severe chronic renal failure.

    h. Postpericardiotomy syndrome. During open heart surgery, the pericardium is incised. Usually, the pericarditis that arises from this injury is short-lived; however, it may be protracted and severe in some patients.

    i. Radiation. Radiation therapy delivered to the chest for thoracic malignancies may cause pericarditis.

  2. Clinical features

    a. Symptoms. The most common symptom in pericarditis is **inspiratory chest pain.**

      (1) The pain is located in the left side and often is lessened when the patient sits up and leans forward.

      (2) Occasionally, the pain may be similar to that of myocardial ischemia and may radiate to the neck and arm.

    b. Physical signs. The **classic sign** of acute pericarditis is the **pericardial friction rub,** which is a scratchy, leathery sound heard during both systole and diastole. Atrial contraction may add a third component to the rub.

  3. Diagnosis

    a. Physical examination. The presence of a **pericardial friction rub** confirms the diagnosis of pericarditis.

b. **Electrocardiography.** Epicardial inflammation produces a diffuse current of injury with S-T–segment elevation throughout the ECG. There is no reciprocal S-T–segment depression, as is seen in acute myocardial infarction. **Depression of the P-R segment is unique to pericarditis.**

c. **Echocardiography.** The echocardiogram frequently demonstrates a pericardial effusion, which helps confirm the diagnosis.

4. **Therapy**

a. **Specific therapy** should be directed toward the cause of the pericarditis, if the cause is known.

b. **Nonsteroidal anti-inflammatory drugs (NSAIDs)** such as **aspirin, indomethacin,** and **ibuprofen** usually are effective in reducing the inflammation and relieving the chest pain.

c. **Steroid therapy.** Intractable cases of pericarditis, as may occur with Dressler's syndrome and postpericardiotomy syndrome, may require glucocorticoid therapy for relief of symptoms.

B. **Pericardial effusion**

1. **Pathophysiology.** The inflammation caused by acute pericarditis often produces exudation of fluid into the pericardial space. When fluid accumulates slowly, the pericardium expands to accommodate it, but when fluid accumulates rapidly, it compresses the heart, thus inhibiting cardiac filling. This latter condition is known as **cardiac tamponade** (see VI C).

2. **Clinical features**

a. **Symptoms.** The mere presence of a pericardial effusion does not cause symptoms. However, symptoms of acute pericarditis may coexist with a pericardial effusion.

b. **Physical signs.** As the effusion accumulates, it acts as a cushion around the heart.

(1) The precordium becomes quiet, palpation of the PMI becomes difficult, and the heart tones become distant and soft.

(2) Although the accumulation of fluid between the layers of pericardium may diminish a pericardial friction rub, a friction rub still may exist in the presence of a large effusion.

3. **Diagnosis**

a. **Electrocardiography.** The ECG demonstrates low voltage; electrical alternans often is present.

b. **Chest radiography.** Cardiac enlargement occurs as the effusion develops. Typically, the cardiac silhouette has a **"water bottle" appearance.** The presence of an extremely enlarged heart without signs of vascular congestion suggests the diagnosis of pericardial effusion.

c. **Echocardiography.** An echocardiogram demonstrating an **echo-free space between the two layers of the pericardium** is diagnostic of a pericardial effusion.

d. **Pericardiocentesis.** The presence of a pericardial effusion may be confirmed by the aspiration of fluid from the pericardial sac. Examination of the fluid helps to establish the cause of the effusion.

(1) The fluid should be sent for a cell count and differential, bacterial and fungal cultures, stains and cultures for *Mycobacterium tuberculosis,* protein content, and LDH content.

(2) An additional aliquot of fluid should be centrifuged and examined for tumor cells.

(3) If collagen vascular disease is suspected, fluid should be tested for antinuclear antibodies (ANAs).

(4) Bloody effusions are characteristic of certain etiologies (e.g., neoplasia, tuberculosis). However, bloody effusions can also occur if the needle is passed too far and ventricular blood is aspirated by mistake. It is possible to distinguish the two because ventricular blood clots, whereas an effusion does not.

    e. Therapy for a pericardial effusion is the same as that for acute pericarditis, but involves aspiration of the effusion as well.

C. Cardiac tamponade

   1. **Definition and pathophysiology.** Cardiac tamponade is a **life-threatening condition** in which a pericardial effusion has developed so rapidly or has become so large that it compresses the heart.

     a. The heart cannot fill adequately, and because the heart can pump out only what it takes in, impaired filling causes a profound reduction in cardiac output.

     b. The external pressure produced by the fluid on the four chambers of the heart is dispersed equally. Because external pressure usually rises to a greater level than the normal cardiac filling pressures, intrapericardial pressure, left and right atrial pressures, and left and right ventricular pressures all become equal in diastole.

   2. **Clinical features**

     a. Symptoms. Most patients with cardiac tamponade complain of **dyspnea, fatigue,** and **orthopnea.**

     b. Physical signs

       (1) Pulsus paradoxus is the normal fall in systolic blood pressure that occurs during inspiration, but in tamponade the finding is exaggerated. A pulsus paradoxus of more than 10 mm Hg occurs in 95% of patients with cardiac tamponade. The presence of pulsus paradoxus implies that stroke volume is falling during inspiration, probably as a result of the following mechanisms:

         (a) Septal shift. During inspiration, right ventricular filling is augmented by negative intrathoracic pressure, which increases venous return. This causes transient enlargement of the right ventricle and pushes the ventricular septum into the left ventricle, thus reducing the size and output of the left ventricle.

         (b) Tensing of the pericardium. Inspiration produces downward traction on the pericardium, further compressing the cardiac structures and reducing left ventricular output.

         (c) Right ventricular enlargement. The enhanced right ventricular filling during inspiration also distends the right ventricle, causing it to take up more room in the pericardial space. This further limits left ventricular filling.

         (d) Negative intrathoracic pressure. During inspiration, the negative pressure inside the chest subtracts pressure from the extrathoracic vasculature, further reducing blood pressure.

         (e) Expansion of the pulmonary vascular bed. The pulmonary vascular bed expands during inspiration, increasing its capacity and, thus, reduces left atrial filling.

       (2) Neck vein distention. The intrapericardial pressure and right atrial pressure are reflected by extreme elevation of the jugular venous pressure. However, Kussmaul's sign (i.e., increased neck vein distention with inspiration) usually is absent in this condition.

       (3) Narrowed pulse pressure. Reduction in left ventricular stroke volume leads to a reduction in systolic pressure; the tachycardia that usually occurs as a compensatory mechanism diminishes diastolic runoff and maintains diastolic pressure. Thus, pulse pressure is narrowed; however, less severe cases of cardiac tamponade may coexist with a normal pulse pressure.

       (4) Shock. The carotid upstroke is diminished in volume, the systolic blood pressure is reduced, and the periphery is cold and clammy because of the vasoconstriction present in reduced cardiac output states.

   3. **Diagnosis.** Elevated neck veins and pulsus paradoxus in a patient exhibiting symptoms of compromised cardiac output strongly suggest the diagnosis. A chest radiograph that shows an enlarged heart, together with an echocardiogram that confirms the presence of a pericardial effusion, make the diagnosis of cardiac tamponade reasonable, especially if clinical signs and symptoms are present. The diagnosis

may be further strengthened by catheterization, which would confirm that left and right atrial pressures are equal.

4. **Therapy.** The only effective therapy for cardiac tamponade is removal of fluid from the pericardial sac. Thus, **emergency pericardiocentesis** is indicated. The use of **pressor agents** and **volume expansion** are of limited benefit until pericardiocentesis can be performed.

D. **Constrictive pericarditis**

1. **Definition.** Constrictive pericarditis is the diffuse thickening of the pericardium in reaction to prior inflammation, which results in reduced distensibility of the cardiac chambers. Cardiac output is limited, and filling pressures are increased to match the external constrictive force placed on the heart by the pericardium.

2. **Etiology.** Most conditions that cause acute pericarditis may lead to chronic constrictive pericarditis.

3. **Clinical features**
   a. **Symptoms.** Most patients with constrictive pericarditis complain of **dyspnea on exertion** as a result of limited cardiac output. Although approximately 50% of patients complain of **orthopnea,** paroxysmal nocturnal dyspnea is rare. Symptoms related to systemic venous hypertension frequently are reported and include **ascites, edema,** and **jaundice.** Thus, the clinical picture typically is dominated by **symptoms of right-sided failure** rather than left-sided failure.
   b. **Physical signs**
      (1) **Jugular venous distention.** The jugular veins are distended, indicating systemic venous hypertension. Neck vein distention increases with inspiration (**Kussmaul's sign**).
      (2) **Carotid pulse.** The carotid upstroke is normal, but the volume may be decreased as a result of decreased stroke volume.
      (3) **Heart sounds.** The heart sounds are distant. Early in diastole, a pericardial knock may be heard, which falls in the same cadence as an S_3 but is higher pitched.
      (4) **Other signs of systemic venous hypertension** frequently present include **ascites, edema, hepatic tenderness,** and **hepatomegaly.**

4. **Diagnosis**
   a. **Electrocardiography.** The ECG shows low voltage in the limb leads. **Atrial arrhythmias** are common.
   b. **Chest radiography** reveals **pericardial calcification** in 50% of patients. This finding is seen as a **radiopaque ring around the heart** in the lateral view. The heart usually is normal in size, although cardiomegaly occasionally is noted.
   c. **Echocardiography.** Although pericardial thickening often can be detected, reliable diagnosis of constrictive pericarditis by echocardiography is difficult.
   d. **Magnetic resonance imaging (MRI)** gated to the cardiac cycle is an imaging technique capable of measuring pericardial thickness.
   e. **Cardiac catheterization** reveals equal pressures in the four cardiac chambers during diastole; in addition, all pressures usually are elevated. A marked **Y descent** is present in the right atrial pressure tracing. Left and right ventricular pressure tracings demonstrate a characteristic **dip** and **plateau** or **"square root"** **sign.**

5. **Therapy.** Surgical removal of the pericardium is curative. However, immediate relief of constrictive symptoms may not occur for up to 6 weeks after **pericardiectomy.**

VII. **CONGENITAL HEART DISEASE IN THE ADULT**

A. **Atrial septal defect**
1. **Classification**
   a. An **ostium secundum atrial septal defect** occurs in the **midportion** of the intraatrial septum and is caused by failure of the septum secundum to form properly.

b. An **ostium primum atrial septal defect** results from improper septation of the en-docardial cushion portion of the septum. It invariably involves the **mitral valve,** which is cleft and often regurgitant.

c. A **sinus venosus–type atrial septal defect** occurs **high in the atrial septum** and frequently is associated with anomalous drainage of one or more of the pulmo-nary veins into the right atrium.

d. Holt-Oram syndrome is characterized by the presence of a **secundum defect** to-gether with **bony abnormalities of the forearms and hands.** Holt-Oram syn-drome is a **hereditary** disease that is transmitted in an autosomal dominant fashion.

2. Pathophysiology

a. Left and right atrial pressures usually are equal in atrial septal defect; thus, no pressure gradient exists between the atria. However, the increased thickness of the left ventricle as compared to the right ventricle makes the left ventricle less compliant and, therefore, harder to fill. Blood flow takes the path of least resis-tance and, thus, is shunted from the left atrium to the right atrium. The net ef-fect is to increase the volume work of the right ventricle.

b. The increased volume pumped through the pulmonary vasculature may lead to architectural changes in the pulmonary vasculature and to the development of irreversible pulmonary hypertension—a serious but rare complication.

3. Clinical features

a. Symptoms. Patients with atrial septal defect may have a **prolonged symptom-free period.** Eventually, symptoms develop and may include **palpitations** as a result of atrial arrhythmias, **fatigue, dyspnea on exertion, orthopnea, frequent respiratory tract infections,** and **symptoms of right ventricular failure.**

b. Physical signs

(1) Wide and fixed splitting of the S_2 is the **classic finding** in atrial septal de-fect. The increased cardiac flow through the right ventricle delays pulmonic valve closure, widening the normal splitting of the S_2. Inspiration produces relatively little change in right-sided flow, so there is little respiratory varia-tion in the splitting of the S_2.

(2) Murmur. Under low pressure, blood flow from the left to the right atrium occurs through a wide aperture and produces no turbulence or murmur. However, the increased pulmonary blood flow in atrial septal defect pro-duces a **systolic ejection murmur,** which is **heard in the pulmonic area.** The increased flow also may produce a **diastolic rumble across the tricus-pid valve** if the left-to-right shunt ratio is greater than 3:1.

(3) Neck vein distention, ascites, and **edema** are indicative of right ventricular failure.

4. Diagnosis

a. Electrocardiography. In ostium secundum defects, incomplete right bundle block and right axis deviation are common findings. Ostium primum defects usually involve the anterior fascicle of the left bundle, producing left anterior hemiblock and left axis deviation.

b. Chest radiography

(1) Increased pulmonary blood flow produces increased pulmonary vascular markings in the lungs, called **shunt vascularity.**

(2) Right ventricular enlargement may encroach on the retrosternal airspace, re-ducing it in the lateral view.

(3) Enlargement of the pulmonary artery segment in the posteroanterior view also may be seen.

c. Echocardiography

(1) The echocardiogram shows enlargement of the right ventricle, and the atrial septal defect itself may be seen in many cases.

(2) A **saline injection,** which carries with it microbubbles of air, shows a **nega-tive-contrast image at the site** of the defect.

(3) Doppler examination of the interatrial septum will demonstrate the abnor-mal presence of left-to-right blood flow across the septum.

    d. Cardiac catheterization

        (1) During cardiac catheterization, the diagnosis can be confirmed by passage of the catheter across the atrial septal defect.

        (2) Left and right atrial pressures usually are equal.

        (3) Oxygen samples drawn from the superior vena cava and right atrium demonstrate a **step-up in oxygen concentration** in the right atrium, as highly oxygenated left atrial blood is shunted into the right atrium. Oxygen saturations can be used to quantitate the magnitude of the left-to-right shunt.

5. Therapy

    a. Surgical correction, which has a low operative mortality rate, is indicated for shunts with a pulmonary-to-systemic flow ratio of greater than 2:1, even in asymptomatic patients. Shunts of this magnitude may lead to the development of pulmonary hypertension, usually become symptomatic, and worsen with age.

    b. Alternatively, several catheter-based devices for defect closure are under investigation.

B. Ventricular septal defect

1. Pathophysiology. In ventricular septal defect, the left ventricle actively propels the blood into the right ventricle, resulting in the taxation of both ventricles and in increased pulmonary blood flow. Pulmonary hypertension is more severe and more frequent in ventricular septal defect than in atrial septal defect.

2. Clinical features. Because most ventricular septal defects lead to symptoms and are corrected in childhood, significant congenital ventricular septal defect rarely is diagnosed for the first time in adulthood.

    a. Symptoms of ventricular septal defect are those of both **left-** and **right-sided congestive heart failure.**

    b. Physical signs

        (1) Displacement of the PMI to the left is indicative of left ventricular enlargement.

        (2) Sternal lift is indicative of right ventricular enlargement.

        (3) Murmur. A **harsh, holosystolic murmur** is heard along the left sternal border. The murmur often is accompanied by a **thrill** and radiates to the right of the sternum.

        (4) Aortic regurgitation. Ventricular septal defects may involve the right coronary cusp of the aortic valve, producing insufficient support for this valve leaflet and, hence, aortic regurgitation. Approximately 6% of patients with ventricular septal defect have signs of aortic insufficiency.

3. Diagnosis

    a. Electrocardiography. The ECG typically shows **biventricular hypertrophy.**

    b. Chest radiography. Cardiac enlargement is the rule. If the shunt is greater than 2:1 in magnitude, **shunt vascularity** usually is present.

    c. Echocardiography. The septal defect frequently can be demonstrated during two-dimensional echocardiography. Left and right ventricular enlargement is seen as well. Doppler examination reveals abnormal blood flow from the left ventricle to the right ventricle.

    d. Cardiac catheterization

        (1) A left ventriculogram obtained in the left anterior oblique position demonstrates flow of contrast from the left ventricle across the septum into the right ventricle.

        (2) During cardiac catheterization, an **oxygen step-up** occurs at the level of the right ventricle. Pulmonary hypertension, if present, can be quantified.

4. Therapy. Because patients with ventricular septal defects are prone to pulmonary vascular complications and bacterial endocarditis, ventricular septal defects with a magnitude of 2:1 or greater should be corrected surgically.

C. **Patent ductus arteriosus**

1. **Pathophysiology.** In patent ductus arteriosus, blood flows from the aorta into the pulmonary artery after the takeoff of the left subclavian artery. Volume overload is imposed on the left ventricle, which must pump blood into both the systemic and pulmonary circulations, and in time may lead to left ventricular failure. The increased pulmonary blood flow created by this lesion may lead to the development of pulmonary hypertension, imposing a pressure overload on the right ventricle.

2. **Physical signs**
   a. **Murmur.** Throughout the cardiac cycle, the vascular resistance and pressure in the pulmonary circuit are lower than pressure in the aorta. Therefore, blood is shunted from left to right in both systole and diastole, and a **continuous murmur** with systolic and diastolic components is heard.
   b. **Pulses.** The presence of a low-pressure, low-resistance pathway allows for increased aortic runoff in diastole, which produces **bounding, full pulses** similar to those found in aortic insufficiency.

3. **Diagnosis**
   a. **Chest radiography** reveals an enlarged cardiac silhouette with the presence of shunt vascularity. In adults, the patent ductus may become calcified, rendering it visible on the chest radiograph.
   b. **Echocardiography** may reveal the patent ductus. Doppler interrogation detects abnormal flow of blood from the aorta to the pulmonary artery.
   c. **Cardiac catheterization**
      (1) During cardiac catheterization, the catheter usually can be passed from the pulmonary artery into the descending aorta, confirming the presence of a patent ductus arteriosus.
      (2) **Oximetry** can be used to quantify the magnitude of the left-to-right shunt.
      (3) **Aortography** demonstrates the flow of contrast from the aorta through the patent ductus into the pulmonary artery.

4. **Therapy.** Surgical closure of the patent ductus is indicated in adults with a shunt ratio of greater than 2:1. Catheter techniques for ductus closure are under investigation.

D. **Coarctation of the aorta** is a stenosis of the aorta, usually at the site of the ductus arteriosus.

1. **Pathophysiology.** Coarctation of the aorta often leads to hypertension.
   a. If severe, the stenosis limits aortic blood flow distal to the constriction. Distal tissues are perfused by an extensive collateral arterial circulation.
   b. While renal blood flow and renal function usually are normal in the adult with coarctation of the aorta, the kidneys still are perfused at a subnormal blood pressure.
   c. Some investigators have found elevated renin levels and activation of the renin–angiotensin system in adults with coarctation, which helps to explain the hypertension.

2. **Clinical features.** If the coarctation does not cause heart failure due to pressure overload in childhood, it may not be detected until it presents as hypertension in the adult.
   a. **Symptoms.** Patients with coarctation may complain of **headache, claudication, and leg fatigue.**
   b. **Physical signs**
      (1) **Blood pressure** determined in the arms usually is elevated, whereas pulses and blood pressure in the legs usually are reduced, representing the gradient across the coarctation.
      (2) **Habitus.** The upper body usually is well developed, while the legs occasionally appear underdeveloped.
      (3) **Murmur.** Typically, a **midsystolic** murmur is heard over the back. If the stenosis is severe, a continuous murmur may be heard. Continuous murmurs also may be heard diffusely over the chest cavity due to increased flow through collateral vessels.

3. **Diagnosis**
   a. **Electrocardiography.** The ECG shows left ventricular hypertrophy.
   b. **Chest radiography. Cardiac enlargement** usually is seen. Dilatation of the aorta proximal and distal to the coarctation with indentation at the site of the coarctation may cause the aorta to assume a **figure "3" appearance.** Dilatation of chest wall arteries forming the collateral pathways produces **rib notching.**
   c. **Cardiac catheterization.** During cardiac catheterization, the gradient across the coarctation can be measured. Aortography also allows visual demonstration of the coarctation.

4. **Therapy. Surgical correction** of the coarctation is standard therapy. **Percutaneous balloon aortoplasty** appears effective in some cases and is under investigation as an alternative to surgery.

5. **Complications. Hypertension, infective endocarditis, dissection of the thoracic aorta,** and **rupture of cerebral (berry) aneurysms** frequently are seen in patients with coarctation of the aorta. Hypertension may persist even after the coarctation is repaired.

E. **Ebstein's anomaly of the tricuspid valve**

1. **Pathophysiology.** In Ebstein's anomaly, the tricuspid valve is situated abnormally low in the right ventricle. Part of the tricuspid valve is tethered directly to the right ventricle. Thus, a portion of the right ventricle actually lies above the AV groove and is "atrialized," reducing the size of the right ventricle and usually resulting in **tricuspid regurgitation.** A **coexistent atrial septal defect** occurs in approximately 75% of cases.

2. **Clinical features**
   a. **Symptoms.** Depending on the degree of tricuspid regurgitation and whether an atrial septal defect exists, a patient's status may **range from asymptomatic to cyanotic.**
      (1) Dyspnea on exertion, peripheral edema, and other **symptoms of right ventricular failure** frequently are encountered.
      (2) Palpitations also are common in this anomaly, which is associated with **Wolff-Parkinson-White (WPW) syndrome** in approximately 10% of patients. WPW syndrome is characterized by abnormal ventricular conduction as the result of a congenital short circuit of the conducting system. Tachyarrhythmias are common.
   b. **Physical signs**
      (1) **Tricuspid regurgitation.** A **large v wave** in the neck veins and a pulsatile liver reflect tricuspid regurgitation.
      (2) **Heart sounds.** Wide splitting of the S_1 and S_2 is heard. Because an S_3 and an S_4 often exist also, a quadruple or quintuple cadence is a common auscultatory finding.
      (3) **Murmur.** The **holosystolic murmur of tricuspid regurgitation** is heard along the sternal border and may be accompanied by a systolic thrill.

3. **Diagnosis**
   a. **Electrocardiography.** The ECG may show evidence of WPW syndrome (a short P-R interval and a slurred QRS upstroke). Other findings include giant P waves and right bundle branch block.
   b. **Echocardiography.** The echocardiogram in Ebstein's anomaly shows delayed closure of the tricuspid valve in relation to the mitral valve. The inferior and leftward displacement of the tricuspid valve usually can be demonstrated.
   c. **Cardiac catheterization.** The simultaneous demonstration of a right atrial pressure tracing with a right ventricular electrogram in the "atrialized" portion of the right ventricle is pathognomonic.

4. **Therapy.** Tricuspid valve replacement and closure of the atrial septal defect may be useful in patients who have developed early signs of right ventricular failure.

F. **Eisenmenger's syndrome**

1. **Pathophysiology.** In Eisenmenger's syndrome, which can occur with any intracardiac shunt, the **left-to-right shunt is reversed** to produce a right-to-left shunt. Reversal occurs as a result of pulmonary vascular disease that leads to increased pulmonary vascular resistance. Increased pulmonary vascular resistance leads to decreased right-sided compliance and increased right-sided pressures, which produce right-to-left shunting.

2. **Clinical features**
   a. **Cyanosis** may be constant or noted only during exercise. **Differential cyanosis** may occur in the presence of a patent ductus arteriosus; the preductal tissues (including the upper trunk) are pink and the postductal tissues are cyanotic.
   b. **Angina.** Patients with Eisenmenger's syndrome may suffer from exertional chest pain, which occurs even in the presence of normal coronary arteries. Reduced myocardial oxygenation and increased right ventricular wall stress may be factors causing the symptom.
   c. **Heart failure.** Dyspnea on exertion, ascites, and peripheral edema are common.

3. **Diagnosis**
   a. **Electrocardiography.** Right ventricular hypertrophy invariably is present.
   b. **Echocardiography. Saline injection** demonstrates right-to-left shunting of microbubbles in the presence of either an atrial or a ventricular septal defect. **Doppler examination** also demonstrates the abnormal right-to-left blood flow at the site of the shunt.
   c. **Hemogram.** Patients with Eisenmenger's syndrome are **polycythemic.** Hemoglobin concentrations in excess of 20 g/dl are common.
   d. **Cardiac catheterization.** Right-sided pressures are extremely elevated. Oximetry is used to quantitate the right-to-left shunt. Administration of 100% oxygen via a rebreathing mask does not significantly correct the arterial desaturation.

4. **Therapy.** Surgical therapy generally is not successful.
   a. **Closure of the shunt site,** which acts as an escape valve for the right ventricle, increases right ventricular pressures and causes worsening of right ventricular failure.
   b. **Phlebotomy** may be necessary to avoid hyperviscosity by maintaining the hemoglobin level at less than 20 g/dl.

VIII. VENOUS THROMBOSIS

A. **Deep venous thrombosis**

1. **Definition.** Deep venous thrombosis occurs when a blood clot forms in the lower extremities or in the pelvic veins. The exact initiating events are unknown. The gravity of deep venous thrombosis stems from the tendency of the thrombi to become pulmonary emboli; this tendency is especially pronounced for clots located above the popliteal fossa.

2. **Predisposing factors**
   a. **Immobilization.** The muscles in the legs act as pumps to maintain venous return from the lower extremities. Inactivity of these muscles leads to **venous stasis,** with subsequent development of **thrombophlebitis.** Stasis is likely to occur during surgery, prolonged bed rest, and prolonged periods in one position.
   b. **Venous incompetence.** Venous valvular incompetence and the presence of varicose veins increase the incidence of thrombophlebitis.
   c. **Congestive heart failure.** In congestive heart failure, cardiac output is reduced, as is venous return from the legs.

   d. Injury. Direct mechanical injury to the lower extremities may lead to blood clot formation and the development of thrombophlebitis.
   e. Hypercoagulable states. Malignancy, estrogen use, and **hyperviscosity syndrome** may produce a hypercoagulable state, increasing the risk of thrombophlebitis.

3. **Clinical features**
   a. Symptoms. The patient usually presents with **unilateral leg pain** and **swelling.**
   b. Physical signs. In general, the physical examination for deep venous thrombosis is unreliable. Tenderness on compression of the calf muscles, pain during dorsiflexion of the foot **(Homans' sign),** and an increase in the circumference of the affected leg by at least 1 cm suggest the presence of deep venous thrombosis.

4. **Diagnosis**
   a. Noninvasive studies. Impedance plethysmography and **Doppler ultrasonography** are useful tests for the detection of deep venous thrombosis.
   b. Invasive studies. Contrast venography currently is the most effective way to demonstrate the area of blood clot. This technique is associated with complications, including adverse reactions to the contrast agent and postvenography thrombophlebitis.

5. **Therapy**
   a. Anticoagulants prevent additional clot formation and allow the body's autolytic system to effectively lyse and heal deep venous thrombosis. Anticoagulation therapy is usually maintained for 3–6 months.
      (1) Anticoagulation with **intravenous heparin** is indicated in the acute treatment of deep venous thrombosis.
      (2) After adequate treatment with heparin, **oral anticoagulation with warfarin** is begun.
   b. Thrombolytic agents result in more rapid resolution of the thrombus and improve late competency of venous valves, helping to prevent future venous stasis.
      (1) Streptokinase, t-PA, and **urokinase** activate the conversion of plasminogen to the autolytic agent, **plasmin.** Whereas heparin can only prevent new clot formation, streptokinase, t-PA and urokinase lyse an already formed clot.
      (2) Bleeding complications with thrombolytic agents tend to be more severe than with anticoagulants. Currently, there is no consensus on whether anticoagulation or thrombolysis is the preferred therapy for deep venous thrombosis; however, anticoagulation is the more common therapy.

6. **Prophylaxis.** There is substantial medical evidence that the incidence of deep venous thrombosis for hospitalized patients can be reduced by the following methods.
   a. Rapid mobilization. Prolonged bed rest should be avoided when possible. The increasingly rapid mobilization of patients following myocardial infarction has significantly reduced the incidence of thromboembolic complications following this disease.
   b. Increasing deep venous flow
      (1) Antithromboembolic stockings compress the superficial veins, thereby increasing deep venous flow and reducing stasis and the incidence of thromboembolism.
      (2) Foot exercises and **avoidance of leg crossing** are further methods of preventing deep venous thrombosis.
   c. Minidose heparin. Intermittent doses of subcutaneous heparin given at 8- to 12-hour intervals inhibit factors X and XI in the clotting cascade without producing overt anticoagulation. This treatment significantly reduces the incidence of deep venous thrombosis in both medical and surgical patients put to bed rest.

B. **Superficial thrombophlebitis.** Unlike deep venous thrombosis, in which a thrombus may break off and become a pulmonary embolism, superficial thrombophlebitis has **little potential for embolic complications.** Patients with superficial thrombophlebitis may present with a painful tender cord that can be easily palpated in the lower extremities. In the absence of concomitant deep venous thrombosis, **anticoagulation is not indicated.** Superficial thrombophlebitis is **treated with elevation of the legs,** heat, and **administration of salicylates.**

IX. CARDIOVASCULAR SYNCOPE

A. **Definition.** Syncope is a sudden loss of consciousness of brief duration.

B. **Pathophysiology.** Cardiovascular syncope occurs when the brain's metabolic needs cannot be met by the available blood supply. Adequate perfusion is dependent on an adequate systemic blood pressure: BP = CO × SVR (where BP = blood pressure, CO = cardiac output, and SVR = systemic vascular resistance). Therefore, a fall in cardiac output or a fall in systemic vascular resistance can precipitate a fall in blood pressure, leading to syncope. Because CO = SV × HR, (where SV = stroke volume and HR = heart rate), either inadequate stroke volume or inadequate heart rate reduces cardiac output, potentially leading to hypotension and syncope.

C. **Etiology**

1. **Reduced cardiac output**
   a. **Bradycardia**
      (1) **Heart block.** A block in the cardiac conduction pathway may prevent the SA nodal electrical signal for ventricular contraction from being transmitted, in turn causing bradycardia. Whether or not syncope occurs depends on whether an alternative, lower pacemaker (e.g., the AV junction) produces an escape rate fast enough to maintain blood pressure.
         (a) **Types of heart block**
            (i) **Complete** heart block indicates that no SA nodal impulses are conducted to the ventricle.
            (ii) **Second-degree** heart block indicates that some SA nodal impulses are conducted while others are not.
         (b) **Causes of AV block** include myocardial infarction, idiopathic degeneration of the conducting system, amyloidosis, sarcoidosis, and drugs that interfere with cardiac conduction (e.g., digitalis, calcium channel blockers and β blockers).
      (2) **Sick sinus syndrome** occurs when there is a deficit in impulse generation from the sinus node, which may lead to bradycardia and syncope.
         (a) Profound sinus bradycardia, sinus arrest or exit block, and the tachycardia–bradycardia syndrome are the arrhythmias that comprise the sick sinus syndrome. The tachycardia–bradycardia syndrome is one of atrial instability where supraventricular tachycardia halts abruptly and is followed by severe bradycardia.
         (b) Sick sinus syndrome may result from ischemic heart disease and idiopathic or inflammatory degeneration of the SA node.
   b. **Impaired stroke volume.** The rhythmic filling and emptying of the left ventricle generates its stroke volume; therefore, conditions that either inhibit left ventricular filling or inhibit left ventricular emptying can severely reduce stroke volume, leading to hypotension and syncope.
      (1) **Conditions that limit left ventricular filling**
         (a) **Obstruction to inflow.** Any mechanical block in the cardiovascular system that inhibits filling of the left ventricle will impair its output. Such obstructions include mitral stenosis, left atrial myxoma, right atrial myxoma, pulmonary embolism, and pulmonic stenosis.
         (b) **Tachycardia.** Both ventricular tachycardia and very rapid supraventricular tachycardia reduce the diastolic filling period of the left ventricle, limiting its filling and reducing its stroke volume. In ventricular tachy-

cardia, the shortened diastolic filling period is compounded by incomplete ventricular relaxation which further limits filling.

(c) **Impaired systemic venous return.** Failure of adequate systemic venous return to the right heart subsequently impairs its output to the left heart, impairing left ventricular stroke volume.

  (i) Typically, impaired venous return occurs when the supine patient assumes the upright posture.

  (ii) Normally, the tendency for gravity-induced venous pooling of blood in the legs is offset by venous vasoconstriction, which helps maintain venous return. However, in the face of dehydration, antihypertensive drugs, or autonomic dysfunction, impaired venous return may produce **orthostatic syncope.** Autonomic dysfunction may be idiopathic, familial, surgically induced or due to diabetes, alcoholism or pyridoxine deficiency.

(2) **Conditions that impair left ventricular emptying.** The left ventricle may be impaired from emptying either as a result of a severe, sudden depression in myocardial contractile function, or as a result of outflow obstruction.

  (a) **Decreased myocardial contractility.** The sudden and severe degree of contractile depression required to cause syncope is almost invariably caused by global ischemia produced by main left or triple-vessel coronary disease or acute myocardial infarction.

  (b) **Obstruction to outflow.** Obstruction of left ventricular outflow that produces syncope is caused by valvular aortic stenosis and hypertrophic obstructive cardiomyopathy.

2. **Reduced total peripheral resistance.** If cardiac output is maintained but total peripheral resistance falls, blood pressure also falls, potentially causing syncope.

  a. An inappropriate fall in total peripheral resistance is usually operative in the **common fainting spell.** Increased blood flow to the skeletal muscles, due to a fall in total peripheral resistance, may divert flow from the brain and result in fainting. Venodilation and relative bradycardia may further compound the **"vasovagal faint"** by reducing venous return and cardiac output.

  b. Reduced total peripheral resistance leading to syncope may also occur in drug-induced, familial, or idiopathic autonomic dysfunction.

D. **Diagnosis.** A single fainting episode or episode of light–headedness occurs in more than 50% of the population at some point in a lifetime. It would be impossible to extensively explore the cause of the event in every such patient. A good history and physical examination should be adequate to exclude potentially serious causes of a single episode of syncope. However, recurrent syncope requires a more extensive workup.

1. **History.** A thorough patient interview can reveal clues that might point to a specific etiology for the patient's recurrent syncope.

  a. A history of palpitations might indicate an arrhythmia.

  b. The observation that syncope occurred upon assumption of an upright position suggests orthostatic hypotension.

  c. A history of chest pain might indicate an ischemic event or pulmonary embolism.

  d. A change in antihypertensive medication or a recent episode of dehydration are additional clues.

2. **Physical examination.** During the physical examination, those maneuvers that might reveal a reason for hypotension and possible syncope should be emphasized.

  a. **Blood pressure**

  (1) The blood pressure should be recorded in both arms in both the supine and the sitting or standing positions.

  (2) Upon assuming an upright posture, it is normal for systolic blood pressure to fall slightly while diastolic pressure increases. There is also usually a slight increase in heart rate.

      (a) A frank fall in systolic and diastolic pressure upon assuming an upright posture may indicate volume depletion or sympathetic compensation that is inadequate to counteract the change in posture.

      (b) A fall in diastolic pressure of more than 10 mm Hg is significant and may suggest an orthostatic etiology of the patient's syncope.

   b. Heart rate and rhythm. The pulse should be examined for an extended period of time in an effort to detect arrhythmia or bradycardia.

   c. Valvular obstruction. The murmurs and physical findings associated with mitral stenosis, aortic stenosis, pulmonic stenosis, or idiopathic hypertrophic subaortic stenosis should be recognized as indications of potentially correctable mechanisms for syncope.

   d. Thromboembolism. Thrombophlebitis in the lower limbs indicates a source of pulmonary emboli, which can cause syncope. Physical evidence that a pulmonary embolus is present includes wheezing, increased intensity of the pulmonary component of the S_2, and jugular venous distention.

3. Electrocardiography. If second- or third-degree AV block is detected, it demonstrates the likely cause of the patient's syncope. Bundle branch block and arrhythmias, or both, on the standard ECG should raise suspicion that heart block or arrhythmia are syncopal etiologies.

4. Holter monitoring. If the patient interview, physical examination, and electrocardiogram point to an arrhythmia as the potential cause for the patient's syncope, Holter monitoring may be performed. This tape recording, which documents each heart beat over a 24-hour period, increases the period of observation for the detection of arrhythmias and constitutes an exceptional piece of positive evidence in arriving at the diagnosis. Unfortunately, because most arrhythmias occur sporadically, most Holter monitor exams are negative even when an arrhythmia is the source of the patient's syncope.

5. Electrophysiologic testing. If the initial workup demonstrates that heart disease is present but fails to demonstrate a specific cause of syncope, electrophysiologic stimulation may provoke the arrhythmia responsible for the patient's syncope. Having established an arrhythmic cause for the patient's syncope, the proper therapy may then be instituted.

E. **Therapy**

1. Therapy of bradyarrhythmias. When a bradyarrhythmia has been established as the cause of the patient's syncope, drug-induced bradycardia should be ruled out as a cause by discontinuing potentially offending drugs. Subsequent insertion of a permanent pacemaker will protect the patient from subsequent syncope.

2. Therapy for tachyarrhythmias

   a. Drug therapy for both ventricular and superventricular tachyarrhythmias that have caused an episode of syncope is clearly indicated [see II D 1 b (3)]. In general, such therapy should be guided by electrophysiologic testing.

   b. Antitachycardia pacemakers or **implantable defibrillators** may be employed to electrically correct arrhythmias if drug therapy fails.

3. Therapy for autonomic dysfunction. If autonomic dysfunction is the cause of orthostatic hypotension and syncope, little can be done to directly treat the underlying cause. Instead, therapies to protect the patient from possible hypotension should be instituted. These include high salt intake to insure volume expansion, support stockings to prevent venous pooling, and atrial pacemaking if an inappropriate lack of tachycardia during hypotension is part of the patient's underlying syndrome.

4. Correction of mechanical obstructions to cardiac inflow or outflow. Any fixed valvular lesion that has caused an episode of syncope should be corrected. If idiopathic hypertrophic subaortic stenosis is determined to be the cause of the syncope, standard therapy with propranolol or verapamil is indicated to reduce the amount of outflow obstruction. If medical therapy fails, myomectomy may be necessary.

STUDY QUESTIONS

DIRECTIONS: Each of the numbered items or incomplete statements in this section is followed by answers or by completions of the statement. Select the ONE lettered answer or completion that is BEST in each case.

1. Which one of the following statements best characterizes the physical signs noted in aortic regurgitation?

(A) A large increase in stroke volume occurs when the condition is acute, producing many of the physical signs present in this disease
(B) Concentric left ventricular hypertrophy is the major compensatory mechanism
(C) A low-pitched, diastolic blowing murmur is heard best when the patient is lying down
(D) The presence of an Austin Flint murmur indicates moderate to severe insufficiency
(E) Quincke's pulse is elicited best in the femoral artery

2. The single most reliable physical sign of congestive heart failure in patients over the age of 40 years is

(A) a third heart sound (S_3)
(B) a fourth heart sound (S_4)
(C) pulmonary rales
(D) ascites
(E) edema

3. Which of the following statements best characterizes tricuspid regurgitation?

(A) Infective endocarditis is a common cause
(B) The murmur heard in tricuspid regurgitation decreases with inspiration
(C) Large a waves in the jugular venous pulse are characteristic
(D) Correction of coexistent left ventricular failure rarely improves the condition
(E) Cardiac catheterization is required for the diagnosis

4. Which of the following physical signs and symptoms is indicative of left ventricular failure?

(A) Neck vein distention
(B) Ascites
(C) Anorexia
(D) Orthopnea
(E) Cardiac edema

5. One hemodynamic abnormality in the pathophysiology of mitral valve stenosis is

(A) increased left ventricular filling
(B) increased left atrial pressure
(C) increased forward cardiac output
(D) decreased right ventricular pressure

6. Which one of the following usually causes irreversible congestive cardiomyopathy?

(A) Endocrinopathies (e.g., thyrotoxicosis)
(B) Metabolic disorders (e.g., hypophosphatemia)
(C) Prolonged ethanol abuse
(D) High-dose doxorubicin therapy

7. Which one of the following is indicative of cardiac tamponade?

(A) Pulsus paradoxus
(B) A wide pulse pressure
(C) Kussmaul's sign (i.e., increased neck vein distention with inspiration)
(D) A forceful left ventricular apex beat

8. Which one of the following statements about variant (Prinzmetal's) angina is true?

(A) S-T segment depression is present on the electrocardiogram (ECG)
(B) An attack of variant angina is most often precipitated by exertion
(C) Variant angina usually results in myocardial infarction
(D) Coronary artery spasm produces variant angina

9. One sign of severe aortic stenosis noted during physical examination is

(A) a harsh, late-peaking holosystolic murmur
(B) a loud aortic component (A_2) of the second heart sound (S_2)
(C) a delayed carotid upstroke
(D) a diastolic rumble
(E) an opening snap

10. The systolic ejection murmur in hypertrophic obstructive cardiomyopathy is diminished when the patient

(A) performs the Valsalva maneuver
(B) lies down
(C) inhales amyl nitrite
(D) stands up
(E) is treated with digoxin

11. The diagnosis of constrictive pericarditis is supported by which one of the following findings?

(A) Neck vein distention that increases during inspiration
(B) Exaggerated first and second heart sounds (S_1 and S_2)
(C) Unequal diastolic pressures in the four chambers of the heart
(D) A predominance of left-sided signs and symptoms over right-sided findings

Questions 12–14

A 35-year-old white woman enters the emergency room complaining of chest pain. The pain is episodic and usually lasts for 5–10 minutes. Sometimes it is related to exercise, but on other occasions, it occurs at rest. The pain does not radiate. The patient is a non-smoker and has no history of hypertension. Two other family members have died of heart disease, one at 50 years of age and the other at 56 years of age. On physical examination the patient is in no acute distress. Her blood pressure is 120/70 and her pulse is 70. Examination of the precordium finds that the point of maximal impulse (PMI) is forceful. There is a II/VI systolic ejection murmur heard along the left sternal border. The murmur increases in intensity when the patient stands up. The electrocardiogram (ECG) shows nonspecific S-T segment and T-wave abnormalities.

12. Which one of the following is the most likely diagnosis?

(A) Innocent flow murmur
(B) Aortic stenosis
(C) Hypertrophic obstructive cardiomyopathy
(D) Mitral stenosis
(E) Pulmonic stenosis

13. Which one of the following tools would be best to use when diagnosing this patient?

(A) Chest x-ray
(B) Cardiac catheterization
(C) Thallium scanning
(D) Echocardiography
(E) Myocardial biopsy

14. The most appropriate therapy for this patient is

(A) immediate surgery
(B) propranolol
(C) vasodilators
(D) digoxin
(E) furosemide

DIRECTIONS: Each set of matching questions in this section consists of a list of four to twenty-six lettered options (some of which may be in figures) followed by several numbered items. For each numbered item, select the ONE lettered option that is most closely associated with it. To avoid spending too much time on matching sets with large numbers of options, it is generally advisable to begin each set by reading the list of options. Then, for each item in the set, try to generate the correct answer and locate it in the option list, rather than evaluating each option individually. Each lettered option may be selected once, more than once, or not at all.

Questions 15–19

(A) Atrial septal defect
(B) Ventricular septal defect
(C) Patent ductus arteriosus
(D) Coarctation of the aorta
(E) Ebstein's anomaly

Match each physical sign of congenital heart disease with the lesion it best characterizes.

15. Absent femoral pulses

16. Fixed, widely split second heart sound (S_2)

17. Quintuple cardiac cadence on auscultation

18. Continuous murmur

19. Holosystolic murmur

Questions 20–24

(A) Mitral stenosis
(B) Mitral regurgitation
(C) Tricuspid regurgitation
(D) Aortic stenosis
(E) Aortic regurgitation

Match each physical sign of valvular heart disease with the lesion it best characterizes.

20. Pulsatile liver C

21. Loud first heart sound (S_1) A

22. Soft, single second heart sound (S_2) D

23. Third heart sound (S_3, or ventricular gallop) B

24. Systolic blood pressure that is 20 mm Hg higher in the leg than in the arm (Hill's sign) E

ANSWERS AND EXPLANATIONS

1. The answer is D [IV C 3 b (2)–(4)]. An Austin Flint murmur (diastolic rumble) probably occurs when a large amount of blood regurgitated from the aortic valve strikes the mitral valve, generating the murmur and indicating a moderate to severe insufficiency. In acute aortic regurgitation, there is little time for ventricular dilatation and, thus, little increase in stroke volume; therefore, many of the signs of aortic regurgitation often are absent when the insufficiency is acute. Eccentric, rather than concentric, hypertrophy is the rule in aortic regurgitation. Eccentric hypertrophy allows for increased chamber size and reestablishment of forward stroke volume. A diastolic blowing murmur is characteristic of aortic insufficiency, but it is high-pitched and best heard when the patient is sitting up and leaning forward. Quincke's pulse is seen in the nail beds.

2. The answer is A [I D 2 e]. A third heart sound (S_3) is the most reliable physical sign of congestive heart failure in individuals who are older than 40 years, although it is a normal finding in some young, healthy athletes. A fourth heart sound (S_4) can be a normal finding in older patients. Pulmonary rales, while often the result of heart failure, may have many noncardiac causes. Ascites and edema can result from hepatic, neoplastic, or local factors not associated with cardiac pathology.

3. The answer is A [IV E 1 a, 3 b (2)–(3), 4, 5]. Infective endocarditis is a common cause of tricuspid regurgitation. The murmur of tricuspid regurgitation typically increases with inspiration. Large v waves are seen in the jugular venous pulse. Because a common cause of right ventricular failure and secondary tricuspid regurgitation is left ventricular failure, correction of left ventricular failure, when present, often is useful in the treatment of tricuspid regurgitation. Diagnosis of tricuspid regurgitation usually is made on the basis of clinical or echocardiographic evidence. Cardiac catheterization rarely is used to make the diagnosis.

4. The answer is D [I D 1 b]. Orthopnea is indicative of left ventricular failure. Orthopnea is defined as dyspnea (i.e., the feeling of breathlessness) that occurs in the recumbent position. Recumbency leads to increased cardiac venous return and, thus, increased left and right ventricular volumes. The increased left ventricular volume results in increased left ventricular filling pressure, which leads to pulmonary congestion and the feeling of breathlessness. Neck vein distention, ascites, anorexia, and cardiac edema all are signs and symptoms of right ventricular failure.

5. The answer is B [IV B 2]. Left ventricular filling is decreased in mitral valve stenosis, and a pressure gradient develops across the stenotic valve, increasing left atrial pressure. With increasing severity, the stenotic mitral valve may seriously decrease forward cardiac output. Because the right ventricle must fill the left ventricle, a stenotic mitral valve imposes a pressure overload on the right ventricle, which must generate enough force to push blood through the constricted valve.

6. The answer is D [V A 2]. Doxorubicin (an antitumor medication) causes irreversible congestive cardiomyopathy when administered in large doses. The most common identifiable cause of cardiomyopathy is alcohol abuse, the cessation of which can lead to significant improvement in ventricular function. Thyrotoxicosis and hypothyroidism are endocrine disorders that have been linked to congestive cardiomyopathy, which is reversible with correction of the underlying endocrinopathy. Metabolic disorders such as hypophosphatemia and hypocalcemia also produce reversible cardiomyopathy.

7. The answer is A [VI C 2 b (1)]. Pulsus paradoxus occurs in 95% of patients with cardiac tamponade. A narrow pulse pressure, as opposed to a wide pulse pressure, is a sign of cardiac tamponade. Impairment of cardiac filling cause a decrease in stroke volume, which produces a narrow pulse pressure and hypotension. Neck veins are elevated due to the increase in pressure that is required to fill the heart, but Kussmaul's sign usually is absent in this condition. The fluid in the pericardium cushions the apex impulse, thereby reducing or obscuring its intensity in cardiac tamponade.

8. The answer is D [III A 5 a (2) (d)]. Variant (Prinzmetal's) angina is caused by coronary artery spasm, which produces total, but transient, coronary occlusion. Although patients with Prinzmetal's angina occasionally have S-T segment depression as well as elevation, it is the S-T segment elevation on which the diagnosis is based. Variant angina usually occurs at rest and often at night. Even in patients who experience repeated attacks of variant angina, myocardial infarction is the exception rather than the rule.

9. The answer is C [IV A 3 b]. A delayed carotid upstroke is the most reliable sign of severe aortic stenosis. The ejection murmur in severe aortic stenosis usually is harsh and peaks late in systole, when outflow from the left ventricle is at a maximum. However, the murmur may be quite soft, because decreased outflow in the later stages of the disease reduces the intensity of the murmur. The aortic component (A_2) of the second heart sound (S_2) usually is soft or absent because motion of the valve is limited. An opening snap occurs in mitral, not aortic, stenosis.

10. The answer is B [V B 4 b (2) (a)–(b)]. The systolic ejection murmur in hypertrophic obstructive cardiomyopathy is diminished when the patient lies down. All actions that decrease left ventricular size (e.g., the Valsalva maneuver and inhalation of amyl nitrite) bring the anterior leaflet of the mitral valve (i.e., the active obstructing body in hypertrophic obstructive cardiomyopathy) closer to the septum and increase the amount of obstruction. This, in turn, increases the intensity of the murmur. Conversely, actions that increase cardiac size by increasing venous return (e.g., lying down or squatting) tend to diminish the intensity of the murmur. Digoxin increases contractility, which tends to worsen outflow obstruction and thus increases the murmur.

11. The answer is A [VI D 3 b (1)–(3)]. In constrictive pericarditis, deep inspiration causes an increase in jugular venous distention (Kussmaul's sign). The first and second heart sounds (S_1 and S_2) are reduced in intensity due to reduced sound transmission through the thickened pericardium. In both constrictive pericarditis and cardiac tamponade, the diastolic pressures are equal in all four chambers of the heart. In most cases of constrictive pericarditis, the clinical findings of right-sided failure are more prominent than those of left-sided failure.

12–14. The answers are: 12-C [V B 4], **13-D** [V B 5 b], **14-B** [V B 6 a]. The most likely diagnosis is hypertrophic cardiomyopathy, as evidenced by the increased intensity of the systolic ejection murmur when the patient stands up. When a patient with hypertrophic cardiomyopathy stands up, blood pools in the legs, decreasing left ventricular size and bringing the anterior leaflet of the mitral valve in closer contact with the hypertrophied ventricular septum. This increases the obstruction and makes the mumur louder. Conversely, innocent flow murmurs and the murmurs associated with pulmonic and aortic stenosis decrease when the patient stands, because the temporary pooling of central volume in the legs decreases forward cardiac output, thereby decreasing turbulent flow in the valve. The murmur of mitral stenosis is a diastolic murmur, not a systolic murmur.

The echocardiogram is a highly effective diagnostic tool in hypertrophic cardiomyopathy, provided the patient can be visualized adequately. Asymmetric hypertrophy of the septum compared to the free cardiac wall confirms the diagnosis. If obstruction is present, there will also be systolic anterior motion of the mitral valve. There are no particular features of hypertrophic cardiomyopathy demonstrable on a chest radiograph. Thallium scintigraphy may show the hypertrophied septum, but this is not the optimum form of imaging. Cardiac catheterization can certainly confirm the diagnosis, but this invasive test needs to be performed in only a minority of patients when echocardiography can not adequately visualize the patient's heart.

Symptoms of hypertrophic cardiomyopathy may be relieved with propranolol, a β-adrenergic blocking agent. By decreasing heart rate, propranolol allows increased left ventricular filling, thereby increasing separation of the anterior leaflet of the mitral valve and the septum and reducing the amount of obstruction.

Unlike valvular aortic stenosis (where death may be imminent after the development of symptoms unless surgery is performed) in hypertrophic cardiomyopathy, there is no evidence that surgery prolongs life. Both digoxin (by increasing the force that contraction) and furosemide (by decreasing left ventricular size) would worsen the obstruction and likely exacerbate the patient's symptoms.

15–19. The answers are: 15-D [VII D 2 b (1)], **16-A** [VII A 3 b (1)], **17-E** [VII E 2 b (2)], **18-C** [VII C 2 a], **19-B** [VII B 2 b (3)]. Coarctation of the aorta is a stenosis of the aorta, distal to which there is limited aortic blood flow. This diminishes transmission of the pulse from the aorta to the distal extremities, usually resulting in absent femoral pulses.

In atrial septel defect, both ventricles fill from a common cardiac reservoir—the combined left and right atria. With inspiration, there is little differential in total pulmonary blood flow; thus, closure of the pulmonic valve does not change in its timing with reference to closure of the aortic valve. The classic finding in atrial septal defect, therefore, is a fixed and widely split second heart sound (S_2).

In Ebstein's anomaly of the tricuspid valve, the first heart sound (S_1) is split and the usual presence of an atrial septal defect causes wide splitting of the S_2. These sounds together with the frequent occurrence of a third heart sound (S_3, or ventricular gallop) or a fourth heart sound (S_4, or atrial gallop) produce a quintuple cadence on auscultation.

In patent ductus arteriosus, the pressure in the aorta is higher than the pressure in the pulmonary artery throughout both systole and diastole. This produces continuous flow from the aorta to the pulmonary artery and, thus, a continuous murmur.

In vetnricular septal defect, left ventricular pressure is higher than right ventricular pressure throughout the systole. Thus, the murmur heard is holosystolic.

20–24. The answers are: 20-C [IV E 3 b (4)], **21-A** [IV B 3 b (4)], **22-D** [IV A 3 b (3)], **23-B** [IV D 3 b (4)], **24-E** [IV C 3 b (4) (b)]. A pulsatile liver often is felt in patients with tricuspid regurgitation as the mechanical effects of right ventricular systole are transmitted back to the hepatic veins.

In mitral stenosis, the mitral valve remains open during most of diastole, due to the pressure gradient across the stenotic mitral valve. Ventricular systole then closes the valve forcibly, with a resultant increase in the intensity of the first heart sound (S_1).

A soft, single second heart sound (S_2) often is noted in aortic stenosis due to the severely impaired motion of the stenotic aortic valve. The redcuced motion cause the aortic component (A_2) of the S_2 to be absent. Thus, only the pulmonic component (P_2) is heard, which is soft.

Although a third heart sound (S_3) could be heard in any cardiac condition, it is most prominently heard in mitral regurgitation, even in patients without congestive heart failure.

In aortic regurgitation, a disproportionate (i.e., 20 mm Hg) increase in systolic blood pressure is noted in the leg as compared with the arm. This finding, called Hill's sign, usually indicates that the aortic regurgitation is severe.

Chapter 2

Pulmonary Diseases

Stanley B. Fiel

I. PULMONARY FUNCTION STUDIES

A. **Introduction.** Tests of pulmonary function provide three basic kinds of information:

1. **Lung volumes** are the volumes of the various intrapulmonary compartments.
   a. **Static lung volumes** reflect the elastic properties of the lungs and chest wall.
   b. **Dynamic lung volumes** reflect the patency of the airways.

2. **The expiratory flow rate** is the maximal rate of airflow during forced expiration.
   a. The rate of airflow is influenced by lung volume and by effort (i.e., force of expiration). Airflow increases with increasing effort, especially at high lung volumes [greater than 75% of the vital capacity (VC)].
   b. Other factors influencing flow rate include the elastic recoil of the lung, small peripheral airway resistance, and the cross-sectional area of larger central airways.

3. **Diffusing capacity (D_L)** is the efficiency of gas transfer from alveoli to pulmonary capillary blood.

B. **Spirometry**

1. **Definition.** Spirometry is a simple, easy test of pulmonary function. The spirometer device plots a tracing (the **spirogram**) of the lung volume against time (in seconds) while the patient takes as deep a breath as possible and then exhales all the inspired air as rapidly and forcefully as possible.

2. **Uses.** Spirometry can aid in distinguishing obstructive from restrictive lung diseases (Table 2-1), and can suggest the severity of functional impairment and its reversibility with treatment. It is useful both diagnostically and as a monitoring tool.

C. **Values obtainable from the spirogram.** Many spirogram measurements are stated as a percentage of **predicted values** that are determined from many normal individuals grouped on the basis of sex, age, and height. The range of normal is 80%–120% of the predicted value.

1. **Tidal volume (V_T)** is the volume of air in one breath during normal quiet breathing. The V_T (normal, 500–800 ml) varies according to effort and level of ventilation. The portion of the V_T that participates in gas exchange is the **alveolar volume (V_A)**; the remainder, approximately 30% of the V_T, is **"wasted"** or **"dead space."**

2. **VC** is the maximal volume of air that can be expelled from the lungs following a maximal inspiration. Because VC decreases progressively with restrictive lung disease, it is useful, in conjunction with D_L (see I E 1), for monitoring the course and response to therapy in a patient with a restrictive lung disorder.

3. **Forced vital capacity (FVC)** is the same as VC, except that the inhalation is performed as rapidly and forcefully as possible. Forced expiration causes the airways to narrow, slowing the rate of expiration.

4. **Forced expiratory volume in 1 second (FEV_1)** is the volume of air forcefully expired during the first second after a deep breath, that is, the portion of the FVC exhaled in 1 second. The FEV_1 primarily reflects the status of large airways. It is often expressed as a percentage of the VC (normal FEV_1 = 75% VC).

TABLE 2-1. Obstructive and Restrictive Lung Disorders

Primarily obstructive ventilatory defects (disorders characterized by reduced flow rates)
Chronic obstructive pulmonary disease
Chronic bronchitis
Pulmonary emphysema
Asthma
Cystic fibrosis
Primarily restrictive ventilatory defects (disorders characterized by reduced lung volumes)
Parenchymal disorders
Alveolar and interstitial processes (e.g., edema, fibrosis, infection)
Large space-occupying lesions
Atelectasis
Resection of pulmonary tissue
Chest wall disease
Obesity
Kyphoscoliosis
Ankylosing spondylitis
Pleural disease
Effusion
Pneumothorax
Fibrothorax
Neuromuscular diseases
Guillain-Barré syndrome
Spinal cord injury
Muscular dystrophies
Poliomyelitis

5. **FEV$_1$/FVC** is the ratio of the FEV$_1$ to FVC, expressed as a percentage (normal, $\geq$ 70%).* The FEV$_1$/FVC is **effort-dependent,** that is, it increases with increasing expiratory effort. The FEV$_1$/FVC ratio is particularly useful in evaluating obstructive disorders but is also helpful in the evaluation of restrictive disorders. If only the FEV$_1$ is low (FEV$_1$/FVC < 70%), obstruction is suggested; if both the FEV$_1$ and FVC are low (FEV$_1$/FVC $\geq$ 70%), restriction is suggested.

6. **FEF$_{25\%-75\%}$** is the forced expiratory flow rate over the middle half of the FVC (i.e., between 25% and 75% of the FVC); it is also called the **maximal mid-expiratory flow rate (MMEFR or MMFR).** The FEF$_{25\%-75\%}$ primarily reflects the status of the small airways, and it is more sensitive than the FEV$_1$ for identifying early airway obstruction. The FEF$_{25\%-75\%}$ is **effort independent.**

D. **Other lung volumes** (Figure 2-1). Obtaining the following values requires the use of spirometry and either helium dilution (which measures the volume of gas in the lungs) or, preferably, body plethysmography (which measures intrathoracic gas volume).

1. **Total lung capacity (TLC)** is the volume of air in the lungs after a maximal inspiratory effort.

2. **Functional residual capacity (FRC)** is the volume of air remaining in the lungs at the end of a normal expiration. The FRC reflects the resting position of the lungs and chest wall; it is the lung volume at which the inward recoil of the lungs is balanced by the outward recoil of the chest wall. The FRC has two components:
a. **The expiratory reserve volume (ERV)** is the amount of the FRC that can be expelled by a maximal expiratory effort.

---

* In this case, percentage is not a percentage of predicted normal.

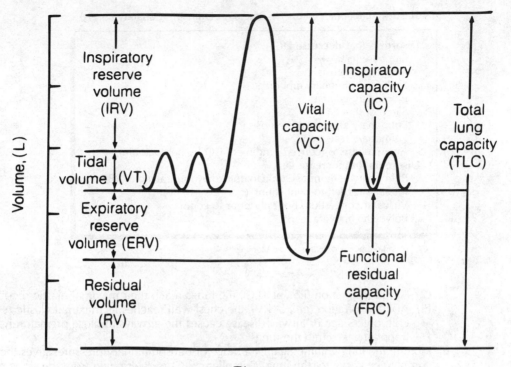

Figure 2-1. The subdivisions of lung volume as recorded by a spirometer. The record is generated on paper calibrated for volume in the vertical direction and time in the horizontal. The term "capacity" is applied to a subdivision composed of two or more volumes.

    b. The residual volume (RV) is the volume of air remaining in the lungs after a maximal expiratory effort (normal, 25%–30% of FRC).

  3. Lung volume relationships are as follow:
    a. TLC = VC + RV
    b. RV = FRC − ERV

E. **Other tests of pulmonary function**

  1. Diffusing capacity of carbon monoxide ($D_{L_{CO}}$). The D_L indicates the adequacy of the alveolar–capillary membrane.
    a. The $D_{L_{CO}}$ is determined by measuring the amount of carbon monoxide (CO) transferred from the alveolar gas to the pulmonary capillary blood after the patient inhales a known amount of CO (0.1%); it is expressed in ml/min/mm Hg.
    b. The $D_{L_{CO}}$ has a number of uses. It helps in distinguishing between asthma, chronic bronchitis, and emphysema. It indicates the severity of emphysema. It provides a useful monitoring tool in sarcoidosis and in interstitial lung disease.
    c. The effects of various disorders on the $D_{L_{CO}}$ are shown in Table 2-2.

  2. Compliance curve. The **elastic properties of the lung** can be assessed from the relationship between a change in lung volume and a change in transpulmonary pressure (the pressure in the alveoli minus the pressure within the pleural space; $P_A - P_{PL}$).
    a. A given volume of air in the lung requires a certain amount of pressure to achieve that degree of inflation. This pressure is a combination of the elastic (inward) recoil of the lung and the elastic (outward) recoil of the chest wall.
      (1) At the normal resting end-expiratory position of the lungs (i.e., at FRC), the elastic recoil of the lung is exactly balanced by the elastic recoil of the chest wall.

TABLE 2-2. Effect of Various Disorders on Diffusing Capacity (D_{LCO})

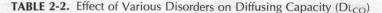

> **Disorders that decrease D_{LCO}**
>   Emphysema
>   Interstitial fibrosis
>   Multiple pulmonary emboli
>   Pulmonary edema
>   Sarcoidosis
>   Pulmonary alveolar proteinosis
>   Pulmonary resection
>   Anemia (due to reduced binding of CO by hemoglobin)
> **Disorders that increase D_{LCO}**
>   Pulmonary hemorrhage (due to uptake by intra-alveolar RBCs)
>   Intracardiac left-to-right shunt
>   Vascular congestion, but only prior to edema
>   Polycythemia vera (early)

CO = carbon monoxide; RBCs = red blood cells.

    (2) At full inspiration (i.e., at TLC), the lungs reach their maximal elastic recoil.
    (3) At full expiration (i.e., at RV), the chest wall reaches its maximal elastic recoil, unless age or airway disease causes the airways to close prematurely, trapping gas within the lungs.

  b. Plotting the lung volume against a range of transpulmonary pressures gives the **compliance curve** for the lung. **Compliance (C)** is determined from the slope of the pressure–volume (P–V) curve over the tidal volume range: C = V/P (normal, 200 ml/cm H_2O).

  c. Changes in lung elastic recoil inversely affect the compliance curve.
    (1) Loss of lung elastic recoil (e.g., in emphysema) increases compliance, shifting the compliance curve to the left.
    (2) Increased lung elastic recoil (e.g., in restrictive lung diseases, such as idiopathic pulmonary fibrosis) decreases compliance, shifting the compliance curve downward and to the right.

  3. Airway resistance (Raw). Measuring Raw primarily reflects the status of large airways, because 80%–90% of the resistance to airflow is in the large central airways.
    a. Raw is usually determined from dynamic lung volumes and expiratory flow rates; when a more accurate measure is needed, body plethysmography is used.
    b. Raw is increased in obstructive lung disease and decreased in restrictive lung disease.

F. **Patterns of pulmonary function impairment**

  1. Obstructive lung disorders
    a. Flow rates. A **reduced FEV_1/FVC** (less than 70%) is the time-honored indicator of obstructive airway disease. However, the FEV_1/FVC may be normal even with considerable peripheral airway obstruction. A reduced $FEF_{25\%-75\%}$ (60% or less of predicted value) may detect airway obstruction when the FEV_1/FVC is normal. However, the range of normal $FEF_{25\%-75\%}$ values is wide.
    b. Lung volumes. Changes in lung volume may be seen in moderate to severe obstructive airway disease.
      (1) Lung volume measurements are useful in identifying hyperinflation due to premature airway closure.
        (a) During a forced expiration, if the terminal airways close before all the air is expelled, hyperinflation results, causing an increase in the FRC, RV, and RV/TLC.
        (b) In small airway disorders, because of air trapping, the RV may increase while the FRC and FEV_1 remain normal.

      (2) In emphysema, the alveolar wall destruction and loss of lung elastic recoil cause an increase in the TLC.

    c. Compliance is increased in emphysema, because lung elastic recoil is reduced.

    d. Raw is increased in obstructive lung disease.

      (1) In intrinsic airway disease, airway inflammation, edema, and smooth muscle spasm cause increased Raw.

      (2) In emphysema, increased Raw is due to loss of elastic support with less distention of the airway.

  2. Restrictive lung disorders

    a. Flow rates. FEV_1/FVC and $FEF_{25\%-75\%}$ may be normal or may be increased due to increased traction on the intrathoracic airway walls.

    b. Lung volumes

      (1) A **reduction in VC and TLC** is the most useful indicator of a restrictive ventilatory defect.

      (2) Lung stiffness in restrictive diseases increases the lung elastic recoil, thus lowering the FRC.

      (3) Chest wall stiffness (e.g., in kyphoscoliosis) lowers lung volumes because it restricts lung expansion.

    c. Compliance is reduced because lung elastic recoil is increased.

    d. Raw is decreased because the elastic forces maintain wider airways at any lung volume.

G. **Arterial blood gases.** The partial pressures of oxygen (**Pa_{O_2}**) and carbon dioxide (**Pa_{CO_2}**) and the **pH** of arterial blood are important in assessing pulmonary function, because these data indicate the status of gas exchange between the lungs and the blood.

  1. Pa_{O_2} and Pa_{CO_2}. The Pa_{O_2} and Pa_{CO_2} show the net effect of lung disease on gas exchange.

    a. The Pa_{O_2} normally decreases with age due to the loss of lung elasticity (normal Pa_{O_2} is approximately 90 mm Hg at age 20 years and approximately 75 mm Hg by age 70 years). A lower than normal Pa_{O_2} indicates hypoxemia. However, tissue oxygenation is not significantly reduced until the Pa_{O_2} decreases to less than approximately 60 mm Hg.

    b. The Pa_{CO_2} (normal, 35–45 mm Hg) reflects alveolar ventilation—**hypercapnia** (respiratory acidosis, a high Pa_{CO_2}) indicates **hypoventilation,** and **hypocapnia** (respiratory alkalosis, a low Pa_{CO_2}) indicates **hyperventilation.**

  2. pH

    a. Comparing the arterial pH (normal, 7.35–7.45) with the Pa_{CO_2} helps to distinguish respiratory from metabolic abnormalities. For example, if the Pa_{CO_2} and pH are related **inversely** (one declining while the other increases), the acid–base imbalance is respiratory.

    b. Clinically, however, results often are not straightforward, being complicated by the nature of the patient's disorders and any medications being taken.

H. **Ventilation–perfusion ($\dot{V}/\dot{Q}$) mismatch** (inequality of pulmonary gas exchange)

  1. $\dot{V}/\dot{Q}$ relationships

    a. Ventilation and blood flow through the lung should match if there is to be adequate uptake of oxygen and adequate elimination of carbon dioxide.

    b. The overall **$\dot{V}/\dot{Q}$ ratio** of the lung is 0.8. Thus, there is a normal **"physiologic $\dot{V}/\dot{Q}$ mismatch,"** equivalent to a 2% **shunting** of pulmonary arterial (mixed venous) blood directly into the pulmonary venous circulation without gas exchange.

  2. Significance of $\dot{V}/\dot{Q}$ mismatch

    a. A **low $\dot{V}/\dot{Q}$ ratio** signifies inadequate ventilation of an adequately perfused area of the lung. The result is a lowered Pa_{O_2} or hypoxemia.

      (1) Unless the alveoli are occluded or fluid filled, the hypoxemia can be corrected by administering oxygen, because the oxygen will reach the areas of alveolar hypoxia.

(2) If an area of the lung has **no alveolar ventilation,** it has no gas exchange at all **($\dot{V}/\dot{Q} = 0$).** The result is **right-to-left shunting** of blood; that is, true venous blood mixes with arterial blood. This form of hypoxemia is refractory to oxygen therapy because the oxygen cannot reach the alveolar–capillary membrane.

(3) Blood coming from well-oxygenated regions of the lung cannot compensate for the low oxygen content of areas with a low $\dot{V}/\dot{Q}$, because the hemoglobin is already fully saturated and its oxygen content cannot be increased.

b. A high $\dot{V}/\dot{Q}$ ratio signifies adequate ventilation of a poorly perfused area of the lung. Oxygen exchange is inefficient because the available hemoglobin can only take up so much oxygen.

(1) If an area of the lung has **no blood flow** at all, it has no gas exchange at all ($\dot{V}/\dot{Q} = \infty$). All of the oxygen going to that area of alveolar dead space is wasted ventilation.

(2) Alveolar dead space results in carbon dioxide retention as well as hypoxia. The hypercapnia stimulates the respiratory center, thereby increasing the work of breathing but also increasing ventilation. Even though this may normalize the P_{CO_2}, it does not improve the lowered P_{O_2}.

c. Typically, in patients with $\dot{V}/\dot{Q}$ abnormalities, the reduction in Pa_{O_2} is much more marked than the increase in Pa_{CO_2}. However, as lung disease progresses, ventilation cannot increase any further. The result is hypoxemia and hypercapnia, that is, acute respiratory failure.

3. Alveolar–arterial oxygen gradient (A-a D_{O_2}) is the difference (i.e., gradient) between the **alveolar** P_{O_2} (the **PA_{O_2}**) and the **arterial** P_{O_2} (the **Pa_{O_2}**). **A decrease in the A-a D_{O_2} reflects an increase in the $\dot{V}/\dot{Q}$ ratio.**

a. Calculating the A-a D_{O_2} can help in distinguishing hypoventilation from other causes of hypoxemia and in suggesting the severity of lung disease.

(1) The PA_{O_2} is calculated from the simplified alveolar gas equation:

$$AV_2 = F_{I_{O_2}} (P_B - P_{H_2O}) - Pa_{CO_2}/R$$

where $F_{I_{O_2}}$ = the fraction (percentage) of oxygen in the inspired air (160 mm Hg for room air at sea level); P_B = atmospheric pressure (760 mm Hg); P_{H_2O} = partial pressure of water vapor (47 mm Hg—included in the formula because inspired air is saturated with water vapor); and R = the respiratory exchange ratio (0.8). Filling in the numbers gives the equation

$$PA_{O_2} = 160(760 - 47) - Pa_{CO_2}/0.8$$

(2) The Pa_{O_2} is determined directly from a blood sample.

b. The Pa_{O_2} is normally 5–15 mm Hg lower than the PA_{O_2} because of the physiologic $\dot{V}/\dot{Q}$ mismatch; the difference increases with age. Thus, the A-a D_{O_2} is normally less than 15 mm Hg and increases with age.

II. CHRONIC OBSTRUCTIVE PULMONARY DISEASE (COPD)

A. Introduction

1. Definition. COPD is defined as a disease state characterized by the presence of airflow obstruction due to chronic bronchitis or emphysema. The airflow is generally progressive, may be accompanied by airway reactivity, and may be partially reversible. COPD is a common disorder usually characterized by progressive obstruction to airflow and a history of inhalation of irritants (e.g., tobacco smoke). COPD also is referred to as **chronic obstructive lung disease (COLD), chronic airways obstruction (CAO),** and, either individually or together, chronic bronchitis and emphysema.

a. Chronic bronchitis can be defined in terms of clinical symptoms (i.e., excessive mucus secretion in the bronchial tree leading to productive cough for at least 3 months during each of 2 successive years).

    b. Emphysema can be described in terms of morbid anatomy (i.e., destruction of alveolar walls and abnormal enlargement of air spaces distal to the terminal nonrespiratory bronchiole).

    c. Many patients have, in varying degrees, a combination of these two entities. Therefore, the more general term COPD is appropriate.

2. The **social and economic consequences** of COPD are staggering. Screening studies of the general population suggest that 5% of individuals have significant airflow obstruction.

3. The **death rate** due to COPD has doubled every 5 years in the past two decades. COPD is the fourth leading cause of death in the United States. Unlike many other diseases (coronary heart disease, stroke, and other cardiovascular diseases) for which there has been a 20%–60% decline in mortality rate over the past 20 years, the incidence of COPD has increased by 70% over the same period.

B. **Etiology.** The precise scientific etiology of COPD is unknown; however, the most important environmental etiologic agent is chronic inhalation of tobacco smoke (Figure 2-2).

1. **Tobacco smoke.** Smoking in **pack years** (the number of years a patient has smoked × the number of packs smoked per day) is directly related to ventilatory dysfunction and pathologic changes in the lung. Smoking stimulates inflammatory cytokines and depresses alveolar macrophages, reduces the functional integrity of pulmonary surfactant, retards mucus transport, enhances the release of lysosomal enzymes, and produces numerous other effects believed to be involved in the pathogenesis of COPD.

2. **Other environmental factors**

    a. The extent that urban and industrial **air pollution** contributes to the pathogenesis of COPD is not entirely known. Studies comparing patients who live in areas of clean air with those who reside in highly polluted areas indicate a higher incidence of COPD in the latter group.

    b. The role of **infections** in the development and progression of COPD is unproven. However, evidence suggests that upper respiratory **viral infections** in childhood may predispose the patient to COPD in adulthood, and viral infec-

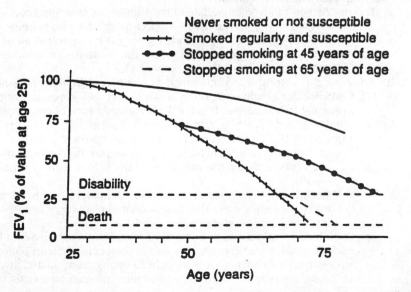

Figure 2-2. Age-related rate of decline in lung function in various patient groups. FEV_1 = forced expiratory volume in 1 second. (Modified with permission from Snider GL, Saling LJ, Renard SI: Chronic bronchitis and emphysema. In Textbook of Respiratory Medicine. Edited by Murray JF and Nadel JA. Philadelphia, WB Saunders, 1994, p 1342.)

tions are frequent precipitating factors in symptomatic exacerbations of COPD. **Bacterial infections** are less clearly implicated.

3. **α_1-Antitrypsin deficiency** is a well-recognized genetic factor predisposing the patient to emphysema.

a. Presumably, this deficiency increases the susceptibility of pulmonary tissue to autodigestion by naturally occurring proteases.

b. Emphysema may develop early in life in individuals with homozygous deficiency. Cigarette smoking accelerates the process. In its pure form (see also Chapter 5 IX C 1), α_1-antitrypsin deficiency presents as hepatic cirrhosis, absence of the α_1-globulin peak on serum protein electrophoresis, negligible amounts of serum α_1-antitrypsin, and advanced panlobular emphysema, predominantly in the base of the lungs.

C. **Pathogenesis.** Evidence suggests that COPD begins in the small airways (i.e., those less than 2 mm in diameter). Normally, these airways contribute only a small amount of the total resistance to airflow in the tracheobronchial tree. In COPD, however, the small airways are the sites of extensive disease and airflow limitation.

1. Histopathologic abnormalities of the small airways are common findings at autopsy in young smokers. This small-airway disease is presumed to progress over approximately 30 years to the characteristic clinical picture of disabling COPD.

2. If young smokers stop smoking, the abnormalities observed in tests of small airway function tend to resolve. It is unclear at what point during the course of the disease that the changes become irreversible and inevitably progress to COPD.

D. **Pathology and pathophysiology.** The pathologic changes of COPD are seen in both the airways and the pulmonary parenchyma.

1. **The bronchitic component**

a. Early in the disease, the small airways demonstrate mucous plugging, inflammation, peribronchiolar fibrosis, narrowing, and obliteration.

b. In established disease, the bronchitic component includes varying degrees of mucous gland hyperplasia, mucosal inflammation and edema, bronchospasm, and impacted secretions. These elements contribute to airway narrowing and increased airway resistance.

2. **The emphysematous, component**

a. The destruction of alveolar walls and the supporting structure produces widely dilated air spaces. The loss of tissue support for the airways is believed to contribute to airway narrowing by a tendency for the unsupported airways to collapse dynamically during expiration to low lung volumes. In addition, the loss of the alveolar capillary membrane reduces $D_{L_{CO}}$.

b. Anatomically, emphysema is classified as either **centrilobular** or **panlobular.**

(1) **Centrilobular emphysema** often is associated with **chronic bronchitis** and **bronchial inflammation.** It is the most common type of emphysema encountered in clinical practice, and it is rare in nonsmokers.

(a) Centrilobular emphysema is believed to represent a destructive lesion of the respiratory bronchiole. It originates at the center of the lobule and is distinct from the periphery of the acinus with its septae and vessels.

(b) Centrilobular emphysema is variable and patchy and has a predilection for upper lung zones. The greatly dilated respiratory bronchioles coalesce and may produce bullous cysts.

(2) **Panlobular emphysema,** in contrast to centrilobular emphysema has little association with chronic bronchitis and is seen commonly in patients with α_1-antitrypsin deficiency. It is thought to evolve from dilated alveolar ducts at the periphery of the lobules to markedly enlarged air spaces.

E. **Clinical features**

1. **Typical history.** COPD is an insidious, long-term process that typically develops as follows.

  a. Mild but asymptomatic changes in the small airways develop in a teenager who smokes.
  b. As an adult, this smoker experiences chronic cough and symptoms that suggest an upper respiratory infection.
  c. By middle age, the smoker has significant bronchial disease characterized by progressive airway obstruction that produces dyspnea on exertion. This occurs in 25%–50% of smokers and frequently goes unrecognized with the patients' more sedentary life-style.
  d. When the smoker's respiratory system is placed under stress from an unrelated health problem, the presence of COPD becomes evident. Pneumonia, surgery, and trauma are common precipitating events.

2. Clinical syndromes
  a. Two classic types of COPD exist and are given various names. Patients with "emphysematous," "dyspneic," or "type A" COPD are referred to as **pink puffers;** those with "bronchitic," "tussive," or "type B" COPD are referred to as **blue bloaters.**
    (1) Pink puffers have predominant emphysema and show symptoms at a relatively advanced age (often greater than 60 years). There is progressive exertional dyspnea, weight loss, and little or no cough and expectoration.
      (a) Pulmonary function testing reveals mild hypoxia, hypocapnia, decreased $D_{L_{CO}}$, only a mild increase in Raw, and little improvement in airflow after treatment with bronchodilators.
      (b) These patients usually undergo a slowly progressive downhill course.
    (2) Blue bloaters have predominant chronic bronchitis and, at a relatively young age, experience chronic cough and expectoration, episodic dyspnea, and weight gain. Wheezing and rhonchi frequently are heard in the chest, and cor pulmonale often develops, accompanied by edema and cyanosis.
      (a) Pulmonary function testing reveals severe hypoxia, hypercapnia, polycythemia, increased Raw, improved airflow after treatment with bronchodilators, and relatively preserved lung volumes and $D_{L_{CO}}$.
      (b) Pathologically, there is minimal emphysema but significant bronchiolitis, bronchitis, mucous gland hyperplasia, and right ventricular hypertrophy. This is in contrast to the pathologic findings in pink puffers, in whom the major finding is emphysema with little or no airway inflammation.
  b. Patients with emphysema have proportional and matched losses of ventilation and perfusion and, hence, are spared severe hypoxia; in contrast, patients with chronic bronchitis have marked $\dot{V}/\dot{Q}$ mismatch, resulting in severe hypoxia. The hypoxia in chronic bronchitis is worsened by the hypercapnia, which may be the result of respiratory muscle fatigue or an acquired or congenital reduction in central respiratory drive.
  c. Although the definitions for the two types of COPD are useful concepts, such pure entities represent extremes of the spectrum of COPD and are rarely encountered. Most COPD patients have a mixture of emphysema and chronic bronchitis.

F. **Diagnosis.** The diagnosis of COPD may be suspected based on the patient's history, symptoms, and physical signs, or it may become obvious through chest radiograph and clinical circumstances.

1. COPD in middle-aged smokers can be diagnosed by spirometric screening.

2. On physical examination, the findings might include hyperinflation, poor diaphragmatic movement, the use of accessory muscles of respiration, and decreased breathing sounds and wheezing on auscultation.

3. The chest x-ray may show hyperinflation, a loss of vascularity, a flattened diaphragm, and a small heart. In addition, patients with chronic bronchitis often show thickened bronchial walls and "dirty" lung fields.

4. Diagnosis should not test solely on the basis of radiographic findings. Objective documentation of expiratory flow obstruction by pulmonary function testing is necessary for the diagnosis of COPD.

G. **Clinical course and prognosis**

1. COPD tends to be a progressive disorder unless there is some form of intervention (i.e., cessation of smoking, removal of other irritants, or medical therapy). Once COPD is well advanced, specific medical therapy may not slow the progression of disease. However, cessation of smoking may alter the decline in pulmonary function in all but far-advanced disease.

2. The FEV_1 declines by approximately 50–75 ml/yr in a typical patient with COPD, as compared with a normal decline of approximately half that rate.

3. Survival is statistically related to the degree of ventilatory function that exists when the patient is first evaluated. For example, among patients with an initial FEV_1 of less than 0.75 L, the 5-year survival rate is 25%, whereas among those with an initial FEV_1 and 1 L, the 5-year survival rate is approximate 50%.

H. **Therapy**

1. **Bronchodilation.** Overall, most patients with COPD show improvement in pulmonary function after sufficient bronchodilator therapy.
   a. COPD is not always an irreversible process. A patient may have airflow reactivity even when pulmonary function studies performed after bronchodilator therapy have indicated nonreversible airflow obstruction. It appears that 15%–20% of COPD patients in this category have reversible airflow obstruction.
   b. The three major classes of bronchodilators are **xanthines** (theophylline-type agents), **β-adrenergic agonists,** and **anticholinergics** (ipratropium bromide). These agents may be used separately or in combination. The newer, selective β-adrenergic agonists offer advantages over the older agents in terms of a longer duration of bronchodilating action (β_2 effect) and reduced cardiac stimulation (β_1 effect).

2. **Corticosteroid therapy.** The use of corticosteroids to treat the bronchospasm associated with COPD is controversial. However, some patients clearly have an asthma-like component to their disease and would likely respond to steroid therapy to some extent. Inhaling corticosteroids via a metered-dose inhaler (MDI) is the preferred route of delivery, although the role of corticosteroids in COPD is not clearly defined.

3. **Sputum mobilization.** Traditional expectorants and mucolytic agents appear to have little beneficial effect in COPD patients. Bland hydrating aerosols and physical therapy may improve bronchial drainage transiently, but the long-term benefit is not known. Postural drainage usually is reserved for patients with bronchiectasis.

4. **Management of infection.** There has been a long-standing empiricism in the use of broad-spectrum antibiotics during exacerbations in patients with COPD. In addition, COPD patients should receive annual vaccination against influenza; a vaccine for pneumococcal infection also should be given.

5. **Pulmonary rehabilitation programs.** Participation in these programs may decrease patient morbidity and improve the quality of life. Patients are instructed in exercise programs aimed at increasing exercise tolerance and respiratory muscle stamina. Counseling and nutritional guidance are also available.

6. **Surgery**
   a. The **resection** of large localized bullae may be of benefit in carefully selected patients.
   b. In the future, lung **transplantation** may offer the ultimate cure; single and double lung transplantations have been performed in patients with COPD with encouraging results.
   c. A new technique, **volume reduction surgery (VRS),** is being evaluated. In pa-

tients with emphysema, the lungs become hyperinflated, the chest wall expands outward, and the diaphragm is flattened, inhibiting respiratory muscle efficiency. VRS most likely works by removing 20%–30% of diseased, poorly functioning lung to create more space for diaphragmatic excursion.

7. **Oxygen.** Oxygen is the only known therapeutic modality in COPD that can improve survival. Its value, however, is only demonstrable in those patients with a Pao_2 of 55 mm Hg or less on room air at rest.

8. **α_1-Antitrypsin.** For those patients with a deficiency of α_1-antitrypsin, replacement therapy is available.

I. **Prevention.** Avoidance of smoking is by far the best means of disease prevention. In addition, patients should avoid chronic exposure to other bronchial irritants. Simple spirometric screening of high-risk patients can help to detect early disease and prevent further deterioration.

J. **Complications of COPD** include cor pulmonale, polycythemia, infection, respiratory failure, bronchogenic carcinoma, nocturnal hypoxia, general disability, and (for unknown reasons) a proclivity for peptic ulcer disease.

1. **Pneumonia** occurring in a COPD patient is of special concern because of its relative severity and its potential for precipitating respiratory failure.

2. **Respiratory failure** may be precipitated by many conditions, including heart failure, sedation, infection, acute bronchospasm, and trauma.

3. Although **bronchogenic carcinoma** is not strictly a complication of COPD, it occurs in COPD patients with high frequency, presumably because of the common denominator of tobacco smoking.

4. Concomitant left ventricular dysfunction appears to be due to independent primary myocardial disease, not pulmonary disease.

III. **ASTHMA**

A. **Definition.** Asthma is a reversible airway obstruction that is characterized by hyperirritability and inflammation of the airways. Substances that have no effect when inhaled by normal individuals can cause bronchoconstriction in patients with asthma. Asthma per se does not cause emphysema or other chronic diseases but alone may be a significant cause of disability. A principal feature of asthma is its extreme variability, both from patient to patient and from time to time in the same patient. Another feature of asthma that is important to its pathophysiology and treatment is the presence of airway inflammation.

B. **Incidence and etiology**

1. Asthma occurs in 3%–8% of the population. Etiologic or pathologic classification of the disease is difficult; however, asthma traditionally is divided into two forms.
   a. An **allergic form,** responsible for most of childhood asthma, is immunologically mediated—it is due to type I (immediate) hypersensitivity to inhaled antigens.
   b. An **intrinsic form** occurs in adults and shows no evidence of immediate hypersensitivity to specific antigens.

2. In patients in whom the evidence of immediate hypersensitivity to antigen is absent or equivocal, most attacks do not appear to be provoked by inhalation of antigens, and there is a poor correlation between the severity of symptoms and the levels of specific antigens circulating as airborne particles. These observations indicate that asthmatic bronchospasm may not necessarily require an immunologically mediated hypersensitivity reaction.

C. Pathogenesis

1. **Biochemical mediators**
   a. The **mediators of immediate hypersensitivity** and their mechanisms of action are discussed in Chapter 7 II A.
   b. **Other biochemical mediators,** including serotonin, prostaglandins, thromboxanes, and endoperoxides, also cause tissue inflammation and may be particularly important in the pathogenesis of **nonallergic** asthma.
   c. The physiologic changes seen in asthma can be directly induced by mediators that diffuse locally to mucous glands, vessels, and smooth muscle. It is clear, however, that the simple release of mediators is not sufficient to cause an asthmatic attack.

2. **Airway hyperirritability**
   a. The tracheobronchial tree of asthmatic individuals appears to have an exaggerated reactivity, sometimes called **nonspecific bronchial hyperreactivity** to distinguish it from the bronchospasm provoked by immunologically specific antigens. The ubiquity of bronchial hyperreactivity has caused pathogenetic theories to shift in focus from the **nature of biochemical mediators** to the **responsiveness of the end organ.**
   b. The mechanism underlying bronchial hyperreactivity is unknown, but a number of factors have been suggested.
      (1) **Muscle reactivity.** A change in the contractile mechanisms of airway smooth muscle may induce hyperreactivity.
      (2) **Autonomic reactivity.** The abnormality may exist in the nerves that regulate the tone of the muscle, not in the muscle itself.
         (a) The **parasympathetic system** appears to mediate the reflex bronchial constriction caused by inhalation of nonspecific irritants such as dust or sulfur dioxide.
         (b) A deficiency in the **sympathetic nervous system** may be responsible for bronchial hyperreactivity.
         (c) A third system of autonomic innervation, the **nonadrenergic inhibitor system,** may exist in the bronchial muscles as it does in the gut, where it seems to inhibit constriction of intestinal smooth muscle. Congenital absence of this system leads to Hirschsprung's disease (see Chapter 5 V C), in which the distal bowel is intensely constricted. A similar deficiency in the airway conceivably could cause recurrent constriction of bronchial smooth muscle.
      (3) **Environmental factors.** Bronchial reactivity is temporarily increased by upper respiratory viral infections and by exposure to pollutants such as ozone, nitrogen dioxide, and industrial fumes. By amplifying the response to the materials released from mast cells, this increased reactivity could be responsible for the exacerbations of asthma seen with viral infections, occupational exposures, and exposure to severe pollution.

D. Pathophysiology

1. Pathophysiologically, asthma is characterized by constriction of airway smooth muscle, hypersecretion of mucus, edema and inflammatory cell infiltration of the airway mucosa, and thickening of the basement membrane underlying the airway epithelium.

2. These pathophysiologic changes are not uniformly distributed. Some airways may display a predominance of bronchospasm, others may be occluded by mucous plugging, and still others may appear unaffected.

E. Clinical features

1. Asthma classically presents as episodic bouts of coughing, dyspnea, chest tightness, and expiratory wheezing. Attacks may be provoked by upper respiratory viral infection, exposure to allergens, emotional stress, and many nonspecific precipitating events.

2. The **symptoms** of asthma exhibit a wide spectrum of severity, reflecting the variability of the underlying airway obstruction. Some patients display only occasional attacks of exertional dyspnea and wheezing, which respond to inhaled bronchodilators alone; other patients have chronic symptoms requiring continuous use of orally inhaled medications. Although this latter group of patients may have irreversible thickening of the airway walls, their illness still is episodic in occurrence.

3. The term **status asthmaticus** usually is reserved for a prolonged, severe asthmatic attack that does not respond to treatment and involves bronchospasm so severe that the patient is at risk for ventilatory failure.
   a. The clinical manifestations of severe asthma include fatigue, a pulse rate of more than 100 bpm, and cyanosis. The use of accessory muscles for respiration frequently is noted.
   b. An inspiratory decrease of more than 20 mm Hg in systolic blood pressure (i.e., **pulsus paradoxus**) indicates gross overinflation of the lung and wide swings in pleural pressure.

F. **Diagnosis**

1. **Physical examination** of an asthmatic patient typically reveals tachycardia, tachypnea with prolonged expiration, overinflation of the chest with poor movement of the diaphragm, and diffuse, high-pitched expiratory wheezing.

2. **Sputum analysis.** Sputum may appear purulent due to an increased eosinophil content or due to an inflammatory response to a viral tracheobronchitis. Sputum smears may reveal **Curschmann's spirals** (i.e., mucus that forms a cast of the small airways) or **Charcot-Leyden crystals** (i.e., breakdown products of the eosinophils).

3. **Hematologic studies** reveal a modest leukocytosis and eosinophilia in both the allergic and intrinsic forms of the disease.

4. **Pulmonary function testing**
   a. The FVC is reduced; the FEV_1/FVC ratio is reduced but may improve after inhalation of a bronchodilator. RV, TLC, and lung compliance usually are increased, and the $D_{L_{CO}}$ frequently is increased.
   b. After symptomatic recovery, TLC and lung compliance return to normal, but the maximal expiratory flow rate may remain reduced at low lung volumes and an abnormal distribution of ventilation may persist, reflecting resistant obstruction of small airways.

5. **Chest x-ray** usually shows nothing more than overinflation. Occasional findings include localized density due to a large mucous plug and the ominous sign of pneumothorax or pneumomediastinum, reflecting the rupture of alveolar tissue caused by high intra-alveolar pressure.

6. **Arterial blood gas studies.** The P_{CO_2} usually is low; that is, less than 36 mm Hg. An increased P_{CO_2} or a normal P_{CO_2} (40 mm Hg) indicates severe obstruction. Arterial hypoxia is common despite the increased ventilation and is due to underventilation of lung segments supplied by narrowed airways (i.e., there is a $\dot{V}/\dot{Q}$ mismatch).

G. **Therapy** is based on an understanding of the underlying pathophysiologic mechanisms. Effective management of asthma relies on four integral components: objective measures of lung function, pharmacologic therapy, environmental measures to control allergens and irritants, and patient education.

1. **Goals of therapy.** The goals of therapy are to:
   a. Maintain near "normal" pulmonary function
   b. Maintain normal activity levels
   c. Prevent chronic and troublesome symptoms (e.g., cough, nocturnal symptoms)
   d. Prevent recurrent exacerbations
   e. Avoid adverse effects from asthma medications

2. Principles of treatment. Asthma is a **chronic condition with acute exacerbations.**
    a. Prevention of exacerbations is particularly important.
    b. Early intervention when treating acute exacerbations of asthma is important to reduce the likelihood of developing severe airway narrowing.
    c. The evidence suggesting the presence of airway inflammation in all asthma subjects indicates that **control of airway inflammation** is a key factor in treating asthma. Morphologic studies show that bronchial infiltration with inflammatory cells is most evident in mild to severe asthma. The increased levels of inflammatory mediators are associated with airway hyperresponsiveness.

3. Pharmacologic therapy
    a. Anti-inflammatory agents (e.g., **corticosteroids, cromolyn sodium, cromolyn-like compounds**) interrupt the development of bronchial inflammation and have a prophylactic or preventive action. They may also modulate ongoing inflammatory reactions. These agents decrease the severity of acute asthma attacks as well as chronic asthma.
        (1) Administration can be oral or via an inhaler.
        (2) Oral or intravenous routes are recommended in acute attacks; aerosolized corticosteroids are for long-term use.
    b. Bronchodilators act principally to dilate the airways by relaxing bronchial smooth muscle. Agents include sympathomimetics, methylxanthines, and anticholinergics.
        (1) Methylxanthines (theophylline) and **sympathomimetics** (β_2 agonists) are used during acute attacks of asthma. Methylxanthines are given intravenously at a loading dose, followed by continuous infusion, and β_2 agonists are inhaled.
        (2) Anticholinergic agents (e.g., ipratropium) are used primarily as supplements to other bronchodilators during acute attacks.

IV. BRONCHIECTASIS, CYSTIC FIBROSIS, AND LUNG ABSCESS

A. Bronchiectasis

1. Definition. Bronchiectasis is a pathologic, irreversible dilatation of the bronchi caused by destruction of the bronchial wall, usually resulting from suppurative infection in an obstructed bronchus.

2. Etiology and pathogenesis
    a. The small bronchi of childhood are most susceptible to bronchial infection and to obstruction by impacted secretions, foreign bodies, or compressing lymph nodes. Seventy-five percent of patients can recall experiencing symptoms of bronchiectasis as early as the age of 5 years.
    b. The most common cause of bronchiectasis is bacterial pneumonia, which may be primary or may be a complication of measles, aspiration of gastric contents or particulate matter, or tumor.
    c. Predisposing conditions include congenital disorders (e.g., congenital cystic disease of the lung, bronchial stenosis, or compression of bronchi by anomalous arteries to the lung), immune deficiencies (e.g., hypogammaglobulinemia or IgA deficiency), and cystic fibrosis.

3. Clinical features. The symptoms of bronchiectasis include a chronic cough productive of purulent sputum, recurrent chest colds or pneumonias, occasional hemoptysis, and pleuritic pain. These symptoms cannot be differentiated from those of chronic suppurative bronchitis. Progressive dyspnea, cyanosis, digital clubbing, and cor pulmonale are seen in advanced cases.

4. Diagnosis
    a. Physical examination reveals rales over the area of involvement on repeated examinations.

  b. Pulmonary function testing produces normal results in mild cases, but, in moderate or severe cases, it may reveal either restrictive or a mixture of restrictive or obstructive ventilatory patterns.

  c. Chest radiography shows peribronchial fibrosis in the involved segment. Segmental lung collapse in areas of bronchiectasis is common.

  d. Bronchography can provide a definitive diagnosis if the patient is stable and not actively infected or coughing up blood. Secretions and clots block the entry of contrast medium, and pneumonia causes temporary dilatation of the bronchi.

  e. Computed tomography (CT) scanning, particularly **high-resolution computed tomography (HRCT),** can often identify bronchiectasis, eliminating the need for bronchoscopy.

5. Therapy. The proper therapy can markedly improve a patient's symptoms.

  a. Medical treatment is the mainstay and consists of therapy with antibiotics on a regular basis (e.g., ampicillin, tetracycline, erythromycin, or as indicated by culture and sensitivity testing), postural drainage, and immunization against influenza and pneumococcal pneumonia.

  b. Surgical resection generally is not effective for eliminating chronic cough and sputum unless the operation is performed in early childhood for single local airway disease.

  c. Bronchodilation may be effective if the obstruction is reversible.

  d. Oxygen therapy is appropriate if PaO_2 levels are depressed.

B. Cystic fibrosis

1. Definition. Cystic fibrosis is an autosomal recessive disease characterized by dysfunction of the exocrine glands, leading to obstruction in such organs as the lungs, pancreas, and gastrointestinal tract. In 99% of cystic fibrosis patients, death is due to respiratory failure, with portal hypertension secondary to biliary cirrhosis accounting for the remainder of deaths.

2. Incidence

  a. An estimated 30,000 cystic fibrosis patients live in the United States. The disease is most common in whites, occurring in 1 of 2000–2500 births, and 5% of the white population are carriers. Because inheritance is recessive and heterozygotes have no disease, a negative family history does not rule out the disease.

  b. Once thought to be unique to children, cystic fibrosis now is recognized as the most common cause of obstructive airway disease among individuals up to age 30 years. The median age of patients with cystic fibrosis has risen from the teens in the 1960s to approximately 30 years in 1995.

3. Etiology and pathogenesis

  a. The genetic abnormality that is responsible for cystic fibrosis has been identified. Most patients with cystic fibrosis have a deletion at position 508 on the long arm of chromosome 7. This deletion produces an abnormal membrane transport protein called **cystic fibrosis transmembrane regulator (CFTR).**

  b. The abnormality in patients with cystic fibrosis seems to be an electrochemical defect in the epithelial cell that involves chloride impermeability and increased sodium resorption. This abnormality leads to the viscid mucus that is observed and the subsequent obstruction of organs served by exocrine glands.

4. Clinical features. The manifestations of cystic fibrosis are varied, with pulmonary abnormalities being the overriding clinical concern.

  a. Pulmonary manifestations

   (1) The earliest pulmonary manifestation is peripheral airway obstruction resulting from plugged bronchi. Repeated bouts of infection lead to a cycle of obstruction, tissue damage, and infection that ultimately progresses to a loss of pulmonary function.

   (2) The predominant organism to colonize the lung is the highly resistant mucoid strain of *Pseudomonas aeruginosa.* Initial infections may be due to *Staphylococcus aureus.* Complete eradication of the organisms is virtually impossible.

(3) Many cystic fibrosis patients develop sinusitis and nasal polyps, and most have clubbing of the digits.

(4) Older children and adolescents have problems referable to the cardiopulmonary system, but most patients die of respiratory complications.

b. Nonpulmonary manifestations also are common and include meconium ileus, malabsorption, fatty infiltration of the liver, focal biliary cirrhosis, glucose intolerance, sterility in the male, and a predilection for heat prostration due to severe salt depletion.

5. Diagnosis

a. Sweat test. An abnormal sweat test is observed in virtually all cases of cystic fibrosis and, in combination with certain clinical hallmarks, confirms the diagnosis.

(1) In patients with cystic fibrosis, the sodium and chloride concentrations in sweat are elevated drastically, while normal concentrations of these ions exist elsewhere. The **quantitative pilocarpine iontophoresis sweat test** defines the upper limit of normal as a sweat chloride concentration of 60 mEq/L.

(2) A positive sweat test is diagnostic of cystic fibrosis in the presence of at least one of the following three criteria:

(a) A reliable family history of cystic fibrosis

(b) Obstructive pulmonary disease

(c) Pancreatic insufficiency

b. Pulmonary function testing shows limitation of maximal expiratory flow rate and an elevated RV. The $D_{L_{CO}}$ is usually within normal limits.

c. Chest radiography reveals striking manifestations that are more pronounced at the apices, particularly on the right. Findings include hyperinflation, cyst formation, atelectasis, bronchiectasis, and segmental infiltration.

6. Therapy

a. In the **early stages** of the disease, therapy must be individualized according to specific clinical manifestations.

(1) Salt depletion is a potential problem in warmer climates.

(2) Nutritional supplementation and pancreatic enzyme replacement often are indicated.

(3) Pulmonary infections may require hospitalization and vigorous treatment with parenteral antibiotics, hydration, humidification, and supplemental oxygen.

b. In the **late stages** of the disease, therapy is aimed at suppressing infection with specific antibiotics, inducing sputum through physical manipulation, and administering supplemental oxygen as required. Dornase-α, a drug that hydrolyzes extracellular DNA and makes sputum less viscous, has been approved for use in cystic fibrosis patients. This drug has been shown to decrease respiratory tract infections and increase pulmonary function.

c. In **end-stage** disease, bilateral lung transplantation (the procedure of choice) can be considered. Results are similar to those obtained with bilateral lung transplantation in other end-stage lung diseases.

d. New therapies aimed at counteracting the pathophysiologic process of cystic fibrosis are being tested and include gene therapy, ion transport manipulation, and administration of anti-inflammatory agents, antibiotics, and antielastases.

7. Complications. Cor pulmonale that is only partially responsive to oxygen therapy develops late in the disease, with all of the manifestations of right-sided heart failure (e.g., hepatomegaly and peripheral edema). Other pulmonary complications of cystic fibrosis include **hemoptysis** and **pneumothorax.**

C. **Lung abscess** (see also Chapter 8 V C 5)

1. Definition. A lung abscess is a localized area of infection within the lung parenchyma that develops from an initial pneumonic stage. The center of the infected area first becomes gangrenous, necrotic, and purulent and then becomes well demarcated from the surrounding lung tissue. The wall of the abscess becomes intensely inflamed and lined with fibrous and granulation tissue and abundant blood vessels.

2. **Etiology.** A solitary lung abscess most commonly results from aspiration of secretions in the upper respiratory tract. Other major but less common causes include bronchial obstruction, bacterial pneumonia, pulmonary embolism with infection, spread from transdiaphragmatic infections, chest trauma, and bacteremic infection.

3. **Clinical features**
   a. Initial symptoms are similar to those of acute pneumonia.
   b. Chronically, lung abscess is associated with constitutional symptoms that include weight loss, low-grade fever, fatigue, and malaise.

4. **Diagnosis**
   a. **Physical examination** may reveal relatively normal findings, although clubbing of the nailbeds occasionally is noted. Amphoric breath sounds may be heard over the abscess cavity.
   b. **Pulmonary function testing** usually is not affected by a lung abscess.
   c. **Bronchoscopy** is indicated when an abscess does not resolve completely with antibiotic therapy, or when the possibility of a malignancy or foreign body in the lung must be ruled out.

5. **Therapy.** The treatment of choice is antibiotics, either penicillin or clindamycin. The total duration of therapy may be 4–8 weeks.

V. ACUTE RESPIRATORY FAILURE

A. **Definition.** Acute respiratory failure is defined as hypoxia (i.e., a PaO_2 of less than 50 mm Hg) with or without associated hypercapnia (i.e., a $PaCO_2$ of more than 45 mm Hg).

B. **Classification.** Acute respiratory failure can be divided into two types.

1. **Type I: respiratory failure without carbon dioxide retention** (i.e., low PaO_2 with low or normal $PaCO_2$). This type of respiratory failure is characterized by marked $\dot{V}/\dot{Q}$ abnormalities and intrapulmonary shunting. Type I respiratory failure occurs in such clinical settings as:
   a. Adult respiratory distress syndrome (ARDS) (see VI)
   b. Diffuse pneumonia (viral and bacterial)
   c. Aspiration pneumonitis
   d. Fat embolism
   e. Pulmonary edema

2. **Type II: respiratory failure with carbon dioxide retention** (i.e., low PaO_2 with elevated $PaCO_2$). Type II respiratory failure, or **ventilatory failure,** has two basic physiologic abnormalities—$\dot{V}/\dot{Q}$ imbalance and inadequate alveolar ventilation. Patients with type II respiratory failure are divided into two categories.
   a. In one category are patients with **intrinsic lung disease** characterized by **both $\dot{V}/\dot{Q}$ imbalance and inadequate alveolar ventilation.** Respiratory failure is precipitated by additional clinical insult, usually infection, which worsens the physiologic abnormalities. Examples of such lung diseases include:
      (1) COPD (chronic bronchitis, emphysema) and cystic fibrosis
      (2) Acute obstructive lung disease (asthma, severe acute bronchitis)
   b. In the other category are patients **with intrinsically normal lungs** but with **inadequate ventilation** due to:
      (1) Disorders of respiratory control [e.g., as a result of drug overdose, central nervous system (CNS) disease, trauma, or cerebrovascular accident]
      (2) Neuromuscular abnormalities (e.g., poliomyelitis, myasthenia gravis, Guillain-Barré syndrome)
      (3) Chest wall trauma

C. **Pathophysiologic mechanisms of hypoxia**

1. $\dot{V}/\dot{Q}$ **imbalance** is the most common pathophysiologic cause of hypoxia. Hypoxia results when alveolar ventilation decreases with respect to perfusion in the lung. Hypoxia resulting from a moderate decrease in the $\dot{V}/\dot{Q}$ ratio can be reversed with relatively small increases in the inspired oxygen concentration (i.e., 24%–40% inspired oxygen).

2. **Intrapulmonary shunting** occurs when ventilation approaches or reaches zero in perfused areas (e.g., due to collapsed or fluid-filled alveoli), so that venous blood is shunted directly to the arterial circulation without first being oxygenated. Hypoxia due to a shunt frequently cannot be corrected, even with 100% inspired oxygen.

3. **Hypoventilation with resulting hypercapnia** may contribute to hypoxia. This represents type II respiratory failure.

4. **An abnormality in the diffusion of oxygen across the alveolar–capillary membrane** may contribute to hypoxia during exercise or in conditions of lowered inspired oxygen content (most commonly due to high altitude, e.g., during a commercial flight). However, the contribution of this mechanism to respiratory failure, if any, is insignificant.

D. **Therapy**

1. **Principles.** In both type I and type II respiratory failure, therapy is directed toward the underlying disease as well as toward the ventilatory and hypoxic components. In addition, the acute and chronic aspects of respiratory failure must be considered. Patients with chronic respiratory failure frequently can tolerate a lower P_{O_2} and a higher P_{CO_2} than those with acute respiratory failure.

2. **Oxygen therapy**
   a. In **type I respiratory failure,** patients may be given high concentrations of inspired oxygen, because carbon dioxide retention is not a risk. Oxygen may be delivered by mask or nasal cannula. Mechanical ventilation (see VI E 1 b) may be required.
   b. In **type II respiratory failure,** treatment depends on the cause.
      (1) When the cause is an exacerbation of COPD, the basis of therapy is controlled administration of oxygen (i.e., low-flow oxygen treatment), with care taken not to increase the P_{aCO_2}. Mechanical ventilation may be needed.
         (a) **Noninvasive mask ventilation** with continuous positive airway pressure (CPAP) or bilevel positive airway pressure (Bipap) has been used with some success, thus avoiding the need for airway intubation.
         (b) Positive end-expiratory pressure (PEEP) usually is not helpful in treating the respiratory failure of COPD.
      (2) Type II respiratory failure that arises from causes other than COPD usually is an indication for either invasive or noninvasive mechanical ventilation.

VI. **ADULT RESPIRATORY DISTRESS SYNDROME (ARDS)**

A. **Definition**

1. **Clinical definition.** ARDS is an important form of acute hypoxic, hypocapnic (i.e., type I) respiratory failure characterized by severe dyspnea, hypoxia, loss of lung compliance, and pulmonary edema. The synonym **"wet lung"** emphasizes the presence of increased extravascular lung water (the basic pathophysiologic mechanism underlying this condition).

2. **Physiologic definition**
   a. There is a ratio of arterial oxygen (P_{aO_2}) to the fraction of inspired oxygen (F_{IO_2}) that is ≤ 200, regardless of whether PEEP is being used.

    b. There is a finding of bilateral pulmonary infiltrates.

    c. There is pulmonary capillary wedge pressure (PCWP) of $\leq$ 18 mm Hg or no clinical evidence of elevated left atrial pressure.

B. **Etiology.** ARDS can be initiated by many different events and conditions, including shock, aspiration of fluid, disseminated intravascular coagulation (DIC), bacterial septicemia, trauma, blood transfusion, pancreatitis, smoke inhalation, and heroin overdose.

C. **Pathogenesis and pathophysiology**

    1. ARDS is precipitated by an insult to the capillary endothelium or alveolar epithelium that results in capillary congestion and interstitial edema, leading to disruption of capillary integrity and the extravasation of fluid, fibrin, red cells, and white cells into the lung interstitium, lymphatics, and, ultimately, the alveoli.

    2. The severe hypoxia in this condition is caused by extreme $\dot{V}/\dot{Q}$ imbalance and the shunting of blood in the fluid-filled areas of the lung.

    3. The lungs stiffen and become less compliant, resulting in difficulty with mechanical ventilation and subsequent high peak airway pressures.

D. **Clinical features and diagnosis.** Symptoms may develop immediately after the insult but usually are delayed 24–48 hours.

    1. Progressive tachypnea usually is the earliest sign, followed by dyspnea.

    2. Physical findings often are absent or limited to bronchial breath sounds and rales.

    3. Pulmonary function and blood gas studies show increased minute ventilation, decreased lung volumes, and acute respiratory alkalosis.

    4. Chest x-ray shows patchy, diffuse bilateral fluffy infiltrates.

    5. Cardiac output usually is increased somewhat, although terminally it may decrease and be accompanied by metabolic acidosis and tissue hypoxia.

E. **Therapy**

    1. **Oxygenation.** The ultimate goal of therapy is to provide adequate tissue oxygenation. Overall tissue oxygenation can be estimated from the mixed venous oxygen content ($C\bar{v}o_2$). In addition, concomitant measurement of cardiac output by thermodilution can aid in the correction of abnormal oxygen transport.

        a. Hypoxia can be corrected by maintaining the Pao_2 at approximately 60–80 mm Hg. This results in about a 90% oxygen saturation, which ensures that tissue oxygen needs are met as long as cardiac output and hemoglobin level are normal.

        b. **Mechanical ventilation** is required by most patients with ARDS.

            (1) **PEEP** commonly is used to increase lung volume (i.e., FRC), reduce intrapulmonary shunt, and improve $\dot{V}/\dot{Q}$ relationships. PEEP may cause barotrauma or a reduced cardiac output. In patients whose cardiac output is compromised, the Pao_2 increases but oxygen delivery to the tissues may decrease. Therefore, it is important to measure mixed venous Po_2 ($M\bar{v}o_2$) and cardiac output when using PEEP.

            (2) Other methods of ventilation, such as **inverse-ratio** and **high-frequency ventilation** may have use in certain situations.

    2. **Other measures.** The underlying disease process must be treated. In addition, patients who require more than 24–48 hours of mechanical ventilation should receive nutritional support, preferably through the gastrointestinal tract.

VII. COR PULMONALE

A. **Definition.** Cor pulmonale refers to disease of the right ventricle that results from pulmonary hypertension secondary to a pulmonary disease. It is characterized by right ventricular dilatation, hypertrophy, and, eventually, failure.

B. **Etiology.** Cor pulmonale can occur in any condition that causes pulmonary hypertension. **Acute cor pulmonale** is most often due to extensive pulmonary embolization. **Chronic cor pulmonale** occurs most often in patients with COPD; stress in these patients may induce acute but reversible exacerbations of the cor pulmonale.

C. Pathophysiology

1. **Mechanisms of pulmonary hypertension**
   a. **Hypoxia and acidosis.** The vasoconstrictive effect of hypoxia is a potent stimulus for the development of pulmonary hypertension. This mechanism may be augmented by acidosis, which also has a direct, although less dramatic, effect on the pulmonary vasculature. The most important aspect of hypoxic vasoconstriction is its potential to be reversed with increased concentrations of inspired oxygen.
   b. **Obliteration or obstruction of the pulmonary vascular bed.** A less common mechanism of pulmonary hypertension, obliteration or obstruction of the pulmonary vascular bed, is seen in recurrent pulmonary embolism, primary pulmonary hypertension (a rare disease of unknown cause), and pulmonary fibrosis. Substantial loss of the pulmonary vascular bed can also result from emphysema or lung surgery.

2. **Development of cor pulmonale**
   a. Although acute hypoxia elicits approximately the same pressor response, each bout of pulmonary hypertension predisposes the patient to progressively higher levels of residual hypertension after recovery.
   b. The resultant sustained pulmonary hypertension causes smooth muscle hypertrophy in the pulmonary arteries and then in the peripheral pulmonary vessels. The pulmonary vascular bed becomes more rigid and less reactive to changes in cardiac output.
   c. This, in turn, affects the performance of the right ventricle, causing right ventricular hypertrophy and right-sided heart failure (i.e., cor pulmonale).
   d. No reliable evidence supports the claim that cor pulmonale causes left ventricular failure.

D. **Clinical features and diagnosis**

1. Early in the course of the disease, patients may demonstrate pulmonary hypertension only in association with exercise.

2. The **physical findings** of peripheral edema, liver enlargement, and neck vein engorgement usually are associated with cor pulmonale but are nonspecific and do not contribute to the diagnosis except in advanced disease.

3. An **oxygen saturation** of less than 85% usually causes pulmonary arterial pressure to increase above 25 mm Hg. Acidosis and exercise cause further elevations.

4. **Roentgenographic findings,** such as widening of the pulmonary arteries, are insensitive and unreliable indicators of pulmonary arterial pressure.

5. **Electrocardiography** shows the appearance of flat or inverted T waves in the right ventricular precordial leads, right axis deviation of greater than 30° in the mean electrical axis of the QRS, transient S-T depression of leads II, III, and aVF, and transient right bundle branch block.

6. **Cardiac catheterization** provides definitive diagnosis but rarely is necessary.

E. **Therapy.** Prevention and treatment of cor pulmonale are focused on correction of hypoxia and acidosis, control of hypervolemia, and improvement of right ventricular failure.

1. **Supplemental oxygen.** The initial steps in the treatment of cor pulmonale are to administer supplemental oxygen and improve the patient's ventilatory status by treating the underlying lung disease. Because many patients are oxygen-sensitive, it is

imperative not to give high-flow oxygen but to give just enough to keep the saturation at approximately 90%.

2. **Diuresis.** Fluid retention is common and can compromise pulmonary gas exchange and heighten pulmonary vascular resistance. Improved oxygenation and salt restriction may control the cor pulmonale, but diuretics frequently are necessary.

3. **Phlebotomy** provides a short-term effect and may be useful when hematocrit is greater than 55%–60%.

4. **Digitalis** has no benefit unless there is left ventricular failure.

5. **Vasodilators** have been used, especially in cor pulmonale associated with obliterative vascular disease or fibrotic lung disease; however, the value of these agents is unknown.

VIII. PULMONARY EMBOLISM

A. **Definition.** In pulmonary embolism, a thrombus arises elsewhere in the body and migrates to the pulmonary vascular tree, where it causes obstruction. Nearly all pulmonary emboli derive from deep venous thrombosis (see Chapter 1 VIII A). Rarely (e.g., in sickle cell disease), pulmonary arterial thrombosis occurs as a primary event without discernible clots elsewhere.

B. **Incidence.** Acute pulmonary embolism is a major cause of morbidity and mortality in the United States. Fully 50% of cases of deep venous thrombosis are complicated by pulmonary embolism. Each year, as many as 650,000 individuals sustain pulmonary emboli, an estimated 150,000 of whom die as a result. (This mortality figure has not changed during the past 25 years.)

C. **Etiology**

1. **Site of thrombus formation.** Stasis in the **iliofemoral venous system** with subsequent **deep venous thrombosis** is the most common precursor of pulmonary embolism. Other common sites of thrombus formation include the **prostatic and pelvic veins.** Except in drug abusers, pulmonary emboli generally do not originate in the upper extremities.

2. **Predisposing factors.** Conditions that increase a patient's risk of venous thrombosis, and, therefore, pulmonary embolism, are discussed in Chapter 1 VIII A 2.

3. **Precipitating factors.** The factors that control the tethering of a thrombus to the wall of a vein and the dislodging of a thrombus into the circulation are not well understood. However, exercise and straining at defecation, with consequent changes in venous flow and pressure, are well-known precipitating events.

D. **Pathophysiology**

1. **Embolization.** When a thrombus breaks off from its site of origin, it is carried through the inferior vena cava and right ventricle to the pulmonary arteries, where it lodges. Pulmonary emboli may occur singly or multiply and vary in size from microscopic particles to large saddle emboli that completely block the major branches of the pulmonary artery.

2. **Hemodynamic consequences**
   a. Obstruction of the pulmonary arteries by the embolus increases resistance to blood flow through the pulmonary circuit and increases right ventricular afterload. When more than 50%–60% of the pulmonary perfusion is impeded, severe pulmonary hypertension, right ventricular strain, and cardiac failure ensue.
   b. The embolism may also cause intrapulmonary reflexes and the release of humoral substances (e.g., histamine, serotonin, prostaglandins), leading to vasocon-

striction throughout the lungs. This vasoconstrictive effect further increases pulmonary vascular resistance and the work of the right ventricle.

c. Fewer than 10% of cases of pulmonary embolism progress to **pulmonary infarction** because the lung parenchyma has three sources of oxygen (i.e., the airways, the bronchial circulation, and the pulmonary circulation).

d. Recurrent pulmonary emboli progressively occlude the pulmonary vascular bed and lead to chronic progressive pulmonary hypertension and, ultimately, **cor pulmonale.**

3. Pulmonary consequences

a. The primary pulmonary consequence of an embolism is $\dot{V}/\dot{Q}$ **mismatch.**

   (1) "Wasted" ventilation ("dead space") occurs in the lung segments where the vascular supply is obstructed and perfusion cannot occur.

   (2) Conversely, overperfusion and diminished vascular resistance in other lung segments cause profound right-to-left intrapulmonary shunting, with inadequate oxygenation of a large portion of perfused blood.

b. Other pulmonary responses include congestive atelectasis of the ischemic segment of the lung, reflex bronchiolar and vascular constriction, and the loss or malfunction of alveolar surfactant.

E. Clinical features and diagnosis

1. Symptoms. The patient may complain of dyspnea at rest and chest pain resembling that of myocardial infarction. Syncope may occur as cardiac output declines. Pulmonary infarction may cause pleuritic pain and hemoptysis.

2. Physical examination

a. Nearly all patients with pulmonary embolism have tachypnea and tachycardia, and many have a low-grade fever.

b. In **massive pulmonary embolism,** the severe physiologic consequences are manifested as cyanosis, peripheral venous engorgement, and hepatic congestion; there may be evidence of cor pulmonale. In **submassive pulmonary embolism,** the less profound hemodynamic changes may be transient, so that hypotension, tachycardia, and hypoxia may not be observed at the time of initial examination.

c. Auscultation reveals percussion dullness and decreased breath sounds over the involved base; findings are usually normal over the remaining lung segments. Occasionally, a pleural friction rub or wheezing is heard.

d. Evidence of deep venous thrombosis is seen in 50% of patients.

3. Chest x-ray. Results are normal in most patients. A few show plate-like atelectasis, a unilaterally high diaphragm, and a small pleural effusion. Occasional findings include a bulging pulmonary artery and a large oligemic lung segment. A wedge-shaped, pleural-based density is typical of a pulmonary infarction.

4. Electrocardiography. The electrocardiogram (ECG) usually is not specific but may help to differentiate between myocardial infarction and pulmonary embolism.

a. The most common finding is sinus tachycardia with or without premature atrial and ventricular contractions. The mean P axis commonly shifts to the right when right-sided pulmonary obstruction is severe and the S wave in lead I and the Q wave in lead III are abnormal.

b. Right ventricular strain may produce intermittent right bundle branch block, P pulmonale (i.e., "peaked" P waves), and marked clockwise rotation of the ECG.

5. Blood gas analysis

a. Hypoxia (indicated by a decrease in P_{O_2}), hyperventilation (indicated by a decrease in P_{CO_2}), and a mild acute respiratory alkalosis (indicated by a low P_{CO_2} and slightly elevated pH) are the classic changes seen in patients with pulmonary embolism. However, they are not specific for pulmonary embolism and pulmonary embolism may occur without these changes.

b. A more sensitive indicator of abnormal gas exchange is the A-a D_{O_2}; a normal gradient essentially rules out pulmonary embolism.

6. **Pulmonary radioisotope scanning**
   a. In **perfusion scanning,** the patient's blood is labeled with a radioactive tracer. Poorly perfused areas of the lung show up as relatively inactive areas on the scan. However, even though normal results virtually exclude the diagnosis, the test is not specific for pulmonary embolism, because pneumonia and COPD can also produce scanning abnormalities.
   b. In **xenon ventilation scanning,** the patient inhales the radioactive tracer. This procedure often is performed in conjunction with perfusion scanning to increase the specificity of the test. Finding well-ventilated but poorly perfused areas suggests pulmonary embolism; finding areas with both perfusion and ventilation defects suggests parenchymal lung disease rather than pulmonary embolism.
   c. Scanning results must be correlated with the patient's clinical picture and with the chest x-ray results. Diagnostic accuracy may be increased by obtaining ventilation and perfusion scans in four positions and then comparing scanning results with concurrent chest x-rays.

7. **Pulmonary angiography** is the standard test for the diagnosis of pulmonary embolism. It is unequivocally diagnostic if emboli are visualized. Although invasive, this test should be performed when ventilation and perfusion scans are equivocal and also when the risks from long-term anticoagulation therapy are greater than usual.

8. When the diagnosis of pulmonary embolism remains in question despite many diagnostic studies, **corroborative evidence** of venous disease in the lower extremities should be sought.
   a. Noninvasive methods include impedance plethysmography, leg and thigh scanning with radioiodinated fibrinogen, and Doppler ultrasonography. However, these techniques can produce false-positive results, and they cannot be used to evaluate pelvic veins.
   b. Contrast venography is helpful in diagnosing occlusion of the pelvic, thigh, and leg veins. This invasive technique is not without morbidity, however; it has been associated with phlebitis, hypersensitivity reactions, and local pain.

F. **Therapy**

1. **Anticoagulants**
   a. Unless contraindicated, the drug of choice for documented or suspected pulmonary embolism is **heparin,** given in doses that maintain the partial thromboplastin time (PTT) at 2 to 2 $\frac{1}{2}$ times the normal value. it is preferably given by continuous intravenous administration.
   b. After anticoagulation with heparin has been achieved for a few days, therapy is changed to **warfarin,** given orally, in doses that maintain the prothrombin time (PT) at 2 to 2 $\frac{1}{2}$ times the normal value or at international normalization ratio (INR) of 2.5–3.0. The oral anticoagulant is continued for 3–6 months. **Oxygen** is given routinely to correct hypoxia, and **bed rest** ordinarily is prescribed until the dyspnea and pain resolve, after which patients can ambulate while remaining on anticoagulant therapy.

2. **Thrombolytic agents.** Fibrinolytic agents are given when rapid lysis of clots is important.
   a. Because thrombolytic agents increase the risk of hemorrhage, they are reserved for use when occlusion has produced right-sided heart failure and hemodynamic instability.
   b. Thrombolytic agents appear to provide long-term physiologic improvement in the pulmonary vascular bed. The long- and short-term mortality rates are unchanged, however.

3. **Surgery**
   a. Inferior vena caval ligation, clipping, and plication and, more recently, percutaneous "umbrella" insertion, are surgical remedies with modest morbidity that preclude embolic recurrence for a short time.

    (1) Collateral venous channels in the pelvis or lower abdomen may develop in patients with chronic vena caval obstruction and may find routes around the obstruction to the pulmonary artery, eventually negating the effectiveness of the surgical procedure.

    (2) Vena caval occlusion should therefore be reserved for patients in whom embolism recurs, despite adequate anticoagulation therapy, and for patients in whom anticoagulants are contraindicated (e.g., patients with active bleeding).

  b. Embolectomy remains an alternative treatment for patients who cannot maintain effective cardiac output. Occasionally, embolectomy is lifesaving, but the overall survival rate is approximately 10%.

4. Prophylactic minidose heparin therapy. Giving small doses of heparin prophylactically has been helpful in preventing pulmonary embolism in certain high-risk patients, with little risk of hemorrhage.

  a. Minidose heparin prophylaxis is particularly applicable for older patients who undergo lower abdominal or pelvic surgery and who are at bed rest postoperatively. It also is helpful for obese surgical patients. The customary regimen is to give subcutaneous heparin 2 hours before surgery and to continue it after surgery until the patient is ambulatory.

  b. It also is recommended for patients at prolonged bed rest because of stroke, myocardial infarction, cardiac failure, or cancer.

  c. Minidose heparin has not been shown to be effective for major orthopedic, prostatic, ocular, or neurosurgical procedures.

IX. DISEASES OF THE PLEURA

A. Pleural effusion

1. Definition. A pleural effusion is an abnormal accumulation of fluid in the pleural space.

2. Etiology and pathogenesis

  a. In health, the pleural cavity contains a small volume of lubricating serous fluid, formed primarily by transudation from the parietal pleura and absorbed primarily by the capillaries and lymphatics.

  b. The balance between formation and removal of this fluid may be compromised by any disorder that increases the pulmonary or systemic venous pressure, lowers the plasma oncotic pressure, increases capillary permeability, or obstructs the lymphatic circulation.

  c. A pleural effusion may be a transudate or an exudate (Table 2-3).

    (1) Transudates are caused by elevated venous pressure or by decreased plasma oncotic pressure; the primary pathologic process does not directly involve the pulmonary surface.

    (2) Exudates are caused by increased permeability of the pleural surface (due to inflammation, trauma, or disease) or by obstruction of the lymphatics.

  d. A pleural effusion may have a noninflammatory or an inflammatory cause.

    (1) Noninflammatory pleural effusions may occur in any condition that causes ascites, obstruction of the venous or lymphatic outflow from the thorax, isolated left- or right-sided congestive heart failure, or a severe reduction in the plasma protein concentration.

    (2) Inflammatory pleural effusions result from inflammation of structures adjacent to the pleural surface.

      (a) The site of inflammation usually is just beneath the visceral pleura within the lung but occasionally is within the mediastinum, diaphragm, or chest wall. Secondary inflammation of larger areas of the pleural surface may result in rapid outpouring of exudate.

TABLE 2-3. Causes of Pleural Effusions

Causes of exudates
  Malignancy (e.g., bronchogenic carcinoma, lymphoma, metastic tumor)
  Inflammatory processes
    Infections (e.g., tuberculosis, pneumonia)
    Pulmonary embolic disease
    Collagen vascular disease (e.g., rheumatoid arthritis)
    Subdiaphragmatic process
    Asbestosis
    Pancreatitis
    Hypothyroidism
  Trauma
Causes of transudates
  Decreased plasma oncotic pressure
  Nephrotic syndrome
  Cirrhosis
  Increased hydrostatic pressure
    Congestive heart failure

        (b) Removal of the fluid by the normal clearing mechanisms may be considerably retarded by inflammatory obstruction of the lymphatics that drain the thorax.

3. **Clinical features and diagnosis**
   a. **Symptoms** result from inflammation of the parietal pleura and compression of the lung.
      (1) Pleuritic pain occurs most commonly with inflammatory effusions and often is accompanied by a friction rub.
          (a) The pain commonly is a sharp, stabbing sensation that is minimal during quiet respiration but intensifies abruptly during full inflation of the lungs.
          (b) Pleuritic pain must be differentiated from the pain of rib fracture, costochondritis, compression of intercostal nerve roots, herpes zoster, acute bronchitis, and various cardiovascular and esophageal conditions.
      (2) Dyspnea can occur if the accumulation of pleural fluid compresses the lung and interferes with the movement of the diaphragm.
   b. **Physical signs.** Fluid usually accumulates first at the base of the lung where the earliest physical signs are noted.
      (1) Auscultation usually reveals a dull to flat percussion and reduced or absent breath sounds over the area of the effusion. An area of **bronchial breathing** sometimes is heard over the adjacent compressed lung and may be accompanied by an altered voice quality or **egophony.**
      (2) The mediastinum usually shifts away from the side of a large effusion unless the mediastinum has become fixed in position by a tumor or unless a portion of the lung on the affected side has become completely atelectatic.
   c. **Radiographic appearance**
      (1) Chest x-ray. The earliest visible signs of effusion on a plain-film radiographs are blunting of the costophrenic angle and blurring of the posterior diaphragm in the lateral view. Posterior–anterior films may show no abnormality if there is less than 300 ml of pleural fluid. A lateral decubitus film may help to differentiate free fluid from previous inflammatory adhesions.
      (2) Diagnostic ultrasound may help to localize the effusion more accurately when complete removal by thoracentesis is difficult.
   d. **Specialized diagnostic procedures**
      (1) Unless a cause has been established, the presence of fluid in the pleural cavity is an indication for **thoracentesis.**

        (a) The fluid should be removed, the gross appearance noted, and specimens sent to the laboratory for examination.

        (b) Routine laboratory procedures include measuring the total protein and lactate dehydrogenase (LDH) content and examining the spun specimen for cells. Bacteriologic and cytologic examinations and analysis for glucose, amylase, and pH provide further information.

    (2) When an inflammatory effusion is suspected or known to be present, **needle biopsy** may be performed at the time of initial thoracentesis.

    (3) When ordinary measures fail to establish a definitive diagnosis and needle biopsy of the pleura is negative, **thoracotomy** or the newer technique of **video-assisted thoracoscopy (VATS)** with exploration of the lung and biopsy of the involved areas of the pleural surface may be essential for accurate diagnosis.

  4. Differential diagnosis. Laboratory data can help in determining the cause of a pleural effusion.

    a. It is useful to establish whether the fluid is an exudate or a transudate (see Table 2-3). The following laboratory data indicate the presence of an **exudate:**

      (1) A protein content of more than 3 g/dl

      (2) A high LDH content

      (3) A pleural fluid–serum LDH ratio of greater than 0.6

      (4) A pleural fluid–serum protein ratio of greater than 0.5

    b. The presence of **gross blood** in the pleural fluid is most common when the effusion is due to tumor, trauma, or pulmonary infarction.

    c. The pleural fluid–serum **glucose** ratio is rarely low when the effusion is caused by tuberculosis or tumor but usually is very low in effusions that are due to rheumatoid arthritis.

    d. The pleural fluid **amylase** level frequently is elevated when the effusion is due to pancreatic disease or rupture of the esophagus, and occasionally is elevated moderately in malignant effusions.

    e. The pH of pleural fluid usually is 7.3 or greater; lower values occasionally are seen in tuberculosis and malignant effusions. A pH of less than 7.2 in a parapneumonic effusion suggests an empyema.

  5. Therapy

    a. Treatment must be directed at the disease causing the effusion. Appropriate therapy may call for chest tube placement, antibiotics, antituberculous therapy, repeated thoracentesis, or chemical pleurodesis to eliminate the pleural space.

    b. Dyspnea may be relieved by a thoracentesis, but this procedure carries the risk of pneumothorax (from pleural puncture) or cardiovascular collapse (from removing too much fluid too quickly).

B. **Empyema**

  1. Definition and clinical features. An empyema is an accumulation of pus in the pleural space; it is an occasional complication of both bacterial pneumonia and lung abscess. The fluid usually is thick and has the appearance of frank pus. As previously stated, pleural fluid with a pH of less than 7.2 strongly suggests an empyema.

  2. Therapy. An empyema almost always requires chest tube drainage as well as antibiotic therapy. If the fluid itself is noninfected, with a relatively low white blood cell (WBC) count and a pH of more than 7.2, the empyema may resolve with systemic antimicrobial therapy. However, after several days without adequate drainage, most empyemas become loculated, so that tube drainage is not effective and rib resection is necessary to allow open drainage.

C. **Pneumothorax**

  1. Definition. Pneumothorax is an accumulation of air or gas in the pleural space. If the accumulation is large enough, the underlying lung parenchyma may become collapsed and functionless.

2. Etiology

a. Pneumothorax is a common medical problem, frequently caused by **trauma. Spontaneous pneumothorax** occurs with the rupture of bullae in an upper lobe. It occurs more frequently in men than in women, and especially in men 20–40 years of age.

b. Pneumothorax also may occur **secondary** to lung involvement in **many diseases,** such as tuberculosis, trauma, malignancy, emphysema, histiocytosis X, interstitial pneumonitis and fibrosis, and pulmonary infarction.

3. Clinical features and diagnosis

a. The major **symptoms** of pneumothorax are **pain** and **dyspnea.** The pain may be either sharp and severe or mild and dull.

b. Physical examination reveals hyperresonance and decreased breath sounds over the involved side.

c. Chest x-rays, if obtained during expiration, may help to demonstrate small pneumothoracic areas, because this technique increases the contrast between the lung and the pleural space.

4. Therapy

a. A small spontaneous pneumothorax often resolves by itself. A more severe or a secondary pneumothorax calls for reexpansion of the lung via placement of an intercostal chest tube and application of appropriate negative pressure. The treatment is continued for 24–48 hours after the lung is reexpanded, so that the pleural space will seal and that pleural adhesions will prevent recurrence.

b. Spontaneous pneumothorax has a tendency to recur, and surgical treatment should be considered after three or more occurrences on a given side. Surgery involves an open thoracotomy and abrasion of the pleural surfaces, which produces symphysis of the parietal and visceral pleurae.

5. Complications. Although pneumothorax is a relatively benign condition, serious complications can result.

a. Bilateral simultaneous pneumothorax is rare but can cause prompt death.

b. Pneumothorax may be accompanied by hemorrhage into the pleural space, which results in **hemopneumothorax.**

c. Tension pneumothorax is a buildup of positive pressure within the pleural space, which rapidly produces severe respiratory embarrassment. Patients undergoing positive-pressure mechanical ventilation are particularly at risk.

(1) Tension pneumothorax presumably results from a ball-valve mechanism at the site of the air leak, which allows air to enter but not leave the pleural space.

(2) This leads to progressive collapse of the lung, a contralateral shift of the mediastinal structures, and reduced blood flow to the right side of the heart, impairing cardiovascular function as well as lung function. Prompt decompression of the involved pleural space is indicated.

D. **Chylothorax.** When the thoracic duct is lacerated or obstructed by trauma or tumor, lymph may accumulate in the pleural space. This condition, termed chylothorax, is identified by a murky appearance of the fluid, demonstration of fat droplets on staining with Sudan III, and a total neutral fat content of more than 0.5 g/dl.

E. **Primary pleural neoplasia**

1. Localized fibrous mesothelioma. This uncommon tumor arises from the pleural surface and most commonly is attached to the visceral pleura.

a. Symptoms

(1) The lesion may cause chest discomfort and dyspnea if it becomes very large; however, most tumors are discovered before these symptoms develop.

(2) The syndrome of **hypertrophic pulmonary osteoarthropathy,** which is associated with arthralgia of the hands, ankles, wrists, and knees and with clubbing of the fingers, may occur secondary to pleural-based tumors.

    b. Diagnosis. Chest x-ray reveals a mass lesion; a pleural effusion occasionally is present.

    c. Therapy is surgical resection, which also relieves the symptoms of the hypertrophic pulmonary osteoarthropathy.

    d. Prognosis. Most of these tumors are benign, and patients have an excellent prognosis. A few of these tumors are malignant, but with favorable courses.

2. Diffuse malignant mesothelioma

    a. Incidence. This malignant tumor occurs over a wide age range, with the average age at onset being 55 years. The incidence is increased in workers exposed to asbestos; generally, the malignancy develops 20 or more years after exposure.

    b. Symptoms and diagnosis. Chest pain and dyspnea are the predominant symptoms. The chest x-ray may reveal pleural thickening, pleural effusion, or both. The diagnosis is difficult to establish by cytologic examination; open pleural biopsy often is necessary.

    c. Therapy involves radiotherapy or chemotherapy; results are uniformly dismal.

X. CHEST WALL DISORDERS

A. **Etiology.** Chest wall disorders can be either mechanical or neuromuscular in origin. They may cause respiratory dysfunction and, in severe cases, respiratory failure.

1. Mechanical disorders affecting the chest wall include scoliosis, obesity-associated hypoventilation, fibrothorax, thoracoplasty, ankylosing spondylitis, and chest wall trauma.

2. Neuromuscular diseases affecting the chest wall are polyneuropathies, motor system diseases, muscular dystrophies, spinal cord injuries, multiple sclerosis, and myasthenia gravis.

B. **Kyphoscoliosis,** the most common and best understood chest wall disease, is used in this discussion as a prototype for the pathophysiology, course, and management of all chest wall disorders.

1. Definition. Kyphoscoliosis is a common skeletal abnormality characterized by posterior curvature (**kyphosis**) and lateral curvature (**scoliosis**) of the spine. These processes, alone or in combination, decrease the volume and mobility of the lung and chest wall.

2. Incidence. Kyphoscoliosis affects 1% of the United States population and occurs predominantly in females. The deformity is clinically significant in 2.3% of affected individuals.

3. Etiology is not clear in 80% of cases. A major known cause is childhood poliomyelitis. Congenital abnormalities with or without bone defects are uncommon.

4. Pathophysiology

    a. Lung volume is reduced in kyphoscoliosis because the chest wall is distorted. The distortion also causes stiffness of the chest wall, increasing the work of breathing and causing decreased total respiratory compliance and reduction of FRC. The pressure–volume compliance curve of the lung is nearly normal, and forced expiratory flow is preserved relative to lung volume.

    b. Gas exchange is impaired in marked kyphoscoliosis: alveolar hypoventilation occurs and Pco_2 rises. The A-a Do_2 is mildly widened because of $\dot{V}/\dot{Q}$ inequality, which results from the compressive effect of atelectasis and inadequate periodic hyperinflation.

    c. Pulmonary hypertension eventually is present at rest as well as during exercise in patients with moderate chest wall deformity and no clinical signs of cardiac dysfunction.

5. **Clinical features and diagnosis**
   a. **Symptoms**
      (1) **Exertional dyspnea** is the outstanding respiratory symptom. The onset and severity of dyspnea correlate with the degree of the spinal angulation, as measured on the chest film. Hypoventilation supervenes in those patients whose deformity is severe.
      (2) Bronchitic symptoms are unusual unless patients have chronic bronchitis or atelectasis.
      (3) **Sequelae of prolonged arterial hypoxia,** including pulmonary hypertension, right ventricular dysfunction, and cor pulmonale, may develop as late manifestations.
   b. **Chest x-ray.** Ribs on the convex portion of the spine are widely spaced and rotated posteriorly, causing a characteristic hump. Ribs on the concave aspect are crowded and displaced anteriorly and encroach on the apex of the secondary curve. The degree of kyphoscoliosis is determined by measuring the angle formed by converging line segments drawn on the upper and lower limbs of the primary spinal curves.

6. **Therapy**
   a. Early identification of kyphoscoliosis in adolescence is the key to prevention of symptomatic disease. **Corrective intervention** should be considered when the angulation is greater than 40°. There are two forms of intervention.
      (1) **Mechanical.** A Milwaukee brace can be applied externally during the early stages of the disease.
      (2) **Surgical.** The Harrington procedure, using metal rods and focal spinal fusion, can be performed, after which the patient wears a plaster of Paris jacket cast for several months. Surgery does not improve the maximal breathing capacity but may improve arterial oxygen and oxygen desaturation. At best, surgery appears to preserve whatever pulmonary function is present at the time of intervention.
   b. Periodic hyperinflation with positive- or negative-pressure devices appears to increase lung compliance and P_{O_2} in outpatients.

7. **Complications.** Respiratory failure and cor pulmonale, the major complications, result from respiratory infections or injudicious use of sedatives, or both.

C. **Chest trauma**

1. **Blunt trauma.** Blunt chest trauma causes injury either by direct application of sudden force to the chest wall and indirect transmission of these forces to the intrathoracic structures or by secondary visceral destruction by chest wall structures.
   a. Injury of extrapulmonary organs often accompanies blunt chest trauma. Disruption of the chest wall may cause rib fractures, hemothorax, pneumothorax, and flail chest. Inertial injury may cause rupture of the bronchial, diaphragmatic, or great blood vessels.
   b. **Flail chest** most commonly results from motor vehicle injury or overzealous cardiac resuscitation. The chest wall, or at least one hemithorax, is rendered unstable by multiple fractures of the ribs, sternum, or costochondral joints.
      (1) The injured portion moves **paradoxically,** that is, inward on inspiration as the intrapleural pressure becomes subatmospheric and outward on expiration as the intrapleural pressure increases toward atmospheric.
      (2) Respiratory failure is treated with volume-cycled mechanical ventilation, pain control, and oxygen supplementation.

2. **Penetrating trauma** is characterized by puncture or laceration of the chest wall and intrathoracic fistulae. Vehicular accidents and knife and missile wounds are the usual causes. Exploratory thoracotomies are indicated for persistent hemothorax and sucking chest wounds and to determine the likelihood of mediastinal, diaphragmatic, or cardiac disruption.

XI. MEDIASTINAL DISEASES

A. **Mediastinal masses.** The mediastinum is divided into three parts: **superior, anterior and middle,** and **posterior.** Mediastinal masses can occur at any age and are characteristic of the mediastinal compartment in which they occur. The lateral chest x-ray often is the most important initial diagnostic measure.

1. **Masses in the superior mediastinum**
   a. **Thymomas** are the most common superior mediastinal masses. They frequently **present** as cough, chest pain, and superior vena caval obstruction. Myasthenia gravis occurs in approximately one third of patients with a thymoma. Red blood cell aplasia and hypogammaglobulinemia are other recognized but rare associations. Surgical excision is recommended.
   b. **Hodgkin's disease** and **non-Hodgkin's lymphomas** rarely present as masses in the superior mediastinum.
   c. **Intrathoracic goiters** may occur, particularly in middle-aged women. They usually are asymptomatic but may cause stridor, hoarseness, or dysphagia.

2. **Masses in the anterior and middle mediastinum**
   a. **Dermoid** cysts appear as dense, homogeneous lobular shadows in the anterior mediastinum, often with calcifications in the walls. Teeth may be recognized within the tumor. Dermoid cysts usually are asymptomatic unless infection or malignant change develops.
   b. **Pleuropericardial cysts** occur in the middle mediastinum at the right cardiophrenic angle, characteristically appearing as smooth, sharply demarcated masses of uniform density.
   c. **Bronchogenic cysts** and **reduplication of the esophagus** are rare causes of middle mediastinal masses.

3. **Masses in the posterior mediastinum. Neurogenic tumors** are the most common mediastinal tumors and characteristically occur in the posterior mediastinum along the paravertebral border. These tumors often are asymptomatic in the adult but may cause chest pain with stridor, breathlessness, cough, and tracheal compression. Horner's syndrome and spinal cord compression also may occur.
   a. Generalized neurofibromatosis occurs in approximately 25% of patients with a primary posterior mediastinal **neurofibroma.**
   b. Catecholamine secretion may be associated with the rare **pheochromocytoma** in the posterior mediastinum and with other neurogenic tumors.

B. **Mediastinitis**

1. **Acute mediastinitis** is a severe, life-threatening illness that most often follows rupture of the esophagus. It may also follow vomiting, dental work, endoscopy, or other trauma and is characterized by fever, chest pain, and variable mediastinal enlargement. The disease progresses rapidly and requires emergency medical and surgical treatment.

2. **Chronic mediastinitis and mediastinal fibrosis.** *Histoplasma* or, rarely, other fungi or mycobacteria, can produce a chronic granulomatous process in the mediastinum, often with extensive scar tissue that contracts to cause narrowing of the trachea, bronchi, vena cava, pulmonary arteries, and pulmonary veins. Mediastinitis that occurs without any known cause is referred to as **idiopathic mediastinal fibrosis.**

C. **Pneumomediastinum** is the presence of air in the mediastinum. Air is presumed to leak from alveoli and to dissect along bronchi to the hilum, from which it may enter the mediastinum. If pressure builds in the mediastinum, air may expand into the neck tissues, producing subcutaneous emphysema. However, if the mediastinal air is confined, the increasing pressure may interfere with circulation. When this occurs, tracheostomy usually is adequate therapy. Intervention is unnecessary in patients without circulatory problems.

XII. DIFFUSE INTERSTITIAL LUNG DISEASE

A. **Definition.** Diffuse interstitial lung disease is a broad term for a group of related disorders all characterized by diffuse inflammatory alveolar infiltration. Regardless of their various causes, these entities share certain clinical, roentgenographic, pathologic, and physiologic characteristics. All begin acutely and progress to a chronic condition; that is, a potentially reversible interstitial pneumonitis progresses to diffuse pulmonary fibrosis.

B. **Etiology**

1. In approximately 50% of cases, interstitial lung disease occurs spontaneously. The terminology for these diseases is varied. In North America, the term **idiopathic pulmonary fibrosis** is favored, whereas, in Great Britain, **cryptogenic fibrosing alveolitis** is preferred.

2. The remaining cases are associated with many known or suspected causes (Table 2-4). Environmental or occupational exposure to a variety of substances is well

TABLE 2-4. Causes of Diffuse Pulmonary Infiltration

Inhaled substances
    Gases (cadmium, mercury)
    Mineral dusts (silica, asbestos)
    Antigens (bacteria, molds, animal protein)
    Aspirated fluid or foreign body
Drug therapy
    Busulfan
    Bleomycin
    Nitrofurantoin
    Gold
    Cyclophosphamide
    Methotrexate
Radiation therapy
Infection
    Recurrent bacterial pneumonia
    Tuberculosis
    Viral infections
Neoplasia
    Bronchoalveolar carcinoma
    Leukemia
    Lymphoma
    Lymphangitic spread
Metabolic disease
    Uremia
Diseases of unknown etiology
    Sarcoidosis
    Collagen vascular (connective tissue) disease
    Goodpasture's syndrome
    Amyloidosis
    Idiopathic pulmonary hemosiderosis
    Pulmonary alveolar proteinosis
    Bronchiolitis obliterans organizing pneumonia

known to induce interstitial pulmonary fibrosis (see XIII); these substances may act as inciting allergens or directly toxic agents. In other cases, interstitial lung disease is associated with connective tissue disease, sarcoidosis, or chronic hypersensitivity pneumonitis.

C. **Pathophysiology and histology**

1. **Stages.** The pathologic changes in these disorders have a highly variable time course, depending on the degree of exposure and on the type of injurious agent. The clinical course may run from a few weeks to many years.
   a. **Acute stage.** The earliest stage of diffuse interstitial lung disease is characterized by acute damage to capillary and alveolar epithelial cells, leading to interstitial and intra-alveolar edema and subsequent formation of hyaline membranes. This stage may either resolve completely or progress to the stage of acute interstitial pneumonia.
   b. **Chronic stage.** In many patients, the disease progresses to a chronic stage, in which extensive deposition or alteration of collagen results in widespread fibrosis. In addition, this stage is marked by smooth muscle hypertrophy and profound disruption of the alveolar spaces, which are lined with atypical cuboidal cells.
   c. **End stage.** The disease eventually progresses until the lung becomes "honeycombed." In this stage, the entire alveolar and capillary network is replaced with fibrous tissue and dilated spaces, the capillary bed is decreased, and the lung has no remaining gas exchange function.

2. **Histologic classification**
   a. Several names have been used in an attempt to describe the various pulmonary changes. A common histologic classification consists of the following five categories:
      (1) Usual interstitial pneumonitis (UIP)
      (2) Desquamative interstitial pneumonitis (DIP)
      (3) Lymphocytic interstitial pneumonitis (LIP)
      (4) Giant cell interstitial pneumonitis (GIP)
      (5) Bronchiolitis obliterans with organizing pneumonia (BOOP)
   b. Many authorities feel that these classifications are somewhat artificial and may represent various stages or different pathways in the progression from acute to end-stage pulmonary fibrosis.
   c. The histologic pattern observed at biopsy depends largely on the stage of the disease at which the specimen is obtained. In addition, because this is a heterogeneous pathologic process, different areas within a given specimen may show varied stages of anatomic alteration.

3. **Effects on pulmonary function**
   a. In the early stage of disease, hypoxia and an increase in the A-a Do_2 occur with exercise. As the disease progresses, resting hypoxia develops. The abnormalities of gas exchange are almost certainly the result of $\dot{V}/\dot{Q}$ abnormalities. Although DL_{CO} usually is decreased as the disease progresses, this becomes significant in causing hypoxia only during exercise, not at rest.
   b. The ventilatory pattern becomes restrictive late in the disease and is characterized by a decrease in all subdivisions of lung volume. Lung compliance is decreased, shifting the pressure–volume compliance curve downward and to the right. Expiratory flow rates (and hence the FEV_1/FVC ratio) usually are well preserved.
   c. The abnormalities in airway function tests that are seen in a number of patients with pulmonary fibrosis indicate that the peripheral airways are significantly involved in this pathologic process.

D. **Clinical features**

1. **Symptoms** of infiltrative lung disease seen most frequently are dyspnea on exertion and nonproductive cough. Increased fatigability, fever, and weight loss also are common.

2. **Physical findings** include tachypnea, digital clubbing, and late inspiratory dry crackle. If the disease is severe, cyanosis and evidence of right ventricular failure also may be present.

E. **Diagnosis.** The clinical, roentgenographic, and physiologic findings strongly suggest the diagnosis of diffuse infiltrative lung disease. Definitive diagnosis requires tissue confirmation, preferably by open-lung biopsy or VATS.

1. **Laboratory findings,** including pulmonary function studies (see XII C 3), usually are nonspecific. Tests for antinuclear antibodies (ANAs), rheumatoid factor, and immunoglobulins may be positive.

2. **Roentgenographic findings. Chest x-ray** usually reveals a diffuse reticulonodular pattern throughout both lung fields that is often more pronounced at the lung bases. In some cases, however, clinical evidence of disease may exist without roentgenographic confirmation.

3. **Open-lung biopsy** is useful in determining the stage of the disease, the appropriate therapy, and the probable prognosis. Whether the disease will respond to therapy appears to correlate well with pathologic evidence of fibrosis. Specimens showing active cellular infiltrates and minimal fibrosis suggest a much better prognosis than those showing extensive fibrosis.

4. Because the histologic changes are heterogeneous, **transbronchial lung biopsy** is of limited usefulness unless there is clear-cut evidence of sarcoid granuloma, infection, or carcinoma.

5. **Bronchoalveolar lavage,** with analysis of the cellular elements retrieved, is a diagnostic procedure that has been used experimentally. It indicates that infiltrative lung disease is associated with an increased number of polymorphonuclear leukocytes, whereas hypersensitivity pneumonitis is associated with an increased number of lymphocytes. It is too nonspecific to be used diagnostically.

F. **Therapy**

1. **Corticosteroids** have been the mainstay of therapy and are clearly indicated when open-lung biopsy reveals an active cellular process without extensive fibrosis. Large doses (e.g., prednisone 1 mg/kg/day) may be used initially, and physiologic and radiographic parameters should be monitored closely. If there is improvement after 6 weeks, the dosage should be tapered gradually, with frequent monitoring to detect physiologic relapse.

2. If no improvement occurs with steroids alone, **immunosuppressive agents** may be advisable, either given alone or in combination with steroids. Azathioprine is the most widely used; cyclophosphamide and chlorambucil also have been used.

G. **Prognosis.** Interstitial lung disease has a variable course.

1. Some cases resolve or arrest spontaneously or after removal of a known causative agent (e.g., a drug or environmental factor).

2. However, progressive interstitial lung disease can be an insidious, devastating disease with considerable morbidity and mortality. The average length of survival after diagnosis is 4–5 years.

XIII. **OCCUPATIONAL LUNG DISEASES**

A. **Introduction.** The respiratory system has continuous, active, contact with the environment. Many respiratory illnesses are caused by inhalation of impure air. To produce lung disease, an injurious inhalant must:

1. Exist in a size and form that is capable of reaching the lower respiratory tract
2. Be deposited on or absorbed into bronchial or alveolar surfaces
3. Remain in the respiratory tract for a sufficient time to produce injury

B. **Pulmonary responses to mineral dusts**

1. **Asbestos-related disease.** Asbestos is the term applied to several naturally occurring fibrous silicates, whose fibers may be long, curled, and flexible, or straight and brittle. Asbestos fibers may cause several distinct types of lesions.

   a. **Asbestosis.** This is a diffuse interstitial cellular and fibrotic reaction of the lung to inhaled asbestos fibers. Affected patients complain of breathlessness, and physical signs include digital clubbing and basilar rales. The chest film shows small lungs containing hazy infiltrates composed of small irregular or linear opacities; lower lung zones are more heavily affected. A restrictive ventilatory impairment and a reduced $D_{L_{CO}}$ are the expected abnormalities.

   b. **Nonneoplastic pleural disorders.** Asbestos may cause pleurisy with effusion, pleural plaques, and diffuse pleural thickening.

   c. **Cancer.** Many years after exposure (latency period), cancer can develop in persons exposed to asbestos at sufficient concentrations.

      (1) **Bronchogenic carcinoma** is a recognized consequence of asbestos exposure, especially in individuals who smoke.

      (2) **Malignant pleural mesotheliomas** (see IX E 2) are rare tumors. They are usually asbestos-related but are not associated with smoking.

2. **Silica-related disease.** Free silica and silicates are abundant components of the earth's crust. To be injurious to the lungs, these particles must exist as respirable aerosols.

   a. **Silicosis** is a diffuse fibrotic reaction of the lungs to inhalation of free crystalline silica (sand, quartz). Inhaled silica particles are ingested by alveolar macrophages, which soon rupture, releasing cytotoxic enzymes along with the engulfed silica particles. The silica is reingested by other macrophages and the cycle continues, stimulating a local fibrotic reaction. The final result is the formation of the relatively acellular **fibrous silicotic nodule** that characterizes this disease.

      (1) **Simple silicosis.** In this stage, the chest x-ray shows numerous small, rounded opacities (isolated nodules) scattered throughout the lungs. Simple silicosis usually is not associated with ventilatory impairment.

      (2) Continued silica exposure causes a progression from simple to complicated silicosis. This progression also may occur because of mycobacterial or mycotic infections.

      (3) **Complicated silicosis.** If the fibrosis continues, isolated nodules may coalesce to form larger masses of fibrotic tissue that distort the lungs. Complicated silicosis can lead to progressive massive fibrosis (PMF) and often produces a mixture of restrictive and obstructive ventilatory impairment.

   b. **Nonfibrotic effects.** Silicates such as talc, kaolin, fuller's earth, and bentonite can produce simple or complicated **pneumoconiosis,** without diffuse pulmonary fibrosis.

3. **Coal workers' pneumoconiosis (CWP, "black lung")**

   a. Although coal dust is less fibrotic than silica, CWP shares with silicosis the x-ray appearance of small, rounded opacities in the simple stage and large, conglomerate masses in the complicated stage. However, simple CWP only occasionally develops into complicated CWP.

   b. **Simple CWP** has no characteristic functional abnormality; a chronic bronchitis probably accounts for most of the respiratory disability in these patients. **Complicated CWP** can lead to PMF, with restrictive ventilatory impairment.

4. **Beryllium-related disease.** Beryllium compounds can produce both acute and chronic lung disease. The acute form is a diffuse pneumonitis that can develop into pulmonary edema. The chronic form is strikingly similar to sarcoidosis, with granulomas throughout the body; it causes progressive loss of respiratory function.

TABLE 2-5. Selected Examples of Hypersensitivity Pneumonitis (Extrinsic Allergic Alveolitis)

Disorder	Responsible Antigen
Farmer's lung	Spores of thermophilic actinomycetes in moldy hay
Bird fancier's lung	Antigens from feathers, excreta, or serum
Mushroom worker's lung	Spores of thermophilic actinomycetes in compost
Malt worker's lung	Spores of *Aspergillus clavatus* in grain
Grain handler's lung disease	Dust derived from the grain weevil
Bagassosis	Thermophilic actinomycetes in sugarcane residue
Humidifier (air conditioner) lung	Thermophilic actinomycetes in humidifiers or air conditioners

5. **Pulmonary response to other mineral dusts.** Some dusts (e.g., tin oxide, iron oxide, barium sulfate), when deposited in the lung, are cleared into aggregations in the pulmonary lobules. These dust collections cause little or no reaction and do not physically interfere with ventilatory function or perfusion.

C. **Pulmonary response to organic dusts (hypersensitivity pneumonitis, extrinsic allergic alveolitis)**

1. **Etiology and pathogenesis.** The inhalation of organic dusts (e.g., fungal spores, thermophilic actinomycetes, and fragments of animal and vegetable matter) causes a diffuse, granulomatous pulmonary parenchymal reaction known as **hypersensitivity pneumonitis** or **extrinsic allergic alveolitis.** Some common examples are listed in Table 2-5. Patients often have antibodies against the offending substances, and the findings suggest a type III hypersensitivity reaction, with tissue damage from the deposition of antigen–antibody complexes. Pathologically, mononuclear interstitial infiltrates and fibrosis predominate.

2. **Clinical features.** Several hours after exposure, patients suffer malaise, fever, and chills, with chest tightness and persistent dry cough. Radiographs obtained during acute attacks show pulmonary infiltrates. Symptoms abate within a few days, but recur with subsequent exposures. Repeated exposures may lead to a fixed restrictive lung disease.

3. **Therapy** includes avoidance of exposure and corticosteroid treatment for acute attacks.

D. **Obstructive airway disease due to inhalants**

1. **Occupational asthma.** Heavy exposure to various occupational inhalants can cause occupational asthma, often without a demonstrable immunologic mechanism. Affected individuals usually are not atopic, and the reaction usually occurs several hours after exposure.
   a. **Etiologic agents** of occupational asthma include:
      (1) Simple inorganic chemicals (e.g., platinum salts)
      (2) Simple organic chemicals (e.g., diisocyanates, formaldehyde, phthalic anhydrides)
      (3) Detergent enzymes derived from *Bacillus subtilis*
      (4) Wood dust, especially western red cedar
      (5) Fungal antigens and grain weevil antigens
      (6) Animal dander and excretions
      (7) Grain and grain contaminants
   b. **Diagnosis and therapy.** The diagnosis is strongly suggested by a history of coughing fits that occur at 2 A.M. or 3 A.M. on workdays but not on weekends or during vacation from work. Direct confirmation by challenge testing is the most convincing demonstration of the causal relationship. Avoidance of expo-

sure is the most effective treatment. Acute attacks may respond to standard asthma medication.

2. Byssinosis is occupational asthma induced by cotton dust; it is seen in textile workers. It is uncertain whether the pathogenic mechanism is immunologic or pharmacologic. At first, the affected worker experiences chest tightness and shortness of breath early in the work week but feels well later in the work week. With years of exposure, the symptoms may last later into the week, until symptoms and signs of chronic fixed airway obstruction finally prevail.

3. Industrial bronchitis. When chronic obstructive bronchitis is caused by occupational inhalants, the disorder is hard to recognize because the symptoms of bronchitis (e.g., chronic cough) are so prevalent in the general population. Identification of an occupational inhalant requires careful and extensive epidemiologic studies. Studies linking chronic bronchitis to exposure to inert dust (e.g., coal dust) as well as foundry and gold mine dust have yielded equivocal results.

E. **Pulmonary response to irritant gases.** Irritant gases inflame the respiratory tract and can cause upper and lower airway disease. In high concentrations, they can cause pulmonary edema.

1. Such agents include ammonia (NH_3), hydrochloric acid (HCl), sulfur dioxide (SO_2), nitrogen dioxide (NO_2), and phosgene (Cl_2CO).

2. Often, there is a latent period of 12–24 hours before the onset of chest symptoms.

3. The pulmonary edema due to any irritant gas is treated with supportive measures and corticosteroids. In some cases, follow-up reveals bronchiolitis obliterans.

XIV. **PULMONARY DISEASES OF UNKNOWN ETIOLOGY.** Except for sarcoidosis, pulmonary diseases of unknown etiology are encountered infrequently by clinicians.

A. **Sarcoidosis**

1. Definition. Sarcoidosis is a multisystem disease characterized by the presence of noncaseating granulomas in various organs. The lungs are involved in more than 90% of reported cases. Sarcoidosis usually presents as mediastinal or hilar lymphadenopathy with pulmonary infiltration, combined with cutaneous or ocular lesions. Less common but important manifestations include peripheral adenopathy, erythema nodosum, arthritis, splenomegaly, hepatomegaly, hypercalcemia, diffuse or localized CNS involvement, and cardiomyopathy. A consistent immunologic feature is depression of delayed-type hypersensitivity.

2. Incidence. Sarcoidosis can occur in either sex at any age but appears most commonly in the third to fifth decades of life. In the United States, the incidence of sarcoidosis is 10- to 18-fold higher in blacks than in whites.

3. Possible etiologic factors. The noncaseating epithelioid granuloma of sarcoidosis suggests a tissue response to some focal insult.
   a. Infectious agents. Clinical and pathologic similarities have suggested a connection with tuberculosis and other mycobacterial disease. However, a failure to identify any infectious agents consistently and lack of an epidemiologic association have made any infectious case unlikely.
   b. Immunologic defects
      (1) Patients with sarcoidosis show impaired cellular immunity characterized by a complete skin anergy to tuberculin and other common skin antigens. The level of circulating T lymphocytes is decreased, possibly due to sequestration in the lung, because bronchoalveolar lavage typically reveals marked increases in these cells.
      (2) The significance of these immunologic abnormalities is unknown. They may represent a fundamentally abnormal immunologic responsiveness, or it

may be that the immunologic changes are secondary phenomena and that the primary pathologic process remains to be discovered.

   (3) Humoral immunity is normal, and susceptibility to infection is not increased.

4. **Pathology**
   a. The fundamental lesion of sarcoidosis is a noncaseating granuloma. This cluster of epithelioid cells is indistinguishable from the granulomas occurring in other diseases such as fungal disease, mycobacterial disease, and Hodgkin's disease.
   b. Giant cells frequently are present and contain several types of inclusions. Lymphocytes and rare plasma cells may be present at the periphery of the granuloma; neutrophils and eosinophils are absent.

5. **Clinical features** vary considerably, depending on the site and extent of involvement.
   a. **Pulmonary involvement**
      (1) **Symptoms.** Fatigue and exertional dyspnea are common. Cough, if present, usually is nonproductive. Hemoptysis is rare. Chest pain occurs infrequently, and pleurisy is uncommon.
      (2) **Pulmonary function testing.** Results may be normal but usually show some impairment of gas exchange and some evidence of lung restriction with reduced VC and D_{LCO}. In many cases, small airway function also is abnormal.
      (3) **Chest x-ray.** Enlarged intrathoracic lymph nodes are seen, particularly early in the course of the disease. Parenchymal manifestations vary from a faint interstitial infiltrate, to well-developed diffuse nodular infiltrates, to varying degrees of lung fibrosis, including honeycombing. The **radiographic staging** of pulmonary involvement in sarcoidosis is as follows:
         (a) **Stage 1:** Bilateral hilar adenopathy and normal lung parenchyma
         (b) **Stage 2:** Bilateral hilar adenopathy and interstitial infiltrate
         (c) **Stage 3:** Interstitial infiltrate only
         (d) **Stage 4:** Fibrosis
   b. **Systemic involvement**
      (1) **Uveitis** is a common presentation and may progress to blindness.
      (2) A variety of infiltrative **skin lesions** occur in one third of patients and often portend chronic progressive sarcoidosis. An exception is **erythema nodosum,** which may occur early in the disease and is associated with a good prognosis.
      (3) **Bone and joint involvement.** Transient polyarthritis is associated with erythema nodosum; a chronic form of arthritis also occurs. Bone involvement may produce cystic destruction and disability.
      (4) **Nervous system involvement** may present as Bell's palsy and other cranial neuropathies, peripheral neuropathies, and (rarely) granulomatous meningitis.
      (5) **Cardiomyopathy** manifests as arrhythmias and conduction disturbances that carry a high risk for sudden death.
      (6) **Liver function abnormalities** may occur.
      (7) **Disturbances in calcium metabolism** (e.g., hypercalciuria, renal stones, and hypercalcemia; see Chapter 6 Part I: XII B 4 b) occur in up to 25% of patients.

6. **Clinical course and prognosis.** The course of sarcoidosis is variable. Granulomas may remain unchanged in tissue for many years, may regress, or may organize, resulting in tissue fibrosis. Chronic inflammation and fibrosis in the lung cause serious structural distortion and loss of function.
   a. In most patients, the disease regresses within 2 years and does not recur. Any tissue destruction that occurs is permanent but usually causes no major disability.
   b. In approximately 25% of patients, the disease is more progressive and causes serious disability. In this more severely affected group, multisystem involvement is common, with skin sarcoidosis and hypercalcemia being particularly prominent. Approximately 5% of patients die of respiratory failure.

7. Diagnosis

a. Sarcoidosis should be suspected in any patient with mediastinal or hilar adenopathy and interstitial lung disease (e.g., pulmonary fibrosis). Erythema nodosum, uveitis, skin lesions, hypercalcemia, multisystem disease, and granulomas of any organ should also suggest sarcoidosis.

b. Diagnostic confirmation requires tissue biopsy demonstrating typical granulomas in a patient with consistent clinical presentations; transbronchial biopsy is often diagnostic. Because sarcoidosis is a diagnosis of exclusion, all tissue samples should be cultured to rule out infectious causes and should be specially stained for identification of fungal disease.

8. Therapy. Corticosteroid administration is the principal treatment for sarcoidosis. However, a decision must be made as to whether a patient's symptoms warrant therapy that has proven hazards.

a. Sarcoidosis that carries a threat of disability should be treated. Indications include symptomatic pulmonary disease, uveitis, hypercalcemia, cardiac sarcoidosis, and neurologic sarcoidosis.

b. The patient must be assessed periodically to determine whether continuation of treatment is warranted. Clinical observation, pulmonary function testing, and chest x-ray frequently are used to evaluate the effectiveness of the therapeutic regimen. However, serum angiotensin converting enzyme (ACE) assay and bronchoalveolar lavage are better indicators of disease activity for use in follow-up.

B. Goodpasture's syndrome (see also Chapter 6 Part I: X G)

1. Definition. Goodpasture's syndrome is a progressive autoimmune disease of the lungs and kidneys that produces intra-alveolar hemorrhage and glomerulonephritis. The disease is rare, occurs at all ages, and is predominant in males.

2. Pathogenesis and pathology

a. Goodpasture's syndrome is caused by an anti-glomerular basement membrane (anti-GBM) antibody, usually IgG, that reacts with glomerular and alveolar basement membranes.

b. Linear deposition of the antibody, characteristic of a type II hypersensitivity reaction, occurs along the basement membrane of glomeruli, alveoli, and capillaries.

   (1) The pathologic result in the lung is diffuse capillary leakage and intra-alveolar hemorrhage but little or no inflammation.

   (2) The renal lesion is a proliferative glomerulonephritis that progresses to renal failure.

3. Clinical features. The patient usually presents with hemoptysis and dyspnea; however, renal failure without pulmonary complaints can be an initial finding, and a history of respiratory illness often precedes the onset of pulmonary hemorrhage.

4. Diagnosis

a. Bilateral alveolar infiltrates on chest x-ray, hypoxia, and a restrictive pattern on pulmonary function testing are characteristic.

b. The diagnosis is confirmed by demonstration of anti-GBM antibody in the serum or in a biopsy specimen from the kidney or lung.

c. **Differential diagnosis** includes Wegener's granulomatosis, systemic lupus erythematosus (SLE), and idiopathic pulmonary hemosiderosis.

   (1) **Wegener's granulomatosis** (see XIV C) usually affects both the upper and lower respiratory tract, and lacks anti-GBM antibody.

   (2) **SLE** (see Chapter 10 VII) is distinguished from Goodpasture's syndrome by the absence of anti-GBM antibody and the findings of free DNA, various ANAs, and depressed serum levels of complement.

   (3) **Idiopathic pulmonary hemosiderosis** is characterized by repeated pulmonary hemorrhage but no nephritis. Death from massive hemorrhage may occur at any time, but prolonged survival with or without symptoms of pulmonary insufficiency is common. Idiopathic pulmonary hemosiderosis has no known immune mechanisms for pathogenesis, and no successful therapy has evolved.

5. Prognosis and therapy

  a. Untreated Goodpasture's syndrome is rapidly fatal as a result of renal failure or asphyxia from pulmonary hemorrhage.

  b. Currently, the combination of plasmapheresis to remove circulating anti-GBM antibodies and immunosuppressive therapy with corticosteroids and alkylating agents appears to give the best results. High-dose corticosteroid therapy often controls episodes of lung hemorrhage but not the progressive renal disease. This treatment does not prevent the ultimately fatal outcome.

  c. Bilateral nephrectomy with hemodialysis or kidney transplantation has been used to control end-stage renal disease.

C. **Wegener's granulomatosis** (see also Chapter 6 Part I: X N 3)

  1. Definition. This disease is the prototype of a group of rare disorders characterized by granulomatous inflammation and necrosis of the lung and other organs. All ages are affected; men are affected more commonly than women.

  a. Wegener originally described the syndrome as a destructive granulomatous infiltration of the upper respiratory tract and lung parenchyma combined with glomerulonephritis.

  b. Today, the disease is recognized as a systemic vasculitis with a predilection for the respiratory tract and kidney. Other commonly involved sites are the skin, joints, and peripheral nerves. Involvement of the eyes, heart, and CNS can also occur.

  c. A variant form affects the respiratory tract, chiefly the lungs, while sparing the kidney.

  2. Pathogenesis and pathology

  a. The pathogenetic mechanism is thought to be an immunologic injury of vessels, with secondary inflammatory changes.

  b. The pathologic lesion is an angiitis of small vessels with characteristic tissue necrosis surrounded by mononuclear inflammatory cells, forming noncaseating granulomas.

    (1) In the lung, this process commonly results in excavation and destruction of the lung parenchyma, causing hemoptysis and pulmonary insufficiency.

    (2) The renal lesion is a focal glomerulonephritis that can progress to renal failure.

  3. Diagnosis. Wegener's granulomatosis is identified by the classic clinical triad of upper and lower respiratory involvement and glomerulonephritis, supported by a positive antineutrophilic cytoplasmic antibody (ANCA) test and biopsy of the involved tissue (see also Chapter 10 IX E).

  4. Prognosis and therapy

  a. The untreated disease is fatal in most patients within 1 month to several years. Some forms of the disease are associated with longer survival rates, particularly those that do not involve active nephritis.

  b. Correct diagnosis is critical because of the remarkable efficacy of **cytotoxic therapy.** Cyclophosphamide alone or with corticosteroids produces rapid reversal of the disease, if introduced early in the course.

D. **Histiocytosis X (eosinophilic granuloma of the lung)**

  1. Definition. Histiocytosis X is a generic term for a group of systemic disorders characterized by various degrees of fibrosis with focal infiltrations of tissue by nonmalignant histiocytes and eosinophils. The disease can be localized to one area (e.g., bone or lung) or it can be widely disseminated. **Eosinophilic granuloma** (of bone or lung) is localized; **Letterer-Siwe disease** and **Hand-Schüller-Christian syndrome** are widespread syndromes.

  2. Incidence. The disease is rare, affects men more commonly than women, and affects children and young adults more commonly than other age groups. An abnormality of the immune system is suspected.

3. **Pathology.** Proliferating histiocytes show cytoplasmic inclusions, the so-called "X bodies." Pulmonary histiocytosis X produces bilateral, reticulonodular infiltrates, with a predilection for the upper lobes and typical progression to cyst formation, fibrosis, and honeycombing.

4. **Clinical features and diagnosis**
   a. **Findings** may include cough, chest pain, dyspnea, fever, spontaneous pneumothorax, and a honeycomb appearance on chest x-ray. Lytic bone disease may be present. A triad of diabetes insipidus, exophthalmos, and bone lesions is seen occasionally.
   b. **Pulmonary function testing** indicates restriction and impaired gas exchange. In advanced cases, severe obstruction may dominate.
   c. **Definitive diagnosis** requires biopsy of involved tissue or electron-microscopic demonstration of X bodies in bronchoalveolar lavage fluid.

5. **Therapy and prognosis.** Corticosteroids are given for pulmonary manifestations, but their efficacy is uncertain. Surgery or radiotherapy is used for localized bone disease. The prognosis is variable—some cases result in death, but spontaneous remissions are common.

E. **Alveolar proteinosis**

1. **Definition.** Alveolar proteinosis is a rare disease characterized by massive accumulations of a phospholipid- and protein-rich substance in alveoli. The interstitium usually is not involved, and there is no underlying disease or other organ involvement. The disorder is more common in men than in women and has been described in all ages.

2. **Pathology.** The substance in the alveoli is closely related to pulmonary surfactant and probably accumulates as a result of impaired clearance. Macrophages engorged with the substance also are present, but other inflammatory cells are lacking.

3. **Clinical features**
   a. **Findings.** Dyspnea, nonproductive cough, pulmonary rales, and cyanosis are common.
   b. **Clinical course and prognosis**
      (1) Patients are predisposed to lung infection, including nocardiosis and fungal infections, possibly because of a functional impairment of alveolar macrophages.
      (2) The disease may progress to respiratory insufficiency and death, but spontaneous resolution is just as common. Pulmonary fibrosis has been described as a late complication.

4. **Diagnosis.** Pulmonary function testing shows a restrictive ventilatory pattern and hypoxia. Chest x-ray shows an alveolar infiltrate, usually in a bilateral perihilar butterfly distribution similar to the pattern seen in pulmonary edema. Lung biopsy is necessary to demonstrate the periodic acid–Schiff (PAS)–positive material in the alveoli.

5. **Therapy.** Patients with minimal symptoms require no therapy. For the dyspneic patient, bronchoalveolar lavage is effective and reverses the physiologic abnormality. Corticosteroids are contraindicated because they increase the risk of infection.

F. **Bronchiolitis obliterans organizing pneumonia (BOOP)**

1. **Definition and pathology.** BOOP, also called cryptogenic organizing pneumonia (COP), is a clinicopathologic syndrome involving granulation tissue within small airways and alveolar ducts. It is associated with chronic inflammation in the surrounding alveoli.

2. **Etiology.** Viral infection, toxic inhalation, rheumatoid arthritis and other collagen-vascular diseases, as well as drugs are some of the potential causes of BOOP.

3. **Clinical features**
   a. BOOP affects both men and women. The mean age at presentation is 58 years; patients range in age from 21 to 80 years.
   b. The disease usually presents as a subacute flu-like illness with coughing, fever, malaise, fatigue, and weight loss. Inspiratory crackles are frequently present.

4. **Diagnosis**
   a. **Chest x-rays** reveal bilateral, diffuse alveolar opacities.
   b. **Pulmonary function testing** shows a restrictive defect.
   c. **Lung biopsy** is the definitive way to make a diagnosis.

5. **Therapy.** In two-thirds of patients, corticosteroid therapy results in rapid and complete recovery.

XV. SLEEP APNEA SYNDROME

A. **Definition.** Sleep apnea is a disorder characterized by repetitive periods of **apnea** (i.e., cessation of breathing) occurring during sleep. A period of more than 10 seconds without air flow is considered to constitute an apneic episode. Patients with this syndrome can have hundreds of such episodes during the course of one night's sleep.

B. **Etiology and pathophysiology.** Sleep apnea may be obstructive, central, or mixed.

1. In **obstructive sleep apnea,** transient obstruction of the upper airway, usually the oropharynx, prevents inspiratory air flow. The obstruction results from loss of tone in the pharyngeal muscles or the genioglossus muscles (which normally cause the tongue to protrude forward from the posterior pharyngeal wall).

2. In **central apnea,** there is no drive to breathe during the apneic episode; that is, there is no signal from the respiratory center to initiate inspiration. Rarely, the cause is a neurologic disorder. Why the drive is absent in other individuals is not known.

3. In **mixed apnea,** patients have episodes of both obstructive and central apnea.

C. **Clinical features**

1. **Symptoms.** Usually, it is the sleep partner who notices the patient's problems. Loud snoring is prominent, and the patient may thrash about during periods of obstructive apnea. During the daytime, patients are overly somnolent and may show personality changes or slowed mentation.

2. **Physical signs.** In patients with **central** apnea, monitoring of the chest wall motion reveals no movement; this corresponds to cessation of air flow and oxygen desaturation. In patients with **obstructive apnea,** chest wall and abdominal movement can be detected during the patient's fruitless attempts to move air through the obstructed airway.

D. **Therapy**

1. **Central apnea.** Treatment is with respiratory stimulants. A phrenic nerve pacemaker may be implanted to electrically stimulate the diaphragm.

2. **Obstructive apnea.** Some patients may respond to respiratory stimulants; others require more drastic measures. These include tracheostomy to bypass the upper airway, nasal continual positive airway pressure (CPAP) to prevent occlusion, or surgery to debulk the posterior pharynx. Patients who are markedly obese may benefit from weight reduction.

E. **Complications.** Serious complications include cardiac arrhythmias, pulmonary hypertension, and unexplained cor pulmonale.

STUDY QUESTIONS

DIRECTIONS: Each of the numbered items or incomplete statements in this section is followed by answers or by completions of the statement. Select the ONE lettered answer or completion that is BEST in each case.

1. Which one of the following findings is virtually always seen in a patient with adult respiratory distress syndrome (ARDS)?

(A) A small localized mass on chest x-ray
(B) Reduced lung compliance
(C) Normal oxygenation with impaired minute ventilation
(D) Increased arterial P_{CO_2}
(E) Pulmonary embolism

2. Shortly after symptoms of an asthmatic attack have resolved, pulmonary function testing is most likely to show

(A) normal values for peak expiratory flow
(B) decreased lung compliance
(C) increased residual volume (RV)
(D) no change in peak expiratory flow after inhalation of a bronchodilator
(E) decreased diffusing capacity ($D_{L_{CO}}$)

3. Which combination of findings provides a definitive diagnosis of cystic fibrosis?

(A) Family history of cystic fibrosis; abnormal pulmonary function
(B) Abnormal pulmonary function; pancreatic insufficiency
(C) Pancreatic insufficiency; high electrolyte concentration in sweat
(D) High electrolyte concentration in serum; abnormal chest x-ray
(E) Abnormal chest x-ray; family history of cystic fibrosis

4. Which one of the following is the best measure of airflow obstruction?

(A) Diffusing capacity ($D_{L_{CO}}$)
(B) Residual volume (RV)
(C) 1-Second forced expiratory volume (FEV_1)
(D) 1-Second forced expiratory volume–forced vital capacity ratio (FEV_1/FVC)
(E) Forced vital capacity (FVC)

5. Which one of the following diagnostic techniques is most specific for pulmonary embolism?

(A) Pulmonary angiography
(B) Ventilation lung scanning
(C) Perfusion lung scanning
(D) Arterial blood gas analysis
(E) Chest x-ray

6. Chronic obstructive pulmonary disease (COPD) is classified as emphysematous or bronchitic, depending on the pathologic changes that occur in the lung. Although these two COPD syndromes rarely exist as pure entities, they can be differentiated on the basis of their clinical presentation. Which one of the following clinical features is common to both the emphysematous and bronchitic types of COPD?

(A) Polycythemia
(B) Improved airflow with bronchodilators
(C) Dyspnea
(D) Chronic cough
(E) Hypercapnia

7. Restrictive ventilatory defects are best characterized by

(A) low lung volumes
(B) a decrease in the 1-second forced expiratory volume–forced vital capacity (FEV_1/FVC) ratio
(C) an increased vital capacity (VC)
(D) a decreased diffusing capacity $D_{L_{CO}}$
(E) an increased airway resistance (R_{AW})

8. A 62-year-old woman who has congestive heart failure develops pneumonia and a large pleural effusion. Thoracentesis is performed in an effort to establish whether the pleural effusion is due to congestive heart failure or pneumonia. Which finding would indicate that the pleural effusion is due to congestive heart failure?

(A) A protein content of 6 g/dl
(B) A pH of 7.13
(C) A glucose content of 20 mg/dl
(D) A lactate dehydrogenase (LDH) content of 100 mg/dl (with a serum LDH level of 420 mg/dl)
(E) A pleural fluid–serum protein ratio of 0.7

DIRECTIONS: Each set of matching questions in this section consists of a list of four to twenty-six lettered options (some of which may be in figures) followed by several numbered items. For each numbered item, select the ONE lettered option that is most closely associated with it. To avoid spending too much time on matching sets with large numbers of options, it is generally advisable to begin each set by reading the list of options. Then, for each item in the set, try to generate the correct answer and locate it in the option list, rather than evaluating each option individually. Each lettered option may be selected once, more than once, or not at all.

Questions 9–13

Match each of the following statements to the pulmonary disease of unknown etiology it best describes.

(A) Sarcoidosis
(B) Goodpasture's syndrome
(C) Wegener's granulomatosis
(D) Alveolar proteinosis
(E) Alveolar microlithiasis

9. This progressive disease of the lungs and kidneys can produce intra-alveolar hemorrhage and glomerulonephritis.

10. Granulomatous inflammation and necrosis of the lung and other organs are characteristic of this disease.

11. This disease is characterized by massive accumulations of a phospholipid-rich material in alveoli.

12. This systemic disease is characterized by the presence of noncaseating granulomas in the lung and other organs.

13. Cardiac involvement in this disease may manifest as arrhythmias and conduction disturbances.

ANSWERS AND EXPLANATIONS

1. The answer is B [VI C–D]. Adult respiratory distress syndrome (ARDS, "wet lung") begins with a disruption of capillary integrity, which leads to extravasation of fluid, fibrin, and protein into the alveoli. As a result, the lungs become wet and stiff (i.e., noncompliant). This condition is characterized by severe hypoxia caused by extreme ventilation–perfusion ($\dot{V}/\dot{Q}$) imbalance and shunting of blood in the fluid-filled areas of the lung. Clinical features include progressive tachypnea; patchy, diffuse, fluffy infiltrates on chest x-ray; increased minute ventilation; and decreased lung volumes. There usually is an absence of specific physical findings.

2. The answer is C [III F 4 a–b]. Patients who have had a recent asthmatic attack, even though asymptomatic, still have residual airflow obstruction that may take a couple of months to disappear. During this time, patients still respond to bronchodilators but show abnormal peak expiratory flow, increased lung compliance, and continued maldistribution of ventilation. Diffusing capacity (D_{LCO}) is decreased in abnormalities of capillary blood volume due to either destruction on the alveolar capillary membrane (e.g., in emphysema) or to a thickened interstitial membrane (e.g., in diffuse interstitial lung disease). Neither of these abnormalities exists in asthma.

3. The answer is C [IV B 5 a (1)–(2) (a)–(c)]. Although chest x-ray and pulmonary function testing reveal abnormalities, the sweat test is the definitive test for cystic fibrosis. In virtually all cases of cystic fibrosis, sodium and chloride concentrations in sweat are increased significantly, while concentrations of these electrolytes are normal elsewhere in the body. In order to make a diagnosis of cystic fibrosis, this defect must be identified. The diagnosis is confirmed by a positive sweat test combined with any one of the following findings: a family history of cystic fibrosis, obstructive pulmonary disease, or pancreatic insufficiency.

4. The answer is D [I F 1 a]. A decrease in the 1-second forced expiratory volume–forced vital capacity (FEV_1/FVC) ratio is the hallmark of airflow obstruction. The FEV_1 is the volume of air forcefully expired during the first second after a maximal inhalation; the FVC is the total volume of air that can be forcibly expelled from the lungs after a maximal inhalation. The FEV_1 is decreased in obstructive as well as restrictive lung disease. The diffusing capacity (D_{LCO}) and the residual volume (RV) do not identify airway obstruction. The D_{LCO} indicates the adequacy of the alveolar–capillary membrane; the RV is the volume of air remaining in the lungs after a maximal expiratory effort.

5. The answer is A [VIII E 7]. Pulmonary angiography is the standard test for the diagnosis of pulmonary embolism. Algorithms have been developed for patients with appropriate clinical data and high-probability results on ventilation and perfusion lung scanning; in such cases, this combined technique has almost the diagnostic accuracy of pulmonary angiography. Abnormal results on arterial blood gas analysis and chest x-ray are too nonspecific to be helpful. When ventilation and perfusion scanning, arterial blood gas analysis, or both produce normal results and the alveolar–arterial P_{O_2} is normal, pulmonary embolism is extremely unlikely.

6. The answer is C [II E 1, 2 A (1)–(2)]. All patients with chronic obstructive pulmonary disease (COPD) experience dyspnea to some degree. The two classic types of COPD—emphysematous and bronchitic—represent extremes of the spectrum and rarely are encountered in their pure form in clinical practice. By definition the emphysematous type of COPD presents at a relatively older age (older than 60 years) and is characterized by progressive exertional dyspnea, weight loss, little or no cough, mild hypoxia, hypocapnia, and only a mild increase in airway resistance (R_{aw}) that shows little improvement with bronchodilation. The bronchitic type of COPD presents at a relatively young age and is characterized by episodic dyspnea, fluid retention, chronic cough, severe hypoxia, hypercapnia, polycythemia, and an increase in R_{aw} that improves with bronchodilation.

7. The answer is A [I F 2]. Restrictive disorders are characterized by low lung volumes. Diffusing capacity ($D_{L_{CO}}$) may or may not be decreased in pulmonary fibrosis, a type of restrictive disease. A decrease in the forced expiratory volume in one second–forced vital capacity (FEV_1/FVC) ratio is the hallmark of obstructive, not restrictive, disease. Vital capacity (VC) and airway resistance (R_{aw}) are decreased in restrictive lung disorders.

8. The answer is D [IX A 2 c; Table 2-3]. With the exception of the lactate dehydrogenase (LDH); findings, all of the pleural fluid findings listed indicate the presence of an exudate. Exudates are caused by inflammation or disease of the pleural surface or by lymphatic obstruction (e.g., due to tuberculosis, lung cancer, or pneumonia). Transudates are caused by elevated systemic or pulmonary venous pressure or by decreased plasma oncotic pressure (e.g., due to congestive heart failure or nephrotic syndrome). Therefore, in establishing the etiology of a pleural effusion, it is useful to determine whether the fluid is a transudate or an exudate. This determination often can be made on the basis of a chemical analysis of the pleural fluid. A pleural fluid protein content of more than 3 g/dl and a LDH content of more than 250 mg/dl usually indicate the presence of an exudate. In addition, an exudate usually is associated with a pleural fluid–serum protein ratio of less than 0.5 and a pleural fluid–serum LDH ratio of less than 0.6. Pleural fluid pH values below 7.2 and a pleural fluid glucose content of less than 20 mg/dl also are associated with inflammatory effusions (exudates).

9–13. The answers are: 9-B [XIV B 1], **10-C** [IXIV C 1], **11-D** [XIV E 1], **12-A** [XIV A 1], **13-A** [XIV A 5 b (5)]. Goodpasture's syndrome is a rare, progressive disease of the lungs and kidneys, which is caused by an anti–glomerular basement membrane (anti-GBM) antibody, usually IgG. The anti-GBM antibody reacts with glomerular and alveolar basement membranes to cause alveolar hemorrhage and glomerulonephritis. There is no evidence of necrotizing granuloma in Goodpasture's syndrome, as there is in Wegener's granulomatosis.

Like Goodpasture's syndrome, Wegener's granulomatosis may involve the kidneys and lungs as well as other organs. This disease is characterized by granulomatous inflammation and necrosis of these organs. Wegener's granulomatosis is regarded as a systemic vasculitis; Goodpasture's syndrome is not.

Alveolar proteinosis is characterized by massive accumulations of a phospholipid-rich material in alveoli. The substance, which is closely related in its chemical and physiologic properties to pulmonary surfactant, may well accumulate as a result of impaired clearance. There is no evidence of vasculitis, granuloma, or renal disease in this entity.

The lesion in sarcoidosis classically is a noncaseating granuloma, which occurs in the lungs as well as other organs. Systemic involvement may be demonstrated as uveitis, skin lesions, polyarthritis (bone and joint involvement), Bell's palsy and other cranial neuropathies (neural involvement), and arrhythmias and conduction disturbances (cardiac involvement).

Chapter 3

Hematologic Diseases

Ronald N. Rubin

I. RED BLOOD CELL DISORDERS

A. Anemia caused by abnormal hemoglobin synthesis and iron metabolism. Hemoglobin, which represents 95% of the total composition of a red blood cell, is a mixture of globin and the iron-containing heme compound, **protoporphyrin.** Any abnormality in hemoglobin synthesis or iron metabolism results in hemoglobin-deficient cells. As a rule, such deficient cells exhibit **hypochromia** (i.e., diminished hemoglobin concentration) and **microcytosis** (i.e., diminished size). Both conditions may be detected using the red blood cell indices available by calculation and the Coulter counter along with an examination of a stained blood smear. Disorders causing this type of anemia fall into four major classes.

1. **Iron deficiency anemia** is the most common form of anemia in the United States, where 20% of adult women are reported to be iron deficient.
   a. **Etiology.** Iron deficiency is most commonly caused by blood loss when the loss of the iron component exceeds dietary intake of iron. Examples include gastrointestinal blood loss from an ulcer or a tumor and menstrual blood loss. Occasionally, in the neonate and young child, new blood formation and subsequent increased iron use exceeds iron intake and results in anemia without concomitant blood loss.
   b. **Clinical manifestations.** The symptoms of iron deficiency anemia, like all anemias, include fatigue and weakness. Symptoms specific to iron deficiency may include epithelial changes, such as brittle nails and atrophic tongue. In addition, the underlying pathology may dominate the symptoms (e.g., in the case of a peptic ulcer).
   c. **Diagnosis.** In the appropriate clinical setting (e.g., in a young woman with excessive menstrual blood loss and anemia), a smear showing hypochromia and microcytosis is adequate for the diagnosis. When more specific tests are needed, a positive diagnosis is made from an absence of marrow iron on bone marrow examination, abnormally low levels of ferritin, and a low serum iron level in association with an elevated total iron-binding capacity.
   d. **Therapy.** Treatment usually involves restoration of the body's iron stores to correct the anemia. As a rule, oral iron in the form of ferrous sulfate suffices; however, for patients who do not tolerate this form, ferrous gluconate and fumarate are available. In difficult cases that are refractory either physiologically or due to an inability to take oral iron, parenteral iron preparations are given. Reticulocytosis occurs 7 days after appropriate treatment; after 3 weeks, the hemoglobin level increases several grams.

2. **Anemia of chronic disease.** This mild to moderate anemia is associated with inflammatory diseases, such as rheumatoid arthritis, serious infections, and carcinoma.
   a. **Pathophysiology**
      (1) Anemia of chronic disease is characterized by hemoglobin levels of 8–10 g/dl, although lower levels are possible. It is unusual for the hemoglobin level to be less than 7 g/dl.
      (2) Patients with this anemia have plentiful iron but diminished iron utilization by the bone marrow. Therefore, inadequate amounts of iron are available to the bone marrow for red blood cell formation despite adequate body stores.
      (3) Another important mechanism for this anemia is an impaired marrow response to erythropoietin.
      (4) Circulating cytokines, such as interleukin-6 (IL-6) or tumor necrosis factor (TNF), which are released as a result of the inflammatory state, are thought to be involved.

    b. Diagnosis is based on confirmation of the following.

      (1) The anemia associated with chronic inflammation is of moderate degree and reveals slight hypochromia and microcytosis.

      (2) The mean corpuscular volume (MCV) is 80–85 μm^3, and the mean corpuscular hemoglobin concentration (MCHC) is 30%–32%.

      (3) If stained, the marrow reveals plentiful iron stores. Also, serum ferritin levels usually are normal or only slightly elevated. Serum iron is lowered as is the total iron-binding capacity, unlike the clinical situation with iron deficiency anemia.

    c. Therapy. Hematinics, including iron, are not effective treatment for this disorder.

      (1) Correction of the underlying disease can lead to reversal of the anemia within 1 month.

      (2) Exogenous erythropoietin can be effective therapy in certain situations, such as perioperatively in rheumatoid patients undergoing joint replacement surgery. Because the inflammatory state induces a relative hyposensitivity to erythropoietin, generous doses may be needed.

3. Sideroblastic anemias

    a. Pathophysiology. These anemias, caused by disorders in the synthesis of the heme moiety of hemoglobin, are characterized by trapped iron in the mitochondria of nucleated red blood cells. Most of the enzymes for protoporphyrin synthesis are located in the nucleated red blood cell mitochondria. Thus, derangements in these pathways cause iron accumulation in the perinuclear mitochondria, which renders this anemia its characteristic morphologic finding of **ringed sideroblasts.** The defective heme synthesis causes diminished hemoglobin levels in these cells; as a result, this cell population is hypochromic and microcytic.

    b. Types. There are two types of sideroblastic anemias.

      (1) Hereditary sideroblastic anemia. This X-linked condition is due to an abnormality in pyridoxine (vitamin B_6) metabolism. It is thought to be a congenital defect in the enzyme **δ-aminolevulinic acid (ALA) synthetase.**

      (2) Acquired sideroblastic anemias are more common than the hereditary type. Lead, alcohol, and the antibacterial drug isoniazid cause sideroblastic anemia by inhibiting enzymes of protoporphyrin synthesis; however, many cases are idiopathic.

    c. Diagnosis. This anemia may be relatively severe in patients older than 60 years and is characterized by hemoglobin levels of 8–10 g/dl. Coulter counter reveals normocytic or even macrocytic cells, but examination of the blood smear shows a dimorphous population with some very small cells. The bone marrow reveals erythroid hyperplasia, and iron staining demonstrates the ringed sideroblasts. Iron studies show elevated ferritin levels and high serum iron levels with high transferrin saturation. Often, some normal or slightly macrocytic cells are seen intermingling with the hypochromic, microcytic cells, and a blood smear revealing such a condition is diagnostic of this anemia.

    d. Therapy

      (1) If a drug such as isoniazid or alcohol is involved, the anemia and sideroblastic changes regress with discontinuation of the agent.

      (2) All patients should be given a trial of **pyridoxine** in high doses; however, in all but the hereditary cases, this usually fails. Often, these patients are transfusion dependent. Acute leukemia develops in a portion (10%) of patients with acquired idiopathic disease. In these patients, the sideroblastic anemia was a preleukemic syndrome.

      (3) Efficacy using **exogenous erythropoietin** to treat this condition is approximately 20%, and this therapy should be tried in transfusion-dependent patients.

4. Thalassemias are genetic disorders characterized by diminished synthesis of one of the globin chains. These diseases are due to abnormalities in the genes that are responsible for synthesis of the globin portion of the hemoglobin molecule. Thalassemias are named according to the deficient chain.

a. **Types**
  (1) **α-Thalassemias.** These disorders are characterized by deficient α-chain synthesis, usually due to deletion of the α-globin gene from the genome. RNA for the α-globin gene is not present in the α-thalassemias. There are four such genes and, thus, four α-thalassemias; these range from a mild, subclinical, asymptomatic anemia to a severe anemia that is fatal in utero. The α-thalassemias are most prevalent in Asian populations.
  (2) **β-Thalassemias.** These disorders are due to the absence or malfunction of the β-globin gene. In the latter case, RNA is present but in reduced amounts or in defective forms. The two β-globin genes in the genome result in two different forms of β-thalassemia. **β-Thalassemia major,** or **Cooley's anemia,** is a severe disease that appears in childhood. Such patients are transfusion dependent. Patients with **β-thalassemia minor,** a mild anemia, are not transfusion dependent and can live full, normal lives. The β-thalassemias are most prevalent in individuals of Mediterranean descent, particularly those from Greece and Italy.
b. **Diagnosis.** The thalassemias should be suspected in an anemic patient who reveals marked abnormalities on blood smear. Such abnormalities include microcytosis, hypochromia, and poikilocytosis (i.e., the presence of bizarrely shaped red blood cells).
  (1) **α-Thalassemia** is most difficult to diagnose when it exists in the carrier state. Patients with the carrier form have a mild microcytic, hypochromic anemia. There is no excess of the non–β-hemoglobins because all chains have α components. Therefore, sophisticated studies are required for definitive diagnosis. In neonates, however, the diagnosis can be made from cord blood tests that show an increase in **Bart's hemoglobin.**
  (2) **β-Thalassemia** resembles iron deficiency anemia except that iron is present in the marrow. The diagnosis is confirmed by quantitative globin measurements that reveal an elevation in the non–β-chains [e.g., hemoglobin A_2 (Hb δ) and fetal hemoglobin (Hb F)].
c. **Therapy** includes chronic red cell transfusions and folic acid supplementation. The regular use of ambulatory iron chelation has slowed the development of iron overload in these patients. In selected patients, bone marrow transplantation has been curative, and this form of therapy likely will be used more frequently in the future.

B. **Macrocytic anemias** are characterized by red blood cells that exceed 100 μm in size. Three major mechanisms are linked to the development of macrocytic anemia.

1. **Accelerated erythropoiesis.** Reticulocytes and young erythrocytes are larger than normal; therefore, individuals with large numbers of reticulocytes have large numbers of circulating cells of great size. A reticulocyte count confirms the diagnosis.

2. **Increased membrane surface area.** Patients with excessive plasma lipids absorb these lipids onto red blood cell surfaces, which creates an enlarged membrane surface area and a macrocytosis in excess of 100 μ. This condition is most common in patients with liver disease and can be diagnosed by a blood smear that reveals the characteristic **target cell** of liver disease (i.e., a round macrocyte with a redundant membrane). Liver disease causes this by diminished hepatic synthesis of lecithin–cholesterol acetyl transferase (LCAT), which results in excess plasma-free cholesterol, which is absorbed onto red blood cell membranes.

3. **Defective DNA synthesis** is the main characteristic of the classic **megaloblastic anemias.** In these conditions, red blood cells cannot produce nucleic acid and so nuclear maturation is arrested. Cytoplasmic maturation proceeds, however, resulting in abnormally large cells. These cells are larger than those seen with accelerated erythropoiesis, and they have an increased membrane surface area. An MCV that exceeds 115 μm^3 is not uncommon.
  a. **Etiology.** Megaloblastic anemias usually are caused by a deficiency of either vitamin B_{12} or folic acid.

    (1) B$_{12}$ deficiency may result from fish tapeworm infestation, strict vegetarian (vegan) diets, or intestinal blind loops with bacterial overgrowth. The most common cause, however, is a lack of the intrinsic factor necessary for vitamin B$_{12}$ absorption into the terminal ileum. This condition leads to classic **pernicious anemia.**

    (2) Folic acid deficiency is caused by dietary deficiency due to inadequate intake, inadequate absorption, or both. This condition is most commonly encountered in alcoholics.

    (3) Drug-induced disorders of DNA synthesis. Certain drugs used to treat cancer (e.g., methotrexate), bacterial infections (e.g., trimethoprim), and parasitic infections (e.g., pyrimethamine) as well as phenytoin interfere with folic acid metabolism and cause megaloblastic anemia and bone marrow changes. These diagnoses can be made easily from patient history.

  b. Clinical manifestations. Patients with megaloblastic anemia have varying degrees of anemia associated with large red blood cells. Because nucleic acid metabolism is necessary for all cellular elements in bone marrow, white blood cells and platelets are diminished. The ineffective erythropoiesis and intramedullary hemolysis associated with this disorder often result in serum **lactate dehydrogenase (LDH)** levels that exceed 500 units/dl. Both red and white blood cells in bone marrow reveal the classic megaloblastic sign of immature, open nuclei in association with mature cytoplasmic components. Blood smear shows characteristic oval macrocytes and hypersegmented polymorphonuclear leukocytes.

  c. Differential diagnosis

    (1) Serum levels of vitamins as well as red blood cell folic acid levels should be measured to determine whether the deficiency is in folic acid or vitamin B$_{12}$.

    (2) Vitamin B$_{12}$ has a neurologic function; therefore, when a macrocytic anemia is associated with neurologic symptoms, particularly posterior column signs and symptoms, vitamin B$_{12}$ deficiency should be suspected. The hallmarks of pernicious anemia are macrocytic anemia, neurologic symptoms and signs, and **atrophic glossitis.**

    (3) The **Schilling test** for the presence of intrinsic factor and intestinal function should be performed to differentiate the cause of vitamin B$_{12}$ deficiency.

  d. Therapy. Specific therapy is determined by the vitamin that is missing. Folic acid alone should never be given in an undiagnosed case of macrocytic anemia; folic acid reverses hematologic signs, but neurologic degeneration continues unabated.

    (1) Patients with pernicious anemia due to vitamin B$_{12}$ deficiency require lifelong treatment with parenteral vitamin B$_{12}$. If reversible causes are found (e.g., intestinal bacterial overgrowth), appropriate measures may reverse the deficiency and obviate the need for permanent vitamin B$_{12}$ therapy.

    (2) Folic acid deficiency is treated with oral preparations of folic acid.

C. **Normochromic, normocytic anemias** represent a vast array of conditions characterized by normal cell size and hemoglobin concentration. These anemias are not related by common pathogenic mechanisms; **classification is by the degree of marrow response to the anemia.**

  1. Anemia associated with impaired marrow response. The following anemias are characterized by normal or low reticulocyte counts.

  a. Hypoplastic, or aplastic anemia, is an intrinsic marrow disease characterized by an absence of stem cells. All myeloid (derived from the bone marrow) cell lines are involved, with a resultant **pancytopenia.** Severe cases of this serious disease are associated with a high mortality rate. Levels of serum erythropoietin are usually elevated proportionately to the degree of anemia. There is little effective medical treatment for this disease. In young patients, bone marrow transplantation techniques are curative in cases in which an appropriate marrow donor is available.

  b. Disorders characterized by infiltration of bone marrow (myelophthisic anemias) include myeloma, carcinoma, and leukoerythroblastosis. Disruption of bone marrow architecture is common; a blood smear that reveals immature white blood cells and nucleated red blood cells is a clue to the presence of these conditions. A bone marrow aspirate and biopsy confirm the diagnosis in such cases.

  c. Anemia due to diminished erythropoietin secretion is the anemia of **chronic renal failure.** Erythropoietin is a protein–lipid molecule required by the marrow for adequate red blood cell formation. With severe kidney disease, the erythropoietin secreted by the kidneys is lost and anemia ensues. The degree of anemia roughly correlates with the degree of renal failure.

    (1) Proper attention to iron and folic acid stores is important in this group of patients, because deficiencies in these nutrients secondarily complicate the anemia of renal failure.

    (2) Erythropoietin has been uniformly effective in raising the hemoglobin to normal or near normal levels in these patients, and this increase in hemoglobin has translated into an enhanced quality of life for these patients.

  d. Other anemias associated with hypoproliferation of bone marrow include those associated with hypothyroidism, hypopituitarism, and liver disease.

2. Anemia associated with appropriately increased red blood cell production. The following anemias are characterized by an increased number of reticulocytes.

  a. Anemia following hemorrhage. An increased reticulocyte count is the normal marrow response in patients who bleed either overtly (eg., with surgery) or covertly (e.g., into the gastrointestinal tract) and have adequate iron stores. This condition can be confused with hemolysis; however, the clinical situation of a postoperative patient with a large resolving hematoma confirms the diagnosis of posthemorrhagic anemia.

  b. Hemolytic anemias represent conditions in which red blood cell survival is shortened. In most cases, the marrow is intrinsically normal; thus, adequate new red blood cells can be made, and the patients have elevated reticulocyte counts. Diagnostic of these anemias are signs of increased red blood cell destruction (e.g., shortened red blood cell half-life, elevated serum LDH, and reduced haptoglobin) combined with signs of accelerated marrow activity (e.g., elevated reticulocyte counts and erythroid hyperplasia in the marrow). The diagnosis of hemolysis should be made first, and the specific cause of the hemolysis sought later. Hemolytic anemia exists in hundreds of forms, which are grouped as follows.

    (1) Hemolytic anemia due to factors extrinsic to the red blood cell

      (a) Autoantibodies can attach to the red blood cell and cause its destruction by the reticuloendothelial system. A classic example is **Coombs-positive hemolytic anemia** due to either warm [immunoglobulin G (IgG)] or cold (IgM) antibodies. This anemia may be idiopathic or may arise as a complication of collagen disease or lymphoma. In severe cases, steroids and splenectomy may be required to control the anemia.

      (b) Exogenous agents, such as malarial organisms, can render the red blood cell liable to hemolysis.

      (c) Abnormalities in the circulation can cause premature destruction of red blood cells. The following are examples of such abnormalities; disorders associated with each condition are cited also.

        (i) Lipid abnormalities (spur-cell anemia in advanced liver disease)

        (ii) Fibrin deposition in the microvasculature with shearing of red blood cells [disseminated intravascular coagulation (DIC) syndrome]

        (iii) Red blood cell damage due to trauma from prosthetic heart valves

    (2) Hemolytic anemia due to factors intrinsic to the red blood cell. These disorders involve congenital abnormalities that render the red blood cell liable to hemolysis.

      (a) Membrane disorders include such conditions as **hereditary spherocytosis.** In this disorder, a defect in the membrane sodium–potassium–ATPase pump causes red blood cell swelling. This results in the characteristic finding on blood smear of small, round, hyperchromic red blood cells without the usual central pallor (i.e., spherocytes). These cells are osmotically fragile and are destroyed in the spleen. Splenectomy usually controls the anemia, although the red blood cell defect remains.

(b) Hemoglobin disorders—hemoglobinopathies. These diseases, of which more than 250 are known, are caused by point mutations in the DNA code related to variation in a single amino acid in the globin chains. Such amino acid changes cause a variety of structural and functional changes in the red blood cell. When amino acid changes occur in the inner hydrophobic structural portions of the hemoglobin molecule, unstable hemoglobin disease with low-grade hemolysis can result (e.g., Hb Zurich). Amino acid changes in the heme–oxygen binding areas of the molecule cause changes in oxygen affinity and give rise to the so-called polycythemic hemoglobinopathies (e.g., Hb Potomac). The most commonly encountered hemoglobinopathies involve amino acid changes near the surface of the globular hemoglobin molecule, which predispose the hemoglobin to polymerization. Such polymerization results in the hemoglobin becoming rigid, with subsequent membrane and cell shape changes. These affected red blood cells become liable to hemolysis.

(i) Hemoglobin S (Hb S). The most common hemoglobinopathy is Hb S, which causes **sickle cell anemia.** This disorder occurs in 1% of African Americans. The disease manifestations result from three major pathophysiologic aspects (Table 3-1). The polymerized hemoglobin severely deforms red blood cells and results in **severe, chronic hemolysis.** This manifests as severe, chronic anemia (with hemoglobin in a range from 5–10 g/dl); predisposition to aplastic crises associated with parvovirus and other infections; and elevated bilirubin levels with almost universal gallstone disease and frequent, chronic ulceration of the legs in the ankle area. **Predisposition to infection** has multiple causes, including splenic autoinfarction and diminished synthesis of opsonizing immunoglobulins. This predisposition results in frequent infections, especially with encapsulated microorganisms such as pneumococci and *Haemophilus* and *Salmonella* species. Occasionally, these infections can be overwhelming, causing sepsis and death within hours of onset. Finally, **acute episodes of pain ("painful crises")** are the principal symptom and cause of morbidity in patients with sickle cell disease. Painful crises are thought to be the result of microvascular occlusion with infarction resulting from local hyperviscosity associated with the rigid, deformed and abnormally adhesive sickle cells.

(ii) Other common hemoglobinopathies that cause less severe sickle syndromes, include hemoglobin C (Hb C), hemoglobin O (Hb O), and mixtures such as hemoglobin SC (Hb SC).

TABLE 3-1. Clinical Manifestations of Sickle Cell Anemia

Related to Chronic Hemolytic Anemia	Related to Abnormal Adhesions, Sickling, and Vaso-occlusion	Related to Increased Susceptibility to Infection
Normocytic anemia	Painful crises	Pneumococcal sepsis
Elevated bilirubin and LDH	Cerebrovascular accident	*Salmonella* sepsis
Gallstone disease	Acute and chronic cardiopulmonary disease (e.g., acute chest syndromes, cor pulmonale)	Osteomyelitis
	Priapism	
	Splenic autoinfarction	
	Skeletal changes (e.g., aseptic necrosis of the hip)	

LDH = lactate dehydrogenase

(iii) Diagnosis is confirmed by hemoglobin electrophoresis, which demonstrates the characteristic changes in mobility caused by specific amino acid changes.

(iv) Therapy, which is still not satisfactory, continues to evolve. **Supportive medical care** remains the cornerstone of effective therapy and includes transfusions when indicated (e.g., during hypoplastic crises and as a means of preventing recurrent strokes), proper fluid management and attention to hydration, and analgesics for the pain of microvascular occlusion. Appropriate **monitoring for** and treatment of the potentially fatal problem of **intercurrent infections** is crucial. In children, prophylactic penicillin has been shown to prevent 80% of potentially lethal cases of pneumococcal bacteremia. Similar generous use of antibiotics and pneumococcal vaccine in adults is recommended as well. Newer directions in therapy have been toward manipulation of the hemoglobin mix within the cell to diminish the propensity to polymerize. Hb F has been found to have an inhibitory effect on sickling. Certain agents stimulate Hb F production. The cytotoxic agent hydroxyurea has been the most extensively studied, and recent data suggest that enhancing Hb F levels using hydroxyurea results in less painful crises in selected cases. Finally, bone marrow transplantation, which results in phenotypic cure, has been reported in patients with coexisting sickle cell anemia and acute leukemia. As the technology of marrow transplantation evolves and becomes safer, such therapy may become an option. Patients with hemoglobinopathies with significant morbidity and mortality rates (e.g., sickle cell anemia) are candidates for **gene transfer therapy** as this technology is developed.

(c) Disorders of the cytoplasm and enzymes occur as congenital hemolytic anemias. A red blood cell lacks a nucleus and mitochondria when it leaves the marrow; therefore, a red blood cell must survive its 120-day life span with its given complement of enzymes. A deficient cell is hemolyzed earlier than a normal cell.

(i) Glucose-6-phosphate dehydrogenase (G6PD) deficiency is an extremely common X-linked disorder; more than 150 subtypes affect more than 100 million individuals worldwide. Deficient individuals are liable to oxidant stress, which occurs with infections and with certain drugs (e.g., sulfa drugs and quinine). Such oxidant stress results in denatured hemoglobin or Heinz bodies, which results in hemolysis of affected red blood cells. A deficiency of G6PD also destroys the reducing capacity of the red blood cells. It is believed that G6PD protects individuals from falciparum malaria; this disease is most common in endemic areas. **Diagnosis** is made by demonstrating Heinz bodies during an acute hemolytic anemia episode or by measuring abnormally low levels of enzyme in the steady state. Enzyme levels should not be measured during a hemolytic episode when they may temporarily become more normal due to destruction of old, extremely deficient cells and due to their replacement by relatively G6PD-rich reticulocytes and neocytes.

(ii) Pyruvate kinase (PK) deficiency is an autosomal recessive example of an enzymopathy. This deficiency is most common in northern European populations. Patients may benefit from splenectomy.

II. **HEMATOCRIT DISORDERS.** Increases in hematocrit are caused by either **increased red blood cell mass** or **decreased plasma volume.** The following discussion deals exclusively with disorders associated with abnormal elevation of hematocrit (i.e., hematocrit of 55% and above).

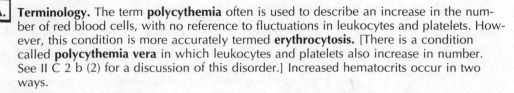

A. **Terminology.** The term **polycythemia** often is used to describe an increase in the number of red blood cells, with no reference to fluctuations in leukocytes and platelets. However, this condition is more accurately termed **erythrocytosis.** [There is a condition called **polycythemia vera** in which leukocytes and platelets also increase in number. See II C 2 b (2) for a discussion of this disorder.] Increased hematocrits occur in two ways.

1. **Relative erythrocytosis** refers to an elevation of hematocrit due to diminished plasma volume; red blood cell mass remains normal in this condition.

2. **Absolute erythrocytosis** refers to an elevation of hematocrit due to a true increase in red blood cell mass.

B. **Pathophysiology.** Blood flow and viscosity are inversely proportional to hematocrit; therefore, an excessively elevated hematocrit can diminish tissue blood flow, decrease tissue oxygen delivery, and increase cardiac work. In extreme cases, this can result in hyperviscosity syndromes.

C. **Classification**

1. **Relative erythrocytosis** exists in two forms.
   a. **Stress erythrocytosis,** or **Gaisböck's syndrome,** occurs predominantly in middle-aged men. This disorder usually is asymptomatic, although it may be associated with increased cardiovascular disease. It is important to differentiate patients with stress erythrocytosis from those with early and subtle manifestations of the much more serious condition polycythemia vera; the former group requires no treatment.
   b. **Erythrocytosis occurs secondary to known causes of contracted plasma volume** (e.g., excessive diuresis; nasogastric drainage; severe gastroenteritis, especially in infants; and burns). These conditions are apparent clinically; therapy includes fluid and plasma replacement with treatment of the underlying condition.

2. **Absolute erythrocytosis** is classified according to the mechanism responsible for increased red blood cell mass.
   a. **Hypoxia**
      (1) **Etiology.** Causes include severe lung disease, severe heart failure, cyanotic heart disease with right-to-left cardiopulmonary shunts, and abnormal hemoglobins with increased oxygen affinity.
      (2) **Pathophysiology.** The red blood cell mass rises secondary to tissue hypoxia, which causes an increase in renal erythropoietin and subsequently a hematocrit elevation.
      (3) **Diagnosis** may be apparent clinically, but blood gas analysis showing arterial oxygen saturation less than 92% and P_{50} analysis (i.e., studies of the oxygen-releasing characteristics of hemoglobin) may be required to confirm the diagnosis.
      (4) **Therapy** is somewhat conjectural, but phlebotomy is a favored treatment for patients with hematocrits that are persistently greater than 55%.
   b. **Neoplasia**
      (1) **Neoplastic erythropoietin sources** cause the red blood cell mass to increase.
         (a) **Etiology.** Causes include hypernephroma and renal cysts; such renal pathology accounts for more than 90% of this type of erythrocytosis. Other tumors include cerebellar hemangioblastoma, hepatoma, and uterine fibroids.
         (b) **Diagnosis** requires radiologic demonstration of the appropriate tumor with intravenous pyelography, computed tomography (CT), or ultrasound techniques. Reasonably accurate assays for erythropoietin are becoming available and demonstrate extremely elevated titers from autonomous erythropoietin secretion by these tumors.
         (c) **Therapy.** Removal of the tumor corrects the hematocrit.

(2) Autonomous bone marrow

(a) In the condition **polycythemia vera,** the bone marrow becomes autonomous and synthesizes cells independently of erythropoietin levels. (Theoretically, erythropoietin levels should be near zero if measured accurately.) Polycythemia vera represents a true neoplasm of the marrow stem cells.

(i) Diagnosis. According to the Polycythemia Vera Study Group, diagnosis is confirmed by the presence of all three of the following **major criteria** or by the first two major criteria and any two of the following **minor criteria.**

The major criteria are elevated red blood cell mass, arterial oxygen saturation exceeding 92%, and splenomegaly.

The minor criteria are leukocytosis, thrombocytosis, elevated leukocyte alkaline phosphatase (LAP), and elevated serum vitamin B_{12} level.

(ii) Therapy involves removal of red blood cells, suppression of marrow function, or both.

Phlebotomy removes red blood cells and should be performed to lower hematocrit to below 50%. If used alone, this is the safest therapy. Marrow suppression is needed when hematocrit control requires frequent phlebotomy or when other cell lines are elevated.

Radioactive phosphorus effectively modulates marrow activity and is well tolerated. This treatment is especially good for elderly patients.

Chemotherapy with the antimetabolite hydroxyurea is used to control many cases of polycythemia vera. Few if any leukemogenic or second malignancy–inducing effects have been encountered with this agent.

(iii) Survival is measured in years and is 7–10 years in most studies. Untreated polycythemia vera, however, has a survival of only 2–3 years. The major causes of morbidity and mortality are thromboembolic and cardiovascular in nature. Leukemic transformation, occurs in 5%–10% of patients.

(b) A pathophysiologically related disorder is **myelofibrosis,** a chronic myeloproliferative disorder characterized by splenomegaly, immature granulocytes and erythrocytes in the blood, distorted tear-drop–shaped red cell forms, and marrow fibrosis.

The disease is a **monoclonal stem cell disease** of primitive hematopoietic stem cells. The **fibrosis** is a secondary event.

Anemia and signs and symptoms of **massive splenomegaly** are the hallmarks of the disease.

Most **therapy is supportive.** In selected cases of true hypersplenism and symptoms from massive splenomegaly, splenectomy is beneficial.

D. **Therapeutic approach** (Table 3-2)

TABLE 3-2. Therapeutic Approach to Elevated Hematocrit Levels

Hematocrit	Significance	Comments
55%–60%	Begin to see decreased cardiac output and oxygen delivery; begin to see decreased cerebral blood flow	Consider elective phlebotomy to lower hematocrit
> 60%	Marked increased in blood viscosity; patient may be overtly symptomatic	Clear indication for phlebotomy; in polycythemia vera, marrow suppression may be needed

III. **WHITE BLOOD CELL DISORDERS.** The white blood cells include lymphocytes, monocytes, eosinophils, basophils, and neutrophils (polymorphonuclear leukocytes). Disorders of white blood cells can be considered in terms of excessive or reduced numbers of cells and in terms of functional abnormality.

A. **Lymphocytes** exist in marrow as well as in the lymphoid tissue of the body. Lymphocyte functions include delayed hypersensitivity, which is performed by T lymphocytes (**T cells),** and antibody production, which is performed by B lymphocytes (**B cells)** and plasma cells.

1. **Lymphopenia** refers to a diminished number of lymphocytes.
   a. **Lymphopenia without significant immune deficiency** is seen in many illnesses that cause elevated serum cortisol levels, such as acute infections and inflammatory states. Also, chemotherapy, radiotherapy, and Hodgkin's disease are associated with lymphopenia. In none of these conditions is antibody production severely affected.
   b. **Congenital lymphopenia with immune deficiency** is associated with specific immune deficiency syndromes.
      (1) **Varieties**
         (a) **B-cell deficiency**
            (i) **Bruton's agammaglobulinemia** is an X-linked disease characterized by recurrent infections with encapsulated organisms and caused by deficient quantities of opsonizing antibody. Although peripheral lymphocyte counts may be normal, specific counting for B cells shows their absence. Also, lymphoid follicles reveal no germinal centers, which are the B-cell areas. Therapy consists of exogenous gamma globulin and plasma via transfusion.
            (ii) **Other B-cell deficiency states** include common variable hypogammaglobulinemia and IgA deficiency.
         (b) **T-cell deficiency. Thymic hypoplasia** (DiGeorge syndrome) is the prototypical T-cell deficiency syndrome. Patients with this condition have variable total lymphocyte counts but low numbers of T cells with absent T-cell function. Recurrent fungal infections are seen in these patients.
         (c) **Deficiency of both B and T cells.** Disorders characterized by diminished numbers of both B and T cells include ataxia–telangiectasia syndrome, Wiskott-Aldrich syndrome of immunodeficiency and thrombocytopenia, and severe combined immunodeficiency disease (SCID).
      (2) **Diagnosis.** For all of the conditions discussed, diagnosis requires the clinical setting of repeated infections combined with:
         (a) Lymphocyte counts of B and T cells, including surface subset markers.
         (b) Measurement of specific immunoglobulin levels
         (c) Demonstration of the absence of specific B-cell areas (i.e., germinal centers and plasma cells) or T-cell areas (i.e., thymus and lymph node medullary cords)
      (3) **Therapy. Bone marrow transplantation** has been curative in many of these conditions.
   c. **Acquired immune deficiency syndrome (AIDS)** is discussed in Chapter 8.

2. **Lymphocytosis** is defined as an excessive number of lymphocytes (i.e., $>5000/\mu$l). The differential diagnosis of absolute lymphocytosis is limited.
   a. **Infection.** Certain infections cause lymphocytosis. In children, both pertussis and acute infectious lymphocytosis may cause counts that exceed 50,000. In adults, lesser elevations are seen with hepatitis and infectious mononucleosis.
   b. **Hematopoietic disorders** associated with lymphocytosis include acute lymphocytic leukemia, chronic lymphocytic leukemia, and certain lymphomas.
      (1) **Chronic lymphocytic leukemia (CLL).** An adult who is older than 50 years and who manifests a mature lymphocytosis most likely has CLL. The cells associated with CLL are mature lymphocytes that accumulate in the body.
         (a) **Diagnosis.** A peripheral blood smear showing a mature lymphocytosis is

adequate. Corroborative findings include marrow infiltration by mature lymphocytes, an enlarged spleen, and lymphadenopathy. Lymphocyte markers can also be determined. The technique of flow cytometry is diagnostic.

    (b) Staging. The CLL tumor burden is related to certain clinical findings, which also have prognostic significance.

        (i) Stage 0 is characterized by peripheral lymphocytosis only. The prognosis for patients with stage 0 CLL is excellent; patients usually survive 10–12 years.

        (ii) Stages 1 and 2. Stage 1 is characterized by peripheral lymphocytosis and lymphadenopathy; stage 2 is characterized by the presence of splenomegaly. Both stages 1 and 2 have intermediate prognoses, with patient survival rate of usually 4–7 years.

        (iii) Stages 3 and 4. Stage 3 is characterized by the presence of anemia and stage 4 by the presence of thrombocytopenia. Both stages 3 and 4 signify marrow failure and have ominous prognoses, with patient survival rate of approximately 18 months.

    (c) Therapy for CLL is conservative. The chance of survival is not significantly improved with any known treatment. Excessive therapy can be harmful.

        (i) Early-stage CLL. As a rule, stages 1 and 2 CLL should not be treated.

        (ii) Late-stage CLL is treated with an alkylating agent (e.g., chlorambucil), with or without steroids. Low-dose total body irradiation also is used. The antimetabolite, fludarabine, is used in patients in whom therapy with alkylating agents fails; it is being evaluated as a frontline agent for treating CLL.

  (2) Certain well-differentiated **lymphomas** also are characterized by an excessive number of lymphocytes in the blood. These disorders are similar to CLL.

  (3) Acute lymphocytic leukemia (ALL) is characterized by maturation arrest in the lymphoid line with tissue infiltration by lymphoblasts. (This disease is discussed in more detail in IV A.)

  3. Monocytosis and monocytopenia. Monocytes are **phagocytic cells** that are an important component of the cellular immune system and that secrete many cytokines, including TNF, all of the interferons, GM–colony-stimulating factor (GM-CSF) and G-CSF.

    a. Isolated monocytopenia does not occur. Monocytopenia in combination with decreases in other cell lines occurs with aplastic anemia, hairy cell leukemia, and steroid use.

    b. Benign monocytosis can occur in many infectious diseases [e.g., tuberculosis, subacute bacterial endocarditis (SBE), cytomegalovirus] and inflammatory diseases (e.g., rheumatoid arthritis and sarcoid). The finding is nonspecific.

    c. Monocytosis can accompany essentially all of the hematologic and lymphatic malignancies.

B. **Basophils, eosinophils, and neutrophils.** Disorders in these cells also are classified according to fluctuations in cell numbers and to functional deficiency.

  1. Basophils. An abnormally increased number of basophils is called **basophilia.** This uncommon condition usually is associated with the myeloproliferative syndromes, particularly chronic myelogenous leukemia (CML).

  2. Eosinophils. An abnormally increased number of eosinophils is called **eosinophilia.** This condition is more common than basophilia and occurs secondary to other disease processes, including:

    a. Neoplasia (e.g., lymphoma and Hodgkin's disease)

    b. Addison's disease

    c. Allergic and atopic disease (most common cause of eosinophilia)

    d. Collagen vascular disease (e.g., necrotizing vasculitis)

    e. Parasitic infestation

3. Neutrophils

a. **Neutrophilia** is an excessively increased number of neutrophils in the blood. The following are causes of neutrophilia.

   (1) Most cases of neutrophilia result from conditions such as infection, tumor, stress, collagen disorders, and steroids; the underlying disease may not be apparent clinically.

   (2) In unusual cases, more than 50,000 neutrophils/μl appear in the blood. These so-called **leukemoid reactions** can be differentiated from the leukemias by the absence of the circulating blast forms and by the finding of elevated LAP values.

   (3) Neutrophilia also results from **neoplastic marrow diseases,** such as polycythemia vera and CML.

   (a) **Diagnosis of CML.** CML is suspected in patients with excessive white blood cell counts and splenomegaly. Peripheral blood smears reveal a spectrum of cell forms ranging from mature polymorphonuclear neutrophils to immature blasts. Two findings confirm the diagnosis: the presence of an abnormal marker chromosome (the **Philadelphia chromosome**) in the marrow precursor cells and very low LAP levels. The fusion protein of the abnormal gene in CML is detectable as is the abnormal genetic material itself.

   (b) **Prognosis of CML.** The median survival rate for CML patients is 3–4 years. Most patients die during the so-called **blast crisis,** when this chronic disorder converts into a highly malignant variety of acute leukemia.

   (i) **Hydroxyurea** is an effective palliative agent that reduces the leukemia cell burden in the chronic phase of CML.

   (ii) α-**Interferon** (α-**IFN**) administered three times weekly also induces remission in many patients. In some cases, it can convert the patient's marrow to Philadelphia chromosome–negative status and may be curative.

   (iii) **Marrow transplantation** is curative and is the therapy of choice for younger patients (see IV D 3).

b. **Neutropenia** is an absolute decrease in the number of circulating neutrophils. Neutropenia occurs rarely as an early manifestation of intrinsic marrow disease (e.g., acute leukemia) but more commonly occurs secondary to exogenous stimuli.

   (1) **Infections.** Certain viral infections (e.g., hepatitis and influenza) and bacterial infections (e.g., typhoid fever) cause neutropenia.

   (2) **Drugs** (e.g., phenothiazines, fluoxetine, and antithyroid medications) are associated with neutropenia and, in severe instances, can cause agranulocytosis. Agranulocytosis is characterized by:

   (a) Profoundly lowered neutrophil counts (i.e., $<500/\mu$l)

   (b) Severe prostration, high fever, and often a necrotic pharyngitis

   (c) Bone marrow showing **maturation arrest** (i.e., large numbers of immature white blood cell forms in an otherwise normal marrow)

   (d) High mortality rates unless treated early and aggressively with support measures and potent bactericidal antibiotics. Use of genetically engineered CSF and other marrow growth factors has been encouraging.

   (3) The **collagen vascular diseases** [e.g., systemic lupus erythematosus (SLE) and RA] have been shown to cause neutropenia via immune destruction of white blood cells.

   (4) **Familial forms of neutropenia** include familial benign chronic neutropenia, cyclic neutropenia, and chronic idiopathic neutropenia. These disorders have good prognoses, although they are associated with increased nuisance infections (e.g., boils) when the neutrophil count is less than $500/\mu$l. They respond well to G-CSF.

   (5) **Chemotherapeutic agents** used in the therapy of malignant disease are the most common cause of neutropenia. Such agents include alkylating agents (e.g., cyclophosphamide), antimetabolites [e.g., methotrexate, 5-fluorouracil

(5-FU), and cytosine arabinoside], and tumor antibiotics (e.g., doxorubicin). Chemotherapy-induced neutropenia can be markedly ameliorated in difficult cases by the judicious use of G-CSF.

c. **Functional disorders** of neutrophils involve a compromised ability to fight infection. These conditions are rare; affected individuals have recurrent infections. The following are prototypical examples.

(1) **Chédiak-Higashi syndrome** is an autosomal recessive disorder characterized by albinism and increased pyogenic infection. Also, neutrophils and other granule-containing cells (e.g., melanosomes) reveal giant, fused, peroxidase-staining granules with decreased ability to kill ingested microbes.

(2) **Chronic granulomatous disease (CGD)** of childhood is an X-linked disorder in neutrophil metabolism characterized by a defect in neutrophil-free radical formation (associated with the oxidative burst and killing activity in neutrophils), resulting in susceptibility to recurrent suppurative infections. This condition often is fatal, and the diagnosis is confirmed by the presence of neutrophils that cannot oxidize nitroblue tetrazolium dye to blue-black from colorless. Bone marrow transplantation has been effective in these cases.

IV. **ACUTE LEUKEMIAS.** These disorders in the maturation of hematopoietic tissue are characterized by the presence of immature leukocytes in the marrow and peripheral blood. The immature cells are arrested in the earliest phases of differentiation and are referred to as **blasts.**

A. **Classification and epidemiology.** It is important both prognostically and therapeutically to distinguish the lymphocytic from the nonlymphocytic (myelogenous) leukemias. Classification of cells involves special histochemical stains (e.g., peroxidase in myelogenous leukemia), marker enzymes (e.g., terminal transferase in acute lymphocytic leukemia), and specific cell-surface antigenic markers; use of these methods in combination allows classification that approaches 95% accuracy. Cytogenetic analysis, marker chromosome defects, and chromosomal banding techniques have even further refined and made more accurate classification of acute leukemias. In addition, such chromosomal groupings appear to identify subgroups within specific leukemia types that have different responses to therapy and different prognoses.

1. **Acute lymphocytic leukemia (ALL)** is common in children: 85% of cases of ALL occur in children, and 90% of leukemia that occurs in children is ALL. Conversely, ALL is not a common leukemia in adults. The ALL cell origin is in the lymphoid line. Techniques such as membrane surface markers and antibody detection of surface antigens have enabled investigators to characterize ALL subsets.

a. The most common ALL variant (comprising 75% of cases) is of B-cell lineage of null variety (i.e., there is absent rosette formation). This variant also expresses the common ALL antigen (CALLA) on the cell surface.

b. T-cell ALL and other less common varieties comprise the remainder of cases.

c. Most ALL varieties express terminal deoxynucleotidyl transferase (TdT), and staining for this enzyme is useful in differentiating ALL from myelogenous leukemias.

d. Differentiating subtypes has prognostic significance in that, for example, T-cell varieties of ALL are more resistant to therapy and have far worse prognoses than common variety B-cell ALL.

2. **Acute myelogenous leukemia (AML),** or **acute nonlymphocytic leukemia (ANLL),** is common in adults, and the incidence increases with age. Specific environmental risks increase AML incidence in populations. They include moderate to high doses of ionizing radiation, chemicals such as benzene and petroleum products, and prior exposure to cytotoxic chemotherapy agents such as alkylating drugs (e.g., cyclophosphamide and chlorambucil). The AML cell of origin probably arises at different levels of hematopoiesis in different patients, which accounts for the clinically well-defined subtypes of AML. In most cases, the AML clone arises from multipotential precursors

TABLE 3-3. French–American–British (FAB) Classification of Acute Myelogenous Leukemia (AML)*

Designation	Description	Comments
M0	Acute myeloid leukemia lacking myeloid differentiation, with reactivity with myeloid antigens or ultrastructural evidence of peroxidase-positive blasts	. . .
M1	Acute myeloid leukemia without maturation	. . .
M2	Acute myeloid leukemia with maturation	. . .
M3	Promyelocytic leukemia	Characterized by abnormal promyelocytes with giant granules; often associated with DIC; prognosis likely better than with other forms of AML
M4	Acute myelomonocytic leukemia	Characterized by cerebriform monoblasts; extramedullary involvement common (e.g., spleen, gums); hyperleukocytosis (>50,000 cells/μl) and CNS involvement common; prognosis worse than most other forms of AML
M5	Acute monocytic leukemia	Characterized by cerebriform monoblasts; extramedullary involvement common (e.g., spleen, gums); hyperleukocytosis (>50,000 cells/μl) and CNS involvement common; prognosis worse than most other forms of AML
M6	Erythroleukemia	Erythroid precursors involved; abnormal multinucleated RBC blasts in marrow
M7	Acute megakaryocytic leukemia	Uncommon variant associated with fibrosis in marrow, bizarre platelets on smear, poor response to therapy, and poor prognosis

CNS = central nervous system; DIC = disseminated intravascular coagulation; RBC = red blood cell.
* As modified by the National Cancer Institute Workshop.

capable of differentiating into granulocyte, erythrocyte, macrophage, or megakaryo-cyte colony-forming units (CFU-GEMM). Therefore, in most patients, lymphoid and erythroid lineages are not involved in the leukemic process. Several different categories of AML with distinctive cellular and clinical characteristics have been long recognized (Table 3-3).

B. **Clinical features** of acute leukemia represent the effects of marrow infiltration by nonmaturing, functionless blast cells, including subsequent bone marrow failure.

1. **Physical findings** include fatigue and pallor (due to anemia); fever and infection (due to neutropenia); petechiae, purpura, and epistaxis (due to thrombocytopenia). Infiltrative symptoms may include splenomegaly, gum hypertrophy, and bone pain.

2. **Laboratory findings** include almost universal pancytopenia and circulating blast forms. Increased cell turnover results in elevated uric acid levels. In promyelocytic

leukemia, DIC is usually present with hypofibrinogenemia and elevated fibrin split products.

C. **Diagnosis.** The diagnosis of acute leukemia is confirmed by the finding of blast infiltration of the bone marrow. Special histochemical stains (e.g., peroxidase, Sudan black), enzyme markers (e.g., TdT), surface antigenic markers, and chromosome cytogenetic studies are performed to identify the specific subtype of leukemia involved.

D. **Therapy** of acute leukemia is complex. **Medical regimens** achieve complete remission in 65%–70% of all patients with de novo AML and appear to cure 25% of these. Therapy carries a 20% early mortality rate and is, therefore, best performed by physicians who are experienced with the drugs used and the supportive care needed to maintain the patient through the induction period and to achieve remissions. **Marrow transplantation** has higher cure rates in patients eligible for this therapy.

  1. **Chemotherapy.** Initial therapy consists of chemotherapeutic ablation of the leukemic cell line. In many cases, especially those of AML, it is necessary to ablate all normal marrow as well. Because normal marrow has a shorter generation time than leukemic blasts, recovery with normal marrow tissue is possible. This initial marrow ablation is termed **induction therapy.**
     a. **ALL induction therapy.** ALL blasts are initially more selectively sensitive to chemotherapy than AML blasts. It often is possible to destroy ALL blasts with some sparing of normal marrow. Thus, induction therapy for ALL is associated with lower morbidity and mortality rates than it is for AML.
        (1) Combinations of vincristine, prednisone, anthracyclines, and L-asparaginase are used to obtain initial remissions.
        (2) Consolidation therapy and a period of less intensive maintenance therapy with agents such as mercaptopurine and methotrexate are effective.
        (3) Treatment of potential sanctuary sites, such as the central nervous system (CNS), is required in many cases of ALL.
        (4) Bone marrow transplantation has a role, usually after initial relapse. Chemotherapy has excellent results in ALL, far superior to those in AML, especially in children younger than 15 years in whom the cure rate approaches 80%. In adults, complete remission rates of 80% can be achieved, usually for longer than 2 years. However, only 15%–20% of these patients remain in remission.
     b. **AML induction therapy** requires ablation of all marrow elements, both blasts and normal tissue. The best available regimen remains cytosine arabinoside and an anthracycline antibiotic. More aggressive administration of cycles of chemotherapy after induction to eliminate residual leukemic cells does prolong the remission duration and is beneficial. Data indicate that:
        (1) AML populations will have a 60%–70% complete response rate to induction regimens.
        (2) With varying postinduction regimens, the median response duration is 12–15 months, with 25%–35% of these patients experiencing 24-month disease-free survival.
        (3) Of the AML population, 15%–25% are alive 2 years after their diagnosis. Some of these will relapse, and some will be "cured."

  2. **Radiotherapy** is used in ALL to sterilize sanctuary sites of late relapse. Such sites are found in the CNS and, possibly, in the testes.

  3. **Bone marrow transplantation** has emerged as definitive, curative therapy for acute leukemia. Bone marrow transplantation usually is used after the first remission has been obtained. The goal of marrow transplantation is to eradicate permanently the residual leukemia and prevent relapse. Ultra–high-dose chemotherapy alone or with radiotherapy prior to marrow transplantation may be given in doses that are not limited by concerns of toxicity to the marrow, because the subsequent marrow infusion and transplantation rescues the patient from the marrow toxicities that these therapies produce.

a. Suitable donors are a prerequisite for successful marrow transplantation. Identical twin donors are optimal but rare. The most common donors (35%) are human leukocyte antigen (HLA)-matched siblings.

b. When no matched donors are available, autologous marrow infusion of harvested and stored remission marrow has accrued improving survival rates. A recent review demonstrated a 48% survival rate at 4 years in patients transplanted in first remission. The major cause of failure is recurrent leukemia after transplantation. Various marrow purging techniques to remove leukemic cells are under study.

c. Graft-versus-host disease (GVHD) is a major obstacle encountered in marrow transplantation. This reaction results from the grafting of immunocompetent donor T cells, which respond to alloantigens expressed on host cells.

   (1) Major target organs are skin (dermatitis), gastrointestinal tract (diarrhea), and liver.

   (2) Therapy may be prolonged and usually consists of some combination of prednisone, cyclosporine, and low-dose azathioprine.

d. Other important post-transplantation factors include the toxicity of the preparative regimens, interstitial pneumonitis, other infections, graft rejection (rare), and hepatic veno-occlusive disease.

4. **Supportive therapy** is extremely important and serves as a prototype for supportive therapy in other forms of neoplasia. The following principles apply to the use of chemotherapy regimens as well as to bone marrow ablation and transplantation.

   a. The **hemoglobin level** should be maintained above 8 g/dl by transfusions of packed red blood cells.

   b. **Hemorrhage is best prevented** by prophylactic transfusion of platelet concentrates. Although serious spontaneous bleeding is unusual unless the platelet count declines below 10,000/μl, most physicians prefer to maintain platelet counts above 20,000/μl. This practice has lowered the incidence of fatal hemorrhage in acute leukemia from 80% to less than 20%.

   c. **Control of infection** is a major determinant of survival of patients being treated for the acute leukemia that is caused by drug-induced neutropenia.

      (1) **Isolation techniques have been tested as a means of avoiding infection.** Totally protected environments decrease incidence of infections but have little impact on remissions and survival. Such environments feature expensive laminar flow rooms, sterilized food, and gut sterilization by nonabsorbable antibiotics. Many physicians do not use these methods but instead maintain strict hand-washing and skin-care techniques, use long-term central catheters to avoid peripheral indwelling lines, and practice strict rectal care to achieve similar results.

      (2) **Infections are treated early and aggressively.** Neutropenic patients (those with polymorphonuclear leukocytes <500/μl) are susceptible to all organisms, especially gram-negative rods and fungi (e.g., *Candida, Aspergillus*).

         (a) Initial temperature elevations require thorough clinical evaluation, vigorous cultures, and immediate and empiric treatment with broad-spectrum bactericidal antibiotic combinations of cephalosporins, aminoglycosides (e.g., tobramycin), and semisynthetic penicillins (e.g., piperacillin).

         (b) Secondary temperature elevations that occur after treatment with potent broad-spectrum antibiotics may require the empiric use of antifungal agents (e.g., amphotericin B). The possible role for prevention of fungal infections with prophylactic triazoles (e.g., fluconazole) is being evaluated.

         (c) Attention to electrolytes and uric acid is required in those patients with high cell turnover and in those receiving multiple antibiotics.

            (i) Treatment with allopurinol and adequate fluids is required for uric acid control.

            (ii) Electrolyte levels, especially the potassium level, must be maintained in patients being given antibiotics.

   d. **Stimulation of marrow recovery** using growth factors made by recombinant DNA technology is finding a role in supportive therapy. Myeloid CSFs have been shown to result in more rapid recovery of polymorphonuclear leukocyte counts in

AML patients treated with either chemotherapy of bone marrow transplantation. G-CSF is administered 3–4 days after discontinuing induction therapy and accelerates recovery of normal myelopoiesis. Whether this maneuver improves the patient's chance of survival is controversial.

E. **Prognosis**

1. The prognosis for children with **ALL is very good;** more than 95% obtain complete remission. Approximately 70%–80% of patients are disease free at 5 years and are likely cured. If relapse occurs, second complete remissions can be obtained in most cases. Patients in second remissions are candidates for marrow transplantation, with 35%–65% survival probability long term.

2. The prognosis for patients with **AML is poor.** Among patients receiving the best care, using current chemotherapy regimens, 75% obtain complete remission and 25% die. Furthermore, the usual duration of remission is only 12–18 months. Although some investigators claim 20% cure rates using intensive postremission therapy, there is little common experience with significant cure rates. In patients younger than 30 years, bone marrow transplantation, both allogeneic and autologous, is the treatment of choice after obtaining a first complete remission. Current results indicate that 50% of young patients with AML who undergo allogeneic bone marrow transplantation experience prolonged disease-free intervals and may be cured. Similar encouraging results are accruing for autologous bone marrow transplantation rates. As better ways to prevent GVHD evolve, the morbidity and mortality rates associated with allogeneic bone marrow transplantation should decline and curability for patients with AML should increase.

V. **DISORDERS OF COAGULATION AND HEMOSTASIS**

A. **General considerations.** Hemostasis requires an intact coagulation system of vascular and tissue components, platelets, and coagulation proteins. Deficiency or disease of any of these components may cause either spontaneous or trauma-related hemorrhage.

1. **History.** A careful history provides clues to the pathogenesis of bleeding. Immediate, mucocutaneous bleeding suggests vascular or platelet disease; delayed deep-tissue bleeding and hemarthrosis suggest coagulation protein deficiency. Genetic transmissions of bleeding disorders (e.g., the X-linked hemophilias) also are elicited by history, as is ingestion of drugs (e.g., aspirin).

2. **Physical findings** aid in differentiation of bleeding syndromes. Mucocutaneous petechiae and purpura suggest platelet disorders; hematomas and hemarthrosis suggest coagulopathy.

3. **Laboratory testing** is vital in the evaluation of bleeding disorders. Single tests rarely provide conclusive results, so various batteries of tests have been developed. The coagulation cascade is shown in Figure 3-1, the interpretation of common tests of hemostasis and blood coagulation is shown in Table 3-4, and the diagnosis of common bleeding disorders based on commonly used tests is shown in Table 3-5.

B. **Disorders of blood vessels and vascular tissues.** The following bleeding disorders result from pathology in the vessel area itself, with secondary leakage of blood. Most of these disorders have as their hallmark a visible and usually palpable skin lesion. Testing performed on patients with these bleeding disorders reveals normal coagulation and, occasionally, increased bleeding times.

1. **Autoimmune (allergic) purpura (Henoch-Schönlein purpura)** occurs most commonly in children and young adults.
   a. **Etiology.** The syndrome is associated with streptococcal infections and drugs (e.g., penicillin).

INTRINSIC SYSTEM

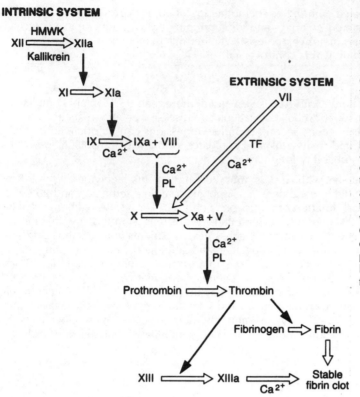

Figure 3-1. The coagulation cascade. Each coagulation factor, when activated, activates the next factor in the series. (Factors are numbered in order of their discovery, not in order of activation.) In the intrinsic system, factor XII is initially activated by an unknown mechanism and subsequently by kallikrein during the contact phase. Alternatively, factor VII and tissue factor can initiate the extrinsic system. Intrinsic and extrinsic pathways each end with activation of factor X, setting off a final, common pathway that ends with formation of the fibrin clot. Open *arrows* indicate conversion of a substrate or a reactant to a product. HMWK = high–molecular-weight kininogen; TF = tissue factor; PL = phospholipid.

TABLE 3-4. Interpretation of Common Tests of Hemostasis and Coagulation

Test	Normal Range (± SD)	Causes of Abnormalities
Platelet count	150–450,000/μl	Thrombocytopenia; thrombocytosis
Bleeding time (template method)	2.0–7.5 min	Thrombocytopenia; von Willebrand's disease; platelet dysfunction; vascular disorders
Partial thromboplastin time Standard Activated	60–90 sec 30–40 sec	Deficiencies or inhibitors of prekallikrein, HMWK; factors VIII, IX, XI, XII; lupus inhibitors; heparin
Plasma prothrombin time	11–14 sec	Deficiencies or inhibitors of factors V, VII, X, prothrombin; lupus inhibitors
Plasma thrombin time	12–20 sec	Hypofibrinogenemia; abnormal fibrinogens; heparin
Fibrinogen assay	160–450 mg/dl	Hypofibrinogenemia; abnormal fibrinogens
Fibrin degradation product assay	<10 μg/ml	DIC; fibrinogenolysis; liver disease

Adapted with permission from Wintrobe MM, et al: *Clinical Hematology*, 8th ed. Philadelphia, Lea and Febiger, 1981, p 1051.
DIC = disseminated intravascular coagulation; HMWK = high–molecular-weight kininogen; SD = standard deviation.

TABLE 3-5. Presumptive Diagnosis of Common Bleeding Disorders by Primary Screening Tests

Platelet Count	Bleeding Time	PTT	PT	Presumptive Diagnosis	Common Etiologies
Decreased	Prolonged	Normal	Normal	Thrombocytopenia	ITP; drugs
Normal	Prolonged	Prolonged	Normal	von Willebrand's disease	. . .
Normal	Prolonged	Normal	Normal	Thrombocytopathy	Drugs; uremia
Normal	Normal	Prolonged	Normal	Coagulopathy of intrinsic pathway	Hemophilia A or hemophilia B; factor VIII and lupus-type inhibitors
Normal	Normal	Prolonged	Prolonged	Coagulopathy of common or multiple pathways	Liver disease; vitamin K deficiency; DIC; heparin
Normal	Normal	Normal	Prolonged	Coagulopathy of extrinsic pathway	Factor VII deficiency
Normal	Normal	Normal	Normal	. . .	Hereditary telangiectasia; allergic purpura

Adapted with permission from Lee GR, et al: *Wintrobe's Clinical Hematology*, 9th ed. Philadelphia, Lea and Febiger, 1993, p 1315.
DIC = disseminated intravascular coagulation; ITP = idiopathic thrombocytopenic purpura; PTT = partial thromboplastin time; PT = prothrombin time.

    b. Clinical signs. Perivascular inflammatory lesions with serosanguinous leakage into the skin, submucosa, and serosa are the hallmark of the disease. The lesions are symmetric and palpable and are usually found on the distal extremities. Bowel lesions may cause gastrointestinal symptoms; joint lesions cause arthritis.

    c. Therapy and prognosis. No specific therapy is uniformly helpful. Prognosis is good, except in the 5%–10% of patients who develop glomerulonephritis.

2. Purpura associated with infections may be due to embolic occlusion of the microvasculature (e.g., endocarditis) or to endothelial injury by the infectious agent (e.g., *Rickettsia*). Biopsy and culture of the material may be helpful.

3. Structural malformations of vessels and vascular tissues are associated with the following conditions.

    a. Scurvy is caused by vitamin C deficiency; collagen synthesis is impaired as a result of this deficiency. Vessel walls with poor collagen support are pliable and easily ruptured.

        (1) Physical findings associated with scurvy include perifollicular petechiae, gum bleeding, and subperiosteal hemorrhages. Bleeding time usually is prolonged.

        (2) Therapy with 1 g/day of vitamin C rapidly corrects all bleeding.

    b. Hereditary hemorrhagic telangiectasia is an autosomal dominant disorder associated with abnormally thin vessel walls and impaired vascular contractility. Such vessels are markedly friable, liable to burst with trauma, and unable to contract appropriately for primary hemostasis.

        (1) Physical findings include small, nodular violaceous lesions on the lips, face, ears, tongue, and gastrointestinal mucosa; these lesions blanch upon pressure. Bleeding is common, especially gastrointestinal bleeding, with resultant iron deficiency anemia.

        (2) Diagnosis involves the association of three factors: recurrent hemorrhage, multiple telangiectases, and familial occurrence.

    c. Diminished collagen synthesis due to **steroid therapy** results in a syndrome of vascular fragility and skin bleeding.

4. Miscellaneous vascular conditions

    a. Paraproteinemias, including cryoglobulinemias and amyloidosis, are associated with skin bleeding. Diagnosis requires demonstration of the paraprotein.

    b. Senile purpura occurs in elderly individuals as a result of degeneration and loss of dermal collagen, elastin, and subcutaneous fat. This disorder is characterized by benign purpura of the arms, thought to be caused by shearing injury to blood vessels from the hypermobility of the skin on the thinned underlying tissue.

C. **Disorders of platelets.** Platelets play a role in the primary arrest of bleeding; abnormalities in these hemostatic components result in prolonged bleeding times and lead to hemorrhagic diathesis. Platelet abnormalities are classified according to disorders of number and function.

1. **Thrombocytopenia** (i.e., decreased numbers of platelets) is the **most common cause of abnormal bleeding.**
   a. **General considerations**
      (1) With a platelet count of less than 100,000/μl, bleeding time (and clinical bleeding, if the hemostatic system is stressed) begins to prolong. Most individuals experience petechiae or purpura with platelet counts between 50,000 and 20,000/μl. More serious spontaneous bleeding (e.g., gastrointestinal, CNS) may occur with platelet count of less than 10,000/μl.
      (2) Thrombocytopenia is an indication for a marrow examination, which reveals the presence of the platelet precursors, **megakaryocytes.** The absence of megakaryocytes indicates platelet production problems. The presence of megakaryocytes indicates either peripheral destruction of platelets or, in the presence of splenomegaly, splenic sequestration of platelets.
   b. **Mechanisms** of thrombocytopenia include impaired platelet production, abnormal platelet pooling, and increased peripheral destruction. Examples, marrow findings, and therapies are summarized in Table 3-6.
      (1) **Impaired platelet production**
         (a) **Etiology**
            (i) Megakaryocytes may be selectively suppressed by certain agents (e.g., thiazide diuretics, ethanol).
            (ii) A special cause of thrombocytopenia due to impaired platelet production is ineffective thrombopoiesis associated with the megaloblastic hematopoiesis seen in vitamin B_{12} and folate deficiencies as well as in cases of myelodysplastic and preleukemic syndromes. Megakaryocytes are present in marrow but are abnormal (megaloblastic or dysplastic) in morphology and function. Their platelets are abnormal and destroyed in the marrow.
            (iii) Another rare cause is amegakaryocytic thrombocytopenia caused by congenital deficiency of megakaryocyte colony-forming units (CFU-Meg).
         (b) **Diagnosis** is confirmed by a bone marrow smear that reveals marrow megakaryocytic hypoplasia.
         (c) **Therapy** involves removal of the offending agent, if possible, or treatment of the underlying disease. Patients have essentially normal platelet half-lives and should be transfused with exogenous platelets if they are thrombocytopenic and bleeding. Thrombocytopenia associated with vitamin B_{12} or folate deficiency is rapidly corrected by therapy with the deficient vitamin.
         (d) **Associated conditions**
            (i) Impaired platelet production is associated with aplastic anemia, myelophthisic processes with replacement of marrow by tumor or fibrosis, and certain rare congenital syndromes (e.g., rubella infection with absent radii).
            (ii) Amegakaryocytic thrombocytopenia has responded to therapies directed against the immune system, including antithymocyte globulin and cyclosporine. In these settings thrombocytopenia is associated with pancytopenia.
      (2) **Abnormal platelet pooling** results when platelets are sequestered from the circulation. **Splenic platelet sequestration** is the most common cause of abnormal platelet pooling.
         (a) **Pathophysiology.** Normally, the spleen holds one third of the circulating platelet pool. As splenomegaly occurs, higher numbers of platelets are sequestered and, thus, are unavailable for hemostasis. In very large spleens,

TABLE 3-6. Mechanisms of Thrombocytopenia

Mechanisms	Marrow Findings	Clinical Conditions	Therapy
Impaired production of platelets	Megakaryocytes reduced or absent	Induced chemically or physically (e.g., chemotherapy, radiation)	Removal of offending agents; supportive
		Aplastic anemia, paroxysmal nocturnal hemoglobinuria, leukemia	Marrow transplatation
		Infection (e.g., viral hepatitis cytomegalovirus, tuberculosis)	Treatment of infection
Ineffective production of platelets	Abnormal and/or dysplastic megakaryocytes	Megaloblastic disorder (vitamin B_{12} deficiency, folate deficiency)	B_{12} or folate supplementation
		Myelodysplasias and myeloproliferative disorders	Treatment of underlying disorder
Enhanced destruction of platelets (immune-mediated)	Increased megakaryocytes	Idiopathic thrombocytopenic purpura	See V C 1 b (3)
		Post-transfusion purpura	Plasmapheresis
		Drug-induced (e.g., rifampin, methicillin, sulfonamides, phenytoin, quinine, quinidine, heparin)	Removal of offending agent
		Lymphomas	Treatment of underlying disorder
		Immune complex disorder (e.g., systemic lupus erythematosus)	Steroids
Enhanced destruction of platelets (not immune-related)	Increased megakaryocytes	Thrombotic thrombocytopenic purpura	Plasmapheresis
		Hemolytic uremic syndrome	Plasmapheresis
		Disseminated intravascular coagulation	Treatment of underlying disorders
		Dilution and cardiopulmonary bypass	Supportive
		Splenomegaly	Usually not required; splenectomy may be necessary occasionally

as much as 90% of the platelet pool may be sequestered; however, platelets in the peripheral circulation do have normal survival times.

(b) **Diagnosis** of hypersplenism is suggested by a moderate thrombocytopenia (platelet counts of less than 40,000/μl are unusual), a bone marrow smear that reveals adequate marrow megakaryocytes, and evidence of significant splenic enlargement.

(c) **Clinical features** in such cases are dominated by the underlying illness causing the splenomegaly (e.g., cirrhosis with portal hypertension).

(d) **Therapy** usually is not required, although splenectomy may correct the problem. Transfused platelets are sequestered in the same ratio and are less effective than in hypoactive marrow states.

(3) **Increased peripheral destruction** of platelets is the **most common form of thrombocytopenia.** Conditions involving increased platelet destruction are characterized by shortened platelet survival and increased numbers of marrow megakaryocytes. **Idiopathic thrombocytopenic purpura (ITP)** is the prototypical immune-mediated thrombocytopenia; no apparent exogenous causes for platelet destruction exist.

(a) **Clinical features.** The **acute variant** of ITP occurs in children between the ages of 2 and 6 years and often occurs after a nonspecific viral illness. The **chronic variant** occurs in young adults, more commonly in young women. All ITP patients show varying degrees of thrombocytopenia, which in some acute cases is severe (i.e., associated with platelet counts of less than 1000/μl), and all show increased megakaryocytes. Other blood findings and cell lines are normal. Patients have mucocutaneous bleeding with petechiae, purpura, mucosal bullae, and excessive bleeding after trauma.

(b) **Diagnosis** requires exclusion of associated illnesses (e.g., SLE) and thrombocytopenia that is induced by drugs (e.g., quinidine). Platelet antibody techniques are available but remain somewhat nonspecific and are not as helpful either diagnostically or as disease monitors as had been hoped.

(c) **Clinical course.** The acute childhood variant often runs its course and resolves within 4–8 weeks; the adult form is more chronic and demonstrates relapses and remissions.

(d) **Therapy** for the acute childhood form usually involves protection from trauma and, in some cases, a short course of steroids. Treatment of adult ITP is more complex and protracted.

  (i) **High doses of steroids** produce complete remission, requiring no further therapy in approximately 35% of cases.

 (ii) **Splenectomy** often is necessary in the remainder of cases and is associated with complete remission.

(iii) **Refractory patients** may require **immunosuppresive therapy** (e.g., with azathioprine and cyclosphosphamide). Although **platelet transfusions** should not be withheld in ITP patients who are bleeding, such exogenous transfusions are less efficacious that in other thrombocytopenic states because of the same short survival of the platelets. An effective therapy that can temporarily elevate platelet counts in an acute crisis is **infusion with intravenous IgG.** The infused IgG apparently competes for and saturates reticuloendothelial binding sites, making fewer of them available for platelet binding and destruction. This maneuver has also gained popularity as a preoperative therapy in ITP patients requiring surgery. **Low doses of cyclosporin** have been effective in small numbers of patients.

(e) **Prognosis.** The overall prognosis is good; only 2%–3% of ITP patients die after 5 years.

2. **Thrombocytopathia** involves platelets that are adequate in number but unable to function properly in hemostasis and in the primary arrest of bleeding.

a. **Description.** Thrombocytopathia is characterized by:
   (1) Platelet-type mucocutaneous bleeding
   (2) Normal platelet counts but prolonged bleeding times
   (3) Demonstrable abnormalities in platelet function testing (e.g., aggregometry)
b. **Etiology**
   (1) **Drug-related platelet dysfunction** is the most common cause of abnormal platelet function.
      (a) **Aspirin** permanently acetylates platelet membranes, impairing the platelet prostaglandin synthesis [e.g., impairing synthesis of thromboxane $A_2(TXA_2)$] required for proper platelet function. Such impaired platelets may prolong bleeding times and cause bruising and increase hemorrhage with trauma. The aspirin-induced platelet lesion permanently alters circulating platelets and lasts until the platelets are replaced by new unaffected ones, usually in 3–7 days.
      (b) **Other anti-inflammatory drugs** (e.g., indomethacin) cause similar dysfunction but differ from aspirin in that their effects are not permanent and disappear when the agent is withdrawn.
   (2) **Uremia-associated dysfunction**
      (a) The **mechanism** is unclear, although data imply that uremic toxins in plasma result in disaggregation of high–molecular-weight polymers of factor VIII that are required for proper platelet function.
      (b) **Therapy.** In bleeding uremic patients, dialysis may evoke a response. Maneuvers to restore normal molecular-weight forms of factor VIII may temporarily correct this dysfunction. These maneuvers include administering factor VIII exogenously as cryoprecipitate and eliciting endogenous increases in factor VIII by giving desmopressin (dDAVP).
   (3) **Congenital forms of platelet dysfunction** include Glanzmann's thrombasthenia (an intrinsic platelet disorder) and von Willebrand's disease (vWD; a congenital absence of the high–molecular-weight forms of factor VIII required for platelet aggregation). Many deficiencies in platelet prostaglandin pathway enzymes have been elucidated in recent years. These are rare autosomal recessive syndromes characterized by bleeding and prolonged bleeding times with normal platelet counts. Refined platelet studies are required for diagnosis.

D. **Disorders of the coagulation system** can be classified as hereditary or acquired. The hereditary forms usually result from deficiency of a single coagulation protein. Although greatly variable in degree, the clinical manifestations of these disorders are somewhat similar. The acquired forms, which are more complex than the hereditary forms, usually result from multiple and mixed deficiencies in the coagulation proteins.

1. The **hereditary coagulopathies** are best exemplified by the disorders of factor VIII.
   a. **Hemophilia A** is the most common hereditary coagulopathy, accounting for 68%–80% of such conditions.
      (1) **Pathogenesis.** Genetically, hemophilia A is transmitted as a classic X-linked recessive trait—the disorder is carried by females and manifested in males. Bleeding results from the absence of VIII^{pro}, the small–molecular-weight, or **procoagulant, portion** of the factor VIII molecule. The large **antigenic portion** of the molecule, VIII^{ag}, is present in normal amounts.
      (2) **Clinical features** vary with the degree of deficiency and are summarized in Table 3-7. The nature of hemorrhage is deep-tissue bleeding with deep hematomas, hemarthrosis, and significant bleeding after stress such as trauma and surgery. Repeated hemarthrosis results in severe disabling arthropathy, which is the clinical hallmark of severe hemophilia A.
      (3) **Diagnosis.** The constellation of spontaneous or unexpected hemorrhage, especially hemarthrosis, in a male patient with an appropriate family history is suggestive. Laboratory tests reveal a prolonged **partial thromboplastin time (PTT),** which is indicative of deficiencies in the intrinsic thromboplastin system; other coagulation tests are normal. The diagnosis is confirmed by factor

TABLE 3-7. Clinical and Laboratory Findings in Hemophilia A and Hemophilia B

Severity	Level of Factor VIII or IX (U/dl)	Partial Thromboplastin Time	Clinical Picture
Severe	0–2	Very prolonged	Hemarthrosis and spontaneous bleeding severe and frequent; crippling common
Moderate	2–5	Prolonged	Hemarthrosis and spontaneous bleeding infrequent; disability uncommon; severe bleeding from injuries and surgery
Mild	5–25	Variable	Hemarthrosis and spontaneous bleeding very unusual; unsuspected and severe bleeding from injuries and surgery
Subclinical	25–49	Usually normal	Bleeding after major trauma or surgery possible; diagnosis often missed

Adapted with permission from Lee GR, et al: *Wintrobe's Clinical Hematology,* 9th ed. Philadelphia, Lea and Febiger, 1993, p 1428.

assay demonstrating low levels of VIII^{pro} and normal levels of VIII^{ag}. Detection of the abnormal gene itself is possible.

(4) **Therapy** is with VIII^{pro} transfusion either in the form of cryoprecipitate or factor VIII concentrates. Traditional multiple-donor VIII concentrates were associated with an unacceptably high incidence of transmitted hepatitis and human immunodeficiency virus (HIV). Newer pasteurized preparations and genetically engineered preparations, which obviate these problems, are widely available. This form of therapy has markedly lessened the mortality and morbidity rates associated with hemophilia A.

b. **von Willebrand's disease (vWD)** is a heterogeneous disorder also involving the factor VIII molecule.

(1) **Pathophysiology.** Genetically, its transmission is variable, but in its most common form, vWD is transmitted as an autosomal dominant trait with variable penetrance. This disorder involves hereditary deficiency or derangement of VIII^{ag} and VIII^{pro}. Because VIII^{ag} serves as a cofactor for platelet adhesion, patients manifest both coagulopathy and abnormal platelet function.

(2) **Clinical features** include immediate, mucocutaneous (i.e., platelet-type) bleeding due to VIII^{ag} deficiency and delayed, deep-tissue, post-trauma (i.e., coagulation-type) bleeding due to VIII^{pro} deficiency. As with hemophilia A, the clinical picture for vWD varies with the degree of deficiency.

(3) **Diagnosis** is suggested by abnormal bleeding of a mixed nature in an individual with an appropriate family history. Laboratory tests show prolonged bleeding time due to decreased platelet function and a frequently prolonged PTT due to VIII^{pro} deficiency. Measurements of factor VIII demonstrate either a combined and equivalent deficiency of VIII^{ag} and VIII^{pro} or a derangement in multimer mixtures of VIII^{ag}. Ristocetin-induced platelet aggregation is abnormal in vWD. Other tests of platelet aggregation are normal.

(4) **Therapy** requires the replacement and coordination of both the antigenic and procoagulant portions of factor VIII. Concentrates are rich in VIII^{pro} but low in VIII^{ag}; therefore, either cryoprecipitate or plasma, which contain both, is the treatment of choice in vWD.

c. **Other hereditary coagulation disorders** are uncommon. Diagnosis requires factor analysis to demonstrate the specific deficiency.

(1) Hemophilia B (factor IX deficiency) is identical to hemophilia A in its genetic features and clinical manifestations. Therapy differs in that either plasma or a purified prothrombin complex (which contains concentrated factors II, VII, IX, and X) is used as a source for factor IX.

(2) Factor XI deficiency is an autosomal recessive coagulopathy with milder clinical manifestations than those of the hemophilias. PTT is prolonged due to low factor XI levels. Plasma serves as adequate replacement therapy.

(3) Factor XII, prekallikrein, and **high–molecular-weight kininogen deficiencies** are unique in that they cause significant prolongations of PTT yet no predisposition to hemorrhage. Diagnosis is suggested by abnormal PTT with no history of bleeding, even with trauma. Factor analysis is necessary to demonstrate the deficient factor.

(4) Deficiencies of all other factors have been described but are rare.

2. The **acquired coagulation disorders** are more complex than the hereditary forms. The acquired coagulopathies usually involve multiple and mixed factor deficiencies and often are complications of other diseases. Coagulation testing shows abnormalities in multiple pathways; often the bleeding severity correlates poorly with coagulation abnormalities seen in laboratory testing.

a. **Vitamin K-dependent–factor deficiency**

(1) Etiology

(a) This coagulopathy occurs with **liver failure** when hepatocyte dysfunction is sufficient to impair the synthesis by the liver of factors II, VII, IX, and X. In such cases, evidence of liver disease is present (i.e., jaundice, transaminase elevation) in addition to the coagulopathy.

(b) Malabsorption of vitamin K can occur with biliary obstruction as well as with intestinal disease (e.g., sprue). Again, coagulopathy merely complicates the obvious clinical picture.

(c) Particularly in intensive care units, **nutritional deficiency** occurs in patients with poor oral intake of vitamin K and in those in whom antibiotics have removed the gastrointestinal flora that serve as an alternate vitamin K source.

(d) Drugs can interfere with vitamin K metabolism, most specifically, the vitamin K antagonist **coumarin,** which is used to treat thrombotic diseases.

(2) Pathophysiology. The liver synthesizes factors II, VII, IX, and X. The final post-translational step in their synthesis renders these proteins functional and requires γ-carboxylation of a minimum of 10 terminal glutamic acid residues, with vitamin K as a cofactor. Interference in this mechanism causes functional deficiency of these clotting proteins.

(3) Diagnosis. Because many clotting factors are deficient, laboratory testing shows **prolonged PTT** and **prothrombin time (PT).** Specific measurements demonstrate the deficiency of factors II, VII, IX, and X.

(4) Therapy for vitamin K–related coagulopathy varies with its cause.

(a) In cases of malabsorption and nutritional deficiency, supplemental (often parenteral) vitamin K corrects the coagulopathy.

(b) In cases of excess coumarin, withdrawal of the offending drug with supplemental vitamin K is efficacious.

(c) In bleeding patients or patients with liver dysfunction who cannot respond to vitamin K, the deficient factors must be administered in the form of plasma.

b. **Disseminated intravascular coagulation (DIC)**

(1) Etiology. DIC is a common acquired coagulopathy that occurs secondary to other disease processes, such as:

(a) Activation of the intrinsic coagulation pathway by endothelial damage (e.g., in gram-negative sepsis, meningococcemia, and viremia)

(b) Activation of the extrinsic pathway by abnormal entry of tissue thromboplastins into the circulation (e.g., in obstetric complications, carcinomatosis, and massive trauma)

(2) Pathophysiology. DIC is initiated by stimuli in the systemic circulation that activate the coagulation mechanism and cause the abnormal formation of excessive systemic thrombin. The thrombin, in turn, causes extensive activation of coagulation in the microcirculation, which consumes many coagulation moieties and activates the fibrinolytic system secondarily.

(3) Clinical features vary depending on the balance between intravascular coagulation and fibrinolysis and factor depletion.

  (a) In florid acute cases (e.g., amniotic fluid embolism), the coagulopathy is dominant and the major symptoms are bleeding and shock.

  (b) In more chronic cases (e.g., carcinomatosis), thrombosis and clotting may predominate.

  (c) Many cases of DIC involve abnormal coagulation parameters but no bleeding or clotting, whereas other cases have a mixture of both bleeding and clotting complications.

(4) Diagnosis. Laboratory tests reveal a complicated picture. Many coagulation factors are consumed in the diffuse clotting process; these factor deficiencies prolong both PT and PTT. Platelet consumption results in thrombocytopenia. Fibrinogen deficiency arises from thrombin-mediated clotting as well as plasmin-mediated fibrinolysis. The secondary fibrinolysis is demonstrated by the presence of high titers of fibrin degradation products (FDP).

(5) Therapy is controversial; however, it is unanimously agreed that addressing the underlying "trigger" disease is paramount. The role of both factor replacements and anticoagulants to impair the ongoing thrombin production is less clear. The author's preference is to administer platelets and plasma to bleeding patients with markedly lowered levels and to reserve heparin for patients with thrombotic complications (e.g., skin infarction, acral gangrene, and recognizable vessel thromboses). Many patients require no specific coagulation therapy.

c. Liver disease results in a complex coagulopathy involving many aspects of clotting.

  (1) Liver disease results in impaired synthesis of vitamin K–dependent clotting proteins, fibrinogen, antithrombin III, plasminogen, and other protein moieties.

  (2) Impaired clearance of FDP and activated coagulation factors may result in a mild DIC-type condition.

  (3) Portal hypertension may result in splenomegaly and excessive platelet pooling with thrombocytopenia.

  (4) The accumulation of FDP causes impaired platelet function (thrombocytopathia).

d. Pathologic inhibitors of coagulation

  (1) The **lupus-type inhibitor** is the most common coagulation inhibitor. Although first described in patients with SLE, lupus inhibitors most often occur with other conditions or idiopathically.

    (a) The inhibitor is an anti-phospholipid that has inhibitory activity at the prothrombin–platelet membrane complex (see Figure 3-1).

    (b) Clinical testing reveals prolonged PT and PTT but little evidence of bleeding. The diagnosis is suggested by demonstrating that patient plasma causes similar abnormalities when mixed with normal plasma, unlike deficiency states in which such mixtures correct the abnormality. The diagnosis can be confirmed by a positive thromboplastin tissue inhibition (TTI) test and antiphospholipid assays.

    (c) Therapy should be directed toward the underlying disease. These patients do not bleed and need not receive coagulation therapy. Thrombosis is a more common complication.

  (2) Specific inhibitors of coagulation are antibodies with specificity for single coagulation proteins. The most common is factor VIII antibody, which arises in 10% of patients with hemophilia who have received factor therapy.

(a) Clinically, such antibodies cause profound bleeding dyscrasias of similar severity to congenital deficiency.

(b) Diagnosis is made by demonstrating a specific factor deficiency that is not corrected by administration of normal plasma.

(c) Therapy is difficult because the antibody also inactivates exogenously administered factors. Steroids and immunosuppressive agents have been used with limited success.

e. **Other acquired coagulation disorders.** Coagulopathy has been associated with amyloidosis (factor X deficiency), the nephrotic syndrome (due to renal wasting of coagulation proteins, especially factor IX), extracorporeal circulation (thought to activate the coagulation system partially and cause low-grade DIC), and massive transfusions (the patient hemorrhages normal blood, but it is replaced with blood bank–derived blood that is poor in coagulation factors and platelets).

VI. ABNORMALITIES RELATED TO HYPERCOAGULABILITY AND INCREASED TENDENCY TO THROMBOSIS

A. **Anatomic abnormalities of vessels and blood flow.** Disorders predisposing the patient to thrombosis related to anatomic abnormalities of vessels and blood flow and not related to intrinsic abnormalities in the blood itself include the following.

1. **Stasis** can occur in conditions such as postoperative states, orthopedic injury, and neurologic diseases. Pathogenetic factors include venodilation and localized areas of reduced clearance of activated procoagulant factors.

2. **Turbulence** (e.g., associated with aneurysms) can damage vascular endothelium and expose blood to the interior of the vessel wall, facilitating endothelial–platelet–coagulation protein interaction.

3. **Trauma** to blood vessels (e.g., vasculitis) can damage and disrupt vessel walls.

B. **Intrinsic blood disorders.** Disorders predisposing to thrombosis related to intrinsic blood disorders that are associated with abnormalities of platelets include the following.

1. Epidemiological evidence suggests that shortened platelet half-life, platelet activation, and enhanced incidence of thrombosis exist in certain common thrombotic medical conditions including **diabetes, atherosclerosis,** and **hypercholesterolemia.** These patients clearly have enhanced thrombotic tendency. It remains unclear, however, whether this tendency results from increased platelet activation or whether the platelet activation is a secondary event resulting from disease-related vascular abnormality.

2. Specific disorders in which primary abnormalities of platelets result in thrombotic tendency include the following:

    a. **Myeloproliferative diseases,** such as polycythemia vera and essential (hemorrhagic) thrombocythemia, especially when the platelet count exceeds $10^6/\mu l$

    b. **Paroxysmal nocturnal hemoglobinuria (PNH),** which is associated with enhanced platelet reactivity and unusual thromboses involving abdominal hepatic veins

    c. **Heparin thrombocytopenia syndrome,** which is associated with thrombosis of venous and arterial sites in patients using heparin. This syndrome has become more commonly recognized.

    (1) Incidence is 1%–5% of patients on heparin therapy. Most data still suggest that this is more common with bovine (beef) than porcine (pork) heparin.

    (2) Pathogenesis involves heparin-dependent antiplatelet IgG antibody.

    (3) Thrombocytopenia precedes thrombosis, so platelet counts should be monitored in heparin patients and heparin discontinued if the platelet count significantly declines. Once thrombosis occurs the mortality rate can range from 10%–50%.

C. **Specific hereditary disorders of enhanced thrombosis associated with abnormalities of plasma proteins** include:

1. **Abnormal fibrinogens** (dysfibrinogens) that are too sensitive to thrombin or that clot too tightly and do not allow for physiologic lysis by plasmin and **abnormal plasminogens** that are unable to dissolve clots physiologically are rare.

2. **Deficiencies of coagulation inhibitors**
   a. **Antithrombin III deficiency** can be quantitative or qualitative. The defect has variable phenotypic penetrance but often causes recurrent venous thrombosis in young patients.
   b. **Protein C deficiency.** Protein C is a vitamin K–dependent factor synthesized by the liver, which inhibits factors VIIIa and Va. The homozygote condition causes purpura fulminans in neonates. Heterozygotes have enhanced venous thrombosis and may be predisposed to skin necrosis when placed on warfarin without concomitant heparin. In **protein C substrate deficiency,** a genetic defect in factor V renders the factor refractory to the inhibitory activity of protein C. This condition may be the most common congenital hypercoaguable state. It is a substrate abnormality, rather than a lack of agonist, that is the cause of "deficiency" and disease.
   c. **Protein S deficiency.** Protein S is a cofactor that facilitates factors VIIIa and Va inhibition by protein C. Its deficiency results in a thrombotic diathesis syndrome similar to protein C deficiency.

D. **Specific acquired disorders of enhanced thrombosis associated with abnormalities of plasma proteins**

1. **Pregnancy and oral contraceptive agents** are associated with statistically increased incidence of stroke, acute myocardial infarction, and venous thrombosis. Pregnancy and oral contraceptives cause elevation in most procoagulant proteins and diminution of most fibrinolytic and inhibitor proteins, thus altering the hemostatic balance in favor of clotting.

2. **Nephrotic syndrome** is associated with urine wasting of antithrombin III and, more importantly, hypoalbuminemia, which probably results in enhanced platelet aggregation.

3. **Lupus inhibitor syndrome.** The presence of the so-called lupus inhibitor, antiphospholipid antibody syndrome is associated with increased thrombosis, especially in SLE patients. This association probably also exists in non-SLE patients. Most cases, however, are not associated with SLE of other underlying conditions. It remains unclear whether the presence of the inhibitor is causative or merely a marker. Lupus inhibitor is becoming one of the more common diagnosable conditions related to hypercoagulability, with an incidence of thrombotic complications ranging from 9% to 28% in affected patients.
   a. **Pathophysiology.** The lupus inhibitor, or antiphospholipid antibodies, or both, interact with the coagulation pathway at the X–V–Ca complex.
   b. **Clinical manifestations.** Despite prolonged clotting times, thrombosis (both arterial and venous), placental dysfunction, and recurrent miscarriage are major symptoms and signs of this disorder. Abnormal bleeding does not occur.
   c. **Diagnosis.** Laboratory findings include prolongation of the PTT and PT that does not reverse when patient plasma is mixed with normal plasma. Diagnosis is confirmed by further demonstrating the inhibitor reaction within the clotting system using the thromboplastin inhibition test (TTI) and dilute Russel venom viper assays.
   d. **Therapy. Aggressive** anticoagulation with warfarin is indicated in cases of lupus inhibitor syndrome accompanied by clinical thrombosis.

4. **Thrombotic thrombocytopenic purpura (TTP)** is associated with apparent premature release of macroaggregated VIII[ag] into plasma by damaged endothelial cells. This abnormal protein causes excessive platelet–endothelial binding, with microthrombi seen in most vascular beds. Plasmapheresis, which removes much of this abnormal protein, is an effective therapy.

TABLE 3-8. Hypercoagulable States

Inherited	Acquired
Antithrombin III deficiency	Pregnancy
Protein C deficiency	Oral contraceptive use
Protein C substrate abnormality	Malignancy (chronic disseminated intravascular coagulation)
Protein S deficiency	Nephrotic syndrome
Abnormal fibrinogens	Lupus anticoagulant and antiphospholipid antibody syndromes
Abnormalities in plasma fibrinolytic system	Heparin- associated thrombocytopenia and thrombosis syndrome
	Myeloproliferative syndromes
	Paroxysmal nocturnal hemoglobinuria

5. **Malignancy associated with chronic DIC (Trousseau's syndrome)** causes enhanced thrombosis of many varieties. The mechanism for enhanced thrombosis is chronic DIC initiated by tumor cells releasing either thromboplastic substances or activating factor XII, or both.

   a. Migratory thrombophlebitis of superficial veins is uniformly associated with chronic DIC in classic Trousseau's syndrome. Common neoplasms are adenocarcinomas of lung, pancreas, stomach, and prostate. This condition requires heparin therapy for control.

   b. Marantic endocarditis is another DIC variant; it results in fibrin vegetation in the heart and recurrent embolization.

   c. Routine deep vein thrombosis and pulmonary embolism are also statistically associated with malignancy.

E. **Diagnostic and therapeutic approach to hypercoagulability**

1. **Diagnostic approach**

   a. Clinical settings in which investigation for a hypercoagulable state is indicated include:

      (1) Family history of documented thromboembolic events

      (2) Age younger than 40 years at onset of thromboembolic events

      (3) Recurrent thromboembolic events

      (4) Unusual sites of thrombosis (e.g., mesenteric or cerebral veins)

      (5) Resistance to standard therapy for thrombosis

   b. Table 3-8 summarizes several causes of hypercoagulabity.

2. **Treatment depends on the underlying cause.**

   a. In myeloproliferative disorders, platelet counts should be lowered to less than $10^6/\mu l$. Hydroxyurea is effective. Occasionally, plateletpheresis is needed.

   b. Vessel abnormalities can be surgically repaired if found at angiography.

   c. Most congenital protein deficiency states, including protein C, are managed with life-long warfarin therapy.

   d. Lupus-inhibitor patients who have manifested thrombosis are managed with warfarin as long as the inhibitor is present.

   e. Hypercoagulability associated with cancer usually requires long-term subcutaneous heparin therapy because warfarin does not control the thrombotic diathesis in these cases. When effective therapy for the tumor is available, as it is for prostate cancer, it temporarily resolves the coagulopathy.

   f. TTP requires plasmapheresis to remove the abnormal factor VIII protein.

STUDY QUESTIONS

DIRECTIONS: Each of the numbered items or incomplete statements in this section is followed by answers or by completions of the statement. Select the ONE lettered answer or completion that is BEST in each case.

1. Thrombocytopenia that is caused by increased platelet destruction is most closely associated with which of the following conditions?

(A) Aplastic anemia
(B) Combination chemotherapy
(C) Acute leukemia
(D) Systemic lupus erythematosus (SLE)
(E) Excessive ethanol intake

2. Increased levels of hemoglobin A_2 (Hb δ) are characteristic of which one of the following disorders?

(A) Sickle cell trait
(B) β-Thalassemia trait
(C) Glucose-6-phosphate dehydrogenase (G6PD) deficiency
(D) Unstable hemoglobin disease
(E) α-Thalassemia trait

3. Which one of the following conditions results in prolongation of the partial thromboplastin time (PTT), but not the prothrombin time (PT)?

(A) Variceal hemorrhage as a result of cirrhosis
(B) Menorrhagia resulting from von Willebrand's disease (vWD)
(C) Therapy with broad-spectrum antibiotics
(D) Therapy with coumarin for phlebitis
(E) Celiac (sprue) disease

4. Which one of the following conditions causes delayed, deep tissue–type bleeding?

(A) Uremia
(B) Hemophilia A
(C) Therapy with aspirin
(D) von Willebrand's disease (vWD)

5. Which one of the following statements regarding patients with idiopathic thrombocytopenic purpura (ITP) is true?

(A) Bone marrow megakaryocytes are generally decreased.
(B) Platelet-associated immunoglobulin G (IgG) is diagnostic.
(C) Splenomegaly and other cytopenias are usually present.
(D) The platelet life span is prolonged.
(E) Splenectomy can be effective therapy.

6. Disseminated intravascular coagulation (DIC) initiated by activation of intrinsic pathway is most likely in which one of the following clinical settings?

(A) Gram-negative bacteremia
(B) Amniotic fluid embolism
(C) Multiple trauma
(D) Promyelocytic leukemia
(E) Trousseau's syndrome

DIRECTIONS: Each of the numbered items or incomplete statements in this section is negativity phrased, as indicated by a capitalized word such as NOT, LEAST, or EXCEPT. Select the ONE lettered answer or completion that is BEST in each case.

7. The LEAST imperative supportive maneuver in the induction phase of acute leukemia is

(A) empiric and aggressive use of broad-spectrum antibiotics
(B) maintenance of platelet counts >20,000/μl
(C) stimulation of marrow recovery by growth factors
(D) vaccination with pneumococcal vaccine and use of immunoglobulins
(E) isolation techniques of varying intensity

8. In blood testing for presumed hypercoagulability, the LEAST specific test is

(A) prothrombin time (PT) and partial thromboplastin time (PTT)
(B) platelet count
(C) antithrombin III level
(D) fibrinogen level
(E) thromboplastin inhibitor assay

DIRECTIONS: Each set of matching questions in this section consists of a list of 4 to 26 lettered options (some of which may be in figures) followed by several numbered items. For each numbered item, select the ONE lettered option that is most closely associated with it. To avoid spending too much time on matching sets with large numbers of options, it is generally advisable to begin each set by reading the list of options. Then, for each item in the set, try to generate the correct answer and locate it in the option list, rather than evaluating each option individually. Each lettered option may be selected once, more than once, or not at all.

Questions 9–13

(A) Acute lymphocytic leukemia (ALL)
(B) Acute myelogenous leukemia (AML)
(C) Both ALL and AML
(D) Neither ALL nor AML

For each description of a clinical situation, select the leukemic state with which it is most closely associated.

9. A 4-year-old patient with pancytopenia and circulating blasts

10. A 60-year-old patient with pancytopenia and circulating blasts

11. A 70%–80% long-term survival (? cure)

12. A patient with bleeding and infection

13. A patient with gum and skin infiltration

Questions 14–17

(A) Protein C deficiency
(B) Paroxysmal nocturnal hemoglobinuria (PNH)
(C) Lupus inhibitor syndrome
(D) Trousseau's syndrome

Match the following clinical vignettes to the most likely diagnosis.

14. A 30-year-old woman with a history of rash and arthritis has deep vein thrombosis. She has had a problem with recurrent abortions.

15. A 45-year-old man, who has been followed up by his physician for 4 years for chronic iron deficiency anemia with unknown source of blood loss, has portal vein thrombosis.

16. A 60-year-old man had deep vein thrombosis of his left leg last month and is being appropriately managed with warfarin. He has symptoms of new clot formation in the right leg as well as a clot in his left forearm.

17. A 67-year-old woman with mitral stenosis is started on warfarin by her cardiologist. On the third day, painful red areas appear on her thigh and breast.

ANSWERS AND EXPLANATIONS

1. The answer is D [V C 1 b (1) (a), (3)]. Systemic lupus erythematosus (SLE) triggers the production of an autoimmune antiplatelet antibody that is directly associated with enhanced platelet destruction. Aplastic anemia, combination chemotherapy, ethanol abuse, and acute leukemia are associated with impaired platelet production due to absent or diminished numbers of megakaryocytes.

2. The answer is B [I A 4]. Increased levels of hemoglobin A_2 (Hb δ) are characteristic of β-Thalassemia trait. Thalassemia syndromes are genetic disorders characterized by diminished synthesis of globin chains due to globin gene defects. Thalassemias are named according to the deficient chain. Thus, β thalassemia is characterized by deficient synthesis of the β chain, which is a component of hemoglobin A (Hb A). In an attempt to compensate, non–Hb A hemoglobins are increased (e.g., Hb A_2, which is composed of α and δ globins, concentration increases). The presence of such hemoglobins in increased amounts aids in the diagnosis of β-thalassemia trait. Because all chains have α components, there is no excess of minor hemoglobins in α-thalassemia trait. In sickle cell states, mutated hemoglobins [e.g., hemoglobin S (Hb S) and hemoglobin C (Hb C)] are present, rather than increased quantities of normal minor hemoglobins. In glucose-6-phosphate dehydrogenase (G6PD) deficiency and unstable hemoglobin disease, hemoglobin becomes oxidized and precipitates as Heinz bodies.

3. The answer is B [V D 2 a (1), (2)]. von Willebrand's disease (vWD) involves factor VIII in the intrinsic pathway and prolongs activated partial thromboplastin time (PTT) and not the prothrombin time (PT). The PT measures the extrinsic coagulation pathway and thus requires normal levels of factor VII for normalcy. Factor VII is synthesized in the liver and requires vitamin K as a cofactor for synthesis. Thus, liver disease (e.g., cirrhosis) diminishes synthesis of factor VII and prolongs PT. Malabsorption of vitamin K, as is seen in sprue, lowers available vitamin K and can prolong PT. Broad-spectrum antibiotics eliminate bowel flora; a secondary source of vitamin K. In patients on these antibiotics, especially

those with poor oral intake (e.g., those in the intensive care unit), lowered vitamin K results in prolonged PT. Coumarin is a vitamin K antagonist, so it directly interferes with factor VII synthesis and prolongs PT. If vitamin K depletion is severe enough in any of these situations, factors II, IX, and X are also affected and the PTT is prolonged; however, only vWD prolongs only the PTT.

4. The answer is B [V D 1 a]. Hemophilia A involves coagulation factor VIII^{pro}; platelet function is not affected in this disease. This results in a coagulation-type bleeding syndrome with delayed, deep tissue–type bleeding. Although the exact mechanism is unclear, uremia is believed to cause platelet dysfunction by toxins that alter the factor VIII antigen polymers required for normal platelet function. Aspirin causes thrombocytopathia by inhibiting synthesis of thromboxane A_2 (TXA_2), a strong inducer of platelet aggregation. von Willebrand's disease (vWD) is a genetic defect involving VIII^{ag}, which is the platelet-supporting portion of factor VIII. This results in defective platelet function much more frequently than coagulation-type bleeding.

5. The answer is C [V C 1 b (3)]. Except when thrombocytopenia has caused chronic bleeding with iron deficiency anemia, isolated thrombocytopenia is the rule in idiopathic thrombocytopenic purpura (ITP). Splenomegaly and other cytopenias are not part of ITP, and their presence should bring the diagnosis into doubt. ITP is the prototypical thrombocytopenia due to increased peripheral destruction. Platelet life span is markedly shortened, and, in response, the bone marrow megakaryocytes are increased. Platelet-associated antibodies can usually be found on platelets and in plasma, although their significance remains controversial. Long-term therapy uses corticosteroids and splenectomy. Immunosuppression may be required in refractory cases.

6. The answer is A [IV A 2; V D 2 b (1), (3)]. Disseminated intravascular coagulation (DIC) is a syndrome in which, by various pathophysiological methods, abnormal thrombin is generated in plasma and initiates diffuse intravascular micro (and occasionally macro) clot formation. Varying initiating events can trigger this process. Gram-negative sepsis causes endothelial damage with activation of factor XII and the intrinsic coagulation pathway of thrombin generation. Amniotic fluid embolism, multiple trauma, carcinomatosis and promyelocytic leukemia all release tissue thromboplastins into the systemic circulation and activate the extrinsic coagulation of thrombin generation.

7. The answer is D [I C 2 b (2) (b) (iv); IV D 4 b, c, d]. Pneumococcal vaccine and exogenous immunoglobulins have been shown to diminish infectious morbidity and mortality in certain hematologic patients (i.e., post-splenectomy, sickle cell anemia and chronic lymphocytic anemia patients), but these role in acute leukemia is limited at best. Humoral immunity is well maintained in acute myelogenous leukemia (AML) patients and partly, if ever requires such exogenous support. The therapy for AML, or acute nonlymphocytic leukemia (ANLL), is aggressive and difficult. It involves the ablation of leukemic tissue but invariably results in ablation of normal marrow tissue as well. Profound and prolonged pancytopenia results. The functions of marrow elements must therefore be supported. The empiric use of broad-spectrum antibiotics in febrile patients with polymorphonuclear leukocytes (PMNs) less than $500/\mu l$ and the use of prophylactic platelet transfusion to maintain platelet counts greater than $20,000/\mu l$ have markedly diminished the incidence of early mortality from infection and bleeding, respectively. Early studies using genetically engineered growth factors indicate their ability to hasten marrow recovery and resolution of cytopenias with similar lessen of infectious and hemorrhagic morbidity. Isolation techniques do have a role in lessening incidence of infection, but controversy remains in regard to the degree of strictness that is most effective.

8. The answer is A [VI E 2; Table 3-8]. Although epidemiological studies have suggested that very shortened prothrombin time (PT) or partial thromboplastin time (PTT) may be associated with a population predisposed to clotting complications, in an individual, such values have little, if any, significance. Very high platelet counts ($>10^6/\mu l$), especially in myeloproliferative diseases, are associated with enhanced thrombosis. The thromboplastin inhibitor assay detects the lupus inhibitor, which is also associated with enhanced clotting. Congenital antithrombin III deficiency is detectable by assaying antithrombin III as are congenital fibrinogen abnormalities. Furthermore, chronic disseminated intravascular coagulation (DIC)

and Trousseau's syndrome of recurrent thrombosis in cancer patients may be detected by discovering a lowered plasma fibrinogen level and high titers of fibrin split products (FSPs).

9–13. The answers are: 9-A [IV A I], **10-B** [IV A 2], **11-A** [IV E 1], **12-C** [IV B 1], **13-B** [IV A 2; Table 3-3]. Acute lymphocytic leukemia (ALL) is predominantly a disease of childhood. Although induction therapy is much easier and more successful with ALL than with acute myelogenous leukemia (AML), ALL often has some component of marrow failure with associated bleeding and infection. With current therapy, remission is obtained in more than 95% of cases; 70%–80% of cases have long-term survival and represent possibly cured patients. AML is most commonly a disease of adults, and its incidence increases with increasing age. Induction therapy is long and difficult to perform, with marrow ablation by chemotherapy associated with almost universal bleeding and infection. Long-term survival is unusual in AML. AML has several subtypes, some of which are characterized by gum and skin infiltration (e.g., monocytic and myelomonocytic leukemias).

14–17. The answers are: 14-C [VI D 3], **15-B** [VI B 2 b], **16-D** [VI D 5], **17-A** [VI C 2 b]. The lupus inhibitor is found in one third of systemic lupus erythematosus (SLE) patients. In lupus patients, the association with thrombosis risk is 10%–15%. In patients without SLE who display a similar inhibitor-type antibody, there is less risk of thrombosis, but the risk is still far in excess of normal.

Paroxysmal nocturnal hemoglobinuria (PNH) is a difficult diagnosis to make, and the disorder can masquerade as chronic iron deficiency (due to urine losses), chronic hemolysis, or both. PNH is associated with increased thrombotic risk and has a tendency to involve intra-abdominal veins.

Recurrent thrombosis associated with adequate warfarin anticoagulation, especially when migratory and involving superficial veins, suggests the presence of chronic disseminated intravascular coagulation (DIC) with an occult adenocarcinoma (Trousseau's syndrome).

Warfarin can, in the early phases of administration, lower the vitamin K–dependent, short half-life protein inhibitor protein C more rapidly and out of balance with the coagulation factors II, VII, IX, and X, thus affecting the hemostatic balance toward clotting. Characteristically, it occurs soon after the initiation of warfarin without concomitant administration of heparin.

Chapter 4

Oncologic Diseases
Donna Glover

I. **TUMOR GROWTH. Uncontrolled growth** distinguishes malignant from normal cells. Typically, the more rapid the growth rate, the more poorly differentiated the tumor.

A. **Patterns of tumor growth.** Proliferating neoplasms may spread in two ways.

1. **Direct invasion** of local tissue

2. **Metastasis** to distant organs
   a. Different types of **tumors vary in their metastatic potential.** For example, cancers of the head and neck tend to remain localized and spread slowly to distant foci. However, rapidly growing carcinomas, such as small-cell lung cancer, are already widely disseminated in most patients at the time of diagnosis.
   b. Each cancer also exhibits a distinct **pattern of spread.** For example, common sites of metastases in breast cancer patients include lung, liver, bone, adrenal glands, skin, and ovary.
   c. Growth is usually more rapid in metastatic sites than in the primary tumor.

B. **Tumor growth rate and prognosis.** Growth rate and patterns of spread are important determinants of both prognosis and the response to particular therapeutic modalities.

1. **Fast-growing neoplasms,** including acute leukemias, small-cell lung carcinoma (SCLC), and lymphomas, are generally highly responsive to chemotherapy and radiation therapy.

2. **Slow-growing tumors,** such as low-grade sarcomas, are less responsive to these modalities. Surgical resection and radiation therapy are more effective treatment options for these neoplasms.

3. Growth rates can be estimated by **flow cytometry** from the percentage of cells in the S phase of the cell cycle. S-phase determination is especially helpful in predicting the prognosis of early-stage breast cancer and in evaluating the necessity for adjuvant therapy in breast cancer patients with negative lymph nodes.

C. **Chromosomal changes and cancer**

1. **Oncogenes** are mutant genes that cause multiple changes in the regulatory controls of the cell. Most oncogenes are derived from **proto-oncogenes,** normal genes that affect cell growth and differentiation but have the potential to become oncogenic following mutations in their DNA sequences.
   a. Oncogenes **induce aberrations** that give the affected cell the characteristics of malignancy (e.g., they may induce changes in cell shape, growth factor secretion, contact inhibition, anchorage independence, or glucose transport). For example,
      (1) Oncogenes can cause tumor cells to acquire growth factor independence in a variety of ways.
         (a) They may cause the tumor cell to secrete mitogenic growth factors that then stimulate growth of the same cell, leading to autostimulation of cell growth.
         (b) They may affect the cytoplasmic pathway that is responsible for picking up signals from cell surface receptors. Proteins of some oncogenes, such as *ras* and *src,* produce mitogenic signals in the cytoplasm that are not dependent on growth factors.
      (2) Certain oncogenes may be silent in normal cells, but, under the influence of specific growth factors, they may become active.

(3) Oncogenes can alter the function or increase the number of growth factor receptors on the surface of cells, leading to aberrant cell proliferation.

b. Single oncogenes are unable to induce the transformation of fully normal cells into fully malignant cells. Each oncogene **induces only a subset of changes** associated with full malignancy.

c. Activation of proto-oncogenes

(1) Point mutations. A point mutation is a single-base change in a gene. In bladder carcinoma, a change in 1 base out of 6000 in the proto-oncogene leads to the structural alteration of a protein. This alteration affects cell metabolism and induces malignancy.

(2) Gene fusion. In chronic myelogenous leukemia (CML), the *abl* proto-oncogene derives its oncogenicity by fusing with a fully unrelated gene, the BCR gene. The protein encoded by the BCR–*abl* hybrid has a different structure and function from the normal *abl* proto-oncogene protein.

(3) Amplification. Differences in the level of expression of encoded proteins can also cause proto-oncogenes to become oncogenic. For example, in childhood neuroblastoma, the amount of the N-*myc* gene is increased from a diploid number to many dozens per cell. N-*myc* gene amplification is associated with a poor prognosis and is a significant factor in the aggressiveness of this tumor.

2. Anti-oncogenes (tumor suppressor genes) function in the normal cell to restrict or repress cellular proliferation. When they are genetically inactivated, tumorigenesis can occur.

a. Inactive alleles of tumor suppressor genes can be acquired in the following two ways:

(1) Somatic mutation

(2) Passage through a germ line, which creates a congenital predisposition to cancer (e.g., as occurs with retinoblastoma)

b. Inactivation of tumor suppressor genes is associated with neuroblastoma, small-cell lung cancer, kidney cancer, colon carcinoma, Wilms' tumor, bladder cancer, osteoblastoma, and liver cancer, among other malignancies.

II. **CANCER STAGING.** This prognostic strategy defines a series of categories or stages, each of which represents a step in the degree of malignancy and aggressiveness of the tumor. The stage of a tumor describes its **size, the extent of regional lymph node spread,** and the **presence or absence of metastases.**

A. **Objectives**

1. Estimating prognosis. The stage of a tumor figures significantly in estimates of prognosis, although it is not always the most influential prognostic variable. All currently used staging systems assign the most favorable prognosis to stage I; higher stages are associated with a progressively poorer prognosis.

2. Determining the best course of therapy. Because the staging of all solid tumors is based largely on the anatomic extent of the disease, staging is critical to the sequence of local, regional, and systemic treatment approaches, as well as to the integration of combined-modality therapies.

3. Facilitating investigation. Staging provides a uniform classification system for comparing data in the clinical literature.

B. **Staging systems.** Staging systems for all solid tumors are based principally on the **anatomic extent of disease.** Differences in tumor biology preclude a universal staging system applicable to all cancers.

1. The **TNM classification system** is the most widely used staging system for carcinomas and sarcomas. This system assigns the tumor to a **T level,** which corresponds to the size and extent of the primary tumor; an **N level,** which describes the degree of nodal involvement; and an **M level,** which describes the presence and extent of distant metastases. Site-specific definitions of TNM stages have been compiled for a wide range of neoplasms.

2. Older classification systems remain in use for a number of sites, including lymphomas and carcinomas of the colon, rectum, prostate, and testicle.

C. **Staging procedures.** Diagnostic and therapeutic procedures differ in their sensitivity to detect cancer. To avoid confusion, staging assignments must specify the type of information used to determine the stage. The American Joint Committee on Cancer (AJCC) has defined the following three levels of staging information.

1. **Clinical staging** uses all available **pretreatment data,** including diagnostic data obtained from physical examination, radiologic or nuclear imaging techniques, laboratory tests, endoscopy, and biopsy or other invasive procedures. The procedures of choice vary with the natural history of the tumor and the details of the clinical presentation.

2. **Pathologic staging** is based on data obtained during surgery and from examination of the resected specimen.

3. **Retreatment staging** is used to restage the tumor prior to additional therapy, following failure of initial treatment.

III. TREATMENT MODALITIES

A. **General principles**

1. Cancer treatment may be either **curative** or **palliative.**
   a. **Curative** procedures aim to eradicate the tumor and imply that the patient will remain disease-free (i.e., will not experience a recurrence) indefinitely.
   b. **Palliative** treatment seeks to prolong life and minimize discomfort when a cure is impossible. Recurrence is an ever-present possibility, although the patient may initially exhibit a robust, or even a complete, response.

2. The treatment program typically includes a combination of surgery, radiation therapy, chemotherapy, and, in some cases, the use of biologic response modifiers.

3. Therapy must be customized to meet the specific needs of the patient. A multidisciplinary approach that coordinates the efforts of the pathologist, oncologist, radiation therapist, and other specialists facilitates the design and implementation of such a plan.

B. **Radiation therapy.** Half of all cancer patients require radiation therapy at some point during the course of their disease.

1. **Applications**
   a. Radiation therapy, either alone or in conjunction with chemotherapy and surgery, is curative in some cancers (e.g., Hodgkin's disease, head and neck cancer).
   b. Radiation therapy also has palliative applications (e.g., relief from metastatic bone pain in advanced breast cancer).

2. Radiation therapy can be used alone or in combination with chemotherapy or surgery.
   a. **Chemotherapy** may be used concurrently or prior to radiation therapy to enhance efficacy.
      (1) For example, the pyrimidine analogue 5-fluorouracil (5-FU) acts as a radiation sensitizer when administered concurrently with radiation therapy.
      (2) However, combined-modality therapy can also contribute to severe toxic-

ity reactions. The **radiation recall effect,** an enhanced or reactivated response in a previously irradiated area precipitated by the concurrent administration of doxorubicin or methotrexate, is a classic example.

b. Radiation therapy may be used **prior to surgery** to inhibit metastasis or induce tumor regression and **postoperatively** to enhance efficacy. Preoperative radiation is associated with an increased incidence of postsurgical complications, including impaired wound healing and fistula formation.

3. **Side effects.** Most patients experience systemic or local side effects, especially those patients receiving curative high-dose radiation (e.g., for the treatment of head or neck cancer).

a. **Time course**
   (1) **Acute side effects,** principally swelling and inflammation, occur within days or weeks of treatment.
   (2) **Chronic effects,** such as fibrosis and scarring, may not be apparent until months or even years after therapy.

b. The **severity** of adverse reactions is a function of the treatment site, the size of the radiation field, the amount of radiation energy, and dosage variables (e.g., total dose, radiation dose per fraction, and dose rate). Side effects can be minimized by:
   (1) Accurately targeting the tumor area using current radiologic techniques [e.g., computed tomography (CT) and magnetic resonance imaging (MRI)]
   (2) Directing radiation to avoid critical organs (e.g., the spinal cord)
   (3) Blocking normal tissue
   (4) Reducing the treatment field over the course of therapy

c. **Systemic effects** of radiation therapy include malaise, fatigue, anorexia, and a depressed blood count. These generalized symptoms are especially common in patients treated concurrently with radiation and chemotherapy.

d. **Skin reactions** occur after high-dose therapy directed to sites on or near the skin surface (e.g., the chest wall after mastectomy) or female reproductive organs (e.g., the vulva). Such reactions are less common after high-energy photon beam therapy. Retreatment or the use of overlapping fields may result in severe and persistent skin reactions.
   (1) **Acute reactions** consist of erythema, dry desquamation with pruritus, and moist desquamation.
   (2) The affected area should be kept as clean and dry as possible. Additional treatment measures include:
      (a) Topical application of vitamin A and D ointment, baby oil, or cornstarch
      (b) Cleansing the area with a 1:1 solution of hydrogen peroxide and normal saline
      (c) Topical application of corticosteroids
   (3) Patients should avoid wearing irritating clothing and being directly exposed to the sun.

e. Reactions of the **oral cavity and pharynx,** such as mucositis, pain, anorexia, xerostomia, and dental caries, occur after high-dose radiation to the head or neck area.
   (1) Strict attention to dental hygiene, topical anesthetics, artificial saliva preparations, and nutritional counseling may be helpful.
   (2) Severe cases may require insertion of a gastric feeding tube or percutaneous gastrostomy.

f. **Gastrointestinal reactions** occur with doses exceeding 4000–5500 cGy.
   (1) **Esophagitis** usually subsides in 7–10 days but predisposes the patient to superimposed *Candida* infections. Treatment measures include use of antacids, a bland diet, and topical anesthetics.
   (2) **Radiation gastritis** or **enteritis** may present as nausea, vomiting, diarrhea, abdominal pain, anorexia, or bleeding. Treatment measures include:
      (a) Antiemetics (e.g., prochlorperazine, trimethobenzamide)

           (b) Antidiarrheals (e.g., diphenoxylate hydrochloride-atropine sulfate, loperamide hydrochloride)

           (c) A bland, low-fat, low-residue, high-gluten diet

           (d) Dietary supplements

       (3) Rectal inflammation may result in bleeding or pain. A low-residue diet, stool softeners, or steroid enemas may give relief.

   g. Radiation pneumonitis, characterized by cough, dyspnea, and chest pain, usually occurs 2–3 months after delivery of radiation to a significant lung volume. Treatment consists of prednisone, 15 mg four times a day. Steroids should be discontinued gradually to avoid recurrence of symptoms.

   h. Central nervous system (CNS) symptoms may occur during therapy or may not appear until weeks or months later.

       (1) Acute symptoms accompanying intracranial irradiation include headache and signs of increased intracranial pressure (ICP); gastrointestinal symptoms (i.e., nausea and vomiting) may also occur. Dexamethasone, 4 mg four times a day, usually provides rapid relief.

       (2) Delayed symptoms include short-term memory loss, visual memory disturbances, and white matter abnormalities, such as calcifications and ventricular dilatation.

       (3) A somnolence syndrome, characterized by hypersomnia and fatigue, has been observed several weeks or months after intracranial irradiation, especially in patients receiving concurrent intrathecal chemotherapy.

   i. Bone marrow suppression may follow large-field irradiation used in the treatment of Hodgkin's disease or pelvic malignancies, especially if the patient is receiving concurrent chemotherapy. Leukopenia or thrombocytopenia may require suspension of therapy; anemia, however, is rare. Hemoglobin values below 9 g/dl require transfusion.

C. Chemotherapy

   1. Introduction. The use of cytotoxic chemotherapy has increased dramatically in the past 3 decades. Combinations of these drugs with surgery, radiation therapy, or both have produced high complete remission rates and enhanced long-term survival in many malignancies.

     a. Chemotherapeutic responses. Chemotherapy is inadequate to control some of the most common adult cancers. In these cases, responses are almost always incomplete and of brief duration, with minimal or no increase in survival. Chemotherapeutic responses are defined as complete responses, partial responses, stable disease, or progression of disease.

       (1) A **complete response** implies complete disappearance of all known tumor without development of any new malignant lesions.

       (2) A **partial response** means a 50% or greater shrinkage in the tumor size.

       (3) Stable disease implies either a less than 50% decrease or a less than 25% increase in the size of all measurable tumor masses.

       (4) Progressive disease implies a greater than or equal to 25% increase in the size of all measurable lesions or the development of a new lesion considered to represent metastatic disease.

     b. Combination chemotherapy regimens use effective drugs that have high response rates for a specific tumor type. Combinations of drugs have different side effects, different mechanisms of cytotoxicity, or both. If drugs share the same side effects, individual drug doses are reduced accordingly. Compared with single-agent therapy, combination chemotherapy increases response rates. By killing cancer cells via more than one mechanism, combination chemotherapy may prevent or delay the development of drug resistance.

     c. The most commonly used chemotherapeutic agents and their mechanisms of action, therapeutic uses, and toxicities are discussed in the following sections (Table 4-1). Specificities of administration, dose modifications, and drug interactions are discussed for particular agents.

   2. Alkylating agents

TABLE 4-1. Classes of Common Chemotherapeutic Agents Used in Oncologic Disease

Alkylating Agents	Vinca Alkaloids	Antibiotics	Antimetabolites	Platinum Analogues	Miscellaneous
Nitrogen mustards	Vincristine	Daunorubicin (daunomycin)	Methotrexate	Cisplatin	Taxol
Mechlorethamine	Vinblastine	Doxorubicin (adriamycin)	5-Fluorouracil (5-FU)	Carboplatin	Etoposide
Ifosfamide	Navelbine	Plicamycin (mithramycin)	Floxuridine (FUdR)		Procarbazine
Cyclophosphamide		Mitomycin	Mercaptopurine (6-MP)		Fludarabine
Chlorambucil		Bleomycin	Cytarabine (Ara-C)		
Melphalan		Mitoxantrone	Thioguanine (6-TG)		
			Pentostatin		
Nitrosoureas					
Carmustine (BCNU)					
Lomustine (CCNU)					
Streptozocin					
Alkyl sulfonates					
Busulfan					
Ethylenimines and methylmelamines					
Thiotepa					
Hexamethylmelamine					
Triazenes					
Dacarbazine (DTIC)					

a. Mechanism of action

  (1) Alkylating agents react strongly with nucleophilic substances and form covalent linkages. The toxic effects of alkylating agents are believed to be related to free radical formation and alkylation of the components of DNA, RNA, and cellular proteins. These reactions have profound effects on DNA replication and transcription and may cause cytotoxicity, mutagenesis, and carcinogenesis.

  (2) Alkylation can take place in proliferating and nonproliferating cells. Therefore, alkylating agents are not cell cycle specific. The proliferating compartment is more sensitive to the killing effects of these drugs.

b. Drug resistance to alkylating agents can occur because of decreased drug accumulation by resistant cells, increased pharmacologic inactivation of alkylating agents, increased repair of alkylating agent–induced damage, and increased intracellular sulfhydryl groups (e.g., free thiols), which compete with other targets (e.g., DNA) to neutralize the drug intracellularly. Patients who fail treatment with one alkylating agent often respond to another.

c. Chemical classes of alkylating agents include nitrogen mustards; nitrosoureas; alkyl sulfonates (busulfan); ethylenimines and methylmelamines; and triazenes (dacarbazine).

d. Therapeutic uses and toxicity are summarized in Tables 4-2 through 4-6.

TABLE 4-2. Nitrogen Mustards

Drug	Therapeutic Uses	Common Toxicities
Mechlorethamine (nitrogen mustard)	Hodgkin's disease; sclerosing agent for pleural effusions; topical dilute solution in mycosis fungoides	Bone marrow suppression; nausea; vomiting; alopecia; infertility; sclerosing agent
Cyclophosphamide (Cytoxan)	Hodgkin's disease; lymphomas; chronic lymphocytic leukemia (CLL); multiple myeloma; breast cancer; small-cell lung cancer; ovarian cancer; pediatric tumors; bone marrow transplantation	Bone marrow suppression; infertility; alopecia; nausea; vomiting; hemorrhagic cystitis (which is prevented by high fluid intake)
Ifosfamide	Soft tissue sarcomas; testicular cancer; ovarian cancer; cervical cancer; lymphomas	Bone marrow suppression; infertility; alopecia; vomiting; central nervous system (CNS) toxicity (which may be reduced by limiting high single doses, reducing narcotic use, reducing antinausea agents and other CNS active drugs)
Melphalan (Alkeran)	Myeloma; macroglobulinemia; formerly used in ovarian and breast cancer	Bone marrow suppression; infertility; nausea; alopecia
Chlorambucil (Leukeran)	CLL; macroglobulinemia; lymphoma	Bone marrow suppression; nausea; alopecia (rare); infertility; skin rash; rarely hepatic toxicity

TABLE 4-3. Nitrosoureas

Drug	Therapeutic Uses	Common Toxicities
Carmustine (BCNU)	Brain tumors; Hodgkin's disease; multiple myeloma; bone marrow transplantation	Bone marrow suppression; nausea; vomiting; mild and reversible liver toxicity; rare lung and kidney damage
Lomustine (CCNU)	Lymphoma; brain tumors; colon cancer	Bone marrow suppression; nausea; vomiting; dermatitis; alopecia; transient hepatotoxicity (usually rare and mild)
Streptozocin	Pancreatic islet cell tumors; carcinoids	Nausea; vomiting; duodenal ulcers; renal toxicity; mild bone marrow suppression; glucose intolerance due to islet cell damage; mild hepatic toxicity

TABLE 4-4. Alkyl Sulfonates

Drug	Therapeutic Uses	Common Toxicities
Busulfan	Chronic myelogenous leukemia; bone marrow transplantation	Bone marrow suppression; infertility; pulmonary fibrosis; skin hyperpigmentation

3. **Vinca (plant) alkaloids and podophyllotoxins**
   a. **Mechanism of action**
      (1) **Vinca alkaloids** appear to crystallize microtubular spindle proteins, leading to an arrest of the cell cycle in mitosis.
      (2) **Podophyllotoxins** cause metaphase arrest by exerting a macromolecular effect on DNA synthesis. They can induce strand breaks in DNA by interacting with topoisomerase II.

TABLE 4-5. Ethylenimines and Methylmelamines

Drug	Therapeutic Uses	Common Toxicities
Thiotepa	Lymphoma; superficial bladder cancer; breast cancer; ovarian cancer; bone marrow transplantation; intrathecal therapy for carcinomatous meningitis	Bone marrow suppression; infertility; nausea and vomiting (rare with low doses)
Hexamethylmelamine	Ovarian cancer; small-cell lung cancer; lymphoma; endometrial cancer; cervical cancer	Nausea; vomiting; bone marrow suppression; infertility; mood changes; peripheral neuropathy; paresthesias; ataxia

TABLE 4-6. Triazenes

Drug	Therapeutic Uses	Common Toxicities
Dacarbazine (DTIC)	Melanoma; sarcomas; Hodgkin's disease	Nausea; vomiting; malaise; low-grade fever; flu-like syndrome; bone marrow suppression; rare hepatic toxicity and diarrhea

    b. Therapeutic uses and toxicity are summarized in Table 4-7.

4. Antibiotics

    a. Mechanism of action. Antitumor antibiotics are natural substances that inhibit DNA and RNA synthesis. They behave as both phase-specific and phase-non-specific agents and exhibit a variety of effects on different phases of the cell cycle.

    b. Therapeutic uses and toxicity are summarized in Table 4-8.

5. Antimetabolites

    a. Mechanism of action. Most antimetabolites are phase-specific and act during the S phase of the cell cycle. Antimetabolites interact with cellular enzymes by:

        (1) Substituting some metabolite that is normally incorporated into a key molecule such as DNA or RNA, thus interfering with cellular function

        (2) Competing with a normal metabolite for occupation of the catalytic site of a key enzyme

        (3) Competing with normal metabolites that act as important enzyme regulatory sites or other important receptors

    b. Therapeutic uses and toxicity are summarized in Table 4-9.

6. Platinum analogues

    a. Mechanism of action. The platinum complexes bind to DNA, forming intrastrand crosslinks. In addition to their reactivity with DNA, the platinum ana-

TABLE 4-7. Vinca Alkaloids

Drug	Therapeutic Uses	Common Toxicities
Vincristine (Oncovin)	Acute lymphocytic leukemia; Hodgkin's disease; lymphoma; Kaposi's sarcoma	Neurotoxicity (the first signs are loss of deep tendon reflexes, decreased distal sensation, and paresthesias); sclerosing agent; alopecia; constipation
Vinblastine (Velban)	Hodgkin's disease; lymphoma; testicular cancer; non–small-cell lung cancer; Kaposi's sarcoma	Bone marrow suppression; nausea; peripheral neuropathy; constipation; a sclerosing agent
Navelbine	Non–small-cell lung cancer; breast cancer; lymphoma	Bone marrow suppression; peripheral neuropathy; mild alopecia; sclerosing agent
Etoposide (VP-16)	Testicular cancer; small-cell lung cancer; non–small-cell lung cancer; lymphomas; sarcomas (pediatric and Kaposi's)	Delayed leukopenia; mild thrombocytopenia; rare nausea; anorexia; diarrhea; rare hypotension with rapid infusions

TABLE 4-8. Antibiotics

Drug	Therapeutic Uses	Common Toxicities
Daunorubicin (daunomycin)	Acute myelogenous leukemia (AML)	Bone marrow suppression; nausea; vomiting; alopecia; sclerosing agent; infertility; cardiomyopathy
Doxorubicin (Adriamycin)	Breast cancer; lymphomas; sarcomas; lung cancer; stomach cancer; thyroid cancer	Bone marrow suppression; nausea; vomiting; mucositis; gastrointestinal toxicity; alopecia; infertility; cardiomyopathy; sclerosing agent
Mitoxantrone (DHAD)	Breast cancer; lymphoma; AML	Myelosuppression; rarely nausea; vomiting; alopecia; elevated liver function tests; occasionally blue urine; cardiotoxicity
Mitomycin (Mutamycin)	Breast cancer; cancer of the stomach, pancreas, colon, cervix, and lung; used as a radiosensitizer with 5-fluorouracil for anal cancer	Bone marrow suppression; sclerosing agent; lung, hepatic, and kidney damage; infertility; hemolytic–uremic syndrome; cardiotoxicity
Bleomycin	Testicular cancer; head and neck cancer; lymphomas; Hodgkin's disease; cervical cancer	Mild myelosuppression; fever; allergic reactions; lung toxicity; skin changes; alopecia; rarely hypotension; sclerosing agent
Plicamycin (mithramycin)	Malignant hypercalcemia; prevents bone resorption by toxic effects on osteoclasts	Nausea; vomiting; bone marrow suppression; hypocalcemia; coagulopathy; liver toxicity; renal toxicity; skin reactions; sclerosing agent

logues also bind to nuclear and cytoplasmic proteins. Cisplatin behaves as a bifunctional alkylating agent.

b. Therapeutic uses and toxicity are summarized in Table 4-10.

7. Miscellaneous agents include paclitaxel (Taxol), procarbazine, and fludarabine (Table 4-11).

D. **Biologic response modifiers** are agents that alter the growth characteristics or antigenicity of a tumor, resulting in a therapeutic enhancement of host response. The mechanism of action may be immunologic or nonimmunologic.

1. Classification. Biologic response modifiers are classified according to the following functional categories.

a. Agents that **restore, augment,** or **modify host immunologic mechanisms** thought to be critical for tumor growth and metastasis [e.g., bacille Calmette-Guérin (BCG), interferon-α (IFN-α)]

b. Cells or cellular products that have direct **cytotoxic** or **cytostatic** effects (e.g., bone marrow transplants, transfusion of T lymphocytes)

c. Agents that alter **metastatic potential** or that effect the **initiation** or **maintenance of neoplastic transformation** (e.g., retinoids)

TABLE 4-9. Antimetabolites

Drug	Therapeutic Uses	Common Toxicities
Methotrexate	Acute lymphocytic leukemia (ALL); osteogenic sarcoma; lymphoma; breast, head, neck, gastric, and bladder cancers; choriocarcinoma; intrathecal use for carcinomatous meningitis	Bone marrow suppression; mucositis; diarrhea; nausea; rare kidney and liver damage. (Toxicities are increased when used with other highly protein-bound drugs. High doses should be given with intravenous leucovorin hydration and alkalinization of the urine)
5-Fluorouracil (5-FU)	Cancers of the breast, colon, stomach, pancreas, head and neck, esophagus, and anus; antitumor activity is increased when it is given with leucovorin	Bone marrow suppression; mucositis; diarrhea; hyperpigmentation; rare cerebellar ataxia; myocardial ischemia
Mercaptopurine (6-MP)	Maintenance therapy for acute leukemia	Bone marrow suppression; nausea; stomatitis; rarely rash; liver toxicity; intrahepatic cholestasis
Cytarabine (ara-C)	Acute myelogenous leukemia (AML); ALL; blastic phase of chronic myelogenous leukemia; preleukemia	Bone marrow suppression; nausea; anorexia; stomatitis; flu-like syndrome; liver toxicity; cerebellar dysfunction
Thioguanine (6-TG)	AML	Bone marrow suppression
Pentostatin	Lymphoma; hairy cell leukemia	Bone marrow suppression; increased renal toxicity; conjunctivitis; fever; hepatotoxicity

2. **BCG,** an attenuated strain of *Mycobacterium bovis,* has demonstrated activity when administered locally in direct contact with tumor cells.
   a. **One successful application** of BCG therapy is in the **treatment of recurrent superficial bladder cancers.** Direct instillation of BCG into the bladder following transurethral resection or fulguration of visible lesions significantly reduces the incidence of recurrent tumors as well as the number of patients ultimately requiring cystectomy for invasive bladder cancer.
   b. **Toxicity** includes local irritation and a flu-like illness, consisting of fever and malaise, which is common in the first 24 hours after administration.

TABLE 4-10. Platinum Analogues

Drug	Therapeutic Uses	Common Toxicities
Cisplatin	Testicular, ovarian, head and neck, lung, bladder, cervix, and esophageal cancer; lymphoma; a radiation sensitizer	Renal toxicity; vomiting; hearing loss; myelosuppression; tinnitus; peripheral neuropathy; hair loss
Carboplatin	Ovarian and lung cancer; other cisplatin-sensitive tumors	Myelosuppression; vomiting; much less nephrotoxicity, neuropathy, and ototoxicity than cisplatin

TABLE 4-11. Miscellaneous Agents

Drug	Therapeutic Uses	Common Toxicities
Taxol	Ovarian, breast, lung, and head and neck cancer	Allergic reactions (which may be prevented by premedication with dexamethasone, Benadryl, and cimetidine); myelosuppression; alopecia; myalgias; flu-like syndrome
Fludarabine	Chronic lymphocytic leukemia; lymphoma	Myelosuppression; flu-like syndrome; nausea; alopecia
Procarbazine	Hodgkin's disease; lymphoma	Neurologic symptoms; hypotensive reactions with tricyclic antidepressants and substances with high tyramine contents; disulfiram-like reaction with alcohol and drugs in nose drops, cough preparations, and local anesthetics; bone marrow depression; nausea; vomiting; peripheral neuropathy; lethargy; rash; central nervous system toxicity

3. **Hematopoietic growth factors** are a family of proteins that regulate the proliferation, differentiation, maturation, and function of blood cells.
   a. The **interleukins IL-1, IL-3, and IL-6** affect totipotential **stem cells,** immature hematopoietic precursors. In addition, these cytokines have widespread physiologic effects on lymphocytes and other organs.
   b. **Colony-stimulating factors** act primarily on differentiated cells. These factors include erythropoietin (EPO), granulocyte colony-stimulating factor (G-CSF), granulocyte macrophage colony-stimulating factor (GM-CSF), and macrophage colony-stimulating factor (M-CSF).
      (1) **EPO,** synthesized by the kidney, is a major regulatory factor of red blood cell (RBC) production. Intravenous administration of EPO results in a marked increase in reticulocyte number and the hematocrit.
         (a) **Therapeutic indications** for EPO include anemia due to renal disease, acquired immune deficiency syndrome (AIDS), and other chronic illnesses; myelodysplastic syndromes; and anemia from chemotherapy associated with decreased EPO production.
         (b) **Side effects.** Rarely, EPO administration is associated with an increase in diastolic blood pressure.
      (2) **GM-CSF** primarily stimulates the production of neutrophils, eosinophils, granulocytes, and monocytes whereas G-CSF stimulates neutrophils and granulocytes.
         (a) **Therapeutic indications.** Both G-CSF and GM-CSF reduce and shorten granulocyte nadirs from chemotherapy, hasten recovery after bone marrow transplantation, and help restore bone marrow function in disease-related or iatrogenic neutropenia. As a result, patients experience fewer febrile episodes and a reduced requirement for antibiotics after chemotherapy and bone marrow transplantation.
         (b) **Side effects.** G-CSF may produce mild to moderate bone or muscle pain or alterations in blood chemistry values. A few patients may develop splenomegaly, headache, flushing, chest discomfort, cutaneous reactions, or hypotension.
4. The **interferons** are a group of proteins and glycoproteins that possess antiviral and antiproliferative activities. They also enhance T-cell and macrophage activity, stimulate the expression of tumor-specific cell surface antigens, modify oncogene expression, and promote cellular differentiation.
   a. **Two types of α-IFN** have been approved for the treatment of hairy-cell leuke-

mia and Kaposi's sarcoma. α-IFN has also been used in CML, non-Hodgkin's lymphoma, renal cell cancer, mycosis fungoides, melanoma, carcinoid tumors, and myeloma: α-IFN improves disease-free and overall survival of patients with high-risk melanoma (i.e., patients with regional node metastases). **Toxic** reactions include a flu-like illness, with fever, chills, malaise, mild leukopenia, and elevation of hepatic enzymes.

  b. **β-interferon (β-IFN)** and **γ-interferon (γ-IFN)** are other antigenic interferons that may have therapeutic potential.

5. **Interleukin-2 (IL-2),** a lymphokine secreted by activated T lymphocytes, modifies the proliferation and function of T and B cells and is essential for the growth of T cells and peripheral blood lymphocytes.

  a. High concentrations of IL-2 stimulate the production of **lymphokine-activated killer (LAK) cells** capable of lysing tumor cells. The administration of of IL-2 and LAK cells, known as **adoptive immunotherapy**, has shown promise in treating malignant melanoma and renal cell cancer.

  b. **Side effects.** IL-2 is associated with severe toxicity, including a capillary leak syndrome, fluid retention, renal failure, pulmonary edema, severe neurologic symptoms, shortness of breath, elevations in serum creatinine and bilirubin, anemia, thrombocytopenia, diarrhea, skin rashes, and fever.

6. **Levamisole** stimulates phagocytosis and chemotaxis.

  a. **Therapeutic effects.** Levamisole restores defective leukocyte migration, increases nucleic acid and protein synthesis, stimulates T cells, and enhances lymphocyte and macrophage cytotoxicity.

  b. **Indications.** When used in conjunction with 5-FU, levamisole significantly reduces the risk of recurrence in stage C colon cancer.

7. **Monoclonal antibodies** are the products of immune B lymphocytes fused with an established myeloma cell line.

  a. Monoclonal antibodies facilitate histopathologic diagnosis. They have particular value in staging leukemias and lymphomas and in differentiating anaplastic tumors.

  b. Short-lived responses to antibody administration have been observed in leukemia, melanoma, and several other malignancies. Possible mechanisms of antitumor activity include:

    (1) Immunologic destruction of tumor cells via complement-mediated cytotoxicity and antibody-dependent cell-mediated cytotoxicity

    (2) Direct inhibition of tumor growth

  c. Antibodies may be used ex vivo to purge autologous bone marrow of residual tumor cells before reinfusion after high-dose cytotoxic chemotherapy.

  d. Monoclonal antibodies also have potential utility as vehicles for the delivery of radioisotopes and chemotherapeutic agents.

  e. **Antiidiotypic antibodies** mimic tumor-specific cell-surface antigens and are undergoing investigation in the development of **tumor vaccines.**

IV. BREAST CANCER

A. **Incidence.** Breast carcinoma has increased in frequency over the last decade. As many as one in nine women will develop breast cancer during her lifetime.

B. **Risk factors**

1. **Family history.** There are at least two hereditary patterns to breast cancer.

  a. **Familial aggregation** is associated with a modest increase in risk and is relatively common. The risk is markedly increased among first-degree relatives.

  b. **True genetic pattern.** Linkage to a specific gene with high penetrance accounts for less than 5% of all cases of breast cancer. Cancer tends to occur at a younger age and is more likely to be bilateral. Multiple family members over three or more generations are affected.

(1) **p53** is a tumor suppressor gene that appears in carriers and patients in Li-Fraumeni families. The gene is located on chromosome 17.

(2) **BRCAI gene,** located on chromosome 17q, is seen in patients with a family history of breast and ovarian cancer.

2. **Early menarche**

3. **Late menopause**

4. **Nulliparity or a first pregnancy after age 30 years**

5. **Fibrocystic breast disease**

6. **Prior history of invasive or noninvasive breast cancers** (intraductal or lobular carcinoma in situ)

7. **Age**

8. **Estrogen replacement therapy (ERT)** is associated with a modest relative risk of breast cancer.

9. **Prolonged use of oral contraceptives** before the first pregnancy

10. **Dietary factors** [e.g., high-fat diet (unproven), alcohol consumption]

C. **Pathology.** Breast cancers are adenocarcinomas.

1. **Classification**
   a. **Papillary carcinomas** (1% of breast cancers) are low-grade, noninvasive intraductal lesions.
   b. **Medullary carcinomas** (5%–10% of breast cancers) are large bulky tumors that have a low-grade infiltrating tendency and are surrounded by lymphocytes.
   c. **Inflammatory carcinomas** (5% of breast cancers) invade the dermal lymphatics and cause skin redness, induration, warmth, and an erysipeloid margin.
   d. **Infiltrating ductal scirrhous carcinomas** (70% of breast cancers) are characterized by nests and cords of tumor cells surrounded by a dense collagenous stroma.

2. **Estrogen receptor (ER) status.** Breast cancer can be classified according to the presence or absence of ERs, cellular proteins found in hormone-responsive tissues. Receptor status can change over the course of the disease. The 20%–30% of breast cancer patients with *erb*B-2 oncogene expression have more aggressive cancers and may have greater drug resistance.
   a. **ER-positive** tumors are more common in postmenopausal patients. Approximately 60% of primary breast cancers have detectable ERs.
   b. **ER-negative** tumors are common in premenopausal patients. One third of patients with ER-negative primary breast cancers develop recurrent tumors that are ER-positive.

D. **Diagnosis**

1. **Early detection.** Routine breast self-examination and screening mammography have led to earlier detection of curable breast cancers.
   a. **Breast self-examination.** All women should be taught the technique of breast self-examination. Such examinations are best performed monthly after the menstrual period, when breast swelling and fibrocystic changes are less likely to interfere with the detection of a lump or mass. More than 80% of breast cancers occur as a painless mass.
   b. **Mammography.** All women between 35 and 40 years old should have a baseline mammogram.
      (1) Depending on the presence of known risk factors, patients should undergo mammography either yearly or every other year between age 40 and 50 years, and yearly after age 50 years.

TABLE 4-12. Staging System for Breast Cancer

Stage	Primary Tumor	Lymph Nodes	Distant Metastases
0	Carcinoma in situ (lobular or intraductal) Paget's disease of nipple	−	−
I	Tumor ≤ 2 cm	−	−
IIA	Tumor ≤ 2 cm	+, but not fixed	−
IIB	Tumor > 2 cm but ≤ 5 cm	− or +, but not fixed	−
III	Tumor > 5 cm Tumor ≤ 5 cm	+ or − fixed nodes	−
IV	Tumor with skin nodules, ulceration, fixation to chest wall, skin or breast edema	Supra- or infra-clavicular nodes	+

+ = positive; − = negative.

    (2) Women with risk factors for breast carcinoma should have a yearly mammogram at an earlier age.

    (3) Most breast cancers are irregular masses or areas associated with microcalcifications.

2. Pretreament evaluation

    a. In addition to a **medical history, physical examination, chest radiograph,** and **routine laboratory tests** (e.g., blood count, liver and renal function values, and serum calcium), all patients with newly diagnosed breast cancer should have a **mammogram to detect multicentricity** or **bilateral involvement.**

    b. Radiologic tests include a bone scan and in advanced breast cancer, a CT or MRI scan of the liver. If the bone scan shows evidence of metastatic disease and radiographs are negative, a CT scan or MRI scan of the bone or a bone biopsy should be performed to determine the correct therapy.

    c. Excisional biopsy is indicated for patients who are good candidates for lumpectomy and breast preservation. **Needle biopsy** may also be helpful for diagnostic purposes before excisional biopsy.

    d. Tumor markers. Patients with metastatic disease may have elevation in CA-15-3 or carcinoembryonic antigen (CEA) tumor markers.

E. **Staging.** Table 4-12 gives the currently used staging system for breast cancer.

F. **Therapy.** The primary goal of therapy is to provide optimal control of the disease in the breast and regional tissues while providing the best possible cosmetic result. Systemic therapy should be given to patients at high risk for metastatic disease to eradicate micrometastases. Patients should be seen by a medical oncologist, radiation therapist, and surgeon to determine the best course of treatment, which may include surgery, radiation therapy, adjuvant chemotherapy, and adjuvant endocrine therapy.

    1. Surgery

        a. The optimal surgical **approach** is determined by the following factors.

        (1) Disease stage

        (2) Tumor size

        (3) Tumor location

        (4) Breast size and configuration

        (5) Number of tumors in the breast

        (6) Available surgical and radiotherapeutic techniques

        (7) Patient preference concerning breast conservation

TABLE 4-13. Contraindications for Breast Conservation Surgery

Large tumor in a small breast (increases likelihood of poor cosmetic results)

Subareolar primary tumors

More than one tumor in the breast

Contraindications to radiotherapy

Advanced disease (i.e., beyond stage II)

Large areas of intraductal disease or microcalcifications

Tumors with an extensive intraductal component (i.e., ≥25% of the primary tumor is in situ and there is at least one focus of breast cancer that is in situ in normal breast tissue and is separate from the breast primary)

　

　b. **Procedures**
　　(1) **Modified radical mastectomy** entails removal of the breast and axillary contents with preservation of the pectoral muscles. Patients may undergo breast reconstruction during surgery or at a later time.
　　(2) **Partial mastectomy,** or **lumpectomy,** involves excision of the tumor and an adjacent rim of normal tissue.
　　　(a) **A level I or II axillary dissection** is performed for adequate staging and local control.
　　　(b) **Level III dissection** should be considered in patients with clinically positive nodes.
　　　(c) Three weeks after surgery, external beam radiation is used, with a boost to the local tumor site.
　　(3) In the past, most patients underwent modified radical mastectomy. Recent data suggest that breast conservation procedures, such as lumpectomy, allow adequate local control of the tumor and improve cosmetic outcome in selected cases; however, not all patients are suitable candidates for breast conservation (Table 4-13).
2. **Radiation therapy**
　a. **Patients treated with lumpectomy and axillary dissection** should receive definitive radiation therapy to the breast and lymphatics if they have positive lymph nodes.
　b. **Patients undergoing mastectomy** should receive postoperative radiation if they have any of the following risk factors for local recurrence.
　　(1) Primary tumor over 5 cm in size
　　(2) More than four positive axillary nodes
　　(3) Tumors involving the margin of surgical resection, invasion of pectoral fascia or muscle, or extranodal extension into the axillary fat
　c. In **patients at a high risk for distant metastases,** radiation therapy can be given concurrently or delayed until the completion of adjuvant chemotherapy. The risk of arm edema is increased by postoperative axillary radiation.
3. **Adjuvant chemotherapy** delays or prevents recurrence and improves survival in patients with positive axillary nodes as well as in some patients with negative axillary nodes.
　a. Table 4-14 lists **recommendations** for adjuvant chemotherapy. Premenopausal patients with positive axillary nodes are most likely to benefit from chemotherapy; such patients experience a 25%–30% reduction in mortality.
　b. **Combination chemotherapy** is superior to single-agent therapy, especially in patients with metastatic breast cancer. Six cycles of therapy or 6 months of treatment are as effective as longer treatment periods.
　c. **Drug regimens.** Maximal doses should be used unless the patient develops significant toxicity.
　　(1) The most popular adjuvant therapy regimen is cyclophosphamide, methotrexate, and 5-FU.

TABLE 4-14. Adjuvant Chemotherapy in Stage I and II Breast Cancer

	Premenopausal	Postmenopausal
Node positive		
Estrogen receptor (ER) negative	CMF × 6 months or CA × 4 months	Controversial, no therapy or tamoxifen × 5 years + 1 year of chemotherapy
ER positive	CMF × 6 months or CA × 4 months	Tamoxifen × 5 years + 1 year of chemotherapy
Node negative,		
Tumor >1 cm, ER negative	CMF × 6 months or CA × 4 months	CMF × 6 months or CA × 4 months ± tamoxifen
ER positive	No therapy or tamoxifen if high S-phase; CMF × 6 months	Tamoxifen alone or, if high S phase, tamoxifen and CMF × 6 months or CA × 4 months
Node negative, tumor ≤1 cm	No therapy	No therapy

CA = cyclophosphamide, adriamycin; CMF = cyclophosphamide, methotrexate, and 5-fluorouracil.

(2) Patients at higher risk for developing recurrent or metastatic disease may be administered cyclophosphamide, doxorubicin, and 5-FU. Response rates for this regimen in patients with metastatic breast cancer range from 65%–80%.

(3) Alternative regimens for patients with metastatic disease include doxorubicin, thiotepa, and vinblastine; high-dose cisplatin; mitomycin; intravenous vinblastine or 5-FU by continuous infusions; cyclophosphamide, methotrexate, and 5-FU; Taxol; and Navelbine.

4. Adjuvant endocrine therapy
  a. Studies of **ovarian ablation by radiation** or **oophorectomy** or chemically by Lupron or Zoladex in premenopausal patients have reported mixed results, with possible long-term benefits in certain subgroups.
  b. Hormonal therapy
    (1) The estrogen antagonist **tamoxifen** is the preferred agent in **postmenopausal patients with positive hormone receptors** (see Table 4-14). In these patients, tamoxifen delays recurrence and improves survival; chemotherapy is about half as effective as tamoxifen.
      (a) The benefit of tamoxifen in premenopausal patients with ER-positive tumors is less clear.
      (b) Patients with ER-negative tumors exhibit little or no response.
    (2) Hormonal therapy for metastatic breast cancer (Table 4-15)
      (a) Hormonal therapy is appropriate for patients with subcutaneous metastases, lymph node involvement, pleural effusions, bone metastases, and nonlymphangitic lung metastases. Patients with liver metastases, lymphangitic disease of the lung, pericardial metastases, or other potentially life-threatening metastases should be treated with chemotherapy.
      (b) Patients with ER-positive primary tumors exhibit response rates of at least 30% to hormone therapy. If the tumor contains both positive estrogen and progesterone receptors, the response rate increases to 75%.
      (c) Patients whose hormone receptor status is unknown may respond to hormone therapy if the tumors are well-differentiated or if 1–2 years have elapsed between occurrence of the primary breast cancer and the development of metastatic disease.

TABLE 4-15. Hormonal Agents Recommended for Metastatic Breast Cancer

Premenopausal patients
  Oophorectomy or radiation therapy to ovaries
  Tamoxifen
  LH-RH antagonists (goserelin acetate, leuprolide acetate)
  Aminoglutethimide and hydrocortisone
  Arimidex
  Fluoxymesterone
Postmenopausal patients
  Tamoxifen
  Megestrol acetate
  Aminoglutethimide
  Arimidex
  Fluoxymesterone
  High-dose estrogen (DES)
  LH-RH antagonists

LH-RH = luteinizing hormone-releasing hormone; DES = diethylstilbestrol.

  (d) Patients with a previous response to hormonal therapy may respond to discontinuation of the original agent and substitution of a second agent listed in Table 4-15.
  (e) Other hormonal therapies include Megace, Arimidex, Halotestin, aminoglutethimide, and luteinizing hormone–releasing hormone (LH-RH) antagonists.

5. **Specific treatment recommendations**
   a. **Intraductal breast cancer** has an excellent prognosis. Because the tumor is noninvasive (i.e., confined to the ducts), careful pathological review can exclude any risk of lymph node involvement or distant metastases.
      (1) Patients may be treated by total mastectomy or by lumpectomy followed by radiation, although this procedure is associated with a slightly higher incidence of second breast primaries.
      (2) Axillary node dissection is controversial; most experts believe it is unnecessary in these patients.
   b. **Lobular carcinoma in situ.** Patients with this noninvasive lesion are at extremely high risk for development of invasive cancer in both breasts. Treatment options include bilateral mastectomy or rigorous observation and follow-up.
   c. **Stage I and II disease.** Most patients with stage I and II breast cancer have the option of either a modified radical mastectomy or breast conservation with lumpectomy, axillary dissection, and postoperative radiation therapy.
   d. **Stage III disease.** Treatment options are determined by tumor resectability.
      (1) **Patients with operable tumors** are treated with modified radical mastectomy and postoperative radiation therapy. These patients may also receive preoperative or postoperative adjuvant chemotherapy.
      (2) **Patients with inoperable stage III disease** have a high rate of local and distant recurrence and poor survival rates.
         (a) A combined-modality approach, using systemic chemotherapy in addition to surgery and radiation, is required.
         (b) In most cases, aggressive combination chemotherapy is initiated after biopsy to reduce tumor bulk, to facilitate local treatment, and to eradicate distant micrometastases.

G. **Prognosis.** Approximately 50% of patients with operable breast cancer develop recurrent disease unless they receive adjuvant chemotherapy or hormone therapy. Prognostic factors include:

1. **Axillary node status.** This status is the most important predictor of recurrence and survival. Seventy percent of patients with negative nodes are disease-free at 10

years. This figure declines to 40% of patients with no more than three positive nodes and 15%–25% of patients with four or more positive nodes.

2. **Histopathology.** Poorly differentiated tumors with high nuclear grades have higher recurrence rates. Tumor size is an important prognostic factor independent of lymph node status. Tumors larger than 5 cm are associated with a decreased survival rate and an increased risk of recurrence.

3. **Hormone receptor status.** Of primary breast cancers, 60%–70% express ERs and 40%–50% express progesterone receptors. Patients with hormone receptor–positive tumors have lower rates of recurrence and prolonged survival rates compared with those with receptor-negative tumors.

4. **S-phase fraction and DNA index.** The S-phase fraction (i.e., the percentage of tumor cells in the S phase of the cell cycle) is proportional to the tumor growth rate. Patients with aneuploid tumors or high S-phase fractions, as determined by flow cytometry, have a poor prognosis compared with those with slow-growing diploid tumors.

5. **Oncogenic expression.** Expression of the HER-2 (c-*erb*B-2, neu) oncogene is associated with a poor prognosis.

6. **Other prognostic factors.** The following prognostic factors have been associated with a poorer prognosis in some studies: cathepsin-D, p53, HER-α/neu (*erb*-B2), epidermal growth factor receptor (EGF-R), TGF-α, pS$_2$, and monoclonal antibody NCRC11.

V. OTHER GYNECOLOGIC MALIGNANCIES

A. Ovarian cancer

1. **Incidence.** Ovarian cancer develops in 1 in 70 women and is the most common cause of death from a gynecologic malignancy. Incidence rates are highest in the industrialized nations.

2. **Risk factors** for ovarian cancer include:
   a. Nulliparity
   b. Fewer than average number of pregnancies or a history of miscarriage
   c. Family history of ovarian cancer
   d. History of endocrine disorders

3. **Diagnosis.** Ovarian cancer is rarely diagnosed before the disease has reached an advanced stage.
   a. **Early detection**
      (1) **Pelvic ultrasound** detects small lesions in the ovary, even those that cannot be palpated during bimanual examination.
      (2) Determination of levels of the **tumor marker CA 125** and an annual **pelvic ultrasound** are recommended for patients with a family history of ovarian cancer.
   b. **Pretreatment evaluation**
      (1) All patients with ovarian cancer should undergo abdominal and pelvic CT scanning, pelvic ultrasound, chest radiograph, intravenous pyelography (IVP), a barium enema, cystoscopy, and flexible sigmoidoscopy.
      (2) Routine blood chemistries, including albumin, magnesium, renal and liver function testing, should be performed. An elevated CA-125 is found in 80%–85% of patients. If a germ cell tumor is suspected, the following tumor markers should be drawn: lactate dehydrogenase (LDH), alpha fetoprotein (AFP), and human chorionic gonadotropin (hCG).
      (3) A careful laparotomy establishes the stage and extent of the disease and may permit the reduction of tumor masses.

TABLE 4-16. International Federation of Gynecology and Obstetrics (FIGO) Classification of Ovarian Carcinoma

Stage	Characteristics
I	Growth limited to the ovaries
IA	Growth limited to one ovary; no ascites No tumor on the external surface; capsule intact Tumor present on the external surface and/or capsule ruptured
IB	Growth limited to both ovaries; no ascites No tumor on the external surface; capsule intact Tumor present on the external surface and/or capsule(s) ruptured
IC	Tumor either stage IA or IB; ascites* present or positive peritoneal washings
II	Growth involving one or both ovaries with pelvic extension
IIA	Extension and/or metastases to the uterus and/or tubes
IIB	Extension to other pelvic tissues
IIC	Tumor either stage IIA or IIB; ascites* present or positive peritoneal washings
III	Growth involving one or both ovaries with intraperitoneal metastases outside the pelvis and/or positive retroperitoneal nodes; tumor limited to the true pelvis with histologically proven malignant extension to small bowel or omentum
IV	Growth involving one or both ovaries with distant metastases; pleural effusion with positive cytology; parenchymal liver metastases

Adapted with permission from Durant JR, Omura GA: Gynecologic neoplasms. In *Medical Oncology.* Edited by Calabresi P, Schein PS, Rosenberg SA. New York, Macmillan, 1985.

* Ascites is peritoneal effusion that, in the opinion of the surgeon, is pathologic or clearly exceeds normal amounts.

      (a) The entire abdominal contents should be explored, and any suspicious lesions should be removed or biopsied.

      (b) In addition to checking the primary tumor for rupture or adherence, the surgeon should note the amount and type of ascites (if present). Samples of fluid should be collected for cytologic analysis via peritoneal washing.

      (c) The para-aortic nodes in the region of the renal hila should be biopsied.

  4. Staging. Table 4-16 lists the staging procedure for primary ovarian carcinoma.

  5. Therapy

    a. Surgery

      (1) Procedures

        (a) Most patients undergo **bilateral salpingo-oophorectomy** and **transabdominal hysterectomy.** All gross residual disease should be resected if possible. In most cases, if a patient has metastatic disease outside the abdominal and pelvic areas, debulking surgery is not indicated.

        (b) Because ovarian cancer frequently spreads throughout the peritoneal cavity and usually is associated with omental and peritoneal seeding, the entire abdominal and pelvic cavities should be explored, a **partial omentectomy** performed, and the pericolic gutters inspected.

      (2) Adjuvant therapy and follow-up

        (a) Patients with stage IA or stage IB disease with well-differentiated or moderately differentiated tumors require no additional adjuvant therapy after surgery. Otherwise, patients should receive adjuvant therapy, which may include **total abdominal radiation therapy, intraperitoneal radioisotopes,** or **chemotherapy.** Advanced ovarian cancer (i.e., stage III or IV) is not curable by surgery alone. However, **reduction** of bulky cancer is associated with an improved response to either radiation or chemotherapy, if the largest residual mass is reduced to less than 2 cm in diameter. Less extensive reductions are not beneficial, even if large amounts of the tumor are removed.

   (b) Second-look surgery. Surgical reexploration following chemotherapy can detect remission, assess response, and allow further cytoreductive surgery in an attempt to prolong survival. Approximately 50% of patients with clinically complete responses have surgically documented complete remissions.

b. Chemotherapy. Systemic chemotherapy results in high response rates in patients with ovarian cancer and increases the likelihood of a cure in patients with resectable disease.

   (1) Drug regimens. The most commonly used agents are cyclophosphamide, cisplatin, carboplatin, hexamethylmelamine, and Taxol. There are few data to support the use of doxorubicin-based regimens. In the past, therapy was with cyclophosphamide and carboplatin or cisplatin, but newer regimens use Taxol with cisplatin or carboplatin.

   (a) Carboplatin (400 mg/m^2) is equivalent in efficacy to cisplatin (100 mg/m^2) and is associated with less peripheral neuropathy and ototoxicity, although it has an increased rate of bone marrow toxicity. Carboplatin may be combined with autologous bone marrow transplantation.

   (b) Taxol is associated with a 30% response rate in patients who have failed to respond to other therapy.

   (2) Treatment of residual disease after induction chemotherapy

   (a) Radiation therapy has consistently failed to prolong survival and is associated with unacceptable rates of bowel toxicity.

   (b) Intraperitoneal chemotherapy is based on the slow peritoneal clearance of many chemotherapeutic agents relative to total body clearance.

   (i) Drugs are administered in large volumes (1–2 L) through semipermanent systems (e.g., catheters).

   (ii) Agents that have been used intraperitoneally in ovarian cancer include methotrexate, 5-FU, carboplatin, and cisplatin.

c. Radiation therapy. For patients with advanced disease, radiation therapy is an option. Success is directly related to the volume of disease at the time of therapy.

6. Prognosis

a. The stage of disease is the most important prognostic factor.

   (1) Patients with distant metastases are rarely cured, even after combination chemotherapy.

   (2) Patients with disease limited to the ovary may be cured with surgery alone.

   (3) Patients with minimal stage III disease have an excellent prognosis with debulking surgery followed by combination chemotherapy, especially if the tumor can be reduced to less than 2 cm in diameter.

b. Histologic grade has greater prognostic significance than type. Borderline tumors, which display nuclear characteristics of malignancy but lack stromal invasion, behave in an indolent fashion.

B. Cervical cancer

1. Incidence. Carcinoma of the cervix was once one of the most common causes of cancer death, but incidence rates have been halved in the past 30 years.

a. This decline in mortality rate is largely attributable to the introduction of the Papanicolaou (Pap) smear for the diagnosis of dysplasia or carcinoma in situ.

b. Invasive cancer is most frequently seen in patients between 45 and 55 years of age from lower socioeconomic groups.

2. Etiology

a. Risk factors for cervical cancer include:

   (1) Early initial sexual activity

(2) Multiple sexual partners

(3) Early age at first pregnancy and multiple pregnancies

(4) History of venereal infection

(5) Oral contraceptive use

b. Recent studies have implicated infection with human papillomavirus (HPV), which causes common genital warts, in the progression of cervical cancer. Several oncogenes have been implicated as well, including overexpression of the c-*myc* oncogene and *ras* oncogene.

3. **Pathology**

a. **Squamous metaplasia** is the precursor of **cervical intraepithelial neoplasia** (CIN), which is subdivided into three grades according to severity.

(1) Grade I (mild to moderate dysplasia)

(2) Grade II (moderate to severe dysplasia)

(3) Grade III (severe dysplasia and carcinoma in situ)

b. Carcinoma in situ exhibits cytologic evidence of neoplasia without invasion of the basement membrane. This stage can persist as long as 3–10 years before progressing to invasive cervical carcinoma.

4. **Diagnosis**

a. **Early detection**

(1) The **Pap smear** is useful for detecting early lesions and has a sensitivity of 90%–95%.

(a) As a preventive measure, women older than 20 years of age should have two consecutive yearly smears; if results are negative, the test should be repeated every 3 years until age 65.

(b) Hemorrhage, inflammatory reactions (e.g., a fungating mass), or invasive cancer may result in a false-negative smear.

(2) Women with epithelial abnormalities in the Pap smear should undergo **cervical biopsy.** Visible lesions necessitate biopsy, regardless of Pap smear findings. If there are no visible lesions, colposcopy (using a binocular microscope and light source) reduces the need for cervical conization.

b. **Pretreatment evaluation** should include chest radiograph, IVP, complete blood count (CBC), liver and renal function studies, and a barium enema in patients with symptoms involving the colon or rectum.

(1) Because of the possibility of upper extension of the tumor, **curettage** of the endocervical canal and endometrium is recommended during the initial evaluation.

(2) A **pelvic CT scan** can define the extent of pelvic disease.

(3) **Cystoscopy** and **rectosigmoidoscopy** should be performed in patients with advanced disease.

(4) Use of **lymphangiography** is controversial.

5. **Staging.** The clinical staging system for cervical cancer is listed in Table 4-17. Clinical staging is often inaccurate, and staging laparotomy studies have shown that approximately 30% of patients have more extensive disease than is suggested by clinical staging procedures.

6. **Therapy.** Cervical cancer in most patients is treated with **surgery, radiation therapy,** or a **combination of both.** Chemotherapy with hydroxyurea may also be prescribed as a radiation sensitizer. Cisplatin has documented activity as a single-agent treatment option.

a. Carcinoma in situ and CIN are usually treated by **total abdominal hysterectomy.** In women desiring to bear children, these lesions can be managed by cervical conization and careful follow-up.

b. Therapy for stage I microinvasive cancer (i.e., an invasion of less than 3 mm in depth) is identical to that for carcinoma in situ. The risk of central recurrence and lymph node metastasis is increased when the tumor exceeds 3–5 mm in depth; in these cases, hysterectomy and pelvic lymphadenectomy are indicated.

TABLE 4-17. International Federation of Gynecology and Obstetrics Classification of Cervical Cancer

Stage	Characteristics
0	Carcinoma in situ intraepithelial carcinoma
I	Carcinoma strictly confined to the cervix
IA	Microinvasive carcinoma
IB	Invasive carcinoma
II	Carcinoma extends beyond the cervix but does not reach the pelvic wall; vaginal involvement limited to the upper two thirds
IIA	Vaginal involvement but no parametrial involvement
IIB	Parametrial involvement
III	Carcinoma extends to the pelvic wall and involves the lower third of the vagina; rectal examination reveals no cancer-free space between the tumor and the pelvic wall; all cases with hydronephrosis or a nonfunctioning kidney should be included, unless these disorders are known to be due to another cause
IIIA	Vaginal involvement (lower third); no extension to the pelvic wall
IIIB	Pelvic wall or parametrial involvement; hydronephrosis or a nonfunctioning kidney
IV	Carcinoma extends beyond the true pelvis or involves the mucosa of the bladder or rectum
IVA	Adjacent organ involvement
IVB	Distant organ involvement

    c. Radical hysterectomy, pelvic lymphadenectomy, and radiation therapy have similar results in stage IB and IIA cancers. Because of the 15%–25% incidence of lymph node metastases, treatment consists of radical hysterectomy and bilateral pelvic lymphadenectomy.

       (1) Postsurgical complications include bladder and urethral dysfunction or fistulas.

       (2) Radiation therapy (brachytherapy and external beam radiation) may be administered after surgery. Adjuvant radiation is indicated after surgery if there is microscopic parametrial extension, lesions of more than 4 cm, nodal metastases, lymphatic or vascular invasion, positive margins, or grade 3 lesions.

    d. Patients with invasion beyond the cervix but without distant metastatic involvement can be managed with either radiation therapy or surgery. If there is parametrial spread (i.e., the tumor extends through the pelvic wall or into the vagina), radiation therapy may be preferred.

  7. Prognosis. The 5-year survival rate for stage I cervical cancer is 75%–90%; for stage II, 50%–70%; for stage III, 30%–35%; and for stage IV, 10%–15%.

    a. Tumor volume is an important prognostic factor within stages. Both the grade and tumor volume within a given grade have prognostic significance. Histologic type has little significance, except for some unusual variants.

    b. The progressive decrease in survival with advancing stages is associated with an increasing **frequency of lymph node metastases.**

    c. Other poor prognostic factors include **tumor grade, depth of invasion,** and **lymphovascular space invasion.**

C. **Endometrial cancer**

  1. Incidence. Carcinoma of the endometrium is the most common gynecologic malignancy, accounting for 9% of all malignant tumors in women. The incidence of endometrial cancer has been steadily increasing since the 1970s. Approximately 34,000 new cases are diagnosed annually, resulting in approximately 3000 cancer deaths.

2. **Risk factors. Obesity, diabetes, hypertension, polycystic ovarian disease, late onset of menopause,** and **unopposed estrogen therapy** are associated with an increased risk of endometrial cancer. Progesterone decreases the risk associated with the use of postmenopausal estrogens. Risk increases with age. Use of combination oral contraceptives appears to decrease risk. Other risk factors include tamoxifen, chronic anovulation, and irregular menses.

3. **Pathology.** Most endometrial cancers are **adenocarcinomas.** Sixty-seven percent are characteristic endometrioid adenocarcinomas, 20% are endometrial adenocarcinomas with focal areas of benign squamous metaplasia, and 13% are adenosquamous carcinomas.

4. **Clinical features and diagnosis**
   a. Most women with endometrial cancer have abnormal uterine bleeding.
   b. Only 15%–20% of cases of endometrial cancer are identified by Pap smear. Diagnostic procedures include biopsy, fractional dilatation and curettage (D and C), endometrial brush, and jet-wash techniques.
   c. **Pretreatment evaluation** includes routine hematologic and blood chemistries, urinalysis, chest radiograph, and occasionally, hysteroscopy or hysterography.
      (1) **CT** and **cystoscopy** should be performed if there is evidence of bladder dysfunction.
      (2) Patients with gastrointestinal symptoms should undergo **proctosigmoidoscopy** and **barium enema.**
      (3) **Lymphangiography** is used to define involvement of the para-aortic nodes in high-risk patients.

5. **Staging.** The staging system for endometrial carcinoma is listed in Table 4-18. Seventy-four percent of patients who are seen have stage I disease; 13%, stage II disease; 9%, stage III disease; and 3%, stage IV disease.

6. **Therapy**
   a. Treatment measures include **surgery, radiation therapy, hormone therapy,** and, occasionally, **chemotherapy.**
      (1) Synthetic progestogens are the most commonly used hormone therapy agents, with response rates of approximately 35%. The probability of response depends on the histologic grade of the tumor and the presence of progesterone receptors. Well-differentiated tumors have the highest response rates.
      (2) Chemotherapy is of little benefit, but some activity has been seen with cyclophosphamide, 5-FU, doxorubicin, hexamethylmelamine, and cisplatin.
   b. **Specific treatment recommendations**
      (1) Adenomatous hyperplasia can be treated with hysterectomy or hormone therapy, depending on the patient's desire for children.
         (a) Continuous combination estrogen and progesterone contraceptive

TABLE 4-18. International Federation of Gynecology and Obstetrics (FIGO) Classification of Endometrial Carcinoma

Stage	Characteristics
0	Carcinoma in situ
I	Carcinoma confined to the corpus
II	Extension to the cervix only
III	Extension outside the uterus but confined to the true pelvis
IV	Extension beyond the true pelvis or invading bladder or rectum

agents or high-dose progestogens are used for hormone therapy. Ovulation can be induced in these patients with clomiphene.

(b) Patients maintained on hormone therapy should be carefully monitored and undergo routine endometrial sampling.

(2) Patients with uncomplicated endometrial carcinoma are treated with total abdominal hysterectomy and bilateral salpingo-oophorectomy. Radiation therapy is sometimes considered for high-risk patients.

(3) In patients with stage IB disease, preoperative intracavitary radiation therapy is followed by total abdominal hysterectomy. High-risk patients may also receive postoperative radiation therapy.

(4) Patients with stage II disease and extensive cervical involvement should be managed with intracavitary brachytherapy, external beam radiation therapy, extrafascial hysterectomy, and bilateral salpingo-oophorectomy.

(5) Patients with pelvic involvement are treated with surgery and radiation therapy.

7. Prognosis

a. The **stage at diagnosis** is the most important prognostic factor. Five-year survival rates range from 76% in stage I disease to 9% in stage IV disease.

b. Other important prognostic factors include the **extent of cervical and myometrial invasion, lymph node involvement** (especially pelvic or para-aortic nodes), and **histologic grade.** Of lesser importance are uterine size, positive peritoneal cytology, cell type, and patient age.

VI. MELANOMA

A. **Incidence.** The incidence of melanoma has increased rapidly in the last several decades; it currently accounts for 2.5% of all newly diagnosed cancers. By the year 2000, it is estimated that malignant melanoma will develop in 1 in 150 Americans.

B. **Risk factors** for melanoma include:

1. **Fair skin** that sunburns easily and tans poorly, **light eyes,** and **blond or red hair**

2. A **history of blistering sunburn** during adolescence

3. **Dysplastic nevus syndrome.** This disorder is characterized by atypical nevi greater than 5 mm in diameter with multiple areas of pigmentation and irregular borders. These lesions may be the precursor of malignant melanoma.

4. **A family history** of malignant melanoma

5. Congenital **hairy nevi** or **xeroderma pigmentosum**

6. A **personal history of melanoma.** A patient with one melanoma has a 900-fold greater risk of developing a second one.

C. **Clinical features and diagnosis.** Any skin lesion that varies in color or that changes in size or shape (especially if it is accompanied by bleeding or scaling) should be biopsied.

1. Most melanomas are **dark brown** or **black;** however, because some are not pigmented (**amelanotic**), changes in an existing maculopapular lesion should not be ignored.

2. Some lesions exhibit a variety of colors, including **red, blue, white,** and **brown.**

3. A persistently pigmented area of the nailbed warrants biopsy to exclude a **subungual melanoma.**

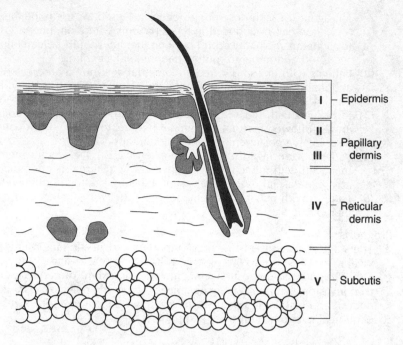

Figure 4-1. Levels of involvement in malignant melanoma. Microstaging of melanomas is based on five levels of invasion, reflecting the depth of tumor penetration. *Level I* (intraepithelial) lesions are confined to the epidermis; *level II* lesions have invaded the papillary layer of the dermis to a depth of 1 mm or less; *level III* lesions reach a depth of 1–2 mm; and *level IV* lesions have progressed beyond 2 mm, well into the reticular dermis. *Level V* lesions have broached the dermis to invade the subcutaneous fat.

D. **Staging.** Figure 4-1 shows the classic microstaging system developed by Clark. Level I lesions are confined to the epidermis and do not metastasize. Lesions that extend into the subcutaneous fat have a much graver prognosis.

E. **Therapy**

1. **Surgery**
   a. **Primary excision.** Lesions that are less than 1 mm in depth can be safely excised with margins of 1 cm. Thicker lesions should be excised with 3-cm margins.
   b. **Nodal dissection.** Elective node dissection is controversial. Some investigators attribute a prophylactic benefit to node dissection in the case of lesions between 1.5 and 3.99 mm in depth. Lymphadenectomy is indicated for patients in whom adenopathy develops.
      (1) In level II patients, radical node dissection yields a 20% cure rate.
      (2) Patients with stage III melanomas (greater than 4 mm thickness) with or without regional spread have a guarded prognosis. Resection of the primary melanoma with in-continuity removal of subcutaneous tissue and fascia over the muscle and the contiguous nodal area is recommended.

2. **Chemotherapy** is of little benefit. Drugs with documented activity include dacarbazine, cisplatin, and the nitrosoureas.
   a. Dacarbazine is considered the best single agent, with a 15% response rate; however, a 30% response rate was observed with tamoxifen and dacarbazine.
   b. The combination of dacarbazine, carmustine, cisplatin, and tamoxifen has a 50% response rate.
   c. Taxol has a 20% response rate.

3. **Biologic response modifiers** have demonstrated antitumor activity in patients with metastatic disease.

a. Interferon has a 15%–20% response rate, primarily in soft tissue and lung metastases. Adjuvant interferon therapy has been shown to improve the disease-free and overall survival rates for stage III patients and those with nodal metastases that are resected.

b. IL-2, combined with LAK cells, has elicited long-term complete responses in patients with metastatic melanoma.

c. Other experimental procedures include **antitumor vaccines** and **monoclonal antibody therapy.**

F. Prognosis

1. The **thickness** of the melanoma, measured from the stratum corneum to the deepest penetration of the tumor, is thought to be the best predictor of the risk of metastatic disease.

   a. The majority of patients with lesions smaller than 0.85 mm in depth are cured by surgical excision.

   b. Ninety-three percent of patients with lesions between 0.85 and 1.69 mm in depth, 70% of those with lesions between 1.7 and 3.6 mm, and 38% of those with lesions deeper than 3.6 mm are ultimately cured.

2. Other prognostic factors include the melanoma site, the patient's age and gender, the degree of ulceration, and the degree of the host lymphocytic response around the primary lesion.

VII. CARCINOMA OF THE LUNG

A. Incidence. The frequency of lung cancer is increasing rapidly. Originally a disease that primarily afflicted men older than age 60 years, lung cancer has become the second most common cause of cancer in women.

B. Etiology. Epidemiologic studies have linked lung cancer to the following factors.

1. **Cigarette smoking.** Research has demonstrated a direct correlation between smoking and lung cancer, with increases in daily cigarette consumption leading to increases in cancer incidence. "Passive smoking" is associated with a small but significant increase in the incidence of lung cancer.

2. **Industrial carcinogens.** Exposure to beryllium, radon, and asbestos has been linked to lung cancer. Cigarette smoking exacerbates the risk associated with such exposure. Smoking and asbestos exposure increase the risk 53-fold.

3. **Air pollutants** (e.g., diesel exhaust, pitch, tar, arsenic, chromium, cadmium, nickel) increase the risk of lung cancer.

4. **Existing lung damage.** Adenocarcinomas of the lung may develop in areas scarred by **tuberculosis** or other lung conditions associated with **fibrosis.** These tumors are called **scar carcinomas.**

5. Patients with **lymphoma** or **malignancies of the head, neck,** and **esophagus** have an increased incidence of lung cancer.

C. Pathology. Four major varieties of lung cancer occur.

1. **Squamous cell carcinomas** were once the most common type of non–small-cell lung cancer, but they have become less common than adenocarcinomas. Squamous cell tumors tend to arise centrally near the hilum where they present as endobronchial disease or as a peripheral lesion.

2. **Adenocarcinoma** is increasing in frequency, especially in women. These lesions are often peripheral, occurring in more distal airways. **Bronchoalveolar cell cancer,** a variant of adenocarcinoma, arises in the alveoli and causes lobular consolidation on the chest radiograph.

3. **Large-cell undifferentiated cancers** account for 5%–10% of all lung cancers. These tumors are usually peripheral lesions.

4. **Small-cell lung carcinoma (SCLC)** arises from neural crest neuroendocrine or amine precursor uptake and decarboxylation (APUD) cells and progresses rapidly without treatment. The average survival time in the absence of treatment is only 2–4 months.

D. **Clinical features**

1. **Local symptoms** of intrathoracic disease include cough, hemoptysis, obstructive pneumonia (due to endobronchial tumors), chest pain, pleural effusion, hoarseness (due to recurrent laryngeal nerve compression by a mediastinal tumor), and superior vena cava syndrome (due to obstruction of the vessel by a mediastinal tumor). Patients with bronchoalveolar cell cancer may have a severe cough productive of clear sputum.

2. **Systemic manifestations** include:
   a. Anorexia and weight loss
   b. Bone pain from distant metastases
   c. Hepatomegaly, tenderness, and fever due to liver involvement
   d. CNS signs or seizures from brain metastases or carcinomatous meningitis
   e. Hypercalcemia from bone metastases or other humoral substances

3. Patients with small-cell carcinoma may present with symptoms of ectopic hormone production or other **paraneoplastic syndromes.**
   a. **Ectopic adrenocorticotropic hormone (ACTH) secretion** causes hypokalemia and muscle wasting.
   b. **Syndrome of inappropriate antidiuretic hormone secretion (SIADH)** results in hyponatremia.

E. **Diagnosis**

1. **Sputum cytology or bronchoscopy** confirms the diagnosis in patients with endobrochial disease. Bronchoscopy also assesses proximal endobronchial tumor extension and the status of the contralateral lung. Bronchoscopy should be done in all patients with centrally located tumors and in selected patients with peripheral tumors.

2. **Transthoracic needle biopsy,** guided by x-ray or CT, is often necessary for the diagnosis of peripheral lesions. The false-negative rate is 15%.

3. **Transbronchial needle aspiration** of mediastinal nodes may obviate the need for more invasive procedures.

4. **Thoracotomy** or **mediastinoscopy** is required in approximately 5%–10% of patients. These invasive procedures are especially useful in the diagnosis of small-cell lung cancer, which grows centrally in the mediastinum rather than endobronchially. Mediastinoscopy or mediastinotomy can also be used to assess the resectability of mediastinal and hilar nodes.

5. **Video-assisted transthorascopic surgery (VATS)** is less invasive than thoracotomy. VATS involves three or four (1- to 2-cm) incisions in the chest wall, diaphragm, lung parenchyma, and mediastinal structures. Visible lesions may be biopsied.

6. **Node biopsy** is used to evaluate suspicious supraclavicular or neck lymph nodes.

7. **CT scans** of the chest, liver, brain, and adrenal glands can establish the **extent of metastatic disease,** including mediastinal node involvement and chest wall invasion.

8. **Radionuclide bone scans** may be used to rule out metastatic disease.

9. **MRI** of the chest is most useful for evaluating spread to cardiovascular organs (e.g., heart, aorta, superior vena cava).

TABLE 4-19. TNM Staging System for Lung Cancer

Stage	Characteristics
Primary tumor (T)	
T_0	No evidence of primary tumor
T_x	Tumor proven by presence of malignant cells in bronchopulmonary secretions, or any tumor that cannot be assessed
T_{is}	Carcinoma in situ
T_1	Tumor ≤3 cm in diameter, no evidence of invasion
T_2	Tumor >3 cm in diameter, or any tumor that either invades the visceral pleura or has associated atelectasis or obstructive pneumonitis extending to the hilar region
T_3	Direct extension into adjacent structure (e.g., pleura or chest wall), involvement of a main bronchus, or associated atelectasis or pneumonitis of an entire lung
Regional lymph nodes (N)	
N_0	No metastases to nodes
N_1	Metastasis to peribronchial or ipsilateral hilar nodes or both
N_2	Metastasis to mediastinal nodes
Distant metastasis (M)	
M_x	Not assessed
M_0	No distant metastases
M_1	Distant metastases present

F. **Staging.** The AJCC TNM staging system for lung cancer is summarized in Table 4-19.

G. **Therapy**

1. **Non–small-cell lung cancer.** Because **surgery is the only curative option** for patients with these cancers, the goals of staging are to evaluate tumor resectability and to determine the extent of disease spread beyond the hemithorax.
   a. **Pretreatment evaluation**
      (1) A tumor is resectable if **thoracotomy** demonstrates that all of the tumor can be completely excised with pathologically negative margins.
      (2) Mediastinoscopy or mediastinotomy should be used only if positive findings will prevent a curative thoracotomy.
   b. **Modalities**
      (1) **Surgery**
         (a) **Operable tumors.** If cardiopulmonary status is compatible with lung resection, surgical options include lobectomy or pneumonectomy depending on the extent of disease. The surgeon should aim to remove the tumor completely with adequate margins of resection, while conserving as much normal lung tissue as possible.
         (b) **Advanced local cancer.** Selected patients may undergo surgical resection with or without chest irradiation.
            (i) Patients with small tumors in the ipsilateral mediastinal nodes or large primary tumors without mediastinal node involvement have 5-year survival rates as high as 35% with a combination of surgery and radiation therapy.
            (ii) **Pancoast's tumor** or tumors of the superior sulcus may also be cured by a combination of surgery and radiation therapy.
      (2) **Radiation therapy**
         (a) Radiation therapy reduces local recurrences in operable stage II tumors.

(b) Patients who cannot tolerate surgery due to insufficient cardiopulmonary reserve should receive chest irradiation. Survival rates at 5 years range from 5%–20% for this group.

(c) **Inoperable or advanced tumors.** Radiation therapy is often used in asymptomatic patients, but survival is, at best, minimally improved. **Palliative therapy** can relieve the symptoms of pain, hemoptysis, superior vena cava syndrome, or pneumonitis that are associated with obstructive lesions. Patients with metastatic disease are also treated with palliative radiation therapy.

(3) **Chemotherapy**

(a) The benefit of adjuvant chemotherapy **in patients with resectable tumors** is uncertain. A recent unconfirmed study suggests that combination chemotherapy using cyclophosphamide, adriamycin, and cisplatin may be superior to immunotherapy in stage II patients who have undergone resection. The median survival time of patients with stage II or III lung cancer who have undergone resection is 22.5 months with chemotherapy, compared with 15.5 months with BCG and levamisole.

(b) Several studies have shown that, in stage III patients, neoadjuvant chemotherapy improves survival. In one study, two courses of cisplatin and vinblastine given before radiation therapy in stage III patients was superior to giving radiation alone. The survival rates were 55% at 1 year (versus 40%), 26% at 2 years (versus 13%), and 23% at 3 years (versus 11%).

(c) **Treatment of metastatic disease.** Combination chemotherapy has a response rate of approximately 10%–30% in patients with metastatic non–small-cell lung cancer. Response rates double in ambulatory patients who have not lost weight. The most commonly used combinations of drugs include:

(i) Carboplatin and Taxol

(ii) Cisplatin and etoposide

(iii) Mitomycin C, vinblastine, and cisplatin

(iv) Navelbine and cisplatin

(v) Ifosfamide, etoposide, and cisplatin

2. **SCLC**

a. **Pretreatment evaluation**

(1) Staging in patients with small-cell cancer aims to differentiate between limited disease and extensive disease.

(a) **Limited disease** is that which is confined to one hemithorax; the entire tumor can be encompassed in a single radiation therapy portal. The highest long-term survival rates (10%–50%) in these patients are obtained with **concurrent chemotherapy and radiation therapy,** especially hyperfractionated radiation therapy and combination chemotherapy.

(b) Patients with **extensive disease** have distant metastases, supraclavicular node involvement, or pleural effusions.

(i) These patients are treated with **combination chemotherapy alone.**

(ii) Radiation therapy has only palliative benefit in patients who have failed to respond to chemotherapy or who have brain metastases.

(2) Staging procedures include chest radiography; CT of the chest, liver, and brain, followed by bone scans or radiography of suspicious areas; and bilateral bone marrow biopsies or aspirates.

b. **Therapy**

(1) **Chemotherapy** is the mainstay of treatment. Active drugs include cisplatin, etoposide, cyclophosphamide, ifosfamide, carboplatin, vincristine, adriamycin, and Taxol. Regimens include etoposide and cisplatin or cyclophosphamide, doxorubicin (Adriamycin), and vincristine (CAV) therapy.

(2) **Prophylactic cranial irradiation** should be considered in responsive patients, especially those with limited disease.

H. **Prognosis**

1. **Non–small-cell lung cancer.** Key prognostic factors include the **extent of tumor dissemination, performance status,** and **weight loss.**
   a. Survival rates range from 40%–50% in stage I disease and from 15%–30% in stage II disease.
   b. Higher rates are observed in patients who undergo extensive mediastinal node sampling.
   c. In advanced cases, radiation therapy alone yields 5-year survival rates of 4%–8%.

2. Long-term survival rates in patients with **limited small-cell carcinoma** vary from 10%–50% after combined chemotherapy and radiation therapy. Extensive disease, however, has a grim prognosis.

VIII. **CANCER OF UNKNOWN PRIMARY SITE (CUPS)**

A. **Incidence.** Patients with CUPS have metastatic carcinoma in the absence of a demonstrable primary site. Approximately 2%–10% of new cancer patients have CUPS. Even at autopsy, the primary site remains obscure in 15%–20% of patients.

B. **Pathology**

1. **Histologic subtypes**
   a. Adenocarcinoma is the most common subtype, occurring in 40%–77% of patients.
   b. Squamous cell carcinomas are present in 5%–15% of patients.
   c. Other cell types include lymphomas, germ cell tumors, melanomas, and sarcomas.
      (1) **Lymphoma** can sometimes be distinguished from undifferentiated carcinoma by special stains such as leukocyte common antigen.
      (2) **Metastatic small-cell endocrine tumors** can be identified by staining for s-100 or neuron-specific enolase.
      (3) **Germ cell tumors** stain positive for AFP or hCG.

2. Light microscopy, electron microscopy, and immunohistochemical techniques may be useful in identifying the histologic subtype or tissue origin.
   a. Visualization of the cellular architecture by **light microscopy** may identify adenocarcinomas, squamous cell carcinomas, melanoma, sarcoma, or lymphoma. However, because CUPS is often anaplastic, differentiation by light microscopy is not always possible.
   b. **Immunohistochemical markers** are an important pathological tool. For example, a positive keratin stain implies that the tumor is of epithelial origin. Table 4-20 lists the immunohistochemical markers that correspond to various cell types.
   c. **Electron microscopy** detects **intracellular bridging,** characteristic of squamous cell carcinomas; **neurosecretory granules,** characteristic of neuroendocrine tumors; **melanosomes,** characteristic of melanoma; and **intracellular structures,** such as myofibrils, characteristic of sarcomas.

C. **Diagnosis.** Because pancreatic, lung, and colon cancers are the most likely primary sources of undifferentiated adenocarcinoma, routine diagnostic procedures include a chest radiograph, fecal occult blood test (accompanied by barium studies in positive cases), and abdominal CT.

1. **Women** should also undergo **mammography, pelvic examination,** and **pelvic ultrasound.**

2. **Prostate-specific antigen levels** should be determined in **men.**

TABLE 4-20. Tumor Markers for Identifying Tissue Origin in Cancer of Unknown Primary Site

Marker	Cell or Tumor Type
Immunohistochemical	
Keratin	Epithelial
Mucin	Adenocarinoma
Estrogen or progesterone receptors	Breast, endometrium, ovary
Acid phosphatase	Prostate
Thyroglobulin	Thyroid
Gremilius	Neuroendocrine
s-100	Sarcoma, melanoma
Vimentin, desmin	Sarcoma
Lymphocyte common antigen	Lymphoma
Serum markers	
Human chorionic gonadotropin (β-hCG)	Germ cell tumor
α-fetoprotein (AFP)	Germ cell tumor, hepatomas
Prostate-specific antigen (PSA)	Prostate
Carcinoembryonic antigen (CEA)	Gastrointestinal malignancies
CA 125	Ovary
CA 15-3	Breast

3. Patients with suspected germ cell carcinomas should also undergo β-hCG and AFP determinations.

D. **Therapy** varies according to the suspected primary site but typically includes palliative radiation therapy or chemotherapy.

1. Slow-growing tumors may merely be monitored at 4- to 8-week intervals.

2. Chemotherapy is an experimental option for **adenocarcinoma.**
   a. The highest response rates have been observed with mitomycin and doxorubicin.
   b. Women with suspected adenocarcinoma in an axillary node should be considered to have stage II breast cancer and be treated accordingly.

3. Patients with **squamous cell carcinoma metastatic to the neck** from an unknown primary site, but no distant metastases, should be treated with neck dissection and radiation therapy to the neck.

4. Young men with **anaplastic tumors of the mediastinum or retroperitoneum** may respond to treatment modalities used for germ cell tumors of the testis, especially if AFP or β-hCG levels are elevated.

E. **Prognosis.** Median survival is only 5–6 months after diagnosis, although there is a broad range and 3%–5% of patients may be alive after 5 years.

IX. **CANCERS OF THE KIDNEY, BLADDER, AND PROSTATE**

A. **Renal cell cancer**

1. **Incidence.** Cancer of the kidney (hypernephroma) accounts for 2%–3% of all cancers. The ratio of affected men to women is 2:3, with an average age of 55–60 years at presentation.

2. **Risk factors.** Patients with von Hippel-Lindau disease or acquired polycystic kidney disease have a higher incidence of renal carcinoma. Familial types of renal

TABLE 4-21. Staging System for Renal Carcinomas

Stage	Characteristics
I	Tumor <2.5 cm in diameter; confined to kidney and capsule
II	Tumor >2.5 cm in diameter; invasion confined to perinephric fat
III	Tumor confined to Gerota's fascia, with involvement of regional lymph nodes, renal vein, or vena cava
IV	Tumor extends beyond Gerota's fascia; distant metastases

cell carcinoma have been associated with abnormalities of chromosome 3 and the common p53 gene.

3. **Pathology**
   a. Most renal tumors are clear-cell carcinomas (adenocarcinomas); however, granular cell tumors, mixed tumors, and aggressive carcinosarcomas (adenocarcinomas with sarcomatous degeneration) also occur. Rarely, tumors arise in renal cysts.
   b. Renal cancers are usually **extremely vascular, readily metastasizing** to the lung, bone, liver, brain, and other sites. Dissemination may also occur when tumor emboli enter the renal vein and inferior vena cava or by nodal spread in the para-aortic, paracaval, hilar, and mediastinal areas.

4. **Clinical features**
   a. Hematuria (40%–70% of patients)
   b. Abdominal mass with flank pain (20%–40% of patients)
   c. Weight loss (30% of patients)
   d. Fever, malaise, night sweats, or anemia (15%–30% of patients)
   e. Paraneoplastic syndromes, including hypercalcemia, polycythemia, or hypertension

5. **Diagnostic procedures** include hematologic studies, IVP, renal ultrasound, and, in some cases, a selective renal arteriogram or venacavogram. Chest radiographs, abdominal CT, and radionuclide bone scans detect the presence of metastases. MRI scans are superior for visualizing a tumor or clot in the renal vein and vena cava.

6. **Staging** follows the classification scheme outlined in Table 4-21.

7. **Therapy**
   a. **Surgery**
      (1) **Radical nephrectomy** with lymph node dissection is the treatment of choice for stage I, stage II, and stage III renal cell carcinomas. Nephrectomy should also be considered for patients with disseminated disease to relieve hematuria and flank pain.
      (2) In certain cases, **selective renal arterial embolization** permits surgical resection or halts life-threatening hematuria.
      (3) Patients with one or two metastatic lesions, indolent tumor growth, and no evidence of progressive metastasis may be candidates for aggressive **surgical resection of metastases.**
   b. **Radiation therapy** has only limited value.
   c. **Chemotherapy** is also relatively ineffective, with transient tumor regression occurring in less than 5% of patients. The most commonly used chemotherapeutic agents are vinblastine and the nitrosoureas.
   d. **Biologic response modifiers**
      (1) α-IFN yields response rates of 13%–20% in patients with soft tissue or lung metastases.
      (2) Recent trials of **IL-2** plus LAK cells are promising, with partial tumor regression reported in 12%–40% of cases. However, the treatment is extremely toxic, and most responses are limited in duration.

8. **Prognosis.** Radical nephrectomy yields a 5-year survival rate in 75% of patients with localized tumors. However, patients with high-grade stage III lesions with vascular invasion have an overall survival rate of only 5%–15%.

B. **Uroepithelial tract carcinomas** (bladder, ureter, and renal pelvis)

1. **Incidence.** These tumors account for roughly 3% of the cancer deaths in the United States. Bladder carcinomas are three times more common in men than in women and usually occur in patients who are 40–70 years of age.

2. **Etiology.** Bladder cancers have been related to **tobacco** as well as certain chemical and biologic carcinogens.
   a. **Occupational carcinogens** in the rubber, dye, printing, and chemical industries have been implicated in bladder carcinoma.
   b. **Saccharin** has been proven to cause bladder tumors in animals, but its role in humans is less clear.
   c. **Schistosomiasis** of the bladder has been strongly correlated with squamous cell carcinoma.
   d. Other etiologic agents include **cyclophosphamide, phenacetin, renal stones, and chronic infection.**

3. **Pathology.** Bladder tumors are generally of transitional cell origin, with the exception of the Oriental schistosome-related variant, which is of squamous cell origin.

4. **Clinical features.** Seventy-five percent of bladder cancer patients present with **hematuria. Bladder irritability** and **infection** are the presenting symptoms in the remaining 25%.

5. **Diagnosis**
   a. **Cystoscopy,** with bimanual palpation and subsequent biopsy, is the definitive diagnostic procedure. This technique is nearly 100% accurate.
   b. **Radiologic procedures** include IVP, pelvic and abdominal CT scans, chest radiograph, bone scan, and retrograde pyelography for renal pelvic or ureteral tumors.
   c. **Laboratory tests** include a CBC and chemistry profile as well as urine cytology and flow cytometry for high-risk patients.

6. **Staging.** Table 4-22 lists the staging system for uroepithelial tumors.

7. **Therapy**
   a. **Surgery**
      (1) **Superficial lesions** (stages O, A, and sometimes B_1) are treated with **endoscopic resection** and **fulguration,** followed by cystoscopy every 3 months. Recurrent or multiple lesions are treated with intravesicular instillation of thiotepa, mitomycin, or BCG.
      (2) **Recurrent cancer, diffuse transitional cell carcinoma in situ,** or **stages B and C invasive cancers** are treated with **radical cystectomy.**
      (3) Tumors of the renal pelvis or ureter are treated by **removal of the affected kidney or ureter.**

TABLE 4-22. Staging System for Uroepithelial Tumors

Stage	Characteristics
0	Superficial mucosal tumors (carcinoma in situ and papillary)
A	Tumor invades the lamina propria
B_1	Tumor confined to <50% of the muscle
B_2	Tumor involves >50% of the muscle
C	Tumor involves the perivesical fat
D	Tumor involves the prostate or lymph nodes

b. Combination chemotherapy with methotrexate, vinblastine, doxorubicin (Adriamycin), and cisplatin (the MVAC regimen) yields response rates of 60%–70%, of which 25%–40% represent complete remissions. The MVAC regimen has also been used in bladder-sparing investigational studies, with or without radiation therapy.

C. **Prostate carcinoma**

1. **Incidence.** Cancer of the prostate accounts for 18% of all new cancers in the United States (approximately 75,000 cases). Incidence rates are higher among blacks and increase with age. At autopsy, the incidence among men older than age 50 years ranges from 14%–46%.

2. **Pathology.** Nearly all prostate cancers are adenocarcinomas.
   a. Prostate adenocarcinomas are classified as **well-, moderately well-,** or **poorly differentiated,** according to the **Gleason prognostic classification system,** which assigns a grade between 0 and 5 to the primary and secondary differentiation patterns.
   b. The majority of prostatic tumors originate in the peripheral zone; only 25% originate in the central zone.
   c. More than 90% of distant metastases involve bone, but soft tissue metastases can also occur in the nodes, lung, and liver.

3. **Clinical features** at presentation include a palpable nodule (observed in more than 50% of patients), dysuria, urinary retention, terminal hematuria, and urinary dribbling, frequency, or urgency.

4. **Diagnosis** remains difficult for early prostatic lesions.
   a. **Screening and diagnosis**
      (1) **Routine physicals. Digital rectal examination** remains the diagnostic gold standard for prostate carcinoma, even though only 10% of the prostatic tumors found as nodules on rectal examination are sufficiently localized for cure.
      (2) **Pathologic examination** of tissue removed for treatment of obstructive prostatic hypertrophy reveals that 10% of cases are malignant.
      (3) The remaining cases, when found, are in advanced stages; often these cancers are **revealed in investigations for metastatic bone disease.**
      (4) **Acid phosphatase levels** detect disease that has penetrated the prostate capsule.
         (a) This test is **abnormal in more than 80% of cases presenting with distant metastases.**
         (b) Phosphatase levels should be obtained before rectal examination or prostate massage, because erroneously high levels have been reported for 1–2 days after such manipulation.
      (5) Recently, levels of **prostate-specific antigen** (PSA) have been advocated as a diagnostic marker, but falsely positive values may occur. If the PSA is more than 10, there is a 66% chance that the biopsy will reveal prostate cancer. If the PSA is between 4 and 10, then 22% of the prostate biopsies will be positive.
      (6) **Transrectal ultrasonography (TRUS)** is most useful for evaluation of prostate size and for the precise biopsy of lesions that are not palpable.
   b. **Confirmation**
      (1) **Needle biopsy,** obtained via the rectum, perineum, or urethra, confirms the diagnosis.
      (2) **Laboratory studies** are used to assess renal function, whereas bone scans, radiographs, IVP, and pelvic or retroperitoneal CT confirm the presence of metastatic disease.

5. **Staging** techniques are crucial to the investigation and proper treatment of prostatic carcinoma.
   a. **Stage A tumors** are unsuspected clinically and are found at autopsy or by examining tissue removed for alleged benign disease. **A₁ (well-differentiated**

with three or fewer foci) tumors have better prognoses than **A₂ (poorly differ-entiated,** or more than three foci) tumors.

b. Stage B tumors are **neoplasms that are confined to the prostate gland.** These are the classic nodules found on rectal examination, which theoretically are curable by surgery, although only 10% of prostate cancers are actually curable by surgery. Many of these nodules already have pelvic node metastases when discovered on rectal examination. Clinically palpable lesions in the prostate are stage B₁ (less than 1.5 cm, involving one lobe) and stage B₂ (more than 1.5 cm, diffuse involvement).

c. Stage C tumors are cancers that have spread beyond the prostate capsule into the pelvis (i.e., to the seminal vesicles) but not to distant sites. These cannot be cured by surgery and account for 40% of new cases.

d. Stage D tumors are cancers that have spread from the prostate area to pelvic lymph nodes, bone, or beyond. Approximately 50% of newly diagnosed cases are stage D on presentation.

6. **Therapy and prognosis** are determined by the stage of disease at diagnosis.
   a. Early disease is treated with radical prostatectomy, external beam radiation, or interstitial implantation radiation therapy.
      (1) Prostatectomy is performed in patients with at least a 10-year life expec-tancy and results in a 10- to 15-year survival rate. Patients with stages A₂, B₁, and B₂ and younger patients with A₁ disease are candidates for surgi-cal cure. Up to 16% of patients presenting with A₁ disease, who are thought to have benign disease, progress.
      (2) Nerve-sparing radical prostatectomy is appropriate for patients with small lesions. This surgical approach preserves normal sexual functioning in 40%–60% of cases, but is associated with a 5%–15% rate of postsurgical urinary incontinence.
      (3) Radiation therapy is used for older patients, those with other medical dis-orders or large prostatic lesions precluding surgery, and for men who wish to retain normal sexual activity. The incidence of impotence with intersti-tial implantation is less than with radical external radiation, which dam-ages the pudendal nerve in as many as 40% of cases. With modern tech-niques, 60–70 Gy provides good local control with minimal morbidity. Radiation is useful in treating metastatic bone disease using external beam or strontium-99 intravenously in patients with widespread disease.
   b. Stage D tumors cannot be cured, so only palliative treatment is available.
      (1) Endocrine therapy is generally the initial mode of treatment.
         (a) In the past, **orchiectomy** and **exogenous estrogens** were used inter-changeably.
            (i) Orchiectomy is preferred in patients with cardiovascular or throm-botic risk.
            (ii) Postsurgical administration of exogenous hormones, such as diethylstilbestrol (DES, 1–3 mg daily), further suppresses testoster-one levels.
         (b) More recent approaches have focused on the LH-RH analogue **leuprol-ide** or Zoladex, either alone or in combination with the anti-androgen **flutamide.** Flutamide and **aminoglutethimide** are an option for patients who fail to respond to primary hormone treatment.
            (i) These hormonal manipulations induce remissions in approxi-mately 50%–80% of patients, although cures are rare.
            (ii) Typically, prostate and soft tissue lesions regress, acid phospha-tase and prostate-specific antigen levels decline to normal values, and bone pain rapidly decreases.
            (iii) The average duration of hormone response is 9–18 months.
         (c) Other hormonal manipulations, such as adrenalectomy, followed by administration of aminoglutethimide or flutamide, may produce tran-sient responses.

(2) **Chemotherapy** is often disappointing. The most frequently used agents are cisplatin, doxorubicin, cyclophosphamide, and 5-FU.

X. TESTICULAR CANCER

A. **Incidence.** Testicular cancer is the most common malignancy in young men and accounts for 1% of all male cancers. The average age at diagnosis is 32 years.

B. **Risk factors** include the presence of a **cryptorchid testicle** and a **prior history** of testicular cancer.

C. **Pathology.** Testicular tumors are classified as **seminomatous** or **nonseminomatous.**

1. **Seminomas** may be further subclassified as **classical, anaplastic,** or **spermatocystic.**

2. Four types of **nonseminomatous tumors** are recognized.
   a. **Embryonal carcinoma**
   b. **Teratoma**
   c. **Yolk sac carcinoma** (also known as **endodermal sinus tumor**)
   d. **Choriocarcinoma**

D. **Clinical features**

1. More than 90%–95% of patients have a **painless, solid testicular swelling.** Occasionally, patients with painful testicular masses are erroneously diagnosed as having epididymitis or orchitis.

2. Para-aortic lymph node involvement can occur as **ureteral obstruction.**

3. Patients may also have **abdominal complaints** from an abdominal mass or **pulmonary symptoms** from multiple nodules.

4. **Gynecomastia** occurs in patients with elevated β-hCG levels.

E. **Diagnosis**

1. **Scrotal ultrasound** may reveal a suspicious intratesticular echogenic focus. Ultrasound can also define penetration of the spermatic cord, epididymis, and scrotum.

2. **Radiological tests** include:
   a. **Chest radiograph**
   b. **CT scans** of the chest, abdomen, and pelvis, as well as the brain (in patients with neurologic symptoms)
   c. **Excretory urography** (to determine the course of the ureter)
   d. **Venacavogram**
   e. **Bipedal lymphangiography,** especially for suspected seminomas
   f. **Isotope scans** of bone

3. **Inguinal exploratory surgery,** including high ligation of the spermatic cord and orchiectomy, is necessary for patients with suspicious scrotal masses.
   a. Vascular control must be achieved before manipulation of the tumor.
   b. Open biopsy and scrotal exploration are contraindicated because of the possibility of tumor spread.

4. **Elevated blood levels of AFP or β-hCG** are diagnostic for nonseminomatous germ cell tumors; most seminoma patients, however, have normal markers.

TABLE 4-23. TNM Classification of Testicular Tumors

Stage	Classification
Primary tumor (T)	
T_x	Primary tumor cannot be assessed or radical orchiectomy cannot be performed
T_0	Histologic scar or no evidence of primary tumor
T_{is}	Intratubular tumor (preinvasive cancer)
T_1	Tumor limited to testis, including rete testis
T_2	Tumor beyond tunica albuginea or into epididymis
T_3	Tumor invades spermatic cord
T_4	Tumor invades scrotum
Regional lymph nodes (N)	
N_1	Single node <2 cm
N_2	Single node >2 cm but <5 cm or multiple nodes <5 cm
N_3	Node >5 cm
Distant metastasis (M)	
M_x	Not assessed
M_0	No distant metastases
M_1	Distant metastases present

Adapted with permission from Frank IN, Graham SD Jr, Nabors WL: Tumor (T), Node (N) Classification Testis Cancer TNM. In *Textbook of Clinical Oncology.* Atlanta, The American Cancer Society, 1991, p 284.

F. **Staging**

1. **Anatomic staging.** The TNM classification for primary testicular tumors, nodal involvement, and distant metastases is outlined in Table 4-23.

2. An older alternative staging system is outlined below.
   a. **Stage A** tumors are confined to the testis.
   b. **Stage B$_1$** exhibits minimal retroperitoneal nodal involvement (fewer than six positive nodes and no nodes greater than 2 cm in diameter).
   c. **Stage B$_2$** is characterized by moderate retroperitoneal adenopathy (more than six positive nodes or any one node between 2 and 5 cm in diameter).
   d. **Stage B$_3$** tumors have massive retroperitoneal nodal involvement or a nodal mass greater than 5 cm.
   e. **Stage C** involves metastasis to nodes above the diaphragm or to distant sites.

G. **Therapy**

1. **Nonseminomatous tumors**
   a. **Clinical stage I disease** limited to the testis may be treated with **orchiectomy** followed by **retroperitoneal lymph node dissection.** Some experts, however, believe that rigorous follow-up to orchiectomy, without surgery, is sufficient.
      (1) In TN_1, TN_2, or M_0-staged patients with nonseminomatous cancer, a seminoma with an elevated AFP level, or a seminoma with persistent β-hCG elevation after orchiectomy, a bilateral retroperitoneal lymph node dissection is carried out.
      (2) Observation is an option for clinical N_0 patients.
   b. Patients with **stage II disease** are treated surgically or with chemotherapy.
      (1) Patients with tumors less than 3 cm in diameter may be treated with node dissection for curative intent.
      (2) Patients with retroperitoneal tumors more than 5 cm in diameter should receive chemotherapy.
      (3) Adjuvant chemotherapy following complete resection is optional. Patients who have proven extranodal extension, any node more than 2 cm in diameter, or at least six positive nodes have a relapse rate following node dis-

section of greater than 50%. With adjuvant chemotherapy, however, the relapse rate approaches zero.

2. **Seminomas**
   a. **Stage I seminomas** are treated with retroperitoneal and pelvic radiation therapy. Following treatment, patients should be reevaluated monthly for the first year, then every 2 months for a second year.
   b. **Stage II seminomas.** Twenty percent of patients with Stage II seminoma have retroperitoneal node metastases.
      (1) Radiation therapy is the treatment of choice for patients with a positive lymphangiogram. Because of bone marrow toxicity from mediastinal radiation therapy, prophylactic radiation to the mediastinum is no longer indicated.
      (2) Patients with retroperitoneal adenopathy have a high relapse rate after radiation therapy. Thus, these patients should receive **chemotherapy.**
   c. **Stage III or IV seminomas (and nonseminomatous germ cell tumors)** are generally treated with high-dose cisplatin in combination with etoposide and bleomycin at 3- to 4-week intervals. Etoposide has replaced vinblastine in combination regimens because of its lower incidence of toxicity.
      (1) Other chemotherapeutic options for patients with recurrent disease include ifosfamide, carboplatin, and vinblastine.
      (2) Surgical removal of residual disease should be considered for patients with refractory disease. Patients with viable residual tumors should receive two additional cycles of chemotherapy. Radiation therapy is indicated for patients with a negative lymphangiogram.
      (3) High-dose chemotherapy with carboplatin and etoposide may be combined with an autologous bone marrow transplant.

H. **Prognosis**

1. **Seminomas.** Patients with stage A and B disease have a cure rate of greater than 90% after radiation therapy. Chemotherapy results in complete response rates ranging from 63%–90%.

2. **Nonseminomatous germ cell tumors.** Complete remission can be obtained in 50%–70% of patients with metastatic disease following chemotherapy alone. Another 10%–15% are disease-free after surgical removal of residual tumor. Relapses occur in 10%–20% of patients within the first 2 years of initial diagnosis and treatment.

3. The probability of complete response to chemotherapy depends on the location and bulk of metastatic disease. Patients with advanced pulmonary or nodal disease exhibit a response rate of 67%, whereas those with advanced organ metastases to the liver or brain have a response rate of only 20%.

XI. **HEAD AND NECK CARCINOMAS**

A. **Incidence.** Head and neck carcinomas account for 5% of the cancers reported each year in the United States. These tumors occur three times more frequently in men than in women. Patients are typically between 50 and 60 years old. The most frequently affected sites are the oral cavity (40%), larynx (25%), oropharynx and hypopharynx (15%), and salivary gland (10%).

B. The following **risk factors** have been associated with an increased incidence of head and neck carcinomas.

1. **Tobacco use.** Cigarette smoking is the major cause of head and neck cancer and relative risk increases with the number of cigarettes smoked per day. Chewing to-

bacco is responsible for a recent increase in the incidence of oral cancer among young adults.

2. Alcohol consumption works in combination with cigarette smoking to increase the incidence of head and neck cancer 10- to 40-fold.

3. Nickel exposure increases the risk of cancers of the nasal cavity and paranasal sinus.

4. Syphilis is associated with an increased incidence of cancer of the tongue.

5. Prolonged sun exposure increases the incidence of lip cancer.

6. The **Epstein-Barr virus** and certain **food dyes** have been linked to nasopharyngeal cancers in Asians.

C. **Pathology.** Most of these tumors (95%) are squamous cell carcinomas, which vary from well-differentiated varieties to invasive, poorly differentiated or undifferentiated varieties. Nodal involvement is a factor of the primary tumor site, size, and degree of differentiation.

1. Tumors of the salivary gland are most commonly of the mixed type, although adenoid cystic carcinomas are not uncommon.

2. Nasopharyngeal cancers may be squamous cell cancers, lymphoepitheliomas, or lymphomas.

D. **Clinical features.** Common symptoms include dysphagia, hoarseness, head or neck pain, ear pain, and neck or head swellings. Large lesions may present with ulcerations or as white patches. Some patients present with adenopathy in the absence of an obvious primary source.

E. **Diagnosis**

1. Detection
   a. Tissue diagnosis relies on biopsy of the non-necrotic portion of the tumor, tumor edge, and adjacent normal mucosa. Open biopsy of the neck nodes should be avoided if head and neck cancer of the squamous cell type is suspected.
   b. Radiologic studies may include:
      (1) Radiographs of the mandible, sinus, or nasopharynx
      (2) CT and MRI scans to evaluate the nasopharynx, thymus, oral cavity, and oral pharynx, and to check nodal involvement
      (3) A barium swallow (in patients with evidence of tumor encroachment on the cervical esophagus)

2. Pretreatment evaluation
   a. A thorough **dental evaluation** is necessary before radiation therapy to help decrease the risk of osteoradionecrosis.
   b. If a mutilating surgical procedure is anticipated, a **prosthodontist** should be consulted to plan reconstructive cosmetic surgery.
   c. Many patients with head and neck cancer are malnourished because of their inability to swallow and chew. All patients should therefore undergo a complete **nutritional assessment** and every attempt should be made to bring the patient into positive nitrogen balance to reduce the complications of treatment.

F. **Therapy.** Small lesions can be treated with curative surgery and radiation therapy. Patients with advanced, unresectable disease can benefit from radiation therapy or combined-modality approaches.

1. Surgery
   a. Primary tumors should be excised with negative margins, which may require skin flaps.
   b. Patients with neck lymph node involvement require **radical neck dissection**

(i.e., dissection of the superficial and deep cervical fascia and close lymph nodes; sternocleidomastoid muscles; internal, external, and jugular veins; spinal accessory nerve; and submandibular glands).

c. Patients with cancers of the oral cavity, oral pharynx, or supraglottic larynx, and no evidence of nodal involvement, are treated with a **functional neck dissection** for better functional and cosmetic results.

d. Surgery is often associated with **morbidity,** including cosmetic deformities, speech impediments, aspiration pneumonia, shoulder droop, and pain.

2. **Radiation therapy.** Most patients are treated with radiation over a 5- to 6-week interval. Side effects include dry mouth, loss of taste, mouth ulcers, osteoradionecrosis of the mandible (which can be prevented by appropriate dental extractions, antibiotics, and fluoride administration), laryngeal edema, and, rarely, hypothyroidism.

3. **Chemotherapy** for locally unresectable or metastatic disease may include cisplatin, infused 5-FU, bleomycin, and methotrexate.

a. New drugs (e.g., carboplatin and trimetrexate) are being tested in clinical trials.

b. **Combination chemotherapy regimens** have reported high response rates in patients with unresectable disease. These patients exhibit response rates as high as 90% after administration of cisplatin and a continuous infusion of 5-FU.

XII. SARCOMAS

A. **Incidence.** Approximately 7000 new sarcomas are diagnosed in the United States each year, constituting 1% of adult malignancies.

B. **Risk factors** include:

1. Exposure to **radiation**

2. Exposure to **chemicals** (e.g., wood preservatives, herbicides, or asbestos)

3. **Genetic abnormalities.** For example, patients with von Recklinghausen's disease have a 10% lifetime risk of development of a neurofibrosarcoma.

4. **Preexisting bone disease.** Osteosarcomas occur in 0.2% of patients with Paget's disease; however, most osteosarcomas occur in patients younger than 20 years of age.

C. **Clinical features**

1. **Soft tissue sarcomas** often present as a **mass, swelling,** or **pain** in the trunk or extremities.

2. Patients with **retroperitoneal tumors** generally experience **weight loss** or **deep-seated pain.**

3. **Bleeding** is the most common presenting feature of **gynecologic** and **gastrointestinal sarcomas.**

4. Most patients with osteosarcomas present with **pain,** a **mass, or both.**

D. **Diagnosis**

1. **Biopsy**

a. A rapidly growing mass or one that exceeds 5 cm in diameter should be regarded with suspicion, especially if it is firm, deep, or fixed.

b. These lesions require a generous incisional biopsy or an excisional biopsy; needle biopsy is usually inadequate.

   c. The biopsy site must be selected carefully to allow for the possibility of limb-sparing surgery.

  2. Imaging procedures include x-rays, MRI, CT, and bone scans.
   a. For soft tissue sarcomas, MRI is superior to CT, providing better definition of soft tissue planes and tumor margins.
   b. MRI or CT and bone scanning are preferred for evaluating bony involvement.
   c. MRI or CT scans of the liver identify hepatic metastases in those patients with visceral sarcomas and in those with extremity sarcomas accompanied by evidence of abnormal hepatic function.

E. **Therapy.** Surgery is the mainstay of therapy, supplemented with radiation therapy or chemotherapy.

  1. Surgery
   a. Definitive resection may consist of extensive surgical excision, including a 2- to 4-cm pathologically documented margin of normal tissue, or conservative resection with documented tumor-free margins, supplemented with radiation therapy. Re-excision should be considered after biopsy if microscopically involved margins are demonstrated.
   b. Limb-sparing surgery can be considered in the majority of patients with extremity sarcomas.
    (1) This procedure is associated with a 90% local control rate and an overall disease-free survival rate of 60%, a success rate that is similar to that found with amputation or radical resection procedures.
    (2) Preoperative intra-arterial chemotherapy and radiation therapy may facilitate limb-sparing surgery in borderline resectable tumors.
   c. Surgeons should avoid seeding the entire surgical field during the procedure. If such seeding occurs, wide excision should be followed by 6600 cGy of radiation therapy.
   d. Surgery offers the chance of a cure for patients with few (i.e., no more than 10–15) pulmonary metastases.

  2. Radiation therapy is used when the tumor margins are less than 2–4 cm or if tumor seeding has occurred. Studies have shown that a combination of limb-sparing surgery and radiation therapy is as effective as amputation.

  3. Chemotherapy
   a. Adjuvant chemotherapy has no clear benefit except in young patients with osteosarcoma and adults with extremity sarcomas. A few studies have reported an increase in disease-free survival rates and overall survival rates with the use of doxorubicin-based combination regimens in extremity sarcomas. Doxorubicin alone appears ineffective.
   b. Advanced sarcomas. Previously treated patients may respond to doxorubicin (15%–35% of patients), dacarbazine (17%), or ifosfamide (20%–40%). Some studies suggest that combination chemotherapy, particularly with doxorubicin and ifosfamide, may be optimal.

F. **Prognosis.** Histologic grade and tumor size are the most important prognostic factors.

  1. Histologic grade is determined by the mitotic rate, nuclear grade, extent of necrosis, nuclear morphology, and cellularity.

  2. Tumor size is an independent prognostic factor. Small (less than 5 cm), completely excised, low-grade lesions rarely recur locally and have a low metastatic rate.

  3. Other factors. Multivariant analysis identified the following factors as being associated with an increased risk of local recurrence: age older than 53 years; presentation with recurrent disease; high-grade, painful mass; limb-sparing surgery; and inadequate surgical margins.

XIII. MULTIPLE MYELOMA (see Chapter 6 Part I: X P)

A. Incidence. Myeloma is a neoplasm of the plasma cells that are derived from B lymphocytes. It is an uncommon neoplasm, accounting for less than 1%–2% of the adult cancers in the United States. The incidence of myeloma increases with advancing age and is twice as common in blacks.

B. Etiology

1. Although no specific underlying causes have been proven, chronic stimulation to the immune system may play a role in the pathogenesis of myeloma. Interestingly, IL-6 can promote the growth of myeloma cells in vitro.

2. Genetic factors, as well as exposure to petroleum, asbestos, laxatives, and radiation may also be important factors.

3. Benign monoclonal gammopathies are suspected precursors to multiple myeloma.

C. Clinical features. With the advent of automated laboratory blood testing, myeloma may be detected earlier.

1. **The major feature** of myeloma is the demonstration of an abnormal monoclonal protein (**M protein**) in the **blood, urine,** or **both.** This M protein usually consists of either one or a combination of the heavy chains (IgG and IgA) and the light chains (κ and λ).
   a. M proteins consisting of the whole immunoglobulin molecules IgG and IgA account for 50% and 25% of the cases, respectively.
   b. M proteins consisting of only light chains account for 25% of cases. In these cases, the M protein is found only in the urine.

2. **Complications** of myeloma include:
   a. Infiltration of the marrow by large numbers of plasma cells, which are usually abnormal
   b. **Weakness, fatigue, infection,** and **bleeding** due to marrow failure
   c. **Osteolytic lesions** due to myeloma-induced bone resorption with subsequent pain and fracture
   d. **Renal abnormalities** due to myeloma infiltration of the kidney, hypercalcemia, toxic effects of light chains on tubules, amyloid deposition, and hyperuricemia
   e. **Recurrent infections** due to acquired hypogammaglobulinemia and leukopenia
   f. **Hypercalcemia** due to myeloma-stimulated osteoclast activity
   g. **Hyperviscosity** due to a high concentration of the M protein, which tends to aggregate

3. The most common clinical finding is the detection of an abnormal M protein, along with a bone marrow examination that shows plasma cell infiltration. The once-common symptoms of **anemia** and **bone pain** are seen less frequently.

D. Diagnosis of myeloma requires the demonstration of:

1. **An abnormal M protein level** (i.e., > 3.5 g/dl) in the serum, urine, or both

2. **Marrow infiltration** by plasma cells (i.e., > 30% plasma cells on bone marrow biopsy)

3. **Additional supportive findings,** including anemia, osteolytic skeletal lesions, renal abnormalities, and hypercalcemia

4. **Plasmacytoma** on tissue biopsy. Because marrow plasmacytosis occurs in many chronic infections or inflammatory processes without an M component, the major difficulty in differential diagnosis is distinguishing myeloma from monoclonal gammopathy of unknown significance (MGUS).

E. **Staging** of myeloma is based on the linear relationship between the easily measured M protein and the cellular tumor burden in myeloma patients.

1. **Stage I myeloma** (low tumor burden) patients have normal calcium and bone films and reveal the following blood data:
   a. Hemoglobulin level > 10 g/dl
   b. IgG level <eq 5 g/dl
   c. IgA level < 3 g/dl

2. **Stage II myeloma** (intermediate tumor burden) patients reveal the following blood data:
   a. Hemoglobulin level = 8.5–10 g/dl
   b. IgG level = 5–7 g/dl
   c. IgA level = 3–5 g/dl

3. **Stage III myeloma** (high tumor burden) patients have hypercalcemia and osteolytic lesions and reveal the following blood data:
   a. Hemoglobin level < 8.5 g/dl
   b. IgG level > 7 g/dl
   c. IgA level > 5 g/dl

F. **Therapy** for myeloma involves several principles.

1. Patients in whom a differential diagnosis of MGUS cannot be excluded and patients with very low-grade **smoldering myeloma** should be examined only at 3- to 6-month intervals for evidence of disease progression.

2. Therapy should be given to patients with bone pain, hypercalcemia, renal failure, bone marrow suppression, and spinal cord compression. Responses are obtained in roughly two thirds of patients.
   a. **Chemotherapy**
      (1) **Agents**
         (a) Classically, **alkylating agents** (e.g., **melphalan**) and **prednisone** are used, although some physicians advocate more aggressive regimens that also contain **doxorubicin, vincristine,** and **nitrosoureas.** The superiority of multiple drug regimens over melphalan and prednisone has not been demonstrated.
            (i) The **vincristine–Adriamycin–dexamethasone (VAD) regimen,** in which vincristine and Adriamycin are administered as a continuous infusion with pulse dexamethasone, can be used as a primary or salvage therapy.
            (ii) When used as salvage therapy, **etoposide, ara-C,** and **dexamethasone** are associated with a 40% response rate, but severe toxicity can occur.
         (b) **Interferon** has been used for maintenance therapy.
      (2) **Toxicity.** Therapy damages marrow and leads to leukemias and excessive secondary marrow diseases in long-term survivors.
      (3) **Evaluation of effectiveness.** When therapy is effective, the M protein levels decline. Therapy can be stopped if the M protein levels become normal or stabilize at 75% below initial levels. Therapy can be resumed when disease progression occurs, although results with retreatment are not as good as those with initial therapy.
   b. **Autologous transplantation** has been performed in more than 300 patients, most of whom have been reinfused with unpurged marrow. The complete remission rate is 20%–30%; 50% of patients who achieve a complete remission are disease-free at 4 years.
   c. **Supportive therapy** is extremely important in the management of myeloma and includes:
      (1) **Radiotherapy** for local bone disease
      (2) **Hydration** and proper **management of hypercalcemia**
      (3) **Orthopedic support** and care

G. **Prognosis** clearly depends on the extent of myeloma at presentation. Patients with smoldering or stage I myeloma may go many years without a need for therapy, whereas patients with stage III myeloma and renal and orthopedic complications do poorly. Mean survival for patients requiring therapy is 2–3 years.

XIV. HODGKIN'S DISEASE

A. **Incidence.** In the United States, 7000–7500 new cases of Hodgkin's disease are reported each year. This neoplasm has a characteristic **bimodal age distribution.**

    1. **A young adult peak** occurs between the ages of 10 and 25 years and is characterized by equal incidence in men and women, a preponderance of nodular sclerosis pathology, and a more benign clinical course.

    2. **A second adult peak** occurs after age 50 years and is characterized by high incidence among men, a preponderance of mixed cellularity, and a more aggressive clinical course.

B. **Etiology**

    1. Clustering of cases in time and place occurs in Hodgkin's disease, suggesting that **viruses or environmental factors may play a role**. However, this clustering is sporadic and has not been substantiated by firm evidence. There have been studies suggesting an association with **Epstein-Barr virus** infection.

    2. Statistical evidence links early-onset Hodgkin's disease with **higher socioeconomic class,** and an increased incidence of Hodgkin's disease among family members suggests a **genetic predisposition**.

C. **Pathology.** There are four major histologic variants of Hodgkin's disease. Of interest, however, is the fact that the precise nature of the truly malignant cell (the binucleate giant cell called the **Reed-Sternberg cell**) remains a point of controversy, despite new techniques that indicate that this cell is more likely derived from the mononuclear phagocyte system than from transformed lymphocytes.

D. **Clinical features and staging.** Hodgkin's disease tends to spread in an orderly fashion from node group to node group. This contiguous nature is in marked contrast to non-Hodgkin's lymphomas, which are multicentric early in their development.

    1. The modified **Ann Arbor classification** used for staging Hodgkin's disease is summarized in Table 4-24.
        a. Hodgkin's disease patients, especially young patients, usually have **asymptomatic swelling of a lymph node**. The B subclassification implies, however, that Hodgkin's disease may present with such **systemic symptoms** as **fever, weight loss,** and **drenching sweats.**
        b. Workup is based on the principle that **early-stage** Hodgkin's disease **can be treated locally** but **late-stage** Hodgkin's disease **requires systemic therapy.** Therefore, patients are aggressively staged to include or exclude stage $IIIA_2$, IIIB, and IV disease. (This staging is far more extensive than staging for non-Hodgkin's lymphomas.)

    2. **Staging procedures** include:
        a. Thorough history and physical examination
        b. Chest radiographs, CT scans of the chest, abdomen, and pelvis, and a lymphangiogram (if a staging laparotomy is to be performed)
        c. Percutaneous bilateral bone marrow biopsies
        d. Gallium 67 (^{67}Ga) scanning
        e. Laparotomy, combined with node sampling, splenectomy, and liver biopsy

TABLE 4-24. Ann Arbor Classification of Hodgkin's Disease

Stage	Characteristics
I	Involvement of a single lymph node region or a single extralymphatic site
II	Involvement of two or more lymph node regions on the same side of the diaphragm
III	Involvement of two or more lymph node regions on both sides of the diaphragm
III$_1$	Involvement limited to the lymphatic structures in the upper abdomen (i.e., spleen or splenic, celiac, or hepatic portal nodes)
III$_2$	Involvement of lower abdominal nodes (i.e., para-aortic, iliac, or mesenteric nodes); possible involvement of the splenic, celiac, or hepatic portal nodes as well
IV	Diffuse or disseminated involvement in extralymphatic organs
Subclassifications	
A	Asymptomatic
B	Unexplained loss of 10% of body weight; unexplained fever of greater than 38°C; night sweats

E. **Therapy** for Hodgkin's disease continues to evolve. However, certain principles have been established and should be firmly adhered to, because **even advanced disease is curable**. Individual variations in treatment should be avoided and, if used, should be limited to well-controlled clinical trials.

1. **Stage I** or **stage II** disease is treated with **extended-field radiotherapy.**

2. **Stage IIIA$_1$** disease is treated with **total nodal radiotherapy**. Patients who relapse after radiotherapy can be successfully given **chemotherapy**. More than 50% of such patients have long-term disease-free survival when such techniques are used.

3. Patients with **stage IIIA$_2$, IIIB,** or **IV** disease require **systemic chemotherapy.** Bone marrow transplants have been used in cases of relapse.
   a. **Regimens**
      (1) Many regimens are available. The classic **MOPP regimen** [i.e., mechlorethamine, vincristine (Oncovin), procarbazine, and prednisone], which is given for at least six cycles plus two additional cycles after complete remission is documented, was the first curative regimen.
      (2) An alternative regimen proven to be more efficacious and less toxic than MOPP consists of BCNU (carmustine), cyclophosphamide, vincristine, procarbazine, and prednisone.
      (3) The **ABVD regimen** [i.e., doxorubicin (Adriamycin), bleomycin, vinblastine, and dacarbazine (DTIC)] has been used as an effective salvage regimen in relapsed patients. Current combination chemotherapy approaches alternate cycles of MOPP with ABVD. The ABVD regimen is at least as effective as MOPP or MOPP and ABVD, and ABVD is associated with reduced risks of secondary malignancies (e.g., leukemia).
   b. **Principles**
      (1) Combined chemotherapy and radiotherapy should not be used routinely until further clinical trials prove the effectiveness of such a regimen.
      (2) Unless chemotherapeutic agents are given in full doses and according to prescribed schedules, their effectiveness can be significantly compromised.
   c. **Side effects**. Both chemotherapy and total nodal irradiation are difficult, toxic, and have many side effects, including severe nausea and vomiting, hypothyroidism, sterility (in some cases), and development of secondary marrow problems, including acute leukemia.

F. **Prognosis** varies mainly with the stage of disease and, to a lesser extent, with histology. Overall, there is a 55%–60% 5-year survival rate with all cases of Hodgkin's disease.

1. Patients with stage I or stage II disease have a 5-year disease-free survival rate exceeding 80%.

2. Patients with stage IIIA disease have roughly a 67% rate of 5-year disease-free survival.

3. Patients with stage $IIIA_2$, IIIB, or IV disease, if treated with chemotherapy, obtain remissions in 80%–95% of cases, with more than 50% of these patients achieving prolonged (i.e., >5 years) disease-free survival.

XV. NON-HODGKIN'S LYMPHOMA

A. **Incidence.** More than 45,000 patients are diagnosed with non-Hodgkin's lymphoma in the United States each year. An increased incidence in older people is attributable to a rising incidence in diffuse large-cell lymphoma. Non-Hodgkin's lymphomas (especially CNS lymphomas) are more common in patients with acquired immunodeficiency states and in patients receiving immunosuppressive drugs, such as renal and heart transplant patients.

B. **Etiology**

1. **Cytogenetic abnormalities,** such as chromosome translocations, are commonly observed in lymphoma cells.

2. **Viral infection**
   a. **The Epstein-Barr virus** has been linked to **Burkitt's lymphoma,** a disease usually found in Africa.
   b. An aggressive T-cell leukemia or lymphoma occurs in Japan and the Caribbean and is associated with human T lymphotropic virus type I **(HTLV-I) infection.**

C. **Pathology.** A number of histologic classification schemes are in use; the one most widely used in the clinical literature is the Rappaport classification system (Table 4-25). The National Cancer Institute classification system (Table 4-26) resulted from a 1982 conference to resolve differences in the various histologic schemes.

TABLE 4-25. The Rappaport Classification of Non-Hodgkin's Lymphomas

Grade	Study Code	Rappaport Classification
Low	A	Diffuse, lymphocytic, well differentiated
	B	Nodular, lymphocytic, poorly differentiated
	C	Nodular, mixed, lymphocytic and histiocytic
Intermediate	D	Nodular, histiocytic
	E	Diffuse, lymphocytic
	F	Diffuse, mixed, lymphocytic and histiocytic
	G	Diffuse, histiocytic
High	H	Diffuse, histiocytic
	I	Diffuse, lymphoblastic
	J	Diffuse, undifferentiated

Adapted with permission from Farvar ML, Eyre H: Histiopathologic classification of non-Hodgkin's lymphoma. In *Textbook of Clinical Oncology.* Atlanta, The American Cancer Society, 1991, p 387.

TABLE 4-26. The United States National Cancer Institute
Classification of the Morphological Subgroups
of Non-Hodgkin's Lymphomas

Low-grade malignant lymphoma
  Small lymphocytic
  Follicular—predominantly small-cleaved cell
  Follicular—mixed (small cleaved and large cell)
Intermediate-grade malignant lymphoma
  Follicular—predominantly large cell
  Diffuse—small-cleaved cell
  Diffuse—mixed (small and large cell)
  Diffuse—large cell
High-grade malignant lymphoma
  Large cell
  Convoluted lymphoblastic
  Small noncleaved cell (Burkitt's)

1. The **low-grade lymphomas** are predominantly B-cell tumors. The **intermediate-grade lymphomas** include both B- and some T-cell lymphomas, whereas **immunoblastic lymphomas** are predominantly B-cell tumors and **lymphoblastic lymphomas** are T-cell types. Most B-cell tumors are monoclonal and produce either a κ or a λ light chain immunoglobulin.

2. **Follicular small-cleaved cell lymphomas** are the most common histologic type, accounting for approximately 40% of cases. These patients have predominantly stage III or IV disease with a high incidence of bone marrow involvement and an indolent course, evolving over many years.

3. **Follicular mixed small-cleaved and large-cell lymphomas** represent 20%–40% of patients. Large cells may account for as much as 25% of the cell population. The lymph node architecture shows distinct nodules, which are usually present throughout the node. Marrow involvement is common. This subtype is indolent but more aggressive than follicular small-cleaved cell lymphoma.

4. **Diffuse large-cell lymphomas** are characterized by large malignant lymphocytes with increased nuclear diameters. These cells have cytologic features of large cleaved or noncleaved follicular cells, with nucleoli, abundant cytoplasm, and frequent mitoses.

5. **Immunoblastic lymphomas** and other high-grade non-Hodgkin's lymphomas include **plasmacytoid, clear-cell,** and **polymorphic** categories. These subtypes are rapidly fatal unless effective treatment is administered promptly.

D. **Clinical features**

1. Most patients are **asymptomatic**. Twenty percent of patients have **fever, night sweats,** or **weight loss**.

2. Patients with indolent lymphomas may have **waxing and waning adenopathy** for several months before diagnosis, although **persistent nodal enlargement** is more common. Extranodal disease most often involves the stomach, lung, and bone, resulting in symptoms characteristic of the affected organ.

E. **Staging and diagnosis**

1. The Ann Arbor staging system used to classify Hodgkin's disease (see Table 4-24) is also used to stage non-Hodgkin's lymphomas.

2. **Staging procedures** include:
   a. An adequate surgical lymph node **biopsy,** examined by an experienced pathologist

   b. Hematologic studies, including a CBC, differential, platelet count, liver and kidney function studies, and uric acid level studies. Serum protein electrophoresis rules out hypogammaglobulinemia or a monoclonal gammopathy.

   c. A complete **history** and **physical examination,** with particular emphasis on all lymph node–bearing areas, including Waldeyer's ring, as well as liver and spleen size

   d. Bilateral bone marrow biopsies and **aspirates**

   e. Radiologic studies, such as chest radiograph; CT of the chest, abdomen, and pelvis; and, rarely, bipedal lymphangiography

   f. Optional procedures, including a staging laparotomy, bone scan or bone radiographs, endoscopy, and liver biopsy

F. **Therapy** usually requires a multidisciplinary approach. Radiation therapy and chemotherapy after surgical biopsy are the most common treatment modalities.

   1. Radiation therapy. Non-Hodgkin's lymphomas are very radiosensitive.

     a. In localized disease, radiation should be targeted to the affected site (4000 cGy to the involved field). The nodal site and draining lymphatics should be included in the radiation field.

     b. Radiation therapy is used **palliatively** in disseminated disease or to "consolidate" a complete response to chemotherapy in areas of bulky disease.

     c. Electron beam therapy has been used in the management of cutaneous lymphomas, such as the early stages of mycosis fungoides.

     d. Stage I indolent lymphomas. Long-term patient follow-up after involved or extended field radiation therapy for localized stage I and II low-grade lymphoma reveals a 10-year relapse-free survival rate of greater than 50%, especially in younger patients.

   2. Chemotherapy

     a. Low-grade indolent lymphomas may not require treatment for many years. When therapy is indicated, **chlorambucil** or **cyclophosphamide,** with or without prednisone, is the agent of choice. Initial results with high-dose chemotherapy followed by autologous marrow transplantation are favorable, but success needs to be measured by long-term follow-up because these patients generally have long-term survival rates, even with less toxic treatment.

     b. Stage I or II intermediate and high-grade lymphomas often respond to combination chemotherapy, with or without radiation therapy. Cure rates approach 80%–90%.

     c. Aggressive intermediate or high-grade lymphomas (e.g., lymphoblastic or Burkitt's lymphoma) require immediate combination chemotherapy. Prophylactic intrathecal chemotherapy may also be given. **Salvage combination chemotherapy** produces second complete or partial remissions, but is rarely curative unless the patient undergoes bone marrow transplantation.

       (1) Common regimens include **CHOP** (cyclophosphamide, doxorubicin, vincristine, and prednisone), **PROMACE-CytaBOM** (cyclophosphamide, doxorubicin, etoposide, prednisone, cytarabine, bleomycin, vincristine, methotrexate, and leukovorin), and **MACOP-B** (methotrexate, leukovorin, doxorubicin, cyclophosphamide, vincristine, bleomycin, and prednisone).

       (2) Because of encouraging results with combination chemotherapy in patients with stage III and IV disease followed by radiation therapy, randomized clinical trials are underway to compare chemotherapy alone and chemotherapy followed by radiation therapy.

       (3) Colony-stimulating factors hasten granulocyte recovery and may permit higher doses and better cure rates.

G. **Prognosis.** Many patients who achieve a complete response, particularly those with diffuse large-cell lymphoma, remain disease-free for an extended period of time and will be cured. Aggressive combination chemotherapy regimens containing doxorubicin have high complete response rates ranging from 40%–80%.

XVI. PARANEOPLASTIC SYNDROMES

A. **Endocrine syndromes** resulting from ectopic polypeptide hormone production are the most common and best understood of the paraneoplastic processes. Many tumors produce more than one biologically active hormone, leading to multiple endocrine paraneoplastic syndromes.

1. **Criteria** for establishing ectopic hormone secretion by tumor cells include:
   a. **Increased hormone levels,** as evidenced by radioimmunoassay or other techniques. However, some patients with elevated hormone levels do not have clinical symptoms.
   b. **Decreased hormone levels after removal or treatment of the tumor**
   c. **Persistent hormone elevation after removal of the normal gland** that secretes the normal hormone
   d. An **arteriovenous gradient for hormone levels** across the tumor vascular bed

2. **Types**
   a. **Ectopic growth hormone (GH) secretion** has been detected in patients with **lung and gastric carcinomas.** The elevated hormone levels may lead to hypertrophic pulmonary osteoarthropathy. Organomegaly may occur with slow-growing carcinoid tumors.
   b. **Ectopic ACTH secretion** was the first paraneoplastic endocrine syndrome described in the literature.
      (1) The most common **tumors associated with ectopic ACTH production** are **small-cell lung cancer** and **atypical carcinoids.** High cortisol levels have also been described in patients with adenocarcinoma and large-cell carcinoma of the lung, other carcinoid tumors, thymoma, neural crest tumors, medullary carcinoma of the thyroid, and bronchial adenomas.
      (2) **Clinical features.** Most patients have **hypokalemia** and **metabolic alkalosis.**
         (a) Patients rarely live long enough for frank Cushing's syndrome to develop. However, diabetes, hypertension, edema, muscle wasting, central obesity, moon facies, and striae may develop in those with extremely high cortisol levels.
         (b) Alterations in mental status, fatigue, and anorexia caused by opiate-like peptide fragments are rare symptoms.
      (3) **Diagnosis** is confirmed by a plasma ACTH level of more than 200 pg/ml, a plasma cortisol level of more than 40 mg/dl without diurnal variation, or a positive dexamethasone suppression test.

B. **Hematologic syndromes** may affect cellular blood elements, the coagulation system, or circulating immunoglobulins.

1. **Paraneoplastic syndromes of cellular blood components**
   a. **Erythrocytosis** occurs in renal cancer and hepatoma.
   b. **Pure red cell aplasia.** Severe anemia due to a complete lack of RBC production is uncommon. However, 50% of patients with pure red cell aplasia have **thymoma.** Many patients with pure red cell aplasia also have other immunologic abnormalities, such as hypogammaglobulinemia, paraproteinemia, positive antinuclear antibodies, or autoimmune hemolytic anemia.
      (1) The **etiology** of red cell aplasia may be related to effects of suppressor T cells on RBC production, leading to a severe reticulocytopenic anemia.
      (2) **Therapy.** In thymoma, surgery or radiation therapy is not uniformly successful in reversing the anemia. **Corticosteroids, splenectomy,** and **immunosuppressive therapy** with cyclophosphamide may be useful.
   c. **Autoimmune hemolytic anemia, or cold agglutinin disease,** is usually caused by an immunoglobulin produced by lymphoma or chronic lymphocytic leukemia cells.
      (1) **RBC** indices may be high or low depending on the reticulocyte response. If the reticulocyte count is high, due to normal marrow function, the in-

dices are normal or high; however, if there is bone marrow suppression, multiple spherocytes are present.

    (2) Therapy. Administration of **prednisone** (1.0–1.5 mg/kg/day) is often effective. **Splenectomy** is also occasionally useful. In most cases, however, neither splenectomy nor corticosteroids are effective for long periods unless the underlying malignancy is effectively treated.

  d. Microangiopathic hemolytic anemia occurs with mucin-producing adenocarcinomas, especially gastric cancer.

    (1) Disseminated intravascular coagulation (DIC) should be excluded by drawing blood to measure fibrinogen and fibrin split products.

    (2) There is no effective **treatment** except treating the underlying tumor. Heparin should not be used unless there is concomitant DIC.

  e. Granulocytosis occurs even in the absence of bone marrow involvement. Other causes of inflammation or infection must be excluded. The most common malignancies associated with granulocytosis include gastric, lung, and pancreatic carcinoma; melanoma; CNS tumors; Hodgkin's disease; and large-cell lymphomas.

  f. Thrombocytosis occurs in as many as one third of all cancer patients. If essential thrombocythemia is present, hydroxyurea should be given to keep the platelet count below 500,000/μl.

  g. Thrombocytopenia is often due to secondary effects of chemotherapy, bone marrow involvement, or radiation therapy, but is also seen in severe microangiopathic hemolytic anemia and DIC. A syndrome resembling autoimmune thrombocytopenia has been described in Hodgkin's disease, lymphoma, some types of leukemia, and certain solid tumors. This form of idiopathic thrombocytopenic purpura is treated with corticosteroids, splenectomy, or immunosuppressive drugs.

2. Paraneoplastic syndromes of the coagulation system

  a. Primary DIC occurs most frequently with mucin-producing adenocarcinomas, such as pancreatic, gastric, lung, prostate, and colon cancers. Both acute and chronic DIC are associated with thrombophlebitis, arterial emboli, endocarditis, circulating inhibitors of coagulation, and abnormal circulating proteins that may precipitate hemorrhagic complications.

    (1) Acute DIC is often observed in acute promyelocytic leukemia, as the result of the release of a procoagulant contained in the abnormal granules of the leukemia promyelocyte.

      (a) Clinical features. Elevation of the prothrombin time (PT) is one of the earliest detectable symptoms along with elevation of fibrin split products and lowered fibrinogen levels. Further decreases in fibrinogen levels and an increase in the partial thromboplastin time occur in more severe cases.

      (b) Therapy. Improved management of acute DIC has led to a better short-term prognosis for most patients.

        (i) Measures include **aggressive transfusion support** to maintain the platelet count between 35,000 and 50,000/μl, **intravenous vitamin K,** and **clotting factor replacement** with fresh-frozen plasma or cryoprecipitate if the fibrinogen level is less than 75 mg/dl.

        (ii) Heparin is controversial, but can be administered cautiously to **refractory patients.**

    (2) Chronic DIC is most common in patients with adenocarcinomas.

      (a) Clinical features include mild prolongations of the PT, high fibrinogen levels, and elevation of the fibrin split products. Patients often have thrombophlebitis or pulmonary emboli.

      (b) Heparin is the treatment of choice; **thrombolytic therapy** may also be considered if there are no contraindications.

  b. Syndromes associated with paraproteins

    (1) Coagulopathy. Abnormal hemostasis and coagulation may develop in patients with plasma cell dysplasias, such as multiple myeloma, due to the ef-

TABLE 4-27. Central Nervous System Paraneoplastic Syndromes and Associated Malignancies

Syndrome	Associated Malignancy
Limbic encephalitis	Small-cell lung cancer
Subacute cellular degeneration	Small-cell lung cancer, ovarian cancer
Myelopathy	
Subacute motor neuropathy	Lymphoma
Subacute sensory neuropathy	Small-cell lung cancer
Sensorimotor polyneuropathy	Small-cell lung carcinoma, Hodgkin's disease
Eaton-Lambert myasthenia	Lung cancer, ovarian cancer
Polymyositis or dermatomyositis	Varied; breast, lung, gastrointestinal, and ovarian carcinomas most common

      fects of paraproteins on normal clotting factors and platelet receptor function. Paraproteins can also inhibit fibrin monomer aggregation and act as inhibitors of factor VIII. If a patient has intractable bleeding, plasmapheresis may be required in combination with chemotherapy.

    (2) Hyperviscosity. In multiple myeloma and macroglobulinemia, patients with a serum viscosity greater than 4.0 (relative to water) may have signs of decreased blood flow, including headaches, dizziness, epistaxis, seizures, hearing loss, altered mental status, and cardiac disease. Treatment consists of prompt plasmapheresis to remove the excessive paraprotein and avoid dehydration, and treatment of the underlying plasma cell dyscrasia.

C. | **CNS syndromes** are rare. The most common (and the malignancies associated with them) are listed in Table 4-27.

DIRECTIONS: Each of the numbered items or incomplete statements in this section is negatively phrased, as indicated by a capitalized word such as NOT, LEAST, or EXCEPT. Select the ONE lettered answer or completion that is BEST in each case.

1. Hodgkin's disease is associated with all of the following treatment-related complications EXCEPT

(A) nausea and vomiting
(B) sterility
(C) hypothyroidism
(D) microangiopathic hemolytic anemia
(E) acute leukemia

2. All of the following therapies are used for metastatic prostate cancer EXCEPT

(A) orchiectomy
(B) leuprolide
(C) estrogen
(D) corticosteroids
(E) somatostatin analogue

3. A patient with nodular lymphoma involving the neck, mediastinum, and retroperitoneum would be expected to require all of the following staging procedures EXCEPT

(A) laparotomy with splenectomy
(B) bone marrow biopsy
(C) computed tomography (CT) of the chest
(D) complete blood count (CBC)
(E) CT of the retroperitoneum

4. Prognostic factors in breast carcinoma include all of the following EXCEPT

(A) estrogen receptor (ER) status
(B) menopausal status
(C) size of primary tumor
(D) percentage of cells in S phase
(E) presence of lymph node metastasis in axillae

5. Patients with renal cell carcinoma may commonly have all of the following symptoms EXCEPT

(A) a palpable mass in the flank area
(B) hematuria, either gross or microscopic
(C) pain in the costovertebral area
(D) anemia and systemic symptoms
(E) renal failure requiring dialysis

6. Factors that have been associated with an increased incidence of head and neck carcinomas include all of the following EXCEPT

(A) alcohol consumption
(B) syphilis
(C) exposure to nickel
(D) hepatitis B virus
(E) tobacco use

7. Complications of multiple myeloma include all of the following EXCEPT

(A) osteolytic lesions
(B) renal failure
(C) hyperviscosity
(D) infections
(E) heart failure

8. True statements concerning adjuvant therapy for breast cancer after initial surgery or radiotherapy include all of the following EXCEPT

(A) premenopausal women show the greatest benefit from adjuvant chemotherapy
(B) adjuvant therapy is effective if started within 1 month of surgery
(C) six months of adjuvant therapy appear to be as effective as longer treatment periods
(D) tamoxifen therapy is particularly beneficial for patients with estrogen receptor (ER)-negative tumors
(E) one of the most popular adjuvant chemotherapy regimens uses methotrexate, 5-fluorouracil (5-FU), and cyclophosphamide

9. Diffuse lymphomas are characterized by all of the following EXCEPT

(A) an increased incidence among patients with immunodeficiency syndromes
(B) a need for aggressive therapy early in the course of disease
(C) a cure rate of 50% with appropriate therapy
(D) a tendency to evolve into acute leukemia

10. An otherwise healthy patient with non–small-cell lung cancer is being evaluated for tumor resectability. Factors that must be considered include all of the following EXCEPT

(A) involvement of lobar fissures
(B) mediastinal node involvement
(C) distant metastases
(D) distance of lesion from the carina

DIRECTIONS: The set of matching questions in this section consists of a list of four to twenty-six lettered options (some of which may be in figures) followed by several numbered items. For each numbered item, select the ONE lettered option that is most closely associated with it. To avoid spending too much time on matching sets with large numbers of options, it is generally advisable to begin each set by reading the list of options. Then, for each item in the set, try to generate the correct answer and locate it in the option list, rather than evaluating each option individually. Each lettered option may be selected once, more than once, or not at all.

Questions 11–15
(A) CA 15–3
(B) CA 125
(C) Prostate-specific antigen
(D) Carcinoembryonic antigen (CEA)
(E) Human chorionic gonadotropin (β-hCG)

Match each of the following tumors with its associated tumor marker.

11. Colon cancer
12. Testicular cancer
13. Ovarian cancer
14. Breast carcinoma
15. Prostate cancer

ANSWERS AND EXPLANATIONS

1. The answer is D [XIV E 3 c]. Microangiopathic hemolytic anemia can occur after long-term use of mitomycin chemotherapy, but mitomycin is not indicated in the treatment of Hodgkin's disease. More common chemotherapeutic regimens for the treatment of Hodgkin's disease include the MOPP regimen [i.e., mechlorethamine, vincristine (Oncovin), procarbazine, and prednisone] and the ABVD regimen [i.e., doxorubicin (Adriamycin), bleomycin, vinblastine, and dacarbazine (DTIC)], both of which have significant gastrointestinal toxicity. Newly available antiemetics can help relieve these side effects. Radiotherapy to the neck area can result in hypothyroidism. Chemotherapy and radiotherapy both can cause sterility and damage marrow stem cells, resulting in an increased risk of secondary acute leukemia.

2. The answer is E [X C 6 b (1) (a)–(b)]. Somatostatin is used to inhibit neuroendocrine secretion in metastatic carcinoid. Orchiectomy, leuprolide, and diethylstilbestrol (DES) in doses sufficient to block androgen production are effective in treating some cases of prostate cancer. Corticosteroids, which suppress adrenal corticosteroid synthesis, are also effective.

3. The answer is A [XV E 2 a–b, d–f]. Because this patient has disease on both sides of the diaphragm, the therapeutic decision likely would not be affected by laparotomy, regardless of further findings with this procedure. A complete blood count (CBC) and bone marrow examination are needed to determine the degree of marrow involvement and reserve if chemotherapy is required. Computed tomography (CT) is an excellent method of evaluating the extent of disease and the patient response to therapy. More than 90% of nodular lymphomas are widely disseminated at diagnosis.

4. The answer is B [IV G 1–4]. Whether a patient is premenopausal or postmenopausal is not a significant prognostic factor in breast cancer, although this information can dictate decisions regarding therapy. Different pathologic subtypes of breast carcinoma carry different prognoses. For example, patients with medullary carcinomas do well, whereas those with inflammatory carcinomas do poorly. The tumor size, the presence or absence of lymph node metastasis in the axillae, and the estrogen receptor (ER) status of the tumor all are independent prognostic variables for the cure rate and the 5- to 10-year survival rate of patients with breast carcinoma. Flow cytometry measures the tumor's DNA index and percentage of cells in S phase. Patients with either aneuploid tumors or a high proliferative index by S phase have poorer prognoses.

5. The answer is E [X A 4]. Renal failure requiring dialysis is usually not a complication of renal cell carcinoma. The classic triad of symptoms that occur in patients with renal cancer consists of anemia, hematuria, and a palpable mass. Although it is uncommon for all three of these to occur simultaneously, most patients (85% or more) have at least one of these symptoms. Anemia and systemic symptoms (e.g., fevers that have no obvious source) also are characteristic of renal cell cancers.

6. The answer is D [XII B 1–4]. Hepatitis B virus is not associated with an increased incidence of head and neck carcinomas. The incidence of squamous cell cancers of the head and neck is related strongly to the use of tobacco and to alcohol consumption, and these factors may have a synergistic effect. Syphilis is associated with an increased incidence of cancer of the tongue. Nickel exposure increases the risk of cancers of the nasal cavity and paranasal sinus.

7. The answer is E [XIII C 2 a–g]. Heart failure is not a complication of multiple myeloma. Patients with multiple myeloma most frequently have an abnormal monoclonal protein (M protein), which is detected in the blood, urine, or both. In the blood, high concentrations of the M protein can lead to hyperviscosity. In addition, the M protein exists in high concentrations in the kidney and acts as a nephrotoxin, contributing (along with hyperuricemia, dehydration, and hypercalcemia) to renal failure in many patients. Myeloma cell-induced bone resorption results in weakened bone, osteolytic lesions, and fractures. The myeloma cells also secrete an osteoclast-stimulating factor, which causes hypercalcemia due to calcium resorption from bone. Myeloma leads to acquired hypogammaglobulinemia, which predisposes patients to infections.

8. The answer is D [IV F 3 a–c, 4 b (1) (b)]. Tamoxifen therapy is most effective in postmenopausal patients with positive hormone receptors. Among breast cancer patients, the most significant benefit from adjuvant chemotherapy occurs in premenopausal women. Although dosage effects have been postulated as the cause of the lesser benefit in postmenopausal women, the precise cause of the difference is unclear. Multiple studies have shown that adjuvant chemotherapy is most effective when begun as soon as possible and no later than 1 month after surgery. In addition, several studies have demonstrated that, if started immediately, 6 months of full-dose adjuvant chemotherapy is as effective as longer regimens. The combination chemotherapeutic regimen of 5-fluorouracil (5-FU), methotrexate, and cyclophosphamide is popular for the adjuvant treatment of breast cancer.

9. The answer is D [XV A, F 2 c]. Acute leukemia is not a complication of diffuse lymphomas. Diffuse lymphomas are complications of congenital as well as acquired immunodeficiencies. For this reason, patients with acquired immune deficiency syndrome are at a greater than normal risk for development of diffuse lymphomas. Also, an increased incidence of lymphoma is seen in transplant patients who have received long-term immunosuppressive therapy. Diffuse lymphomas have aggressive and unfavorable histologies; these diseases require immediate and intensive therapy if responses and cures are expected. With proper therapy, some of the complete responders have prolonged disease-free survival and may be considered cured.

10. The answer is A [VIII G 1 a–b]. Involvement of more than one lobe should not preclude surgery in a patient who otherwise is an acceptable medical candidate for lung resection. However, invasion of mediastinal structures does preclude adequate surgical removal. Distant metastases eliminate the possibility of cure with local resection. Inadequate resection margins result after surgery for tumors that are less than 2 cm from the carina.

11–15. The answers are: 11-D [Table 4-20], **12-E** [XI E 4], **13-B** [Table 4-20], **14-A** [Table 4-20], **15-C** [X C 4 a (5)]. Carcinoembryonic antigen (CEA) is elevated in patients with metastatic or recurrent colon cancer and is often elevated in patients with newly diagnosed operable disease. It is often elevated in adenocarcinomas including gastrointestinal adenocarcinomas and breast cancer.

Testicular cancer of the nonseminomatous germ cell type is often associated with elevations in human chorionic gonadotropin (β-hCG) and α-fetoprotein (AFP).

CA 125 is a reliable marker for ovarian cancer. Patients with elevation of this marker often have residual disease found at second-look surgery.

CA 15-3 is a new tumor marker that often correlates with the activity of disease in patients with metastatic breast cancer.

Examination of prostate-specific antigen levels can lead to the detection of prostate cancer.

Chapter 5

Gastrointestinal Diseases

Anthony J. DiMarino, Jr.

I. **DISEASES OF THE ESOPHAGUS.** The esophagus is basically an organ of transport, with no significant absorptive or secretory function.

A. **Features common to clinical disorders**

1. **Dysphagia,** or difficulty in swallowing, is a symptom often described as a **sticking sensation.**
   a. **Dysphagia for solids** indicates an esophageal obstruction as a result of:
      (1) Carcinoma
      (2) An esophageal web or ring
      (3) Benign esophageal stricture
      (4) Dysphagia lusoria, which occurs when an anomalous blood vessel (usually the right subclavian artery) crosses behind the esophagus
   b. **Dysphagia for solids and liquids** indicates an esophageal abnormality as a result of motor dysfunction, such as:
      (1) Scleroderma
      (2) Achalasia
      (3) Symptomatic diffuse esophageal spasm
   c. **Transfer dysphagia** indicates a difficulty in initiating swallowing and is often associated with a neuromuscular disorder of the pharynx or proximal esophagus (e.g., after a cerebrovascular accident), proximal muscle weakness of the pharynx or esophagus (e.g., polymyositis), or other neuromuscular disorders (myasthenia gravis, myotonia dystrophica, or Parkinson's disease).

2. **Odynophagia,** or pain on swallowing, may be due to:
   a. **Motor disorders** of the esophagus, especially achalasia and diffuse esophageal spasm
   b. **Mucosal disruption** caused by ingestion of lye or other caustic agents, severe peptic esophagitis, severe infections of the esophagus [e.g., human immunodeficiency virus (HIV), candidal esophagitis, herpetic esophagitis, cytomegalovirus (CMV), and *Mycobacterium avium-intracellulare*], drug-induced esophagitis (e.g., drugs including potassium chloride tablets, tetracycline preparations, clindamycin, quinidine, iron supplements and ascorbic acid tablets), and radiation esophagitis

3. **Heartburn** is a substernal burning sensation that radiates in an orad direction and may be initiated by bending forward. This is a specific symptom of gastroesophageal reflux.

B. **Specific disorders**

1. **Reflux esophagitis** is caused by the recurrent reflux of gastric contents into the distal esophagus.
   a. **Etiology and pathogenesis**
      (1) **Lower esophageal sphincter (LES) dysfunction.** Normally, the LES blocks reflux of gastric juice into the esophagus. Reflux esophagitis is thought to stem from a defect in this LES mechanism, such as:
         (a) Decreased resting LES pressure
         (b) Prolonged or repeated intermittent relaxation of the LES
         (c) Transient increase in abdominal pressure
      (2) **Secondary causes** of reflux esophagitis should always be suspected and corrected if possible. The following conditions appear to decrease LES pressure:

    (a) Pregnancy. Especially during the last trimester, heartburn may be severe and probably is caused by progesterone's inhibitory effects on the LES.

    (b) Drugs that may decrease the LES pressure as a side effect of smooth muscle relaxation include:

        (i) Anticholinergic agents

        (ii) β_2-adrenergic agonists and theophylline used to treat asthma and chronic bronchitis

        (iii) Calcium channel-blocking agents and nitrates

    (c) Scleroderma that weakens the esophageal smooth muscle and the LES region may be a cause of severe reflux esophagitis.

    (d) Surgical vagotomy also may produce anatomic alterations that lead to reflux esophagitis.

b. Clinical features

  (1) Heartburn is a specific symptom of gastroesophageal regurgitation.

  (2) Dysphagia in the esophagitis patient generally is for solids and may indicate a developing stricture.

  (3) Anemia may occur if recurrent esophageal bleeding is present.

c. Diagnosis. Several tests have been proposed for the diagnosis of reflux esophagitis.

  (1) Barium swallow and upper gastrointestinal series. This is the least sensitive test. Generally, it is positive only in severe gastroesophageal reflux with a very weakened LES or in the presence of esophageal ulceration.

  (2) Acid-reflux test. This test involves monitoring intraesophageal pH after instilling 300 ml of 0.1 N hydrochloric acid (HCl) into the stomach. The acid-reflux test probably is a very sensitive test; however, it is an invasive test that requires positioning a pH tube in the distal esophagus.

  (3) Acid-perfusion test (Bernstein test). This test is intended to reproduce the pain associated with reflux and involves esophageal perfusion of 0.1 N HCl alternately with normal saline solution.

  (4) Twenty-four hour pH monitoring measures the number of episodes and length of time that the distal esophageal pH is less than 4.0.

  (5) Scintigraphy involves the introduction of technetium 99 (^{99}Tc) into the stomach followed by abdominal compression and radiographic counting over the esophagus. This noninvasive technique can demonstrate reflux as well as provide a useful quantitative measure of its presence.

  (6) Endoscopy with biopsy is especially helpful in ruling out associated peptic ulcer disease.

  (7) Esophageal manometry is useful in evaluating LES pressure. Pressures consistently measured at less than one third of the lower limit of normal usually are associated with significant reflux. This technique is especially useful in the preoperative evaluation of esophageal reflux when a fundoplication is contemplated.

d. Therapy

  (1) Increasing the reflux barrier may be accomplished by:

    (a) Measures such as elevating the head of the bed 2–4 inches and avoiding eating for 3 hours before bedtime

    (b) Administration of alginic acid and antacid combinations

    (c) Administration of drugs that increase LES tone (e.g., bethanechol, metoclopramide, domperidone, cisapride)

    (d) Antireflux surgery, especially Nissen fundoplication

  (2) Decreasing gastric acid effects may be accomplished by:

    (a) Administration of antacids

    (b) Administration of histamine$_2$ (H$_2$)-receptor antagonists (e.g., cimetidine, famotidine, ranitidine, nizatidine)

    (c) Administration of hydrogen/potassium (H$^+$/K$^+$) proton pump adenosine triphosphatase (ATPase) blockers (proton pump inhibitors) such as omeprazole or lansoprazole

(3) Maintaining LES pressure. The following agents decrease LES pressure and should be avoided:
  (a) Anticholinergic agents
  (b) β-adrenergic drugs
  (c) Calcium channel-blocking agents
  (d) Chocolate
  (e) Fats
  (f) Nicotine (smoking)
  (g) Nitrates
  (h) Xanthine and its derivatives (e.g., caffeine)
  (i) Peppermint

e. Complications
  (1) Benign esophageal stricture probably occurs in a small portion of all reflux esophagitis cases and is best diagnosed by a bolus barium swallow, endoscopy with biopsy, or cytology.
  (2) Esophageal ulceration may be accompanied by hemorrhage; however, the primary symptom is severe and unrelenting pain.
  (3) Reflux-induced laryngitis is a common cause of recurrent hoarseness in adults.
  (4) Pulmonary aspiration is a serious sequela of reflux esophagitis. Patients older than 30 years of age who develop repeated pneumonia or asthma should be evaluated for esophageal reflux.
  (5) Barrett's esophagus refers to a condition in which columnar epithelium replaces the normal squamous epithelium of the esophagus, possibly as a result of continuous inflammation. This is considered a premalignant state, with a 40-fold increased risk of adenocarcinoma and is probably responsible for the increased incidence of adenocarcinoma of the esophagus.

2. Obstructive esophageal conditions
  a. Carcinoma. Adenocarcinoma is almost equal to squamous cell carcinoma of the esophagus in incidence in the United States. Carcinoma occurs predominantly in men and with varying incidence throughout the world. The population of the United States is considered at low risk; esophageal cancer occurs in only 4 of 100,000 individuals.
    (1) Etiology. Certain factors appear to increase the risk of esophageal cancer.
      (a) Tobacco smoking may increase the risk two to four times.
      (b) Alcohol consumption has been shown to increase the risk up to 12 times in France. Alcohol and tobacco appear to have an additive effect.
      (c) Geographic factors. Incidence levels were found to be 400 times greater in certain regions in China and Iran and may be attributable to a diet that includes increased amounts of pickled food, nitrosamines, and molds and decreased amounts of selenium and fresh fruits and vegetables.
      (d) Vitamin deficiency, especially of vitamins A and C, may be associated with an increased risk for esophageal cancer.
      (e) Lye ingestion is associated with the development of esophageal cancer many years after exposure.
      (f) Achalasia may be associated with a 10% risk of subsequent carcinomas.
      (g) Barrett's esophagus [see I B 1 e (5)]. Adenocarcinoma eventually may develop in 10% of patients with Barrett's esophagus.
      (h) Tylosis–hyperkeratosis of the palms and soles. More than 80% of patients with this autosomal dominant condition develop squamous cell carcinoma of the esophagus.
      (i) Celiac sprue
    (2) Clinical features
      (a) Progressive dysphagia for solids indicates the presence of an ongoing obstructive lesion. Usually, when the esophageal lumen narrows to 1.2 cm or less, a **persistent dysphagia** for solid food is observed.

    (b) Pain usually signifies extension of the tumor beyond the wall of the esophagus.

    (c) Dysphagia for liquids, cough, hoarseness, and **weight loss** generally are symptoms of advanced esophageal carcinoma.

  (3) Diagnosis

    (a) Barium x-ray with a barium-coated bolus (e.g., bread or a marshmallow) should be done when obstructive dysphagia is suspected.

    (b) Endoscopy with biopsy and cytologic study, if performed together, establishes a diagnosis in approximately 90% of cases and is the diagnostic procedure of choice.

    (c) Computed tomography (CT) and **bronchoscopy** should be used to evaluate the presence and extent of nodal metastases and bronchial invasion.

  (4) Therapy

    (a) Surgery generally is performed if the lesion is in the lower one third or in the distal portion of the middle one third of the esophagus. Surgery restores esophageal patency, but 5-year cure rates average only 5%–10%.

    (b) Radiotherapy is prescribed for lesions located in the proximal part of the middle one third or in the upper one third of the esophagus. Approximately 6000 cGy usually are administered.

    (c) Esophageal bougienage or **stent therapy** with Silastic tubes may be used in certain cases to maintain esophageal patency.

    (d) Lasers are being used to vaporize tumors to the extent that a lumen is established.

    (e) Chemotherapy has not been shown to prolong life significantly in controlled trials, but new regimens combining radiotherapy and chemotherapy have shown encouraging results in initial studies.

b. Benign esophageal stricture may be a sequela of prolonged reflux esophagitis. Heartburn may lessen as solid-food dysphagia worsens with progression of the stricture. Diagnosis is established by a bolus barium swallow and endoscopy. Treatment generally is with tapered bougies or with balloon dilatation catheters.

c. Esophageal webs seen in the upper one third of the esophagus may be due to a failure of complete embryologic recanalization. Webs in this area also may be associated with iron deficiency anemia in the **Plummer-Vinson (Paterson-Kelly) syndrome.** Effective treatment of this syndrome includes administering iron for the anemia and using an esophageal bougie to fracture the webs.

d. Esophageal rings most commonly occur at the squamocolumnar junction and are called **Schatzki's rings.** Dysphagia for solids often is intermittent in this condition, especially if the narrowest point of the esophagus measures between 1.2 and 2 cm. Esophageal bougienage often is effective therapy.

3. Esophageal motor disorders

a. Oropharyngeal dysphagia (transfer dysphagia) is a descriptive term applied to a disorder of the neuromuscular apparatus of the distal pharynx and upper esophagus. Symptoms include difficulty in initiating swallowing, nasal regurgitation, and cough with pulmonary aspiration. The types of disorders associated with oropharyngeal dysphagia include:

  (1) Cerebrovascular accident, which may be the most common of these disorders and usually is due to transient brain stem edema

  (2) Myasthenia gravis

  (3) Myotonic dystrophy

  (4) Polymyositis

  (5) Bulbar poliomyelitis

  (6) Parkinson's disease

  (7) Multiple sclerosis

  (8) Amyotrophic lateral sclerosis

  (9) Hypothyroidism

b. Symptomatic diffuse esophageal spasm (SDES)

 (1) Pathology. Although occasional reports have described an esophageal muscular hypertrophy, these are not consistent. Most investigators think that a neural defect exists. LES abnormalities (similar to achalasia), with incomplete relaxation, have been described in 30% of cases, and documented progression to classic achalasia lends credence to a neural pathogenesis.

 (2) Clinical features

  (a) Dysphagia for both solids and liquids occurs.

  (b) Odynophagia can occur, especially after ingestion of solids or liquids of extremely hot or cold temperature.

  (c) Spontaneous chest pain similar to angina pectoris may be noted. Nocturnal pain, which is often described, is relieved by the smooth muscle relaxant nitroglycerin (the same treatment prescribed for anginal pain). The ability of nitroglycerin to provide relief may further confuse the diagnosis.

 (3) Diagnosis is based on clinical evidence.

  (a) Radiography may reveal a corkscrew-shaped esophagus.

  (b) Esophageal manometry should reveal:

   (i) High-amplitude, repetitive, simultaneous contractions in approximately 30% of the basal state or after ergonovine or edrophonium stimulation (not a routinely performed test). (In a variant of SDES called the **nutcracker esophagus,** high-amplitude prolonged contractions may be associated with chest pain.)

   (ii) Several normal peristaltic sequences to differentiate SDES from achalasia

   (iii) Incomplete relaxation of the LES in approximately 30% of patients

  (c) Balloon distention of the esophageal lumen can be used as a stimulus. A smaller than normal amount of air or water insufflation of the balloon indicates a lower threshold for pain.

 (4) Therapy is successful in approximately 50% of cases and includes:

  (a) Anticholinergic agents

  (b) Nitrates (short- or long-acting)

  (c) Calcium channel-blocking agents

  (d) Esophageal bougienage

  (e) Hydralazine to decrease peristaltic amplitude

  (f) Surgery with a longitudinal esophageal myotomy (in severe, incapacitating cases only)

c. Achalasia

 (1) Incidence. Achalasia occurs in approximately 1 in 100,000 individuals in the United States and equally in both sexes. The most common age of onset is between 20 and 40 years.

 (2) Pathology. A neural defect is suggested by decreased ganglion cells, with fibrosis and scarring in Auerbach's plexus. **Wallerian degeneration** is suggested by examination of vagal esophageal fibers. The dorsal vagal nucleus also is abnormal. Supersensitivity to cholinergic stimulation and exogenous gastrin is described.

 (3) Clinical features include:

  (a) Dysphagia for solids and liquids in 95%–100% of patients

  (b) Weight loss in 90% of patients

  (c) Chest pain, which is severe in approximately 60% of patients

  (d) Nocturnal cough in approximately 30% of patients, indicating possible overflow aspiration of unemptied esophageal contents and, in such cases, the need for immediate treatment

  (e) Recurrent bronchitis or pneumonia, both of which are serious complications, in approximately 7%–8% of patients

 (4) Diagnosis is made by excluding malignancy (i.e., carcinoma or lymphoma) at the esophagogastric junction, which may mimic achalasia ("secondary achalasia"). Secondary achalasia may be characterized by greater weight loss, shorter duration of symptoms, and less esophageal dilatation in an older person.

(a) **Radiography** may reveal a flaccid, dilated, fluid-filled esophagus with a beak-like tapering over the LES region.

(b) **Manometry** is the most sensitive diagnostic method and should reveal:

(i) Absence of normal peristalsis in the entire esophagus

(ii) Elevated LES pressure

(iii) Incomplete relaxation of the LES, which probably accounts for the major clinical findings because there is a persistent obstructing barrier after swallowing

(5) **Therapy**

(a) **Drugs.** Nitrates, anticholinergic agents, β-adrenergic agonists, and calcium channel-blocking agents are effective in less than 50% of patients. Prostaglandins may hold promise as future forms of therapy.

(b) **Pneumatic dilation** is effective in 70%–90% of patients, has a mortality rate of approximately 0.2%, and has a perforation rate of about 2%–3%.

(c) **Endoscopic injection of botulinum toxin** into the LES results in decreased LES pressure and decreased dysphagia in 70%–80% of patients.

(d) **Surgical therapy**

(i) The favored procedure is a **Heller myotomy,** which has a 65%–90% success rate and a 3%–4% surgical complication rate. For operations that do not incorporate an antireflux procedure, the rate of postoperative reflux may increase to 25%–30% after several years.

(ii) **Endoscopic myotomy** is undergoing clinical trials.

d. **Systemic sclerosis (scleroderma)** is a systemic collagen vascular disease involving the skin in 98% of cases. The esophagus is found to be abnormal in 75% of autopsies and in 80% of cases studied manometrically.

(1) **Pathology.** The early esophageal effects are thought to be neural because no anatomic abnormality of the smooth muscle can be identified at a time when marked weakness of the esophagus is noted. The strong association with Raynaud's phenomenon, which also is believed to have a neural basis, is consistent with this theory. A late defect may include a disuse type of atrophy of the circular smooth muscle elements of the esophagus; the longitudinal muscular layers remain intact.

(2) **Clinical features** include:

(a) Dysphagia for solids and liquids

(b) Severe heartburn in approximately 50% of patients

(c) Esophageal stricture in approximately 25% of long-term survivors

(3) **Diagnosis**

(a) **Radiography.** Supine esophagography may reveal poor esophageal emptying due to an absence of peristalsis.

(b) **Manometry,** the most reliable diagnostic technique, reveals:

(i) Decreased LES pressure

(ii) Very weak, low-amplitude peristaltic contractions in the distal smooth muscle portion (lower two thirds) of the esophagus

(4) **Therapy.** The esophageal disorder is treated with antireflux measures (see I B 1 d).

4. **Other esophageal disorders**

a. **Diverticula**

(1) **Zenker's diverticulum** is a mucosal herniation (not a true diverticulum) above the cricopharyngeal region; obstructive symptoms may occur if

there is incomplete emptying of this diverticulum. Large diverticula are treated surgically.

   (2) Traction diverticula occur in the mid and distal regions and are thought to be secondary to an adjacent inflammatory process, such as tuberculosis.

   (3) Epiphrenic diverticula occur in the distal esophagus, above the LES, and often are asymptomatic.

b. Infections. Bacterial and viral sources of esophageal infection are common, but several infectious agents are of particular interest.

   (1) Candidal esophagitis usually occurs in diabetic patients, immunocompromised hosts (e.g., patients infected with HIV or patients on cancer chemotherapy or undergoing steroid treatment), and in those with poor esophageal emptying (e.g., patients with achalasia or severe stricture). Odynophagia is a major symptom, and diagnosis is made by endoscopy and cytologic studies. Treatment is with nystatin, ketoconazole, fluconazole, or, in resistant cases, low doses of amphotericin B.

   (2) Herpes simplex virus (HSV) may cause esophagitis in immunocompromised hosts. The esophagitis is characterized by relatively small, isolated ulcers. Biopsy of the ulcerating edges may show characteristic multinucleated cells with nuclear inclusions. Treatment is with vidarabine or acyclovir.

   (3) CMV infection of the esophagus is often seen in immunocompromised patients and may produce very large ulcerations of the esophagus. Intranuclear inclusion bodies are observed on biopsy and treatment is with ganciclovir.

   (4) HIV esophagitis may result in a diffuse inflammatory esophagitis. Treatment of isolated acquired immune deficiency syndrome (AIDS) esophagitis is with steroids.

c. Esophageal burns. Ingestion of caustic agents (i.e., strong alkali or acid) can cause serious esophageal burns. Ingestion of lye or detergents such as chlorine bleach is a common suicidal gesture in adults and a common accident in children. Emergency endoscopy should be performed to assess the extent of damage. Steroids and broad-spectrum antibiotics are recommended initially in management of esophageal burns. Long-term sequelae in survivors may include esophageal stricture and esophageal carcinoma.

d. Esophageal tears are seen most commonly after vomiting (75% of cases), straining, or coughing.

   (1) A mucosal tear **(Mallory-Weiss syndrome)** produces significant hematemesis after an initial nonbloody vomitus. Surgery is required in less than 10% of these cases.

   (2) A rupture of the esophagus **(Boerhaave's syndrome)** usually occurs above the esophagogastric junction. Air in the left mediastinal region suggests the diagnosis, and immediate surgical intervention is necessary if the patient is to survive.

e. Paraesophageal hernia. Unlike the much more common and clinically insignificant hiatal hernia, a paraesophageal hernia may lead to gastric vascular compromise. The esophagogastric junction traverses the diaphragm in the appropriate location. The body of the stomach then travels above the diaphragm, and gastric volvulus with incarceration may occur. Surgery may be necessary to alleviate symptoms of pain, upper gastrointestinal bleeding, and ischemia.

f. Pill-induced esophagitis is often caused by medications such as aspirin, other nonsteroidal anti-inflammatory agents, potassium chloride tablets, iron preparations, quinidine, and certain antibiotics. These medications are often temporarily lodged in the esophagus, because of either inadequate liquid with swallowing or a relative narrowing of the esophagus. Severe erosions and strictures may develop in a minority of cases. Treatment is symptomatic.

II. DISEASES OF THE STOMACH

A. Gastritis

1. **Acute gastritis** is an inflammation of the gastric mucosa, which may be diffuse or localized and usually is self-limited.
   a. **Etiology**
      (1) **Drugs** that can damage the mucosal barrier and lead to back-diffusion of acid and pepsin include:
         (a) Aspirin and similar nonsteroidal anti-inflammatory agents
         (b) Alcohol, which may produce an additive effect with aspirin
      (2) **Accidental ingestion of caustic substances,** such as strong alkali (e.g., lye), strong acid [e.g., sulfuric acid (H_2SO_4) and HCl], or fixatives [e.g., formaldehyde and trinitrophenol (picric acid)], can be fatal. Patients who survive the ingestion of such corrosives sustain injuries that leave considerable scars and subsequent antral narrowing.
      (3) **Stress** related to severe illness, especially illness involving many organ systems, causes acute gastritis. Ischemia and gastric acid, even at normal levels, may be involved. Antacids, H_2-receptor antagonists, proton pump inhibitors, and cytoprotective agents (e.g., sucralfate, prostaglandins) may be effective as prophylactic or therapeutic agents in cases of stress-induced gastritis.
      (4) **Infections**
         (a) *Helicobacter pylori* infectious gastritis (see III C 4)
         (b) **Phlegmonous gastritis,** bacterial invasion of the stomach wall, is a rare but fatal condition most commonly caused by streptococci; however, it also has been associated with staphylococci.
         (c) **Infections with CMV, herpesvirus, M. avium-intracellulare, Candida, T. pallidum,** and **M. tuberculosis** have been associated with gastritis, especially in immunocompromised patients.
   b. **Clinical features,** which are absent in 30% of patients, include:
      (1) **Epigastric burning** and **pain, nausea,** and **vomiting**
      (2) **Gastrointestinal bleeding,** which may be severe and associated with hematemesis and shock
   c. **Diagnosis** is made in most cases on the basis of endoscopic visualization with or without biopsy. Congestion, friability, superficial ulceration, and petechiae frequently are seen in the gastric mucosa.
   d. **Therapy** begins with removal of offending agents. Antacids, antiviral and antifungal agents, H_2-receptor antagonists, proton pump inhibitors, and surface-acting agents (e.g., sucralfate) are useful as well. Patients with acute hemorrhagic gastritis usually respond to fluid or blood replacement combined with a regimen of antacids, H_2-receptor antagonists, and omeprazole or lansoprazole, which keep the gastric pH above 3.5. Surgery rarely is necessary for these patients and is associated with high morbidity and mortality rates.

2. **Chronic gastritis** is characterized by a superficial lymphocyte infiltrate in the lamina propria.
   a. **Etiology.** Chronic gastritis can be caused by:
      (1) Prolonged use of alcohol, aspirin, and other irritating drugs
      (2) Radiation or thermal injury
      (3) Immunologic factors
      (4) Infections (e.g., *H. pylori*)
   b. **Types**
      (1) **Chronic type A gastritis** involves the fundus and body of the stomach; the antrum is spared. This type of gastritis is associated with parietal cell antibodies, high serum gastrin levels, and pernicious anemia.
      (2) **Chronic type B gastritis** involves the antrum of the stomach; the body and fundus are relatively spared. Gastrin cell antibodies have been detected in some patients with this gastritis. More commonly, reflux of duo-

denal or biliary secretions or *H. pylori* infections are linked causatively to type B gastritis.

c. **Clinical features** may be few in patients with chronic gastritis. Type A gastritis is associated with hypochlorhydria or achlorhydria, whereas type B gastritis is associated with normal acid levels. Hypothyroidism, diabetes mellitus, and vitiligo occur more frequently with type A than with type B gastritis.

d. **Clinical course.** Data suggest that these lesions may remain unchanged for several years. Gastric atrophy develops in approximately 50% of patients with superficial gastritis over 10–20 years. There is an increased association with gastric polyps, gastric ulcer, and gastric cancer in both types of chronic gastritis, with type B being associated with a higher incidence of gastric cancer than type A.

e. **Therapy** usually is unnecessary; however, conditions associated with gastritis (e.g., pernicious anemia, *H. pylori* infections, hypothyroidism, and diabetes) should be treated accordingly. Some authors suggest yearly gastric cytologic analysis as a means of diagnosing an early cancer in affected patients.

3. **Special types of gastritis**

a. ***H. pylori*** infectious gastritis is caused by a gram-negative, spiral-shaped bacterium that survives in the acidic milieu of the stomach by producing urease, which liberates ammonia. Chronic gastritis involving *H. pylori* has been associated with 80%–90% of duodenal ulcer patients (see III C 4) and with 60%–70% of gastric ulcer patients. It has been associated with mucosa-associated lymphatic tissue (MALT)-type gastric lymphoma and implicated in adenocarcinoma of the stomach.

b. **Eosinophilic gastroenteritis** refers to the infiltration of eosinophils into the gastric antrum, small bowel, or both. This infiltration, which is believed to be immunologically mediated, causes thickening of the intestinal wall with subsequent antral obstruction. Peripheral eosinophilia may occur. Differentiation from other infiltrative diseases (e.g., tuberculosis, sarcoidosis, lymphoma, syphilis, histoplasmosis, Crohn's disease, and carcinoma) may be difficult and depends on endoscopic biopsy. Corticosteroid therapy has been successful in providing a prolonged remission.

c. **Granulomatous gastritis** is an infiltrative disease characterized by noncaseating granulomas, with or without giant cells. Crohn's disease, sarcoidosis, beryllium poisoning, or idiopathic causes may result in granulomatous gastritis. Gastric outlet obstruction is common. Treatment with steroids or surgery is often required.

d. **Hypertrophic gastritis** is an uncommon condition associated with massive enlargement of the gastric folds.

(1) **Clinical features.** In its most extreme form (i.e., Ménétrier's disease), there is hyposecretion of gastric acid, protein loss from the stomach, peripheral edema, weight loss, and abdominal pain.

(2) **Diagnosis** is made by endoscopy and biopsy, often with a suction apparatus.

(a) On biopsy, gastric mucous cells are hyperplastic, and inflammatory cells are present in some patients.

(b) Lymphoma, amyloid infiltration, carcinoma, and Zollinger-Ellison syndrome also can cause large rugal folds and should be excluded.

(c) A type of hypersecretory hypertrophic gastritis is similar to Ménétrier's disease but is associated with high acid output and hyperplasia of parietal gastric cells.

(3) **Therapy** includes anticholinergic agents, which appear to close the tight junctions between cells and decrease protein loss, H_2-receptor antagonists, and steroids. Surgery (gastric resection) is reserved for intractable cases.

B. **Gastric neoplasms**

1. **Gastric carcinoma**

a. **Incidence.** The most common cancer in the United States 70 years ago, gastric carcinoma continues to decline in incidence in this country. The incidence of gastric cancer remains high, however, in Japan and eastern Europe, and it appears to be inversely related to the incidence of carcinoma of the colon. Recently, there has been an increased incidence of fundic gastric adenocarcinoma associated with young, middle-class, white men. Gastric carcinoma is twice as common in men as it is in women and usually occurs in patients who are 50–75 years of age. The incidence is highest among individuals of low socioeconomic classes.

b. Pathogenesis. Although the cause of gastric carcinoma is unknown, certain relationships have been observed. A 20% higher incidence of gastric cancer among family members and a higher incidence among individuals with blood group A suggest that there is a genetic component. Tobacco use, vitamin C deficiency, and consumption of preserved foods (especially salted or smoked foods) and nitrosamines also are thought to play etiologic roles. Premalignant conditions include:

    (1) Pernicious anemia

    (2) Atrophic gastritis

    (3) Postgastrectomy, especially 10–20 years after Billroth II resection

    (4) Gastric polyps, which have approximately a 40% incidence of malignancy if they are adenomatous and larger than 2 cm in diameter[*]

    (5) Immunodeficiency disorders, especially common variable immunodeficiency[†]

    (6) *H. pylori* infection

c. Clinical features

    (1) Weight loss and **anorexia** are observed in approximately 70%–80% of patients.

    (2) Epigastric pain is described by approximately 70% of patients.

    (3) Several other symptoms may be noted, including early satiety, vomiting, and weakness and fatigue secondary to chronic blood loss and anemia.

        (a) Early satiety is particularly common in patients with **linitis plastica,** because the gastric wall does not distend normally.

        (b) Vomiting often is a result of pyloric obstruction by the tumor mass but also can result from impaired gastric motility.

        (c) Gross gastrointestinal bleeding is rare in gastric carcinomas, occurring in less than 10% of patients. Dysphagia can occur if the lesion is near the esophagogastric junction.

        (d) A palpable, left supraclavicular (Virchow's) node may indicate metastatic disease.

d. Diagnosis may be established by the following procedures.

    (1) Upper gastrointestinal series can reveal a mass, ulcer, or thickened, nondistensible "leather bottle" stomach (linitis plastica). The simultaneous use of air contrast techniques enhances the diagnostic accuracy of radiographs.

    (2) Endoscopy with biopsy and brush cytology has a 95%–99% accuracy rate in diagnosing gastric cancer.

    (3) Increased serum carcinoembryonic antigen (CEA) levels as well as elevated 2-glucuronidase levels in gastric secretions may be seen in gastric carcinoma patients. Achlorhydria in response to maximum stimulation and in the presence of a gastric ulcer almost always indicates malignant ulceration.

e. Therapy

    (1) Surgery is the treatment of choice but is associated with a 5-year survival rate of only approximately 12%. If the disease is superficial, as it often is in Japan, the survival rate may be as high as 70%. Cancer in a gastric ulcer has a slightly better prognosis, with approximately a 30%–50% 5-year survival rate.

---

[*] Most gastric polyps are hyperplastic and not thought to be premalignant.
[†] In one series, 33% of such patients developed gastric cancer.

(2) Chemotherapy has a 25%–40% response rate, but little improvement in survival rate has been described.

2. Lymphomas
  a. True gastric lymphoma usually occurs as a bulky mass associated with large, thickened gastric folds. Pain is the most common presenting symptom. Histologic examination usually shows diffuse histiocytic non-Hodgkin's lymphoma, but non-Hodgkin's lymphomas of all types are more common than Hodgkin's disease in the stomach. Gastric lymphoma, especially of the MALT type, has been strongly associated with *H. pylori* infection.
    (1) Diagnosis. Gastric lymphoma should be differentiated from Ménétrier's disease, Zollinger-Ellison syndrome, and hypertrophic gastritis. Diagnosis is confirmed by biopsy, either at endoscopy with a suction apparatus or at surgery.
    (2) Therapy. Surgery and localized radiotherapy are the generally accepted forms of therapy, with 5-year survival rates approaching 50% in non-Hodgkin's lymphoma patients whose lymphoma is confined to the stomach. Chemotherapy is valuable in patients with systemic disease. If *H. pylori* lymphoma is identified, treatment of the *H. pylori* alone may lead to resolution.
  b. Gastric pseudolymphoma is a condition that may occur after therapy with certain drugs, especially phenytoin. Often associated with gastric ulceration and granulation, it does not usually perforate. No mass is noted, and the lymphocytic infiltrate has germinal centers.

3. Other gastric tumors (stromal tumors)
  a. Benign leiomyomas usually are less than 4 cm in diameter and occur in the distal antrum. A central ulceration occasionally occurs and may necessitate excision for recurrent upper gastrointestinal bleeding.
  b. Leiomyosarcomas, which account for approximately 1% of all gastric malignancies, are similar to gastric lymphomas in treatment procedures and 5-year survival rates. Generally, leiomyosarcomas of the stomach exceed 4 cm in diameter.
  c. Rare gastric malignancies, such as **fibrosarcomas, neurogenic sarcomas,** and **metastatic carcinomas** (especially from breast and lung carcinomas and melanoma), must be differentiated from primary gastric carcinoma.

C. **Disorders of gastric emptying**

1. Pyloric stenosis
  a. Acquired pyloric stenosis occurs transiently, due to edema from peptic ulcer disease, or chronically, due to pyloric scarring from recurrent ulcer disease or neoplasm.
  b. Congenital pyloric stenosis usually presents in infancy.
    (1) Incidence. Congenital pyloric stenosis occurs in approximately 2–4 of 1000 births and usually is seen in firstborn male children. There is a familial incidence.
    (2) Clinical features include postprandial projectile vomiting of nonbilious material, dehydration, and weight loss. Visible peristalsis may be noted, with a mass palpated in the epigastrium.
    (3) Diagnosis is based on radiographic demonstration. A plain film reveals air in the stomach, and a barium swallow confirms the diagnosis.
    (4) Therapy is by surgery (Ramstedt operation) and consists of a myotomy of the circular muscle of the pylorus.

2. Gastric bezoars are collections of nondigestible substances that sometimes form and cannot pass through the pylorus. Trichobezoars are composed of hair, and phytobezoars are composed of plant fibers. Bezoars generally are seen in patients who have undergone previous gastric surgery or in mentally retarded individuals who consume nondigestible substances. The symptoms include those of gastric-outlet obstruction and bleeding from superficial ulcerations. It is important to exclude a gastric mass or cancer, and the diagnosis can be established endoscopically. Bezoars sometimes can be enzymatically dissolved with papain, acetylcysteine, or cellulase; otherwise, endoscopic or surgical removal is necessary.

3. **Gastric diverticula** occur on the posterior wall of the stomach in approximately 75% of cases and usually are within 2 cm of the esophagogastric junction. Unless they bleed or perforate, these congenital lesions are asymptomatic. **Pseudodiverticula,** seen most commonly in the antrum, are scarred remnants of previous peptic disease.

4. **Gastric volvulus** may occur due to weak ligamentous attachments or may be secondary to a paraesophageal hernia, an intrinsic gastric lesion, or an adjacent mass. Diagnosis is supported by the finding of two separate fluid levels in the left upper quadrant and by a lack of barium passage into the pylorus. Therapy consists of temporary nasogastric suction. Recurrent or acute volvulus with gastric vascular compromise may require surgery.

5. **Gastroparesis** is a disorder of gastric emptying that is not caused by an obstruction. The diagnosis should not be made until mechanical obstruction has been ruled out by an upper gastrointestinal series or by endoscopy. Gastroparesis most frequently is caused by insulin-dependent diabetes mellitus (IDDM) of longer than 10 years' duration. Other conditions associated with gastroparesis include systemic sclerosis, postvagotomy states, and therapy with anticholinergic agents. In diabetes, loss of gastric phase III activity is noted on electrical recordings, with other signs of diabetic visceral neuropathy often being seen as well. Treatment with prokinetic agents such as metoclopramide, domperidone, erythromycin, or cisapride has been effective.

III. PEPTIC ULCER DISEASE

A. **Introduction.** Peptic ulcer disease refers to a group of disorders of the gastrointestinal tract. The disorders are similar in that they all involve areas of discrete tissue destruction caused by acid and pepsin. Peptic ulcers occur most commonly in the stomach or proximal duodenum, less commonly in the distal esophagus, and rarely in the small intestine. (Peptic ulcers in the distal small intestine usually are associated with a Meckel's diverticulum that contains gastric mucosa.) In general, the clinical features and treatment of peptic ulcer disease are similar regardless of location, although peptic esophagitis caused by reflux of gastric contents has some unique features (see I B 1).

B. **Incidence.** Peptic ulcer disease occurs more commonly in men than in women. Duodenal ulcers are three times more common than gastric ulcers and occur approximately 10 years earlier; the peak incidence for duodenal ulcers is at approximately 40 years of age, as opposed to 50 years of age for gastric ulcers. The relapse rate at 1 year is approximately 80% for patients with duodenal ulcers; patients with gastric ulcers have a 33% chance that subsequent duodenal ulcers will develop.

C. **Pathogenesis.** Acid and pepsin are necessary for an ulcer to develop; however, several factors, especially *H. pylori* infection, are thought to contribute to the pathogenesis.

1. **Social factors**
   a. **Tobacco smoking** increases the risk of development of peptic ulcer disease. Smoking also increases the morbidity and mortality rates and decreases the healing rate for peptic ulcers. The mechanism may be a decrease in pancreatic bicarbonate secretion and, therefore, a lowered alkaline level in the duodenum, an increase in gastric emptying with a lowered duodenal pH, an increase in serum pepsinogen I secretion, or a decrease in pyloric sphincter pressure with an increased reflux into the stomach.

b. Drugs. Ulcers develop in approximately 30% of arthritis patients who take high doses of aspirin. Other nonsteroidal anti-inflammatory drugs have been incriminated, with an antiprostaglandin effect suggested as an underlying factor in this group of drugs. Steroids also are thought to break the mucosal barrier and may double the risk of peptic ulcer disease.

c. Alcohol compromises the mucosal barrier and increases gastric acid secretion.

2. Physiologic factors

a. Gastric acid, although essential for ulcer production, generally is measured at normal or decreased levels in gastric ulcer patients. Many investigators attribute this to an increase in the back-diffusion of hydrogen ion (H^+) into the mucosa or submucosa. Slightly elevated levels of gastric acid are noted in the basal and stimulated states in duodenal ulcer patients.

b. Serum gastrin. In duodenal ulcer patients, serum gastrin levels are normal during fasting and increased in the postprandial state. In gastric ulcer patients, both fasting and postprandial levels of serum gastrin are higher than normal.

3. Genetic factors

a. First-degree relatives of gastric ulcer patients have three times the risk of development of gastric ulcers as the general population. Similarly, the risk of duodenal ulcer is increased in the first-degree relatives of duodenal ulcer patients.

b. An increased incidence of duodenal ulcer also has been documented among individuals with blood group O, individuals who demonstrate elevated serum levels of pepsinogen I, and those who are nonsecretors of blood group substances.

4. Infectious etiology

a. *H. pylori* has been identified on cultures of the gastric antrum in 90% of patients with duodenal ulcer disease or antral type B gastritis, and the association for patients with gastric ulcer disease is 60%–70%. In addition, there is an increased association of *H. pylori* infections with MALT lymphomas of the stomach and gastric cancer.

b. Pathophysiology. *H. pylori* is found on gastric epithelium and does not penetrate the cell. It has secretory immunoglobulin A (IgA) and host immunoglobulin (IgG) specificity. If it is a primary offender, it may act as a "barrier breaker," allowing acid back-diffusion and peptic ulcer disease to develop. *H. pylori* elaborates ammonia, which damages cell surfaces, and liberates a number of other inflammatory cell recruiting factors and adhesion molecules.

c. Diagnosis. *H. pylori* liberates urease, and a biopsy of the gastric antrum may change a pH color monitor. A urea breath test using carbon 13 (^{13}C)- or ^{14}C-labeled urea measures exhaled labeled carbon dioxide. Supplemented culture medium (starch, blood, or charcoal) may be optimal under microaerophilic conditions at 37°C. Warthin-Starry silver, Giemsa, or hematoxylin and eosin stains may show the organism in an extracellular location. Antibodies to *H. pylori* detected by enzyme-linked immunosorbent assay demonstrate active or prior infection.

d. Treatment is with amoxicillin, doxycycline with metronidazole, and a bismuth preparation for 2 weeks. Newer approaches have included clarithromycin and proton pump inhibitors.

e. Outcome. Studies have shown a decreased relapse rate in duodenal ulcers treated with antibiotics and bismuth as compared with H_2 blockers.

5. Associated diseases

a. Some patients with **multiple endocrine neoplasia, type I (MEN I),** present with gastrin-secreting tumors. This probably accounts for the reported association of duodenal ulcer disease with hyperparathyroidism.

b. Antral atrophic gastritis may be caused by back-diffusion of bile through the pylorus; it is associated with a high incidence of gastric ulcers.

c. Patients with **rheumatoid arthritis** have an increased risk of ulcer disease, which probably is secondary to the drugs used for treatment.

d. Chronic obstructive pulmonary disease (COPD) has been found in a significant number of gastric ulcer patients.

   e. Hepatic cirrhosis and **chronic renal failure** are demonstrated in a significant
      number of duodenal ulcer patients.

6. **Psychosomatic factors** include chronic anxiety and type "A" personality.

D. **Clinical features**

1. **Pain** is the predominant symptom, although it may be absent in 25% of gastric
   ulcer patients. The pain characteristically is described as an epigastric burning sensation and may be accompanied by bloating or nausea. Eating may exacerbate the
   pain in gastric ulcer patients, whereas in duodenal ulcer patients, the pain usually
   is diminished by eating, only to recur 2–3 hours later. Pain may awaken patients
   from sleep, especially those with duodenal ulcers.

2. **Upper gastrointestinal hemorrhage** may be the presenting sign of peptic ulcer disease, and anemia from chronic blood loss may be seen.

3. Less common symptoms include:
   a. **Repeated vomiting,** which may indicate gastric-outlet obstruction
   b. **Weight loss,** which is somewhat more common with gastric ulcer

E. **Diagnosis.** Because the patient may complain of only vague symptoms, a high index
   of suspicion is needed.

1. **Radiography** is a useful screening tool; however, an upper gastrointestinal series
   may miss up to 30% of gastric ulcers, and scarring of the duodenal bulb from
   chronic or recurrent ulcer disease may make radiographic interpretation difficult.
   Double-contrast techniques may improve diagnostic accuracy. Duodenal ulcers always are benign; however, gastric ulcers may be benign or malignant. Radiographic criteria for benign gastric ulcers include:
   a. Ulcer crater extending beyond the gastric wall
   b. Gastric folds radiating into the base of the ulcer
   c. Thick radiolucent collar of edema (Hampton's line) surrounding the ulcer base
   d. Smooth, regular, round or ovoid ulcer crater
   e. Pliable and normally distensible gastric wall in the area of the ulcer

2. **Endoscopy** may be used as the primary diagnostic maneuver or to confirm a radiographic diagnosis. Because 5% of gastric ulcers that occur in the United States are
   malignant, many authors advocate endoscopy with multiple biopsies at the margin
   of the ulcer and simultaneous cytologic brushings for the evaluation of all gastric
   ulcers, with subsequent endoscopy in 6–8 weeks to document healing.

3. **Gastric acid analysis** may be helpful to distinguish benign from malignant gastric
   ulcers. Because benign ulcers rarely exist in the setting of achlorhydria, the absence of acid should prompt further workup with gastric biopsies and cytologic
   studies. Although gastric ulcers in the presence of achlorhydria nearly always
   are malignant, most malignant ulcers are found in stomachs with normal acid
   secretion.

F. **Therapy** is virtually the same for esophageal, gastric, and duodenal ulcers.

1. **Intensive antacids** have been shown to promote the healing of gastric and duodenal ulcers. The healing rates, which are approximately 70%–80% at 4 weeks, appear equal to those of the H_2-receptor antagonists and are considerably better than
   the healing rates with placebo (45%). The timing of antacids is important, and dosage varies according to the neutralizing capacity of the specific antacid. Calcium-
   containing antacids are no longer recommended because they produce an acid rebound due to calcium-stimulated gastrin release. Magnesium may accumulate to
   toxic levels in renal failure patients taking magnesium-containing antacids. In all
   patients, the most common side effect of these medications is diarrhea, which can
   be avoided by placing patients on alternating doses of magnesium- and aluminum-
   containing antacids.

2. **H$_2$-receptor antagonists** are the mainstay of treatment because of patient convenience, sustained acid reduction, and increased healing rates with diminished relapse rates.
   a. **Cimetidine, ranitidine,** and **famotidine (nizatidine)** decrease recurrence with bedtime dosing.
   b. **Side effects** of these H$_2$-receptor antagonists are few. Cimetidine affects the cytochrome P-450 system, so decreased dosages are advised for patients taking warfarin, diazepam, theophylline, and other drugs that affect the cytochrome P-450 system. Compared with other H$_2$-receptor antagonists, large doses of cimetidine may slightly increase the risk of central nervous system (CNS) side effects or gynecomastia.

3. **Antibiotics** are used to treat *H. pylori* infection. Regimens typically involve combinations of an antibiotic (e.g., metronidazole, amoxicillin, tetracycline preparations, clarithromycin), a bismuth-containing product, and a proton-pump inhibitor (double or triple therapy). Treatment is for approximately 2 weeks with a 70%–90% response rate, depending on the regimen selected.

4. **Anticholinergic agents** have a limited therapeutic role as they decrease meal-stimulated acid secretion by only approximately 30%. These agents may be used to delay gastric emptying of antacids, especially at night. More selective anticholinergic agents, such as pirenzepine, may be more useful.

5. **Diet.** There is no proof that bland diets promote healing in peptic ulcer disease. In fact, milk may be harmful because it increases acid secretion, probably by calcium- and protein-stimulated gastrin release. Caffeine and alcohol stimulate gastric acid secretion and, therefore, should be restricted in acute cases. Decaffeinated coffee also may stimulate acid release. Ulcer patients who smoke should be urged to decrease or stop smoking.

6. **Other therapeutic agents**
   a. **Sucralfate** is a nonsystemic agent, which, in the presence of an acid pH, coats the ulcer bed and promotes healing. Sucralfate is as effective as H$_2$-receptor antagonists and antacids and has no significant side effects.
   b. **Carbenoxolone** is useful but slightly less effective than H$_2$-receptor antagonists in healing peptic ulcers. This derivative of the licorice root decreases gastric permeability to H$^+$, decreases the peptic activity of gastric juice, and increases the life span of gastric epithelial cells with a thickening of the gastric mucosa. The major drawback of carbenoxolone is its aldosterone-like effect of sodium and water retention.
   c. **Bismuth** has both ulcer-insulating and pepsin-inactivating properties but does not decrease gastric acid production. Healing rates are slightly better in gastric than in duodenal ulcer patients, and the overall rate of adverse reaction is low. In *H. pylori*–associated disease, bismuth may cause the organisms to dislodge from gastric epithelial cells. Milk and antacids may interfere with its action and should be avoided for 1 hour before and after ingestion of bismuth.
   d. **Prostaglandin E$_2$ (PGE$_2$)** and **PGF$_2$** may have a cytoprotective effect on gastric mucosa. These agents also increase gastric blood flow and decrease gastrin-stimulated acid secretion. A PGE$_2$ analogue, **misoprostol,** has been shown to be effective in treating peptic ulcer disease and has been released for use in preventing gastric ulcers in patients taking nonsteroidal anti-inflammatory drugs. The major side effects of prostaglandins are diarrhea and nausea.
   e. **Tricyclic antidepressants** (e.g., doxepin) have been proven effective in treating peptic ulcers, probably because of their H$_2$-receptor antagonist effects.
   f. **Proton pump inhibitors** (e.g., omeprazole, lansoprazole) are approved for treatment of reflux esophagitis and duodenal ulcers. These compounds irreversibly block proton pump function and markedly decrease acid production. This class of powerful drugs has been shown to cause carcinoid tumors in rats given very high doses of these drugs for more than 2 years.

7. **Gastric irradiation** decreases acid production for approximately 1 year and may

play a role in treating recurrent disease in elderly patients who cannot tolerate drugs or surgery.

8. **Surgery** is effective therapy for peptic ulcer disease and reduces recurrence rates to a low percentage.
   a. **Procedures.** The most commonly performed operation is **distal subtotal gastrectomy,** with wedge resection of a gastric ulcer if one is present. **Vagotomy with drainage (V + D)** and **vagotomy with antrectomy (V + A)** are the usual procedures for complicated peptic ulcer disease. V + D is associated with a higher recurrence rate (approximately 7%–15%) than V + A (3%), but it is associated with less postoperative weight loss. A proximal selective vagotomy appears to lessen postoperative complications.
   b. **Indications.** The high incidence of postoperative complications, regardless of the type of procedure, has limited the role of surgery to **treatment of complications** (including acute emergencies) and **intractable cases.**

G. **Complications**

1. **Hemorrhage** occurs in 20% of patients and is the most serious complication, having a 10% mortality rate. If blood requirements exceed 3 U in 24 hours for longer than 48–72 hours or if in-hospital rebleeding occurs, surgical intervention is indicated. Repeated bleeding episodes occur in approximately 30%–40% of cases and may require surgery.

2. **Perforation** occurs in approximately 5%–10% of all peptic ulcers and is far more common with duodenal ulcers than with gastric ulcers. Of ulcers that perforate, 10% bleed simultaneously. Symptoms and signs include intense pain, a rigid abdomen, decreased bowel sounds, and direct or rebound tenderness. This catastrophic complication is confirmed in approximately 75%–85% of cases by an erect abdominal radiograph showing free air under the diaphragm. Most cases require immediate surgical intervention, but selected patients have been treated successfully with nasogastric suction and antibiotics.

3. **Gastric-outlet obstruction** occurs in approximately 5%–10% of ulcer patients. Of these, 80% of the cases are caused by recurrent duodenal ulcer disease, with prepyloric or pyloric channel ulcers being less common causes. Early satiety, epigastric fullness, nausea, and vomiting of undigested food (frequently ingested several hours earlier) suggest the diagnosis. Weight loss is common. Physical examination may reveal a succussion splash. The diagnosis is confirmed by aspiration of greater than 300 ml of gastric contents more than 3 hours after a meal or by a positive saline load test. Treatment consists of nasogastric aspiration for at least 72 hours, with close attention to replacement of H^+, Na^+, chloride ion (Cl^-), and potassium ion (K^+). Approximately 25%–40% of patients require surgery because 20%–40% of medically treated patients have recurrent obstruction.

4. **Penetration** into an adjacent organ usually is a complication of posterior duodenal ulcers, with penetration into the pancreas. Pain usually is sudden in onset and radiates to the back. Serum amylase and lipase levels frequently are elevated. Treatment is with surgery.

H. **Postsurgical complications**

1. **Stomal ulceration** after surgery may indicate an unrecognized hypersecretory state (e.g., Zollinger-Ellison syndrome, retained gastric antrum, or incomplete vagotomy). The diagnosis of a stomal ulcer is best made by endoscopy. Treatment is with long-term H_2-receptor antagonists, and repeat surgery may be necessary.

2. **Afferent loop obstruction** is a rare complication. The patient usually complains of bloating and vomiting of a clear or bilious material approximately 30–60 minutes after eating. The diagnosis is suggested by the failure of orally ingested barium to enter the loop or by the retention inside the loop of technetium-iminodiacetic acid (Tc-HIDA), which is cleared by the liver and biliary system after intravenous injec-

tion but does not enter the gastrointestinal tract. Bacterial overgrowth can occur, and surgical revision of the afferent loop may be necessary.

3. **Alkaline gastritis** often is seen endoscopically in patients who have undergone antrectomy or subtotal gastrectomy. Gastritis often is asymptomatic but may cause nausea, vomiting, weight loss, and epigastric pain. Diagnosis may be aided by measurement of HIDA-labeled bile refluxing back into the stomach. Because the gastritis is secondary to this increased reflux of duodenal secretions into the stomach, patients may require surgery (a Roux-en-Y anastomosis) to divert these secretions farther down the gastrointestinal tract. Some cases may be treated effectively with substances that bind bile acids (e.g., aluminum-containing antacids and cholestyramine) or with sucralfate.

4. **Dumping syndrome** is a nonspecific term that refers to a variety of postprandial symptoms.
   a. **Early dumping syndrome** occurs approximately 30 minutes after a meal and is associated with dizziness, flushing, diaphoresis, and palpitations. These symptoms have been ascribed to osmotic shifts of fluid or release of massive amounts of intestinal hormones as food empties rapidly from the stomach. The early dumping syndrome can be minimized by decreasing the carbohydrate content of meals and by avoiding liquids with meals. Synthetic somatostatin has been used in resistant cases.
   b. **Late dumping syndrome** occurs several hours after a meal and is characterized by dizziness, weakness, and drowsiness. This syndrome may be due to reactive hypoglycemia.

5. **Nutritional problems**
   a. **Anemia** occurs in approximately 25% of patients after surgery for peptic ulcer disease. Factors that may contribute to iron deficiency include low-grade blood loss from alkaline pouch gastritis, diversion of iron away from its preferential absorption site (i.e., the duodenum), and lack of gastric acid needed for conversion of iron to the preferred form for absorption (i.e., Fe^{3+}). A lack of intrinsic factor leads to vitamin B_{12} deficiency in patients who have undergone a substantial gastric resection.
   b. **Weight loss** occurs in approximately 50% of postoperative patients but is not severe unless a large gastric resection has been performed.
   c. **Significant steatorrhea** usually indicates a secondary problem (e.g., bacterial overgrowth or unmasked celiac disease), although 50% of patients have an increase in stool fat secondary to rapid transit and poor mixing of food with bile salts and pancreatic enzymes.
   d. **Bone thinning** may be due to decreased absorption of vitamin D and calcium.

6. **Gastric pouch cancer** rates are two to four times greater in ulcer patients who have undergone surgery than in patients whose ulcers are treated medically, especially 15–20 years after Billroth II gastric resection.

I. **Zollinger-Ellison syndrome** refers to a non–beta islet cell tumor that produces gastrin and is associated with gastric acid hypersecretion and peptic ulcer disease. The tumors are biologically malignant in 60% of cases and most commonly involve the pancreas. Other tumor sites include the stomach, duodenum, spleen, and lymph nodes. Tumor size varies from 2 mm to 20 cm. Approximately 10% of the patients with Zollinger-Ellison syndrome have a resectable lesion.

1. **Clinical features**
   a. **Pain** from peptic ulcer disease is common in Zollinger-Ellison syndrome. In approximately 75% of cases, the ulcers are located in the duodenal bulb. The remaining cases involve ulcers in the distal duodenum or jejunum or ulcers in multiple locations.
   b. **Diarrhea** occurs in approximately 50% of cases due to gastric acid hypersecretion. The high acid levels may damage the small intestinal mucosa, inactivate pancreatic lipase, and precipitate bile acids, causing steatorrhea. The high gas-

trin levels cause incomplete Na^+ and water absorption and increase intestinal motility. In addition, the volume of gastric secretion alone may cause diarrhea.
 c. **Endocrine abnormalities.** Zollinger-Ellison syndrome commonly is associated with other endocrinopathies. Approximately 20% of these patients have hyperparathyroidism. Pituitary, adrenal, ovarian, and thyroid tumors also have been reported with Zollinger-Ellison syndrome. A distinct syndrome of pancreatic, pituitary, and parathyroid tumors (i.e., MEN I) shows an autosomal dominant pattern of inheritance.

2. **Diagnosis** is made based on the following findings.
 a. **Gastrin levels.** Patients demonstrate elevated basal-state gastrin levels that do not increase 1 hour after a meal. Gastrin levels increase (rather than decline) by 200 units after intravenous secretin administration and increase markedly (rather than modestly) after intravenous calcium administration.
 b. **Gastric acid output.** Patients with Zollinger-Ellison syndrome often have basal gastric acid output rates of more than 10 mEq/hr and basal-to-peak output ratios of greater than 0.6.
 c. **Angiography** may be helpful because gastrin-secreting tumors may be highly vascular.

3. **Therapy**
 a. **Surgical**
  (1) **Total gastrectomy** is the traditional therapy. The 10-year survival rate of 50% with this procedure is thought to be attributable mainly to the slow-growing nature of this lesion. Most of the late deaths are caused by metastatic disease.
  (2) **Tumor localization,** which involves sampling gastrin levels through cannulation of multiple pancreatic and abdominal veins, may be useful. This technique offers the hope of surgical cure in cases of multiple primary tumors and in cases involving a tumor that is too small to be visualized by ordinary means.
 b. **Medical**
  (1) **Proton pump inhibitors** are probably the medical treatment of choice.
  (2) **H_2-receptor antagonists** in combination with **anticholinergic agents** have been used, especially in conjunction with a V + D procedure. Patients who have been unresponsive to H_2-receptor blockade may become responsive as a result of surgery.

J. **Other disorders of the stomach**

1. **Portal hypertensive gastropathy** is the term given to diffuse submucosal dilatation of gastric vessels that may rupture; it accounts for upper gastrointestinal bleeding in approximately 10% of patients with portal hypertension. A diffuse but irregular pattern of red spots or linear streaks produces a characteristic pattern at endoscopy. Treatment with β-blockade or bicap (electrocautery) or laser therapy to the gastric wall may decrease rebleeding.

2. **Dieulafoy's ulcer** is a difficult-to-diagnose vascular lesion generally seen in the gastric fundus; it may be a cause of significant recurrent upper gastrointestinal bleeding. Men older than 50 years of age are most commonly affected. The lesion appears as an exposed arterial defect with no or minimal mucosal ulceration. Endoscopy with laser or bicap treatment is effective in stopping the bleeding, but angiography or surgery is often necessary because of the difficulty of identifying the small vascular defect during endoscopy.

IV. **DISEASES OF THE SMALL INTESTINE**

A. **Intestinal obstruction** is a term used to denote failure of passage of intestinal contents and may be due to mechanical obstruction or adynamic ileus.

1. **Mechanical obstruction**
   a. **Etiology**
      (1) **Extrinsic causes** include:
         (a) Adhesions from prior surgery
         (b) Incarcerated hernia
         (c) Metastatic tumors
         (d) Volvulus
         (e) Endometriosis
         (f) Nonsteroidal anti-inflammatory drug–induced strictures (often multiple)
      (2) **Intramural causes** include:
         (a) Hematomas from trauma
         (b) Strictures
         (c) Intramural tumors
      (3) **Intraluminal causes** include:
         (a) Epithelial tumors (especially colonic)
         (b) Intussusception
         (c) Foreign bodies
   b. **Clinical features** include:
      (1) Crampy pain that waxes and wanes in intensity
      (2) High-pitched bowel sounds with rushes and tinkles
      (3) Constipation and obstipation
      (4) Vomiting, which is more prominent in proximal intestinal obstruction
      (5) Distention, which is more prominent in distal intestinal obstruction
      (6) Intestinal ischemia, leading first to edema, then to petechial hemorrhages, and finally to necrosis and gangrene[*]
   c. **Diagnosis** usually is made with plain and upright abdominal radiographs. Characteristic air–fluid levels exist above the area of obstruction, and no air is seen in the rectum. A barium enema may be useful in diagnosing colonic obstruction. Reflux of barium into the small bowel also may be helpful in the diagnosis of low, small bowel obstruction.
   d. **Therapy** includes:
      (1) Replacement of fluid and electrolytes
      (2) Intestinal decompression with nasogastric suction or small bowel intubation
      (3) Surgery, which usually is required for definitive treatment of the underlying problem

2. **Adynamic,** or **paralytic, ileus** is a nonobstructive lack of propulsion through the intestinal tract.
   a. **Etiology.** Adynamic ileus commonly is linked to the following conditions:
      (1) Recent abdominal surgery, which results in ileus that usually is transient (lasting 2–3 days)
      (2) Electrolyte imbalance, especially hypokalemia
      (3) Chemical or bacterial peritonitis
      (4) Severe intra-abdominal inflammation, such as pancreatitis and cholecystitis
      (5) Systemic illness, such as pneumonia
   b. **Clinical features.** Physical examination shows a distended abdomen and diminished bowel sounds.
   c. **Diagnosis.** Radiographs show diffuse intestinal gas and air in the rectum.
   d. **Therapy** includes:
      (1) Bowel rest and placement of a nasogastric tube
      (2) Correction of underlying causes

---

[*]This is secondary to increased intraluminal pressure occurring after 6–12 hours of obstruction, when absorption ceases and secretion commences.

B. **Intestinal pseudo-obstruction** is a rare but important entity characterized by apparently recurrent episodes of mechanical obstruction but with no demonstrable source of obstruction.

1. **Classification.** Pseudo-obstruction can exist with or without an underlying condition.
   a. **Secondary pseudo-obstruction.** Pseudo-obstruction occurs secondary to many conditions that affect either the smooth muscle of the gastrointestinal tract or the neurologic and hormonal control of intestinal motility.
      (1) Underlying diseases that involve the smooth muscle include collagen vascular disease (especially scleroderma), amyloidosis, and myotonic dystrophy.
      (2) Underlying neurologic diseases include Chagas' disease, Parkinson's disease, and Hirschsprung's disease.
      (3) Underlying endocrine disorders include hypothyroidism, diabetes mellitus, hypoparathyroidism, and pheochromocytoma.
      (4) Drugs that depress intestinal smooth muscle function include phenothiazines, tricyclic antidepressants, ganglionic blockers, and clonidine.
      (5) Nontropical sprue and ceroid deposits in the bowel (mahogany bowel) are rare causes of pseudo-obstruction.
   b. **Primary pseudo-obstruction** occurs in two forms.
      (1) Hereditary **hollow visceral myopathy** is a vacuolization and atrophy of intestinal smooth muscle. This disorder, which is transmitted as an autosomal dominant trait, also affects esophageal and urinary tract smooth muscle.
      (2) An **autonomic nervous system abnormality** has been described in some families with primary pseudo-obstruction. There may be a decrease in total myenteric plexus neurons or neuronal eosinophilic intranuclear inclusions. Possible symptoms include orthostatic hypotension, ataxic gait, dysarthria, and absent deep tendon reflexes.

2. **Diagnosis** is made by rigorously excluding causes of mechanical obstruction while documenting abnormal motility.
   a. **Esophageal manometry** showing normal or low LES pressure with decreased amplitude of peristalsis distally indicates the smooth muscle vacuolization type of pseudo-obstruction. Incomplete relaxation of the LES with absent peristalsis and repetitive esophageal contractions may indicate an autonomic nervous system abnormality.
   b. **Radionuclide gastric emptying scans** may show delayed emptying.
   c. **Barium studies** yield nonspecific findings. Most patients show dilated areas of the intestine.

3. **Therapy** is supportive during acute exacerbations. Cholinergic agents and prokinetic agents have been used with limited success, and surgery should be avoided. Home parenteral hyperalimentation may be required for nutritional support. Intestinal stasis with bacterial overgrowth should be treated with antibiotics.

C. **Small bowel diverticula**

1. **Duodenal diverticula** usually are found incidentally during an upper gastrointestinal series, at endoscopy, or at autopsy. They occur most frequently in the proximal duodenum, within 1–2 cm of the papilla of Vater, and are asymptomatic in most patients, although duodenal diverticula may rarely cause upper gastrointestinal bleeding. In some cases, the common bile duct empties directly into the diverticulum, and common bile duct obstruction may occur due to anatomic interference with emptying.

2. **Jejunal diverticula** probably are acquired rather than congenital and usually are asymptomatic. Jejunal diverticula may lead to malabsorption secondary to bile salt deconjugation when stasis is sufficient to allow an increase in small bowel bacteria. This leads to diarrhea, steatorrhea, weight loss, and anemia. Hypochlorhydria

or achlorhydria also may be present. Continuous or alternating antimicrobial therapy often corrects malabsorption, although surgical removal of multiple diverticula or of a single large diverticulum may be necessary in refractory cases.

3. **Meckel's diverticulum** is a common congenital structural defect, which represents the remnant of the vitelline duct. It is found in approximately 2% of autopsies and usually is located in the terminal ileum within 60 cm of the ileocecal valve. Meckel's diverticula average 5–7 cm in length and may be quite large. Approximately one third of Meckel's diverticula contain gastric mucosa, which may produce acid. Diverticulitis, ulceration, bleeding, perforation, and obstruction are complications that require surgical intervention and frequently mimic the symptoms of acute appendicitis. Because of the presence of gastric mucosa, the diagnosis sometimes can be made by means of pertechnetate scanning after H_2-receptor blockade.

D. **Diarrhea** is defined as an increase in stool frequency and volume. The stool usually is liquid, and 24-hour output exceeds 250 g. The patient may experience lower abdominal crampy pain and fecal urgency.

1. **Classification.** Pathophysiologic criteria are used to classify diarrhea as one of three distinct types.
   a. **Secretory diarrhea**
      (1) **Pathophysiology.** Secretory diarrhea occurs when the secretion of fluid and electrolytes is increased or when the normal absorptive capacity of the bowel is decreased. In some cases, increased secretion is caused by activation of the adenyl cyclase–cyclic adenosine 3′,5′-monophosphate (cAMP) system in mucosal cells.
         (a) Agents that activate the adenyl cyclase–cAMP system include cholera toxin, heat-labile *Escherichia coli* toxin, *Salmonella* enterotoxin, and vasoactive intestinal polypeptide (VIP).
         (b) Agents that probably do not activate the adenyl cyclase–cAMP system include heat-stable *E. coli* toxin, a variety of other bacterial enterotoxins (e.g., those produced by *Clostridium perfringens, Pseudomonas aeruginosa,* and *Klebsiella pneumoniae*), castor oil, and phenolphthalein.
         (c) Chronic secretory diarrhea is seen in the pancreatic cholera syndrome with VIP secretion, in medullary carcinoma of the thyroid gland with calcitonin secretion, in carcinoid syndrome with serotonin secretion, and in villous adenoma of the rectum.
      (2) **Diagnosis** of secretory diarrhea is based on the demonstration of persistent diarrhea in the absence of food intake and by the lack of a gap between total stool osmolarity and two times the sum of stool Na^+ and K^+ concentrations.
      (3) **Therapy** includes fluid and electrolyte support while the cause of the diarrhea is being determined. In general, diarrhea secondary to bacterial enterotoxin is self-limited. Any contributing exogenous agent (e.g., phenolphthalein and castor oil) must be withdrawn.
   b. **Osmotic diarrhea** is caused by the presence of nonabsorbable substances in the intestine, with the secondary accumulation of fluid and electrolytes. Such nonabsorbable substances include lactose in the patient with lactase deficiency, laxatives (e.g., magnesium citrate and sodium phosphate), and foodstuffs in a patient with malabsorption. The diagnosis is suggested by the absence of diarrhea after a 48- to 72-hour fast (with concurrent intravenous fluid replacement). There is a gap of greater than 40 between total stool osmolarity and two times the sum of stool Na^+ and K^+ concentrations.
   c. **Abnormal intestinal motility** causes or contributes to the diarrhea seen in diabetes, irritable bowel syndrome, postvagotomy states, carcinoid syndrome, and hyperthyroidism. Mechanisms of abnormal intestinal motility include the following:
      (1) If small bowel peristalsis is too rapid, an abnormally large amount of fluid and partially digested foodstuffs may be delivered to the colon.

(2) Extremely slow peristalsis may allow bacterial overgrowth to occur and bile salt deconjugation to cause secondary malabsorption.

(3) Rapid colonic motility may not allow adequate time for the colon to absorb fluid delivered to the cecum. (Normally, 90% of the fluid is absorbed.)

2. Diagnosis

a. Tests performed on stool samples include:

(1) Culture and sensitivity testing to detect a pathogenic bacterial strain. A positive stool culture is found for 40% of patients who have white blood cells in the stool and fever.

(2) Microscopic examination to identify ova and parasites (three samples should be sent to increase yield)

(3) Guaiac testing to detect occult blood

(4) Sudan staining to detect fat droplets

(5) Wright or **methylene blue staining** to detect white blood cells, which are indicative of invasive infectious causes of diarrhea[*]

(6) Testing for the presence of *Clostridium difficile* in stool

b. Proctosigmoidoscopy also is performed, especially to exclude or confirm a diagnosis of inflammatory bowel disease.

3. Other causes of persistent diarrhea

a. Irritable bowel syndrome is an intestinal motor disorder of unknown cause.

(1) Pathophysiology. Studies of colonic myoelectric activity show an increased incidence of 3 cycles per minute of slow-wave activity among patients with irritable bowel syndrome (i.e., 40% as compared with 10% in normal individuals). Intestinal contractions after a meal or a cholecystokinin injection are more likely to be in the 3 cycle per minute range when compared with the intestinal contractions of normal individuals. The colonic spike activity is delayed from 40 minutes to 70–90 minutes postprandially. The abnormal slow-wave activity may indicate an intrinsic myogenic defect, and the prolonged postprandial spike and contractile activity may indicate a neural or hormonal abnormality. Irritable bowel syndrome is six to eight times more common in women than men, which also suggests a hormonal mechanism.

(2) Clinical features include alternating diarrhea and constipation with postprandial pain but usually no weight loss, gastrointestinal bleeding, protracted nausea, vomiting, or fever. Diarrhea, if present, generally is characterized by a 24-hour output of less than 500 ml. Neither pain nor diarrhea awakens the patient from sleep.

(3) Diagnosis is made based on the exclusion of other gastrointestinal conditions with appropriate tests, including stool culture, guaiac testing, and radiographs. The value of colonic myoelectric testing to establish a diagnosis of irritable bowel syndrome is controversial.

(4) Therapy includes stool bulking agents, antispasmodics, and patient reassurance.

b. Disaccharidase deficiency (i.e., deficiency of the enzymes required to split nonabsorbable disaccharides into absorbable monosaccharides) is a cause of osmotic diarrhea.

(1) Sucrase and **isomaltase deficiencies** are rare, occurring in 0.2% of the population. These deficiencies usually present as watery diarrhea in infancy.

(2) Lactase deficiency usually is not complete (i.e., patients have some enzyme activity) and presents after puberty. It affects 60%–80% of blacks

---

[*]Toxigenic *E. coli,* viruses, Norwalk agent, and *Giardia lamblia* are not invasive. Irritable bowel syndrome, malabsorption syndrome, and laxative abuse do not cause pus in the stool. *Staphylococcus aureus, C. perfringens,* and *Entamoeba histolytica* also may be present with fecal leukocytes.

and occurs to a lesser extent in Asian and Mediterranean populations. Symptoms of lactase deficiency include abdominal bloating, cramping, and watery diarrhea after milk ingestion. Diagnosis can be made by measuring the increase in serum glucose in response to orally administered lactose, with an increase of 20 mg/dl expected after an oral lactose intake of 50–100 mg. Lactose breath tests measure increased H^+ excretion from colonic bacterial digestion of lactose. A relative lactase deficiency may occur after an acute episode of viral enteritis or in association with celiac disease, Whipple's disease, or cystic fibrosis.

c. Incontinence is a disturbing symptom that patients may find difficult to discuss with a physician. It is often not true diarrhea but is associated with inflammatory diseases of the anal canal (e.g., acute gonococcal proctitis, Crohn's disease, and ulcerative colitis) or with systemic neuromuscular diseases (e.g., diabetes mellitus and scleroderma). Incontinence also may be a complication of anal surgery (e.g., fistulectomy and hemorrhoidectomy).

d. Laxative abuse is an increasing cause of diarrhea, which may be associated with psychiatric problems and a desire to lose weight. The type of laxative ingested determines the clinical features. Osmotic diarrhea is caused by magnesium sulfate, nonabsorbable sugars (e.g., lactulose), and sodium phosphate. Dihydroxy bile salts, castor oil, and dioctyl sodium sulfosuccinate (docusate sodium) cause secretory diarrhea. (These secretory agents as well as bisacodyl and phenolphthalein may increase PGE synthesis, thereby reducing or reversing water flux from the intestinal lumen into the blood.) Surreptitious laxative use is difficult to document except in cases of phenolphthalein use, in which alkalinization of a stool or urine sample by the addition of sodium hydroxide causes the color of the sample to change to pink.

e. Systemic mastocytosis is characterized by mast cell proliferation in the skin, bones, lymph nodes, and parenchymal organs. Eighty percent of the patients have gastrointestinal symptoms that include nausea, vomiting, and recurrent episodes of diarrhea and abdominal pain. Pruritus, flushing, tachycardia, hypotensive episodes, and headaches may also be seen on an episodic basis. Heparin, also liberated from mast cells, can contribute to gastrointestinal hemorrhage from peptic ulcer disease, which is related to histamine-induced hyperchlorhydria.

    (1) Diagnosis is suggested when jejunal biopsies show large numbers of mast cells in the lamina propria, muscularis mucosa, and submucosa with normal or mild villous atrophy. The classic dermatologic finding is that of urticaria pigmentosa associated with systemic mastocytosis.

    (2) Treatment has been with agents to block both H_1 and H_2 receptors, anticholinergics, and, occasionally, steroids.

4. Infectious causes of diarrhea include the bacteria listed in Table 5-1, which cause food poisoning. Some organisms, such as *C. difficile* and *Entamoeba histolytica*, primarily attach to the colon and rectum, respectively.

a. *E. coli* is the most common cause of **traveler's diarrhea,** which is the often severe diarrhea that occurs within 2 weeks of a visit to a tropical area. Traveler's diarrhea usually is self-limited.

    (1) A toxigenic, heat-labile *E. coli* can activate cAMP or cyclic guanosine 3′, 5′-monophosphate (cGMP) to cause a secretory diarrhea that may be bloody. Species of *Shigella, Salmonella,* and *Campylobacter* as well as *E. histolytica* and *Giardia lamblia* are other known causes of traveler's diarrhea.

    (2) Trimethoprim–sulfamethoxazole combinations, bismuth subsalicylate, quinolone antibiotics, and oxytetracycline preparations have been shown to be effective in prevention and treatment.

b. *G. lamblia,* a flagellate protozoan, is the most common cause of **water-borne infectious diarrhea** in the United States. It also is common in developing nations because of sewage contamination of drinking water. Infected patients may be asymptomatic, have mild diarrhea, or have a prolonged illness characterized

TABLE 5-1. Bacterial Food Poisoning Syndromes

Organism	Incubation Period	Symptoms	Sources of Contamination	Pathogenic Mechanisms	Comments
Staphylococcus aureus	2–8 hours	SP, SV, D	Meat and dairy food	Toxin	Sudden onset; intense vomiting; no therapy needed in most cases
Bacillus cereus	2–8 hours	SP, SV, SD	Reheated fried rice	Tissue invasion	Early vomiting, later diarrhea; recovery within 24 hours
Clostridium perfringens	8–14 hours	V, SD	Reheated meat	Toxin	Profuse diarrhea
Vibrio parahaemolyticus	6 hours–4 days	V, SD, F	Saltwater seafood	Toxin; tissue invasion	Outbreaks usually associated with ingestion of oysters, clams, and crabs
Salmonella species	8–48 hours	V, SD, F, H, systemic disease	Food	Mild tissue invasion; possible toxin	Diarrhea with low-grade fever; carrier state possible; should not be treated
Pathogenic *Escherichia coli*	1–3 days	SD	Food and water	Toxin; tissue invasion	Traveler's diarrhea; prophylaxis or therapy with trimethoprim–sulfa combinations, bismuth subsalicylate, or doxycycline
Hemorrhagic *E. coli*, serotype 0157:H7	1–7 days	SP, SD, B	Raw beef; unprocessed milk; water	Toxin; tissue invasion	Severe pain and bloody diarrhea; may be associated with hemolytic–uremic syndrome, or TTP; high mortality rate; therapy with amoxicillin or quinolones
Vibrio cholerae	1–3 days	V, SD	Poor hygiene	Toxin	Life-threatening diarrhea; therapy is intravenous replacement of fluid and electrolytes; epidemic occurrence
Shigella species (mild cases)	1–3 days	SD, F, B	Fecal–oral spread; flies	Toxin; tissue invasion	Therapy with ampicillin, trimethoprim–sulfamethoxazole, or chloramphenicol
Clostridium botulinum	1–4 days	V, H, RE	Canned foods	Toxin	Severe CNS symptoms; ventilatory support needed; high mortality rate
Campylobacter fetus	2–10 days	SD, B	Fecal–oral spread; pets	Tissue invasion	Bloody diarrhea, especially in children; therapy with erythromycin
Clostridium difficile	?	SD, F, B	Fecal–oral spread	Toxin	Postantibiotic diarrhea; therapy with vancomycin or metronidazole
Yersinia enterocolitica	?	SP, SD, B	Fecal–oral spread; pets	Tissue invasion; possible toxin	May be seen with polyarthritis in children; therapy with tetracycline

S = severe; P = abdominal pain; V = vomiting; D = diarrhea; F = fever; B = blood in stool; H = headache; RE = respiratory embarrassment; CNS = central nervous system; TTP = thrombotic thrombocytopenic purpura.

by malabsorption, diarrhea, bloating, and crampy abdominal pain. Because the organism preferentially resides in the upper small intestine, the diagnosis can be made by demonstration of trophozoites in duodenal aspirates, although examination of stools for cysts and trophozoites is a good screening test. Treatment with metronidazole or quinacrine usually is successful.

c. **Viruses** commonly cause **acute self-limited diarrhea.** Although many different viruses may cause gastroenteritis, causes of viral gastroenteritis that can be identified with certainty are the **Norwalk agent** (probably a parvovirus) and the **rotavirus.**

d. *Salmonella.* Salmonellosis can be highly variable in its presentation. Gastroenteritis, the most common form of salmonellosis, is an acute self-limited diarrheal syndrome with crampy abdominal pain and fever. Enteric fever is a severe illness primarily caused by *Salmonella typhi* or *Salmonella paratyphi* but is also seen with infection by other types of salmonella. Clinical manifestations include prolonged fever, abdominal pain, rash, and diarrhea. Salmonellal septicemia may be seen in patients with osteomyelitis, mycotic aneurysms, or abscesses with no evidence or history of gastrointestinal disease. Salmonellosis is diagnosed using stool and blood culturing techniques. Because a prolonged carrier state may be induced, patients with gastroenteritis are not given antibiotics. In severe infection, ampicillin, trimethoprim–sulfamethoxazole, or chloramphenicol is used.

e. *Shigella.* Shigellosis is characterized by acute diarrhea with fever and crampy abdominal pain. If left untreated, the disease progresses to a chronic bloody diarrhea without fever but with weight loss and debilitation, which may last for weeks. Diagnosis is made by positive stool culture. In contrast to that for salmonellosis, antibiotic therapy for shigellosis offers symptomatic improvement, with decreased duration of excretion of the organism.

f. *Campylobacter* infection is the most common cause of bacterial diarrhea in the United States. Symptoms include diarrhea, which may be bloody, and fever. Diagnosis is made by positive stool culture but requires special media and handling. Treatment is with erythromycin because the organism is resistant to most other commonly used antibiotics.

g. *Cryptosporidium.* Cryptosporidiosis is a protozoal infection seen commonly in immunocompromised patients such as those with AIDS. This diarrheal syndrome rarely occurs in normal individuals, except in a self-limited fashion, particularly in animal (calf) handlers. The diarrhea is watery, profuse, and debilitating. Diagnosis is made by a modified acid-fast stain of stool. No effective therapy is available, although spiramycin may provide temporary relief.

h. *Isospora belli* infection occurs similarly to cryptosporidiosis. Treatment is with trimethoprim–sulfamethoxazole.

i. *E. histolytica* causes bloody dysentery with fever. Diagnosis is by serologic and stool analysis. Treatment is with metronidazole or iodoquinol.

j. **Hemorrhagic *E. coli* serotype 0157:H7** produces Shiga toxin and causes bloody diarrhea. Hemorrhagic *E. coli* serotype 0157:H7 infection may be associated with hemolytic–uremic syndrome or thrombotic thrombocytopenic purpura. Transmission may occur through ingestion of poorly cooked beef, unprocessed milk, or apple cider made in mills where poorly washed fruit is contaminated with infected animal feces.

5. **Nonbacterial food poisoning**
   a. **Fish poisoning** is caused by ichthyosarcotoxins (toxins found in the flesh of poisonous fish).
      (1) **Ciguatera poisoning** is acquired from certain bottom-dwelling fish found in temperate and tropical coastal zones. Ingestion of such fish is followed in 30 minutes to 30 hours by nausea, vomiting, diarrhea, and paresthesia or numbness of the lips, tongue, and limbs. Treatment is supportive.
      (2) **Scombroid poisoning** is acquired from certain fish species (usually tuna, mackerel, bluefish, herring, and bonito) that are susceptible to the production of a heat-stable toxin by the action of *Proteus morganii.* Symptoms re-

semble those of a histamine reaction and include flushing, headache, dizziness, abdominal cramping, vomiting, and diarrhea. The symptoms appear soon after ingestion and last 4–6 hours. Cooking does not inactivate the toxin once it is formed. Antihistamines may be used for symptomatic relief.

    (3) Tetraodon poisoning. Puffer fish produce a neurotoxin termed tetrodotoxin, which may cause paresthesia of the face and extremities with nausea, vomiting, and diarrhea. Ventilator support may be necessary.

  b. Mushroom poisoning occurs after ingestion of any of the 50 species of mushrooms known to be toxic to humans. *Amanita verna, Amanita virosa,* and *Amanita phalloides* account for most cases of mushroom poisoning. Nausea, vomiting, fever, diarrhea, and abdominal pain develop 6–24 hours after ingestion; 1–4 days later, hepatic and renal insufficiency may develop with subsequent coagulopathy, heart failure, convulsions, and coma. Mushroom poisoning has a mortality rate of 40%–90%.

    (1) Diagnosis is made by history of ingestion or by detection of mushroom toxins in the gastric aspirate.

    (2) Treatment is supportive. Thioctic acid may be curative and should be administered promptly.

E. **Malabsorption** of food or nutrients results from a defect at any step of the digestive process or in any of the organs that participate in normal digestion. The clinical features vary widely because malabsorption may involve a single nutrient or multiple nutrients.

  1. Etiology

    a. Maldigestion refers to a defect either in intraluminal hydrolysis of triglycerides or in micelle formation, which results from the following conditions:

      (1) Pancreatic insufficiency due to chronic pancreatitis, pancreatic carcinoma, or cystic fibrosis

      (2) Deficiency of conjugated bile salts due to cholestatic or obstructive liver disease (e.g., cholangiocarcinoma)

      (3) Bile salt deconjugation due to bacterial overgrowth in blind loops (after Billroth II gastrectomy) or in jejunal diverticula or in association with enterocolonic fistulae or motility disorders (e.g., scleroderma and pseudo-obstruction)

      (4) Inadequate mixing of gastric contents with bile salts and pancreatic enzymes as a result of previous gastric surgery, especially Billroth II gastrectomy

    b. Intrinsic small bowel disease

      (1) Celiac disease causes flattening of the villi and inflammatory cell infiltration in the lamina propria (see IV E 4 c).

      (2) Whipple's disease, a systemic disease that may be infectious in origin, causes mucosal damage and lymphatic obstruction (see IV E 4 d).

      (3) Collagenous sprue refers to the deposition of a collagenous substance in the lamina propria in a patient who otherwise has the clinical and histologic features of celiac disease. Fifty percent of patients with collagenous sprue are responsive to steroids.

      (4) Nongranulomatous ulcerative ileojejunitis is a rare condition of unknown etiology characterized by fever, weight loss, crampy abdominal pain, bloating, and diarrhea. Intestinal ulcerations may occur, and splenomegaly is noted in 20% of cases. Despite therapeutic attempts with steroids and immunosuppressive drugs or surgery, the clinical course often is relentless and the prognosis poor.

      (5) Eosinophilic gastroenteritis is characterized by peripheral eosinophilia and infiltration of the wall of the stomach, small intestine, or colon by mature eosinophils. Many patients present with a specific food allergy and other allergic disorders such as asthma, eczema, and allergic rhinitis, and some patients show symptoms of gastritis. Diagnosis is made by biopsy of the gastric antrum or small bowel, which reveals the eosinophilic infiltration. Steroid therapy may induce a prolonged remission. Elimination diets to remove possible allergens have been successful in some patients.

(6) **Amyloidosis** (either primary or secondary) may affect the small intestine in 70% of cases by amyloid infiltration of the submucosa. Altered motility that allows bacterial overgrowth also may contribute to malabsorption. Gastrointestinal bleeding (occult) may be observed in approximately 25% of cases. Diagnosis is made by biopsy (usually of a rectal valve or stomach) with special stains (e.g., Congo red). Treatment primarily is supportive. A trial of antibiotics for bacterial overgrowth may be given.

(7) **Crohn's disease** may cause malabsorption by mucosal damage, by multiple strictures with bacterial overgrowth, or as a result of the need for multiple bowel resections (see IV G).

c. **Inadequate absorptive surface** results from extensive small bowel resection, usually for Crohn's disease or vascular compromise of the small intestine. Resection of up to 50% of the small intestine is well tolerated if the remaining bowel is normal, and survival is possible following more extensive resection but requires careful management. If the proximal small bowel is resected, calcium, folic acid, and iron may not be absorbed; tetany may result. If the ileum is removed, bile acid and vitamin B_{12} absorption is impaired greatly. Hepatic dysfunction, oxalate kidney stones, and increased gastric acid secretion are common complications of extensive bowel resection. D-Lactic acidosis is a rare but life-threatening complication. Initial therapy includes intravenous fluid and electrolyte administration or parenteral hyperalimentation. Oral feedings should include medium-chain triglycerides (MCT oil), fat-soluble vitamins, and iron. Intramuscular vitamin B_{12} injections and antidiarrheal agents (to slow the transit time) may be needed. Cholestyramine resin may bind nonabsorbed bile salts and lessen the diarrhea; however, this drug also depletes the total body bile salt pool and usually is not used if more than 100 cm of distal ileum has been resected.

d. **Lymphatic obstruction**

(1) **Intestinal lymphangiectasia** may be primary (congenital) or secondary to intestinal tuberculosis, Whipple's disease, trauma, neoplasia, or retroperitoneal fibrosis. In advanced disease, dilated lymphatic channels rupture and leak into the intestinal lumen causing lymphopenia, low serum protein levels, and massive peripheral edema. Small bowel biopsy reveals the characteristic dilated lymphatics. Treatment is with low-fat diet and medium-chain triglyceride supplementation.

(2) **Intestinal lymphoma** may mimic Crohn's disease or adult celiac disease both clinically and radiographically. Clues to the differential diagnosis include persistent fevers and a short duration of symptoms. Enlarged lymph nodes or hepatosplenomegaly may be found on physical examination, and CT may reveal enlarged retroperitoneal nodes. Diagnosis often is made only after surgical biopsy. Therapy includes local resection and radiotherapy. Chemotherapy is used for disseminated disease.

e. **Multiple defects** contribute to malabsorption in the following settings.

(1) **After gastrectomy.** Malabsorption can result following Billroth II gastrectomy, when poor mixing of gastric contents with pancreatic enzymes and stasis in the afferent loop with bacterial overgrowth are present. Therapy includes surgical correction of the afferent loop and broad-spectrum antibiotics.

(2) **Radiation enteritis** interferes with the blood supply to the intestine. Bacterial overgrowth also may occur secondary to the radiation-induced intestinal stricture. Lymphatic obstruction due to edema or fibrosis also may be a part of the syndrome.

(3) **Diabetes mellitus.** Altered gut motility from diabetic neuropathy, bacterial overgrowth, and exocrine pancreatic insufficiency all have been implicated as mechanisms of diabetes mellitus–induced malabsorption.

f. Other causes of malabsorption

(1) Abetalipoproteinemia is a rare disease with neurologic manifestations (e.g., ataxia, nystagmus, incoordination, and retinitis pigmentosa), morphologically abnormal "spiny" red blood cells, low serum cholesterol and triglyceride levels, and low serum betalipoprotein levels. Steatorrhea occurs because apoprotein B, which is necessary for normal chylomicron formation, is lacking in intestinal cells. Fat is found in the epithelial cells on small bowel biopsy. Treatment with MCT oil bypasses the absorption defect. Fat-soluble vitamin supplementation also may be required.

(2) Infections can cause malabsorption and may be viral, bacterial, or parasitic.

(a) Viral and **bacterial enteritis** may cause temporary malabsorption secondary to disaccharidase deficiency, mucosal damage, or both.

(b) Tropical sprue is an endemic malabsorption disorder occurring in the tropics. It is thought to have an infectious etiology because travelers are susceptible to the disease, and treatment with tetracycline usually is effective.

(c) Other infectious causes of malabsorption include hookworm, tapeworm, strongyloidiasis, and *Capillaria philippinensis* (roundworm) infection, which are common outside the United States, and giardiasis, which is relatively common in the United States.

(3) Chronic intestinal ischemia may cause malabsorption when two of the three major intestinal vessels—the celiac artery, superior mesenteric artery, and the inferior mesenteric artery—are occluded (as can be shown angiographically). Symptoms usually are weight loss and crampy postprandial pain, with bloody diarrhea occasionally being present. Vascular surgery has resulted in improvement in several series.

(4) Hypogammaglobulinemia may cause malabsorption, especially if it is associated with serum IgA, serum IgG, or intestinal IgA deficiency. Intestinal and serum IgM also may be increased. Small bowel biopsy shows absence of plasma cells. Nodular lymphoid hyperplasia may be seen in the distal small bowel on radiograph, and *G. lamblia* may be detected in stool or duodenal aspirate. There is an increased risk of intestinal lymphomas and gastric cancer in these patients. Treatment of the giardiasis with metronidazole or quinacrine may improve absorption. Common variable immunodeficiency is treated with intravenous gammaglobulin. A decrease in intestinal infections has been described after intravenous gammaglobulin treatment.

(5) Metastatic carcinoid syndrome is associated with an increased production of 5-hydroxytryptamine (serotonin), which causes increased gastrointestinal motility. Methysergide, cyproheptadine, or somatostatin may be used for therapy if surgical resection is not possible.

(6) Hypoparathyroidism may present as steatorrhea. The mechanism by which parathormone affects fat absorption is unknown, but vitamin D–dependent calcium absorption may play a role.

(7) Drugs that may cause malabsorption include neomycin, kanamycin, bacitracin, and polymyxin. Phenytoin causes a selective folic acid malabsorption.

2. Clinical features are variable. Patients may present with some or all of the following clinical manifestations:

a. Passage of abnormal stools, which are greasy, soft, bulky, and foul smelling and may float in the toilet because of their increased gas content; a film of grease or oil droplets may be seen on the surface of the water

b. Weight loss, which may be severe and involve marked muscle wasting

c. Edema and ascites secondary to hypoalbuminemia

d. Anemia secondary to altered absorption of iron, vitamin B_{12}, folate, or a combination of these

    e. Bone pain or fractures from vitamin D deficiency

    f. Paresthesias or tetany from calcium deficiency

    g. Bleeding from vitamin K deficiency

3. Diagnosis is based on clinical evidence, with confirmation by laboratory tests.

    a. Stool fat analysis may be qualitative or quantitative. A positive Sudan stain indicates excretion of greater than 15 g of fat per day in the stool. A 72-hour fecal fat collection can be used to quantify the amount of fat absorption. Normally, an individual absorbs 93%–95% of all dietary fat ingested. Pancreatic disease often is associated with fecal fat excretion in excess of 20–30 g/day on a 100 g/day fat diet.

    b. D-Xylose absorption testing. Because D-xylose, a five-carbon sugar, does not require enzymatic degradation or micelle formation for absorption, it can be used to measure intestinal mucosal integrity. After a 25-g oral dose, a 5-hour urine collection should contain at least 4–5 g of D-xylose. Alternatively, a 2-hour serum sample may be used.

    c. Testing for unabsorbed carbohydrate. Lowered stool pH occurs when unabsorbed carbohydrates reach the colon and bacterial fermentation occurs. This is particularly common in lactase deficiency but also may be seen in celiac disease and short bowel syndrome.

    d. Pancreatic function testing involves measuring the bicarbonate and total fluid output from the duodenum after secretin stimulation or using pancreatic chymotrypsin (the bentiromide test) to release para-aminobenzoic acid (PABA), which is excreted in the urine. Less than 60% urinary excretion of PABA suggests pancreatic insufficiency.

    e. Measurement of serum carotene levels. Because vitamin A is fat soluble and the serum carotene level is a reflection of vitamin A metabolism, a low serum carotene level with normal vitamin A intake may be a useful screening test for fat malabsorption.

    f. Bacterial overgrowth testing

        (1) Direct culture of jejunal aspirates yielding greater than 10^5 organisms/ml of aspirate is considered abnormal. The diagnosis is strongly suggested by the presence of fastidious anaerobes (clostridia and bacteroides), facultative anaerobes (lactobacilli and enterococci), or coliforms.

        (2) Bile acid breath tests are becoming more popular. The tests are based on the fact that bacteria deconjugate ^{14}C-labeled glycine-cholate before it can be absorbed. ^{14}C-glycine then is metabolized to $^{14}CO_2$, which is exhaled and measured in the breath of patients with bacterial overgrowth.

        (3) Measurement of tryptophan metabolites. Elevated urinary levels of indican and 5-hydroxyindoleacetic acid are due to increased metabolism of tryptophan. This test is not specific, however, because abnormal levels of tryptophan metabolites also are obtained in carcinoid syndrome and Whipple's disease.

    g. Small bowel x-ray, especially by the intubated air contrast technique, may be useful. Pooling or flocculation of barium does not occur as frequently as with previous barium techniques but, if noted, suggests celiac disease. Thick folds may be seen in Whipple's disease, lymphoma, amyloidosis, radiation enteritis, Zollinger-Ellison syndrome, and eosinophilic enteritis, and a pseudo-Whipple's appearance is observed in patients with AIDS enteropathy.

    h. The **Schilling test** is used to diagnose vitamin B_{12} malabsorption.

        (1) An abnormal first-stage Schilling test (administration of radiolabeled vitamin B_{12} only) with a normal second-stage Schilling test (administration of a complex of vitamin B_{12} and intrinsic factor) indicates gastric defects such as pernicious anemia and lack of intrinsic factor due to gastric resection. The second-stage test may be abnormal due to bacterial overgrowth or to resection or inflammation of the terminal ileum, which is the site of absorption. Severe celiac disease also may cause an abnormal second-stage test.

        (2) In severe pancreatic insufficiency, pancreatic proteases are not present in sufficient quantity to cleave B_{12} from gastrin R proteins. In the third stage of the test, labeled B_{12} absorption is improved after pancreatic enzymes are given orally to the patient at the time of the testing procedure.

    i. Small bowel biopsy is essential for the diagnosis of many cases of malabsorption. In properly prepared specimens, normal villous crypt ratios are 3:1 or 4:1. Flattening of the villi with inflammatory cell infiltration is characteristic of celiac disease, but flattened villi alone may be seen in infectious enteritis, giardiasis, lymphoma, and bacterial overgrowth.

  4. Characteristics and management of specific causes of malabsorption

    a. Pancreatic insufficiency may be due to chronic pancreatitis, pancreatic carcinoma, or cystic fibrosis. Bentiromide test or pancreatic secretin test results may be abnormal. Treatment is pancreatic enzyme replacement. H_2-receptor antagonists may increase the potency of enzymes when given 1 hour before meals because acid may inactivate the exogenous enzymes.

    b. Bacterial overgrowth may be due to altered motility (e.g., in diabetes, amyloidosis, intestinal pseudo-obstruction), small bowel diverticula, strictures (e.g., in lymphoma and Crohn's disease), or blind loops after Billroth II gastrectomy. Surgical correction of the anatomic problems may be considered, but treatment with antibiotics frequently is successful. Ampicillin, amoxicillin and clavulanate potassium, tetracycline, or chloramphenicol may be used. Some patients require continuous therapy, and, in these cases, antibiotics should be rotated.

    c. Celiac disease (nontropical sprue)

      (1) Although the **etiology** and **pathogenesis** are not fully understood, it is clear that an abnormal sensitivity to gluten, a protein component of wheat, causes damage to the intestinal mucosa of these patients. The importance of genetic factors is demonstrated by abnormal small bowel biopsies in 10%–15% of first-degree relatives of patients. In addition, 60%–90% of celiac patients have human leukocyte antigen B8 (HLA-B8) and HLA-DW3 compared with 20%–30% of the general population. An additional B lymphocyte antigen is present in 70%–80% of celiac patients as compared with 15% of the general population. Together, these factors may contribute to a binding of gliadin—the offensive protein component in gluten—to intestinal epithelial cells and, hence, to the immunogenicity of the bound product. Celiac patients have proximal intestinal involvement with a relative sparing of the distal ileum.

      (2) Clinical features include diarrhea, steatorrhea, weight loss, and abdominal bloating. Symptoms may begin in childhood and then lessen, only to reappear in the third to sixth decade of life. Iron deficiency anemia unassociated with gastrointestinal blood loss may be seen because iron is preferentially absorbed in the more severely involved proximal small intestine.

      (3) Diagnosis requires small bowel biopsy, which shows villous atrophy, crypt hypertrophy, and cuboidal change in the epithelial cells. Inflammatory cell infiltration in the lamina propria at endoscopy may reveal "scalloped folds" in the proximal duodenum. Antigliadin antibodies (IgG, IgA) are elevated in 90% of patients, especially in those who have not received treatment. Antireticulum and antiendomysial antibodies, which may decrease or disappear with treatment, are thought by many to be more specific, although less sensitive, for celiac disease.

      (4) Therapy is based on withdrawal of gluten from the diet by eliminating wheat, rye, barley, and oats. Only corn and rice flour are permitted. Although clinical response to gluten withdrawal often is dramatic and may be seen in a few days, histologic recovery demonstrated on repeat small bowel biopsy may be delayed for months and, in up to 50% of patients, may never be demonstrated. In severely ill patients, steroids may be of short-term benefit.

      (5) Complications

        (a) Lymphoma or **carcinoma** (especially esophageal) occurs in approximately 10%–15% of cases, and lymphoma is twice as common as carcinoma.

(b) **Intestinal ulcers** or **strictures** may be late complications in some patients with celiac disease.

(c) **Dermatitis herpetiformis** is a skin lesion characterized by papular vesicular eruptions and pruritus. Most patients have an abnormal intestinal biopsy showing villous atrophy, and the skin lesions may respond to gluten withdrawal.

(d) **Collagenous sprue** may develop with a thick band of collagen (< 10–15 microns in diameter) in the lamina propria and is extremely resistant to medical therapy.

d. Whipple's disease is a systemic disorder most commonly occurring in middle-aged men.

(1) The **etiology** and **pathogenesis** of Whipple's disease are not completely understood. Numerous small gram-positive cocci are seen in macrophages in individual organs. Recently, a gram-positive actinomycete called *Tropheryma whippelli* was identified as the infectious agent.

(2) **Clinical features** depend on organ involvement. In the intestine, periodic acid–Schiff (PAS)-positive macrophages (i.e., macrophages that contain bacilli) are found in the lamina propria. The mesenteric lymph nodes, heart, spleen, lungs, and CNS also may be involved. Malabsorption is caused by mucosal damage and lymphatic obstruction. Fever occurs in one third to one half of patients. Arthralgia and arthritis are present in 60% of patients and may precede the gastrointestinal symptoms.

(3) **Diagnosis** is made by intestinal biopsy with a PAS stain. A small bowel radiograph may reveal thickened folds. In rare cases, the disease is focal and the biopsy is normal.

(4) **Therapy** with penicillin, ampicillin, or tetracycline is required for at least 4–6 months and may be continued intermittently (i.e., every other day) thereafter. The relapse rate is approximately 10%.

F. **Protein-losing enteropathy (PLE)** refers to the excessive loss of serum proteins into the gastrointestinal tract. Three types of disorders may cause PLE.

1. Mucosal ulceration causes leakage of protein at the ulcer site and results from the following conditions:
   a. Malignant disease involving the gastrointestinal tract
   b. Multiple peptic ulcers
   c. Nongranulomatous ileojejunitis

2. Mucosal disease without ulceration but with altered metabolism or cell turnover leads to increased permeability to protein. Such diseases include:
   a. Ménétrier's disease
   b. Celiac disease
   c. Whipple's disease
   d. Infectious enteritis

3. Lymph flow obstruction causes increased lymphatic pressure and protein leakage. Lymphatic obstruction results from the following conditions:
   a. Lymphoma
   b. Intestinal lymphangiectasia
   c. Cardiac disease, such as constrictive pericarditis and tricuspid valve disease
   d. *C. philippinensis* infection

G. **Crohn's disease (regional enteritis)** is a chronic granulomatous disease that may occur anywhere in the gastrointestinal tract from the mouth to the anus. The ileum most often is involved, with more than 50% of Crohn's disease patients having ileocolitis. The first peak of incidence occurs between the ages of 12 and 30 years; a secondary peak occurs at age 50 years.

1. Etiology
   a. Genetic factors appear to play a role, with an increased incidence of disease noted in monozygotic twins and siblings. Approximately 17% of patients with Crohn's disease have first-degree relatives with the disease. Men are affected

more often than women, and the disease is more common among Jews. Compared with the general population, Jewish men have six times the risk for development of Crohn's disease.

   b. Infectious agents have been postulated but never identified as a cause of Crohn's disease. An inflammatory response can be induced in the footpads and intestinal walls of mice by injecting an extract of Crohn's disease tissue, and this may reflect a small transmissible agent, such as an RNA virus or a cell wall–defective bacteria. A mycobacterium has been proposed as an etiologic agent.

   c. An **immunologic mechanism** is the most prominent theory. Abnormal numbers, subsets, and functions of T cells have been identified in cases of Crohn's disease. Hyperresponsive immune function, rather than abnormal function, is characteristic of an unrestricted response to inflammation. Recently, a defect in the ability of intestinal epithelial cells to produce normal amounts of suppressor T (Ts) cells (CD8 cells) has been noted.

2. Pathologic features include:

   a. Marked thickening of the involved intestinal wall with transmural inflammation

   b. Enlarged and matted mesenteric lymph nodes

   c. Focal granulomas in 50% of specimens

   d. Deep serpiginous or linear ulcerations leading to cobblestoning and fistula formation

   e. Stricture formation secondary to scarring

   f. Alternating areas of normal and involved mucosa

3. Clinical features are characterized by periodic exacerbations and remissions.

   a. Pain often is colicky, especially in the lower abdomen, and may be increased after meals due to the obstructive nature of the pathologic process.

   b. Systemic symptoms are common and include fever, weight loss, malaise, and anorexia.

   c. Diarrhea is the usual presenting symptom.

   d. Intestinal obstruction is the presenting symptom in approximately 25% of cases. Massive gastrointestinal bleeding may be a presenting symptom in 2%–3% of cases.

   e. Extraintestinal manifestations are numerous.

   (1) Anemia as well as growth or sexual retardation probably are due to inadequate caloric intake.

   (2) Hepatobiliary disorders include fatty liver, pericholangitis, nonspecific hepatitis, cirrhosis, and sclerosing cholangitis. There is an increased risk of gallstones. Liver enzyme or liver biopsy abnormalities occur in 50%–70% of Crohn's disease patients.

   (3) Renal disorders include right ureteral obstruction secondary to contiguous bowel involvement and nephrolithiasis. An increase in calcium oxalate stones is due to increased oxalate absorption, and an increase in uric acid stones is ascribed to increased cell turnover and a concentrated acid urine.

   (4) Peripheral arthritis occurs in 10%–12% of patients and ankylosing spondylitis in 2%–10%.

   (5) Skin problems include erythema nodosum and, rarely, pyoderma gangrenosum.

   (6) Episcleritis or uveitis may occur in 3%–10% of patients.

   f. Fistulas to the skin or other organs occur in approximately 20% of patients. Perianal fistulas or abscesses are especially common in Crohn's colitis.

4. Diagnosis is based on clinical signs and symptoms combined with characteristic radiographic findings, including deep (collar button) ulcerations, long strictured segments (string sign), and skip areas. Colonoscopy may be helpful when there is colonic involvement, and biopsies may show granuloma formation. Laboratory studies are not specific for Crohn's disease but may show multifactorial anemia, leukocytosis, an increased sedimentation rate, and evidence of malabsorption or protein loss. The differential diagnosis includes lymphoma, tuberculosis, radiation enteritis, and *Yersinia* infection (especially in acute enteritis).

5. **Therapy** is symptomatic. No specific therapy or cure exists.
    a. **Supportive measures** include short-term, broad-spectrum antibiotics, antidiarrheal agents, bowel rest with intravenous fluid support, enteral nutrition with tube feedings, total parenteral nutrition, and vitamin supplementation.
    b. **Medical treatment**
        (1) **Sulfasalazine** or 5-aminosalicylic acid preparations in doses of 3–4 g/day may be used alone or in combination with corticosteroids to treat acute disease. This may be more effective in Crohn's colitis. Ethyl cellulose-coated oral 5-aminosalicylic acid preparations may be useful in small bowel disease.
        (2) **Vitamin B_{12} injections** are indicated when ileal disease causes malabsorption of this nutrient.
        (3) **Increased oral calcium, vitamin D,** or **both** may be helpful in patients with calcium oxalate stones by binding oxalate in the bowel and decreasing urinary oxalate.
        (4) **Metronidazole, oral quinolone antibiotics,** or **both** may be effective in treatment of perineal and perianal fistulas.
        (5) **Corticosteroids** have been proven effective by the National Cooperative Crohn's Disease Study, especially in patients with small bowel disease. When remission is obtained, the dosage should be tapered gradually.
        (6) **6-Mercaptopurine, azathioprine,** and **methotrexate** have also been used. **Cyclosporine** may be useful as a down-regulator of the immune system.
    c. **Surgery** may be necessary for recurrent intestinal obstruction, enterocutaneous fistulas, and perforation and for growth retardation that does not respond to increased caloric intake. The recurrence rate after initial resection may be as high as 80% within 15 years, especially with initial small bowel involvement.

H. **Small bowel tumors**

1. **Malignant tumors** of the small intestine are rare and include **adenocarcinomas, carcinoid tumors, lymphomas, and leiomyosarcomas.**
    a. **Etiology and pathogenesis.** Some small bowel malignancies arise de novo, but many are related to underlying conditions such as Crohn's disease and celiac disease. Rarely, these malignancies arise from the polyps of Peutz-Jeghers syndrome, familial polyposis, and Gardner's syndrome. A particular type of lymphoma called Mediterranean lymphoma is endemic to the Middle East. Patients with celiac disease may have a 10%–15% incidence of small bowel malignancy, usually lymphoma.
    b. **Pathology.** Adenocarcinoma is especially common in the proximal small bowel; lymphomas and carcinoid tumors primarily occur in the appendix and ileum. The most common primary small bowel tumor is symptomatic carcinoid, which usually is found in the appendix. Small bowel tumors may be metastatic from the breast, kidney, ovary, and testis as well as from melanoma.
    c. **Clinical features** include bleeding, obstruction, and malabsorption. Carcinoid tumors of the appendix may occur as acute appendicitis but usually are asymptomatic. Rarely, appendiceal carcinoid tumors are metastatic to the liver and, in such cases, may cause carcinoid syndrome, which is characterized by flushing and diarrhea.
    d. **Therapy and prognosis.** Surgery is the treatment of choice, but the prognosis is poor, especially for adenocarcinomas. Lymphomas and leiomyosarcomas have a better prognosis if they are localized to a small segment of the bowel. Radiotherapy and chemotherapy are used postoperatively to treat systemic lymphomas. Carcinoid tumors grow slowly, and patients may survive for many years even if the disease is metastatic. Foregut carcinoids respond to streptozocin in approximately 50% of cases. Somatostatin often decreases the flushing and diarrhea in metastatic carcinoid tumors.

2. **Benign tumors** of the small intestine include **adenomas, lipomas,** and **leiomyomas,** which may be associated with obstruction or bleeding but usually are asymptomatic.

I. **Acute appendicitis** is a common and curable cause of an acute abdomen, which occurs at any age and in both sexes but most often occurs in males between 10 and 30 years of age.

1. **Pathogenesis.** It is believed that the primary event is an obstruction of the appendiceal lumen by a fecalith, inflammation, foreign body, or neoplasm. After obstruction of the lumen, increased intraluminal pressure and infection may cause appendiceal necrosis and perforation.

2. **Clinical features** include pain in the right lower quadrant, which initially is vague but becomes localized to McBurney's point, peritoneal signs, fever, and leukocytosis in the 10,000–20,000 range. Rectal tenderness is common in pelvic appendicitis, and retrocecal appendicitis causes psoas muscle pain on hip extension. Patients at the extremes of age, greatly obese patients, and patients taking corticosteroids may have nonspecific complaints and a relatively benign physical examination. Thus, a high index of clinical suspicion must be maintained in these cases.

3. **Diagnosis**
   a. **Differential diagnoses** includes acute gastroenteritis, mesenteric adenitis, Meckel's diverticulum, and Crohn's disease. In young women, ovarian torsion, ruptured ovarian cyst, and pelvic inflammatory disease (PID) should be considered. In elderly patients, diverticulitis, cholecystitis, incarcerated hernia, cecal carcinoma, and mesenteric thrombosis should be ruled out.
   b. **Diagnostic modalities.** In difficult-to-diagnose cases, a **barium enema** may be used to identify lack of filling of the appendix. A **CT scan** will reveal a masslike effect in the right lower quadrant. On **ultrasound,** a classic "bull's-eye" appearance of the right lower quadrant is felt to be relatively diagnostic of appendicitis.

4. **Therapy** is **surgery,** which should be performed as early as possible to prevent perforation.

V. **DISEASES OF THE COLON**

A. **Constipation**

1. **Simple constipation** is the result of delayed transit of intestinal contents. The highly refined, low-fiber diets of western nations probably contribute to this problem. Although the epidemiologic definition of constipation is less than three stools per week, individual differences exist. Treatment of simple constipation is directed toward increasing intestinal bulk by increasing dietary fiber content with fruits, vegetables, and bulking agents such as psyllium hydrophilic colloids, which trap water and electrolytes within the bowel lumen. Long-term use of potent laxatives should be avoided because they may result in destruction of colonic intramural nerve plexuses and cathartic colon.

2. **Constipation** may occur with a variety of diseases, including ulcerative proctitis, rectal fissures or abscesses, and rectal strictures as well as the varied causes of diffusely decreased intestinal activity discussed in IV A and B. Irritable bowel syndrome, which may present as either constipation or diarrhea, is discussed in IV D 3 a.

B. **Colonic diverticula** are outpouchings of the mucosa only and, therefore, are not true diverticula. In the United States, colonic diverticula occur in approximately 50% of individuals older than 60 years of age.

1. **Pathogenesis.** In western nations, colonic diverticula have been linked to low-fiber diets. Diets low in fiber and bulk are thought to cause an increased intraluminal pressure, particularly in the narrow sigmoid colon. (This belief is based on LaPlace's law, which states that the smaller the radius of a cylinder, the greater the pressure generated at a given tension.) Eventually, the increased intraluminal pres-

sure causes a mucosal herniation at the site of a perforating arteriole carrying blood from the serosal surface to the mucosa.

2. **Clinical features** often are absent in uncomplicated colonic diverticula; however, patients may complain of crampy abdominal pain in the left lower quadrant, with alternating diarrhea and constipation. Often, there is relief of these symptoms after bowel movement.

3. **Therapy** is aimed at increasing stool bulk, thereby decreasing intraluminal pressure with high-fiber foods and hydrophilic colloids. Often this results in symptomatic improvement, probably by regulating bowel frequency. Anticholinergic agents sometimes are used but have not been proven effective.

4. **Complications**
    a. **Diverticulitis** occurs in approximately 25% of patients with diverticulosis. Generally, there is a microperforation (rarely a free perforation) with peridiverticular abscess. Symptoms include left lower abdominal pain, fever, and constipation. Because of the characteristic leukocytosis and left lower abdominal tenderness on physical examination, this condition sometimes is called **left-sided appendicitis.** Treatment with antibiotics, intravenous fluids, and bowel rest (i.e., nothing taken by mouth) is effective in most cases. Metronidazole and ciprofloxacin are used most commonly. Severely ill or toxic patients, however, may require additional antibiotics for adequate coverage of *Pseudomonas* and anaerobes. If an abscess occurs, a fistula to the bladder or vagina may develop.
    b. **Bleeding** occurs in approximately 20%–25% of cases and usually is brisk, painless, and not associated with straining. Blood transfusion may be necessary. In most cases, bleeding stops spontaneously with only supportive therapy. Arteriography or rapid-sequence nuclear scanning using technetium sulfur colloid or technetium-labeled erythrocytes may localize the bleeding portion of the colon and allow segmental surgical resection, if necessary.

C. **Hirschsprung's disease** is a congenital cause of megacolon that occurs in 1 of 5000 live births and is more common in males.

1. **Etiology.** Hirschsprung's disease is caused by incomplete caudad migration of neural crest cells, which renders the internal anal sphincter and a variable segment of the rectum and sigmoid without innervation. The involved segment constitutes a functional obstruction, and the normal proximal colon becomes dilated.

2. **Clinical features.** The disease may occur in infancy as meconium ileus, intestinal obstruction, or severe constipation, or it may occur in later life with milder symptoms.

3. **Diagnosis.** Physical examination reveals the absence of stool in the rectum, and barium enema shows a narrowed (diseased) segment with a dilated proximal colon (normal segment) in approximately 75% of cases. Anal manometry is a good screening test for this disease and reveals a lack of reflex relaxation in the internal anal sphincter upon rectal distention. The absence of ganglion cells on a full-thickness rectal biopsy is diagnostic.

4. **Therapy.** Treatment is surgical.

D. **Ulcerative colitis** is a chronic inflammatory disease of the colonic mucosa and submucosa. Ulcerative colitis and Crohn's disease share some features and, despite their dissimilarities, often are placed together under the generic heading of inflammatory bowel disease. Ulcerative colitis occurs in 2–7 of 100,000 individuals, and females are affected more commonly than males. The major peak of incidence occurs between the ages of 15 and 30 years, with a lesser peak between the ages of 50 and 65 years.

1. **Etiology and pathogenesis** are similar to those of Crohn's disease (see IV G). Family members have an increased risk for the development of inflammatory bowel disease; approximately 15%–17% of patients have a first-degree relative with inflammatory bowel disease. Viral, bacterial, and immunologic theories (similar to those

for Crohn's disease) have been proposed, and Jews have a twofold to fourfold increased incidence. Whereas smoking increases the risk for the development of Crohn's disease, it decreases the risk of the development of ulcerative colitis to approximately half that of the general population. There is an increased risk of the development of ulcerative colitis in patients who have recently discontinued smoking. Ulcerative colitis patients who are HLA-B27 positive have a strong association with arthritis, and especially with ankylosing spondylitis.

2. **Pathology.** The hallmarks of ulcerative colitis are the microabscesses of the crypts of Lieberkühn, which are seen in approximately 70% of cases. The inflammatory response generally is limited to the mucosa. Macroscopic ulcerations are noted with confluence of the inflammatory response. Pseudopolyps occur when normal mucosa is isolated by severe ulcerations, but there are no skip areas. The rectum and distal colon most commonly are involved. Pancolitis is seen in 25% of cases. Ulcerative colitis with rectal sparing is extremely uncommon.

3. **Clinical features** are mild when the disease is limited to the rectum (ulcerative proctitis). Moderate-to-severe symptoms may occur with extensive disease, particularly pancolitis, and include bloody diarrhea, weight loss, fever, left lower abdominal cramping pain, and nocturnal passage of a small volume of blood and mucus. Fulminant disease occurs in 15% of cases.

4. **Diagnosis** is based on clinical presentations along with the exclusion of infectious, parasitic, and neoplastic etiologic factors.
   a. **Stool examination** reveals mucus, blood, and white blood cells without parasites or bacterial pathogens. It is important to rule out the usual causes of dysentery, including *Salmonella, Shigella, Campylobacter,* pathogenic *E. coli* (especially *E. coli* 0157:H7), amebiasis, or *C. difficile* infection.
   b. **Proctosigmoidoscopy** reveals friability, edema, and hyperemia of the mucosa. Ulcerations and a mucopurulent exudate may be present. Islands of normal tissue may have the appearance of pseudopolyps. Numerous biopsy samples should be obtained.
   c. **Barium enema** should not be performed in a severely ill or toxic patient. If the symptoms are subacute, a barium radiograph after minimal preparation may reveal lack of haustral markings, fine serrations (compatible with small ulcerations), large ulcerations, and pseudopolyps.

5. **Therapy** varies with the severity and extent of disease.
   a. In acute flares, **bowel rest with intravenous fluids** may be useful for short periods. Total parenteral nutrition allows prolonged bowel rest with repletion of vitamins, minerals, electrolytes, and calories in the form of carbohydrate, protein, and fat.
   b. **Sulfasalazine** and **5-aminosalicylic acid** have been shown to induce remission and decrease relapse rates in ulcerative colitis patients. The active moiety may be the antiprostaglandin substance 5-aminosalicylic acid which is released in the colon by bacteria. Side effects include headache, nausea, rash, and agranulocytosis. 5-Aminosalicylic acid enemas are effective in left-sided colitis.
   c. **Corticosteroids,** which are administered by enema (especially in distal disease such as ulcerative proctitis) or systemically, may be effective in inducing remission. Prednisone is given in dosages of 20–60 mg/day, and adrenocorticotropic hormone is administered in dosages of 40–80 U/24 hr.
   d. In mild to moderate cases without evidence of toxic megacolon, **antidiarrheal agents, anticholinergic agents,** and **sedation** may be used cautiously.
   e. **Immunosuppressive agents** such as 6-mercaptopurine, azathioprine, cyclosporine, methotrexate, and hydroxychloroquine have been tried in the hopes of avoiding or delaying emergent surgery.
   f. **Surgery (total colectomy)** is reserved for:
      (1) Toxic megacolon that is unresponsive to 24–72 hours of intensive conservative medical measures
      (2) Perforation
      (3) Massive hemorrhage that is unresponsive to conservative treatment (rare)

(4) Carcinoma

(5) Suspected carcinoma in colonic strictures

(6) Growth failure in adolescents, which is unresponsive to conservative treatment

(7) Dysplasia noted on biopsy at the time of sigmoidoscopy or colonoscopy, which should be done routinely for screening in long-standing diseases

(8) Cure, especially after 10 years of disease because of the increased risk of cancer. The ileoanal anastomotic procedure that strips the colonic mucosa and avoids the need for a permanent colostomy has become widespread.

6. **Complications.** The systemic complications noted for Crohn's disease (see IV G 3 e) often occur in ulcerative colitis. There are additional complications of ulcerative colitis, which usually are not seen in Crohn's disease.

   a. **Toxic megacolon** refers to an acute dilatation of the colon (usually the transverse portion) to a diameter in excess of 6 cm. This complication of ulcerative colitis probably is due to severe inflammation, which affects large segments of the colonic musculature as well as neural control of the colon. Anticholinergic and antidiarrheal medications also may contribute. Patients usually are severely ill, with high fever, abdominal pain, and a marked leukocytosis. Treatment is intensive medical therapy for 48–72 hours. Patients who do not respond should undergo an emergency total colectomy.

   b. **Carcinoma** of the colon is associated with long-standing disease of great extent (usually pancolitis). At 10 years, the risk of carcinoma is 10% and may increase to 20% at 20 years and 40% at 25–30 years. The malignancies often are multicentric and aggressive. Strictured areas of the colon present a particularly difficult problem because of the difficulty in differentiating intensive inflammatory disease from ischemic narrowing or carcinoma. Yearly colonoscopic examinations with biopsy samples obtained every 10–20 cm should be performed in patients who have had ulcerative colitis for longer than 8–10 years. If high-grade dysplasia is noted, a prophylactic total colectomy should be considered.

7. **Prognosis.** Mortality rates are approximately 20% in toxic megacolon, with higher rates noted in patients older than 60 years. Approximately 10% of patients do not experience a recurrent attack after the initial onset of disease. Continuous symptoms occur in 10% of patients. Approximately 70%–80% of patients have recurrent remissions and relapses, and approximately 20% of patients eventually require total colectomy.

E. **Angiodysplasia** refers to small vascular abnormalities, which usually are seen in the ascending colon or cecum in patients older than 60 years of age. Involvement of the small bowel or stomach also has been reported but is less common. Associations with aortic stenosis and chronic renal insufficiency have been reported.

1. **Pathogenesis.** Angiodysplasia is believed to result from obstruction of intestinal capillaries and venules as these vessels pass through the muscularis.

2. **Clinical features.** Most patients are asymptomatic, but the abnormal vessels are a common cause of painless lower gastrointestinal bleeding in older individuals.

3. **Diagnosis** may be made by angiographic or colonoscopic demonstration of intraluminal extravasation of blood during the acute episode.

4. **Therapy.** Bleeding usually can be managed conservatively with colonoscopic heater probe or laser treatment, but a right colon resection occasionally is needed for recurrent or massive bleeding. Estrogen treatment has decreased bleeding in some patients.

F. **Endometriosis** involves the colon in approximately 10% of cases. Symptoms include pain or rectal bleeding during menses. A barium enema often reveals extrinsic compression of the rectosigmoid or descending colon. Treatment is hormonal. Rarely, surgery is necessary to alleviate obstruction, pain, or recurrent bleeding.

G. **Tumors of the colon**

1. **Benign tumors.** There are several histologic types of benign colonic polyps. **Adenomatous polyps** are considered to be precursors of adenocarcinoma, and the risk for adenocarcinoma increases when the polyps are larger than 2 cm, villous rather than tubular, and sessile rather than pedunculated. Approximately 5%–10% of individuals older than age 40 years have colonic polyps, but most of these are small hyperplastic lesions that carry no malignant potential. Other benign tumors include leiomyomas, lipomas, and fibromas.

   a. **Clinical features.** Rectal bleeding occurs and may be microscopic or macroscopic. Large polyps may cause symptoms of an incomplete intestinal obstruction with occasional crampy abdominal pain.

   b. **Diagnosis** is made using an air contrast barium enema, endoscopic visualization of the colon, or both procedures.

   c. **Therapy**

      (1) Therapy for pedunculated lesions is colonoscopic removal with snare electrocautery. Sessile lesions may require surgical excision.

      (2) Because carcinoma occurring in an adenomatous polyp may be focal, careful histologic sectioning of the entire polyp, not just a biopsy, is necessary to exclude carcinoma. If malignancy invades the stalk of a polyp, a segmental resection of the colon is indicated to rule out lymphatic spread.

      (3) Synchronous polyps occur in 20% of cases, and metachronous lesions occur in approximately 30% of cases. Therefore, an air contrast barium enema, full colonoscopy, or both should be performed at the time a polyp is first identified and every 3 years thereafter. A yearly stool Hemoccult test also should be performed.

      (4) First-degree relatives of a patient with colonic polyps or carcinoma have approximately a fourfold to fivefold increased risk of development of a similar lesion. The daily use of aspirin or other nonsteroidal anti-inflammatory drugs may be associated with decreased polyp formation.

2. **Hereditary polyposis syndromes**

   a. **Familial polyposis** is an autosomal dominant syndrome characterized by adenomas of the colon. Allelic loss in chromosome 5q21 was named the adenoadenomatous polyposis coli (*APC*) gene and can be detected in peripheral blood leukocytes of patients with familial polyposis of the colon.

      (1) Hundreds of adenomatous polyps of the large intestine or cancer of the periampullary region of the small bowel is noted in patients and should be evaluated periodically with esophagogastric duodenoscopy.

      (2) When osteomas or soft tissue tumors (lipomas, fibromas, desmoid tumors of the mesentery) are present, this condition is called **Gardner's syndrome.**

      (3) Colonic malignancy develops by age 40 years in 80%–90% of patients. A subtotal resection of the colon with close subsequent observation should be performed by age 30 years. Sulindac therapy has led to regression of polyps in several patients.

   b. **Peutz-Jeghers syndrome** is an autosomal dominant polyposis syndrome with mucocutaneous pigmentation, particularly of the buccal mucosa. The polyps are hamartomas, not adenomas, which carry a low risk for malignant transformation and may be present in the stomach and small bowel as well as in the colon. Patients may have recurrent gastrointestinal bleeding.

   c. **Turcot syndrome** refers to pancolonic adenomas with malignant CNS tumors. This autosomal dominant polyposis syndrome has a high risk of malignancy.

   d. **Juvenile polyposis** is an autosomal dominant syndrome with gastrointestinal bleeding from polyps of the colon, small bowel, and stomach. The risk of malignancy is slightly increased in later life.

   e. **Cronkhite-Canada syndrome** is a rare association of intestinal polyps with alopecia, hyperpigmentation, and a lack of fingernails. No conclusive inheritance pattern has been noted.

   f. **Cowden's disease** is a rare autosomal dominant condition characterized by multiple hamartomas of the face, other parts of the skin (acral keratoses), or mouth. Breast lesions (fibrocystic disease or cancer) occur in approximately 50% of patients. Thyroid abnormalities, including goiter or cancer, occur in 10%–15% of patients. There is no increased risk of cancer associated with the gastrointestinal hamartomatous polyps.

3. **Adenocarcinoma** of the colon has been steadily increasing in frequency in the United States and ranks second to lung cancer in men and second to breast cancer in women as the major life-threatening malignancy.

   a. **Epidemiology.** The incidence of colorectal carcinomas is increased in developed countries, especially those with a diet high in red meat and low in fiber. In the United States, the incidence is decreased in Seventh-Day Adventists who practice strict vegetarianism, which also suggests an association with diet. In addition, asbestos workers, machinists, and factory woodworkers have a higher incidence of colorectal carcinomas than the general population.

   b. **Etiology**

      (1) **Diet** has been the focus of most etiologic studies. The increased amounts of red meat and animal fat in the diet in the United States promotes the growth of bacterial strains that produce carcinogens in the colonic lumen. Bile salts also may contribute to this process. Vitamins A, C, and E in certain foods may inactivate the carcinogens, and broccoli, turnips, and cauliflower induce benzpyrene hydroxylase, which also may inactivate ingested carcinogens.

      (2) **Genetic factors.** The role of genetic factors is demonstrated by familial polyposis syndromes and by the fact that first-degree relatives of patients with carcinoma or polyps have a threefold to fivefold increased risk of development of colorectal carcinoma. Hereditary polyposis syndromes account for approximately 1% of colorectal cancer yearly, with hereditary non-polyposis cancer (HNP) family syndromes accounting for 5%–10%.

         (a) **HNP type I** is an autosomal dominant inherited condition characterized by cancer of the colon in younger patients. HNP often develops before the patient reaches 45 years of age and often involves the ascending colon.

         (b) **HNP type II** is associated with carcinoma of the endometrium, ovary, ureter, renal pelvis, stomach, pancreas, and biliary tree, and otherwise is similar to HNP type I.

      (3) **Other risk factors** include:

         (a) Ulcerative colitis, especially pancolitis and disease of greater than 10 years' duration (10% risk)

         (b) Prior history of colon cancer or adenoma (10% risk)

         (c) Familial polyposis syndrome

         (d) History of female genital or breast cancer

         (e) History of juvenile polyps

         (f) Family cancer syndromes

         (g) Immunodeficiency diseases

   c. **Clinical features** vary, depending on the location and size of the tumor. Tumors in the left colon, especially those in the distal 25 cm, may occur as obstruction. Right colon tumors frequently occur as iron deficiency anemia and fatigue. Other common symptoms include a change in bowel habit, a decrease in stool size, obvious blood in the stool, and crampy abdominal pain. Metastatic disease usually involves the liver; however, the bone, lung, and brain also may be affected.

   d. **Diagnosis**

      (1) Diagnosis is made by colonoscopy or air contrast barium enema demonstration of polyps or tumors followed by endoscopic visualization with biopsy and cytologic study. The air contrast barium enema is far more sensitive than the single contrast examination. Despite these techniques, it can be difficult to differentiate the tumor from diverticulitis, benign stricture, and Crohn's disease.

(2) High-risk patients should have frequent stool guaiac testing and thorough evaluation of unexplained blood loss.

(3) CEA determinations, although not useful for screening purposes, may be used for periodic follow-up in patients with a history of carcinoma of the colon, with an increasing titer being indicative of recurrent or metastatic disease.

e. **Therapy** is excision of the tumor. Although focal carcinoma without stalk invasion in a polyp can be cured by colonoscopic snare cautery, most tumors require segmental resection of the bowel along with the omentum and regional lymph nodes. Radiation may be used preoperatively and in patients with recurrent disease. Rectal tumors traditionally have been treated with abdominal perineal resections, but recent studies suggest that local excision, radiotherapy, and fulguration may offer excellent results with a decreased risk. Chemotherapy has been disappointing, with only a 15%–20% response rate. When administered by intrahepatic artery perfusion, however, chemotherapy may be useful for decreasing pain in patients with liver metastasis. Adjunctive chemotherapy with levamisole and 5-fluorouracil (5-FU) may prolong life, especially in patients with positive lymph nodes (stage C carcinoma in the Dukes classification system).

f. **Prognosis.** The overall 10-year survival rate is 45% and has not changed significantly over the past several years.

(1) **Dukes' classification A and B.** Cancer confined to the mucosa is often detected by Hemoccult testing or sigmoidoscopy and is associated with an 80%–90% survival rate.

(2) **Dukes' classification C.** Cancer that is limited to the regional lymph nodes is associated with a 50%–60% survival rate.

(3) **Dukes' classification D.** Cancer that has metastasized to distant organs is associated with a survival rate of less than 25%.

H. **Collagenous colitis** is a recently described syndrome of chronic watery diarrhea, especially seen in middle-aged women. Laboratory data are usually normal, except 50% of patients may have an increase in erythrocyte sedimentation rate. Hypoalbuminemia and mild steatorrhea have been reported. Colonoscopic examination findings are normal, but biopsy reveals a thick layer of subepithelial collagen deposition, which is greater than 15 μ in thickness (normal collagen deposition is less than 5 μ). Treatment is with antidiarrheal agents, sulfasalazine, steroids, or all three. Microscopic colitis, marked by a lymphocytic infiltrate, is probably an early stage of collagenous colitis.

I. **Pseudomembranous colitis** is an acute, potentially severe disease of the colon characterized by exudative plaques that cover the intestinal mucosa.

1. **Pathogenesis.** The disease is caused by an enterotoxin produced by *C. difficile,* an anaerobic bacterium. It is thought that antibiotic therapy may "select out" the *C. difficile* organism, allowing proliferation and toxin production. Symptoms begin 3 days to 4 weeks after initiating antibiotic therapy. Virtually all antibiotics have been associated with this disease, but clindamycin, ampicillin, and the cephalosporins are the most common offenders.

2. **Clinical features** include watery diarrhea, crampy abdominal pain, lower abdominal tenderness, and fever. Leukocytosis is common. Dehydration and electrolyte disturbances may develop in severely ill patients. Toxic megacolon and colonic perforation are rare but are serious complications that may require surgical intervention. Approximately 20% of patients have a relapse after primary treatment.

3. **Diagnosis** is made by demonstration of *C. difficile* toxin in the stool or by sigmoidoscopic visualization of the characteristic yellow-white plaques in an erythematous and edematous mucosa. Biopsy of the plaques shows a mucinous, fibrinous, polymorphonuclear exudate. Most patients have disease throughout the colon; however, the disease may be confined to the right colon, and, in such cases, sigmoidoscopic findings are negative.

4. Therapy. The first step in treatment is to discontinue unnecessary antibiotics, which results in improvement in most patients. Cholestyramine may be used to bind the toxin. The organism is sensitive to vancomycin, bacitracin, and metronidazole.

J. **Cloacogenic carcinoma** accounts for 2.5% of all anorectal carcinomas. It is a carcinoma of the transitional epithelium of the region of the dentate line in the anal canal. It occurs at the junction of the ectoderm and entodermal cloaca—the blind caudal extension of the hindgut. It is more common in women, with a 3:1 ratio, and it is most common in the 55- to 70-year-old age-group. Treatment is with radiation and then surgery.

K. **Volvulus of the colon** generally involves either the sigmoid colon (slightly more common) or the cecal region. Sigmoid volvulus usually occurs in individuals older than 60 years of age who live in nursing homes, have CNS disease, or take antimotility drugs. Men are more susceptible, especially men with chronic constipation. Cecal volvulus commonly follows previous surgery. Acute cases require emergency colonoscopy or barium enema. Surgical resection may be necessary in 70%–90% of cases.

L. **Cytomegalovirus (CMV) colitis** is often seen in patients with AIDS, severe diabetes, renal failure, or inflammatory bowel disease. Bloody diarrhea may occur due to a deeply ulcerated colon. Intranuclear inclusion bodies may be noted on biopsy. The ulcers of CMV colitis may lead to perforation. Ganciclovir has been used for treatment in some cases.

VI. DISEASES OF THE RECTUM AND ANUS

A. **Ulcerative proctitis** is a localized form of ulcerative colitis, which has a better prognosis and a greatly decreased risk of malignancy as compared with ulcerative colitis.

1. Clinical features. Symptoms include diarrhea, rectal bleeding, and tenesmus; only rarely do fever, weight loss, and the systemic complications of ulcerative colitis occur.

2. Diagnosis is made by ruling out other causes of proctitis, especially infection, and by documenting the absence of inflammation above the rectum by sigmoidoscopy.

3. Therapy. Sulfasalazine, rectal corticosteroids, and 5-aminosalicylic acid enemas often are effective treatment.

4. Outcome. In approximately 15%–20% of cases, ulcerative proctitis progresses to diffuse ulcerative colitis.

B. **Infectious proctitis**

1. Venereal diseases that cause infectious proctitis include syphilis, gonorrhea, lymphogranuloma venereum, and herpes simplex. These diseases are especially common in homosexual men who may have multiple simultaneous infections.

　　a. Syphilis of the rectum almost always is primary syphilis. The chancre, which is painless, appears 10–90 days after exposure. Diagnosis is made by dark-field examination of discharge from the chancre and by serologic testing, although the Venereal Disease Research Laboratories (VDRL) test does not become positive until 1–2 weeks after the appearance of the chancre.

　　b. Gonorrhea may be asymptomatic or may cause rectal bleeding and diarrhea. Diagnosis is made by culturing the organism.

　　c. Lymphogranuloma venereum is caused by one strain of *Chlamydia trachomatis,* a gram-negative obligate intracellular bacterium. When left untreated, the acute proctitis may develop into a chronic destructive inflammation with late stricture formation. The organism is difficult to culture, although culture in yolk sacs and tissue cultures are possible. Serologic diagnosis generally is more available. Titers of greater than or equal to 1:16 are highly suggestive of current infection.

    d. Herpes simplex may cause constipation, hematochezia, severe anorectal pain, tenesmus, and mucopurulent discharge from the rectum. Bladder dysfunction with impotence may be present. Rectal biopsy demonstrates intranuclear inclusions. The symptoms subside spontaneously but may recur.

  2. Amebiasis (i.e., infection with *E. histolytica*) may be present as a diffuse colitis or extraintestinal disease (e.g., meningitis and liver abscess), or it may be confined to the rectosigmoid, especially in homosexual men. Symptoms range from mild diarrhea to bloody dysentery. Diagnosis is made by demonstrating the organism in the stool or in sigmoidoscopic biopsies of the characteristic flask-shaped ulcers. Treatment with metronidazole or iodoquinone may be useful.

C. **Solitary rectal ulcer** is a syndrome consisting of a superficial ulceration of unknown cause combined with passage of mucus or blood and dull rectal pain. The ulcers usually are 2 cm in diameter and located 7–10 cm from the anal verge. They are multiple in 25% of patients. A weakness in the rectal sling musculature may be a contributing cause. Diagnosis is made by excluding other causes of rectal ulcers, including infections, inflammatory bowel disease, and carcinoma. Treatment is supportive.

D. **Hemorrhoids** are dilated internal or external veins of the hemorrhoidal plexus located in the lower rectum. In the United States, 60%–70% of the population experience symptoms of hemorrhoids at some time. Signs and symptoms include perianal pruritus, rectal bleeding (especially small amounts on the toilet tissue or bright droplets into the toilet bowl), anal pain, and a palpable mass in the anal region. The diagnosis is made by anoscopy or sigmoidoscopy. Treatment is with stool softeners, supportive care with heat or antiedema measures, or surgery. Internal hemorrhoids may be tied with rubber banding or resected with laser or bicap electrocautery techniques.

E. **Anal fissures, abscesses,** and **fistulas** are tears, infections, and hollow channels from the rectum to the perianal skin, respectively. Locally applied heat, sitz baths, and antibiotics may be effective. Occasionally, however, it is necessary to drain surgically or to excise an abscess or a fistulous tract.

F. **Pruritus** of the perianal skin has many causes, including infection (bacterial, fungal, or parasitic), localized anorectal disease (e.g., fistulas and fissures), dermatologic diseases (e.g., psoriasis and eczema), poor hygiene, diarrhea, and systemic diseases such as diabetes mellitus. The underlying condition should be treated. In addition, local care with careful cleaning following defecation and nightly application of hydrocortisone cream may be helpful in controlling symptoms.

G. **Squamous cell carcinoma** of the anus is a rare malignancy that presents as bleeding, pain, a mass, and change in bowel habits. Treatment is surgical, and the 5-year survival rate is 60%.

H. **Cloacogenic carcinoma** is described in V J.

VII. DISEASES OF THE PANCREAS

A. **Acute pancreatitis**

  1. Etiology

    a. Common causes. Approximately 70% of cases of acute pancreatitis that occur in the United States are due to either alcohol abuse or gallstones.

(1) In alcoholic pancreatitis, proteinaceous plugs develop in the pancreatic ducts and calcify in the body of the pancreas, leading to stasis and atrophy of distal segments. Alcoholic pancreatitis is most common in men who have ingested large amounts of alcohol over a period of at least 10 years.

(2) In gallstone pancreatitis, the passage of a common duct stone (or multiple small stones, or even microlithiasis) may initiate reflux of biliary or intestinal contents into the pancreatic gland.

b. Less common causes of acute pancreatitis include:

(1) Postoperative pancreatitis, which may be severe and is especially common after hepatobiliary tract surgery

(2) Abdominal trauma

(3) Hyperlipidemia, types I and V (increased chylomicrons). Dietary and medical treatment of hypertriglyceridemia reduces recurrences.

(4) Drugs such as azathioprine, 6-mercaptopurine, estrogens, thiazides, furosemide, sulfonamides, tetracyclines, corticosteroids, valproic acid, pentamidine, and 2–3 dideoxyinosine

(5) Hypercalcemia

(6) Uremia

(7) Peptic ulcer disease, with penetration into the pancreas

(8) Cystic fibrosis (in rare cases)

(9) Endoscopic retrograde cholangiopancreatography (ERCP)

(10) Viral infections, especially mumps, coxsackievirus B

(11) Vascular insufficiency

(12) Pancreatic cancer, probably by localized ductal obstruction

(13) Hereditary pancreatitis, which may be inherited in an autosomal dominant pattern and carries an increased risk for development of pancreatic carcinoma

(14) Ampullary lesions or duodenal disease involving the ampulla and periampullary regions

(15) Pancreas divisum, in which the main portion of the pancreas drains into the smaller accessory duct (see VII B 1 c)

(16) The bite of a certain scorpion (*Tityus trinitatis*), which causes increased pancreatic enzyme secretion and may be associated with pancreatitis

(17) Idiopathic causes

2. Clinical features include:

a. Abdominal pain, which often is a steady or severe pain in the periumbilical region and may radiate to the back

b. Nausea and vomiting, which occur in 70% of cases

c. Abdominal tenderness, usually without guarding or rebound

d. Diminished or absent bowel sounds

e. Epigastric fullness or mass, which usually is found late in the course of the disease

f. Retroperitoneal bleeding, causing a hematoma at the umbilicus **(Cullen's sign)** or flank **(Turner's sign),** which is seen in hemorrhagic pancreatitis

3. Diagnosis usually is based on characteristic clinical presentations, especially in a patient with a history of previous pancreatitis.

a. Elevated serum amylase levels almost always exist during an acute attack but also may be due to perforated ulcer, intestinal infarction, obstruction, ruptured ectopic pregnancy, amylase-producing tumors, salivary gland disease, and decreased amylase clearance due to amylase–globulin complexes (macroamylase) or renal disease. All amylase-producing tumors (e.g., lung and ovary) are salivary-amylase–type tumors. Amylase may be falsely low in hyperlipidemic pancreatitis.

b. Elevated serum lipase levels also are found in acute attacks. Increased serum trypsinogen levels may be helpful in difficult-to-diagnose cases.

c. The amylase-to-creatinine clearance ratio may be elevated above the normal range of 1%–4% in acute pancreatitis; however, this ratio also is elevated post-operatively, in diabetic ketoacidosis, and in burn patients.

d. Abdominal radiographs may reveal a localized ileus (sentinel loop) in the small bowel region adjacent to the pancreas.

4. Therapy is supportive and includes intravenous administration of fluids and analgesics and bowel rest. Morphine may cause sphincter of Oddi spasm and should be avoided. Nasogastric suction often is used to drain gastric secretions and thereby limit pancreatic stimulation; however, the effectiveness of this procedure has not been proven. Intravenous hyperalimentation, which does not stimulate exocrine pancreatic release, may be used in protracted illness. If an impacted gallstone causes pancreatitis, then ERCP, sphincterotomy, and stone removal is the treatment of choice.

5. Complications account for the 10% mortality rate associated with acute pancreatitis and include the following conditions.

    a. Hemorrhagic pancreatitis is considered an extension of edematous pancreatitis due to chemical mediators (e.g., elastase), which leads to retroperitoneal hemorrhage and widespread tissue necrosis. Hemorrhagic pancreatitis is more common after trauma, postoperative pancreatitis, and the initial attack of acute pancreatitis and may require peritoneal lavage or surgical intervention for placement of drains. Blood may be present in the peritoneal cavity. The diagnosis is suggested by a declining hematocrit in a severely ill patient. An elevated methemalbumin level also may be observed.

    b. Adult respiratory distress syndrome is due to increased alveolar capillary permeability and may cause severe hypoxia requiring mechanical ventilation.

    c. Pancreatic abscess is suggested when high fever, elevated serum amylase levels, and leukocytosis persist beyond 7–10 days. Gas shadows in the region of the pancreas may be revealed by an abdominal flat plate or by CT. Treatment includes surgical drainage and antibiotics.

    d. Pancreatic pseudocyst refers to a collection of fluid and debris within the pancreas or in a space lined by the pancreas and other adjacent structures. Diagnosis is made by ultrasonography. Approximately 50% of pseudocysts (usually smaller ones) resolve spontaneously. Those persisting beyond 6–10 weeks require drainage to avoid potentially serious complications such as hemorrhage and rupture.

    e. Pancreatic ascites may occur due to a leaking pseudocyst with pancreatic ductal destruction. The diagnosis is suggested by very high serum amylase levels in peritoneal fluid. Conservative therapy with total parenteral nutrition and repeated paracentesis may lead to resolution, but pancreatic resection may be necessary in intractable cases.

B. **Chronic pancreatitis** results in permanent structural damage of pancreatic tissue.

1. Etiology. Most of the causes of acute pancreatitis in the United States also can result in chronic pancreatitis. A notable exception is gallstones, which cause only recurrent acute attacks of pancreatitis.

    a. Alcohol abuse accounts for 90% of cases of chronic pancreatitis in adults.

    b. Cystic fibrosis is the most common cause of chronic disease in children.

    c. In pancreas divisum, which results from a congenital failure of the dorsal and ventral pancreas to fuse (approximately 5% of people), the main portion of the pancreas may drain through the small accessory duct of Santorini, not the large duct of Wirsung. Chronic obstruction to drainage and pancreatitis may occur in approximately one third of patients with this drainage. Pancreas divisum remains controversial as a cause of chronic pancreatitis.

2. Clinical features

    a. Pain, the usual presenting symptom, typically occurs in the epigastrium after eating and radiates to the back.

    b. Malabsorption occurs in association with steatorrhea and weight loss.

    c. Jaundice occurs due to edema and fibrosis in the pancreatic head and causes obstruction of the pancreatic portion of the common bile duct.

d. Diabetes is common; however, ketoacidosis, nephropathy, and diabetic vascular disease rarely occur.

3. **Diagnosis** is suggested by the development of continuous pain and signs of pancreatic insufficiency in a patient with known recurrent pancreatitis, especially when due to alcohol ingestion. Specific tests include:
   a. Abdominal radiographs, which reveals pancreatic calcification in 30%–40% of cases
   b. Secretin-stimulation testing with duodenal intubation and aspiration, which reveals a low bicarbonate concentration in the pancreatic secretion and low enzyme output
   c. ERCP, which shows diffuse ductal dilatation with an irregular, beaded ("chain of lakes") appearance

4. **Therapy** is aimed at controlling the manifestations of the disease because the underlying damage to the gland is permanent. In addition, agents that may promote further damage (e.g., alcohol) should be withdrawn.
   a. Control of pain may require narcotic analgesics, but care must be taken to avoid addiction. With abstinence from alcohol over a period of time, some patients experience a lessening of pain.
   b. Replacement of pancreatic enzymes may be indicated for the treatment of steatorrhea or for the relief of pain. Antacids or H_2-receptor antagonists may increase the effectiveness of oral enzyme preparations.
   c. Insulin may be needed in advanced cases.
   d. MCTs, which are more easily absorbed than longer-chain fatty acids, are often given.
   e. Treatment of pancreas divisum may be to enlarge the accessory duct surgically or endoscopically.
   f. Surgery is a last resort and generally is used for severe pain or recurrent, severe attacks. Subtotal (80%) pancreatectomy and the Puestow procedure (i.e., anastomosis of the pancreatic duct lengthwise to a loop of the jejunum) are used most commonly.

C. **Neoplastic cystic lesions** of the pancreas include serous and mucinous cystadenomas and adenocarcinomas. These lesions are true cysts of the pancreas, with multiple small cysts (serous) or large cysts (mucinous). These are not seen to communicate with the pancreatic duct on ERCP. They do not contain amylase, and the serum amylase level is usually normal (as discussed, the serum amylase level is elevated in approximately 60%–75% of cases of pseudocysts). These lesions are more common in women, and most affected individuals experience weight loss and have no prior history of pancreatitis. Angiography usually reveals hypervascularity, and treatment is surgical removal—often with complete cure.

D. **Adenocarcinoma** of the pancreas accounts for more than 90% of pancreatic malignancies. The adenocarcinoma is pancreatic ductal in approximately 95% of patients. This tumor has been increasing in incidence during the twentieth century and is second to colon carcinoma as the leading cause of gastrointestinal cancer–related death. Men are affected more commonly than women, and the average age at presentation is 55–65 years. Seventy percent of adenocarcinoma of the pancreas occurs in the head of the pancreas, with 30% occurring in the body or tail.

1. **Etiology.** The risk of pancreatic carcinoma is significantly increased in patients with hereditary pancreatitis and in smokers, and the risk is slightly increased in diabetic patients. A recent study suggests that long-term exposure to the insecticide DDT may be associated with an increased risk of pancreatic cancer. Chronic pancreatitis is also a known predisposing cause for pancreatic cancer.

2. **Clinical features**
   a. **Common symptoms.** Approximately 75% of patients have pain that has been present for 3–4 months by the time of diagnosis. The pain typically is postprandial epigastric or periumbilical discomfort, which radiates to the back and is re-

lieved by sitting up or bending both knees. Jaundice is present in approximately 65% of patients, and weight loss occurs in 60% of patients. Diarrhea and steatorrhea also are somewhat common. The gallbladder may be palpable (Courvoisier's sign) in some patients. A palpable epigastric mass may be found on physical examination.

  b. Less common symptoms include unexplained thrombophlebitis (Trousseau's sign), depression, the new onset of diabetes mellitus, or acute pancreatitis.

3. **Diagnosis** often requires a high index of suspicion in the patient with constant epigastric or periumbilical distress.

  a. **Laboratory tests** reveal an elevated serum alkaline phosphatase level in 80% of patients, which often is due to hepatic metastasis but may be due to compression of the pancreatic portion of the common bile duct. Elevated levels of CEA, lactate dehydrogenase, and serum glutamic–oxaloacetic transaminase (SGOT) also are common. Jaundice is found in 65% of patients, and 25% of patients have high serum amylase levels. CA19-9, a tumor marker, has been associated with carcinoma of the pancreas. Although not useful as a screening test, it has an approximate 80% sensitivity and 90% specificity for carcinoma of the pancreas and may be a marker for recurrent diseases or metastasis after primary resection.

  b. An **upper gastrointestinal series** may reveal a widened loop or an "inverted 3 sign" due to indentation by the pancreas along the medial aspect of the duodenum.

  c. **CT** and **ultrasonography** of the pancreas demonstrate a mass in 75%–80% of patients.

  d. **ERCP** is abnormal in approximately 85%–90% of patients and generally shows a discrete stricture in the main pancreatic duct with proximal dilatation.

  e. **Endoscopic ultrasound (EUS)** may be more sensitive than extracorporeal ultrasound.

  f. **Angiography** may reveal displacement or encasement of the pancreatic or duodenal arteries. The venous phase may be especially useful if the superior mesenteric vein or splenic vein is occluded.

  g. **Secretin-stimulation testing** may reveal a decrease in the volume of pancreatic secretion but normal enzyme and bicarbonate concentrations.

  h. **Chiba (skinny) needle biopsy** under the guidance of CT or ultrasonography may be used to obtain cytologic specimens and is positive for malignancy in 80%–90% of patients.

4. **Therapy and prognosis.** The overall 5-year survival rate for patients with pancreatic carcinoma is less than 5%.

  a. **Surgery** is the mainstay of therapy, but only 15% of patients are candidates for curative resection. The **Whipple procedure** (resection of the pancreas with excision of the common bile duct and duodenum) has a 20% surgical mortality rate and a 5% 5-year survival rate. Palliative biliary and gastrointestinal bypass surgery may provide relief of pruritus, jaundice, and symptoms of gastric-outlet obstruction.

  b. **Chemotherapy** has a 15%–20% response rate but does not prolong survival.

  c. **Radiotherapy** decreases the size of the tumor mass in approximately 60%–70% of patients and can be used for palliation. Preoperative chemotherapy and radiation protocols are being used to increase resectability.

5. **Islet cell tumors** account for 5% of pancreatic adenocarcinomas. They may be multicentric, and they tend to grow slower than tumors of ductular origin. Islet cell tumors frequently are associated with endocrine adenomas in the pituitary and parathyroid glands (e.g., in MEN I syndrome).

  a. **Gastrinoma** causes the Zollinger-Ellison syndrome (III I).

  b. **Insulinoma** is characterized by inappropriately high insulin levels in the presence of hypoglycemia. Because only 10%–15% of insulinomas are malignant, surgical resection is the treatment of choice. Synthetic somatostatin may be an effective treatment.

  c. **Glucagonoma** is found in patients with a syndrome of diabetes mellitus, weight loss, anemia, and a characteristic rash (migratory necrolytic erythema). Most glucagonomas are malignant, but surgical debulking may provide symptomatic improvement. Streptozocin is the most commonly used chemotherapeutic agent. Somatostatin may be used.

d. **Somatostatinoma** usually occurs in association with the triad of diabetes, steatorrhea, and gallstones. Approximately 50% of patients have a positive family history of islet cell tumors. The diagnosis usually is made either incidentally at surgery for another problem (e.g., cholecystitis) or late in the course of the disease when metastatic disease is present. Streptozocin therapy has been effective in a small number of patients.

e. **VIPoma** (also called **pancreatic cholera, Verner-Morrison syndrome,** and the **watery diarrhea, hypokalemia,** and **achlorhydria syndrome**) is a tumor of non-α, non-β islet cells that secrete vasoactive intestinal peptide (VIP), which causes watery diarrhea. Solitary lesions may be cured by surgical resection. Some patients are responsive to corticosteroids, and streptozocin has been used successfully in patients with metastatic disease. Synthetic somatostatin may also be used.

VIII. DISEASES OF THE BILIARY TRACT

A. **Gallstones** are extremely common, occurring in 15%–20% of the population of the United States.

1. **Types**
   a. **Cholesterol gallstones.** Most gallstones that occur in western populations are composed primarily of cholesterol, which is thought to precipitate from supersaturated bile, especially at night when bile is concentrated in the gallbladder. For women, the risk of cholesterol gallstones increases with age, use of oral contraceptives (at least during the first 5 years of use), rapid weight loss, family history of diabetes mellitus, and ileal disease (Crohn's disease) or ileal resection resulting in a decreased bile salt pool.
   b. **Pigmented gallstones,** composed primarily of calcium bilirubinate, are found in patients with chronic hemolysis (e.g., sickle cell disease) as well as in Asian populations. In Asia, biliary infection with β-glucuronidase–producing organisms leads to increased amounts of poorly soluble deconjugated bilirubin in bile.

2. **Therapy.** One third to one half of patients with gallstones are asymptomatic and should be treated expectantly. Surgical removal of asymptomatic gallstones is unnecessary except in diabetic patients in whom the risk of acute cholecystitis with complications is high.

B. **Acute cholecystitis**

1. **Etiology.** In 90%–95% of cases, acute cholecystitis is caused by obstruction of the cystic duct by an impacted gallstone, which leads to edema of the gallbladder wall with submucosal hemorrhage and mucosal ulceration. Polymorphonuclear infiltration is a later event and probably is due to the low bacterial count of the obstructed gallbladder. Acalculous cholecystitis may occur secondary to salmonellosis, polyarteritis nodosa, sepsis, and trauma.

2. **Clinical features**
   a. An attack of acute cholecystitis starts with crampy pain in the epigastrium or right upper quadrant, which may radiate to the back near the right scapular tip (biliary colic). The pain is thought to be generated by ductal obstruction and often is postprandial, typically subsiding within several hours.
   b. An elevated temperature or white blood cell count, fever, nausea, vomiting, and ileus also may be present.

    c. Right upper quadrant tenderness precipitated by deep inspiration during palpation of the right upper quadrant is known as **Murphy's sign.**

    d. Jaundice occurs in 20% of patients and is thought to be due to common duct stones or edema of the common bile duct.

3. Diagnosis is suggested by the characteristic clinical picture, especially in a patient known to have gallstones.

    a. Most gallstones consist of cholesterol and are radiolucent; 10%–15% of gallstones contain enough calcium to appear radiopaque.

    b. Although gallbladder ultrasonography can show the presence of stones (i.e., the fluid-filled gallbladder appears lucent, whereas the stones within it are sono-opaque and cast shadows), this test cannot be used to demonstrate cystic duct obstruction.

    c. Failure to visualize the gallbladder during radionuclide scanning following an intravenous injection of iminodiacetic acid (HIDA scanning) strongly suggests cystic duct obstruction.

    d. Cystic duct obstruction is also suggested when oral cholecystography fails to visualize the gallbladder, but cholecystography is as reliable as HIDA scanning.

4. Therapy

    a. Supportive treatment. Therapy initially is supportive, with intravenous fluid replacement and nasogastric suction for 24–48 hours. Later, the gallbladder may be removed surgically.

    b. Dissolution. Cholesterol stones in patients who are not operative candidates may be treated with **ursodeoxycholic acid** or **chenodeoxycholic acid** to dissolve the stones. If several small stones are present and floating, a 50%–70% chance of dissolving the stones may be expected over a period of 12–24 months.

    c. Lithotripsy may be tried if the gallbladder is functional, the stone mass is less than 3.0 cm, and the patient has no acute symptoms (approximately 20%–25% of patients).

    d. Percutaneous introduction of methylterbutaline ether has also been used in patients who refuse cholecystectomy.

    e. Laparoscopic cholecystectomy may allow gallbladder removal on a ''same-day surgery'' basis in many cases.

5. Complications generally require surgical intervention.

    a. Empyema refers to a pus-filled gallbladder. Patients may be toxic and are at high risk for perforation.

    b. Perforation

        (1) Localized perforation occurs several days to 1 week after the onset of acute cholecystitis and leads to a pericholecystic abscess.

        (2) Free perforation into the abdominal cavity, which has a 25% mortality rate, occurs early in the clinical course, probably because inflammation in the early stages is insufficient to wall off the abscess.

        (3) Perforation into an adjacent organ may involve the duodenum, jejunum, colon, or stomach. If a large stone is passed into the lumen, intestinal obstruction (gallstone ileus) may result.

    c. Emphysematous cholecystitis is due to gas-forming bacteria (often clostridia, *E. coli,* or streptococci) in the gallbladder lumen and wall. Men are affected more commonly than women, and 20%–30% of patients have diabetes mellitus. Early surgical intervention is indicated to prevent perforation.

    d. Postcholecystectomy syndrome refers to abdominal pain that persists after cholecystectomy. The usual cause is an initially mistaken diagnosis, with pain persisting from the underlying process (e.g., pancreatic disease and irritable bowel syndrome). Some patients may have common duct stones.

C. **Chronic cholecystitis** is a clinical term used to describe a condition of recurrent subacute symptoms due to gallstones. Patients with chronic cholecystitis show wide variability in the thickening and fibrosis of the gallbladder wall and in the inflammatory infiltrate. The diagnosis is based on failure to visualize the gallbladder with oral cholecystography. After ruling out other sources of chronic abdominal pain (e.g., peptic ulcer disease, pancreatitis, and irritable bowel syndrome), a cholecystectomy may be performed to relieve symptoms.

D. **Choledocholithiasis**

1. **Pathophysiology.** Choledocholithiasis usually occurs when a gallstone is passed into the common duct from the gallbladder or when a gallstone that was missed during operative cholangiography or common duct exploration is retained. Occasionally, a stone forms de novo in the common duct, especially when there is stasis from ductal obstruction.

2. **Clinical features.** Symptoms frequently are intermittent and include colicky pain in the right upper quadrant, fever, chills, and jaundice accompanied by elevated serum levels of alkaline phosphatase and the transaminases. Sepsis may result from ascending cholangitis, which is a closed-space infection.

3. **Therapy.** Antibiotics are given as needed to control infection, but definitive treatment consists of surgical removal of the stone or endoscopic sphincterotomy and stone extraction. Patients who are poor surgical risks and in whom there is access to the biliary tree (i.e., with a T tube) may be treated by infusion of monooctanoin to dissolve the stones or by extracorporeal shock wave lithotripsy.

E. **Biliary dyskinesia** is a clinical syndrome of right upper quadrant symptoms, and it is similar to chronic calculous cholecystitis, although not associated with the structural abnormality of the biliary tree often seen after cholecystectomy.

1. **Pathophysiology.** An abnormality of biliary motor function is proposed, and manometric findings may reveal elevated basal sphincter of Oddi pressure (usually 35 mm Hg greater than intraduodenal pressure), a paradoxical contraction of the sphincter of Oddi after cholecystokinin injection, or both.

2. **Therapy.** Patients may respond to smooth muscle relaxants (e.g., nitrates and calcium channel-blocking agents) or to endoscopic or surgical sphincterotomy of the sphincter of Oddi.

F. **Biliary stricture**

1. **Pathophysiology.** Biliary stricture is a narrowing of the common bile duct generally due to surgical injury or scarring subsequent to exploration of the common bile duct. Rarely, trauma or choledocholithiasis may result in a biliary stricture.

2. **Clinical features.** Patients usually have intermittent obstructive jaundice several weeks to months after biliary tract surgery. Cholangiography demonstrates the presence of a smooth concentric narrowing of the duct, with proximal dilatation being a common finding.

3. **Therapy.** The usual treatment is surgical anastomosis of the dilated proximal end of the bile duct to the intestine, but some patients may undergo percutaneous transhepatic or endoscopic balloon dilatation with biliary stent placement.

G. **Sclerosing cholangitis,** a rare disease that causes progressive narrowing of the bile ducts, generally is diagnosed in the third or fourth decade of life and is three times more common in men than in women.

1. **Clinical features.** Approximately 70% of patients have inflammatory bowel disease (usually ulcerative colitis), but the biliary and intestinal diseases have independent clinical courses. The usual presenting symptom is pruritus. There is an increased risk of cholangiocarcinoma in such patients.

2. **Diagnosis.** Early diagnosis is possible in asymptomatic patients who show marked elevation of serum alkaline phosphatase levels on routine biochemical screening. ERCP or percutaneous cholangiography should establish the diagnosis.

3. Therapy

a. **Medical treatment.** Corticosteroids, ursodeoxycholic acid, methotrexate, long-term antibiotics, or varying combinations of these medications have been used with varying success.

b. **Surgical treatment.** Surgical anastomosis of the diseased duct to the intestine may be difficult or impossible, but liver transplantation is a consideration in many patients. Endoscopic or percutaneous dilatation of strictures is possible in some cases.

H. **Oriental cholangitis** is a disease of Asian populations or first-generation immigrants from Asia. Incidence rates for men and women are equal. The etiologic factors may be bile stasis (often associated with parasitic infestation) and a low protein diet. The disease is characterized by recurrent right upper quadrant pain, fever, jaundice, and bile duct pigmented stones. Infected bile is often found at surgery. Treatment is with surgery and surgical drainage of the bile ducts.

I. **Cystic malformation of the bile ducts**

1. **Choledochal cysts** occur as jaundice, cholangitis, or a large cyst filled with numerous stones. Diagnosis may be made by cholangiography. Surgery is used to excise the cyst or to anastomose the cyst to the intestine.

2. **Caroli's disease** is characterized by saccular dilatation of the intrahepatic ducts, which may be associated with right upper quadrant pain, cholangitis, or both due to ductal stone formation. Hepatic fibrosis with portal hypertension may develop, especially in patients with medullary sponge kidney. Recently, cholangiocarcinoma has been reported in congenital biliary cysts (up to 30%), especially if stones are present in the cyst. Surgical decompression occasionally is helpful, and antibiotics are used during acute episodes of cholangitis.

J. **Tumors of the gallbladder**

1. **Adenocarcinoma** of the gallbladder is a disease of older women. The tumor affects three times as many women as it does men, and the average age at diagnosis is 65–75 years. Although most patients have associated gallstones, cancer develops in less than 1% of all patients with stones. Symptoms generally mimic those of acute or chronic cholecystitis. On physical examination, a mass may be palpable in the right upper quadrant, and obstructive jaundice may be seen secondary to local spread of the tumor to the common bile duct. A calcified gallbladder may be seen on abdominal radiographs. An operation consisting of cholecystectomy, lymph node dissection, and removal of a small portion of the adjacent liver is indicated if no obvious metastatic disease is found, but prognosis generally is poor.

2. **Benign tumors** of the gallbladder include abnormalities of the mucosal lining (e.g., adenomatous hyperplasia, cholesterolosis, and cholesterol polyps), cystic changes in the glands, and papillary adenomas. These lesions usually are asymptomatic. In some patients with no other demonstrable causes for abdominal pain, however, cholecystectomy has provided relief of symptoms.

K. **Tumors of the bile duct.** Adenocarcinoma of the bile duct (cholangiocarcinoma) is a disease of older men and is not associated with gallstones.

1. **Etiology.** An increased risk is observed in patients with ulcerative colitis who have sclerosing cholangitis and in patients exposed to benzene or toluene derivatives. Parasitic infection, especially with *Clonorchis,* of the biliary system has been linked to the high rate of cholangiocarcinoma in Asian populations.

2. **Pathology.** Most tumors are of the scirrhous or papillary type. An extensive desmoplastic reaction may make diagnosis difficult. Two thirds of the tumors are located in the common bile duct or at the bifurcation of the common hepatic duct **(Klatskin tumors).**

3. **Clinical features.** Jaundice, with or without pain, is present in most patients, and weight loss also is common. Pruritus may be severe. Common duct tumors causing obstruction distal to the cystic duct result in a palpable gallbladder that is not tender.

4. **Laboratory data.** Serum alkaline phosphatase levels are markedly increased as are direct and total bilirubin levels. Serum transaminase levels show smaller increases and generally are less than 200 mg/dl.

5. **Diagnosis.** Dilatation of the intrahepatic ducts is revealed by ultrasonography or CT, and percutaneous cholangiography or ERCP findings generally suggest the diagnosis. The differential diagnosis includes pancreatic carcinoma, choledocholithiasis, biliary stricture, and sclerosing cholangitis.

6. **Therapy.** Surgery is the treatment of choice for approachable lesions; however, most hepatic duct tumors are not surgically resectable. A pancreaticoduodenectomy (Whipple procedure) may be used to treat distal lesions that have no obvious tumor extension. Palliative procedures include biliary bypass surgery and stenting tubes left in at the time of the percutaneous cholangiography. Frequent replacement of these tubes may be necessary because they are prone to blockage. Cure is rare and is achieved in only 10% of patients, but, because the tumors are slow growing, palliative bypass surgery or stenting may offer patients several years of symptomatic relief.

IX. DISEASES OF THE LIVER

A. **Acute liver disease** (Table 5-2)

1. **Acute viral hepatitis,** one of the most common health problems in the world, is caused by any one of several viruses.
   a. **Etiology**
      (1) **Hepatitis A** is an RNA virus transmitted primarily by the fecal–oral route. The incubation period is 2–6 weeks. Acute infection is anicteric in 50% of cases. Hepatitis A does not lead to chronic disease or to a carrier state.
      (2) **Hepatitis B** is a DNA virus transmitted parenterally. Individuals at high risk include intravenous drug abusers, homosexual men, and those exposed to blood and blood products (e.g., patients and health professionals in dialysis units). The incubation period ranges from 1 to 6 months. Chronic disease or a persistent carrier state develops in approximately 10% of patients.
      (3) **Hepatitis C** is an RNA virus that may account for 90% of post-transfusion hepatitis. The modes of transmission (parenteral, sexual, and perhaps perinatal) are similar to those of hepatitis B. The incubation period is 2 weeks to 6 months. Chronic hepatitis develops in up to 30%–50% of patients. Of these, approximately 50% have chronic active hepatitis, and cirrhosis goes on to develop in many.
      (4) **Non-A, non-B, non-C hepatitis** may be caused by more than one virus. The incubation period is similar to that of hepatitis C (2 weeks to 6 months). Most cases previously designated as non-A, non-B hepatitis are designated as hepatitis C. Cases that are not accounted for by hepatitis C, and so are designated as non-A, non-B hepatitis, may progress to chronic hepatitis, as occurs in hepatitis C.
      (5) **Delta hepatitis (hepatitis D)** is caused by a small, defective RNA virus (delta agent) that is infectious only in the presence of hepatitis B infection because it relies on hepatitis B proteins for replication. It can, therefore, complicate acute hepatitis B infection but is seen more commonly as a "super infection" with an increase in abnormal liver function tests in a patient with chronic hepatitis B. Delta hepatitis generally has a chronic, severe clinical course.

TABLE 5-2. Comparison of Viral Hepatitis Types A, B, C, Delta, and E

	Hepatitis A	Hepatitis B	Hepatitis C	Delta Agent (Hepatitis D)	Hepatitis E	Hepatitis G
Type of Virus	RNA	DNA	RNA	RNA (hepatitis B required for replication)	RNA	RNA
Incidence of Positive Antibody in the United States (%)	40	10	2–3	Low	Very low	Low
Incidence after Blood Transfusion (%)	0 to extremely rare	10–20	60–90	?	...	...
Incubation Period	2–6 weeks	1–6 months	2–24 weeks	1–6 months	2–8 weeks	2–24 weeks
Infectivity Stage	Last 3 weeks of inoculation to 1–2 weeks after jaundice occurs	During hepatitis B surface antigen positivity	?	?	?	
Complications	Fulminant hepatitis (rare)	Fulminant hepatitis (rare but more common than with hepatitis A); chronic active hepatitis	Fulminant hepatitis (rare but more common than with hepatitis A); chronic active hepatitis	Present in 20%–50% of cases of fulminant hepatitis and/or chronic active hepatitis	Fulminant hepatitis in pregnant women with 10%–20% mortality	Chronic carrier states; fulminant hepatitis
Mechanism of Spread	Fecal–oral	Parenteral	Parenteral	Parenteral	Fecal–oral	Parenteral
Prevention	Pooled immune serum globulin; vaccination	Hepatitis B immune globulin; vaccination	Pooled immune serum globulin	?	Good hygiene	?
Carrier State	Rare, if ever	1%–2%	Yes (50% of patients)	?	?	Yes

(6) **Hepatitis E** is a small RNA virus (possibly a calicivirus) that has been described in cases of acute hepatitis in Mexico, Asia, and Africa. It has a short incubation period and is probably waterborne. The mortality rate in pregnant women may be 10%–20%.

(7) **Hepatitis G** is a recently described RNA virus that is transmitted parenterally and accounts for approximately 15% of non-A, non-B, non-C cases of chronic hepatitis. It may also be associated with fulminant hepatitis.

(8) **Other viruses** that can cause acute hepatitis include the Epstein-Barr virus, CMV, HSV, and those causing yellow fever and rubella.

b. **Pathology.** The lesions of acute viral hepatitis are similar regardless of etiology and include mononuclear cell infiltration, cellular ballooning and necrosis, and condensed cytoplasm with pyknotic nuclei (acidophilic bodies).

c. **Clinical features** of viral hepatitis include:

(1) Malaise, anorexia, and fatigue

(2) Arthritis and urticaria, which are especially common in hepatitis B, are ascribed to circulating immune complexes

(3) Influenza-like syndrome, which is especially common in hepatitis A

(4) Jaundice (with dark urine or light stools), which is seen in 50% of cases

(5) Hepatic enlargement or tenderness

(6) Splenomegaly, which occurs in 20% of patients

d. **Diagnosis** of acute viral hepatitis is based on the clinical features as well as such laboratory findings as elevated levels of the transaminases [i.e., SGOT (AST) and serum glutamic–pyruvic transaminase (SGPT or ALT)], serum bilirubin, and serum alkaline phosphatase. In addition, the increase in bilirubin exceeds the increase in alkaline phosphatase.

(1) In hepatitis A, the IgM antibody is elevated early in the course, followed by an elevation of the IgG antibody in 2–3 months.

(2) In hepatitis B, a positive surface antigen usually is diagnostic. However, because this is an early finding, it may be necessary to follow the increase of IgM anticore and later of antisurface antibodies to document acute infection (Figure 5-1).

(3) Hepatitis C can be diagnosed using techniques that detect viral RNA.

(4) Delta hepatitis may be diagnosed by an elevated delta antibody titer, often with the disappearance of B surface antigen from the serum. A persistently high or slowly falling hepatitis delta antibody is seen in chronic states.

(5) Hepatitis E serologic testing has recently been described.

e. **Therapy** is supportive and includes intravenous fluids to provide hydration, correct electrolyte abnormalities, and provide caloric intake if nausea and vomiting are present. Vitamin K should be given if the prothrombin time is elevated. Interferon is useful in certain cases of hepatitis B and C (those with low viral loads), but relapse rates are high.

f. **Clinical course and complications.** Nearly all cases of acute viral hepatitis are benign, with most patients demonstrating normal results on liver function testing by 8–10 weeks. Complications may occur, however, and include the following conditions.

(1) **Fulminant hepatitis** is a rare complication of hepatitis A but occurs in 1%–2% of patients with hepatitis B and hepatitis C. It is an especially common complication of delta agent superinfection in patients with chronic hepatitis B antigenemia. Patients usually have progressive jaundice, hepatic encephalopathy, and ascites. Hepatorenal syndrome is common. Elevated prothrombin time is an early sign. The initially elevated serum transaminase levels later decline, and liver size decreases as a result of necrosis of the liver parenchyma. The mortality rate varies with age and approaches 90%–100%, especially in patients older than 60 years of age.

(2) **Chronic persistent hepatitis** may occur after hepatitis B, hepatitis C, hepatitis G, or non-A, non-B, non-C hepatitis and is defined as elevated serum transaminase levels for a period of more than 6 months. Liver biopsy

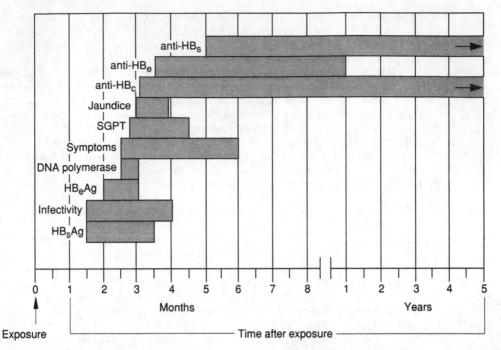

FIGURE 5-1. Typical clinical course of acute hepatitis B. Recombinant and pooled-plasma vaccines against hepatitis B do not transmit active hepatitis B surface antigen (*Hb_sAg*) and do not contain hepatitis B e antigen (*Hb_eAg*) or hepatitis core antigen. Consequently, the serologic profile of a vaccinated individual consists of hepatitis B surface antibody (*anti-HB_s*) only. *SGPT* = serum glutamic–pyruvic transaminase; *anti-HB_c* = hepatitis B core antibody; *anti-HB_e* = anti-hepatitis B e antibody.

shows a periportal lymphocytic infiltrate but no extension beyond the portal limiting triad and no fibrosis. Most patients are asymptomatic, although some report fatigue, anorexia, and abdominal pain. Results of liver function testing are only mildly abnormal. The clinical course is benign.

 (3) Chronic active hepatitis is another complication of hepatitis B and hepatitis C, in which serum transaminase levels are elevated for a period of more than 6 months. Pathologically, there is inflammation, necrosis, and fibrosis bridging portal areas or between portal areas and central veins. The disease may progress to cirrhosis, and, on physical examination, patients may have splenomegaly, spider angiomata, caput medusae, and other signs of chronic liver disease. There is no consistently effective treatment, but trials of α-interferon and other antiviral agents, such as the protease inhibitor lamivudine, have produced promising results. Liver biopsy is necessary for diagnosis.

 (4) A **chronic carrier state** for hepatitis B surface antigen exists in 0.2% of the population of the United States. A carrier state also may exist for hepatitis C because blood donated by apparently normal individuals may transmit this disease when transfused. Carriers of hepatitis B or C virus may have an increased risk of hepatoma.

 (5) Cholestatic hepatitis may occur and is characterized by the alkaline phosphatase level elevated disproportionately to the transaminase level. The clinical course is typical of acute viral hepatitis, but this presentation must be differentiated from biliary tract obstruction.

 (6) Aplastic anemia is seen rarely after acute viral hepatitis. The mortality rate is high, and no treatment has been proven effective.

g. Prevention

 (1) Immune serum globulin is effective when administered after exposure to hepatitis A and also may be partially protective against hepatitis B and hepatitis C.

TABLE 5-3. Agents of Drug-Induced Liver Disease

Drugs Causing Direct Toxicity	Drugs Causing Altered Metabolism	Drugs Causing Immune-Mediated Reactions			
		Viral Hepatitis-Like	Granulomatous Hepatitis	Inflammatory Cholestasis	Chronic Active Hepatitis
Acetaminophen	Androgens	Halothane	Allopurinol	Chlorpromazine	Acetaminophen
Amiodarone	Corticosteroids (?)	Isoniazid	Hydralazine	Chlorpropamide	Aspirin
Aspirin	Estrogens	Oxacillin	Phenylbutazone	Erythromycin estolate	Isoniazid
Alcohol	Ethanol	Phenytoin	Phenytoin	Propylthiouracil	Methyldopa
Carbon tetrachloride	Intraveous tetracycline	Sulfonamides	Quinidine	Thiazides	Nitrofurantoin
Heavy metals		Valproic acid	Sulfa drugs		Oxyphenisatin
Methotrexate					
Mushroom toxins (phalloidin and phallin)					
Niacin					
Phosphorus					

(2) **Hepatitis B immune globulin,** which is immunoglobulin containing high titers of antibody to hepatitis B, conveys passive immunity and is recommended after confirmed exposure to hepatitis B (e.g., from skin puncture by a contaminated needle).

(3) **Vaccines**

    (a) **Hepatitis A vaccine.** An effective vaccine for prevention of hepatitis A is available.

    (b) **Hepatitis B vaccine,** a preparation of the surface antigen, conveys active immunity and is recommended for individuals at high risk, such as dialysis patients, medical personnel with frequent exposure to blood products, and individuals who are hepatitis B antibody–negative and who have had confirmed exposure to hepatitis B. Infants are routinely vaccinated.

2. **Drug-induced liver disease** may follow exposure to virtually any drug and manifests as a variety of clinical syndromes and histologic findings. Any drug may induce liver disease that overlaps two or more categories of disease mechanisms (Table 5-3).

    a. **Direct toxicity** by a chemical (e.g., carbon tetrachloride) or a metabolite (e.g., acetaminophen) usually represents a dose-related injury. Niacin may cause a dose-related toxicity at greater than 3 g/day in crystalline form or 1–2 g/day in sustained-release form. Acetaminophen overdose can be treated with *N*-acetylcysteine, which binds to the toxic metabolite and provides cysteine for glutathione synthesis, or intravenous cimetidine, which decreases cytochrome P-450 activity and prevents conversion of acetaminophen to its toxic metabolite. Small doses of acetaminophen (3–14 g) ingested with alcohol may induce hepatic necrosis marked by high levels of hepatic aspartate aminotransferase (3000–24,000 IU). Such cases have a high mortality rate.

    b. **Indirect toxicity.** Liver disease may result from interference with the metabolism of bilirubin (e.g., by estrogens and androgens) or with protein synthesis (e.g., by intravenous tetracycline, which causes microvesicular fat accumulation in hepatocytes).

    c. **Immunologic drug reactions** can cause a variety of syndromes, including cholestatic jaundice (a syndrome mimicking acute viral hepatitis), a condition with a histologic picture indistinguishable from chronic active hepatitis, and granulomatous hepatitis. Skin rashes, eosinophilia, and fever may be present. In some cases, it has been postulated that a drug or metabolite binds to the liver cell membrane and acts as a **hapten.**

(1) **Isoniazid** causes a clinical condition that is similar to viral hepatitis and has been shown to be related to a metabolite.

(2) **Halothane** and other fluorinated anesthetics frequently cause only mild hepatitis or postoperative fever after first exposure but may cause fulminant hepatitis and death on reexposure.

(3) **Chlorpromazine** and **chlorpropamide** cause cholestatic jaundice. An inflammatory infiltrate that frequently includes eosinophils is shown on liver biopsy.

(4) **Diphenylhydantoin** causes a serum sickness–like syndrome, which may result in massive hepatic necrosis and death.

(5) **Methyldopa** may cause the clinical and histologic findings of chronic active hepatitis, and some authors believe that a metabolite is responsible.

(6) **Excess intake of vitamin A** (20,000–40,000 U/day) for years may cause cholestatic hepatic injury. Vitamin A is deposited in the Ito cells of the liver, and large deposits compress the sinusoids. Serum bilirubin and alkaline phosphatase levels may be elevated, prothrombin time may increase, and hepatic enzyme activity may be relatively normal. Over time, cirrhosis may result.

3. **Alcoholic liver disease** refers to the group of liver disorders caused by acute and chronic alcoholism. Acute effects include alcoholic fatty liver and alcoholic hepatitis. Chronic alcoholism is a major cause of cirrhosis of the liver, which is discussed in IX B 2 b. In the United States, alcoholic liver disease represents the fourth most common cause of death of adults 35–55 years old. It appears that alcohol consumption of less than 80 g/day in men and 40 g/day in (nonpregnant) women generally is not associated with alcoholic liver disease.

   a. **Alcoholic fatty liver** occurs because alcohol alters normal lipid metabolism. Most patients have hepatomegaly but otherwise are asymptomatic unless they have other systemic problems related to alcohol use (e.g., pancreatitis and delirium tremens). Laboratory abnormalities include increases in γ-glutamyl transpeptidase, serum transaminases, and alkaline phosphatase. Histologic examination shows large-droplet fatty change in the liver. The prognosis is excellent for patients who completely abstain from alcohol consumption.

   b. **Alcoholic hepatitis** is an acute syndrome that generally occurs in the setting of heavy alcohol consumption. Many patients are reported to have ingested more than 100 g of alcohol daily for more than 1 year. (Approximately 100 g of alcohol are contained in 8 ounces of 100-proof whiskey, in 30 ounces of wine, and in eight 12-ounce cans of beer.) The role of decreased vitamin and protein intake is controversial.

      (1) **Clinical features** include fever, jaundice, hepatomegaly, and liver tenderness. Ascites, encephalopathy, and variceal bleeding occasionally are present.

      (2) **Laboratory data** include leukocytosis, increased AST (usually less than 350 IU/ml), elevated serum bilirubin, decreased serum albumin, and a modest increase in serum alkaline phosphatase. Occasionally, a cholestatic phase is present with marked elevations in the alkaline phosphatase and direct bilirubin. The ALT almost always is lower than the AST due to decreased pyridoxine intake and conversion to pyridoxal phosphate. Alcohol-induced thrombocytopenia is present in 10% of patients.

      (3) **Diagnosis** is based on liver biopsy that reveals large-droplet fatty liver, polymorphonuclear infiltration, alcoholic hyaline (Mallory bodies), hepatocyte necrosis, and, occasionally, sclerosis of central veins.

      (4) **Therapy** is supportive and includes a daily diet of 2500–3000 kcal with supplemental B vitamins (especially thiamine) and folate. Absolute abstinence from alcohol is crucial. Propylthiouracil and corticosteroids have a controversial therapeutic role but may be useful in severe cases.

4. **Nonalcoholic steatohepatitis** is often associated with obesity, diabetes mellitus, intravenous hyperalimentation, or jejunoileal bypass surgery. The liver is fatty on biopsy, and Mallory bodies are occasionally observed. There is a modest increase in

transaminase levels (twofold to fourfold above normal). Although initially thought to be benign, prolonged steatohepatitis may lead to cirrhosis. Treatment is with removal of the offending agent or, in the case of obesity, weight loss. Loss of approximately 10% of body fat may result in decreased hepatic enzyme elevation.

B. **Chronic liver disease**

1. **Chronic active hepatitis** most commonly is caused by viral infection or drugs. When not associated with either of these etiologies, chronic active hepatitis generally is thought to be immunologically mediated, although an immunologic mechanism has not been proven. This form of chronic active hepatitis sometimes is called lupoid hepatitis (but idiopathic autoimmune hepatitis is the more appropriate term), because the typical patient is a young woman with elevated antinuclear antibody.

   a. **Clinical features** include malaise, fatigue, and vasculitis. As the disease progresses, the clinical picture is dominated by manifestations of chronic liver disease, including ascites, encephalopathy, and variceal bleeding.

   b. **Diagnosis** is based on liver biopsy that shows piecemeal necrosis and bridging fibrosis. The serum transaminases are persistently elevated to levels that often are 10 times the normal levels. Elevated antinuclear antibody is present in 50% of patients, and anti–smooth muscle antibody is found in 75%.

   c. **Therapy** with high-dose corticosteroids, azathioprine, or both is beneficial in the immune-mediated type of chronic hepatitis but usually not in the drug- and virus-associated diseases. Interferon (3–5 million units three times weekly) has been shown to decrease evidence of hepatitis B and C viral activity in 30%–60% of cases. Lamivudine may eliminate or decrease hepatitis B virus activity, but recurrence may occur after withdrawal of therapy. Studies with ribavirin and α-interferon are ongoing. Treatment of the idiopathic autoimmune type of chronic active hepatitis is continued until the serum transaminase levels decline to less than twice the normal levels and a repeat liver biopsy shows resolution of the inflammation (generally after a period of more than 1–2 years).

2. **Cirrhosis of the liver**

   a. **Overview of pathology.** Two basic types of liver cirrhosis occur, but the sine qua non of all cirrhotic liver disease is the presence of fibrosis with the formation of nodules that lack a central vein.

      (1) **Chronic sclerosing cirrhosis** is characterized by minimal regenerative activity of the hepatocytes, resulting in fibrosis without substantial nodule formation. The liver is small and hard.

      (2) **Nodular cirrhosis** is characterized by regenerative activity and the appearance of numerous fine nodules. The liver initially may be quite large.

   b. **Alcohol-induced cirrhosis.** Chronic alcohol abuse causes cirrhosis of the liver (Laennec's cirrhosis), which, in most cases, is thought to be a sequela of alcoholic hepatitis. The clinical features of alcohol-induced cirrhosis reflect impaired blood flow through the liver due to obstruction by fibrotic bands, resulting in portal hypertension, and to a decrease in hepatocytes available for metabolic functions. Long-term alcohol use also may be directly toxic to the testis, resulting in testicular atrophy and impotence. These effects are compounded in men by increased peripheral levels of estrogens, which cause spider angiomata, gynecomastia, and palmar erythema. Complications of alcohol-induced cirrhosis are as follow.

      (1) **Ascites**

         (a) **Pathogenesis.** Increased back pressure into capillaries as well as decreased oncotic pressure because of decreased albumin synthesis allow accumulation of a transudative fluid in the peritoneal cavity. In addition, increased circulating aldosterone (possibly secondary to altered liver metabolism) contributes to Na^+ and water retention.

         (b) **Diagnosis** may be obvious on physical examination if fluid accumulation is large. Ultrasonography is effective for detecting small amounts of fluid. Paracentesis, which may require guidance through ultrasonography, yields a straw-colored fluid with less than 2.5 g/dl of protein, a white blood cell count of less than 300/μl (usually mononuclear), a normal glucose level, and a low serum amylase level. A serum albumin to ascites albumin greater than 1.1 g/dl is indicative of portal hypertension.

(c) Therapy is based on sodium restriction (usually 500 mg/24 hr) and bed rest (to decrease endogenous aldosterone production). Fluid restriction may be necessary if hyponatremia develops. Aldosterone antagonists (e.g., spironolactone) and other mild diuretics are used if initial measures fail. Large-volume paracentesis can be used, and 10 g of albumin should be replaced intravenously for each 1 L of ascitic fluid removed. Because peritoneal lymphatics have a limited ability to mobilize ascites, weight loss should be limited to 2 lb/day unless peripheral edema exists. Surgical shunting (Le Veen or Denver shunt) can be useful in recalcitrant cases, but bacteremia and disseminated intravascular coagulation (DIC) are potential complications of these shunts. Placement of a **transjugular intrahepatic portosystemic (TIP) shunt** to connect the hepatic and portal veins can reduce portal hypertension and relieve ascites.

(d) Complications include respiratory compromise and rupture of the umbilicus in cases of massive ascites. Infection of even a small amount of fluid (e.g., due to spontaneous bacterial peritonitis) can be fatal.

(2) Varices occur due to the development of collateral vessels that bypass the obstructed liver. Varices are common in the esophagus and somewhat less common in the stomach and hemorrhoidal plexus.

(a) Diagnosis of esophagogastric varices may be suggested by an upper gastrointestinal series but is best made by endoscopy. Endoscopy is essential in the acutely bleeding patient because the mortality rate is high (40%–50% for each episode of bleeding) and early treatment can be lifesaving.

(b) Short-term therapy with vasopressin by continuous intravenous infusion (usually in conjunction with nitroglycerin to decrease complications) is effective in 60% of patients. Somatostatin has been used acutely. Balloon tamponade with a Sengstaken-Blakemore tube controls bleeding in 80% of patients but is associated with a risk of aspiration and esophageal rupture. Emergency surgery has a 50% mortality rate. Endoscopic sclerotherapy or endoscopic rubber banding is effective in approximately 80%–90% of acute cases. A TIP shunt can stop variceal bleeding.

(c) Long-term therapy to reduce the chance of rebleeding includes multiple endoscopic sclerotherapy or variceal rubber banding procedures to obliterate all varices and nonselective β-adrenergic blockers (e.g., propranolol, nadolol) to reduce portal pressure. Surgical portal decompression decreases the frequency of bleeding but does not increase survival rates because there is increased encephalopathy and liver failure. In Japan, devascularization of the distal esophagus and proximal stomach (Sugiura procedure) has been effective. Liver transplantation is reserved for good-risk alcohol-abstinent individuals.

(3) Portosystemic encephalopathy is a reversible neurologic syndrome characterized by mood changes, confusion, drowsiness, disorientation, and coma.

(a) Etiology. The primary cause of hepatic encephalopathy is unclear. Elevated ammonia levels are found in the blood. More recently implicated, however, are false neurotransmitters and elevated levels of mercaptans and fatty acids. Increased levels of endogenous benzodiazepine substances may be noted. In addition, increased levels of aromatic amino acids and decreased levels of branched-chain amino acids are found in the blood, brain, and urine. Secondary causes of hepatic encephalopathy are thought to include:

(i) Azotemia, due to increased nitrogen load

      (ii) Constipation, which causes increased ammonia production and absorption due to prolonged contact of intestinal contents with the gastrointestinal tract

      (iii) Increased dietary protein, which causes increased production of ammonia and other nitrogenous wastes

      (iv) Gastrointestinal bleeding, which delivers a protein load to the gastrointestinal tract

      (v) Hypokalemia

      (vi) Alkalosis, which together with hypokalemia leads to impaired renal excretion of ammonia and to increased transfer of ammonia across the blood–brain barrier

      (vii) Infection, which leads to increased tissue catabolism and increased protein load

      (viii) Sedatives, whose direct depressant effect on the brain is compounded by decreased hepatic catabolism of the drugs

  (b) Therapy includes reversal of any of the secondary causes. In addition:

      (i) Lactulose effectively decreases colonic pH and traps ammonium ion (NH_4^+) in the gastrointestinal tract. It also is an effective cathartic.

      (ii) Neomycin decreases intestinal flora, which convert gastrointestinal proteins into ammonia.

      (iii) Dietary protein should be limited to less than 40 g/day.

      (iv) The use of branched-chain amino acids, although academically appealing, may not improve encephalopathy.

(4) Hepatorenal syndrome is a progressive renal failure that occurs in patients with severe liver disease. It is a functional renal failure because the kidneys are morphologically normal and function well when transplanted into normal recipients. The mortality rate in hepatorenal syndrome is 90%–100%.

  (a) Etiology. Although the exact mechanism of hepatorenal syndrome is not known, several factors are implicated, including:

      (i) Afferent arteriolar vasoconstriction, which leads to increased renal vascular constriction

      (ii) Relative shunting of blood from the cortex to the medulla of the kidney

      (iii) Decreased glomerular filtration rate

      (iv) Decreased renal blood flow

  (b) Diagnosis is suggested by the combination of oliguria (i.e., urine output of less than 300 ml/24 hr) with increasing blood urea nitrogen and creatinine concentrations in a patient with severe liver disease. Additional laboratory findings include urinary Na^+ concentration of less than 10 mEq/L and benign urine sediment. It is important to rule out other causes of oliguria (e.g., acute tubular necrosis, hypovolemia, and urinary tract obstruction).

  (c) Therapy generally is unsuccessful. A fluid challenge should be given to all patients to rule out hypovolemia. Success occasionally has been reported with Le Veen or Denver shunts, portacaval shunts, or liver transplantation. No drugs have been shown to be beneficial.

(5) Coagulation defects usually are due to decreased hepatic synthesis of clotting factors. In addition, splenomegaly may contribute to thrombocytopenia.

(6) Hepatopulmonary syndrome is a hypoxic state most likely caused by intrapulmonary vascular shunting (effectively, a right to left shunt). Exercise or standing-induced hypoxia is noted and clubbing may be present in severe cases. This syndrome is probably present in 30% of patients with cirrhosis and may be severe in 10% of patients.

c. Nonalcoholic cirrhosis may be caused by a variety of disease processes and toxins but, in general, has clinical features that are similar to those of alcohol-induced cirrhosis.

(1) Primary biliary cirrhosis is a disease of unknown etiology. The usual patient age at diagnosis is 40–60 years, and 90% of patients are women.

    (a) Pathogenesis. The mechanism of primary biliary cirrhosis is thought to be immunologic and involves inflammatory destruction of small intrahepatic biliary ducts. Early histologic changes include lymphocytic infiltration and periductal granuloma formation. Later in the disease process, the portal areas may show an absence of ducts.

    (b) Clinical features

        (i) There is a lack of symptoms early in the course of this disease. However, an early diagnosis often is suspected on the basis of a marked increase in the alkaline phosphatase level noted on routine biochemical screening.

        (ii) The first symptom usually is pruritus, which may be devastatingly severe, especially at night.

        (iii) Jaundice occurs in later stages of the disease, as do osteopenia (in 25% of patients) and xanthomas (in approximately 10% of patients).

        (iv) In addition, primary biliary cirrhosis is associated with such conditions as Sjögren's syndrome (in 75% of patients), the presence of antithyroid antibody (in 25% of patients), rheumatoid arthritis (in 5% of patients), and the CREST syndrome—calcinosis, Raynaud's phenomenon, esophageal motility dysfunction, sclerodactyly, and telangiectasia—(in 3% of patients).

    (c) Diagnosis is made by the constellation of increased serum cholesterol, markedly increased alkaline phosphatase (four to six times the normal level), increased direct bilirubin, and the presence of a positive antimitochondrial antibody, which is found in more than 90% of patients. The liver biopsy shows characteristic changes. Extrahepatic biliary obstruction must be ruled out.

    (d) Therapy is supportive and includes administration of antipruritic agents and supplementation of vitamins D and K and calcium as well as aminobiphosphonate for prevention of osteoporosis. MCTs, which do not require bile salt micelles for adsorption, may be used as a dietary supplement. The pruritus may respond to cholestyramine, which binds bile salts in the intestine. Results have been achieved with certain drugs (i.e., azathioprine, chlorambucil, colchicine, methotrexate). Perhaps the most promising medical treatment is ursodeoxycholic acid, which may improve hepatic structure and function if initiated before advanced stages of the disease. Intravenous naloxone therapy may be useful for severe pruritus. Standard definitive surgery is liver transplantation, with 5-year survival rates of 70% in most series.

(2) Secondary biliary cirrhosis usually occurs after several years of biliary tract obstruction.

    (a) Etiology includes common bile duct stones, common duct strictures, cholangiocarcinoma, ampullar carcinoma, sclerosing cholangitis, and chronic pancreatitis with compression of the common duct as it traverses the pancreatic head.

    (b) Clinical features are similar to those of primary biliary cirrhosis but may be superseded by manifestations of the underlying disease. In addition, patients may develop cholangitis with shaking chills, fever, leukocytosis, and jaundice. Antimitochondrial antibodies usually are not present.

    (c) Therapy is aimed at relieving the obstruction and includes surgery, external drainage, and placement of an indwelling stent.

d. Cardiac cirrhosis is a rare, late manifestation of severe prolonged right ventricular failure, which is most often seen with rheumatic heart disease (either mitral or aortic stenosis with tricuspid regurgitation). Constrictive pericarditis and severe cardiomyopathy also may be associated with cardiac cirrhosis. Clinical features include an enlarged liver, ascites, and splenomegaly. Prothrombin time often is prolonged and precludes the use of anticoagulants in treatment of the valvular lesion. Prognosis depends on the course of the cardiac disease.

e. **Other causes of cirrhosis** include Wilson's disease, α_1-antitrypsin deficiency, hemochromatosis, drug-induced liver disease, and virus-induced cirrhosis of the liver.

f. **Vascular problems mimicking cirrhosis**
   (1) **Budd-Chiari syndrome,** or **hepatic vein thrombosis,** is associated with hypercoagulable states, pregnancy, tumors, abdominal trauma, and use of oral contraceptives. Patients usually have ascites, and liver biopsy shows centrilobular congestion. Doppler ultrasound examination may show decreased or absent flow in the hepatic vein. Attempts to catheterize the hepatic vein often are unsuccessful, and the mortality rate is 50%–90%. In acute Budd-Chiari syndrome (within 1 week of onset) treatment with streptokinase or thromboplastin activating factor may be beneficial. Side-to-side portacaval shunts may prolong survival. Liver transplantation may be required.
   (2) **Splenic vein thrombosis** is due to abdominal trauma, pancreatitis, and tumor. Although the portal vein remains patent, gastric varices develop as splenic vein collaterals. Both esophageal and gastric varices develop in 15% of cases. Diagnosis is made by angiography, and therapy with splenectomy is curative.
   (3) **Veno-occlusive disease,** a disease of small hepatic vessels, may follow hepatic radiation (greater than 3500 cGy), azathioprine therapy, or ingestion of certain types of Jamaican tea. After bone marrow transplantation, veno-occlusive disease is seen in approximately 20% of patients.

g. **Nodular transformation of the liver** is a noncirrhotic cause of portal hypertension characterized by the unexplained development of small nodules, especially in the perihilar area. Recurrent variceal bleeding may occur.

3. **Liver abscess**
   a. **Amebic liver abscess.** Of the six *Entamoeba* species found in the human colon, *E. histolytica* is the only true pathogen. In the United States, homosexual men and institutionalized individuals are at greatest risk for amebic liver abscess. This disease also is common where diarrheal disease due to *E. histolytica* is endemic.
      (1) **Clinical features** include right upper quadrant pain and fever. Pleuritic pain, chills, and night sweats also may be noted. There is a history of intestinal amebiasis in 50% of patients.
      (2) **Laboratory data.** More than 50% of patients have elevated white blood cell counts ($>20,000/\mu l$), serum transaminase levels, and serum bilirubin levels. Serum alkaline phosphatase levels are abnormal in approximately 80% of affected individuals.
      (3) **Diagnosis** is suggested by a filling defect demonstrated in the liver through the use of gallium scanning. Ultrasonography and CT also may be helpful in the diagnosis of amebic liver abscess. Aspiration of a cystic cavity may reveal "anchovy paste" fluid with trophozoites. Serologic tests (e.g., the indirect hemagglutination and gel diffusion tests) are positive in 95% of cases.
      (4) **Therapy** with amebicides (e.g., metronidazole, chloroquine, and diiodohydroxyquin) may be effective alone or may be combined with CT-directed aspiration of the abscess cavity. Liver scanning should be continued until healing occurs.
      (5) **Complications** include rupture of the cyst into the pleural space, lung, bowel, and retroperitoneum. Rarely, a cyst extends to the body surface.
   b. **Pyogenic liver abscess** usually is due to biliary tract disease, including acute cholecystitis and cholangitis. Other infections (e.g., appendicitis and diverticulitis) as well as intrinsic hepatic lesions also are important causes. In 10% of cases, the etiologic factor cannot be determined. Approximately 70% of ab-

scesses contain mixed flora; the most commonly found organisms are anaerobes, *E. coli, Klebsiella* species, *Staphylococcus aureus,* and streptococci.

(1) **Clinical features** include fever, chills, right upper quadrant pain, anorexia, and nausea. Pleuritic pain occasionally occurs, and weight loss is common. Tender hepatomegaly is present in 50% of cases. The alkaline phosphatase level is elevated in approximately 80% of patients, jaundice is present in approximately 33%, and blood cultures are positive in 40%. CT combined with liver scanning, ultrasonography, or both can be used to detect an abscess greater than 2 cm.

(2) **Diagnosis** is suggested by the clinical presentation and can be confirmed by CT- or ultrasonography-guided aspiration.

(3) **Therapy.** Antibiotics, with or without external drainage, frequently are successful and necessary for multiple small abscesses. Treatment usually is continued for 4–6 weeks. Occasionally, surgical drainage is required.

c. **Focal hepatic candidiasis** is an entity consisting of hepatic and splenic granulomas containing *Candida albicans* hyphae in immunocompromised hosts. Most patients have previously received cytosine arabinoside for acute leukemia.

(1) **Clinical features** include a fever of unknown origin in an immunocompromised host. Signs of oropharyngeal candidiasis may be present, and there may be right upper quadrant pain or tenderness.

(2) **Diagnosis** is made by **liver biopsy.** At laparotomy or laparoscopy, small white nodules less than 5 mm in width are seen. Liver function abnormalities include modest bilirubin and enzyme elevation with an increase in alkaline phosphatase.

(3) **Therapy** consists of systemic amphotericin B, often in conjunction with fluconazole.

4. **Hepatic cysts**

a. **Solitary cysts,** generally found in the right lobe of the liver, usually are asymptomatic but may cause pain and fever secondary to bleeding, infection, or rupture.

b. **Polycystic liver disease** is the presence of multiple cysts that range from several millimeters to greater than 10–15 cm in diameter. Like solitary cysts, most cysts in polycystic liver disease are asymptomatic except in cases involving hemorrhage, infection, or rupture. Renal cysts are found in 50% of patients; cysts also may be found in the pancreas, spleen, and lungs. Results of liver function testing usually are normal, although mild elevation of serum alkaline phosphatase levels may be seen. Surgical aspiration or decompression occasionally is necessary.

c. **Hydatid cysts.** This disease is most common in Greece, France, Italy, South America, and Iceland and may be found elsewhere in the descendants of individuals from these regions.

(1) **Etiology.** Hydatid cysts are formed when the infecting organism (i.e., *Echinococcus granulosus* or *Echinococcus multilocularis*) is ingested and travels via the portal circulation to the liver.

(2) **Clinical features.** The cyst usually enlarges for 10–20 years after the initial infection before becoming symptomatic. There is calcification of a solitary cyst (seen in 50% of patients) and the presence of daughter cysts within a larger cyst.

(3) **Diagnosis** is made by positive complement fixation or indirect hemagglutination tests. Eosinophilia is occasionally seen. Liver biopsy and aspiration are not suggested because leakage may cause fatal anaphylaxis.

(4) **Therapy** is surgical.

(5) **Complications** include rupture, infection, hemorrhage, and slow leakage causing allergic manifestations.

d. **Peliosis hepatis** is a rare condition involving multiple blood-filled hepatic cysts. The liver often has a mottled blue appearance. Rupture with bleeding may be fatal. There is an association between this condition and tuberculosis, therapy with androgenic steroids, and the use of oral contraceptives. There is also an association with AIDS patients, especially those with angiomatosis (*Rochenellia*). Progressive hepatomegaly with liver failure may occur. CT scanning may reveal multiple defects. Percutaneous liver biopsy reveals characteristic changes but is dangerous because of the vascular nature of the lesions.

5. Granulomatous hepatitis

   a. Etiology. Granulomatous hepatitis most often is secondary to systemic infections (e.g., tuberculosis), sarcoidosis, fungal infections, syphilis, and viral infections (e.g., infectious mononucleosis, CMV infection, and varicella). Q fever, parasitic diseases, Hodgkin's disease, and beryllium toxicity also may cause granulomatous hepatitis. In addition, granulomatous hepatitis may be a manifestation of drug reactions involving phenylbutazone, sulfa drugs, hydralazine, or allopurinol. Occasionally, no cause can be found.

   b. Clinical features. Symptoms include weakness, fatigue, markedly increased erythrocyte sedimentation rate, and fever.

   c. Diagnosis is made by liver biopsy.

   d. Therapy for the secondary form of granulomatous hepatitis includes withdrawal of the offending agent and treatment of the underlying lesion. The idiopathic form may respond to corticosteroid therapy.

C. **Systemic diseases with prominent liver involvement**

   1. α_1-Antitrypsin deficiency is a genetic defect of the glycoprotein that normally inhibits proteolytic enzymes such as trypsin, chymotrypsin, and elastase. There are 24 alleles in the protease inhibitor (Pi) system. Ninety percent of the population of the United States is phenotype PiMM. The 22 genotype is homozygous for the disease state, and patients have less than 20% of normal serum levels of α_1-antitrypsin. Individuals with phenotype PiMZ have approximately 50%–60% of normal levels. Homozygotes (PiZZ) usually have liver disease in childhood. Liver disease may develop in PiSZ or PiMZ heterozygotes, especially those who smoke, and COPD may develop in them as adults (see Chapter 2 II B). Disease does not develop in all individuals with the abnormal genotypes. Diagnosis is made based on a decreased α_1-globulin level observed on a protein electrophoresis, a decreased α_1-antitrypsin level in the serum, and by Pi typing. Liver biopsy reveals diastase-resistant PAS-positive globules in portal areas. There is no effective therapy. Liver transplantation may be used in advanced cases.

   2. Amyloidosis involves the liver in 50% of cases. Patients have hepatomegaly on physical examination but usually are asymptomatic. Results of liver function testing often are normal but may reveal a marked elevation of serum alkaline phosphatase.

   3. Hemochromatosis is an inherited disorder (thought to be autosomal recessive) in which increased absorption of iron leads to iron deposition in the liver, heart, pancreas, and other organs. Men are more commonly affected than women (at a ratio of 8:1). In the United States, approximately 8%–9% of the population are heterozygotes and 1 in every 220 are homozygotes, making hemochromatosis one of the most common genetic liver diseases.

   a. Clinical features include hepatomegaly, hyperpigmentation, and abnormalities of the cardiac conduction system, testes, and joints. Fifty percent of the patients have abdominal pain. Cirrhosis and diabetes also may develop.

   b. Laboratory findings include elevated levels of serum transaminases, increased serum iron with elevated percent saturation (generally greater than 80%), and high serum level of ferritin. HLA haplotypes associated with primary hemochromatosis include A3, B7, and B14. Liver biopsy shows iron deposits in both hepatocytes and Kupffer cells. This finding rules out secondary iron overload (hemosiderosis) in which iron is deposited in Kupffer cells alone. A skin or intestinal biopsy as well as an analysis of family members for elevated iron, total iron-binding capacity, or ferritin levels also may be helpful in the differential diagnosis. Screening family members for the elevated HLA haplotypes may be used. CT or magnetic resonance imaging (MRI) of the liver shows characteristic changes.

c. Therapy. Repeated phlebotomy (usually once or twice weekly for several months or years) decreases total body iron stores, which may be at 10 times the normal level. Phlebotomy is continued until anemia develops or serum iron and ferritin levels normalize. Untreated patients have an increased risk of hepatoma.

d. Prognosis. If hemochromatosis is diagnosed before cirrhosis develops, the prognosis with treatment is good (80% survival at 15 years). If cirrhosis or diabetes mellitus is present at the time of diagnosis, or if the iron stores do not decrease to normal levels after 18 months of treatment, the prognosis is not as favorable. Patients with hemochromatosis and cirrhosis have approximately a 220-fold increased risk of liver cancer.

4. **Sarcoidosis.** Approximately 70% of patients with sarcoidosis have granulomas in the liver. Patients usually do not have symptoms referable to the liver but may have increased serum alkaline phosphatase levels. Forty percent of patients have hepatomegaly. A liver biopsy showing noncaseating granulomas may aid in the diagnosis.

5. **Wilson's disease** is an autosomal recessive disease characterized by excessive copper deposition, which, if untreated, may lead to fulminant hepatic failure. Copper also is deposited in the brain, kidney, and cornea; copper depositions in the cornea cause **Kayser-Fleischer rings.** CNS disease may be prominent if the diagnosis is made in adulthood. Diagnosis is suggested by decreased serum ceruloplasmin levels, and increased urinary copper excretion (>100 μg/24 hr); it is confirmed by an increased hepatic copper concentration in a liver biopsy sample. Treatment is with d-penicillamine and chelating agents. Hepatic transplantation has been used for fulminant hepatic failure.

6. **Liver disease of pregnancy**
   a. **Cholestasis** usually is seen in the last trimester of pregnancy and is benign. Patients may complain of pruritus and jaundice, and all symptoms disappear rapidly after delivery of the baby. The syndrome is thought to be mediated by estrogens, progesterone, or both, and subsequent use of oral contraceptives or pregnancy may cause a recurrence of symptoms. Recently, ursodeoxycholic acid therapy has relieved pruritus and allowed the delay of delivery for greater fetal maturity.
   b. **Acute fatty liver** is a severe disease usually occurring in a primigravida in the last trimester of pregnancy. Fulminant liver failure may develop, and an association with toxemia has been reported. Prognosis is poor but is improved by prompt delivery. Pathologic changes in the liver include small-droplet fatty change similar to that seen in fatty liver induced by tetracycline and valproic acid.
   c. **HELLP syndrome** is characterized by hemolysis, elevated liver enzymes, and a low platelet count. It is often seen in the third trimester of pregnancy and is associated with toxemia in approximately 50% of patients. Abdominal pain and vomiting may be severe. The treatment is delivery of the baby.
   d. **Hepatic rupture.** Rarely, there may be hepatic rupture after necrosis of the liver occurs in eclamptic patients in their last trimester. Patients with hepatic rupture have generally been older and multiparous.

D. **Inherited disorders of bilirubin metabolism**

1. **Gilbert's syndrome** is an essentially benign condition that occurs in approximately 7% of the population of the United States. Decreased uridine diphosphate (UDP) glucuronyl transferase activity leads to mild unconjugated hyperbilirubinemia (usually less than 3 mg/dl), which increases after fasting.

2. **Crigler-Najjar syndrome** exists in two forms:
   a. **Type I** is rare and is characterized by an absence of hepatic UDP glucuronyl transferase activity. Patients usually die in infancy.
   b. **Type II** also is rare and is characterized by markedly diminished hepatic UDP glucuronyl transferase activity, leading to unconjugated hyperbilirubinemia in

the range of 5–25 mg/dl. Phenobarbital may be used to induce microsomal enzyme activity. In most cases, there are no clinical sequelae.

3. **Rotor's syndrome** is a rare autosomal recessive condition. Impaired transport of conjugated bilirubin out of the hepatocyte leads to conjugated hyperbilirubinemia in the range of 2–10 mg/dl. The liver biopsy is normal, and the clinical course is benign.

4. **Dubin-Johnson syndrome** is similar to Rotor's syndrome, except that liver biopsy shows the accumulation of a dark pigment within hepatocytes. The elevated serum bilirubin may respond somewhat to phenobarbital therapy.

5. **Alagille's syndrome** is one of various types of familial intrahepatic cholestasis syndromes. Alagille's syndrome is an autosomal dominant syndrome that is generally identified in infants younger than 3 months of age. It is associated with congenital heart disease (ventricular or atrial septal defects), bony defects (butterfly vertebra or spina bifida), and renal or biliary tree anomalies. There are classic cholestatic laboratory test findings, and few bile ducts are seen on liver biopsy. Most patients have mild disease, but cirrhosis develops later in approximately 10% of these patients.

E. **Tumors of the liver**

1. **Benign tumors**
   a. **Hepatic adenomas** usually occur in women of childbearing age and are more common in those who use oral contraceptives.
      (1) **Clinical features** may be completely absent. Some patients report right upper quadrant fullness. Occasionally, spontaneous rupture of the adenoma leads to intra-abdominal hemorrhage, which is fatal in 25% of patients.
      (2) **Diagnosis** is made by demonstration of a hepatic mass by CT and a cold spot through liver scanning. Results of liver function testing are normal, and serum α-fetoprotein is normal. Because the tumors are hypervascular, liver biopsy is not suggested.
      (3) **Therapy** includes discontinuing the use of oral contraceptives and monitoring tumor size to document regression. If regression does not occur, the tumor should be removed surgically to prevent rupture.
   b. **Focal nodular hyperplasia** also occurs primarily in women; the theory that this lesion is associated with oral contraceptive use is controversial. The lesion is composed of central connective tissue with radiating septa, which divide the mass into nodules. Liver scanning may not reveal an abnormality because all the elements of liver tissue, including Kupffer cells, are present. However, CT and angiography demonstrate a hypervascular mass. The clinical course is benign. There is no potential for malignant transformation, and hemorrhage, rupture, and necrosis are rare.
   c. **Hemangiomas** are the most common benign tumors of the liver and are found at autopsy in 5%–7% of patients. Women are affected more commonly than men.
      (1) **Clinical features** usually are absent. Large lesions may be associated with thrombocytopenia and hypofibrinogenemia, especially in infants. Hemangiomas also may be associated with telangiectasia of other organs.
      (2) **Diagnosis** is made by angiography, rapid-sequence CT, MRI, or SPECT liver scan. Abdominal radiographs may show calcification. Liver scanning shows a cold spot, which ultrasonography reveals a solid mass. Hemangiomas usually are single but may be multiple.
      (3) **Therapy** usually is not necessary. However, corticosteroid therapy, radiotherapy, and embolization all have been shown to be effective in decreasing the size of large hemangiomas.

2. **Malignant tumors**
   a. **Primary hepatocellular carcinoma (hepatoma)** occurs five times more frequently in men than in women and accounts for approximately 2.5% of all malignancies in the United States. In parts of South Africa and Asia, hepatoma

may account for 50% of all carcinomas. The peak age of incidence is 40–60 years.

(1) **Etiology** is not known, but the following risk factors are noted.

    (a) **Cirrhosis** is present in 75%–90% of patients. Patients with a history of postnecrotic or alcohol-induced cirrhosis, hemochromatosis, or α_1-antitrypsin deficiency are at higher risk than patients with a history of primary biliary cirrhosis, cardiac cirrhosis, or Wilson's disease. Patients with a history of hemochromatosis have a risk for hepatoma increased 220 times if cirrhosis is present. Children with hereditary tyrosinemia have a 40% risk of hepatoma.

    (b) **Previous infection with hepatitis B or C.** Serologic markers are found in a high percentage of patients with hepatoma. It is thought that the risk of hepatoma is increased 20-fold by infection with hepatitis B.

    (c) **Aflatoxin,** which is produced by the mold *Aspergillus flavus,* is a common contaminant of grain and peanuts in parts of Africa where there is a high incidence of hepatoma.

    (d) **Long-term androgen therapy** has been linked to the incidence of hepatoma.

    (e) **Schistosomiasis** and **clonorchiasis** are endemic in parts of the world where hepatoma is common (i.e., Africa and Japan).

(2) **Clinical features** include:

    (a) Hepatomegaly

    (b) Hepatic bruit or friction rub.

    (c) Ascites, which may be bloody (50% of patients)

    (d) Nonspecific symptoms such as malaise, anorexia, weight loss, and abdominal pain (approximately 33% of patients)

    (e) Clinical deterioration or sudden increase in the serum alkaline phosphatase in an otherwise stable cirrhotic patient

(3) **Diagnosis**

    (a) **Liver function testing** shows an elevated serum alkaline phosphatase level with only a modest elevation of the serum transaminases.

    (b) **Gallium scanning** reveals focal **filling defects.**

    (c) **Elevated α-fetoprotein.** The α-fetoprotein level is elevated in 75% of patients in the United States and in 85%–90% of patients in Africa and Japan.

    (d) **Angiography** reveals a hypervascular mass with a **tumor blush.**

    (e) **Liver biopsy** can be used to confirm the diagnosis but should be performed with caution because of the vascular nature of the lesions.

(4) **Therapy.** No effective treatment exists, and average survival is less than 6 months after the time of diagnosis.

    (a) **Surgery** can be attempted if the tumor is confined to one lobe of the liver, and it is associated with a 5-year survival rate of less than 10%. If the lesion is localized and less than 3 cm in diameter, a 50% success rate for resectional surgery has been reported. **Transplantation** with adjuvant chemotherapy may be undertaken if invasion of the major vessels has not occurred. Results are not clear.

    (b) Patients only rarely respond to **radiotherapy** or **chemotherapy,** although radiolabeled transferrin treatment has been recently reported to be effective in certain cases.

b. **Angiosarcoma** is a rare vascular tumor, accounting for 2% of hepatic malignancies. Angiosarcoma generally is seen in men aged 50–70 years.

(1) **Etiology.** There is a strong correlation between the incidence of angiosarcoma and a history of exposure to vinyl chloride, arsenic, or Thorotrast (a radiologic contrast medium no longer in use). The tumor may be discovered as late as 10–25 years after exposure.

(2) **Clinical features** are nonspecific. This tumor has a tendency to rupture or bleed spontaneously, and hemoperitoneum is noted in 15% of patients.

(3) **Diagnosis** is based on liver function tests showing an elevated serum alkaline phosphatase level, liver scanning showing a defect, and arteriography

showing a vascular tumor. Because fatal hemorrhage has been reported after closed liver biopsy, an open procedure always should be used to obtain tissue for definitive diagnosis.

c. **Metastatic disease** is much more common than primary hepatic malignancy. Only lymph nodes are more commonly involved by metastatic disease than the liver. Up to 50% of patients dying from malignant disease have liver involvement. The most common primary tumors showing spread to the liver are carcinomas of the gastrointestinal tract, malignant melanoma, and carcinomas of the pancreas, lung, breast, kidney, and ovary. Ocular malignant melanomas most commonly metastasize to the liver. In addition, lymphoma commonly involves the liver.

(1) **Clinical features** include fever, right upper quadrant pain, and hepatomegaly. A friction rub may be present over the liver. Jaundice may be directly due to hepatic involvement or to nodal compression in the porta hepatis (especially in colonic, breast, and bronchogenic carcinomas and in lymphoma).

(2) **Diagnosis** is suggested by an elevated serum alkaline phosphatase level and by abnormal findings obtained through ultrasonography, liver scanning, CT portography, or MRI; the diagnosis is confirmed by liver biopsy. A blind biopsy is positive in 65% of patients, and yield can be increased by making multiple passes and by using guidance by CT or ultrasonography. Aspiration cytology also can be used to establish the diagnosis.

(3) **Therapy** depends only on the underlying tumor type. Lymphoma may respond to systemic radiation and chemotherapy, and malignancies of the breast and ovary may respond to hormone manipulation. Perfusion of chemotherapeutic agents directly into the hepatic artery may be useful for some tumors. Occasionally, patients with solitary metastatic lesions may be cured by resection or by the use of cryosurgery. The outlook for most patients with metastatic disease, however, is grim, with a median survival of 3 months.

X. DISEASES OF THE PERITONEUM, MESENTERY, AND ABDOMINAL VASCULATURE

A. Diseases of the peritoneum

1. **Ascites** refers to the accumulation of fluid in the peritoneal cavity.
   a. **Pathogenesis.** The following mechanisms lead to ascites formation:
      (1) **Increased hydrostatic pressure,** which may be due to:
         (a) Cirrhosis
         (b) Hepatic vein occlusion (Budd-Chiari syndrome)
         (c) Inferior vena cava obstruction
         (d) Constrictive pericarditis
         (e) Congestive heart failure
      (2) **Decreased colloid osmotic pressure,** which may result from:
         (a) End-stage liver disease with poor protein synthesis
         (b) Nephrotic syndrome with protein loss
         (c) Malnutrition
         (d) Protein-losing enteropathy
      (3) **Increased permeability of peritoneal capillaries,** which may result from:
         (a) Tuberculous peritonitis
         (b) Bacterial peritonitis
         (c) Malignant disease of the peritoneum
      (4) **Leakage of fluid into the peritoneal cavity,** leading to:
         (a) Bile ascites
         (b) Pancreatic ascites (usually secondary to a leaking pseudocyst)

       (c) Chylous ascites (secondary to lymphatic duct disruption due to lymphoma or trauma)

       (d) Urine ascites

    (5) Miscellaneous causes, including:

       (a) Myxedema

       (b) Ovarian disease (Meigs' syndrome)

       (c) Chronic hemodialysis

b. Diagnosis. The presence of ascites usually is indicated on physical examination by abdominal distention, a fluid wave, or shifting dullness. Abdominal ultrasonography can reliably detect small amounts of fluid. Paracentesis can be performed with or without guidance by ultrasonography, and the ascitic fluid should be analyzed.

    (1) Total protein content greater than 2.5 g/dl is diagnostic of exudative ascites, which usually is seen in tumors, infections, and myxedema. If the serum albumin level minus the ascitic albumin level is less than 1, a tumor rather than infection may be the cause of the ascites.

    (2) The amylase concentration is elevated in pancreatic ascites.

    (3) The triglyceride concentration is elevated in chylous ascites.

    (4) Cytologic findings are frequently positive in malignancy.

    (5) A white blood cell count greater than $250/\mu l$ is suggestive of infection. If most cells are polymorphonuclear, bacterial infection should be suspected. When mononuclear cells predominate, tuberculosis or fungal infection is likely.

    (6) A red cell count greater than $50,000/\mu l$ denotes hemorrhagic ascites, which usually is due to malignancy, tuberculosis, or trauma. Hemorrhagic pancreatitis, a ruptured aortic aneurysm, and a ruptured hepatic adenoma may cause frank bleeding into the peritoneal cavity.

    (7) Gram staining and culture document bacterial infection.

    (8) A pH of less than 7 suggests bacterial infection.

c. Therapy depends on the underlying cause. Transudative ascites may be treated with bed rest, Na^+ restriction, and careful use of diuretics. Paracentesis of up to 1 L of fluid may provide relief of acute respiratory embarrassment secondary to tense ascites. Removal of more than 1 L at a time may lead to hypovolemia and shock, unless 10 g of albumin are replaced intravenously for each 1 L of ascitic fluid removed. A Le Veen or Denver shunt may be used for intractable or malignant ascites, but these shunts introduce high risks of infection and DIC. The TIPS procedure also has been shown to be useful in treating refractory ascites.

2. Bacterial peritonitis

  a. Pathogenesis

    (1) Primary or **spontaneous bacterial peritonitis** usually develops in the setting of preexisting ascites.

    (2) Secondary or **acute bacterial peritonitis** usually results from a perforated viscus, a ruptured appendix, an intestinal infarction, or ulcerative colitis.

  b. Clinical features include:

    (1) Abdominal pain, with or without guarding and rebound

    (2) Fever

    (3) Leukocytosis

    (4) Paralytic ileus

  c. Diagnosis

    (1) Paracentesis aids in determining whether the fluid is exudative or transudative, has an elevated white blood cell count (a predominance of polymorphonuclear cells is diagnostic), and can be cultured to identify the infecting organism. Inoculating an anaerobic culture tube with freshly drawn ascitic fluid (i.e., at the patient's bedside) and inoculation of blood culture bottles are often useful. If the initial ascitic fluid total protein content is less than 1.0 mg/dl, patients have an increased risk for spontaneous bacterial peritonitis.

    (2) Radiographic examination reveals free air under the diaphragm in the presence of a perforated viscus, may show a nonspecific ileus, or may show a hazy appearance consistent with ascites.

d. Therapy
   (1) Supportive measures include intravenous administration of fluids, correction of electrolyte abnormalities, and nasogastric suction.
   (2) Antimicrobial therapy includes ampicillin and an aminoglycoside to cover gram-negative organisms, pneumococcus, and other streptococci. (Anaerobes also are common offenders.)
   (3) Surgical intervention is necessary in cases of secondary bacterial peritonitis.

3. Other causes of peritonitis
   a. Bile peritonitis
      (1) Pathogenesis. Bile spillage into the peritoneal cavity (e.g., from a ruptured gallbladder or gallbladder puncture during liver biopsy) results in a chemical peritonitis.
      (2) Clinical features include severe abdominal pain and shock secondary to exudation of fluid from the damaged peritoneum.
      (3) Therapy is surgical after patients have been stabilized with intravenous volume replacement and correction of electrolyte abnormalities.
   b. Starch peritonitis
      (1) Pathogenesis. Approximately 2–4 weeks after abdominal surgery, granulomatous peritonitis develops if the peritoneal cavity has been contaminated with surgical glove powder (starch), lint from surgical drapes, particles of suture material, or talc.
      (2) Clinical features include abdominal pain, distention, tenderness, and fullness.
      (3) Diagnosis. Examination of the ascitic fluid under a polarized microscope shows starch granules termed **maltese crosses.** Laparoscopy reveals studding of the peritoneal surface.
      (4) Therapy is with corticosteroids or nonsteroidal anti-inflammatory agents.
   c. Gonococcal peritonitis (Fitz-Hugh-Curtis syndrome) usually is seen in young women and is due to an ascending infection originating in the pelvis. Chlamydia recently has been reported to cause an identical syndrome.
      (1) Clinical features, which mimic those of acute cholecystitis, include abdominal pain, fever, and right upper quadrant peritoneal signs. Occasionally, a hepatic friction rub is present.
      (2) Diagnosis. Laboratory tests show an elevated white blood cell count and mild abnormalities in liver function. Pelvic examination may reveal adnexal tenderness, and culture of cervical mucus usually is positive. Laparoscopy shows **violin-string adhesions** from the liver to either the right adnexa or the abdominal wall.
      (3) Therapy is ceftriaxone. If chlamydia also is present, tetracycline is given.

4. Subphrenic abscess refers to a collection of pus located inferior to the diaphragm and above the liver, spleen, or stomach.
   a. Pathogenesis. Abscess formation usually is a complication of diverticulitis, a ruptured appendix, a perforated ulcer, or an abdominal wound with peritoneal soiling. Occasionally, an abscess is seen after uncomplicated abdominal surgery.
   b. Clinical features include fever, leukocytosis, and abdominal and shoulder pain.
   c. Diagnosis may be suggested by a radiograph showing elevation of one hemidiaphragm but usually requires demonstration of the abscess cavity by CT or ultrasonography.
   d. Therapy is surgical drainage and broad-spectrum antibiotics to combat gram-negative as well as anaerobic organisms.

5. Tumors of the peritoneum
   a. Metastatic lesions are the most common peritoneal tumors. The primary lesion usually is adenocarcinoma of the gastrointestinal tract, pancreas, or ovary. However, sarcomas, lymphomas, leukemias, and carcinoid tumors all may involve the peritoneum.
      (1) Diagnosis is made by paracentesis showing an exudative fluid with a mod-

erately increased lymphocyte count and positive cytologic findings. Needle biopsy of the peritoneum also may be used.

(2) **Therapy** is directed at the underlying malignancy. Intraperitoneal injection of a sclerosing agent occasionally may be helpful.

b. Mesothelioma is seen most commonly in men older than 50 years of age and is associated with asbestos exposure.

(1) **Clinical features** include abdominal distention, abdominal pain, nausea, vomiting, and weight loss.

(2) **Diagnosis** requires demonstration of malignant cells through paracentesis with cytologic testing, needle biopsy, or laparotomy with biopsy.

(3) **Therapy** includes radiotherapy, chemotherapy, or both, but patient response usually is poor.

c. Pseudomyxoma peritonei is a rare condition characterized by the presence of thick gelatinous material in the peritoneal cavity.

(1) **Pathogenesis.** This condition results from the rupture of either an appendiceal mucocele or an ovarian mucinous cystadenoma. Some authors have reported the presence of low-grade malignancy in a high percentage of the underlying tumors.

(2) **Clinical features** include increasing abdominal girth without shifting dullness in an otherwise healthy individual.

(3) **Diagnosis** often requires laparotomy.

(4) **Therapy** is surgical removal of the mucinous material and underlying tumor.

B. **Diseases of the mesentery**

1. Mesenteric panniculitis (mesenteric Weber-Christian disease) is a rare condition usually seen in older men, which causes inflammation and fibrosis of the mesentery.

a. Pathogenesis is thought to involve overgrowth of normal fat tissue in the mesentery with subsequent degeneration, necrosis, and progression to fibrosis and scar formation. The initiating event may be ischemia, infection, or trauma.

b. Clinical features include crampy abdominal pain, fever, weight loss, nausea, and vomiting. Lymphatic obstruction may develop with resultant ascites, steatorrhea, and PLE.

c. Diagnosis requires laparotomy, which reveals a thickened fibrotic mesentery with fat necrosis and infiltration by foamy macrophages.

d. Therapy with corticosteroids or immunosuppressive drugs has varying results. In many patients, the process appears to be self-limited, and the prognosis is excellent.

2. Mesenteric cysts are congenital anomalies of the mesenteric lymphatic system, which occur as slowly enlarging, painless, round, smooth, mobile masses. Treatment is drainage or excision. Mesenteric cysts are benign but rarely may cause symptoms due to rupture, bleeding, or torsion.

3. Mesenteric adenitis generally is seen in children and young adults and mimics acute appendicitis.

a. Etiology. Mesenteric adenitis usually is caused by a viral infection; however, many cases are due to *Yersinia* infection.

b. Clinical features are abdominal pain (which may be severe), nausea, vomiting, and fever. Some patients have additional evidence of a viral infection (e.g., pharyngitis and myalgia).

c. Diagnosis usually is made at laparotomy for presumed appendicitis.

d. Therapy includes antibiotics, if *Yersinia* is identified, and supportive care.

C. **Diseases of the abdominal vasculature**

1. Abdominal aortic aneurysm usually manifests as an asymptomatic pulsatile mass, but some patients have abdominal pain, back pain, and leg ischemia. The cause usually is atherosclerosis. Leakage of blood into surrounding tissues with associated abdominal, back, or flank pain may precede overt rupture by several weeks. Rupture into the duodenum—occurring as massive gastrointestinal hemorrhage—or into the abdomen may be catastrophic. Treatment is surgical, with replacement of the aneurysm with an aortic graft made of Dacron or some other synthetic material. Postoperative aortoenteric fistulas with erosion of the graft into the duodenum (usually in the setting of an infected graft) may be seen several years after aneurysmectomy and may result in fatal bleeding if not recognized early.

2. **Acute mesenteric ischemia** is a classic syndrome of decreased blood supply, usually involving the superior mesenteric artery. Patients have advanced arteriosclerotic cardiovascular disease, often with a history of congestive failure, acute myocardial infarction, cerebrovascular disease, or peripherovascular disease. Many patients have taken splanchnic constricting agents such as digoxin. Embolic disease (which affects 25% of patients) often is associated with unstable cardiac rhythms. Thrombosis and nonocclusive mesenteric ischemia are the leading causes of acute mesenteric ischemic syndromes, each accounting for 25% of cases. Mesenteric venous infarction and inferior mesenteric arterial disease account for the rest of the cases.

   a. **Clinical features.** Sudden severe periumbilical pain is the most common symptom. A benign but hypoperistaltic abdomen is observed. Anteroposterior (flat plate) radiograph of the abdomen often shows normal findings, but may show separation of bowel loops or "thumbprinting" (submucosal hemorrhage and edema).

   b. **Diagnosis** is supported by an increased white blood cell count (often greater than 20,000/μl) and is confirmed by abdominal angiography. Doppler ultrasonography also may show decreased flow through the superior mesenteric arterial or celiac tree.

   c. **Therapy** is surgical removal of the embolus or thrombus, although occasionally antithrombotic agents, balloon angioplasty of narrowed vessels, or bypass surgery is used.

3. **Chronic mesenteric ischemia** usually is seen only when there is significant occlusion of two of the three major splanchnic arteries. The syndrome usually is seen in older patients with a history of cardiovascular disease.

   a. **Clinical features** include intermittent crampy abdominal pain occurring 15–30 minutes after eating and lasting several hours. Because of the association of pain with eating, patients characteristically become fearful of eating and decrease their intake to the point of substantial weight loss. Physical examination frequently discloses evidence of peripheral vascular disease, but there are no specific findings indicating intestinal ischemia. The presence or absence of an abdominal bruit is not helpful.

   b. **Diagnosis** is difficult and must be based on strong clinical suspicion combined with angiographic demonstration of significant narrowing (greater than 50%) of two of the three major splanchnic arteries.

   c. **Therapy** is surgical vascular reconstruction. Vasodilators have not been shown to be effective.

4. **Ischemic colitis** is due to a lack of arterial blood to the colon. Although any portion of the colon may be affected, the most common site is the left colon and, in particular, the so-called "watershed area" at the splenic flexure. This area is vulnerable because it is the site where the superior mesenteric arterial supply ends and the inferior mesenteric arterial supply begins. The rectum usually is spared because it has a generous blood supply.

   a. **Clinical features** include bloody diarrhea, lower abdominal pain, and occasional vomiting. Infarction rarely occurs. The older adult who has a history of heart disease or abdominal aortic aneurysm surgery (with ligation of the inferior mesenteric artery) is particularly susceptible.

   b. **Diagnosis** is suggested by negative findings for other causes of bloody diarrhea in the elderly population (i.e., polyp, carcinoma, diverticulosis, and angiodysplasia). The white blood cell count may be elevated to approximately 20,000/μl. A flat-plate radiograph of the abdomen may show thumbprinting. A barium enema is a safe study and may reveal diffuse submucosal change. Generally, sigmoidoscopy reveals only bloody fluid.

  c. Therapy is supportive with bowel rest, intravenous fluids, blood replacement, and antibiotics to prevent secondary invasion.

  d. Prognosis generally is good. Late strictures may develop, which could require balloon dilation or surgery.

5. **Vasculitis.** Involvement of the mesenteric vessels by polyarteritis nodosa, lupus erythematosus, or rheumatoid vasculitis mimics arterial embolization (causing bowel infarction) or chronic mesenteric ischemia. The diagnosis is suggested by the systemic features of the disease. Surgery is required for acute infarction. Otherwise, medical treatment with corticosteroids, immunosuppressive agents, or both frequently is effective.

6. **Splenic infarction** is characterized by severe abdominal pain in young patients (younger than 40 years) who have primary hematologic disease (sickle cell disease, leukemia, lymphoma), or in older patients (40 years or older) who have embolic diseases. An abscess may develop with hemorrhage or rupture. Diagnosis is suggested by CT or spleen scan with ^{99}Tc and treatment is surgical.

DIRECTIONS: Each of the numbered items or incomplete statements in this section is followed by answers or by completions of the statement. Select the **ONE** lettered answer or completion that is **BEST** in each case.

1. Which of the following esophageal disorders is best characterized by dysphagia for both solids and liquids?

(A) Esophageal carcinoma
(B) Achalasia
(C) Schatzki's rings
(D) Benign esophageal stricture
(E) Barrett's esophagus

2. The incidence of squamous cell carcinoma of the esophagus compared with the incidence of adenocarcinoma of the esophagus is best estimated at a ratio of

(A) 500:1
(B) 200:1
(C) 50:1
(D) 1:1
(E) 0.5:1

3. Which of the following drugs can cause granulomatous hepatitis?

(A) Alcohol
(B) Acetaminophen
(C) Phenytoin
(D) Methyldopa
(E) Amiodarone

4. Which one of the following statements regarding the esophageal webs of Plummer-Vinson (Paterson-Kelly) syndrome is true?

(A) They are caused by folate deficiency
(B) They are located in the distal esophagus
(C) They cause gastroesophageal reflux
(D) Treatment includes esophageal bougienage
(E) They are elevated iron stores in the blood

5. Which one of the following drugs exacerbates reflux esophagitis?

(A) Chlorpropamide
(B) Metoclopramide
(C) Theophylline
(D) Cisapride
(E) Omeprazole

6. Odynophagia is often associated with

(A) scleroderma
(B) esophageal varices
(C) herpes simplex virus (HSV) infection
(D) achalasia
(E) Schatzki's rings

7. Which of the following are risk factors for esophageal carcinoma?

(A) Vitamin E deficiency, achalasia, alcohol consumption
(B) Achalasia, tylosis–hyperkeratosis, tobacco smoking
(C) Ingestion of carbonated beverages, lye ingestion, vitamin A deficiency
(D) Barrett's esophagus, benign esophageal stricture, vitamin C deficiency
(E) A diet high in pickled foods, Asian descent, female

8. Which of the following statements about irritable bowel syndrome is true?

(A) Lactase deficiency is the preferred term
(B) An underlying neuromuscular or hormonal defect is likely
(C) An underlying immunologic defect is likely
(D) The syndrome may be a premalignant state
(E) Incontinence is a common clinical feature

9. The serologic profile of an individual who has had recombinant hepatitis B vaccine includes positive test results for

(A) hepatitis B surface antigen (HB$_s$Ag)
(B) hepatitis B core antibody (anti-HB$_c$)
(C) hepatitis B e antibody (anti-HB$_e$)
(D) hepatitis B surface antibody (anti-HB$_s$)
(E) anti-HB$_c$ and anti-HB$_s$

10. The most common site of origin of the tumor associated with the Zollinger-Ellison syndrome is

(A) stomach
(B) duodenum
(C) lymph nodes
(D) spleen
(E) pancreas

11. The most common site for ischemic colitis to occur is

(A) splenic flexure
(B) cecum
(C) rectum
(D) sigmoid colon
(E) hepatic flexure

12. The triad of diabetes, gallstones, and steatorrhea is associated with which one of the following?

(A) Gastrinomas
(B) Somatostatinomas
(C) VIPomas
(D) Glucagonomas
(E) Insulinomas

13. Hepatitis B and C share which one of the following epidemiologic characteristics?

(A) Associated with the development of chronic hepatitis in 50% of patients
(B) Active infection is associated with a high mortality rate
(C) Vaccination provides adequate protection against disease
(D) Rare in intravenous drug abusers
(E) Places patient at increased risk for hepatoma

14. Nonbloody diarrhea is associated with which one of the following?

(A) Shigella infection
(B) *Escherichia coli* serotype 0157:H7 infection
(C) Ulcerative colitis
(D) *Giardia lamblia* infection
(E) Colonic ischemia

15. Polypoid lesions of which disease are highly associated with malignancy?

(A) Ulcerative colitis
(B) Crohn's disease
(C) Gardner's syndrome
(D) Peutz-Jeghers syndrome
(E) Juvenile polyposis

16. Which one of the following is characteristic of celiac disease?

(A) Prominent villi on small bowel biopsy
(B) Elevated antigliadin antibody titers
(C) Improvement of symptoms with increased intake of barley and oats
(D) Increased risk of lymphoma in 0.1% of patients
(E) Distal intestinal involvement

17. Right lower quadrant pain, fever, leukocytosis, McBurney's point localization of pain, and at times rectal tenderness is most associated with

(A) diverticulitis
(B) ulcerative colitis
(C) appendicitis
(D) tubo-ovarian abscess
(E) cholecystitis

18. Chronic type A gastritis is associated with

(A) parietal cell antibody
(B) decreased serum gastrin level
(C) *Helicobacter pylori* infection
(D) antral involvement
(E) nonsteroidal anti-inflammatory drugs

19. Which one of the following is associated with nonalcoholic steatohepatitis?

(A) Amiodarone therapy
(B) Thin body habitus
(C) Phenytoin sodium therapy
(D) Right hemicolectomy
(E) Normal transaminases

20. Gastroparesis (delayed gastric emptying) may be caused by

(A) cholinergic drug therapy
(B) duodenal ulcer
(C) diabetes insipidus
(D) scleroderma
(E) gastric varices

21. Which one of the following is a radiographic feature of benign gastric ulcers?

(A) An ulcer crater that is irregular in shape
(B) Absence of edema surrounding the ulcer base
(C) Gastric folds radiating into the center crater
(D) Intimate association with a gastric mass
(E) Lack of ulcer crater extension beyond the gastric wall

22. A complete small bowel obstruction might be suspected in a patient with

(A) hypoactive bowel sounds
(B) pain out of proportion to physical examination
(C) crampy abdominal pain that waxes and wanes
(D) diarrhea
(E) a flat, rigid abdomen

23. Which one of the following findings is diagnostic for malabsorptive syndrome?

(A) Prominent villi on small intestine biopsy
(B) 3 g of D-xylose in a 5-hour urine collection
(C) High carotene level with normal vitamin A intake
(D) 4 g of fat on a 72-hour fecal fat collection
(E) Negative Sudan stain

24. Adenomatous polyps of the colon represent an increased risk for cancer when

(A) they are of tubular histology
(B) they are associated with active bleeding
(C) they are larger than 2 cm in diameter
(D) they are pedunculated
(E) the patient is younger than 50 years of age

25. Which one of the following statements regarding spontaneous (primary) bacterial peritonitis is true?

(A) It is more likely when ascitic fluid total protein exceeds 1.0 mg/dl
(B) It develops in the setting of preexisting ascites
(C) The ascitic polymorphonuclear count is less than 100 cells/μl
(D) It is often associated with aspergillosis
(E) It is associated with a perforated viscus

26. Acute mesenteric ischemia is commonly associated with which one of the following?

(A) A normal white blood cell count
(B) Involvement of the inferior mesenteric artery
(C) Constipation
(D) A definitive clinical presentation
(E) Lack of a significant medical history

ANSWERS AND EXPLANATIONS

1. The answer is B [I A 1 b (2), B 2 c]. Esophageal motor disorders, such as achalasia, are characterized by dysphagia for both solids and liquids. Obstructive esophageal conditions, such as carcinoma, stricture, and Schatzki's rings, cause dysphagia for solids but allow free passage of liquids. The dysphagia associated with Schatzki's rings is intermittent; in carcinoma and stricture, however, the dysphagia is constant. Barrett's esophagus is the replacement of normal squamous epithelium with columnar epithelium; there is no dysphagia present unless an ulceration or stricture complicates this condition.

2. The answer is D [I B 2 a]. Over the past 5 years, the incidence of adenocarcinoma of the esophagus almost equals the incidence of squamous cell carcinoma of the esophagus. An increase in the incidence of Barrett's esophagus is likely responsible for the increased incidence of adenocarcinoma.

3. The answer is C [Table 5-3]. Phenytoin (as well as allopurinol, hydralazine, phenylbutazone, quinidine, and sulfa drugs) can cause granulomatous hepatitis. Alcohol, acetaminophen, and amiodarone cause direct effects on the liver. Acetaminophen and methyldopa each can cause a chronic active hepatitis.

4. The answer is D [I B 2 c]. Esophageal webs are seen in the upper third of the esophagus and may be caused by failure of complete embryological recannulation or by mucosal proliferation secondary to iron deficiency—the Plummer-Vinson (Paterson-Kelly) syndrome. Because of the associated iron deficiency, treatment includes iron supplementation in addition to fracturing the webs with an esophageal bougie.

5. The answer is C [I B 1 a (2)]. Theophylline, a β-adrenergic drug used as a bronchodilator for treating asthma and chronic bronchitis, is a smooth muscle relaxing agent that exacerbates reflux esophagitis. Other smooth muscle relaxing agents that can exacerbate gastroesophageal reflux disease include diltiazem, isosorbide dinitrate, and atropine. Metoclopramide and cisapride are both prokinetic

agents that have constricting effect on the lower esophageal sphincter (LES) and improve gastric emptying. Omeprazole, a proton pump inhibitor, is helpful in the management of resistant gastroesophageal reflux disease. Chlorpropamide is an oral hypoglycemic agent that has no effect on the LES.

6. The answer is C [I A 2, B 4 b]. Odynophagia, or pain on swallowing, may be caused by motor disorders of the esophagus (e.g., diffuse esophageal spasm) or mucosal disruption (e.g., as a result of infection or drug-induced esophagitis). The most important infectious agents are *Candida,* herpes simplex virus (HSV), cytomegalovirus (CMV), and HIV. These infections are commonly seen in immunocompromised hosts. Severe gastroesophageal reflux with ulcerative esophagitis and radiation esophagitis can lead to severe odynophagia as well. Drugs that may cause mucosal disruption include potassium chloride tablets, tetracycline preparations, clindamycin, quinidine, ascorbic acid, and iron sulfate. Scleroderma is a motor disorder that affects the smooth muscle portion of the esophagus, causing weak, simultaneous, and ineffective peristalsis. Dysphagia is usually the only symptom. Schatzki's rings are benign esophageal strictures primarily seen in the distal esophagus, in which dysphagia is the only symptom present. Esophageal varices caused by portal hypertension are generally found incidentally at the time of upper endoscopy or when acute upper gastrointestinal bleeding is present.

7. The answer is B [I B 2 a]. Achalasia, tylosis–hyperkeratosis, and tobacco smoking are risk factors for esophageal carcinoma. Tobacco smoking can increase risk two- to fourfold. Achalasia is associated with a 10% risk of subsequent carcinomas. Tylosis, which is characterized by hyperkeratosis of the palms and soles, is associated with an incidence of squamous cell carcinoma that exceeds 80%. Other risk factors for esophageal cancer include diet (high in pickled foods, nitrosamines, and molds and low in selenium, fresh fruits, and vegetables); geographic factors (incidence is high in certain regions of China and

Iran); vitamin A and C deficiency; a history of lye ingestion; Barrett's esophagus; celiac sprue; and alcohol consumption. Consumption of carbonated beverages, vitamin E deficiency, benign esophageal stricture, gender, and Asian descent are not risk factors.

8. The answer is B [IV D 3 a]. Irritable bowel syndrome, a common cause of alternating diarrhea and constipation, is a functional disorder of motility that probably involves a neuromuscular or hormonal defect. Lactase deficiency is a separate entity that may contribute to irritable bowel syndrome but also may be totally unrelated. There is no evidence of an immunologic defect, and the syndrome is not considered a premalignant state. Incontinence is a symptom of altered anorectal physiology seen with inflammatory diseases of the anal canal and with systemic neuromuscular disorders, such as diabetes or scleroderma; whereas incontinence occasionally may be seen with explosive diarrhea, incontinence is not a common feature of irritable bowel syndrome and should suggest a systemic disorder.

9. The answer is D [IX A 1 d; Figure 5-1]. The vaccine against hepatitis B, in either the recombinant or the pooled plasma form, does not contain hepatitis B e or hepatitis B core antigen. Therefore, the antibody produced is simply that against hepatitis surface antigen. Because no active surface antigen is transmitted, test results for hepatitis B surface antigenemia are negative.

10. The answer is E [III I]. The Zollinger-Ellison syndrome is a non–beta islet cell tumor that produces gastrin and is associated with gastric acid hypersecretion and peptic ulcer disease. Tumors are biologically malignant in 60% of cases, and the most common site involved is the pancreas. Tumor size ranges from 2 mm to 20 cm.

11. The answer is A [X C 4]. Ischemic colitis is caused by a lack of arterial blood supply to the colon. Although any portion of the colon may be affected, the most common site is the left colon and, in particular, the so-called "watershed" area at the splenic flexure.

12. The answer is B [VII D 5 d]. Somatostatinomas are associated with the clinical triad of diabetes, steatorrhea, and gallstones. Gastrinomas, which cause Zollinger-Ellison syndrome, are associated with recurrent peptic ulcer disease, diarrhea, and multiple endocrine neoplasia, type I (MEN-I) syndrome in 20% of patients. VIPoma (pancreatic cholera, Verner-Morrison syndrome, and the watery diarrhea, hypokalemia and achlorhydria syndrome) is a non-α, non-β islet cell tumor that secretes vasoactive intestinal peptide (VIP), leading to watery diarrhea. Glucagonomas are characterized by a syndrome of diabetes mellitus, weight loss, anemia, and a rash (migratory necrolytic erythema). Insulinomas are characterized by high insulin levels in the presence of hypoglycemia.

13. The answer is E [IX A 1 f (4)]. Patients who are chronic carriers of hepatitis B and those with chronic active hepatitis B and C infection are at increased risk for developing hepatoma. Hepatitis B is parenterally transmitted, putting intravenous drug abusers, homosexual men, and those exposed to blood or blood products at risk. There is a 10% risk of chronic disease or becoming a chronic carrier. Hepatitis C is transmitted through parenteral, sexual, and perhaps perinatal methods and accounts for 90% of posttransfusion hepatitis. Approximately 30%–50% of patients develop chronic hepatitis. Fulminant hepatitis B is associated with a high mortality rate whereas fulminant hepatitis C rarely occurs. Vaccination provides adequate protection against hepatitis B; however, currently there is no hepatitis C vaccine.

14. The answer is D [IV D 4 b, e, j; V D; X C 4; Table 5-1]. *Giardia lamblia* is the most common cause of water-borne infectious diarrhea in the United States. The organism preferentially resides in the upper small intestine and infected patients may be asymptomatic, have mild diarrhea, or develop a prolonged illness characterized by malabsorption, diarrhea, bloathing, and crampy abdominal pain. Organisms such as *Shigella* and *Escherichia coli* serotype 0157:H7 are invasive organisms that can cause fever, crampy abdominal pain, and bloody diarrhea. Ulcerative colitis is an inflammatory bowel disease characterized by bloody diarrhea. Colonic ischemia is characterized by the acute the onset of crampy abdominal pain and bloody diarrhea caused by a low-flow state to the colon.

15. The answer is C [V G 2]. Gardner's syndrome, characterized by familial adenomatous polyposis associated with osteomas or soft tissue tumors, has an extremely high risk for the development of colorectal cancer. Juvenile polyposis commonly leads to gastrointestinal bleeding from polyps of the colon, small bowel, and stomach, and the risk of malignancy is slightly increased later in life. Peutz-Jeghers syndrome is characterized by mucocutaneous pigmentation of the buccal mucosa and hamartomatous polyps in the stomach, small bowel, and colon. These polyps carry a very low risk for malignant transformation. Both ulcerative colitis and Crohn's disease do carry an increased risk of colon cancer, but these disorders are not associated with adenomatous colonic polyps.

16. The answer is B [IV E 4 c]. Celiac (nontropical) sprue is a disease characterized by abnormal sensitivity to gluten, a protein component of wheat. Celiac patients have proximal intestinal involvement with relative sparing of the distal ileum. Proximal small bowel biopsy will reveal flat villi. Antigliadin antibodies (IgG and IgA) are elevated in 90% of patients, and long-term complications of lymphoma and carcinoma occur in 10% of patients.

17. The answer is C [IV I]. Acute appendicitis most often occurs in males between the ages of 10 and 30 years. Clinical features include right lower quadrant (McBurney's point) pain, fever, and leukocytosis. Differential diagnoses include acute gastroenteritis, mesenteric adenitis, Meckel's diverticulum, Crohn's disease, ovarian torsion, ruptured ovarian cyst, pelvic inflammatory disease (PID), and, in elderly patients, diverticulitis, cholecystitis, incarcerated hernia, and mesenteric thrombosis.

18. The answer is A [II A 2 b (1)]. Chronic type A gastritis is most likely immunologically mediated, an assumption that is based on the serologic finding of parietal cell antibody. Parietal cells are gastric acid–producing cells located in the body and fundus (but not the antrum) of the stomach. As a result of parietal cell damage, chronic type A gastritis is characterized by hypo- or achlorhydria, and because there is little or no gastric acid to shut down production of gastrin, serum gastrin levels are high. Intrinsic factor also is produced by parietal cells and, therefore, vitamin B_{12} deficiency is common in these patients. Vitamin B_{12} deficiency accounts for the common finding of pernicious anemia in chronic type A gastritis. Type B gastritis predominantly involves the antrum and is most often caused by *Helicobacter pylori* infection and chronic

administration of nonsteroidal anti-inflammatory drugs.

19. The answer is A [IX A 4]. Nonalcoholic steatohepatitis is often associated with obesity, diabetes mellitus, intravenous hyperalimentation, jejunoileal bypass surgery, and drugs such as amiodarone. The liver is fatty on biopsy, and Mallory bodies are occasionally noted. Laboratory examination may reveal a two- to fourfold increase in transaminase levels. Initially thought to be a benign condition, prolonged steatohepatitis may lead to cirrhosis. Treatment consists of reducing risk factors; for example, loss of 10% of body weight has been associated with a marked improvement of transaminase levels in obese patients.

20. The answer is D [II C 5]. Gastroparesis is a disorder of gastric emptying and is not associated with mechanical obstruction. It is most frequently associated with a greater than 10-year history of insulin-dependent diabetes mellitus (IDDM). Other conditions associated with gastroparesis include systemic sclerosis, postvagotomy states, and the use of anticholinergic agents. Prokinetic agents (e.g., metoclopramide, domperidone, erythromycin, cisapride) have been used to treat gastroparesis. Gastric varices have no effect on gastric emptying.

21. The answer is C [III E 1]. Although endoscopy and biopsy are required to confirm that a gastric ulcer is either benign or malignant, an upper gastrointestinal series can provide useful diagnostic information. Radiographic criteria for benign gastric ulcers include an ulcer crater that extends beyond the gastric wall; gastric folds radiating into the base of the ulcer; Hampton's line (collar of edema surrounding the ulcer base); a smooth, regular, round or ovoid ulcer crater; and pliable and normal distensibility of the gastric wall in the area of the ulcer. Malignant ulcers appear to be irregular in shape and, at times, are clearly associated with a gastric mass.

22. The answer is C [IV A 1 b]. Mechanical intestinal obstruction may be the result of extrinsic, intramural, or intraluminal causes. Symptoms include crampy abdominal pain that waxes and wanes, obstipation or constipation, nausea and vomiting, and abdominal distention. Physical examination of the abdomen reveals high-pitched bowel sounds and rushes and tinkles, as well as marked abdominal distention and tympany on percussion. Pain out of proportion to the physical examination is most suggestive of acute mesenteric ischemia.

23. The answer is B [IV E 3 a, b, e, i]. After a 25-g oral dose of D-xylose, a 5-hour urine collection should contain at least 5 g of D-xylose. The finding of less than 4–5 g of D-xylose in the stool is indicative of malabsorption syndrome. Flat villi with inflammatory cell infiltration on small bowel biopsy are characterized by celiac disease. The serum carotene level is a reflection of vitamin A metabolism. Because vitamin A is a fat-soluble vitamin, a low serum carotene level with normal vitamin A intake may be useful in screening for fat malabsorption. A positive Sudan stain is indicative of an underlying malabsorptive process. However, the gold standard test for fat malabsorption is a 72-hour stool collection for fecal fat. The coefficient of fat absorption in the small intestine is 7%. As a result, a patient consuming a 100-g fat diet should have no more than 7 g of fat in the stool each day; more than 7 g of fat would be consistent with a malabsorption syndrome.

24. The answer is C [V G 1]. Adenomatous polyps that represent an increased risk for adenocarcinoma are greater than 2 cm in diameter, villous rather than tubular, and sessile rather than pedunculated. There is no associa-

tion with increased risk related to bleeding or patient age.

25. The answer is B [X A 2]. Spontaneous (primary) bacterial peritonitis develops in a setting of preexisting ascites. Clinical features include abdominal pain, fever, leukocytosis, and paralytic ileus. The initial ascitic fluid total protein count is less than 1.0 mg/dl. The absolute polymorphonuclear count in the ascitic fluid is generally greater than 250 cells/μl. Bacterial peritonitis associated with a perforated viscus is secondary bacterial peritonitis.

26. The answer is D [X C 2]. Acute mesenteric ischemia is a classic syndrome characterized by decreased blood supply; usually the superior mesenteric artery is involved. In general, patients have comorbid conditions, such as atherosclerotic cardiovascular disease, congestive heart failure, acute myocardial infarction, cerebrovascular disease, or peripheral vascular disease. Clinical presentation is the basis of diagnosis. Symptoms include sudden, severe periumbilical pain with a benign physical examination (symptoms are out of proportion to the physical examination). Abdominal radiographs may show separation of bowel loops or "thumbprinting." The leukocyte count is generally greater than 20,000 cells/μl and metabolic acidosis is present.

Chapter 6

Renal Diseases, Fluid and Electrolyte Disorders, and Hypertension

Stanley Goldfarb
Fuad N. Ziyadeh

PART I: RENAL DISEASES

I. CLINICAL ASSESSMENT OF RENAL FUNCTION

A. Urinalysis

1. **Urine color** normally is yellow.
   a. **Darkening** on standing may be seen with some diseases (e.g., porphyria) and with certain drugs (e.g., methyldopa).
   b. **Red-orange-brown urine** may be seen with hematuria, hemoglobinuria, and myoglobinuria and with certain drugs (e.g. , phenothiazines).

2. **Urine chemistry.** Qualitative chemical analysis of urine is performed with commercially available **dipsticks.**
   a. **Blood** usually is not present in normal urine. Intact erythrocytes, hemoglobin, and myoglobin all produce positive test results.
   b. **Glucose** usually is not present in normal urine above 0.3 g/24 hr.
   c. **Ketone bodies** are present in the urine of healthy individuals only during fasting. Sodium nitroprusside reagent detects acetoacetate but not β-hydroxybutyrate.
   d. **Protein** usually is not present in normal urine above 150 mg/24 hr. The dipstick detects only albumin, not immunoglobulins or light chain polypeptides, which must be assayed using acid precipitation.
   e. **Bilirubin** is not present in normal urine. If elevated in blood, water-soluble conjugated bilirubin is filtered and present in urine.
   f. **Urine pH** can be maximally acidified below a pH of 5.0 and maximally alkalinized above a pH of 7.5.

3. **Urine concentration and dilution** are measured by either specific gravity (normal = 1.000–1.025) or osmolality (normal = 50–1000 mOsm/kg urine). Many factors can affect urine concentration and dilution.

4. **Urinary sediment** of formed elements is prepared by centrifugation of urine at 2000 RPM for 10 minutes. The sediment from 12 ml of urine is resuspended in 1 ml of supernatant and is examined microscopically.
   a. **Crystals** that are seen in acid urine include cystine and uric acid; those found in alkaline urine include calcium phosphate and calcium oxalate.
   b. **Cells** that are found in various disease states include erythrocytes, leukocytes, and epithelial cells (i.e., renal tubular, transitional, or squamous).
   c. **Bacteria** may be seen and are best confirmed with Gram staining of the sediment.
   d. **Casts** are cylindrical elements formed in disease states associated with low intrarenal urine flow or heavy proteinuria. The cast is a protein coagulum, which is formed in the renal tubule and traps any tubular luminal contents within its matrix. Casts are named for the elements recognized within them, such as:
      (1) Red cell cast
      (2) White cell cast
      (3) Renal tubular cell cast

        (4) Granular cast
        (5) Hyaline cast
        (6) Waxy cast

B. **Renal function testing**

1. **Glomerular filtration rate (GFR)** is a measure of the amount of plasma ultrafiltrate derived from blood in a specified time period. (A normal GFR is 115–125 ml/min.) In most kidney diseases, the GFR is an accurate index of overall renal function.

2. **Urine concentrating ability** is determined by measuring urine osmolality after 18–24 hours of water deprivation and again after the administration of 5 units of **vasopressin.** Under these conditions, urine reaches an osmolality of 900 mOsm/kg (or a specific gravity of 1.023) in 90% of normal individuals.

3. **Urine diluting ability** is determined by measuring urine osmolality and volume 5 hours after a water load of 20 ml/kg body weight. Urine reaches an osmolality of 100 mOsm/kg (or a specific gravity of 1.003), and urine volume exceeds 80% of the water load in normal individuals.

4. **Renal urine acidification.** Fasting urine pH normally is below 5.5. Acidification can be tested by administering 100 mg ammonium chloride/kg body weight to decrease plasma bicarbonate concentration below 20 mEq/L. Urine normally acidifies (i.e., urine pH drops below 5.5) under these conditions.

C. **Radiography**

1. Plain-film radiography, tomography, ultrasonography, and computed tomography (CT) are useful noninvasive techniques for determining renal size and the presence of obstruction, stones, or mass lesions.

2. Intravenous urography and arteriography may also help to define intrarenal morphology.

D. **Renal biopsy**

1. **Indications** for renal biopsy include acute renal failure of unknown etiology or abnormal course, delayed recovery from acute renal failure, and a poorly functioning or deteriorating renal allograft. Also, renal biopsy occasionally may be indicated in cases of nephrotic syndrome and diabetes and in defining the progression of lupus nephritis.

2. **Contraindications** for renal biopsy include diastolic blood pressure exceeding 100 mm Hg, infection at the biopsy site, and abnormal blood coagulation.

II. **ACUTE RENAL FAILURE** is defined as sudden, rapid, but potentially reversible deterioration in renal function sufficient to cause nitrogenous waste accumulation in body fluids.

A. **Etiology.** Causes of acute renal failure may be prerenal, postrenal, or parenchymal (Table 6-1).

B. **Clinical features**

1. **Azotemia.** Rising blood urea nitrogen (BUN) and serum creatinine levels are the most readily available laboratory signs of a decrease in GFR. These biochemical changes may be independent of clinical symptoms. Confounding variables that influence BUN and creatinine must be considered before renal failure is confirmed.
    a. BUN level is affected by rates of urea production, a function of the amount of dietary protein or protein breakdown (e.g., catabolic drugs or tissue injury), and by resorption of gastrointestinal or soft-tissue hemorrhage.

TABLE 6-1. Causes of Acute Renal Failure

Classification	Pathophysiology	Example
Prerenal	Severe extracellular volume depletion	Gastrointestinal bleeding
	Decreased renal perfusion	Congestive heart failure
	Renal arterial obstruction	Renal embolus
Postrenal*	Intratubular obstruction	Acute urate nephropathy
	Intrarenal pelvic obstruction	Staghorn calculus
	Ureteropelvic obstruction	Kidney stone
	Ureteral obstruction	Stone, clot, compression by extrarenal lymph nodes
	Bladder outlet obstruction	Prostatic hypertrophy
Renal parenchymal	Acute tubular necrosis	Sepsis
	Nephrotoxicity	Aminoglycoside antibiotics, radiocontrast dyes
	Intrinsic renal diseases Glomerulonephritis	Poststreptococcal glomerulonephritis
	Tubulointerstitial nephritis	Drug-induced
	Vasculitis	Wegener's granulomatosis

* Must be bilateral, except in patients with only one kidney, when it is unilateral.

    b. Creatinine level is affected by endogenous creatinine production (increased by breakdown of muscle tissue), by renal creatinine secretion (which is blocked by such drugs as cimetidine and trimethoprim), and by noncreatinine chromogens (usually drugs) that cause measurement errors.

  2. Derangement of urine volume
    a. Anuria (i.e., a urine output of less than 100 ml/day) usually is an ominous sign; however, urine volume per se confers very little diagnostic specificity.
    b. Oliguria is defined as a urine output (generally less than 400 ml/day) that is insufficient to excrete the daily osmolar load. Although most patients with acute renal failure are oliguric, 25%–50% of such patients are not and produce more than 800 ml of urine daily.
    c. Polyuria. Patients may have acutely rising BUN and serum creatinine levels, yet produce more than 3 L of urine daily. This condition may represent a less severe form of acute renal failure, with preservation of small amounts of glomerular filtration in the presence of tubular damage. Patients with partial urinary tract obstruction frequently present with polyuria.

C. Diagnosis
  1. Patient history. Acute renal failure usually results from several, often synergistic, renal injuries. A patient history should include information concerning:
    a. Recent surgical and radiographic procedures
    b. Past and present use of medications
    c. Allergies
    d. Underlying chronic renal disease
    e. Family history of renal disease
  2. Physical examination. The physical examination should be organized so as to parallel the differential diagnosis.
    a. Prerenal failure is suggested by clinical signs of:
      (1) Intravascular volume depletion (e.g., orthostatic changes in blood pressure and pulse and poor skin turgor)

       (2) Congestive heart failure (e.g., elevated jugular venous pressure, a third heart sound, dependent edema, and pulmonary rales)

    b. **Acute allergic interstitial nephritis** is suggested by signs of allergy (e.g., periorbital edema, eosinophilia, maculopapular rash, and wheezing).

    c. **Lower urinary tract obstruction** is suggested by a suprapubic or flank mass or symptoms of bladder dysfunction (e.g., hesitancy, urgency).

  3. Urinalysis

    a. Microscopic examination of urinary sediment provides information for the differential diagnosis.

      (1) The presence of few formed elements or only **hyaline casts** is suggestive of prerenal or postrenal failure.

      (2) An abundance of **erythrocytes** is uncommon in the absence of calculi, trauma, infection, or tumor.

      (3) An abundance of **leukocytes** may signify infection, immune-mediated inflammation, or an allergic reaction somewhere in the urinary tract.

      (4) **Eosinophiluria** occurs in up to 95% of patients with acute allergic interstitial nephritis. Hansel's stain often is needed to distinguish eosinophils from neutrophils in urine.

      (5) **Brownish pigmented cellular casts** and many renal tubular epithelial cells are observed in 75% of patients with acute tubular necrosis (ATN). Pigmented casts without erythrocytes in the sediment from urine with a positive dipstick for occult blood indicate either hemoglobinuria or myoglobinuria.

      (6) **Red blood cell casts** suggest the possibility of acute glomerulonephritis.

    b. **Urine culture** should be performed in all patients with acute renal failure.

    c. **Urine and blood chemistries.** Several biochemical indices aid in the evaluation of acute renal failure. Mainly, these tests distinguish acute oliguria due to prerenal azotemia from that due to parenchymal renal disease (ATN), on the basis that renal tubular function is preserved in the former condition and severely disturbed in the latter. All of these biochemical measures have limitations; their value is recognized when they are used adjunctively, not exclusively.

      (1) The **renal failure index** is the ratio of the urine sodium concentration to the urine-to-plasma creatinine ratio expressed as a percentage $[U_{Na}/(U_{Cr}/P_{Cr}) \times 100]$. Generally, values below 1% are consistent with prerenal failure but may be seen in ATN following cardiac surgery, whereas values above 1% indicate ATN.

      (2) The **fractional excretion of sodium** is the ratio of the urine-to-plasma sodium ratio to the urine-to-plasma creatinine ratio expressed as a percentage $[(U_{Na}/P_{Na})/(U_{Cr}/P_{Cr}) \times 100]$. Values below 1% suggest prerenal failure, and values above 1% suggest ATN.

      (3) **Abnormal blood chemistries** occasionally aid in the diagnosis of renal failure. A BUN-to-serum creatinine ratio above 20 is common in prerenal azotemia.

  4. Radiography

    a. **Ultrasonography** is the method of choice for identifying the presence of two kidneys, for evaluating kidney size and shape, and for detecting **hydronephrosis** or **hydroureter.** Kidneys measure 10%–20% smaller by ultrasonography than by intravenous urography. Renal calculi, abdominal aneurysms, and renal vein thrombosis sometimes are detected by ultrasonography.

    b. **Isotopic flow scans** are marginally useful in evaluating the degree of renal perfusion and the presence of obstructive uropathy. Particularly useful is the radiopharmaceutical agent **diethylenetriamine pentaacetic acid (DTPA),** which is excreted only when there is free flow. Scanning using hippurate is useful in assessing if tubular function is intact. Isotopic scans are most helpful in evaluating the function of the renal allograft.

    c. **Computed axial tomography (CAT)** scans are especially useful in evaluating the nature of **cystic masses** (i.e., whether they are benign or malignant).

    d. **Retrograde pyelography** is performed by injecting contrast material into the ureteral orifice during cystoscopic examination. This method should be performed only after intravenous urography has been attempted. Specific indications for retrograde study include:

(1) Cases of suspected obstructive uropathy, in which the kidneys and collecting system are not visible with urography

(2) Cases in which adequate detail of ureteral and renal pelvic anatomy is not obtained with urography

5. Biopsy. The histologic severity and clinical course of acute renal failure usually do not correlate well; therefore, biopsy is relevant in only a selected group of candidates. It is reserved for patients in whom the cause of nephrotic syndrome is sought or in whom an acute inflammatory lesion such as vasculitis is suspected and requires cytotoxic therapy for treatment. (Patients who follow a classic laboratory and clinical course of ATN usually do not benefit from renal biopsy.)

6. Cystoscopy is indicated in all cases of urethral obstruction and in some cases of ureteral obstruction.

D. **Clinical course**

1. Stages. Acute renal failure due to ATN typically occurs in three stages: **azotemic, diuretic,** and **recovery.** The initial, azotemic stage can be either oliguric or nonoliguric.

2. Morbidity and mortality rates are affected by the presence of oliguria.

a. Gastrointestinal bleeding, septicemia, metabolic acidemia, and neurologic abnormalities are more common in oliguric patients than in nonoliguric patients.

b. The mortality rate for oliguric patients is 50%, whereas that for nonoliguric patients is only 26%.

3. Prognosis is affected by both the severity of the underlying disease and the clinical setting in which acute renal failure occurs. For example, the mortality rate among patients with ATN is 60% when ATN is a result of surgery or trauma, 30% when it occurs as a complication of medical illness, and 10%–15% when pregnancy is involved. Ischemia-associated ATN has nearly twice the mortality risk of nephrotoxic ATN. Patients with no complicating factors who survive an episode of acute renal failure have a 90% chance of complete recovery of kidney function.

E. **Therapy**

1. Preliminary measures

a. Exclusion of reversible causes. Obstruction should be relieved, nephrotoxic drugs should be withdrawn, infection should be treated, and electrolyte derangements should be corrected.

b. Correction of prerenal factors. Intravascular volume and cardiac performance should be optimized.

c. Maintenance of urine output. Although the prognostic importance of oliguria is debated, management of the nonoliguric patient is clearly easier than management of the oliguric patient. Hemodynamic parameters and intravascular volume should be optimized. Loop diuretics may be useful to convert the oliguric form of ATN to the nonoliguric form.

2. Conservative measures

a. Fluid and electrolyte management. Patients with acute renal failure are catabolic and usually lose 0.3 kg of body weight daily. Weight gain or stability usually indicates salt and water retention.

(1) Total oral and intravenous water administration should equal daily **sensible losses** (via urine, stool, and nasogastric or surgical tube drainage) plus estimated **insensible** (i.e., respiratory and dermal) losses, which usually equal 400–500 ml/day.

(2) Combined dietary and intravenous sodium and potassium intake should not exceed the measured 24-hour urinary losses of these electrolytes.

    (3) Sodium bicarbonate should be administered if acidemia becomes severe (i.e., if serum bicarbonate concentration drops below 16 mEq/L).

    (4) Oral phosphate-binding antacids (e.g., aluminum hydroxide) should be given if the serum phosphate concentration exceeds 6.0 mg/dl.

    (5) Magnesium-containing drugs (e.g., magnesium citrate and magnesium hydroxide–containing antacids) should be withheld.

  b. Dietary management. Adequate caloric intake is essential for patients with renal failure. Generally, sufficient calories reflect a diet that provides 40–60 g of protein and 35–50 kcal/kg lean body weight. In some patients, severe catabolism occurs and protein supplementation to achieve 1.25 g of protein/kg body weight is required to maintain nitrogen balance.

3. Drug usage. A patient who develops renal failure abruptly shows only a 1.0 mg/dl/day increase in serum creatinine because endogenous creatinine production remains constant. Therefore, it is impossible to calculate appropriate drug doses based on a patient's serum creatinine level until a new steady state is achieved. Pharmacokinetic measurement of serum drug levels often is necessary for safe drug use.

4. Dialysis is indicated in the management of progressive renal failure that leads to severe uremia, intractable acidemia, hyperkalemia, or volume overload. In addition to the dialysis modalities in chronic renal failure patients (hemodialysis, peritoneal dialysis), **chronic arteriovenous hemofiltration with or without dialysis (CAVH or CAVHS)** or **chronic venovenous hemofiltration (CVVH)** are highly effective forms of ultrafiltration, or dialysis. These modalities utilize highly permeable membranes, which allow the dialysis or filtration processes to occur at very low hydrostatic pressures and flows so that the patient's own blood pressure can provide the driving force for the procedure.

F. Complications

1. Intravascular overload is recognized by weight gain, hypertension, elevated central venous pressure (as indicated by internal jugular vein distention), and pulmonary or peripheral edema.

2. Hyperkalemia (i.e., serum potassium concentration > 5.5 mEq/L) develops as a result of decreased renal excretion combined with tissue necrosis or hemolysis.

3. Hyponatremia (i.e., serum sodium concentration < 135 mEq/L) results from excessive water intake in the face of excretory failure.

4. Hyperphosphatemia (i.e., serum phosphate concentration > 5.5 mg/dl) results from ongoing phosphorous intake in the face of excretory failure or tissue necrosis.

5. Hypocalcemia (i.e., serum calcium concentration < 8.5 mg/dl) results from decreased 1,25-hydroxy vitamin D levels, hyperphosphatemia, or hypoalbuminemia.

6. Hypercalcemia (i.e., serum calcium concentration > 10.5 mg/dl) may occur during the recovery phase following rhabdomyolysis-induced acute renal failure. (This complication is rare.)

7. Acidemia (i.e., arterial blood pH < 7.35) is associated with sepsis or severe heart failure.

8. Hyperuricemia does not require therapy unless the serum uric acid concentration exceeds 15 mg/dl.

9. Bleeding may occur secondary to platelet dysfunction and coagulopathy associated with sepsis.

10. Seizures are related to uremia.

11. Chronic renal failure. A modest decline in filtration may exist in 10% of patients for several months following acute renal failure. In patients with underlying renal disease who experience acute renal failure, progression to chronic renal failure is relatively likely.

III. **CHRONIC RENAL FAILURE** is defined as a substantial and irreversible reduction in renal function over a period of months to less than 20% of normal.

A. **Etiology**

1. **Prerenal causes** of chronic renal failure include severe, long-standing renal artery stenosis and bilateral renal arterial embolism.

2. **Renal causes** include chronic glomerulonephritis, chronic tubulointerstitial nephritis, systemic lupus erythematosus (SLE), diabetes, amyloidosis, hypertension, cystic diseases, neoplasia, and radiation nephritis.

3. **Postrenal causes** derive from long-standing urinary obstruction.

B. **Clinical features** are highly variable. The following constellation of signs and symptoms is referred to as **uremia.**

1. **Neurologic signs** of lethargy, somnolence, confusion, and neuromuscular irritability develop either gradually or abruptly.

2. **Cardiovascular signs** of hypertension, congestive heart failure, and pericarditis also may be precipitous.

3. **Gastrointestinal signs,** particularly anorexia, nausea, and vomiting, are very common.

4. **Metabolic signs** can either be nonspecific (e.g., fatigue, pruritus, and sleep disturbances) or be referable to a specific defect (e.g., bone pain from secondary hyperparathyroidism).

C. **Diagnosis.** The important aim of the diagnostic approach is to establish the chronicity of the renal disease as well as the potential etiologies. Specific approaches are provided in the discussions of specific etiologies.

D. **Therapy**

1. **Dietary restrictions** are vital to the proper care of patients with chronic renal failure in order to reduce symptoms and, possibly, retard the progression of renal failure. Dietary protein is restricted to 0.6 g/kg lean body weight, and dietary sodium is restricted to 4 g/day unless residual urine output obligates greater daily losses. (In these cases, urine sodium concentration should be measured and replaced, but not exceeded, in the diet.) Dietary intake of potassium, magnesium, and phosphorus is restricted, and a fluid intake limit is established based on daily losses.

2. **Renal replacement therapy** is necessary for the maintenance care of end-stage renal disease.
   a. **Indications** include clinical uremia, severe azotemia (i.e., GFR < 10 ml/min), intractable hyperkalemia or acidemia, and intravascular volume overload.
   b. **Modalities** include hemodialysis, peritoneal dialysis, and renal allograft transplantation.

E. **Complications** arise in the course of chronic renal failure and during long-term renal replacement therapy. (A more detailed discussion of renal replacement therapy and the complications associated with this treatment appears in Part I: IV).

1. **Hematologic disorders** include severe anemia and bleeding.

2. **Cardiovascular disorders** include hypertension, pericarditis, cardiomyopathy, arrhythmias, and congestive heart failure.

3. **Neuromuscular disorders** include generalized seizures, confusion, lethargy, emotional lability, myopathy, peripheral neuropathy, and syndromes related to nerve compression (e.g., carpal tunnel syndrome).

4. **Gastrointestinal disorders** include ulcers, gastroduodenitis, colitis, and angiomas of the entire gastrointestinal tract.

5. **Endocrine disorders** include secondary hyperparathyroidism, clinically euthyroid hypothyroxinemia, hyperprolactinemia, altered pituitary and gonadal function (amenorrhea and impotence), and gynecomastia.

6. **Immune system disturbances** include lymphocytopenia, anergy, increased serum anticomplement activity, and abnormal monocyte motility. Increased vulnerability to infectious diseases remains unproven.

7. **Metabolic disorders** include renal osteodystrophy (osteitis fibrosa and osteomalacia) and altered drug metabolism.

IV. MEDICAL COMPLICATIONS OF RENAL REPLACEMENT THERAPY

A. **Introduction.** Renal replacement therapy in patients with chronic renal failure is indicated for uremia (especially pericarditis, neuropathy, and osteodystrophy); intractable hyperkalemia, acidemia, and congestive heart failure; extracellular fluid volume overload that is unresponsive to diuretics; and certain intoxications and poisonings. The choice of modality (i.e., hemodialysis, peritoneal dialysis, or renal transplantation) is based on patient age, underlying diseases, complicating medical conditions, patient preference and motivation, and the practical considerations relating to donor availability and to available sites of peritoneal or vascular dialysis access.

B. **Hemodialysis** is a renal replacement therapy involving **extracorporeal circulation** of blood through a dialysis membrane–containing unit via a surgically constructed vascular fistula or a temporary or permanent external catheter. Percutaneous puncture and cannulation of the vascular access are required at each treatment. Blood and dialysate are separated by the semipermeable membrane, which allows solutes and water to move from blood to dialysate along concentration and osmotic pressure gradients. Complications of hemodialysis can develop at any stage of the procedure, with various manifestations and etiologies (Table 6-2).

TABLE 6-2. Complications of Dialysis—Their Manifestations or Etiologies

Acute Complication	Manifestations or Etiologies
Improper dialyzer preparation	Contamination by preservative (formalin), air bubbles, or bacteria, embolism, sepsis, or membrane rupture
Improper water treatment	Excess calcium, magnesium, aluminum, fluoride, or copper; improper cleansing of municipal water supplies, which may lead to chloramine poisoning and severe hemolysis
Equipment failure	Power failure, air leaks, blood loss from line separation, hypo- or hyperthemia due to improperly warmed dialysate
Allergic reactions	Urticaria, anaphylaxis in response to material in tubing or dialyzer (e.g., sterilants)
Vascular access problems	Bleeding from puncture sites, suture lines, aneurysmal dilatation, endovascular infection
Anticoagulant complications	Local access bleeding, gastrointestinal bleeding
Transfusion complications	Hemosiderosis, hepatitis
Hypotension	Induced by acute volume shifts or true volume depletion; acetate in dialysis fluid, which may induce vasodilatation; autonomic dysfunction secondary to uremic neuropathy
Cardiac arrhythmias	During and following treatment; premature ventricular contractions are commonest form
Dialysis dysequilibrium	Headache, nausea, vomiting, muscle aches, and cramps

C. **Peritoneal dialysis** is a renal replacement therapy involving instillation of 1–3 L of sterile dialysate into the peritoneal cavity via a surgically planted catheter and drainage of the dialysate after a specified **dwell period.** Frequent, brief exchanges (i.e., forty-eight 1-hour exchanges) may be done weekly in-center. Longer exchanges (i.e., four 6-hour exchanges) also are effective and may be done on a continuous ambulatory basis daily or with an automated cycler at night. Maintenance peritoneal dialysis also is associated with specific complications.

1. **Excessive removal of fluid** may result in hypotension, light-headedness, weakness, or syncope.

2. **Catheter-related complications** include occlusion (usually by fibrinous debris), infection, malposition, and, rarely, fracture.

3. **Dialysate-related complications** that develop if dialysate is too rapidly infused or inadequately warmed include abdominal or back pain, nausea, and vomiting.

4. **Peritonitis** is the most serious complication occurring in chronic peritoneal dialysis patients. Infection develops by inoculation through or around the catheter or by contamination of dialysate.
   a. Recurrent peritonitis is associated with high morbidity rates, frequent hospital stays, and considerable expense. Peritoneal fibrosis and loss of dialysis efficiency can complicate multiple recurrent infections and may constitute criteria for withdrawal from this form of therapy.
   b. Treatment of peritonitis is with parenteral and intraperitoneal antibiotics.
   c. Newer catheter configurations (y sets) have markedly reduced the incidence of dialysis-induced peritonitis.

D. **Renal allograft transplantation** may be performed from a donor to a recipient if these individuals are **histocompatible.** Histocompatibility is measured by determination of **human leukocyte antigen (HLA)** types, **mixed lymphocyte reactivity (MLR),** and **blood group** types. Donor kidneys may be from a living relative or from a cadaver with no evidence of infectious disease, specifically, bacteremia, hepatitis, acquired immune deficiency syndrome (AIDS), cytomegalovirus (CMV), syphilis, or malaria. Transplant recipients are given maintenance immunosuppressive agents (e.g., prednisone, azathioprine, cyclosporine, or cyclophosphamide) to prevent graft rejection. Complications of transplantation derive from several sources.

1. **Immunosuppressive disorders** include leukopenia (alkylating agents), hepatitis and vaso-occlusive disease (azathioprine), cystitis (cyclophosphamide), diabetes, obesity, cataracts, and, possibly, peptic ulcer disease, avascular necrosis of bone, and pancreatitis (prednisone). Nephrotoxicity, tremors, hirsutism, and hypertension are complications of cyclosporine.

2. **Secondary hypertension** may develop from extracellular fluid overload (prednisone), high renin secretion from native kidneys, vascular stenosis of the graft from anastomotic stricture or extrinsic compression by lymphocele or urinoma, rejection, recurrent glomerular disease, ureteral obstruction, or hypercalcemia. Coincident primary (essential) hypertension also may develop.

3. **Infection** may occur at any time following transplantation by common pathogens as well as by opportunistic organisms.
   a. Common infections include urinary tract infection (60% of patients), pneumonia (20% of patients), wound or cannula infection, hepatitis, and sepsis.
   b. Uncommon infections encountered in transplant recipients include CMV-associated pneumonia, hepatitis, retinitis, encephalitis, or mononucleosis syndrome; *Cryptococcus* infection; *Listeria monocytogenes* meningitis (usually occurring 6 months post-transplant); *Pneumocystis carinii* infection, and *Legionella pneumophila* infection.

4. **Rejection** may be **hyperacute** (immediate and intraoperative), **acute** (occurring 4–60 days following transplantation), or **chronic** (occurring later than 60 days following transplantation).

    a. Acute rejection is associated with fever, decreased creatinine clearance, oligu-ria, sodium retention, graft enlargement and tenderness, hypertension, and pro-teinuria. Treatment for acute rejection may include high-dose corticosteroids, al-kylating agents, cyclosporine, antilymphocyte globulin, monoclonal antibodies directed against cytotoxic lymphocytes, and, occasionally, transplant (graft) nephrectomy.

    b. Chronic rejection is clinically less dramatic and can be suspected on the basis of decreased creatinine clearance, low-grade fever, increased proteinuria, hyper-chloremic metabolic acidosis, hypertension, oliguria, weight gain, and edema. About 5% of allografts are lost due to chronic rejection that occurs within 5 years of transplantation. Chronic rejection occurs in the majority of grafts with time, and there is no therapy.

5. Malignancy develops in 2%–7% of transplant recipients, a rate that is 100 times greater than the malignancy rate in healthy, age-matched individuals.

    a. Cancer of the skin and lips, lymphomas [especially of the central nervous sys-tem (CNS)], cervical carcinoma, lung carcinoma, head and neck cancer, and colon carcinoma account for the majority of tumors, in order of frequency.

    b. The average time for malignancy to develop is 40 months but may range from 1–158 months. Lymphomas develop sooner (within 27 months of transplanta-tion).

V. PROTEINURIA

A. Definition. Normal adults excrete less than 150 mg of protein in a 24-hour period, the major component of which is **small-molecular-weight proteins.** Urinary protein excre-tion exceeding 150 mg/24 hr is termed **proteinuria.** Small-molecular-weight proteins are excreted at an increased rate if proximal reabsorptive function is impaired (as in tu-bular proteinuria). Albumin is excreted in the urine at a rate of less than 25 mg/day. Higher rates suggest an abnormality in glomerular barrier function, which normally precludes the albumin molecule from crossing the glomerular basement membrane (GBM). An excretion rate greater than 500 mg/day is detectable with routine screening methods and is termed **albuminuria.**

B. Etiology

1. Orthostatic proteinuria refers to an increase in urinary protein that is detected only when the patient has been standing. The 24-hour urinary protein output tends to re-main constant at about 0.5–2.5 g/24 hr, renal function remains normal, and the prognosis is excellent.

2. Tubulointerstitial nephritis. In addition to albumin, tubular proteins such as **Tamm-Horsfall protein** and **β_2-microglobulin** are excreted. Tubulointerstitial ne-phritis is typically seen in patients with drug-induced disease, chronic inflamma-tory disease (e.g., sarcoidosis), or analgesic nephropathy.

3. Glomerulonephritis typically produces albuminuria (>2 g/24 hr). Nephrotic syn-drome (hypoalbuminemia, edema, and hyperlipidemia) occurs when protein excre-tion exceeds 3 g/24 hr.

C. Diagnosis

1. Urinalysis

    a. Screening tests for proteinuria include urine dipsticks (albumin only) and **sulfosalicylic acid precipitation** (albumin, paraproteins, immunoglobulins, and amyloid).

    b. Quantitative, 24-hour testing for urinary protein is essential, particularly in low-volume/high-concentration states (e.g., congestive heart failure).

    c. Lipiduria is suggested by oval fat bodies on microscopic study.

2. **Urine and blood chemistries** should include quantitative protein measurement and urine protein electrophoresis. Elevated blood lipids and hypoalbuminemia support a diagnosis of nephrotic syndrome.

3. **Biopsy** is indicated in the evaluation of patients with significant proteinuria and nephrotic syndrome when no obvious cause is identified by noninvasive means. Pathologic study should include electron microscopy, immunofluorescence, and the use of special stains (e.g., Congo red for amyloid).

D. **Therapy**

1. **Orthostatic proteinuria.** Treatment is not required.

2. **Tubulointerstitial proteinuria.** The underlying disorder must be identified and treated.

3. **Glomerulonephritic proteinuria.** The underlying disorder should be treated. Angiotensin-converting enzyme (ACE) inhibitors are useful for controlling proteinuria associated with glomerular disease. Supportive therapy includes diuretics, antilipemic agents, and dietary manipulation.

E. **Complications** include consequences of hyperlipidemia (atherosclerosis and coronary artery disease), vitamin D deficiency (bone disease), loss of coagulation proteins (thrombosis), and salt retention (congestive heart failure). It has been suggested that patients with nephrotic syndrome are more susceptible to bacterial infections, particularly spontaneous bacterial peritonitis in children.

VI. HEMATURIA

A. **Definition.** Normal adults excrete 500,000–2,000,000 erythrocytes/24 hr, which amounts to less than 3 erythrocytes per high-power field of resuspended urinary sediment.

B. **Etiology.** Causes of hematuria are summarized in Table 6-3.

TABLE 6-3. Causes of Hematuria

Etiology	Clinical Features
Glomerulonephritis Diffuse (e.g., SLE, vasculitis)	Gross or microscopic hematuria, abnormal proteinuria, red blood cell casts, dysmorphic red cells by phase-contrast microscopy
Focal (e.g., I_gA nephritis, thin basement membrane disease)	Gross or microscopic hematuria without proteinuria, dysmorphic red cells by phase-contrast microscopy
Vascular disease	Gross or microscopic hematuria without proteinuria, isomorphic red cells by phase-contrast microscopy
Tumors (e.g., hypernephroma, bladder cancer)	Isomorphic red cells by phase-contrast microscopy
Trauma	Isomorphic red cells by phase-contrast microscopy
Kidney stones	Isomorphic red cells by phase-contrast microscopy
Systemic coagulopathies	Isomorphic red cells by phase-contrast microscopy

SLE = systemic lupus erythematosus.

C. **Diagnosis**

1. **Urinalysis**
   a. Dipstick testing can differentiate hematuria from pigmenturia (i.e., hemoglobin-uria or myoglobinuria). A positive **orthotolidine test** in the absence of micro-scopically detected erythrocytes practically confirms the diagnosis of pigmenturia.
   b. Urine culture should be performed routinely.

2. **Radiography**
   a. Intravenous urography can demonstrate renal masses, cysts, vascular malforma-tions, papillary necrosis, ureteral stricture or obstruction by calculus, bladder tumor, and ureteral deviation.
   b. Special studies (e.g., angiography and nuclear scanning) occasionally are of value in delineating mass lesions.

3. **Biopsy** occasionally may assist in making a diagnosis of **renal hematuria with thin basement membranes** or in characterizing the lesion of a primary glomerular disease.

4. **Cystoscopy** is indicated in the evaluation of hematuria when physical examination, urinalysis, and intravenous urography fail to reveal the cause.

D. **Therapy**

1. The underlying disorder must be identified and treated.

2. Urine volume should be maintained to prevent clots and obstruction in the lower urinary tract.

E. **Complications**

1. **Iron deficiency anemia** may, in a rare case, complicate chronic, significant hematuria.

2. **Lower urinary tract clots** can induce obstruction.

VII. NEPHROLITHIASIS

A. **Definition. Renal calculi** or **stones** arise due to papillary calcification or precipitation in urine of organized crystalline bodies of calcium salts, uric acid, cystine, or struvite. The etiologies of nephrolithiasis are given in Table 6-4.

TABLE 6-4. Etiology of Nephrolithiasis

Stone Type	Etiology or Associated Condition
Calcium phosphate stones	Hyperparathyroidism, distal renal tubular acidosis, idio-pathic hypercalciuria, and medullary sponge kidney
Calcium oxalate stones	Idiopathic hypercalciuria, excess diet oxalate, vitamin C abuse, small bowel diseases, primary hyperoxaluria, and hy-percalcemia; 50% of patients have no identifiable abnor-mality
Uric acid stones	Persistently concentrated and acid urine, hyperuricosuria, hyperuricemia (in gout), and excess dietary purine
Cystine stones	Cystinuria
Struvite stones (triple phosphate, or magnesium–ammonium–calcium phosphate)	Urinary tract infection (chronic or recurrent) by urease-pro-ducing bacteria such as *Proteus, Providencia, Klebsiella, Pseudomonas, Serratia,* and *Enterobacter* species

B. **Clinical features** may vary considerably.

1. **Occult passage** of small, asymptomatic stones may occur. More frequently, however, asymptomatic renal stones are identified radiographically during evaluation for other, unrelated conditions.

2. **Hematuria** virtually always accompanies stone movement within the urinary tract and may be microscopic or gross. Hematuria may occur with or without pain.

3. **Frequency** and **dysuria** are common complaints of patients with stones lodged in the intravesical segment of the distal ureter and may be mistaken for the symptoms of **cystitis.** Dysuria also occurs during the passage of **sludge.**

4. **Abdominal pain, tenesmus,** and **rectal pain** may occur with a stone in the renal pelvis and often are accompanied by nausea and vomiting.

5. **Renal colic,** with flank pain radiating to the inguinal ligament, urethra, labia, testis, or penis, is typical of a stone in the midureter.

6. **Acute obstruction** by a stone may occur, generating renal colic. **Subacute obstruction** may occur with few or no symptoms.

7. **Infection** often complicates stone disease and usually produces flank or back pain, fever, and chills, particularly with urinary obstruction.

C. **Diagnosis**

1. **Patient history** should identify other family members with stone disease as well as the patient's past and present use of drugs and vitamins (particularly vitamins A, D, and C).

2. **Physical examination.** Acute renal colic must be differentiated from other causes of abdominal, pelvic, and back pain.

3. **Urinalysis** provides data in all cases.
   a. Urine pH is inappropriately high in renal tubular acidosis, favoring calcium phosphate stone formation. Low urine volume with low urine pH is a risk factor for uric acid stones.
   b. Crystals often are found appropriate to urine pH, with **acid urine** containing crystals of uric acid and cystine and **alkaline urine** containing crystals of calcium phosphate and struvite.
   c. Bacteriuria may signal infection-related stones; in such patients, urine culture should be performed.

4. **Urine** and **blood chemistries** are critical to the metabolic evaluation of the patient with nephrolithiasis.
   a. A blood sample should be examined for levels of electrolytes, creatinine, BUN, calcium, phosphate, and uric acid.
   b. A 24-hour urine collection should be studied for urine volume and pH and levels of calcium, phosphate, uric acid, oxalate, creatinine, sodium, potassium, and cystine.

5. **Radiography**
   a. **Plain abdominal films** are useful for identifying the composition of renal stones. Calcium stones are intensely radiopaque; cystine, struvite (infection-induced), and mixed uric acid–calcium stones are moderately radiopaque. Abdominal films also help to localize stones, and serial films indicate disease activity as reflected by increases in stone size and number.
   b. **Intravenous urography** is necessary for evaluating radiolucent stones (uric acid) and obstruction of urine flow.
   c. **Ultrasonography** and **CT** may be useful in some cases.

6. **Cystoscopy** is indicated for the detection and removal of bladder calculi and for the removal of ureteral stones lodged near the ureterovesical junction.

7. **Stone analysis.** All efforts should be made to strain urine and capture stones for chemical analysis. Stone analysis is the definitive tool for ascertaining the status of the stone (passed or retained) and its composition.

D. **Therapy**

1. **Medical therapy** is predicated on the identified metabolic disorder. In all circumstances, however, a urine volume of more than 2 L/day should be achieved.
   a. **Calcium phosphate stones.** Primary hyperparathyroidism should be treated promptly by parathyroidectomy; distal tubular acidosis requires independent evaluation; and idiopathic hypercalciuria is treated with diuretics (thiazides or amiloride) or oral neutral potassium phosphate.
   b. **Calcium oxalate stones.** Therapy includes dietary restriction of oxalate-rich food, elimination of large doses (i.e., > 500 mg/day) of ascorbic acid, and administration of hypocalciuric diuretics (thiazides or amiloride) or oral neutral potassium phosphate. Oral administration of potassium citrate may be useful in increasing the urinary excretion of citrate, a major urinary chelator of ionized calcium and an inhibitor of calcium oxalate crystal growth.
   c. **Uric acid stones.** Therapy includes administration of oral sodium bicarbonate to maintain an alkaline urine (i.e., a urine pH > 7) and, in selected patients, restriction of dietary purine or administration of allopurinol.
   d. **Cystine stones.** Sodium bicarbonate is administered to keep urine pH above 7.5, and acetazolamide is given at bedtime to maintain urine alkalinity during the night. Urine output should be maintained at more than 4 L/day. Noncompliant patients and those with severe or refractory stone disease may be candidates for oral D-penicillamine or intrarenal stone dissolution by alkaline or acetylcysteine irrigation.
   e. **Struvite stones.** Treatment is aimed at maintaining urinary asepsis, which may require antibiotics.

2. **Extracorporeal shock wave lithotripsy.** Electrically induced shock waves generated in a water bath are focused on the stone, leading to its in situ dissolution. This technique is safe and effective; moreover, it does not involve surgery. Its use in very large staghorn calculi may be somewhat limited because percutaneous extraction may be required to augment the noninvasive lithotripsy approach.

3. **Surgical removal** is rarely required but is indicated for obstructing stones if there is infection proximal to the stone or if the stone is radiographically determined to be too large to pass spontaneously. Staghorn calculi should be removed if renal function is in jeopardy.

VIII. URINARY TRACT OBSTRUCTION

A. **Introduction.** An obstruction in the urinary tract may occur at any point between the renal tubules and the urethra. Urinary obstruction may be acute or chronic, unilateral or bilateral, and partial or complete. Chronic urinary obstruction often is partial and may be asymptomatic, particularly in slowly progressive cases. The consequences of urinary obstruction include structural changes in the lower urinary tract as a result of increases in pressure opposing normal urine flow **(obstructive uropathy)**, gross dilatation of the calyces and collecting system of the affected kidney **(hydronephrosis)**, and, ultimately, renal parenchymal damage **(obstructive nephropathy)**.

B. **Etiology.** The causes of urinary obstruction can be divided into **mechanical** causes, which may be intrinsic or extrinsic, and **functional** causes.

1. **Intrinsic mechanical causes**
   a. **Intrarenal tubular obstruction** results from precipitation of uric acid, sulfonamide, or paraprotein crystals.
   b. **Extrarenal pelvic** or **ureteral obstruction** is caused by calculus, thrombus, papillary necrosis, or tumor.
   c. **Structural lesions of the ureter or bladder** include stricture, tumor, urethral valves, ureteroceles, and foreign body.

2. Extrinsic mechanical causes

a. Compression. Urinary obstruction can result from compression by:

(1) Prostatic hypertrophy or carcinoma

(2) Uterine prolapse or tumor

(3) Ovarian abscess, cyst, or tumor

(4) Endometriosis

(5) Pregnancy

(6) Enlarged or aneurysmal pelvic vessels

(7) Retroperitoneal tumor, infection, lymphadenopathy, or fibrosis

b. Surgical misadventures that result in obstruction include accidental ureteral ligation.

3. Functional causes. Ureteral or bladder dysfunction results from myelodysplasia, injury or congenital defect of the spinal cord, tabes dorsalis, diabetes mellitus, multiple sclerosis, and autonomic neuropathy including drug-induced neuropathy (e.g., due to disopyramide).

C. **Clinical features** vary depending on the site of the obstruction and the speed with which the obstruction develops.

1. An absence of symptoms often occurs in chronic, slowly advancing obstructive disease. The clinical picture often is overshadowed by signs of the primary disease (e.g., in a case of metastatic tumor or surgical complications) until biochemical evidence of renal impairment develops.

2. Pain and renal enlargement (abdominal or flank mass) usually are present in acute obstruction. The pain characteristically is a steady crescendo, is most severe in the flank, and radiates toward the ipsilateral testis or labium.

3. Urinary symptoms predominate in obstructive disease of the bladder or urethra. Hesitancy, decreased force of urinary stream, urinary frequency, and dribbling are common in the context of obstruction.

4. Renal functional impairment typically is expressed as tubular defects in acid and potassium transport as well as defective tubular responsiveness to hormone action. Clinically, hyperkalemia, mild acidemia, and polyuria precede azotemia, which may progress to renal failure.

D. **Diagnosis**

1. Urinalysis varies but may reveal inappropriately dilute urine, hematuria (in cases of obstruction due to calculus or tumor), or bacteriuria. Because infection often complicates obstruction, causing serious detriment to renal function, urine culture is essential. Examination of the urinary sediment often shows no abnormality but may reveal crystals of uric acid or sulfonamide.

2. Blood chemistries usually are not diagnostic but are helpful in assessing the severity of impaired renal function.

3. Radiography provides the clinical sine qua non of obstruction. Ultrasonography or CT reliably detects evidence of hydronephrosis, such as calyceal blunting and dilatation of the renal pelvis, ureter, or both. Intravenous urography may fail to visualize the kidneys if the GFR is decreased substantially. Retrograde urography occasionally may help to identify unilateral (particularly partial) ureteral obstruction. Nuclear scanning of the kidney often is specific enough to confirm the diagnosis.

E. **Therapy**

1. Relief of obstruction is paramount and should be appropriate to the structural nature of the occluding lesion. Methods include surgery, percutaneous nephrostomy, ureteral stent, and nephroscopic stone removal.

2. Medical management following relief of obstruction is aimed at correcting postobstructive diuresis. Many factors contribute to this diuresis, including the excretion of solute (urea) that was retained during the period of obstruction and the impaired concentrating ability that usually exists in the recently obstructed kidney. Management during this period involves careful, adequate fluid replacement with frequent assessment of body weight, intravascular volume, and blood and urine electrolyte concentration.

F. Complications

1. **Infection,** particularly in the context of obstructing calculi, must be detected and promptly treated to prevent extensive pyelonephritis, perirenal abscess, and sepsis.

2. **Hypertension** may complicate obstruction and occurs secondary to both intravascular volume expansion and ischemic stimulation of renin secretion.

3. **Polycythemia** has been reported in association with hydronephrosis and is purportedly due to increased erythropoietin release.

4. **Persistent tubular defects** may continue beyond 1 year following relief of obstruction. Impaired concentrating ability and limited excretion of a potassium load are the most common defects.

5. **Chronic renal failure** can develop from obstructive disease, most commonly with long-standing obstruction or with complicating urinary tract infection.

IX. URINARY TRACT INFECTION

A. Definition. Urinary tract infections are defined in terms of the involved urinary structures, such as:

1. **Cystitis** (inflammation of the bladder)

2. **Urethritis** (inflammation of the urethra)

3. **Pyelonephritis** (inflammation of renal tubules and interstitium)

4. **Prostatitis** (inflammation of the prostate gland)

B. Etiology. A clinical urinary tract infection occasionally develops from simple inoculation of the lower urinary tract during instrumentation or sexual intercourse. More commonly, however, other risk factors are present and increase the likelihood that inoculation will progress to clinical infection.

1. **Agents of infection**
   a. **Common agents** of urinary tract infection include *Escherichia coli, Proteus, Klebsiella, Enterobacter, Pseudomonas, Serratia,* enterococci, *Candida, Neisseria gonorrhoeae, Trichomonas vaginalis,* and herpes simplex virus (HSV).
   b. **Uncommon agents** include *Staphylococcus* and mycobacteria that cause tuberculosis.
   c. **Rare agents** include *Nocardia, Actinomyces, Brucella,* adenovirus, and *Torulopsis.*

2. **Routes of inoculation**
   a. **Urethral inoculation** is very common among women, particularly those with vaginal and periurethral colonization by virulent bacteria. Local trauma, either mechanical (e.g., intercourse) or biologic (e.g., vaginitis and intertrigo), can predispose to superinfection of the periurethral mucosa. Surgery, particularly cystoscopy, can contaminate the bladder urine.
   b. **Hematogenous spread.** It is extremely unusual for gram-negative bacterial sepsis to induce pyelonephritis in the absence of other risk factors.

3. **Risk factors**
   a. **Obstruction** that induces urinary stasis and impairs host defenses (i.e., via decreased renal blood flow and decreased delivery of leukocytes and antibodies) is a crucial predisposing factor.

    b. **Vesicoureteral reflux** may promote ascending infection in several ways, including increased delivery of bacteria, increased size of the inoculum, incomplete bladder emptying, altered renal hemodynamics, and, possibly, altered host defenses.

    c. **Instrumentation,** particularly the use of urinary drainage (Foley) catheters, frequently is associated with significant bacteriuria.

    d. **Pregnancy** is clearly associated with altered ureteral smooth muscle function and a higher incidence of asymptomatic bacteriuria. The asymptomatic bacteriuria noted in pregnant women is more likely to progress to pyelonephritis than the one that occurs in nonpregnant women.

    e. **Diabetes mellitus** is associated with a high rate of infection. Part of this risk is mediated through neurogenic bladder disturbances, and part is due to other immune disorders in diabetes.

    f. **Immune deficiency,** whether it is congenital, acquired, or drug-induced, increases the risk of urinary infection in concert with the generally increased patient susceptibility.

C. Clinical features

1. **Symptoms of lower tract infection** include urinary frequency, dysuria, burning, suprapubic pain, malodorous or cloudy urine, and continence difficulties. These symptoms (in any combination) are most common in urethritis, prostatitis (with or without perineal pain and ejaculatory pain), and cystitis.

2. **Symptoms of acute pyelonephritis** (parenchymal renal infection) include flank pain, fever, malaise, and any symptoms of lower tract infection.

3. **Septic shock** is frequently seen in elderly or institutionalized patients. Presenting signs include hypothermia, mental status alterations, syncope, and coma.

D. Diagnosis

1. **Urinalysis** of fresh, unspun urine should be performed. The identification of 1 bacterium per high-power field (400x) is indicative of a colony growth on culture of more than 10^5 colonies/ml. Analysis of the centrifuged sediment usually reveals leukocyturia (neutrophils) and bacteriuria. Gram staining of the urinary sediment is routine and may additionally characterize the offending organism, allowing more specific therapy before culture results are known. Microscopic hematuria is common.

2. **Routine urine culture** is the definitive method of diagnosis. A clean-catch, midstream specimen should be submitted for plating within 3 hours; the specimen should be refrigerated if any delay is anticipated. Unquestionably, the growth of more than 10^5 colonies/ml in the presence of symptoms signifies infection worthy of treatment. The diagnostic significance of culture growth below this level is debated. However, a growth of less than 10^5 colonies/ml may warrant therapy under appropriate clinical circumstances, such as severe symptoms, a history of partial antibiotic treatment, known recurrent infections, any suspicion about the accuracy of the laboratory report, and the presence of renal calculi.

3. **Special urine cultures** must be ordered specifically.
    a. In patients with typical symptoms but repeatedly negative routine cultures **(urethral syndrome),** infection by *Ureaplasma* or *Chlamydia* should be suspected and the laboratory instructed to search for these organisms.
    b. **HSV** requires special culture methods, and *N. gonorrhoeae* requires immediate inoculation on Thayer-Martin (chocolate agar) media and carbon dioxide incubation.
    c. Sterile pyuria, even in the asymptomatic patient, should arouse suspicion of **renal tuberculosis.** A first morning urine specimen is best for detecting this condition.

4. **Blood chemistries** provide little information but occasionally demonstrate leukocytosis.

5. **Radiography.** Intravenous urography is helpful in the evaluation of infection complicating chronic vesicoureteral reflux, obstruction, calculi, and chronic pyelonephritis. Voiding cystourethrography and retrograde ureterography occasionally are indicated in the evaluation of recurrent infections, particularly in children.

E. Therapy

1. **Antibiotics.** Initial antibacterial therapy is selected on the basis of the urinalysis and an understanding of the epidemiology and bacteriology of the infection. The appropriateness of this therapy must be confirmed by culture and sensitivity testing in refractory, relapsing, and atypical cases.

   a. **Uncomplicated lower tract infection** may be treated with a 3-day course of amoxicillin (3.0 g orally) or trimethoprim–sulfamethoxazole (320 mg/1.6 g orally). Special recommendations exist for gonorrhea, syphilis, and trichomoniasis.

   b. **Relapsing urinary tract infection and pyelonephritis** should be treated for 14 days. Clinically stable patients may be treated at home with trimethoprim–sulfamethoxazole (80 mg/400 mg orally, twice daily) or a first-generation cephalosporin.

   c. **Prostatitis** must be treated for at least 14 days with antibiotics that penetrate and remain active in prostatic tissue and fluid (e.g., trimethoprim and carbenicillin).

   d. **Recurrent infections.** Typical regimens include trimethoprim–sulfamethoxazole (40 mg/200 mg orally, once daily), methenamine mandelate (500 mg orally, four times daily), and sulfisoxazole (500 mg orally, once daily). Use of agents such as ciprofloxacin (500 mg daily) may result in sterilization of the urine.

   e. **Catheter-associated bacteriuria** in the acutely catheterized patient usually resolves following removal of the catheter. Failure to do so or the development of symptoms within 12–24 hours necessitates appropriate antibacterial therapy.

2. **Corrective surgery** is indicated for the removal of calculi and for the repair of obstructing anatomic lesions.

F. Complications

1. **Abscess formation,** in either the kidney parenchyma or the surrounding retroperitoneal space, often complicates infection proximal to unrelieved obstruction. Persistent systemic symptoms and resistant bacteriuria should prompt diagnostic study using ultrasonography or CT.

2. **Xanthogranulomatous pyelonephritis** is a form of chronic bacterial infection characterized by granuloma formation with lipid-laden macrophages, often in a nonfunctioning kidney. *Proteus mirabilis* is the organism most frequently recovered from renal abscess fluid. There is a history of nephrolithiasis in three quarters of patients, and in many cases a staghorn calculus is identified at surgery.

3. **Emphysematous pyelonephritis** is a rare, life-threatening complication of bacterial pyelonephritis. Seen most frequently in diabetics, this disease is characterized by gas-forming bacterial infection.

4. **Chronic renal failure.** Chronic pyelonephritis can lead to end-stage renal disease, particularly if it coexists with renal calculi or obstruction. Most cases of chronic renal failure due to chronic pyelonephritis are not bacterial in origin but represent a broad spectrum of chronic tubulointerstitial disease.

X. GLOMERULAR DISEASE

A. Hereditary nephritis (Alport's syndrome)

1. **Inheritance and incidence.** Hereditary nephritis is inherited as an X-linked or autosomal dominant trait with variable penetrance. Recent studies have shown that the

disease is caused by a defect in a basement membrane protein (type IV collagen) gene.

2. Clinical features
   a. **Hematuria, red cell casts, pyuria, proteinuria,** and **progressive renal failure** occur with variable severity. Renal failure is more common in men.
   b. **High-frequency sensorineural hearing loss,** often without clinically significant deafness, is characteristic.

3. Therapy and prognosis. No treatment is successful in slowing or preventing the renal failure, and prognosis is variable. Occasionally, patients with Alport's syndrome who undergo renal transplantation develop anti-basement membrane antibody disease (Goodpasture's syndrome) if the normal type IV collagen of the transplanted kidney is recognized as a "foreign" antigen by the Alport host.

B. **Minimal change disease (lipoid nephrosis, nil lesion nephrotic syndrome)**

1. Incidence. Minimal change disease accounts for three quarters of cases of idiopathic nephrotic syndrome in children but only one quarter of cases in adults.

2. Pathology is scant and nonspecific. Fusion of epithelial foot processes is seen with electron microscopy, but this lesion is common to all proteinuric states.

3. Clinical features
   a. **Nephrotic syndrome** is the typical presentation by patients of all ages.
   b. Hypertension occurs in 10% of children and in 35% of adults.
   c. Hematuria is uncommon.
   d. Azotemia develops in 23% of children and in 34% of adults.

4. Therapy
   a. **Glucocorticoids.** The remission rate with adequate steroid treatment (i.e., 1–2 mg/kg/day for 4–8 weeks) is 90% for both children and adults. Prolonged remission is seen in 10%–60% of patients; however, relapse is common and is multiple in 25%–50% of patients. Relapses typically are responsive to steroids, with only 5% of initially steroid-responsive patients developing steroid resistance or dependence.
   b. **Cytotoxic agents** (e.g., cyclophosphamide, chlorambucil) have been effective in steroid-resistant and multiple relapsing cases. Occasionally, steroid-resistant patients gain steroid sensitivity following therapy with cytotoxic alkylating agents. The possibility of gonadal (chromosomal) damage caused by these drugs must be carefully considered.

5. Prognosis. Minimal change disease is associated with low mortality rates (i.e., 10% among adults and 1.5% among children), with only 10% of deaths caused by renal failure.

C. **Membranous glomerulonephritis**

1. Etiology
   a. **Primary (idiopathic) membranous glomerulonephritis** accounts for 30%–50% of cases of idiopathic nephrotic syndrome in adults but less than 1% of cases in children.
   b. **Secondary membranous glomerulonephritis** may occur with a variety of underlying conditions, including:
      (1) **Infection** (e.g., chronic hepatitis B or hepatitis C, syphilis, malaria, schistosomiasis, filariasis)
      (2) **Rheumatic disease** (e.g., SLE)
      (3) **Neoplasm** (e.g., carcinoma of the lung, colon, stomach, breast, and kidney; non-Hodgkin's lymphoma; leukemia; Wilms' tumor)
      (4) **Drug therapy** (e.g., with mercury, gold, D-penicillamine, captopril)

2. Pathology. The stages of membranous glomerulonephritis are defined by the following characteristic findings.

   a. Stage I: Normal appearance by light microscopy; subepithelial electron-dense deposits by electron microscopy

   b. Stage II: Spike-like projections of basement membrane material by light microscopy (best visualized with a silver impregnation stain); variable basement membrane thickening

   c. Stage III: Thick GBM, with a "moth-eaten" or "Swiss-cheese" appearance due to encirclement of immune deposits by spike-like projections of normal GBM

   d. Stage IV: Thickening of the capillary wall, with areas of segmental or global glomerulosclerosis; possible tubulointerstitial fibrosis

3. Clinical features. More than 85% of adults present with proteinuria (> 3 g/day/ 1.73 m^2 body surface area). The GFR usually is normal at diagnosis and often remains normal for 4–5 years thereafter.

4. Clinical course. Membranous glomerulonephritis has a variable course. About 20%–30% of patients achieve a lasting spontaneous remission, 20%–30% develop variable degrees of persistent proteinuria and nonuremic azotemia, and the remainder advance to end-stage renal disease, usually over a 5-year period. Male patients, those with heavy proteinuria (> 10 g/day) and those who do not respond with a remission in proteinuria have a worse prognosis.

5. Therapy with glucocorticoids or cytotoxic agents has been proven effective, but the unpredictable outcome of this disease makes the evaluation of therapy difficult. A recently described protocol using alternating cycles of chlorambucil and prednisone is effective in halting progression to end-stage renal failure in patients with nephrotic syndrome and mild renal insufficiency. Patients treated with cytotoxic drugs are more likely to experience remission of proteinuria.

6. Complications may intervene, causing an abrupt decrease in renal function.

   a. A **hypercoagulable state** exists in nephrotic patients. Renal vein thrombosis is a recognized problem; pulmonary embolism and arterial thrombosis also have been described.

   b. Intravascular volume depletion secondary to vigorous diuretic administration leads to decreased renal blood flow.

   c. Hypertension, obstruction, or **infection** may impair filtration in patients with membranous glomerulonephritis.

D. | **Mesangial proliferative glomerulonephritis**

1. Etiology is unknown.

2. Pathology. The mesangial proliferative lesion in glomerulonephritis is a global and diffuse increase in the number of mesangial cells and in the mesangial matrix.

3. Clinical features may include asymptomatic proteinuria or hematuria. Although 24-hour urinary protein excretion can exceed 3.0 g, the complete nephrotic syndrome is inconsistently seen. One-third of patients are hypertensive at the time of diagnosis. Creatinine clearance is reduced in only 25% of patients at presentation. Serum complement component levels are normal.

4. Clinical course. Mesangial proliferative glomerulonephritis has an extremely variable course.

5. Therapy with high-dose (1–2 mg/kg/day) glucocorticoids has been reported to be effective in remission induction. Some steroid failures respond to treatment with cyclophosphamide or chlorambucil.

E. | **Membranoproliferative glomerulonephritis**

1. Incidence and etiology

   a. Collectively, the disorders in this group account for 41% of cases of idiopathic nephrotic syndrome in children and 30% of cases in adults. Males and females are affected equally.

   b. Membranoproliferative glomerulonephritis may be idiopathic or secondary to SLE, cryoglobulinemia, or chronic viral or bacterial infection.

2. **Pathology.** There are three pathologic types of membranoproliferative glomerulonephritis, each with distinct features.
   a. **Type I** is characterized by an intact GBM, subendothelial and mesangial deposits, significant mesangial prominence with matrix interposition, and immunofluorescent positivity for immunoglobulin G (IgG), complement components (C1q, C4, and C2), and properdin.
   b. **Type II** (also called **dense deposit disease**) is characterized by intramembranous and subepithelial deposits ("humps") in 50% of cases, mesangial deposits, moderate mesangial prominence with interposition, and immunofluorescent positivity for IgG, C3, and properdin.
   c. **Type III** is characterized by features of true membranous glomerulonephritis and features of type I membranoproliferative glomerulonephritis.

3. **Clinical features.** This glomerulonephritis has a highly variable presentation.
   a. Rapid progression to renal failure with edema and severe hypertension (acute nephritis) has been described.
   b. **Hypocomplementemia** is the most characteristic laboratory finding but is not universally present. The degree of C3 depression may be used as a rough guide to disease activity.

4. **Clinical course.** Chronic glomerulonephritis with end-stage renal disease develops in most cases.

5. **Therapy** rarely is effective, although occasional reports claim some benefit of treatment with steroids, alkylating agents, antiplatelet agents, or anticoagulants.

F. **Focal glomerulosclerosis**

1. **Incidence and etiology**
   a. Focal glomerulosclerosis accounts for 5%–12% of cases of idiopathic nephrotic syndrome in adults and is the most common cause of steroid-resistant nephrotic syndrome in children.
   b. The etiology is unknown. Focal glomerulosclerosis is seen occasionally in the context of AIDS, heroin and other intravascular drug use, and chronic vesicoureteral reflux, but the causal relationships are uncertain.

2. **Pathology.** The hallmark lesion of focal and segmental glomerulosclerosis evolves through several stages, including mild mesangial prominence, loss of glomerular cellularity, and collapse of capillary loops.

3. **Clinical features and diagnosis**
   a. **Nephrotic syndrome** is the most common clinical presentation. Hypertension and renal failure occur infrequently in childhood but become more prevalent with advancing age.
   b. There are no specific laboratory findings. Proteinuria tends to be heavy (i.e., > 15 g/24 hr), and the biochemical derangements of nephrotic syndrome are accordingly severe.

4. **Therapy**
   a. Focal glomerulosclerosis is reported to recur in 30%–40% of renal allografts within 3 weeks to 1 year following transplantation.
   b. Recent studies suggest prolonged glucocorticoid therapy (i.e., 6 months or longer) may lead to remission of proteinuria.

G. **Goodpasture's syndrome** (see also Chapter 2 XIV B)

1. **Definition.** Goodpasture's syndrome refers to a group of illnesses defined by the following triad of findings: **glomerulonephritis** (usually crescentic), **pulmonary hemorrhage,** and **antiglomerular basement membrane (anti-GBM) antibody.** The renal and pulmonary components may be severe or clinically silent. The presence of the anti-GBM antibody, however, has become the sine qua non of the diagnosis. Although many systemic illnesses include renal disease and pulmonary hemorrhage [e.g., SLE (see Part I: X M), necrotizing vasculitis (see Part I: X N), Wegener's granu-

lomatosis (see Part I: X N 3), Henoch-Schönlein purpura (see Part I: X K), cryoglobulinemia (see Part I: X O), thrombotic thrombocytopenic purpura (TTP; see Part I: XIV D), legionnaires' disease, and renal disease complicated by pulmonary embolism or congestive heart failure], only those illnesses with detectable anti-GBM antibody are considered bona fide Goodpasture's syndrome.

2. **Clinical features and diagnosis**
   a. **Clinical presentation** is highly variable.
      (1) **Generalized, systemic symptoms** may precede organ-specific complaints. Fever and myalgia are common.
      (2) **Renal involvement** usually is in the form of rapidly progressive renal failure. Proteinuria usually is mild, and the urinary sediment contains erythrocytes and red cell casts. This "nephritic" picture may be mild or severe.
      (3) **Pulmonary manifestations** include radiographic infiltrates, hemoptysis, cough, and dyspnea. The lung disease usually precedes kidney disease by a period of days to weeks.
   b. **Laboratory findings**
      (1) The most important finding is evidence of circulating IgG anti-GBM antibody, which is present in more than 90% of patients.
      (2) The pathologic appearance of the kidney is typically that of a crescentic, proliferative glomerulonephritis. Crescents involve 80%–100% of glomeruli and are highly cellular.

3. **Clinical course.** Like the clinical presentation, the course of Goodpasture's syndrome is variable, ranging from minor recurrent pulmonary hemorrhage for years until an abnormal urinary sediment prompts measurement of anti-GBM antibody to abrupt-onset, fulminant disease, complete renal failure, and asphyxiation by massive pulmonary bleeding over a period of hours to days.

4. **Therapy.** Several methods of therapy appear to benefit patients with Goodpasture's syndrome. However, poor prognostic indicators include oligo-anuria, serum creatinine above 6 mg/ml for many weeks, and advanced histopathologic lesions.
   a. There have been a variety of successful but uncontrolled clinical trials involving combinations of corticosteroids and alkylating immunosuppressive agents.
   b. A promising approach to pulmonary hemorrhage has been intensive, daily plasmapheresis combined with chemotherapy.

H. **Idiopathic crescentic glomerulonephritis** is a pathologically defined entity that typically presents as a rapidly progressive deterioration of renal function. It is imperative to recognize that other lesions may induce the clinical syndrome of **rapidly progressive glomerulonephritis.** This section considers only the idiopathic cases, that is, those cases not due to other crescentic glomerular diseases. However, it is important to consider the many other diseases that can produce this condition (Table 6-5).

1. **Incidence and etiology.** Idiopathic crescentic glomerulonephritis accounts for about one-third of all cases of crescentic glomerulonephritis. Males are affected twice as frequently as females.

2. **Clinical features.** Idiopathic crescentic glomerulonephritis presents as abrupt-onset renal failure, with rapid loss of renal function (in less than 3 months), frequently normal blood pressure, and normal kidney size. Nonspecific symptoms (e.g., weakness, nausea, cough, weight loss, fever, myalgia, and arthralgia) often announce the disease. With the exception of lung involvement, extrarenal involvement is rare.
   a. **Renal manifestations.** Approximately 50% of patients are oliguric and azotemic at the time of presentation.
   b. **Pulmonary manifestations.** Transient, mild pulmonary infiltrates or hemoptysis is seen in half of patients.

3. **Diagnosis.** There are no diagnostic laboratory findings; however, when intrarenal vasculitis is the cause of the glomerulonephritis, the antineutrophilic cytoplasmic antibody (ANCA) test will be positive. The diagnosis is based on the discovery of epithelial crescents in a majority of glomeruli in the renal biopsy specimen.

TABLE 6-5. Causes of Acute Renal Failure with Crescentic Glomerulonephritis

---

In primary glomerular diseases

Primary (idiopathic) diffuse crescentic glomerulonephritis

   Type I: anti-GBM antibody disease **without** pulmonary hemorrhage

   Type II: immune complex disease

   Type III: unknown pathogenesis—diffuse crescent superimposed on other primary glomerular
      disease

Mesangiocapillary glomerulonephritis (especially type II)

Membranous glomerulonephritis with or without superimposed anti-GBM antibody disease

IgA nephropathy (Berger's disease)

Focal and segmental glomerulosclerosis

In association with infectious diseases

Poststreptococcal glomerulonephritis

Infective endocarditis

Occult visceral bacterial sepsis

Other infections (e.g., hepatitis B)

In association with multisystem diseases

SLE

Goodpasture's syndrome (anti-GBM antibody disease with pulmonary hemorrhage)

Henoch-Schönlein purpura—disseminated vasculitis

Wegener's granulomatosis

Microscopic polyarteritis (hypersensitivity angiitis)

Other variants

Cryoimmunoglobulinemia (mixed, essential)

Relapsing polychondritis

Lung cancer, lymphoma

Anti-GBM = anti-glomerular basement membrane; IgA = immunoglobulin A; SLE = systemic lupus erythematosus.

    4. Clinical course and prognosis are very bleak. Renal failure requiring renal replacement therapy develops in 3–6 months in more than 50% of patients.

    5. Therapy. No controlled experimental data are available to support a standard therapeutic approach to idiopathic crescentic glomerulonephritis. Favorable results have been reported in isolated cases using many different treatments, including pulse corticosteroids, alkylating agents, plasmapheresis, and anticoagulant or antiplatelet drugs.

I. **Postinfectious glomerulonephritis** is an acute glomerulonephritis that occurs with a variety of local or systemic infections. (Glomerulonephritis that is associated with infective endocarditis and visceral abscess is discussed in Part I: X Q.) Postinfectious glomerulonephritis has been described as a sequela of disease caused by viruses, fungi, protozoa, and helminths. The prototypical postinfectious glomerulonephritis, however, is **poststreptococcal glomerulonephritis,** which is the subject of the remainder of this section.

    1. Incidence and etiology

        a. Poststreptococcal glomerulonephritis primarily affects school-aged children. The disease is rare before 2 years of age, but has been reported in adults. Males are affected twice as often as females.

        b. Preceding infection with nephritogenic strains of Group A β-hemolytic streptococci (particularly type 12) is the rule, although positive culture of the organism is demonstrated in less than 20% of cases at the time of renal disease. The site of infection (i.e., the skin or pharynx) appears to vary with the geographic area of study. The latent period between infection and clinical glomerular disease is 7–15 days; rarely, it lasts as long as 3 weeks.

2. Pathology. Poststreptococcal glomerulonephritis is a diffuse proliferative disease with mesangial and endothelial hypercellularity. Electron-dense deposits (subepithelial "humps") and foot process fusion are seen by electron microscopy. Immunofluorescence often identifies granular deposits of C3 along the capillary basement membrane.

3. Clinical features and diagnosis

   a. The typical clinical presentation is a sudden onset of hematuria and edema. Nephrotic syndrome develops in less than 15% of patients.

   b. The characteristic, but not diagnostic, laboratory profile is azotemia, hypocomplementemia (CH_{50} or C3), hematuria, leukocyturia, and proteinuria. Supporting data include elevated titers of antistreptolysin O, antihyaluronidase, and anti-deoxyribonuclease B antibodies, all of which suggest preceding streptococcal infection.

4. Clinical course and diagnosis

   a. The typical course of acute poststreptococcal glomerulonephritis is recovery, particularly among children. The acute nephritis resolves with amelioration of edema and hypertension 1–3 weeks after onset. Proteinuria may persist for several months, exacerbated by erect posture and exercise. Microscopic hematuria similarly disappears slowly over a period of several months.

   b. The long-term prognosis is controversial. Some patients advance to end-stage renal disease. Factors associated with this poor prognosis are severe oliguria or anuria, crescents in the biopsy specimen, persistent heavy proteinuria, and relatively older age. Persistence of hypocomplementemia and progressive renal failure may, however, indicate an alternative diagnosis (e.g., membranoproliferative glomerulonephritis).

5. Therapy. Hypertension must be treated aggressively, particularly in children, who develop florid hypertensive encephalopathy at normal adult blood pressures. Furosemide or bumetanide will likely be required for the underlying edema-inducing disease. Antibiotic use is controversial, although a 10-day course of penicillin in the nonallergic patient is safe enough for routine use. Prophylaxis following poststreptococcal glomerulonephritis is not indicated because recurrences are exceedingly rare.

J. **IgA glomerulonephritis (Berger's disease)**

1. Definition and incidence. The disease is characterized by mesangial deposits of IgA in renal biopsies from patients with recurrent hematuria but normal renal function. The incidence of this disease varies remarkably with geographic location, and men are affected three to four times as frequently as women.

2. Pathology is characteristic.

   a. Diffuse, sometimes irregularly distributed IgA deposits are seen in the mesangium. IgM or IgG also may be present.

   b. Focal and segmental glomerulonephritis with mesangial proliferation is common. Mesangial prominence may be the only pathologic finding.

3. Clinical features and diagnosis. The patients, who usually are between 20 and 40 years of age, most commonly present with recurrent, often macroscopic hematuria but a normal GFR and normal tubular function. Biopsies from normal-appearing skin have immunofluorescent positivity for IgA in 50% of cases. Measuring serum IgA levels is not useful.

4. Clinical course and prognosis are variable.

   a. The 20-year survival rate is about 50%.

   b. A minority of patients progress to renal failure. Factors that predict a poor prognosis include advanced age at disease onset, heavy proteinuria, hypertension, and the presence of crescents or segmental sclerosis on renal biopsy.

5. **Therapy.** No evidence suggests that any specific therapy is beneficial.

K. Henoch-Schönlein purpura

1. **Definition.** Henoch-Schönlein purpura is a systemic disease characterized by purpura (which may be slight and go unnoticed), arthritis, abdominal pain, bloody diarrhea, and nephritis.

2. **Incidence.** Henoch-Schönlein purpura affects mainly children. Clinical nephritis affects 30% of patients, but almost all patients have an abnormal kidney biopsy.

3. **Pathology.** The histopathology ranges from mild, diffuse mesangial prominence to focal and segmental proliferative glomerulonephritis on a background of diffuse mesangial proliferation. The hallmark of Henoch-Schönlein purpura is the invariable immunofluorescent positivity for IgA in the mesangium.

4. **Clinical features and diagnosis**
   a. The clinical presentation often is preceded by an infection [caused by a virus (e.g., herpes zoster), mycoplasma, or streptococcus], vaccination, an insect bite, or drug administration. Rash usually develops early and evolves from morbilliform to purpuric. The legs and buttocks are affected most commonly. Arthritis typically is mild and nondeforming. Gastrointestinal bleeding and pain may dominate the presentation.
   b. Laboratory findings are exceedingly nonspecific, although elevated serum IgA is reported frequently. Serum complement component levels usually are normal.

5. **Clinical course and prognosis**
   a. The clinical course is variable. Patients with recurrent purpura, heavy proteinuria, and clinically severe nephritis at the time of presentation and patients whose biopsies show epithelial crescent formation tend to fare poorly.
   b. Among all children with systemic Henoch-Schönlein purpura, the 15-year survival rate is 90%. By 10 years, however, 15% of these patients have persisting disease and 8% have renal impairment. Among adults, 50% heal completely, 15% progress to renal failure, and approximately 35% have persistent disease.

6. **Therapy.** Several treatment methods have been attempted (e.g., immunosuppression, steroid therapy, and anticoagulation) but without proven benefit.

L. Diabetic nephropathy

1. **Incidence.** End-stage renal disease develops in 5%–15% of all patients with diabetes. Among patients with juvenile-onset diabetes, 35% develop renal disease within 20 years of the onset of diabetes. Among new patients considered for maintenance renal replacement therapy (largely chronic hemodialysis), at least 30% have chronic renal failure secondary to diabetes.

2. **Pathogenesis**
   a. The evolution of diabetic nephropathy is symptomatically quiet until late in the disease process. Early in diabetes, the GFR often is above normal. This early hyperfiltration may be most striking in those patients who will subsequently develop glomerular damage.
   b. Initially, **microalbuminuria** (the loss of small amounts of protein, typically below dipstick detection levels) occurs. After 15–20 years of diabetes, **proteinuria** develops. After 3–5 years of proteinuria, **nephrotic syndrome** often develops, as does **azotemia. End-stage renal disease** occurs 1–5 years after the onset of azotemia.

3. **Pathology.** Two major pathologic lesions are associated with diabetes.
   a. **Diffuse glomerulosclerosis** is characterized by an eosinophilic thickening of the mesangium and basement membrane.
   b. **Nodular glomerulosclerosis,** also known as **Kimmelstiel-Wilson syndrome,** consists of round nodules that are homogeneous at the center and have circumfer-

ential layering of nuclei. These nodules often are multiple within a given glomerulus and may be confluent. Nodular glomerulosclerosis is specific for diabetes, but it is found in only 50% of patients with diabetic nephropathy.

4. Laboratory findings are indicative of a slowly declining GFR.

5. Clinical course. Factors that accelerate renal deterioration include hypertension, urinary obstruction, infection, the administration of nephrotoxic drugs, and the use of intravenous radiocontrast material.

6. Therapy
   a. Treatment of diabetic nephropathy is supportive.
   (1) There is little evidence linking tight control of blood glucose to moderation of renal disease, and only in those patients with the earliest lesions (microalbuminuria).
   (2) Restriction of dietary protein (i.e., to 40 g/day) has been advocated as a means of preserving remnant nephron integrity in slowly progressive renal diseases such as diabetes.
   (3) Recent studies advocate ACE inhibitor therapy for patients with insulin-dependent diabetes and renal dysfunction (including albuminuria or a reduced GFR).
   (4) Avoidance of nephrotoxins, treatment of high blood pressure, and surveillance for urinary obstruction (neurogenic bladder) are prudent conservative measures.
   b. End-stage renal disease is treated using the established modalities.
   (1) Patients who undergo transplantation of a kidney from a living relative have a better 5-year survival rate than those who undergo chronic hemodialysis.
   (2) Several dialysis treatment centers have reported good results using continuous ambulatory peritoneal dialysis in patients with diabetes. Insulin may be given intraperitoneally, by which improved diabetic control appears possible.

M. **Lupus nephritis** refers to a spectrum of renal pathology. Presently, four major lesions and three superimposed (secondary) lesions are recognized.

1. Major lesions
   a. Focal proliferative lupus nephritis develops during the first year of clinical lupus in 50% of patients.
   (1) Pathology. The lesion is sharply delineated segmental endothelial and mesangial cell proliferation, which usually affects less than 50% of all glomeruli.
   (2) Clinical features and diagnosis
      (a) Proteinuria is seen in almost all cases; however, nephrotic syndrome is rare. Hematuria is common, and mild renal insufficiency is seen occasionally. Hypertension is not present.
      (b) Serologic findings include positive fluorescent antinuclear antibody (ANA) and modest elevations in anti-DNA antibodies. Complement components (C3 and C4) are at normal or decreased levels.
   (3) Clinical course and prognosis
      (a) Remission, as measured by cessation of proteinuria, is seen in about 50% of patients. Relapses commonly occur with extrarenal flares of systemic lupus. Transition to other forms of the disease (e.g., diffuse proliferative or membranous lupus nephritis) occurs in at least 20% of patients.
      (b) Renal failure is rare unless the disease progresses to diffuse proliferative lupus nephritis.
      (c) The 5-year mortality rate is 10%.
   b. Diffuse proliferative lupus nephritis most commonly develops within the first year of clinical lupus.
   (1) Pathology. Mesangial and endothelial cell proliferation affect most glomeruli with varying severity. Capillary lumina are obliterated, and crescents af-

fect up to 30% of glomeruli. Deposits of IgG, C3, C4, and C1q are diffuse. IgA and IgM deposits also are seen frequently.

(2) Clinical features and diagnosis

  (a) Proteinuria and hematuria are universal; more than 50% of patients present with nephrotic syndrome. Eventually, almost all patients become nephrotic. Azotemia is common early in the course of the disease and may be severe. Hypertension occurs in a minority of cases.

  (b) Serologic findings include positive fluorescent ANA, highly elevated anti-DNA antibodies, and depressed levels of C3 and C4. Cryoglobulinemia develops in some cases.

(3) Clinical course and prognosis

  (a) Remission of the nephrotic syndrome is seen in 33% of patients and sometimes is sustained. Transition to mesangial lupus nephritis occurs occasionally in association with clinical remission.

  (b) The 5-year mortality rate is 50%. Death results from uremia or active systemic lupus, which frequently is complicated by infection. Hypertension and renal failure may occur as sequelae even after long periods of clinical remission.

c. Membranous lupus nephritis develops during the first year of clinical lupus in about 50% of patients.

(1) Pathology. The histopathologic pattern of membranous lupus nephritis is very similar to that of idiopathic membranous glomerulonephritis (see Part I: X C 2).

(2) Clinical features and diagnosis

  (a) Proteinuria is seen in all patients; hematuria is common as well. Nephrotic syndrome is seen at presentation in 50% of patients and ultimately occurs in 80% of patients. Hypertension and renal insufficiency are rare at the outset of membranous lupus nephritis.

  (b) Serologic findings include positive fluorescent ANA, normal or only mildly elevated anti-DNA antibodies, and normal or decreased levels of C3 and C4.

(3) Clinical course and prognosis

  (a) Remission from nephrotic syndrome is seen in 33% of patients, but relapses are common. Transition to focal or diffuse proliferative lupus nephritis has been reported but is rare.

  (b) The 5-year mortality rate is 10% for patients who develop hypertension and renal insufficiency during persistent nephrotic syndrome.

d. Mesangial lupus nephritis may occur as the earliest form of lupus nephritis.

(1) Pathology. Biopsy shows mesangial prominence with an increase in matrix and in the number of mesangial cells.

(2) Clinical features and diagnosis

  (a) The complete spectrum of clinical findings is not fully known. Many patients are asymptomatic or present with only mild urinary abnormalities.

  (b) Serologic findings include positive fluorescent ANA, mild anti-DNA antibody elevations, and normal or mildly decreased C3 and C4 levels.

(3) Clinical course and prognosis

  (a) Urinary abnormalities may remit, and transition to diffuse proliferative or membranous lupus nephritis occurs in 15% of patients.

  (b) This mesangial lesion is associated with clinical progression only if there is transition to a less favorable histology.

2. Superimposed lesions

a. Glomerulosclerosis is a secondary lesion that is seen most commonly in diffuse proliferative lupus nephritis with a protracted course. Progressive glomerulosclerosis may be a cause of renal failure in patients whose systemic lupus remits.

b. Interstitial lupus nephritis usually coexists with glomerular disease but may develop alone.

        (1) Pathologically, this lesion is characterized by intense, mononuclear interstitial infiltration, tubular damage, and interstitial fibrosis.

        (2) IgG and C3 are identified in peritubular capillaries and in tubular basement membranes. Parallel electron-dense deposits are seen.

        (3) Clinical disorders of tubular function (e.g., disorders of potassium excretion, acid excretion, and urine concentration and dilution) are seen in addition to variable, nonselective proteinuria.

    c. Necrotizing vasculitis usually complicates diffuse proliferative lupus nephritis and presents as rapidly accelerating hypertension and renal failure. Histopathologically, an acellular necrosis of vessel walls is seen with proteinaceous occlusive thrombi.

  3. Therapy. Criteria for therapy are not rigidly established. The response of membranous lupus nephritis to therapy varies among reported series. Because of the poor prognosis associated with diffuse proliferative lupus nephritis, this lesion currently is treated—even in cases with few clinical signs or symptoms of renal disease.

    a. Regimens of **glucocorticoid therapy** vary. Induction therapy with oral prednisone (1–2 mg/kg/day) and pulse intravenous methylprednisolone (1–2 g/day) has been described.

    b. Cytotoxic drugs (e.g., cyclophosphamide), when added to steroids, often induce remission, preserve or improve renal function, or both.

N. **Vasculitis**

  1. Introduction. The kidney frequently is involved in systemic vasculitis, although the actual incidence is unknown. The spectrum of renal syndromes associated with vasculitis ranges from modest "microscopic" involvement of arterioles, venules, and capillaries (a syndrome referred to as **hypersensitivity vasculitis**) to extensive "classic" involvement of medium-sized vessels (a syndrome referred to as **polyarteritis nodosa**).

  2. Polyarteritis nodosa

    a. Etiology. This type of vasculitis may be primary (idiopathic) or secondary to drugs, viral infections (e.g., hepatitis B), or rheumatic diseases (e.g., lupus and rheumatoid vasculitis).

    b. Pathology. The kidneys show a focal necrotizing arteritis in vessels ranging in size from the renal artery to the interlobular veins.

    c. Clinical features and diagnosis

        (1) The clinical presentation often is vague, consisting of low-grade fever, myalgia, arthralgia, and weight loss.

        (2) The laboratory findings are numerous and, although nonspecific, frequently suggest the diagnosis of polyarteritis nodosa when considered collectively (see Table 10-9).

        (3) The diagnosis can be confirmed by renal angiography, which shows multiple small aneurysms with segmental infarctions.

    d. Clinical course and prognosis. Progression to organ destruction or death is the expected outcome.

    e. Therapy with daily high-dose glucocorticoids and daily cyclophosphamide (1–3 mg/kg/ day) has increased the 1-year survival rate to greater than 80%.

  3. Wegener's granulomatosis (see also Chapter 2 XIV C) is a special case of vasculitis (necrotizing granulomatous vasculitis) with renal involvement. The disease affects patients of all ages but is more common in middle-aged men.

    a. Pathology. The characteristic and diagnostic lesion of necrotizing vasculitis and granulomatous inflammation is most reliably discovered in pulmonary or upper airway biopsy material. Often, a focal and segmental necrotizing vasculitis and glomerulitis are found with few (if any) immune deposits.

    b. Clinical features and diagnosis

        (1) Wegener's granulomatosis affects the kidney and upper respiratory tract, including the nose, throat, and bronchi. Ulcerative vasculitic lesions, including nasal septal perforation, are the most recognizable presenting signs.

(2) The hematologic and serologic features of Wegener's granulomatosis extensively overlap those of polyarteritis nodosa. ANCAs are present in the serum of most patients and may help in diagnosing the disease and in monitoring response to therapy.

c. **Clinical course.** Wegener's granulomatosis has a variable course. Long-term remissions are seen occasionally with therapy. Death usually results from renal failure, sepsis, hemorrhage, or disseminated intravascular coagulation (DIC).

d. **Therapy** with daily high-dose glucocorticoids and daily cyclophosphamide (1–3 mg/kg/day) has increased the 1-year survival rate from less than 20% to greater than 80%.

O. Cryoglobulins and cryoglobulinemia

1. **Cryoglobulins** are proteins that precipitate at low temperatures and dissolve on rewarming. Three types of cryoglobulins are defined:
   a. **Type I:** Monoclonal cryoglobulins
   b. **Type II:** Mixed cryoglobulins that include a monoclonal component with antibody activity against polyclonal IgG
   c. **Type III:** Mixed cryoglobulins in which both components are polyclonal

2. **Cryoglobulinemia** (i.e., the presence of cryoglobulins in the blood) occurs in a variety of clinically dissimilar conditions. Renal disease is associated primarily with types I and II and probably has an immune complex–mediated pathophysiology.
   a. **Clinical features**
      (1) **Type I cryoglobulinemia** is associated with hematologic malignancies. Heavy proteinuria, hematuria, and, occasionally, anuria are seen. The histologic lesion usually is a membranoproliferative glomerulonephritis.
      (2) **Type II cryoglobulinemia** is associated with a syndrome of immune-complex vasculitis; approximately 50% of patients have renal disease. The wide spectrum of clinical signs varies greatly in severity. Hypertension, azotemia, and anuria are poor prognostic signs. Endocapillary proliferation and mesangial prominence are common pathologic features.
      (3) **Type III cryoglobulinemia** may be associated with a variety of other diseases, with or without renal disease, including SLE, hepatitis B or C, and systemic infections.
   b. **Diagnosis** involves the detection, characterization, and quantitation of cryoglobulins in serum.
   c. **Therapy** in idiopathic cases is not standardized. Encouraging results have been obtained with plasmapheresis.

P. Multiple myeloma (see also Chapter 4 XIII)

1. **Definition.** Multiple myeloma represents a neoplastic transformation of a monoclonal B lymphocyte into a plasma cell, which produces excessive quantities of immunoglobulin or immunoglobulin fragment (paraprotein). More than 50% of patients with multiple myeloma die from complications of renal failure, and a much higher percentage of multiple myeloma patients have some form of renal involvement.

2. **Pathology.** The many mechanisms of renal injury in multiple myeloma have different effects on the kidney (Table 6-6).

3. **Clinical features and diagnosis**
   a. The clinical presentation of renal disease in multiple myeloma often is subtle. Anemia and bone pain in the presence of any form of abnormal urinary finding should prompt evaluation for myeloma. Slowly progressive renal insufficiency is typical; however, acute renal failure may be seen in certain circumstances (e.g., in the presence of hypercalcemia).
   b. Many chemical abnormalities are seen commonly in multiple myeloma. Pseudohyponatremia develops secondary to the presence of large quantities of paraprotein, altering the nonaqueous phase of plasma. The anion gap is low and occasionally is negative because of the positive charges on the immunoglobulin

TABLE 6-6. Mechanisms of Renal Injury in Multiple Myeloma

Mechanism of Renal Injury	Effect on the Kidney
Bence Jones proteinuria	Direct tubular toxicity
	Intratubular obstruction by cast formation
Amyloidosis	Glomerular and tubular amyloid deposits
Hypercalcemia	Renal vasoconstriction
	Calcium–phosphate deposition
Hyperuricemia	Acute urate deposition and tubular obstruction
Hyperviscosity	Vascular occlusion
Light chain nephropathy	Glomerular occlusion

molecules. Urine protein concentration is increased, reflecting excretion of the huge paraprotein burden. As mentioned earlier, dipstick measurement for protein is insensitive to immunoglobulin and often gives false-negative results. Thus, acid precipitation with sulfosalicylic acid is required.

4. **Therapy and prognosis.** Although no specific therapy exists for the renal disease, chemotherapy for the malignancy, meticulous regulation of intravascular volume and electrolyte status, and dialysis (when necessary) may prolong life.

Q. **Glomerulonephritis in infective endocarditis** represents the prototypical bacterial illness that may lead to the induction of glomerulonephritis, presumably through an immune-complex mechanism. Glomerulonephritis is thought to occur by similar means in visceral abscess and in infections arising from extracorporeal circulation devices (shunt nephritis). It is possible that any endovascular infection can produce this glomerulonephritis.

1. **Pathology.** The histologic severity ranges from mild mesangial proliferation to severe crescentic glomerulonephritis.

2. **Clinical features.** About 15% of patients with infective endocarditis develop renal involvement. Nonimmune mechanisms of injury include septic emboli, ischemic ATN with severe congestive heart failure, and, indirectly, antibiotic nephrotoxicity. Immune-complex glomerulonephritis presents with hematuria, red cell casts in the urine, and azotemia.

3. **Therapy.** There is no specific therapy for the renal disease. Except in fairly advanced cases, successful treatment of the underlying infection usually leads to resolution of the renal disease.

XI. **RENAL CYSTIC DISEASE**

A. **Adult polycystic kidney disease**

1. **Definition, etiology, and incidence.** Adult polycystic kidney disease represents the most common cause of renal failure and death in adults with renal cystic disease. It accounts for approximately 10% of all patients on maintenance dialysis.
    a. Inherited as an autosomal dominant trait, adult polycystic kidney disease achieves 100% gene penetrance by the time the patient is 80 years of age. The affected gene is on chromosome 16 in the majority of cases.
    b. Men and women are affected equally.
    c. Adult polycystic kidney disease must be distinguished from **childhood (autosomal recessive) polycystic kidney disease,** which is universally fatal by the third decade of life, and the **congenital multicystic variant of renal dysplasia.**

2. **Clinical features**
   a. The typical presentation of enlarging flank or abdominal masses, abdominal pain, and slowly progressive renal failure becomes clinically evident by the fourth decade of life, and renal replacement therapy becomes necessary within 10 years of the onset of symptoms. Family history is positive in more than 75% of cases. Associated clinical findings may include hypertension, polyuria and nocturia, erythrocytosis, and nephrolithiasis.
   b. Hepatic cysts are demonstrated in 33% of cases; however, liver insufficiency is rare, unlike in the childhood form.
   c. Intracranial (berry) aneurysms occur in 12% of patients. In some series, 6% of all patients with berry aneurysms have adult polycystic kidney disease.

3. **Diagnosis** is made most easily on the basis of specific ultrasonographic findings. Coincident findings include hematuria, impaired urine concentrating ability, and low-grade proteinuria. Heavy proteinuria, persistent hematuria, and pyuria should be investigated because they rarely occur in uncomplicated adult polycystic kidney disease.

4. **Therapy** is restricted to the treatment of end-stage renal disease as it develops. Genetic counseling is important because 50% of offspring are affected. Women with adult polycystic kidney disease are not at an increased risk for fetal demise or hypertension during pregnancy except as contributed by existing renal insufficiency.

B. **Nephronophthisis (medullary cystic disease)**

1. **Definition and incidence.** Medullary cystic disease is the most common cause of end-stage renal disease in children and adolescents.

2. **Pathology.** The kidney is small in medullary cystic disease, which distinguishes this disease from polycystic and multicystic diseases. Cysts may be located at the corticomedullary junction or in the medulla. Acystic forms have been described. Interstitial fibrosis is prominent, but calcification does not occur.

3. **Clinical features.** Loss of urine concentrating ability and failure to conserve sodium appropriately are almost invariable early signs of disease. The initial presentation often includes polyuria, polydipsia, and enuresis, although an azotemic presentation also is common. Progression to renal failure is a constant clinical feature.

4. **Therapy** is aimed at maintaining sodium and water homeostasis during the evolution of disease. Genetic counseling may be appropriate in disease that is clearly familial. The possibility of subclinical disease in siblings must be considered when a donor is being selected for transplantation.

C. **Medullary sponge kidney**

1. **Definition and incidence.** Medullary sponge kidney is not a true cystic disease but rather an ectasia of the renal collecting tubule. This common problem is identified in 1 of every 200 urograms in a large series.

2. **Prognosis** is excellent; many patients have no detectable impairment of renal function. Hypercalciuria is common, as are subtle defects in the ability to concentrate and acidify the urine. Nephrocalcinosis, of variable severity, is found in 50% of cases.

D. **Simple renal cyst**

1. **Definition and incidence.** The simple cyst is the most common renal cystic disease; at least half of all individuals older than 50 years of age have one or more macroscopic renal cysts. Renal cysts may be solitary or multiple and unilateral or bilateral. They usually are located in the cortex and bulge through the renal capsule, but they may occur in the medulla. Large renal cysts are more common among adults, and multilocular cysts are rare.

2. **Clinical features.** Symptoms are rare; simple cysts usually are diagnosed during patient evaluation for other problems. Bleeding and infection stimulate the cyst wall to thicken, and calcareous plaques often form within the cyst wall.

3. **Clinical course.** Simple cysts usually are static, although regression may occur from one radiographic assessment to the next. Solitary cysts may undergo malignant degeneration, although this finding is rare. Hemorrhagic cysts are more likely to contain a neoplasm than nonhemorrhagic cysts (i.e., in up to 30% of cases as compared to less than 1% of cases). Multiple simple cysts may develop in end-stage renal disease in patients who have undergone hemodialysis for longer than 7 years.

4. **Diagnosis** may be made by CT, ultrasonography, urography, or angiography. Cyst puncture (for fluid aspiration and cytology) and contrast radiology should be performed in patients with large cysts with abnormal ultrasonographic appearance.

5. **Therapy.** In the absence of infection or tumor, no specific therapy is indicated for this benign disease.

XII. TUBULOINTERSTITIAL DISEASE

A. Acute interstitial nephritis

1. **Definition.** Acute interstitial nephritis appears to be a kidney-based hypersensitivity reaction, usually caused by a drug. Although the true incidence of acute interstitial nephritis is unknown, several hundred cases have been formally reported, and an increasing awareness of this disease has come with increased case recognition.

2. **Etiology.** Drugs implicated in the pathogenesis of acute interstitial nephritis include β-lactam antibiotics (e.g., methicillin, oxacillin, and cephalothin) and other antibiotics (e.g., sulfonamides); nonsteroidal anti-inflammatory drugs (NSAIDs; e.g., ibuprofen, indomethacin, fenoprofen, and tolmetin); diuretics (e.g., thiazides and furosemide); and many other unrelated drugs (e.g., phenytoin, cimetidine, sulfinpyrazone, methyldopa, and phenobarbital).

3. **Clinical features.** The typical presentation is the development of acute renal failure with fever, rash, and eosinophilia.

4. **Diagnosis**
   a. **Urinalysis** classically shows mild or no proteinuria, microscopic hematuria, pyuria, and eosinophiluria. Some patients with acute interstitial nephritis due to NSAIDs present with nephrotic syndrome characterized by urinary protein excretion exceeding 3.0 g/24 hr.
   b. **Biopsy** shows patchy, irregular interstitial infiltration with inflammatory cells. Monocytes and lymphocytes are constant findings. Eosinophils may be abundant or completely absent. Fibrosis is extremely unusual and should suggest underlying or preexisting renal disease. Rarely, acute interstitial nephritis may progress to a chronic interstitial nephritis, and fibrosis may be prominent. Glomeruli are normal or show only mild mesangial prominence.

5. **Therapy** includes discontinuation of the etiologic drug and initiation of supportive measures (e.g., dietary restrictions, blood pressure management, and acute dialysis). The value of glucocorticoid therapy is unclear; however, the use of steroids may be justified in patients with severe or rapidly progressive renal insufficiency.

6. **Prognosis** is excellent provided that the offending drug is promptly withdrawn. Recovery time varies and may be prolonged in oliguric patients and in patients with extensive interstitial cellular infiltrates. Temporary dialysis may be needed. Rarely, patients progress to end-stage renal disease.

B. Chronic interstitial nephritis.
In general, the clinical features common to these interstitial diseases include relative preservation of glomerular function until late in the disease but an impairment of tubular functions (e.g., urine concentration, dilution, and acidification and potassium excretion) early in the course of the disease.

1. **Drug-related nephropathy**
   a. **Analgesic nephropathy** is the prototypical drug-related chronic interstitial nephritis.
      (1) Analgesic nephropathy occurs more commonly in women than in men. Patients usually are older than 45 years of age and from low socioeconomic classes. Patients often complain of frequent headaches or have coincident psychiatric disease.
      (2) Intravenous urography reveals abnormality in more than 90% of cases, and papillary necrosis is seen in more than 50%. Half of the patients are hypertensive, and anemia is common and often out of proportion to the degree of clinically apparent renal disease.
      (3) Several agents have been implicated (e.g., acetaminophen, phenacetin, and aspirin), but none has been specifically proven culpable. The risk for analgesic nephropathy appears to be increased in patients who use more than 3 g/day of such agents.
      (4) Treatment of progressive analgesic nephropathy is supportive. Removal of the inciting agent may arrest the deterioration of renal function.
   b. **Gold nephropathy** is a frequent and important complication of parenteral gold therapy for rheumatoid arthritis. Gold accumulation leads to immune-complex membranous glomerulonephritis and nephrotic syndrome. Cessation of gold therapy at the first sign of proteinuria is recommended and often results in regression of signs of renal disease. It is not yet known if oral gold preparations are equally nephrotoxic.
   c. **Lithium nephrotoxicity.** Lithium carbonate, used in the treatment of bipolar disorder, is filtered freely and undergoes significant (i.e., 60%–70%) reabsorption in the proximal tubules. Lithium toxicity results in antidiuretic hormone (ADH)–unresponsive nephrogenic diabetes insipidus, incomplete distal renal tubular acidosis, and, rarely, azotemia.
   d. **NSAIDs** have been associated with a variety of clinical renal disorders (see Part II of this chapter for effects on electrolyte metabolism). Table 6-7 gives the mechanism for NSAID-induced disorders.

2. **Toxin-related nephropathy**
   a. **Cadmium nephropathy.** Cadmium is a highly toxic by-product of zinc production, which has numerous industrial applications. During long-term exposure, cadmium accumulates in the kidney whereas blood and urine cadmium concentrations remain normal. Cadmium probably leads to end-stage renal disease, although the true incidence is unknown.
   b. **Lead nephropathy (saturnine gout)** is a well-recognized sequela of chronic lead intoxication.
      (1) The earliest cases of lead intoxication involved miners, paint manufacturers, and distillers of "moonshine" liquor. Lead poisoning also has been reported in children who have ingested lead-based paint. Individuals who re-

TABLE 6-7. Mechanisms for NSAID-Induced Disorders

NSAID-Induced Disorder	Mechanism
Nephrotic syndrome	Severe interstitial nephritis; histologically normal glomeruli
Decreased GFR	Renal vasoconstriction, especially in patients with preexisting renal disease, congestive heart failure, or cirrhosis; patients treated with triamterene at particular risk
Papillary necrosis	Unknown
Edema	Primary renal sodium retention due to prostaglandin inhibition, especially in patients with underlying congestive heart failure

GFR = glomerular filtration rate; NSAID = nonsteroidal anti-inflammatory drug.

cover from acute lead poisoning occasionally are found later to be victims of chronic lead-related renal disease.

(2) Clinical manifestations of lead nephropathy include a reduced GFR, reduced renal plasma flow (RPF), minimal or no proteinuria, normal urinary sediment, hyperuricemia and low urate clearance, and, occasionally, hypertension, hyperkalemia, and acidemia.

(3) Treatment includes removal of lead exposure and chelation therapy with sodium or calcium **ethylenediaminetetraacetic acid (EDTA) or D-penicillamine** (in appropriate cases).

c. **Copper nephrotoxicity** is rare but occasionally is seen in Wilson's disease. Clinically, copper nephropathy may resemble cadmium nephropathy (proximal tubular disease) or ATN. **D-Penicillamine** is the treatment of choice.

d. **Mercury nephropathy.** Mercury is associated with several renal lesions, including membranous and proliferative glomerular disease with nephrotic syndrome, proximal tubular atrophy and Fanconi's syndrome with the development of chronic renal failure, and oliguric ATN. Chelation therapy with **British antilewisite (BAL, dimercaprol)** and hemodialysis may reduce mortality if initiated promptly (i.e., within 48 hours following exposure).

3. **Crystalline nephropathy**
   a. **Uric acid** produces renal injury in three ways.
      (1) **Uric acid stones** may develop in concentrated acid urine.
      (2) **Acute uric acid nephropathy** (acute crystalline obstruction of renal tubules) may accompany sudden or extreme elevations in serum uric acid (i.e., serum levels exceeding 25 mg/dl), as occurs in **tumor lysis syndrome.**
      (3) **Gouty nephropathy,** a syndrome of interstitial fibrosis and decreased renal function, may be related to cortical microtophi and a nephrotoxic influence of hyperuricemia in some gouty patients. Lead nephropathy (saturnine gout) may account for a significant percentage of patients with renal insufficiency and gout.
   b. **Oxalic acid** also produces tubulointerstitial disease. Elevated urine levels of oxalic acid may lead to the formation of calcium oxalate stones or may mimic the syndrome of acute uric acid nephropathy (acute crystalline obstruction). **Primary hyperoxaluria** is an inherited disease of oxalate overproduction, which terminates in renal failure with extensive deposition of oxalate crystals throughout the body (a condition termed **oxalosis). Ethylene glycol poisoning** may lead to renal failure in part by the hyperoxaluria that results from the metabolism of ethylene glycol to oxalate. The use of **methoxyflurane** in anesthesia has been linked to an increased oxalate production with resultant nephrotoxicity. Increased oxalate absorption often is seen following ileojejunal bypass surgery for obesity and may lead to nephrocalcinosis. Mild hyperoxaluria may result from pyridoxine or thiamine deficiency.

4. **Miscellaneous nephropathies**
   a. **Amyloidosis**
      (1) **Definition and classification.** Amyloidosis is a disorder of unknown etiology, which involves the deposition of eosinophilic, amorphous material. The major classifications of amyloidosis are **primary amyloidosis** (occurring without pre- or coexisting illness), **secondary amyloidosis** (occurring in the presence of chronic inflammatory disease), and **heredofamilial amyloidosis.**
      (2) **Clinical features.** Amyloid deposition may be focal and restricted to the kidneys or systemic and generalized. Proteinuria is universal, with nephrotic syndrome developing in 76% of patients. Hypertension occurs in 50% of patients. Kidney size occasionally is increased but decreases with advanced disease.
      (3) **Clinical course.** Progressive deterioration of renal function is the rule.
      (4) **Diagnosis** is unequivocally established by biopsy demonstrating amyloid protein by green birefringence with Congo red stain.
      (5) **Therapy.** There is no effective treatment for primary amyloidosis, although alkylating agents and colchicine have been advocated. Treatment of second-

ary amyloidosis is limited to the treatment of the underlying inflammatory disease. Amyloidosis recurs in the transplanted kidney.

b. Sarcoidosis (see also Chapter 2 XIV A)

    (1) Definition. Sarcoidosis is a granulomatous disease of unknown etiology. Renal involvement may be secondary to noncaseating granulomatous replacement of the renal interstitium.

    (2) Clinical features. Renal size usually is normal, and mild nonselective proteinuria is common. Hypercalcemia, hypercalciuria, or both frequently complicate sarcoidosis as a result of increased synthesis of 1,25-dihydroxycholecalciferol [1,25-$(OH)_2D_3$].

    (3) Clinical course. The hypercalcemia may induce acute renal failure, and the hypercalciuria may lead to nephrocalcinosis or calcium nephrolithiasis. Hyperglobulinemia, when present, may be associated with distal renal tubular acidosis. Although glomerulonephritis has been noted among patients with sarcoidosis, the existence of a true sarcoid glomerulopathy is not fully established.

    (4) Therapy. Steroids are indicated for the management of hypercalcemia.

C. Renal papillary necrosis

1. **Definition.** Renal papillary necrosis results from ischemic necrosis of the renal medulla or renal papillae. There are two forms. The papillary form involves the entire papilla, whereas the medullary form begins with focal areas of infarction in the inner medullary zone.

2. **Etiologic factors.** Conditions associated with renal papillary necrosis include diabetes mellitus, urinary tract obstruction, severe pyelonephritis, analgesic abuse, sickle cell hemoglobinopathy, extreme hypoxia and intravascular volume depletion in infants, and renal allograft rejection.

3. **Clinical features.** The clinical presentation of renal papillary necrosis varies with the stage and extent of disease. Patients with sickle cell trait may have completely asymptomatic renal papillary necrosis, which is discovered incidentally during urography for unrelated complaints. Infection frequently complicates renal papillary necrosis and leads to clinical pyelonephritis. The necrotic papillae may be sloughed and produce typical ureteral colic or ureteral obstruction. Azotemia is an uncommon presenting sign.

4. **Clinical course.** The course of renal papillary necrosis is a function of the underlying disease. End-stage renal disease may develop, particularly among diabetics.

5. **Diagnosis.** Intravenous urography can establish the diagnosis of both forms of renal papillary necrosis. Radiographically, the affected calyces appear irregular and fuzzy early in the disease process. As the lesion progresses, sequestration of the necrotic tissue leads to sinus formation and the appearance of a sinus tract or arc shadow on the urogram. In advanced renal papillary necrosis, the sequestrum may be sloughed and surrounded by contrast material—the so-called ring sign. Calcification, calicectasis, and medullary cavities may be present in this stage.

6. **Therapy** includes relief of obstruction, prevention and prompt eradication of infection, and control of pain (colic). Surgery occasionally is necessary to control hemorrhage or to relieve obstruction.

XIII. RENAL TRANSPORT DEFECTS

A. Meliturias. Excessive quantities of **sugars** may gain access to the urine because of an increase in filtered load (as in the hyperglycemia of diabetes mellitus) or failure of appropriate reabsorption in the nephron.

1. **Primary renal glycosuria** is an autosomal recessive disorder recognized from birth by constant glycosuria in the absence of abnormal carbohydrate metabolism (i.e., hyperglycemia, ketosis, and other meliturias). Two variants are described. Both are associated with a reduction in either the amount of or affinity for the renal transport protein for glucose.

2. **Other meliturias are recognized.**
   a. **Essential pentosuria (L-xylulosuria),** an autosomal recessive defect in the metabolism of glucuronic acid, affects primarily Jews. L-Xylulosuria occurs secondary to a deficiency of nicotinamide–adenine dinucleotide phosphate (NADP)-linked xylitol dehydrogenase.
   b. **Essential fructosuria** also is an autosomal recessive error of metabolism, which is a result of defective phosphofructokinase activity.

B. **Aminoacidurias**

1. **Cystinuria** is an autosomal recessive defect in the transport of cystine, lysine, ornithine, and arginine. The low solubility of cystine accounts for the symptoms and complications of cystinuria in that it predisposes to the formation of renal cystine stones, which may lead to renal failure. Therapy consists of a lifelong alkaline diuresis to prevent stone formation. D-Penicillamine is required in many cases (see VII D).

2. **Dibasic aminoaciduria** is a selective defect in lysine, ornithine, and arginine (but not cystine) transport. Autosomal recessive and dominant forms are recognized. Symptoms include amino acid–induced diarrhea, malnutrition, hyperammonemia, and growth and mental retardation. Therapy consists of a low-protein diet.

3. **Iminoglycinuria** is a benign, autosomal recessive disorder of proline, hydroxyproline, and glycine transport.

4. **Hartnup disease** is an autosomal recessive defect in the transport of neutral α-amino acids. Hartnup disease patients have a reduced ability to convert tryptophan to niacin, resulting in pellagra—a syndrome characterized by photosensitive erythema, cerebellar ataxia, neuropsychiatric symptoms, and delirium. Therapy is oral nicotinamide.

C. **Fanconi's syndrome**

1. **Definition.** Fanconi's syndrome refers to a collection of proximal tubular defects, which may exist in varying number and degree of severity and which may be inherited or acquired.

2. **Etiology**
   a. **Inherited causes** of Fanconi's syndrome include cystinosis, Lowe's syndrome, Wilson's disease, tyrosinemia, galactosemia, glycogenosis, and fructose intolerance.
   b. **Acquired causes** of Fanconi's syndrome include transplant dysfunction, myeloma, Sjögren's syndrome, hyperparathyroidism, potassium depletion, amyloidosis, nephrotic syndrome, interstitial nephritis, heavy metal toxicity, and outdated tetracycline.
   c. An **idiopathic** form of Fanconi's syndrome also exists.

3. **Clinical features and course**
   a. Symptoms and signs of Fanconi's syndrome include glycosuria, aminoaciduria, phosphaturia, bicarbonaturia, vasopressin-resistant polyuria, rickets or osteoporosis, short stature, and uremia.
   b. The natural history of Fanconi's syndrome depends heavily on the course and prognosis of the underlying disease or diseases.

4. **Therapy** is designed to replace lost urinary solutes and to correct the underlying disease or diseases. Phosphate, vitamin D, and bicarbonate should be given when indicated by laboratory and clinical data.

XIV. RENAL VASCULAR DISEASE

A. **Ischemic nephropathy.** Occlusive disease of the renal arterial system encompasses a broad spectrum of clinical syndromes and pathophysiology. Arterial blood flow may be interrupted by in situ thrombosis or by embolism from distant endovascular sites. Occlusion may be sudden and complete or gradual, with resultant functional renal artery stenosis.

1. **Etiology**
   a. **Renal arterial thrombosis** may develop spontaneously in the context of atherosclerosis, aneurysm, arteritis, hypercoagulable states, sickle cell disease, and thrombotic microangiopathy. Thrombosis also may develop as a complication of external trauma, instrumentation with angiography catheters, arterial surgery, and renal allograft transplantation.
   b. **Renal arterial embolism** may be caused by a clot, tumor fragment, or infectious coagulum.
      (1) **Cardiac conditions** that may lead to renal arterial embolism include a dilated left atrium, artificial heart valves, myocardial infarction, infective endocarditis, marantic endocarditis, and myxoma.
      (2) **Noncardiac conditions** that may cause renal arterial embolism include atheromatous plaques and paradoxical, fat, or tumor embolism.
   c. **Cholesterol emboli** may occur spontaneously or follow vascular surgery or radiography. Acute renal failure may be the only manifestation of disease. Occasionally, skin lesions such as petechiae or livedo reticularis may be seen. Pathology of the skin or kidney reveals cholesterol clefts in small and medium-sized vessels. There is no specific therapy, but the disorder may spontaneously regress, leaving the patient with adequate residual kidney function.
   d. **Progressive renal atherosclerosis.** A large number (perhaps more than 20%) of patients with end-stage renal failure have angiographically significant renal artery stenosis. A smaller but unknown proportion have renal insufficiency as a result of the atherosclerotic process. Studies are underway to determine the optimal strategies for identifying and treating these patients. The risks of contrast-dye associated acute renal failure, cholesterol embolization, and acute renal artery dissection have prevented many clinicians from suggesting an aggressive approach in most patients. Intervention is indicated in those with severe, uncontrollable hypertension, and in those patients with diffuse vascular disease with clearly progressive renal insufficiency.

2. **Clinical features and diagnosis**
   a. Acute, complete renal arterial occlusion usually presents as flank pain, hematuria, fever, nausea, tissue necrosis [as evidenced by elevated lactate dehydrogenase (LDH) and serum glutamic-oxaloacetic transaminase (SGOT)], and acute renal failure. The diagnosis is confirmed using radionuclide scanning or angiography. Bilateral occlusion and occlusion of a solitary functioning kidney produce severe anuric acute renal failure.
   b. Chronic or segmental occlusion produces symptoms and signs commensurate with the degree of ischemic damage including progressive renal failure.

3. **Therapy**
   a. Therapy for renal arterial thrombosis is surgical removal of the clot to restore renal blood flow. Best results are obtained when the operation is conducted within 48–72 hours following the onset of disease.
   b. Therapy for renal arterial embolism, which usually is diffuse and involves large numbers of smaller arterial branches, is anticoagulation with heparin and resolution of the underlying focus of emboli.
   c. Therapy for ischemic nephropathy may involve angioplasty, stent placement, or surgical revascularization.

B. **Renal vein thrombosis.** Obstruction of renal venous drainage by a clot may be caused by extension of clots in the vena cava, invasion of the renal vein by tumor, severe dehydration in infants, renal amyloidosis, and certain glomerular diseases associated with nephrotic syndrome, particularly membranous glomerulonephritis.

1. **Clinical features and diagnosis.** Slowly evolving renal vein thrombosis may be completely asymptomatic, whereas acute renal vein thrombosis may produce pain, hematuria, costovertebral angle tenderness, and, ultimately, signs of worsening renal function. The affected kidney appears to be enlarged when visualized with the aid of intravenous urography. Selective venography is diagnostic. New techniques such as Doppler ultrasonography may be particularly useful as a noninvasive approach to diagnosis.

2. **Clinical course.** Renal vein thrombosis generally is not a cause of glomerular disease. Renal vein thrombosis may develop during nephrosis because of loss of anticoagulant proteins and procoagulant deactivators in the urine protein.

3. **Therapy** is controversial, as is the belief that renal vein thrombosis predisposes to pulmonary embolism. Current therapy is long-term (3–6 months) anticoagulation with warfarin sodium. Longer treatment is recommended if embolic phenomena occur.

C. **Renal artery stenosis.** In experimental animals, it has been clearly shown that partial reduction in the luminal size of one or both renal arteries produces renovascular hypertension, which is mediated in most cases by increased renin production with resultant activation of angiotensin and aldosterone. In humans, renal artery stenosis is a recognized cause of renovascular hypertension. However, the coincidence of radiographically demonstrated renal artery stenosis and clinically demonstrated renovascular hypertension does not establish a causal relationship.

1. **Etiology**
   a. Among prepubertal children, the primary lesion responsible for renal artery stenosis is **medial fibromuscular dysplasia.**
   b. Adults over 50 years of age suffer **renal artery atherosclerosis,** which is twice as common in men as in women.
   c. Rare causes include **Takayasu's arteritis, arterial wall disease** (e.g., hematoma, dissecting aneurysm, tumor), and **external arterial compression** due to tumor, fibrosis, or cyst.

2. **Clinical features** include a nearly continuous abdominal or flank bruit, hypokalemia, mild metabolic alkalosis, and asymmetric kidney size. None of these is a constant finding, and often there is no feature to distinguish renal artery stenosis from essential hypertension.

3. **Diagnosis.** Diagnostic strategies vary according to clinical suspicion.
   a. **Rapid-sequence intravenous urography** shows disparity in renal length and a delayed and persistent nephrogram on the affected side.
   b. **Renal angiography** (either standard or digital subtraction) is appropriate if surgical repair is contemplated or a definitive diagnosis is required. Stenotic segments are reliably identified by this study.
   c. **Renal vein renin studies.** Proof that angiographically demonstrated renal artery stenosis is etiologically important is difficult to obtain. Finding that the renal vein renin from the affected side is 1.5 times greater than that from the unaffected side is helpful, but patients may respond to treatment without this biochemical finding. Although volume depletion and furosemide administration increase this test's sensitivity, up to 30% of renal vein renin studies may be misleading or nondiagnostic. The ultimate diagnosis relies on demonstration of normal blood pressure with correction of the renal artery stenosis.

4. **Therapy.** Therapeutic options are antihypertensive drugs, percutaneous transluminal angioplasty (PCTA), and surgical repair of the affected vessel.

D. **Microangiopathy: hemolytic–uremic syndrome** and **thrombotic thrombocytopenic purpura (TTP).** As members of the disease group termed microangiopathic hemolytic anemia, hemolytic–uremic syndrome and TTP are similar clinical syndromes that share features with DIC, malignant hypertension, postpartum renal failure, sepsis, and systemic sclerosis.

1. Clinical features

    a. TTP characteristically presents as fever, microangiopathic hemolytic anemia, thrombocytopenia, fluctuating neurologic signs, purpura, and renal failure. Gastrointestinal involvement (e.g., mucosal bleeding and jaundice) is common. The course usually is fulminant; more than 50% of patients die within 6 weeks of the onset of TTP.

    b. Hemolytic–uremic syndrome is primarily a pediatric disorder characterized by microangiopathic hemolytic anemia, thrombocytopenia, and acute renal failure. The disorder may occur in epidemics and has been reported to follow shigellosis. Hemolytic–uremic syndrome usually has a sudden and dramatic onset, with renal failure the dominant clinical feature. As in TTP, other organ systems may be involved. Renal function returns in most patients who recover from systemic disease, but relapses have been reported.

2. Diagnosis

    a. Laboratory findings are similar in both disorders.

        (1) Anemia is a constant finding, occurring in association with a variety of structurally damaged red cells in the peripheral circulation. The reticulocyte count and fibrin split products are elevated, leukocytosis is common, and the serum LDH and indirect bilirubin levels are elevated. Thrombocytopenia is severe (i.e., < 20,000 platelets/μl). The bone marrow shows erythroid hyperplasia with adequate or increased megakaryocytes. Azotemia is common, and the degree of renal failure is characteristically severe.

        (2) Urinalysis shows hematuria, pyuria, hemoglobinuria, and granular cysts.

        (3) Microbiologic studies may reveal verotoxin-producing *E. coli* as the cause, particularly in epidemics.

    b. Renal biopsy findings also are similar. Arterioles and small arteries are occluded by eosinophilic, hyaline thrombi containing fibrin and platelet aggregates, which cause impressive vascular dilatation. Microinfarcts commonly occur, but without inflammatory infiltrates or signs of vasculitis. Renal lesions are focal and almost completely confined to the arterial side.

3. Therapy. Controlled trials comparing individual treatment programs have not been performed. Therapeutic methods currently in use include antiplatelet drugs (e.g., aspirin, sulfinpyrazone, and dipyridamole), glucocorticoids, exchange transfusion, plasmapheresis, and, rarely, splenectomy.

4. Prognosis has improved with modern therapy. Untreated TTP is almost universally fatal within 1 year. However, 1-year survival rates for treated patients range from 40%–80%. Less than 5% of patients with hemolytic–uremic syndrome die within 1 month.

E. **Systemic sclerosis (scleroderma)** is a generalized disturbance of connective and vascular tissue that leads to fibrosis of the affected tissue. Systemic sclerosis may be a very localized disease (called **morphea**) or a lethal, systemic disease. Renal involvement is a common cause of morbidity and death. The incidence of renal involvement in systemic sclerosis is not solidly established but, based on autopsy series, is estimated to range from 42%–80%. Clinical evidence of renal involvement (i.e., azotemia, hypertension, and active urinary sediment) is seen in about 45% of systemic sclerosis patients. In one study, subtle vascular and hemodynamic abnormalities were seen in 80% of patients.

1. Clinical features and course

    a. Acute renal disease occurs in the context of rapidly accelerating generalized disease activity, with prominent malignant hypertension. Renal failure can ensue precipitously if the blood pressure is uncontrolled. Pathologically, acute renal disease is quite similar to other microangiopathic diseases. The interlobular arteries show marked intimal thickening and mucoid proliferation, which may lead to cortical necrosis. Glomerular changes usually are mild and nonspecific, often consisting of only mesangial prominence. Interstitial edema with some mononuclear infiltrate is common. Unlike isolated malignant hypertension, systemic sclerosis does not primarily affect arterioles but does produce adventitial fibrosis.

   b. Chronic renal disease may be present in systemic sclerosis patients with little or no clinical signs of renal involvement. Kidney size usually is normal, and the earliest sign of disease is proteinuria, which is noted in 30% of patients. Nephrotic syndrome is rare, and hematuria, urinary casts, and pyuria usually are absent. Hypertension complicates chronic renal disease frequently (i.e., in 25%–50% of patients) and is a harbinger of impending deterioration of renal function. Renal failure occasionally develops in systemic sclerosis patients who have neither proteinuria nor hypertension.

2. **Therapy**

   a. Treatment of acute renal disease is, to a large degree, the control of accelerated hypertension. Captopril, enalapril, minoxidil, and nitroprusside may be required. Propranolol and furosemide are frequently used adjunctive agents.

   b. Treatment of chronic renal disease is less clear-cut. It is not known whether some vasoactive therapy during early, nonazotemic, nonhypertensive stages of the disease is protective. Similarly, the role of treatment for patients with abnormal renal biopsies but no clinical renal disease is unclear.

F. **Sickle cell nephropathy**

1. **Pathology**

   a. Sickle cell trait and sickle cell disease are associated with a variety of renal complications. The renal medulla is relatively anoxic and hyperosmolar—factors that favor erythrocyte sickling. Most damage occurs in the renal papillae.

   b. Medullary infarction resulting from occluded (sickled) vessels produces a spectrum of tubular disorders, including impaired urine concentration. Because the injury is located in the renal papillae, these patients behave as though they have been papillectomized. Papillary necrosis also is seen. Patients with sickle cell trait are affected less severely than those with sickle cell disease.

2. **Clinical features**

   a. Impaired secretion of potassium and hydrogen ion occurs, and a frequent biochemical finding is hyperkalemia with a hyperchloremic (normal anion gap) metabolic acidosis (see Part II: IV D 2).

   b. Hematuria represents the most dramatic of the renal abnormalities in sickle cell disease. Although it is usually self-limited, life-threatening exsanguination occurs in rare cases.

   c. Glomerular disease, including nephrotic syndrome, has been documented in sickle cell disease. Membranoproliferative-like lesions have been reported, as has typical membranous glomerulonephritis.

3. **Clinical course.** Although frequently the GFR is supranormal early in the course of sickle cell nephropathy, gradual deterioration of renal function is common. Progression to end-stage renal disease occurs in some cases.

4. **Therapy**

   a. Careful fluid management to maintain adequate intravascular volume, both during crises and at other times, clearly is important. Volume depletion is injurious to renal function and is more likely to occur because of the urine concentrating defect.

   b. Patients who are prone to hyperkalemia or acidosis should be advised to reduce their dietary intake of potassium and protein.

   c. Hemodialysis is useful and does not increase the number or severity of crises or alter the transfusion requirement in most patients.

   d. Kidney allografts are susceptible to sickle cell damage.

G. **Radiation nephritis.** High doses of ionizing radiation are destructive to the kidney and urinary tract. Delivery of at least 2000 rads (radiation-absorbed dose) over a period of several weeks can induce disease. Radiation-induced nephritis most commonly results from inadvertent exposure during radiotherapy for abdominal or retroperitoneal tumor.

1. **Immediate radiation nephrotoxicity** results in decreased renal blood flow, with tubular function and blood pressure remaining normal.

2. **Acute radiation nephritis** develops 6–12 months after exposure. Clinical signs are edema, hypertension, headache, exertional dyspnea, anemia, cylindruria, proteinuria, and microscopic hematuria. Death occurs in nearly 50% of patients as a result of severe azotemia and hypertension. Patients who recover from the acute phase may have some persistent proteinuria.

3. **Chronic radiation nephritis** may follow acute radiation nephritis or develop de novo up to 10 years following exposure. Clinical signs are fairly nonspecific and include fatigue, nocturia, hypertension, hyperuricemia with clinical gout, uremia, anemia, proteinuria, cylindruria, and hyposthenuria.

XV. THE KIDNEY IN PREGNANCY

A. General physiologic effects

1. Under the hormonal influence of pregnancy, renal size increases by 1 cm or more (radiographically); the renal pelvis, calyces, and ureters dilate, as in hydronephrosis; the GFR and RPF increase 25%–40%; a primary respiratory alkalosis develops; and the osmostat resets downward. Uric acid clearance nearly doubles and renal excretion of glucose increases, whereas blood glucose levels remain normal.

2. Clinically, the enlargement of the collecting system should not be mistaken for obstruction. The serum creatinine and BUN values decrease to less than 0.8 mg/dl and 13 mg/dl, respectively. Serum bicarbonate concentration is 4–5 mEq/L lower than in the pregravid state, and serum osmolality is 10 mOsm/kg lower, with a corresponding drop of 5 mEq/L in serum sodium concentration. The serum uric acid is reduced to 3–4 mg/dl, and 24-hour urine glucose may exceed 20 g at term in the absence of diabetes.

B. Urinary tract infections that occur in pregnant women frequently are attributable to the rich nutrient content of the urine and to the urinary stasis resulting from ureteral dilatation. (There is some concern that asymptomatic bacteriuria increases the rate of prematurity, particularly if there is kidney involvement.)

1. **Incidence**
   a. **Symptomatic bacteriuria** represents the most common renal problem seen by obstetricians. Although asymptomatic bacteriuria occurs with equal frequency in pregnant and nonpregnant women (i.e., in 4%–7% of all women), clinical infection (i.e., cystitis or pyelonephritis) develops in 40% of pregnant women.
   b. **Acute bacterial interstitial nephritis** occurs in 1%–2% of pregnant women, with signs and symptoms that are comparable to those seen in nonpregnant women. Lower tract infection also presents with typical symptoms.

2. **Laboratory findings and diagnosis** are the same in both pregnant and nonpregnant women.

3. **Therapy.** Although an overwhelming majority of pregnant women respond well to antibiotic therapy without fetal morbidity, antibiotic therapy must be chosen with respect to possible toxic effects on the fetus.
   a. **Agents of choice.** Sulfonamides displace albumin-bound bilirubin and may cause kernicterus; tetracycline has obvious dental and osseous toxicity. **Ampicillin** is the drug of choice when no allergy exists. **Cephalosporins** are also safe.
   b. **Duration of treatment.** Asymptomatic bacteriuria should be treated for 10–14 days. Clinical pyelonephritis should be treated for 6 weeks, owing to the very high rate of relapse.

C. **Acute renal failure** complicates 1 in 2000–5000 pregnancies and has a bimodal pattern of occurrence. The first peak occurs in the first trimester and is related to septic abortion. The second peak occurs between 34 and 40 weeks' gestation and is related to preeclampsia, hemorrhage, and intravascular volume depletion.

1. **Clinical conditions**
   a. **Cortical necrosis** is a special cause of acute renal failure complicating pregnancy. Acute cortical necrosis accounts for 5% of cases of acute renal failure in the general population but 10%–30% of cases among pregnant women. Cortical necrosis may complicate any phase of pregnancy, particularly with abruptio placentae. The necrosis can be patchy or extensive. Some women recover variable amounts of renal function; however, most cases ultimately progress to end-stage renal disease.
   b. **Idiopathic postpartum renal failure** is a rare cause of renal failure peculiar to pregnancy. These patients present several weeks after an uncomplicated delivery with renal failure and severe hypertension. The exact etiology is unknown; however, the pathologic lesion strikingly resembles the hemolytic–uremic syndrome/TTP complex. It is unknown whether a virus, retained placental tissue, or drugs induce this condition by deranging coagulation or endothelial cell function. Dilatation and curettage to remove any placental fragments is worth consideration. Some patients improve with anticoagulation.

2. **Prognosis.** Pregnancy-related acute renal failure has a better outlook for recovery than renal failure that is induced by medical or surgical complications. Nonetheless, maternal mortality is significant, ranging from 10%–25%.

D. **Hypertension.** Blood pressure declines early in pregnancy, reaching diastolic levels that are 15 mm lower than prepregnancy levels by 22 weeks' gestation. Blood pressure then rises gradually to prepregnancy values by term. This blood pressure drop is accompanied by a constant cardiac output, which suggests decreased peripheral resistance as a mechanism.

1. **Clinical conditions.** Hypertensive disorders of pregnancy are classified for clinical purposes as follows:
   a. **Preeclampsia–eclampsia** (see Part I: XV E)
   b. **Chronic hypertension,** which, in most women, is essential hypertension recognized before pregnancy. A secondary cause rarely is present and may, as in the case of pheochromocytoma, result in disastrously high maternal mortality. A standard evaluation for hypertension should be conducted in women who have high blood pressure and contemplate pregnancy.
   c. **Chronic hypertension with superimposed preeclampsia**
   d. **Late or transient hypertension,** which, in most cases, occurs in the third trimester and resolves within 10 days of delivery but tends to recur in subsequent pregnancies. Many of these women may ultimately develop essential hypertension.

2. **Therapy.** The treatment of hypertension during pregnancy is very difficult. Overly enthusiastic lowering of maternal blood pressure may diminish uteroplacental blood flow, leading to fetal compromise. Diastolic blood pressures above 100 mm Hg in noneclamptic women are best treated with **hydralazine, methyldopa,** or **calcium channel blockers.**
   a. For many reasons, some of which remain controversial, diuretics should not be used routinely.
   b. ACE inhibitors (e.g., captopril) are contraindicated for pregnant women because they reduce placental blood flow and induce acute renal failure in the fetus, renal agenesis, and other deformities.

E. **Preeclampsia–eclampsia (toxemia of pregnancy)** is primarily, but not exclusively, a disease of young primiparas.

1. **Definition.** Preeclampsia is a syndrome of **hypertension** (frequently malignant), **proteinuria, edema,** and, in its extreme, a **microangiopathic hemolytic anemia** with

vascular endothelial destruction. The hallmark of this disease is the **labile vaso-spasm,** reflecting a vascular sensitivity to the pressor effects of endogenous peptides and catecholamines. Blood pressure may fluctuate widely, but sustained 4- to 6-hour periods of hypertension are reliable signs of disease. Preeclampsia that is associated with maternal convulsions and coma is referred to as **eclampsia.**

2. **Pathology.** The renal histopathology is glomerular capillary endotheliosis, with swelling of capillary endothelial cells in the absence of hypercellularity. Vacuolization is common.

3. **Clinical features and diagnosis.** The initial clinical presentation may be mild or severe; however, sustained hypertension newly appearing in the third trimester of a first pregnancy is a suitable criterion for a presumptive diagnosis of preeclampsia. Untreated, fulminant preeclampsia progresses rapidly to maternal convulsions, anuric renal failure, and death.

4. **Therapy** includes hospitalization and bed rest, prompt delivery if the fetus is mature, parenteral magnesium sulfate for impending convulsions, and careful titration of blood pressure to a diastolic range of 95–105 mm Hg. Ganglionic blockers induce meconium ileus in the fetus and are to be avoided. Diuretics are not recommended.

PART II: FLUID AND ELECTROLYTE DISORDERS

I. WATER METABOLISM

A. Normal physiology

1. **Regulation of water intake.** Increased thirst is the normal response to water loss. The neural center that controls the release of **antidiuretic hormone (ADH)** is anatomically close to the thirst center and responds to increased body fluid tonicity.
   a. **Tonicity** refers to the shift of water through biomembranes produced by osmotically active particles such as glucose and sodium. Urea exerts virtually no tonicity because it easily crosses all membranes and produces no osmotic shift of water.
   b. **Osmolality** is a function of the number of molecules in solution independent of effects on water movement.

2. **Regulation of water output**
   a. **Proximal tubular reabsorption.** Of the 200 L/day of water that are filtered at the glomerulus, 125 L are reabsorbed in the proximal tubule.
   b. **Osmotic gradient formation in the medulla.** Glomerular filtrate not reabsorbed in the proximal tubule enters the loop of Henle, where active sodium reabsorption without water reabsorption causes dilution of the urine and increases the concentration of solutes in the medullary interstitium.
   c. **Collecting tubular transport.** Water that reaches the collecting tubule either is excreted (if ADH is absent, causing the tubule to be impermeable to water) or is reabsorbed (if ADH is present, causing the tubule to be permeable to water). Thus, ADH affects the osmolality of urine, which may range from 1200 mOsm/kg to 50 mOsm/kg.

B. Hyponatremia

1. **Definition.** Hyponatremia refers to serum sodium concentration of less than 135 mEq/L. The name, however, is somewhat misleading, because hyponatremia is usually a problem of too much water, not too little sodium. In fact, the sodium content of the body may be increased, decreased, or relatively unchanged. Hypotonicity al-

ways implies hyponatremia. The opposite is not always true: hyponatremia can co-exist with isotonicity or hypertonicity in addition to hypotonicity.

    a. Pseudohyponatremia (isotonic hyponatremia) is a laboratory artifact that occurs in the setting of extreme hyperlipidemia or hyperproteinemia. If the laboratory uses an instrument that reports sodium content per unit volume of total plasma rather than sodium content per volume of the aqueous phase, then significant elevations in plasma lipids or γ-globulins can cause the reported sodium concentration to be artificially low. This artifact can be obviated by using an ion selective electrode that measures sodium ion concentration in the aqueous phase.

    b. Hypertonic hyponatremia results from the shift of water from the intracellular fluid to the extracellular fluid, which is caused by the presence of osmotically active particles (e.g., glucose) in the extracellular fluid space. Serum sodium concentration is reduced, but the osmolality of the extracellular fluid is normal or even above normal.

    c. True hyponatremia (hypotonic hyponatremia) is clinically significant when the serum sodium concentration is less than 125 mEq/L and the serum osmolality is less than 250 mOsm/kg.

2. Etiology

    a. Decreased renal water excretion

        (1) Decreased GFR. A decrease in the filtered load of water to less than 10% of normal results in a clinically significant decrease in the ability of the kidney to excrete water.

        (2) Increased proximal tubular reabsorption. An increase in proximal tubular reabsorption of filtered fluid from the normal 65% to more than 90% may impair the capacity of the kidney to excrete water. Increased proximal tubular reabsorption occurs when the kidney is hypoperfused (e.g., in states of excessive fluid loss from diarrhea or vomiting). Decreased effective renal perfusion in diseases such as congestive heart failure, cirrhosis, or nephrotic syndrome also stimulates proximal tubular reabsorption. This group of disorders is characterized by a low urine sodium concentration, indicating increased renal absorption of sodium, high BUN, and the physical finding of either true volume depletion or one of the edematous conditions.

        (3) Increased collecting tubular reabsorption of water is induced by nonosmotically stimulated ADH secretion. This condition is characterized by relatively normal urine sodium excretion (if intake is normal), a high urine osmolality, and signs of body water expansion resulting from retention of excessively ingested water.

    b. Increased fluid intake. Fluid intake in excess of 1 L/hr exceeds normal excretory capacity and leads to hyponatremia. This situation is seen in patients who are given excessive hyponatric intravenous fluids and in psychiatric patients who drink excessively.

    c. Syndrome of inappropriate ADH secretion (SIADH) results from nonosmotically stimulated ADH release associated with the following disorders.

        (1) Tumor. Several tumors have been reported to produce an ADH-like peptide, most notably oat cell carcinoma of the lung.

        (2) CNS disease. Excessive ADH release has been documented in postseizure patients as well as in those with cerebral trauma, brain tumors, and psychiatric disturbances.

        (3) Pulmonary disease. SIADH has been described with pulmonary tumors, infections, and bronchospastic disease. The mechanism is believed to be stimulation of the so-called **J receptors** in the pulmonary circulation, leading to pituitary ADH release.

        (4) Hypopituitarism. Individuals with glucocorticoid deficiency as a result of impaired adrenocorticotropic hormone (ACTH) release may have excessive ADH release, resulting from the loss of glucocorticoid tonic inhibition of ADH release. Primary adrenal insufficiency involving both glucocorticoid and mineralocorticoid production may be associated with a syndrome of renal sodium wasting, which exacerbates the hyponatremia.

(5) Drug-induced SIADH. Drugs that may produce SIADH include chlorprop-amide and clofibrate, both of which may increase ADH release as well as sensitize the renal tubule to the effects of ADH. Thiazide diuretics, which may directly lead to ADH release, also may cause hyponatremia through ex-cessive renal sodium excretion or through potassium depletion. CNS-active drugs such as carbamazepine also produce SIADH.

(6) Idiopathic SIADH. Elderly patients may have no apparent reason for SIADH and yet maintain sustained hyponatremia. This condition may be related to the increase in ADH release that occurs with advancing age.

(7) Reset osmostat, a variant of SIADH, occurs in chronically ill and malnour-ished patients in whom the serum sodium concentration is reset at a low value (approximately 125 mEq/L), thus maintaining an abnormally low serum osmolality. This new set point for osmolality is termed a "reset osmo-stat." These patients are able to maintain water balance, albeit at constant low serum osmolality: increased water intake leads to inhibition of ADH re-lease, dilution of the urine, and excretion of the water load; water restriction triggers ADH release but at a lower plasma osmolality than normal individu-als and leads to increased urine osmolality and water retention.

3. Clinical features. CNS dysfunction may develop as the tonicity of the extracellular fluid falls and water diffuses down an osmotic gradient into the brain cells, leading to cellular edema. Sustained hyponatremia at a serum sodium concentration below 125 mEq/L may lead to permanent CNS dysfunction. Acute hyponatremia with a de-crease in serum sodium concentration below 125 mEq/L over a period of hours al-most always is associated with acute CNS disturbances such as obtundation, coma, seizures, and death if untreated.

4. Diagnosis
   a. Physical examination may reveal:
   (1) Volume depletion (e.g., in cases related to drugs such as diuretics)
   (2) Volume expansion (e.g., in cases related to cirrhosis or congestive heart failure)
   b. Laboratory data
   (1) Urine osmolality is greater than 50–100 mOsm/kg in the presence of plasma hypotonicity.
   (2) Urine sodium concentration is high when plasma volume is expanded in SIADH but is low when effective arterial blood volume is reduced, as in edematous conditions. A urine sodium concentration less than 20 mEq/L strongly argues against SIADH.
   c. Water loading test. When an intravascularly volume-expanded individual is given 20 ml water/kg orally or intravenously over a period of 20–40 minutes, the normal response is excretion of 80% of this water load within 4 hours and re-duction of urine osmolality to below 100 mOsm/kg. Failure to achieve these ef-fects suggests an impairment in the kidney's ability to excrete water.

5. Therapy
   a. Fluid restriction. All patients who are severely hyponatremic should reduce free water intake to approximately 700 ml/day.
   b. Inhibition of water reabsorption
   (1) Demeclocycline has been shown to alter ADH-induced water flow in the collecting tubule. This drug must be given in doses of 600–1200 mg/day and requires 4–5 days to achieve its peak action. Demeclocycline cannot be administered to patients with liver disease, heart failure, or kidney disease since it may accumulate to toxic levels in these conditions.
   (2) Furosemide. Acute administration of furosemide combined with large amounts of saline may lead to increased water excretion. This effect is rela-tively transient and can be achieved only with acute infusions of furosemide.
   c. Hypertonic infusions. The infusion of 3% sodium chloride rapidly raises the to-nicity of the extracellular fluid. (Serum sodium concentration should not increase faster than 2 mEq/L/hr.) Because extracellular fluid expansion may lead to pulmo-nary edema, hypertonic saline usually is given in combination with bumetanide

or furosemide and should be used only in the treatment of symptomatic patients. Elevation of serum sodium concentration to 125 mEq/L usually alleviates the dangers of brain edema. The amount of hypertonic saline (in mEq) needed to raise the serum sodium concentration ($[Na^+]$) is calculated using the following equation:

$$(\text{normal serum } [Na^+] - \text{current serum } [Na^+]) \times \text{total body water}$$

6. **Complications**
   a. **Acute hyponatremia.** Acute reduction of serum osmolality can produce intracranial hypertension and brain damage, particularly if the serum sodium concentration falls below 125 mEq/L over a period of hours.
   b. **Chronic hyponatremia.** It has been postulated that chronic hyponatremia (serum sodium concentration of < 125 mEq/L) may lead to alterations in cognitive function, but this theory remains controversial.

C. **Hypernatremia**

1. **Definition.** Hypernatremia refers to serum sodium concentration that is above normal. Clinically significant effects are produced at serum sodium levels greater than 155 mEq/L. Hypernatremia always implies hypertonicity of all body fluids because the rise in the extracellular fluid osmolality obligates movement of water from the intracellular space, producing increased intracellular osmotic activity and cell dehydration.

2. **Etiology**
   a. **Extrarenal causes**
      (1) **Decreased fluid intake.** Adequate water intake is required to maintain the tonicity of body fluids in the face of continuous water losses through the skin as well as losses through the urine and gastrointestinal tract. In cool environments, this intake equals approximately 700 ml/day. If intake is less than external losses, body fluid osmolality rises.
      (2) **Increased skin losses.** Profuse sweating may lead to excess water losses through the skin. In addition, burns and other widespread inflammatory lesions of the skin may cause marked fluid losses.
      (3) **Increased gastrointestinal losses.** Diarrhea and protracted vomiting also may result in water deficits.
   b. **Renal causes**
      (1) **Osmotic diuresis.** The presence of osmotically active, nonreabsorbable solute in the glomerular filtrate prevents water and sodium reabsorption and leads to increased renal water losses. Hyperglycemia with glycosuria is a common cause of osmotic diuresis. Since water losses are relatively greater than sodium losses, the serum sodium concentration rises progressively during osmotic diuresis.
      (2) **Decreased ADH effect**
         (a) **Central diabetes insipidus** (i.e., failure of ADH synthesis or release) may occur in the following settings.
            (i) **Tumor.** ADH deficiency may occur either through direct invasion of the neurohypophysis or through increased intracranial pressure compressing the brain stem.
            (ii) **Histiocytosis,** particularly Hand-Schüller-Christian disease, has a predilection for neurohyophyseal involvement, producing ADH deficiency.
            (iii) Sarcoidosis also may involve the neurohypophysis, producing diabetes insipidus.
            (iv) **Trauma.** Classically after resection of the pituitary stalk, a phase of acute ADH release is followed by a prolonged period of central diabetes insipidus.
         (b) **Nephrogenic diabetes insipidus** (i.e., failure of renal water conservation despite high levels of plasma ADH) may occur in the following settings.
            (i) **Renal disease.** Structural disease impairs the integrity of the renal medulla and, thereby, the urine concentrating ability.

(ii) **Hypercalcemia.** Elevation of serum calcium concentration above 12 mg/dl may impair urine concentrating ability, most likely as a result of increased medullary blood flow and dissipation of medullary hypertonicity.

(iii) **Hypokalemia.** Reduction of serum potassium concentration below 3.5 mEq/L leads to a direct stimulation of thirst and a mild impairment of urine concentrating ability.

(iv) **Lithium ingestion** blocks ADH-stimulated osmotic water flow in the collecting tubule.

(v) **Demeclocycline therapy.** This tetracycline antibiotic alters ADH-induced water flow through a direct effect on the cell membrane.

(vi) **Sickle cell anemia.** Reduced medullary blood flow produced by sickling erythrocytes within the vasa recta also may impair urine concentrating ability.

(vii) **Urinary tract obstruction** and the **postobstructive state** are associated with nephrogenic diabetes insipidus.

3. **Clinical features**
   a. **CNS disorders.** Generalized CNS depression, including obtundation, coma, and seizures, develops in young children and elderly patients. Intracerebral and subarachnoid hemorrhage may occur if shrinkage of brain volume leads to tears in the bridging veins.
   b. **Extracellular volume depletion.** Although two-thirds of water deficits are derived from the intracellular fluid, extracellular fluid volume contracts mildly also.
   c. **Abnormal urine output.** If the kidneys cause water losses, polyuria (i.e., urine output that is inappropriately high given the level of plasma osmolality or extracellular fluid volume) may be present. If the kidneys are normal and water losses are extrarenal, urine volume typically is reduced.

4. **Diagnosis**
   a. **Dehydration test.** Urine concentrating ability may be tested after overnight dehydration to determine whether a patient has renal water wasting.
      (1) Water deprivation begins at 8:00 P.M. and lasts 14 hours, after which the urine osmolality should exceed 800 mOsm/kg. The patient then is given a subcutaneous dose of ADH as 5 units aqueous vasopressin. The urine osmolality should not be further increased by this maneuver.
      (2) However, if the urine osmolality is less than 800 mOsm/kg after water deprivation or if it increases by greater than 15% after ADH administration, some degree of ADH deficiency is present.
      (3) If the urine osmolality does not exceed 300 mOsm/kg after water deprivation and there is no further increase after ADH administration, some form of nephrogenic diabetes insipidus is present.
   b. **Plasma ADH assay.** In nephrogenic diabetes insipidus, the urine osmolality may not be a true reflection of ADH release, and, thus, plasma ADH levels should be measured.
   c. **Assay of urine osmolality and composition**
      (1) It is useful to measure the solute composition of the urine in the evaluation of polyuria. Urine osmolality less than 150 mOsm/L suggests a primary defect in water conservation. Urine osmolality greater than 150 mOsm/L during polyuria suggests an osmotic diuresis.
      (2) After measuring urine osmolality, the urine should be analyzed for sodium, glucose, and urea to determine the etiology of the diuresis. A urine pH greater than 6 may indicate bicarbonate diuresis.
   d. **Physical examination** generally is not useful in determining the etiology and pathogenesis of polyuria.

5. **Therapy**
   a. **Free water** may be administered orally, which is the preferred route, or intravenously as a 5% dextrose solution. Infusion of a fluid with a tonicity less than 150 mOsm/L is dangerous and may lead to acute hemolysis.
   b. **Vasopressin** may be administered in several different forms. Currently, the agent

TABLE 6-8. Other Hormones and Their Reactions to Sodium Handling

Hormone	Action on Sodium Transport
Atrial natriuretic peptide	Inhibits renal reabsorption (collecting duct)
Dopamine	Intrarenally generated; inhibits proximal tubule sodium reabsorption
Prostaglandins	Intrarenally generated; inhibit tubular sodium reabsorption and vasodilate the kidney

of choice for treatment of ADH deficiency is **1-deamino-8-D-arginine vasopressin (dDAVP** or **desmopressin),** which may be administered as a nasal spray in a dose of 10–20 μg every 12 hours.

   c. Thiazide diuretics stimulate proximal tubular reabsorption of sodium and water as a result of volume depletion. This action reduces the delivery of fluid to the distal nephron and, thereby, reduces the degree of polyuria. Thiazides are useful as adjunct therapy in patients with nephrogenic diabetes insipidus.

   d. Other drugs, such as clofibrate, carbamazepine, and chlorpropamide, enhance the renal tubular effects of ADH and, possibly, contribute to the stimulation of ADH release in certain settings.

6. Complications. Diseases of water conservation are dangerous only if patients are not allowed access to water. In such settings, severe volume depletion and cellular dehydration may occur.

II. SODIUM METABOLISM

A. **Normal physiology.** Sodium is the primary osmotic component of the extracellular fluid, which contains approximately 3000 mEq of sodium. The sodium content of the extracellular fluid determines the volume of that space and the "fullness," or effective volume, of the systemic circulation. A less than 1% change in renal sodium excretion can produce major changes in extracellular fluid volume.

   1. Renal handling. Approximately 30,000 mEq/day of sodium are filtered at the glomerulus. If sodium intake is approximately 200–300 mEq/day, the entire glomerular filtrate of sodium must be reabsorbed, less 1% (typical amount of ingested sodium), in order to maintain sodium homeostasis. Although only 10%–15% of the glomerular filtrate is reabsorbed in the distal tubule and collecting duct, this site is the major regulator for determining final urine sodium composition.

   2. Hormonal regulation. Aldosterone stimulates sodium reabsorption in the cortical collecting duct. Other hormones may alter renal tubular handling of sodium, but none is as well studied as aldosterone. Aldosterone release from the adrenal gland is governed by the **renin-angiotensin system.**

     a. Renin is an enzyme that catalyzes the conversion of **angiotensinogen** to the decapeptide **angiotensin I** (in plasma). Angiotensin I is converted to the octapeptide **angiotensin II** (in the lung and kidney) by angiotensin-converting enzyme. Angiotensin II is a potent vasoconstrictive agent as well as a potent stimulus for increased aldosterone release from the adrenal gland.

     b. Renin secretion by the kidney is stimulated by renal hypoperfusion, adrenergic stimulation, and circulating catecholamines. Renin is released from the **juxtaglomerular apparatus,** which is located between the afferent and the efferent arterioles of the glomeruli.

     c. Other hormones that regulate sodium handling are listed in Table 6-8.

B. **Edema**

1. **Definition**
   a. Edema generally is defined as an increase in the interstitial compartment of the extracellular fluid.
      (1) Normally, the extracellular fluid volume equals approximately 14 L and accounts for one-third of the total body water. About 25% of the extracellular fluid is represented by plasma volume and is contained within the circulation. The other 75% or 11 L is represented by the interstitial fluid between cells.
      (2) If the interstitial fluid volume increases by approximately 2 L, clinically evident edema may result; edema may be **observable** (as **swelling**) or **palpable** (as **pitting**).
   b. Although edema generally is a function of increased extracellular fluid volume, in some instances increased transcapillary hydrostatic pressure (e.g., as occurs in the portal circulation in cirrhosis) also may contribute to edema.

2. **Pathophysiology.** Edema, or the pathologic increase in extracellular fluid volume, primarily is a function of excessive renal tubular reabsorption of sodium. Decreased renal perfusion (e.g., as occurs in congestive heart failure with reduced cardiac output, in cirrhosis with reduced effective arterial blood volume, and in the nephrotic syndrome) is the proximate cause of the increased renal sodium reabsorption, which represents the body's attempt to maintain adequate effective arterial blood volume.

3. **Etiology**
   a. **Congestive heart failure.** When cardiac output is reduced, effective arterial blood volume is decreased as well. The decrease in effective arterial blood volume triggers the release of renin and aldosterone, leading to stimulation of distal tubular reabsorption of sodium. Additionally, alterations in renal hemodynamics stimulate an increase in the proximal tubular reabsorption of sodium.
   b. **Cirrhosis.** The primary cause of sodium retention in liver disease may be ascites formation as a result of high pressure in the portal circulation. Portal hypertension leads to intravascular fluid volume depletion and secondary renal sodium retention. When hypoalbuminemia occurs, effective arterial blood volume drops, stimulating renal sodium retention. Secondary hyperaldosteronism is common and is caused by intravascular volume contraction as well as impaired hepatic clearance of aldosterone; these factors lead to stimulation of distal tubular reabsorption of sodium. A primary increase in renal sodium reabsorption may occur in cirrhosis.
   c. **Nephrotic syndrome.** Hypoalbuminemia leads to reduced effective arterial blood volume, as a result of renal protein losses, which stimulates renal tubular reabsorption of sodium.
   d. **Chronic renal failure.** When the GFR falls to less than 10 ml/min, the kidney is unable to filter and, therefore, excrete a normally ingested sodium load, which leads to edema.
   e. **Excessive mineralocorticoid activity.** Tumors of the adrenal gland and tumors that secrete large amounts of adrenocorticotropic hormone (ACTH) may be associated with marked sodium retention.

4. **Clinical features**
   a. **Peripheral edema.** Sodium retention may manifest as swelling in the dependent regions of the body.
   b. **Pulmonary edema.** If pulmonary venous pressure acutely rises above 18 mm Hg, pulmonary edema may develop.

5. **Diagnosis**
   a. **Physical examination.** Peripheral edema may be identified by the persistence of an indentation following palpation of the soft tissues in the dependent areas. Pulmonary edema is identified by the physical findings of rales or wheezes or by chest x-ray.
   b. **Urine sodium assay** reveals a urine sodium level that is less than sodium intake and that usually is significantly less than 20 mEq/L.

6. Therapy

a. Dietary sodium restriction is essential for the management of edema. A sodium intake of 1 g (23 mEq)/day is the lowest practical intake level that can be achieved.

b. Diuretics. Several diuretic agents are useful for increasing sodium excretion.

   (1) Loop diuretics, such as furosemide and bumetanide, are particularly effective. Side effects of these drugs include intravascular volume depletion, hypokalemia, metabolic alkalosis, and hypomagnesemia.

   (2) Thiazide diuretics, such as hydrochlorothiazide, inhibit sodium reabsorption in the distal convoluted tubule. They can be used effectively although they are less potent than loop diuretics. Side effects are similar to those of loop diuretics.

   (3) Potassium-sparing diuretics, such as amiloride and triamterene, act primarily to block sodium reabsorption and secondarily to block potassium secretion in the distal tubule. Use of these agents may lead to potassium retention and increased sodium excretion.

   (4) Aldosterone antagonists. Spironolactone is a competitive aldosterone antagonist, the use of which also leads to potassium retention and increased sodium excretion.

III. POTASSIUM METABOLISM

A. **Normal physiology.** Potassium is a primary cationic component of the intracellular fluid, which contains approximately 3000 mEq of potassium. In comparison, the extracellular fluid contains very little potassium—about 65 mEq. The ratio of extracellular to intracellular potassium concentration is an important determinant of electrical activity in excitable membranes (e.g., the cardiac conduction system and somatic nerve endings). The normal dietary potassium intake of 60–90 mEq/day must be excreted by the kidney to preserve potassium homeostasis. Also, dietary potassium intake must be taken up rapidly by cells in preparation for renal excretion; otherwise, the serum potassium rapidly rises to life-threatening levels.

1. **Extrarenal handling.** Cellular uptake of potassium is influenced by the following extrarenal factors.

   a. Insulin. High insulin levels stimulate cellular uptake of potassium.

   b. Epinephrine. This β_2-active catecholamine directly stimulates cellular uptake of potassium. This action may be particularly important during severe exertion, when serum potassium levels rise because of muscle ischemia.

   c. Total body potassium. Individuals with a high total body potassium content may have a reduced capacity for cellular uptake of potassium.

2. **Renal handling.** Most urine potassium is the result of distal tubular secretion. Several factors are known to alter potassium secretion.

   a. Aldosterone secretion. Aldosterone directly stimulates potassium secretion and sodium reabsorption in the collecting tubule of the kidney.

   b. Sodium reabsorption. The delivery of fluid and sodium to the collecting tubule also stimulates potassium secretion. This mechanism accounts for the increased potassium secretion caused by diuretics, which act at more proximal sites in the nephron to block sodium reabsorption.

B. **Hypokalemia**

1. **Definition.** Hypokalemia is defined as serum potassium concentration of less than 3.5 mEq/L. Since most of the potassium content of the body is within cells and cell potassium concentration is about 155 mEq/L, cell potassium can be severely depleted without causing large changes in serum potassium.

2. **Etiology.** Hypokalemia can result from extrarenal or renal causes.
   a. **Extrarenal causes**
      (1) **Dietary deficiency and gastrointestinal losses**
         (a) **Inadequate dietary intake.** Because potassium conservation in the kidney is limited, a severe reduction of intake to less than 10 mEq/day can lead to a large negative potassium balance and hypokalemia.
         (b) **Diarrhea** can lead to severe potassium depletion as the potassium content of diarrheal fluid may be as high as 100 mEq/L.
         (c) **Vomiting.** Although the potassium content of vomitus is relatively small, the secondary effect of intravascular volume depletion—which produces secondary hyperaldosteronism—stimulates renal potassium excretion.
      (2) **Potassium redistribution**
         (a) **Insulin administration.** A therapeutic or replacement dose of insulin can drive potassium into cells, producing acute hypokalemia.
         (b) **Epinephrine infusions** also can produce acute hypokalemia by an independent action involving β_2-receptors.
         (c) **Folic acid and vitamin B_{12} therapy** for patients with megaloblastic anemia stimulates cell proliferation and produces acute hypokalemia as potassium is used in cell synthesis. This effect also may be seen in patients with rapidly growing tumors.
         (d) **Acute alkalemia.** Infusion of large amounts of bicarbonate stimulates potassium entry into cells in exchange for hydrogen ion.
         (e) **Hypokalemic periodic paralysis.** In this rare syndrome, potassium levels fall acutely—without a loss of potassium from the body—prior to episodes of paralysis. This syndrome commonly is associated with thyroid disease in Asians and probably represents a defect in catecholamine sensitivity.
   b. **Renal causes.** Any hyperactivity of the normal components of renal potassium excretion can produce a negative potassium balance via increased renal losses.
      (1) **Drug-induced renal losses**
         (a) **Diuretics** that act proximal to the site of potassium secretion stimulate urinary excretion of potassium by increasing the delivery of sodium and fluid to the distal tubules.
         (b) **Penicillins.** Carbenicillin and ticarcillin act as nonreabsorbable anions in the distal tubule and, thereby, stimulate potassium secretion. Significant hypokalemia is commonly seen.
         (c) **Gentamicin.** Tubular defects with magnesium wasting and secondary potassium wasting occasionally may be seen in patients treated with large doses of gentamicin.
         (d) **Amphotericin B.** This antifungal agent causes damage to the apical membrane of the renal tubular cell, thus increasing potassium loss from the cell. Hypokalemia is a sign of amphotericin toxicity in the kidney.
      (2) **Hormone-induced renal losses**
         (a) **Primary hyperaldosteronism**
            (i) **Primary adrenal adenomas** are associated with hypokalemia, hypertension, and metabolic alkalosis.
            (ii) **Diffuse bilateral adrenal hyperplasia** may be associated with a milder hypokalemia than is seen with primary adrenal adenoma.
            (iii) **Ectopic ACTH syndrome.** Massive mineralocorticoid increase and renal potassium wasting may occur in patients with oat cell lung carcinoma (a tumor that produces and secretes ACTH).
            (iv) **Exogenous mineralocorticoid**
               Licorice ingestion. Licorice produced in Europe (anise) contains a mineralocorticoid-like component, **glycyrrhetinic acid,** the ingestion of which may lead to the development of hypokalemia with hypertension and metabolic alkalosis.
               Tobacco chewing. Certain tobacco compounds also contain a mineralocorticoid-like constituent, and the use of such tobacco

may cause the development of hypokalemia and metabolic alkalosis.

(b) Secondary hyperaldosteronism

    (i) Renin-secreting tumor. This rare entity, diagnosed by arteriography, is characterized by intrarenal tumors of the juxtaglomerular apparatus. Severe hypertension and hypokalemia may occur.

    (ii) Renal artery stenosis may be associated with hypokalemia and hypertension as a result of secondary hyperaldosteronism produced by hyperreninemia.

    (iii) Malignant hypertension. Severe underperfusion of the kidney may occur in malignant hypertension and may lead to hyperreninemia, secondary hyperaldosteronism, and hypokalemia.

    (iv) Disorders with reduced effective arterial blood volume produce only mild hypokalemia despite hyperreninemia and hyperaldosteronism. Reduced tubular flow rate reduces potassium secretion.

        In **congestive heart failure,** secondary hyperaldosteronism may develop, causing mild hypokalemia even in the absence of diuretic use.

        In **cirrhosis,** severe hypokalemia is common because of poor diet (low intake) and secondary hyperaldosteronism.

(3) Potassium loss due to primary renal tubular disorders

    (a) Renal tubular acidosis is characterized by potassium wasting, which may be secondary to sodium depletion and metabolic acidosis or directly attributable to tubular defects in potassium conservation. Potassium wasting is a feature of distal (type I) as well as proximal (type II) renal tubular acidosis of any etiology.

    (b) Bartter's syndrome occurs in children as well as in adults and is characterized by renal potassium wasting, metabolic alkalosis, and polyuria. Blood pressure usually is normal or reduced, but renin and aldosterone levels are very high. The pathogenesis is not well understood, but a primary defect in renal conservation of sodium chloride is considered a likely cause.

    (c) Chronic magnesium depletion produces a syndrome of renal tubular potassium wasting without other associated defects in ion transport. The potassium wasting can be severe and is unresponsive to potassium repletion until magnesium deficits have been corrected.

(4) Potassium loss due to surreptitious diuretic use is associated with a clinical presentation identical to that of Bartter's syndrome, including hypokalemia, magnesium wasting, metabolic alkalosis, hyperreninemia, and hyperaldosteronism.

3. Clinical features

  a. Neuromuscular disorders. Potassium depletion may cause weakness and paralysis.

  b. Cardiac disorders. Arrhythmia, particularly in the presence of digitalis intoxication, is a hallmark of severe hypokalemia.

  c. Endocrine disorders. Hypokalemia is associated with abnormalities in pancreatic insulin release. Glucose intolerance has been shown to worsen as a result of diuretic-induced hypokalemia.

  d. Polyuria. The polyuria of hypokalemia is a function of polydipsia as well as impaired ADH action.

4. Diagnosis

  a. Physical examination. The presence or absence of hypertension is a useful differentiating feature in the approach to the patient with hypokalemia.

    (1) If the patient is hypertensive, the hypokalemia may be caused by excessive mineralocorticoid activity. Since many hypertensive patients are treated with diuretics, any hypokalemia could be a side effect of such therapy.

    (2) If the patient is normotensive, the hypokalemia represents either a gastrointestinal or a primary renal loss of potassium.

b. Serum electrolyte assay rarely is useful for evaluating the specific cause of hypokalemia. An exception is the finding of combined acidosis and hypokalemia, which suggests renal tubular acidosis.

c. Urine potassium assay. Urine potassium levels below 20 mEq/L suggest extrarenal potassium losses, whereas levels exceeding 30 mEq/L suggest renal losses.

d. Renin–aldosterone axis assay

(1) Noninvasive tests

(a) Renin stimulation test. This test is used to determine whether excessive mineralocorticoid activity is due to excessive renin production or to a primary adrenal disorder. To evaluate renin production, 40 mg of furosemide are administered; then plasma renin is measured in both the supine and upright positions.

(i) In normal individuals, renin levels are increased several-fold following furosemide administration, and the levels increase further when the individual assumes the upright position.

(ii) In individuals with renin suppression due to extracellular fluid volume expansion secondary to excessive mineralocorticoid activity, renin levels are suppressed following furosemide administration and are not stimulated when the individual assumes the upright position.

(b) Aldosterone suppression test. To document that aldosterone production is independent of normal inhibitory stimuli, 1–2 L of saline are infused; then plasma aldosterone is measured in both the supine and upright positions. Individuals whose aldosterone levels are not suppressed to below normal values may have primary aldosterone overproduction.

(2) Invasive tests include measurement of bilateral renal venous renin as well as adrenal venous aldosterone and cortisol concentrations. This information is necessary to establish a definitive diagnosis of primary aldosteronism and to define the presence of unilateral or bilateral adrenal disease. The hypertension associated with bilateral adrenal hyperplasia does not respond to adrenalectomy, whereas hypertension of aldosteronoma is responsive to tumor removal.

e. Urine chloride assay. In cases of mineralocorticoid excess, Bartter's syndrome, and diuretic abuse, urine chloride levels tend to be elevated in the presence of metabolic alkalosis and hypokalemia. The absence of elevated urine chloride levels is highly suggestive of gastrointestinal potassium losses.

f. Diuretic assay. If Bartter's syndrome is suspected, the urine must be analyzed for chloride and diuretics, including loop-active agents and thiazides, before a diagnosis of a primary tubular disorder can be established. Such diuretic assays are commercially available.

5. Therapy. In many cases, hypokalemia can be corrected by administration of potassium salts.

a. Forms of potassium salts. Potassium may be administered with a variety of anions. Potassium chloride is the preferred form of therapy since many patients have concurrent chloride deficits. In cases of hypokalemia with coincident renal tubular acidosis, potassium citrate, potassium lactate, or potassium gluconate may be given.

b. Routes of administration. Potassium may be given intravenously or orally.

(1) Intravenous potassium solutions should not exceed a concentration of 60 mEq/L, and the rate of administration should not exceed 60 mEq/hr. Normally, potassium deficits are on the order of 300–1000 mEq/L. These deficits should be replaced slowly, over days, except when digitalis intoxication or life-threatening arrhythmias are present.

(2) Oral potassium is absorbed effectively and should be substituted for intravenous potassium whenever possible. Several potassium salts may be given in wax matrix capsules, which avoid the problem of gastrointestinal ulceration caused by the earlier enteric-coated potassium preparations. A variety of potassium salts also are available as liquid suspensions.

c. **Chronic potassium therapy.** The need for potassium supplementation in mildly hypokalemic patients receiving diuretics is debated. However, serum potassium levels probably should be maintained above 3.5 mEq/L. This level may be accomplished with oral potassium supplementation. Although some foods are high in potassium, it is difficult to overcome these deficits solely by ingesting potassium-rich food.

C. **Hyperkalemia**

1. **Definition.** Hyperkalemia is defined as serum potassium concentration greater than 5.5 mEq/L.

2. **Etiology. Pseudohyperkalemia** may be caused by release of potassium from coagulated cells and platelets after blood is withdrawn for analysis. Measurement of plasma potassium is required to eliminate this artifact. **True hyperkalemia** may result from extrarenal or renal causes.
   a. **Extrarenal causes**
      (1) **Insulin deficiency.** Hyperkalemia in diabetic patients may be due to a lack of insulin and to the presence of associated renal and adrenal abnormalities.
      (2) **Cell lysis syndromes.** Acute cell necrosis following either chemotherapy or a massive crushing injury **(rhabdomyolysis)** produces hyperkalemia by rapid cellular release of potassium.
      (3) **Succinylcholine therapy.** The muscle relaxant succinylcholine may produce hyperkalemia in susceptible individuals with generalized muscle or neurologic disease.
      (4) **Hyperkalemic periodic paralysis** is a rare and poorly understood syndrome that may be associated with an acute shift of extracellular potassium. [The hypokalemic form of this syndrome, which is more common, is discussed in Part II: III B 2 a (2) (e).]
      (5) **Hyperosmolality.** Acute increases in extracellular fluid osmotic activity may produce a transcellular shift of potassium and hyperkalemia. Diabetic patients given intravenous glucose on the suspicion of hypoglycemia may develop this entity if hyperglycemia occurs in the setting of insulin deficiency.
      (6) **Acidosis.** Mineral acidosis, not organic acidosis, may be associated with an acute shift of potassium from the intracellular to the extracellular fluid as hydrogen ions and chloride ions enter cells.
   b. **Renal causes.** The renal capacity to excrete potassium is approximately 500–1000 mEq/day, which is 10–20 times the normal intake. Any impairment of the normal components of renal potassium excretion may reduce this excretory capacity so that normal intake may produce hyperkalemia.
      (1) **Severe renal failure.** When the GFR falls to below 10 ml/min, hyperkalemia may occur, even with normal intake. At a GFR above this level, hyperkalemia is not a result of glomerular insufficiency per se but is the result of a specific disorder in tubular potassium transport or an extrarenal potassium disturbance.
      (2) **Aldosterone insufficiency.** Aldosterone is the major hormonal determinant of renal potassium secretion.
         (a) **Acquired aldosterone deficiency** may occur as a result of renal disease that is associated with reduced renin production. (Recall that renin is an enzyme that cleaves precursor molecules to produce the aldosterone secretagogue, angiotensin II.) Primary adrenal disease also may be associated with reduced aldosterone production. Aldosterone deficiency due to impaired renin production or adrenal disease may be produced by:
            (i) Interstitial renal disease
            (ii) Lead nephropathy
            (iii) Diabetic nephropathy*
            (iv) Obstructive uropathy

---

* Insulin deficiency in this condition may potentiate the hyperkalemia.

(v) Angiotensin antagonist therapy

(vi) Addison's disease

(b) Inherited aldosterone deficiency. Several adrenal enzyme defects associated with deficiency of the 17- or 21-hydroxylase enzymes may be associated with aldosterone deficiency.

(c) Drug-induced aldosterone deficiency. NSAIDs act to reduce renin secretion and may produce hyperkalemia through aldosterone deficiency.

(3) Aldosterone resistance. The following conditions are characterized by tubular defects associated with elevated aldosterone levels but impaired potassium secretion.

(a) Sickle cell nephropathy

(b) SLE

(c) Amyloidosis

(d) Interstitial renal disease

(e) Obstructive nephropathy

(f) Hereditary aldosterone resistance

(g) Use of triamterene, amiloride, or spironolactone

3. Clinical features

a. Neuromuscular disorders. By altering transmembrane electrical potential, severe hyperkalemia may alter muscle function or neuromuscular transmission, leading to severe weakness or paralysis.

b. Cardiac disorders. Cardiac arrhythmias may occur at any level above normal but generally are noted only when serum potassium concentration exceeds 6 mEq/L. As serum potassium level rises, a series of electrocardiographic changes may be seen, including:

(1) Prolongation of the P-R interval

(2) T-wave peaking

(3) Prolongation of the QRS interval

(4) Ventricular tachycardias, ventricular fibrillation, and asystole

4. Diagnosis

a. Elimination of pseudohyperkalemia. In vitro lysis of erythrocytes, leukocytes, or platelets can produce hyperkalemia as a result of intracellular potassium release (pseudohyperkalemia). All hyperkalemic patients should be checked for pseudohyperkalemia by measuring both plasma and serum potassium concentrations and by inspecting the serum for discoloration suggesting hemolysis.

b. Urine potassium assay. Although only a rough correlation exists between urine and serum potassium levels, hyperkalemia induced by increased intake or increased cell lysis should be associated with urine potassium levels exceeding 50 mEq/L. Values less than 30 mEq/L in the setting of hyperkalemia suggest impaired renal secretion of potassium.

c. Renin–aldosterone axis assay. In certain patients, evaluation of aldosterone and renin levels may help to define the etiology of hyperkalemia.

5. Therapy for hyperkalemia is divided into acute and chronic phases.

a. Acute antagonism and redistribution

(1) Calcium. The intravenous administration of 1–2 ampules of calcium chloride acutely antagonizes the cardiac effects of hyperkalemia. Electrocardiographic changes may transiently improve, but serum potassium level remains elevated.

(2) Glucose and insulin. The intravenous infusion of 25 g (1 ampule) of dextrose plus 15 units of insulin lowers serum potassium within 10–15 minutes.

(3) Sodium bicarbonate. The intravenous infusion of 44 mEq (1 ampule) of sodium bicarbonate acutely stimulates cellular uptake of potassium.

(4) β_2**-adrenergic agonists,** given by inhalation or intravenously, rapidly induce potassium uptake into cells, but they are not uniformly effective.

b. Acute removal

(1) Diuretics. Furosemide, bumetanide, and, especially, acetazolamide increase potassium excretion in individuals with adequate renal function.

(2) Aldosterone. The administration of aldosterone as either desoxycorticosterone acetate (15–20 mg/day, intramuscularly) or fludrocortisone acetate (0.2–0.6 mg/day, orally) may increase potassium excretion. Acute administration of desoxycorticosterone acetate in individuals who are aldosterone deficient may also act, in hours, to increase potassium excretion.

    (3) Dialysis. A 4-hour hemodialysis treatment effectively removes potassium and lowers the serum potassium level by approximately 40%–50%. Peritoneal dialysis is less effective, but the acute administration of glucose that accompanies infusion of the dialysate stimulates cellular uptake of potassium.

    (4) Cation-exchange resins. The administration of sodium polystyrene sulfonate binds potassium in the gastrointestinal tract. About 2 mEq of sodium are exchanged for every 1 mEq of potassium removed, so that a substantial sodium load may result. Sorbitol is administered orally to prevent severe constipation. Cation-exchange resins can remove 50–100 mEq of potassium over a 6-hour period and may be given orally or rectally.

  c. Chronic removal. After the acute removal of potassium, potassium homeostasis may be maintained with any of the following agents.

    (1) Aldosterone may be administered in the forms and dosages described above in Part II: III C 5 b (2).

    (2) Diuretics. Furosemide or acetazolamide may be used in combination with fludrocortisone acetate to increase potassium excretion.

    (3) Cation-exchange resins may be given on a chronic basis to increase gastrointestinal excretion of metabolism.

IV. ACID–BASE METABOLISM

A. Normal physiology. Acid–base balance refers to the maintenance of the hydrogen ion concentration of body fluids by three control systems: body buffers (e.g., bicarbonate), the lungs, and the kidneys. Because hydrogen ions (protons) are highly reactive species, even slight changes in hydrogen ion concentration can cause marked alterations in physiologic processes.

  1. Hydrogen ion concentration and pH. The hydrogen ion concentration of body fluids is low compared with the concentrations of other ions. It is more convenient, therefore, to express the concentration as **pH**, or the **negative logarithm of hydrogen ion concentration**. The pH of the extracellular fluid is maintained at about 7.4. Although it cannot be measured directly, the pH of the intracellular fluid most likely is between 7.0 and 7.2.

  2. Generation and elimination of hydrogen ion. Normal metabolic processes generate large amounts of carbonic as well as noncarbonic (nonvolatile) acids, which enter the body fluids and must be buffered and eliminated.

    a. Carbonic acid. Hydrogen ions are produced through complete oxidation of glucose and fatty acids to carbonic acid. Upon dehydration, carbonic acid forms a volatile end product (carbon dioxide), which can be eliminated by the lungs.

    b. Nonvolatile acid is produced through incomplete metabolism of glucose and fatty acids to organic acids (e.g., acetoacetic and β-hydroxybutyric acids) as well as metabolism of proteins such as methionine and phosphoprotein to sulfuric and phosphoric acids, respectively. Approximately 1 mEq of nonvolatile acid per kg of body weight is produced daily and is excreted primarily by the kidneys.

  3. Henderson-Hasselbalch equation. The bicarbonate–carbonic acid (HCO_3^-/CO_2) system is the major buffer component of the extracellular fluid. Acid–base disturbances often are characterized in terms of changes in either the bicarbonate (base) or dissolved carbon dioxide (acid) component of this buffer pair. The classic expression of acid–base state is based on the Henderson-Hasselbalch equation, which relates three variables—pH, carbon dioxide tension (P_{CO_2}), and plasma bicarbonate concentration ($[HCO_3^-]$)—and two constants—pK and S—as:

$$pH = pK + \log \frac{[HCO_3^-]}{S \times P_{CO_2}}$$

where: pK = the negative logarithm of the dissociation constant for carbonic acid (6.1), and S = the solubility constant for carbon dioxide in plasma (0.03 mmol/L/mm Hg). Normally, the plasma $[HCO_3^-]$ is 24 mmol/L and the arterial P_{CO_2} is 40 mm Hg. Thus:

$$pH = 6.1 + \log \frac{24}{1.2} = 7.4$$

4. **Respiratory regulation of arterial P_{CO_2}.** By regulating the rate of alveolar ventilation, the lungs may retain or excrete carbon dioxide and in this way regulate the "acid" component of the bicarbonate buffer system.

5. **Renal regulation of plasma bicarbonate content.** There are two important aspects of hydrogen ion metabolism in the kidney: the reabsorption of bicarbonate ion and the secretion of hydrogen ion.
   a. **Reabsorption of bicarbonate ion.** Approximately 4300 mEq of bicarbonate are filtered daily at the glomerulus, virtually all of which is reabsorbed into the proximal tubules. The remaining minute portion of the filtered bicarbonate is reabsorbed into the distal and collecting tubules. Proximal tubular reabsorption of bicarbonate occurs indirectly by the following process.
      (1) Filtered bicarbonate ion together with secreted hydrogen ion form carbonic acid within the tubular lumen. Sodium ion reabsorption is linked to this secretion of hydrogen ion to maintain electroneutrality.
      (2) Carbonic anhydrase in the brush border of the proximal tubule catalyzes the dehydration of carbonic acid to carbon dioxide and water. Being readily diffusible, carbon dioxide diffuses into the proximal tubular cell, where intracellular carbonic anhydrase catalyzes its rehydration to carbonic acid.
      (3) The bicarbonate ion formed by the dissociation of carbonic acid is passively reabsorbed into the peritubular blood along with equimolar amounts of sodium ion, which is actively transported into the peritubular blood. The hydrogen ion formed by the dissociation of carbonic acid within the cell serves as a source of another hydrogen ion to be secreted.
   b. **Addition of "new" bicarbonate.** In addition to conserving bicarbonate, the kidneys add newly synthesized bicarbonate to the plasma **via secretion of hydrogen ion.** This process replenishes the bicarbonate used to buffer acid produced by incomplete metabolism of neutral foodstuffs and by metabolism of acid precursors in the diet.
      (1) The addition of new bicarbonate does not involve the bicarbonate reabsorbed into the proximal tubule but, rather, the bicarbonate generated within the distal tubular cell via the hydration of carbon dioxide and the dissociation of carbonic acid. This process is similar to that for the reabsorption of the filtered bicarbonate; however, the formed bicarbonate in the cell is "new."
      (2) The renal contribution of new bicarbonate is accompanied by the excretion of an equivalent amount of acid in the urine in the form of titratable acid, ammonium ion, or both.
         (a) **Titratable acid formation and secretion.** The exchange of hydrogen ion for sodium ion converts dibasic sodium phosphate or sulfate in the glomerular filtrate into monobasic sodium phosphate or sulfate, which is excreted in the urine as titratable acid. The hydrogen ion secreted into the distal tubules, therefore, can react with filtered phosphate rather than filtered bicarbonate.
         (b) **Ammonia formation and secretion.** Unlike phosphate, ammonia enters the tubular lumen by tubular synthesis and secretion, rather than filtration. Ammonia is synthesized in the proximal tubule as a product of glutamine metabolism, and then it diffuses across the renal parenchyma to be secreted into the lumen of the collecting tubules. Virtually all of the

nonpolar ammonia that enters the tubular lumen immediately combines with hydrogen ion to form ammonium ion, which is nondiffusible because it is lipid insoluble. The renal excretion of ammonium ion results in the addition of bicarbonate to the plasma.

6. **Concept of compensation.** Compensation can be defined as the physiologic response to an alteration in either the **respiratory** or **metabolic** (renal) component of acid–base balance in order to restore the body pH value toward normal. Physiologic compensation generally is not complete. In the Henderson-Hasselbalch equation, changes in the "numerator" (metabolic component) are associated with secondary changes in the "denominator" (respiratory component), which restore the log ratio toward 24:1.2 (i.e., 20:1) and, therefore, restore pH toward normal. Conversely, changes in the respiratory component are associated with compensatory changes in the metabolic component in order to restore pH toward normal.

B. **Respiratory acidosis**

1. **Definition.** Respiratory acidosis is characterized by an increased **blood Pco_2** (i.e., to a value greater than 40 mm Hg) and a decreased blood pH (i.e., acidemia).

2. **Etiology.** Respiratory acidosis is associated with a reduced capacity to excrete **carbon dioxide** via the lungs. Causes include all disorders that reduce pulmonary function and carbon dioxide clearance.
   a. **Primary pulmonary disease** that is associated with alveolar–arterial mismatch may lead to carbon dioxide retention, usually as a late manifestation.
   b. **Neuromuscular disease.** Any weakness of the pulmonary musculature that leads to reduced ventilation (e.g., myasthenia gravis) may produce carbon dioxide retention.
   c. **Primary CNS dysfunction.** Any severe injury to the brain stem may be associated with reduced ventilatory drive and carbon dioxide retention.
   d. **Drug-induced hypoventilation.** Any agent that causes severe depression of CNS or neuromuscular function may be associated with respiratory acidosis.

3. **Clinical features**
   a. **CNS disorders.** Because blood flow to the brain is regulated by blood Pco_2, respiratory acidosis is associated with increased blood flow to the brain and increased cerebrospinal fluid (CSF) pressure. These effects may lead to a variety of symptoms of generalized CNS depression.
   b. **Cardiac disorders.** The acidemia in respiratory acidosis is associated with reduced cardiac output and pulmonary hypertension (effects that may lead to critically reduced blood flow to vital organs).

4. **Diagnosis**
   a. **Acute respiratory acidosis.** Acute carbon dioxide retention leads to an increase in blood Pco_2 with minimal change in plasma bicarbonate content. For each 10 mm Hg rise in Pco_2, the plasma bicarbonate level increases by approximately 1 mEq/L and the blood pH decreases by approximately 0.08. Serum electrolyte levels are close to normal in individuals with acute respiratory acidosis.
   b. **Chronic respiratory acidosis.** After 2–5 days, renal compensation (i.e., increased hydrogen ion secretion and bicarbonate production in the distal nephron) occurs; that is, the plasma bicarbonate level steadily increases. Arterial blood gas analysis shows that for each 10 mm Hg rise in Pco_2, the plasma bicarbonate level increases by 3–4 mEq/L and the blood pH decreases by 0.03.

5. **Therapy**
   a. **Correction of the underlying disorder.** Attempts should be made to correct muscular dysfunction or reversible pulmonary disease, if either is the cause of the respiratory acidosis. In the case of drug-induced hypoventilation, vigorous attempts should be made to clear the offending agent from the body.
   b. **Respiratory therapy.** A blood Pco_2 of more than 60 mm Hg may be an indication for assisted ventilation if CNS or pulmonary muscular depression is severe.

C. **Respiratory alkalosis**

1. **Definition.** Respiratory alkalosis is characterized by a decreased blood Pco_2 and an increased blood pH (alkalemia).

2. **Etiology.** Respiratory alkalosis is associated with excessive elimination of carbon dioxide via the lungs. Causes include any disorders associated with inappropriately increased ventilatory rate and carbon dioxide clearance.
   a. **Anxiety** (hysterical hyperventilation) is the most common cause of respiratory alkalosis.
   b. **Salicylate intoxication** initially causes overstimulation of the respiratory center, resulting in respiratory alkalosis. Metabolic acidosis may develop from the salicylate load, which enhances the hyperventilation.
   c. **Hypoxia.** Any disorder associated with decreased oxygen tension (Po_2) of blood may lead to an increased respiratory rate and, thus, respiratory alkalosis.
   d. **Intrathoracic disorders.** Any inflammatory or space-occupying lesion in the lung may be associated with primary stimulation of ventilatory rate, leading to a low Pco_2. Such conditions include:
      (1) Pulmonary embolism
      (2) Pneumonia
      (3) Asthma
      (4) Pulmonary fibrosis
   e. **Primary CNS dysfunction.** CNS disorders that may be associated with inappropriate stimulation of ventilation include:
      (1) Cerebrovascular accident (CVA)
      (2) Tumor
      (3) Infection
      (4) Trauma
   f. **Gram-negative septicemia.** An early manifestation of gram-negative septicemia or bacteremia is a primary stimulation of ventilation with respiratory alkalosis. The mechanism is unknown.
   g. **Liver insufficiency.** The most common acid–base disorder in liver disease is primary respiratory alkalosis through a direct CNS effect.
   h. **Pregnancy.** Primary stimulation of ventilation is typically seen throughout pregnancy.

3. **Clinical features.** Acute alkalemia may be associated with several organ system disorders.
   a. **CNS disorders.** A generalized feeling of anxiety may be present and may progress to more severe obtundation and even precoma.
   b. **Neuromuscular disorders.** Acute alkalemia may produce a tetany-like syndrome, which may be indistinguishable from that of acute hypocalcemia.

4. **Diagnosis**
   a. **Acute respiratory alkalosis.** Increased respiratory rate leads to a loss of carbon dioxide via the lungs, which in turn increases the blood pH. For each 10 mm Hg decrease in blood Pco_2 acutely, the plasma bicarbonate level decreases by 2 mEq/L and the blood pH increases by 0.08.
   b. **Chronic respiratory alkalosis.** Within hours after an acute decrease in arterial Pco_2, hydrogen ion secretion in the distal nephron decreases, leading to a decrease in plasma bicarbonate. For each 10 mm Hg decrease in blood Pco_2 chronically, the plasma bicarbonate level decreases by 5–6 mEq/L and the blood pH increases by only about 0.02. Serum chloride level also is elevated.

5. **Therapy.** The primary goal of therapy is to correct the underlying disorder. Use of carbon dioxide–enriched breathing mixtures or controlled ventilation may be required in cases of severe respiratory alkalosis (pH > 7.6).

D. **Metabolic acidosis**

1. **Definition.** Metabolic acidosis is characterized by a decreased blood pH and a decreased plasma bicarbonate concentration. This condition may be caused by one of

two basic mechanisms: the loss of bicarbonate or the accumulation of an acid other than carbonic acid (e.g., lactic acid).

2. **Etiology.** The causes of metabolic acidosis may be divided into those associated with a normal anion gap and those associated with an increased anion gap. **The anion gap reflects the concentrations of those anions that actually are present in serum but are routinely undetermined,** including negatively charged plasma proteins (mainly albumin), phosphates, sulfate, and organic acids (e.g., lactic acid). The anion gap represents the difference between the concentration of unmeasured anions and cations. It can be calculated as follows:

$$\text{Anion gap (mEq/L)} = [Na^+] - ([Cl^-] + [HCO_3^-])$$

The normal value is 10 ± 4 mEq/L. An increase in the anion gap represents an increase in one of these moieties, usually organic acids. No change in the anion gap, with decreases in both plasma bicarbonate concentration and serum pH, suggests a primary loss of bicarbonate or the addition of mineral acid.

a. **Metabolic acidosis with an increased anion gap**
   (1) **Ketoacidosis** refers to a condition of increased **ketone body** (ketoacid) formation, which leads to titration of bicarbonate and consequent metabolic acidosis. Ketoacidosis occurs as a complication of diabetes mellitus, prolonged starvation, and prolonged alcohol abuse.
   (2) **Lactic acidosis.** Decreased oxygen delivery to tissues results in increased lactate production, with accompanying severe metabolic acidosis. Lactic acidosis is a characteristic feature of many conditions associated with low tissue perfusion (e.g., shock and sepsis).
   (3) **Renal failure.** Metabolic acidosis results from the inability of the kidney to excrete the daily hydrogen ion load, derived from food and metabolism, as a result of a decline in ammonium excretion resulting from decreased renal mass. The acidosis of renal failure is characterized by either a normal or elevated anion gap, depending on the severity of the renal failure. In either case, the serum bicarbonate is reduced due to the titration by the retained hydrogen ions.
       (a) The anion gap is elevated only when the GFR is severely reduced (less than 15 ml/min) because the anions (sulfates and phosphates) that accompany the retained hydrogen ions cannot be filtered.
       (b) In mild to moderate renal failure (GFR = 15–40 ml/min) these anions are freely excreted and do not accumulate, resulting in metabolic acidosis with normal anion gap.
   (4) **Intoxication.** The ingestion of a variety of chemical agents may result in the accumulation of organic acids (e.g., lactic acid). Such intoxicants include:
       (a) Salicylate
       (b) Methanol
       (c) Ethylene glycol

b. **Metabolic acidosis with a normal anion gap (hyperchloremic metabolic acidosis)**
   (1) **Renal loss of bicarbonate** may result from the following conditions.
       (a) **Proximal tubular acidosis** is characterized by decreased proximal tubular reabsorption of bicarbonate leading to excessive urinary excretion of bicarbonate. Causes include cystinosis, multiple myeloma, heavy metal poisoning, Wilson's disease, and nephrotic syndrome.
       (b) **Distal tubular acidosis** is characterized by a decreased distal tubular capacity for hydrogen ion secretion and, therefore, the inability to generate new bicarbonate. Causes include amphotericin B toxicity, SLE, obstructive uropathy, Sjögren's syndrome, and other hyperglobulinemic conditions.
       (c) **Hyperkalemic renal tubular acidosis.** Hyperkalemia, particularly that associated with hyporeninemic hypoaldosteronism, is characterized by reduced ammonia excretion, reduced bicabonate production, and, thus, the inability to buffer nonvolatile acids derived from the diet. Acidosis

(i.e., reduced plasma bicarbonate) is due to reduced ammonia production and, therefore, reduced capacity to excrete hydrogen ion and to generate "new" bicarbonate [see Part II: IV A 5 a (3), b (2)].

   (d) Moderate renal insufficiency. The decline in ammonium excretion resulting from decreased renal mass causes a decrease in net acid excretion and, therefore, a decrease in serum bicarbonate concentration. Recall that when the GFR is 15–40 ml/min, anions such as sulfate and phosphate are freely excreted in the urine and do not accumulate, resulting in a normal anion gap.

   (e) Carbon anhydrase inhibition. Drugs such as acetazolamide (a diuretic) and mafenide (a topical treatment for burns) inhibit the action of carbonic anhydrase and thereby reduce proximal tubular reabsorption of bicarbonate.

(2) Gastrointestinal loss of bicarbonate also produces this syndrome and may occur because of:

   (a) Diarrhea

   (b) Pancreatic fistulas

   (c) Ureterosigmoidostomy

3. **Clinical features of metabolic acidosis** usually are related to the underlying disorder. A blood pH of less than 7.2 may lead to reduced cardiac output. Acidosis also may be associated with resistance to the vasoconstrictive action of catecholamines, resulting in hypotension. Kussmaul's (deep and rhythmic) respiration may be prominent as the ventilatory rate increases in response to the fall in serum pH.

4. **Diagnosis**

   a. Serum electrolyte assay shows a decreased bicarbonate and a variable chloride content, depending on whether the acidosis is associated with a normal or an increased anion gap.

   b. Arterial blood gas analysis also demonstrates a decreased bicarbonate level, with a compensatory decrease in blood P_{CO_2}. Winters' formula predicts that, in pure metabolic acidosis, the P_{CO_2} should be 1.5 times the bicarbonate concentration plus 8 ± 2 mm Hg. Variance from this predicted response to pure metabolic acidosis suggests a complicating respiratory dysfunction. (A P_{CO_2} that is lower than predicted suggests primary respiratory alkalosis; a P_{CO_2} that is higher than predicted suggests a disorder of pulmonary function, leading to inappropriate carbon dioxide retention.)

5. **Therapy.** Metabolic acidosis may be treated with alkali when the blood pH is less than 7.2, with therapy aimed at elevating the pH above this point. Sodium bicarbonate is the preferred alkali.

   a. The required amount of bicarbonate can be calculated on the basis that bicarbonate occupies a space that accounts for approximately 50% of body weight. Thus, the amount of sodium bicarbonate needed to raise the plasma bicarbonate from 6 mEq/L to 13 mEq/L is calculated as: 7 mEq/L × 0.5 × kg of body weight. This number is an approximation, and measurements of plasma bicarbonate and blood pH must be repeated in patients so treated.

   b. Underestimation of bicarbonate can occur if bicarbonate losses persist during administration or if ongoing acid production is sufficiently rapid to consume administered bicarbonate in a buffering reaction (lactic acidosis). In the presence of proximal tubular acidosis, the chronic bicarbonate requirement is 2–4 mg/kg/day.

E. Metabolic alkalosis

1. **Definition.** Metabolic alkalosis is characterized by an increased blood pH and an increased plasma bicarbonate concentration.

2. **Etiology.** Increased plasma bicarbonate levels result from either **increased endogenous production of bicarbonate** (in the stomach or kidney), with reduced renal excretion, or **exogenous administration of bicarbonate or other alkali**. Metabolic alkalosis depends on both the factors that initiate alkalemia (generation phase) and

those that maintain it (maintenance phase). Since the renal capacity for bicarbonate excretion is several thousand mEq/day, it is clear that some impairment in renal bicarbonate excretion is mandatory for the maintenance of metabolic alkalosis and a sustained rise in plasma bicarbonate.

    a. Excessive mineralocorticoid action on the distal convoluted tubule and collecting tubule stimulates hydrogen ion secretion, thereby raising the plasma bicarbonate level. This occurs in all cases of primary or secondary hyperaldosteronism.

    b. Vomiting. Loss of gastric hydrochloric acid by any means causes an increase in plasma bicarbonate because the source of hydrogen ion for gastric secretion is the dehydration of carbonic acid within the parietal cells. The concomitant decrease in extracellular fluid volume produced by vomiting, plus the chloride deficits, reduces the GFR and increases the rate of proximal tubular reabsorption of sodium and bicarbonate to maintain the metabolic alkalosis. Potassium deficits also develop because of renal potassium wasting, which may potentiate increased proximal tubular reabsorption of bicarbonate. Secondary hyperaldosteronism due to extracellular volume depletion also contributes to urinary potassium wasting.

    c. Diuretics. Inhibition of sodium chloride reabsorption leads to increased flow rate and, therefore, increased hydrogen ion secretion in the distal convoluted tubule and collecting tubule. Increased hydrogen ion secretion causes increased generation of bicarbonate. The volume depletion produced by the sodium deficits following diuretic use reduces the GFR, stimulates proximal tubular reabsorption of bicarbonate, and maintains metabolic alkalosis. Secondary hyperaldosteronism due to volume depletion causes urinary potassium wasting and also contributes to maintenance of metabolic alkalosis by stimulating hydrogen secretion in the distal segments of the nephron.

    d. Administration of alkali, either as sodium bicarbonate (e.g., during cardiac resuscitation) or as organic ions (e.g., lactate, citrate, and acetate, which are metabolically converted to bicarbonate by hepatic action), results in an increased plasma bicarbonate level. However, unless renal reabsorption of bicarbonate is stimulated, plasma bicarbonate is not sustained at an elevated level.

    e. Rapid correction of hypercapnia. Following sustained respiratory acidosis, renal bicarbonate production is elevated as a compensatory event by a stimulation of hydrogen ion secretion. If arterial Pco_2 then is acutely reduced by mechanical ventilation, a transient state of hyperbicarbonatemia and elevated blood pH ensues (a condition termed **posthypercapnic metabolic alkalosis**).

3. Clinical features of metabolic alkalosis generally are dominated by the underlying disease state. However, symptoms of tetany may be the most pronounced clinical features.

4. Diagnosis

    a. Serum electrolyte assay shows an increased bicarbonate level and a decreased chloride level. Hypokalemia is a frequent finding.

    b. Arterial blood gas analysis reveals an elevated bicarbonate level and a compensatory increase in Pco_2 value. Because a decrease in ventilation is required to elevate Pco_2, hypoxia also may result.

    c. Urinary indices are useful in the diagnosis of metabolic alkalosis. If extracellular fluid volume contraction is not present (e.g., due to excessive mineralocorticoid activity) or if renal reabsorption of sodium chloride is inhibited (e.g., due to diuretic use), urine chloride levels are elevated. If extracellular fluid volume depletion also is present (e.g., due to vomiting), urine chloride level typically is too low to be measured. Rarely, severe potassium depletion (i.e., serum potassium concentration of < 2 mEq/L) is associated with urinary chloride wasting in the presence of extracellular fluid volume depletion.

5. Therapy involves correction of the underlying disease state as well as reduction of renal avidity for bicarbonate. The latter effect is accomplished by extracellular volume expansion with sodium chloride–containing solutions.

    a. The metabolic alkalosis caused by excessive mineralocorticoid activity is highly dependent on potassium depletion. Administration of potassium chloride corrects this disorder.

b. In individuals who have posthypercapnic metabolic alkalosis, judicious administration of acetazolamide or other inhibitors of proximal tubular bicarbonate reabsorption is an adjunct to therapy.

V. CALCIUM METABOLISM

A. Normal physiology

1. Calcium exists in serum in three forms. About 40% of serum calcium is bound to protein, about 5%–15% is complexed with anions such as citrate and phosphate, and the remaining portion is unbound, ionized calcium. The ionized component of serum calcium is the most important clinically. For example, hypoalbuminemia lowers serum calcium by reducing the protein-bound component; the ionized calcium concentration, however, is unaffected by hypoalbuminemia, and the patient is asymptomatic.

2. Ionized calcium homeostasis is maintained by a balance of calcium input into the blood from the gastrointestinal tract and bone and calcium output from the blood into the urine and lower gastrointestinal tract. Calcium transport across the gastrointestinal tract is influenced strongly by **1,25-dihydroxycholecalciferol [1,25-(OH)$_2$D$_3$, or calcitriol],** which is the active metabolite of vitamin D. **Parathyroid hormone (PTH)** raises serum calcium by increasing calcium release from bone, by reducing renal excretion of calcium, and by stimulating renal activation of vitamin D to calcitriol. This is the second of two steps in the metabolic activation of dietary vitamin D. The first step takes place in the liver, and the product is **25-hydroxycholecalciferol** [25-(OH)D$_3$, or **calcifediol**]. Serum calcium level is the principal regulator of PTH release.

B. **Hypocalcemia** is defined as a serum calcium concentration less than 8.5 mg/dl. **Hypoalbuminemia** lowers the total serum calcium by reducing the protein-bound component. Generally, the total serum calcium level is decreased 0.8 mg/dl for each 1 g/L decrement in serum albumin. However, **PTH deficiency** is the primary determinant of hypocalcemia. For a complete discussion of hypocalcemia, see Chapter 9 III B.

C. **Hypercalcemia** results from disorders that cause either increased gastrointestinal absorption or increased bone resorption of calcium. Normal serum calcium level may reach 10.5 mg/dl in men and 10.2 mg/dl in women. Higher values may indicate true hypercalcemia, but serum protein level also must be monitored to confirm that an increased level of protein does not explain the increased total serum calcium. **Hyperparathyroidism** is the result of oversecretion of PTH, which in turn causes hypercalcemia. A full discussion of hypercalcemia can be found in Chapter 9 III A.

VI. PHOSPHATE METABOLISM

A. Normal physiology

1. **Phosphate function.** Phosphate may be the single most important dynamic constituent required for cellular activity. Virtually all bodily functions are powered by the high-energy phosphate bonds of adenosine triphosphate (ATP). In addition, phosphate is the major anion and chief buffer of the intracellular fluid. Its primary role in the renal excretion of hydrogen ion makes phosphate a major constituent of acid–base metabolism as well.

2. **Phosphate distribution.** About 85% of the total body store of phosphate is in bone. Phosphate also is found in the intracellular and extracellular fluid compartments. Plasma phosphate exists primarily in the form of inorganic phosphate, the majority of which is free (not bound to protein).

   The inorganic phosphate content of the extracellular fluid is a prime determinant of intracellular inorganic phosphate, which is the source of phosphate for ATP. Intracellular phosphate deficits may result in reduced cell energy production and, therefore, generalized cell dysfunction.

3. **Phosphate homeostasis** involves the balance of phosphate intake and phosphate output ("external" balance) as well as the maintenance of normal phosphate distribution within the body ("internal" balance).
   a. **External phosphate balance.** Normal dietary intake of phosphate is 1200 mg/day, which is provided primarily by dairy products, and normal phosphate excretion is 1200 mg/day (800 mg in the urine and 400 mg in the stool). The gastrointestinal tract is a passive component of external phosphate balance, whereas renal phosphate handling is closely regulated.
      (1) Normally, 90% of filtered phosphate is reabsorbed in the proximal tubule, with only a minute portion reabsorbed distally. The main regulator of renal phosphate handling is PTH. A high PTH level inhibits phosphate reabsorption, and a low PTH level stimulates it.
      (2) PTH-independent control of renal phosphate reabsorption also is exerted by dietary phosphate content and other hormones such as calcitonin, thyroid hormone, and growth hormone (GH). A decrease in phosphate intake stimulates proximal tubular reabsorption of phosphate.
   b. **Internal phosphate balance** also is regulated because intracellular phosphate levels are 200–300 mg/dl and extracellular levels are 3–4 mg/dl. Increased insulin or β-adrenergic agonist levels, hydrogen ion shifts, and intracellular metabolic disturbances all alter the phosphate distribution in the body.

B. | **Hypophosphatemia**

1. **Etiology.** Hypophosphatemia can result from extrarenal or renal loss of phosphate.
   a. **Extrarenal causes**
      (1) **Dietary deficiency and gastrointestinal losses**
         (a) **Inadequate dietary intake.** Most food contains some phosphate. Inadequate dietary intake of phosphate is unusual and only occurs under specific iatrogenic circumstances.
         (b) **Antacid abuse.** Large amounts of calcium salts (e.g., acetate, carbonate) and aluminum- or magnesium-containing antacids bind phosphate in the gastrointestinal tract, increase gastrointestinal phosphate losses, and may produce hypophosphatemia.
         (c) **Starvation.** During prolonged starvation, cell breakdown liberates phosphate into the extracellular fluid. The amount of phosphate in remaining, intact cells, however, is preserved at normal levels. As urinary plus stool loss of liberated, extracellular phosphate exceeds dietary intake, negative phosphate balance occurs. Although hypophosphatemia does not follow immediately, severe phosphate deficits may develop upon refeeding as cellular uptake of phosphate is stimulated by new cell growth and macromolecule synthesis.
      (2) **Redistribution of body phosphate**
         (a) **Increased glycolysis.** Any condition associated with increased glycolysis within cells causes organic phosphate compounds to accumulate as the phosphorylated carbon residues in the Embden-Meyerhof pathway, with depletion of intracellular organic phosphate. Serum phosphate level falls as phosphate diffuses into cells, causing hypophosphatemia. Reduction of intracellular inorganic phosphate through this mechanism may be drastic and lead to ATP depletion and, thus, reduced cellular energy. In uncomplicated cases, phosphorylated compounds are metabolized

through the Krebs cycle, causing ATP repletion. With more severe phosphate depletion, ATP deficits may lead to cell dysfunction, such as rhabdomyolysis.

(b) **Respiratory alkalosis.** Hyperventilation is associated with reduced serum phosphate because of increased cellular uptake of phosphate. Glycolysis within cells is stimulated by acute elevation of cellular pH. Acute respiratory alkalosis causes hypophosphatemia by enhancing phosphate uptake into cells.

(c) **Sepsis.** Hypophosphatemia is a known concomitant of gram-negative sepsis and may coexist (although independently) with hypophosphatemia because of respiratory alkalosis.

(d) **Epinephrine** also stimulates cellular uptake of phosphate. This effect is independent of cellular phosphate uptake due to insulin-mediated glycolysis or to other alterations of glucose metabolism.

b. **Renal causes**

(1) **Excess PTH.** Any condition associated with normal renal function but elevated PTH levels can produce renal phosphate wasting. This disorder may occur with primary hyperparathyroidism as well as the various states of secondary hyperparathyroidism.

(2) **Primary renal tubular defects.** Conditions such as cystinosis, heavy metal poisoning, multiple myeloma, and Wilson's disease may be associated with generalized proximal tubular defects (Fanconi's syndrome) and renal phosphate wasting.

(3) **Specific transport defects for phosphate** have been designated as **hypophosphatemic vitamin D–resistant rickets,** which may be familial or sporadic and exists in both child-onset and adult-onset forms. In each of these conditions, decreased phosphate transport in the proximal tubule produces excessive renal phosphate wasting.

(4) **Glycosuria.** Phosphate and glucose compete for transport in the proximal tubule. All glycosuric conditions are associated with excessive renal losses of phosphate.

2. **Clinical features**

a. **CNS disorders.** Cellular ATP deficiency may produce obtundation, coma, and seizures. Peripheral neuropathy and Guillain-Barré syndrome also have been described.

b. **Hematologic disorders.** Hemolytic anemia due to cellular ATP depletion and abnormal membrane integrity has been described but is rare. Thrombocytopenia, reduced platelet function, and reduced white cell phagocytic activity have been described but are of uncertain clinical significance.

c. **Muscular disorders.** Dysfunction of skeletal muscle has been described and attributed to ATP deficits. Acute rhabdomyolysis may be particularly prevalent in alcoholic patients who are acutely hypophosphatemic. Paralysis of respiratory muscles with respiratory failure also may be seen.

d. **Bone disorders.** Increased bone resorption with abnormal mineralization occurs in chronic hypophosphatemia.

3. **Diagnosis.** Hypophosphatemia causes complete elimination of phosphate from the urine. A urine phosphate level of more than 100 mg/L strongly suggests renal **phosphate wasting**. A low urine phosphate level suggests antacid-induced phosphate depletion or increased cellular uptake of phosphate. Glucose infusion with secondary insulin release is the cause of hypophosphatemia in most hospitalized patients.

4. **Therapy.** All hypophosphatemic patients should be treated. In general, this therapy involves correction of the underlying condition, such as discontinuation of glucose infusions. In individuals with severe hypophosphatemia and preexisting phosphate depletion (e.g., alcoholic patients), symptomatic hypophosphatemia should be treated with phosphate supplementation. Oral phosphate is preferred, and 1500–2000 mg/day may be given in divided doses. If the patient is comatose or is unable to take oral phosphate, intravenous phosphate may be administered twice daily in 250-mg doses, if serum phosphate is less than 1 mg/dl, provided that serum

phosphate measurements are taken at 12-hour intervals. Infusion of phosphate must be discontinued if the serum phosphate level rises to 1.5 mg/dl.

5. **Complications.** The greatest danger of hypophosphatemia lies in the injudicious administration of intravenous phosphate. Acute hypocalcemia due to the formation of calcium phosphate may lead to shock, acute renal failure, and death. For this reason, intravenous phosphate should be administered only when specific clinical disturbances are clearly attributable to hypophosphatemia.

C. **Hyperphosphatemia**

1. **Etiology**
   a. **Renal failure.** Since the kidney is the main regulator of serum phosphate level, renal failure commonly is associated with hyperphosphatemia. This disorder is not seen until the GFR has decreased to 25% of normal. Serum phosphate level generally does not exceed 10 mg/dl in renal failure. Values exceeding 10 mg/dl suggest an additional etiologic factor.
   b. **Cell lysis syndromes**
      (1) **Rhabdomyolysis.** Acute muscle breakdown of any etiology is associated with the release of cellular phosphate and, therefore, hyperphosphatemia. Severe hyperphosphatemia (i.e., a serum phosphate concentration >25 mg/dl) may be seen in cases associated with acute renal failure.
      (2) **Tumor lysis syndrome.** Malignant disorders associated with a high sensitivity to chemotherapy or radiotherapy result in rapid cell death from such treatments. This syndrome may lead to massive release of phosphate and other intracellular substances into the extracellular fluid. Severe hypocalcemia, cardiovascular collapse, and renal failure due to calcium, urate, and phosphate deposition in the kidney have been described in this condition.
   c. **Exogenous phosphate administration** by any route (i.e., via intravenous infusion, by mouth, or via phosphate enemas) may result in severe and unpredictable hyperphosphatemia.
   d. **Hypoparathyroidism.** Since the level of PTH determines the rate of renal phosphate handling, any condition associated with parathyroid insufficiency or a lack of organ response to PTH may be characterized by hyperphosphatemia.
   e. **Tumoral calcinosis** is a rare disorder characterized by hyperphosphatemia, soft-tissue calcified masses, and normocalcemia. Rather than a disorder of calcium metabolism, this condition is due to a specific increase in the renal reabsorption of phosphate. Tumoral calcinosis may represent a heritable condition.
   f. **Miscellaneous causes.** GH excess, hyperthyroidism, and sickle cell anemia are associated with hyperphosphatemia from excessive renal reabsorption of phosphate. However, this finding is of no clinical significance in these disorders.

2. **Clinical features.** Hypocalcemia, hypotension, and renal failure may be seen in severe hyperphosphatemia. Milder cases, typically seen in chronic renal failure, are associated with secondary hyperparathyroidism. The treatment of hypercalcemia with phosphate may result in cardiac and renal calcification.

3. **Diagnosis.** Hyperphosphatemia in the absence of renal insufficiency is due to hypoparathyroidism, cell lysis, or tumoral calcinosis. The etiologic diagnosis of hyperphosphatemia is made on the basis of the patient history, physical examination, and laboratory data.

4. **Therapy.** Acute hyperphosphatemia may be a medical emergency that requires immediate therapy. In cases of tumor lysis syndrome, acute hemodialysis may be necessary and is an effective treatment. Administration of large amounts of phosphate-binding gels may be useful in the long-term treatment of hyperphosphatemic conditions.

VII. **MAGNESIUM METABOLISM**

A. **Normal physiology.** Magnesium is the second most abundant intracellular cation. (Potassium is the most abundant.)

1. **Magnesium distribution.** More than 50% of the total body store of magnesium is in bone, with most of the remaining portion found in soft tissues, mainly muscle. Less than 1% of body magnesium is in the extracellular fluid, 20%–30% of which is bound to protein and the rest existing as free cation.

2. **Magnesium homeostasis.** Magnesium is absorbed into the small intestine, but this process is primarily unregulated. During dietary deprivation of magnesium, stool magnesium losses result in hypomagnesemia. The kidney efficiently conserves magnesium during dietary deprivation and excretes any excess magnesium due to excessive intake.

B. Hypomagnesemia

1. **Definition.** Clinically important hypomagnesemia occurs when serum magnesium concentration falls below 1.0 mEq/L, although it has been proposed that even mild degrees of hypomagnesemia may be associated with a variety of clinical disorders.

2. **Etiology**
   a. **Extrarenal causes**
      (1) **Dietary deficiency and gastrointestinal losses**
         (a) **Inadequate dietary intake.** Nutritional hypomagnesemia may develop after prolonged starvation as well as postoperatively.
         (b) **Malabsorption.** Generalized malabsorption syndrome, chronic diarrhea, diffuse bowel injury, and chronic laxative abuse all are associated with reduced gastrointestinal absorption of magnesium. Since gut losses of magnesium can occur even in an individual with a normal gastrointestinal tract, any disorder associated with reduced magnesium intake can result in hypomagnesemia.
      (2) **Redistribution of body magnesium.** Acute cellular uptake of magnesium has been described in individuals who are in alcohol withdrawal. Also, following parathyroidectomy for severe osteitis fibrosa cystica, acute bone formation may cause rapid accumulation of magnesium and calcium in bone and consequent hypomagnesemia.
   b. **Renal causes**
      (1) **Primary tubular disorders.** A number of tubular disorders, including Bartter's syndrome, renal tubular acidosis, and postobstructive diuresis, are characterized by a defect in renal magnesium conservation and hypomagnesemia. Hypomagnesemia also may develop in patients following renal transplantation.
      (2) **Drug-induced tubular losses.** Diuretics such as thiazides, furosemide, and ethacrynic acid typically produce varied degrees of hypomagnesemia. Even small doses of the chemotherapeutic agent cisplatin produce marked renal magnesium wasting and clinically severe hypomagnesemia. Gentamicin and amphotericin B also may produce a toxic injury to the renal tubule, with magnesium and potassium wasting occurring in the absence of reduced GFR.
      (3) **Hormone-induced tubular losses.** Hyperaldosteronism is associated with magnesium wasting, although the renal tubular mechanism responsible is unknown. Since PTH is an important determinant of renal tubular magnesium handling, hypoparathyroidism is associated with renal magnesium wasting and hypomagnesemia.
      (4) **Ion- or nutrient-induced tubular losses.** Because calcium and magnesium compete for transport in the ascending limb of the loop of Henle, hypercalcemia is associated with reduced renal magnesium transport. Phosphate depletion, alcohol consumption, or both are associated with decreased renal reabsorption of magnesium, but the mechanisms are unknown.

3. **Clinical features.** Muscle twitching, tremor, and muscle weakness are commonly seen. These physical signs are due to the direct effect of magnesium on neuromuscular function as well as the hypocalcemic effect of hypomagnesemia. Severe chronic hypomagnesemia leads to decreased glandular secretion of PTH as well as impaired bone response to PTH, and both of these effects lead to hypocalcemia. Also, hypomagnesemia produces a defect in renal potassium reabsorption, which eventually

produces potassium depletion. Thus, all of the clinical signs of hypocalcemia and hypokalemia may be seen in hypomagnesemic patients. The clinical presentation of hypokalemia and hypomagnesemia includes cardiac arrhythmias, particularly in the patient given digitalis.

4. **Therapy.** In most patients, magnesium deficits can be repleted by a normal diet. If ongoing losses occur, magnesium supplementation is necessary. Even in severe magnesium deficiency, however, 50% of an administered dose of magnesium is excreted in the urine. Symptomatic deficits usually amount to 1–2 mmol/kg of body weight. If oral magnesium therapy is required, magnesium oxide, given four times daily in doses of 250–500 mg, generally is tolerated and has 25%–50% absorption. If parenteral therapy is necessary, 12 ml (25 mmol) of 50% magnesium sulfate in 1 L of 5% dextrose in water (D5W) are given over 3 hours, and 40 mmol in 2 L of D5W are given over the remainder of the 24-hour period. An additional 25 mmol of magnesium sulfate in 1 L of D5W are given daily for the subsequent 3 days.

C. Hypermagnesemia

1. **Etiology.** Since the kidneys can excrete several hundred mEq of magnesium each day, hypermagnesemia usually is iatrogenic and occurs, in a sustained fashion, only in patients who have impaired renal function and ingest magnesium as either laxatives or antacids. Acute magnesium intoxication may occur in women who are treated for toxemia of pregnancy with intravenous magnesium salts that are administered at an excessive rate. Muscular paralysis can develop at serum magnesium levels of 10 mg/dl.

2. **Therapy.** Calcium ion is a direct antagonist of magnesium and should be given to patients who are seriously ill with magnesium intoxication. Hemodialysis may be required following cessation of magnesium therapy.

PART III: HYPERTENSION

I. GENERAL CONSIDERATIONS

A. **Definition.** Hypertension is present when the blood pressure exceeds 140/90 mm Hg at several determinations. This is an arbitrary definition because a diastolic pressure of even 85 mm Hg may be associated with increased cardiovascular morbidity and mortality. The relative importance of systolic versus diastolic hypertension has not been completely established, but many studies suggest that systolic blood pressure elevation is as, if not more, significant than diastolic blood pressure elevation as a risk factor for a variety of cardiovascular diseases.

1. **Primary (essential) hypertension** is hypertension that has no known cause. Primary hypertension accounts for 70%–95% of cases of hypertension.

2. **Secondary hypertension** is attributable to a diagnosable disease and accounts for the remainder of cases of hypertension.

B. Diagnosis

1. Blood pressure should be measured with a **loosely fitting cuff.** The width of the cuff should equal at least 50% of the length of the upper arm. Initially, blood pressure should be **determined in each arm** to be sure that arterial obstruction in the upper extremity is not falsely lowering the distal arm arterial pressure.

2. Blood pressure may be quite elevated at times of stress; in fact, in some patients, merely being in a physician's office may induce transient hypertension. **Multiple determinations over several visits** and some form of **home** or **workplace monitoring**

should be conducted prior to initiating pharmacologic therapy in hypertensive patients.

C. **Consequences of hypertension.** In general, the mortality rate over 20 years among patients with a systolic blood pressure of greater than 160 mm Hg or a diastolic blood pressure of greater than 100 mm Hg increases 100% in those who are untreated.

1. **Stroke.** Patients with a systolic blood pressure of greater than 160 mm Hg have a fourfold increased risk of stroke if untreated.

2. **Coronary artery disease.** Patients with a diastolic pressure of greater than 95 mm Hg have a more than twofold increased risk of coronary artery disease as compared with normotensive patients. The beneficial response to therapy is not as well defined as it is for stroke, however.

3. **Congestive heart failure.** Patients with blood pressure of greater than 160/95 mm Hg have a fourfold increased incidence of congestive heart failure. In 75% of patients with congestive heart failure, hypertension occurs at some time during the course of their illness. Thickening and hypertrophy of the left ventricle as a result of hypertension may produce congestive heart failure as a result of diastolic dysfunction.

II. **MECHANISMS OF HYPERTENSION**

A. **Primary hypertension**

1. **Abnormal cardiac and peripheral hemodynamics.** Blood pressure is the product of cardiac output and total peripheral resistance; thus, in order for hypertension to occur, there must be an elevation in cardiac output, total peripheral resistance, or both.
   a. An abnormality in peripheral resistance is a contributing factor in most cases of hypertension.
   b. Many patients with hypertension have either persistently elevated cardiac output or elevated total peripheral resistance early in the course of the disease.

2. **Impaired pressure natriuresis**
   a. In normal individuals, an elevation in blood pressure leads to an alteration in intrarenal hemodynamics and physical forces that results in natriuresis. This, in turn, causes a diuresis, a decrease in total extracellular volume, and a fall in blood pressure.
   b. In patients with essential hypertension, the kidney fails to respond normally to elevated arterial pressure and natriuresis is impaired. The homeostatic abnormality may either cause or help sustain the elevated arterial pressure.
   c. The cause of the failure of normal pressure natriuresis is unknown. Hormonal factors, abnormalities in the structure and activity of transport proteins (e.g., the sodium–hydrogen exchanger in the renal tubule), and autonomic nervous system activity have all been implicated experimentally and on a clinical basis.

3. **Baroreceptor resetting.** In hypertensive patients, baroreceptors in the carotid arteries and aorta are "reset" so that higher pressures are required to exert an influence toward lowering blood pressure.

4. **Abnormalities in the renin-angiotensin-aldosterone system.** There is increasing evidence that abnormalities in each component of this complex system may contribute to the pathogenesis of hypertension in many patients with hypertension. For instance, recent experimental studies using gene transfer techniques show that mice with increased gene expression for the angiotensinogen gene are hypertensive.

5. **Abnormalities in other vasoregulatory systems**
   a. **Endothelin,** a peptide produced in many organs and tissues, is a vasoconstrictor with potency several times greater than that of norepinephrine.
   b. **Atrial natriuretic peptide (ANP),** derived from cardiac muscle, may play a role in

normal vascular regulation as a vasodilator and may contribute to extracellular volume homeostasis and blood pressure control in states of mineralocorticoid excess by enhancing sodium excretion.

c. **Endothelium-derived relaxation factor (EDRF)** is thought to be **nitric oxide,** a gas derived from arginine metabolism that is crucial in a number of vasoregulatory phenomena. Defects in this system are thought to contribute to the hypertension associated with pregnancy.

B. **Secondary hypertension.** In 5%–10% of patients with hypertension, the hypertension is secondary to an identifiable disorder in the endocrine system or the autonomic nervous system.

1. **Renovascular hypertension** (see also Part I: XIV C) is an important cause of secondary hypertension. In this disorder, hypertension is the result of a complex interplay between activation of the renin-angiotensin-aldosterone system and the sympathetic nervous system. The pattern of endocrine stimulation may also depend on whether the vascular lesions are unilateral or bilateral.

   a. Initially, high angiotensin II levels lead to vasoconstriction and expanded extracellular fluid volume as aldosterone release is stimulated.

   b. With time, volume expansion may lead to suppression of total renal renin production so that circulating renin values may be normal in spite of the elevated blood pressure. This may explain why unstimulated plasma renin levels are not a good index of the presence of renovascular hypertension in all cases and why some patients (e.g., those with unilateral vascular lesions) may not even demonstrate increased renin secretion.

      (1) The normal levels of renin, which are inappropriate in the presence of hypertension and an expanded extracellular fluid volume, sustain the hypertension.

      (2) In addition, during this chronic phase, increased sympathetic nervous system activity resulting from chronic angiotensin II stimulation contributes to hypertension.

2. **Renal parenchymal diseases.** Hypertension frequently accompanies a variety of renal diseases, highlighting the important contribution of renal endocrine and excretory function in the regulation of blood pressure.

   a. **Altered excretory function.** Defects in the renal excretion of salt and water no doubt contribute to the pathogenesis of hypertension in patients with advanced renal failure. In patients maintained on hemodialysis or peritoneal dialysis, modest reductions in extracellular fluid volume can produce a striking reduction in arterial blood pressure.

   b. **Altered renin-angiotensin-aldosterone activity.** Ischemic changes resulting from intrarenal scarring may activate the renin-angiotensin system and contribute to hypertension in patients with early or advanced renal failure.

3. **Endocrinologic causes**

   a. **Oral contraceptives** cause hypertension in approximately 5% of patients who use them. Hypertension occurs as a result of estrogen-induced increases in angiotensinogen synthesis in the liver. Reduced estrogen levels or the addition of progesterone may ameliorate this complication.

   b. **Mineralocorticoid excess syndromes.** Mineralocorticoid excess leads to hypertension by inducing sodium and water retention, leading to expansion of the extracellular fluid volume. The hypertension is often accompanied by hypokalemia, because mineralocorticoids promote renal potassium excretion in the collecting duct of the nephron. A variety of disorders produce mineralocorticoid excess states.

      (1) **Primary hyperaldosteronism.** Tumors of the adrenal gland, which are common on autopsy, are functionally active in 1%–3% of patients, leading to mineralocorticoid excess. Tumors may be unilateral or bilateral, or the excess may result from a diffuse bilateral hyperplasia of the adrenal zona glomerulosa.

      (2) **Glucocorticoid-remediable hyperaldosteronism.** In rare patients, a defect in adrenal development leads to the synthesis of aldosterone in the adrenal

gland under the influence of ACTH. A gene rearrangement allows expression of ACTH-responsive aldosterone synthase in the zona fasciculata rather than the zona glomerulosa, leading to the production of large amounts of mineralocorticoid hormone. Treatment with dexamethasone suppresses this abnormal pathway. This disorder should be suspected in patients with a family history of hypertension and hypokalemia.

(3) **Exogenous hypermineralocorticoidism.** Some patients may develop striking mineralocorticoid excess hypertension from the ingestion of **glycyrrhetinic acid,** a substance found in European licorice and in some forms of chewing tobacco. Glycyrrhetinic acid blocks the action of 11β-hydroxysteroid dehydrogenase (an enzyme that prevents glucocorticoid binding to receptors in the renal distal tubule), resulting in a high mineralocorticoid state. Patients present with hypertension, hypokalemia, and low renin and aldosterone levels.

(4) **Cushing's syndrome.** Glucocorticoid excess resulting from exogenous glucocorticoid therapy, a pituitary tumor, or an adrenal adenoma produces hypertension in approximately 80% of patients with Cushing's syndrome. Hypertension may occur because cortisol has mineralocorticoid-like effects and, therefore, leads to the retention of sodium and water. However, many patients with Cushing's syndrome and hypertension do not manifest a low renin state as would be expected in primary mineralocorticoidism, implying that other mechanisms may contribute to the hypertension as well.

(5) **Liddle's syndrome** is a familial disorder transmitted as an autosomal dominant form of hypertension. It presents as hypertension and hypokalemia with low renin and aldosterone levels. The cause is a genetic defect in the β subunit of the sodium channel in the apical membrane of the distal renal tubule. This defect mimics the action of mineralocorticoid hormones to enhance sodium entry in the distal nephron, thereby enhancing sodium absorption, increasing potassium excretion, and expanding the extracellular fluid volume, leading to an elevated arterial blood pressure.

c. **Pheochromocytoma.** This tumor of the adrenal medulla increases the secretion of catecholamines, leading to hypertension. Approximately 50% of patients have episodic hypertension; the rest have constant hypertension.

d. **Miscellaneous causes. Acromegaly, hyperparathyroidism,** and **hyperthyroidism** also may produce hypertension. **Coarctation of the aorta,** as noted in Chapter 1 VII D, is a correctable cause of hypertension.

III. APPROACH TO THE HYPERTENSIVE PATIENT. The majority of patients with hypertension have essential hypertension; therefore, the expense, risk, and inconvenience of screening for secondary causes of hypertension should be reserved for a minority of patients suspected of having one of the following disorders.

A. Renovascular hypertension

1. Renovascular hypertension **secondary to atherosclerosis of the renal artery** should be suspected in the following patients:
   a. Patients with severe hypertension associated with advanced hypertensive retinopathy
   b. Patients with hypertension and severe peripheral vascular disease
   c. Patients with hypertension and sudden deterioration in renal function (with or without the recent introduction of ACE inhibitor therapy)
   d. Patients with a known disparity in renal size or function

2. Renovascular hypertension **secondary to fibromuscular dysplasia** should be suspected in young women with severe hypertension, systolic and diastolic abdominal bruits, or a strong family history of hypertension.

B. Hypermineralocorticoid states should be suspected in patients with persistent hypokalemia and hypertension. There is no doubt that these disorders are underdiagnosed because many patients with proven mineralocorticoid excess states are normokalemic. Nevertheless, persistent and unexplained hypokalemia remains the most typical sign.

1. **Primary hyperaldosteronism.** The diagnosis rests on finding patients with hypokalemia and hypertension and proving that hyperaldosteronism causes both disorders.
    a. Patients who have unexplained hypokalemia and hypertension should have their **24-hour urinary excretion rate for aldosterone** measured while consuming a 150-mEq sodium diet. If the aldosterone value is elevated and plasma renin is low, an **abdominal CT scan** should be performed to determine if a surgically correctable (i.e., adenomatous) form of hyperaldosteronism is present.
        (1) Surgery will relieve hypertension and hypokalemia in over 70% of patients if adenoma is the cause. Surgery will not cure hypertension in patients with bilateral hyperplasia, but the hypokalemia will remit.
        (2) Although hypokalemia may not be found in some patients with primary hyperaldosteronism, patients with hypokalemia are more likely to have a positive response to surgery so the finding of spontaneous hypokalemia remains a reasonable screening tool.
    b. **Trial glucocorticoid therapy.** Patients with a family history of hypertension should undergo a trial of glucocorticoid therapy to determine whether glucocorticoid-remediable hyperaldosteronism is present.
    c. **Selective adrenal venography and sampling for lateralizing aldosterone levels** may be performed in some patients.

2. **Pheochromocytoma** should be suspected in hypertensive patients who experience episodes of flushing, diaphoresis, weight loss, and diarrhea.
    a. **Measurement of urinary catecholamines and catecholamine metabolites** (including metanephrine and vanillylmandelic acid) is useful in making the diagnosis.
    b. **CT scanning** should be used to locate the tumor in the adrenal medulla.

3. **Coarctation of the aorta** should be suspected in any young patient with hypertension when the blood pressure in the leg is at least 20 mm Hg greater than that in the arm.

IV. THERAPY OF HYPERTENSION

A. **Goals of therapy.** Therapy of hypertension is aimed at reducing the diastolic blood pressure to less than 90 mm Hg and the systolic blood pressure to less than 150 mm Hg.

B. **Indications for therapy.** Some physicians withhold therapy as long as there is no end-organ involvement and observe the patient for 1–2 years because many patients return to a normotensive state spontaneously; however, it is currently believed that most patients with a blood pressure of greater than 140/95 mm Hg should be treated. In patients with borderline hypertension, controversy exists about the risks versus the benefits of therapy, but most clinicians believe that the benefits of therapy predominate and that all patients with an elevated blood pressure should receive treatment to restore the values to normal.

C. **Types of therapy**

1. **Nonpharmacologic measures**
    a. **Sodium restriction** alone may be sufficient to lower blood pressure in many hypertensive patients, particularly those with a high sodium intake. Limitation of sodium intake to no more than 2 g/day has been shown to reduce blood pressure significantly in susceptible patients.
    b. **Weight reduction** in obese patients also significantly reduces blood pressure.
    c. **Limitation of alcohol consumption.** Alcohol potentiates the action of catecholamines and may exacerbate hypertension in susceptible individuals.

2. **Pharmacologic therapy.** Therapeutic regimens that are simple to follow often have the best patient compliance. In choosing an antihypertensive regimen, consideration should be given not only to side effects, but also to the number of medications and doses per day that the patient must take.

   a. **Diuretics,** which often are the first line of antihypertensive therapy, initially reduce extracellular fluid volume; after weeks, a continued reduction cannot be measured yet blood pressure is maintained at a lower level primarily due to decreased vascular resistance. The exact mechanism whereby diuretics reduce peripheral vascular resistance is unknown.

      (1) **Agents**

         (a) **Thiazide diuretics** (e.g., **hydrochlorothiazide, chlorothiazide, metolazone**) are more effective antihypertensive agents than the loop diuretics (e.g., furosemide, bumetanide, torsemide, ethacrynic acid).

         (b) **Potassium-sparing diuretics** (e.g., **amiloride, triamterene**) act in the distal nephron and collecting tubule and are useful in the therapy of hypermineralocorticoid states.

         (c) **Spironolactone** is a competitive inhibitor of aldosterone.

      (2) **Side effects** of diuretic therapy include hypokalemia, hyperglycemia, hyperlipidemia, hyperuricemia, hypercalcemia (thiazides only), and prerenal azotemia; therefore, periodic laboratory determination of potassium and BUN levels is indicated during diuretic therapy. Uric acid should be monitored periodically in patients with a history of gout. Recent studies implicate hypokalemia caused by diuretics as an important risk factor for unexplained sudden death, a catastrophic complication that can be avoided by potassium supplementation or use of potassium-sparing diuretics.

   b. **β-Adrenergic blocking agents** reduce cardiac output and renin release. However, it is not clear that these are the primary mechanisms by which β blockers reduce blood pressure. The combination of a β blocker and a diuretic agent reduces the diastolic blood pressure to below 90 mm Hg in approximately 80% of patients with mild to moderate hypertension.

      (1) **Agents.** β blockers currently approved for the treatment of hypertension include **propranolol, nadolol, metoprolol, atenolol, timolol, betaxolol, carteolol, pindolol, acebutolol,** and **labetalol.** Labetalol is also an α-adrenergic antagonist.

      (2) **Side effects** of β blockade include bronchospasm, bradycardia, a worsening of existing congestive heart failure, occasional impotence, fatigue, depression, and nightmares.

   c. **Centrally acting adrenergic antagonists.** These agents inhibit sympathetic outflow from the CNS by stimulating central α-adrenoreceptors, reducing peripheral resistance and blood pressure.

      (1) **Agents. Methyldopa, clonidine, guanabenz,** and **guanfacine** are the commonly used centrally acting drugs.

      (2) **Side effects** of methyldopa include somnolence, orthostatic hypotension, Coombs'-positive hemolytic anemia, impotence, and hepatic injury. With clonidine, the major but rare side effect is a rebound phenomenon that produces severe hypertension after withdrawal of the drug.

   d. **Peripherally acting sympathetic nerve antagonists** cause blood pressure to fall by reducing catecholamine release from peripheral sympathetic nerves.

      (1) **Agents.** The most commonly used drugs in this category are reserpine and guanethidine. **Reserpine** depletes nerve storage vesicles of norepinephrine and, thus, limits norepinephrine secretion. **Guanethidine** directly inhibits the release of norepinephrine from adrenergic neurons.

      (2) **Side effects.** The major side effect of reserpine is depression; it also may increase the incidence of gastric ulceration. Orthostatic hypotension is the most common side effect with guanethidine therapy.

   e. **α-Adrenergic blocking agents** pharmacologically antagonize norepinephrine's stimulation of adrenergic receptors, reducing blood pressure by reducing total peripheral resistance. **Prazosin, terazosin,** and **phenoxybenzamine** are the most commonly used α blockers.

    f. Calcium channel antagonists. By modulating calcium release in smooth muscle, calcium blockers reduce smooth muscle tone, thereby acting to produce vasodilatation. The subsequent reduction in total peripheral resistance reduces blood pressure. Calcium channel blockers may also reduce cardiac output by decreasing venous return and the inotropic state.

        (1) Agents. Currently, the dihydropyridines (i.e., **nifedipine, nicardipine, isradipine, felodipine, nimodipine,** and **nitrendipine**), **diltiazem,** and **verapamil** are approved for antihypertensive therapy.

        (2) Side effects. Dihydropyridines may cause headache, flushing, and peripheral edema. Verapamil, and to a lesser extent, diltiazem have cardiodepressant actions, unlike the dihydropyridines, making their use problematic in patients with congestive heart failure. Recent studies have suggested an increased risk of coronary events in patients receiving calcium channel blockers, but it is premature to stop using these valuable agents, particularly in patients with underlying coronary artery disease and hypertension.

    g. Direct vasodilators dilate arteries and arterioles, reducing blood pressure by reducing total peripheral resistance. They are particularly effective when used with a β blocker that inhibits the reflex tachycardia caused by direct vasodilation.

        (1) Agents. Hydralazine and **minoxidil** are the most commonly used direct vasodilators.

        (2) Side effects. The major side effects of hydralazine are headache and a lupus-like syndrome; the latter is reversed when the drug is discontinued. The major side effects of minoxidil are orthostatic hypotension and facial hirsutism.

    h. ACE inhibitors block the conversion of angiotensin I to angiotensin II (a vasoconstrictor) and, thus, reduce total peripheral resistance. In addition, aldosterone production is decreased, reducing the retention of sodium and water.

        (1) Agents include **captopril, enalapril, fosinopril, benazepril, quinapril, ramipril,** and **lisinopril.**

        (2) Side effects. The major side effects with captopril are rashes, leukopenia and, cough, which typically disappears with discontinuation of the drug. Hyperkalemia may occasionally occur as a result of reduced aldosterone secretion. Because angiotensin II serves to maintain the GFR during states of reduced renal blood flow (by maintaining a high vascular resistance in the post-glomerular vessels), the use of ACE inhibitors in patients with compromised renal blood flow may lead to a form of acute renal failure. Reduction in dose or discontinuation of drug is usually sufficient to reverse the fall in GFR.

    i. Angiotensin II-receptor antagonists. This newly introduced class of drugs promises to provide the benefits of blockade of the angiotensin system without some of the annoying side effects, particularly cough. The place of these agents in the clinician's approach to the treatment of hypertension remains to be determined.

D. Therapeutic strategies

    1. First-line therapy. Various agents are now considered appropriate for initial antihypertensive therapy. While many physicians still begin therapy with a diuretic, β blockers, ACE inhibitors, or calcium channel blockers are also appropriate initial drugs. At best, only 75% of patients will have an optimal control of blood pressure with monotherapy.

    2. Second-line therapy

        a. Rather than complicating therapy by adding several drugs in a stepwise fashion, many physicians sequentially try various agents until one agent emerges as effective monotherapy.

        b. Alternatively, submaximal doses of two or three antihypertensive agents added in a stepwise fashion have been advocated as a successful approach. The addition of 12.5 or 25 mg of hydrochlorothiazide will potentiate the action of a number of antihypertensive agents, particularly the ACE inhibitors and the angiotensin II-receptor antagonists. If the blood pressure is still uncontrolled, the use of multiple drug regimens or the addition of direct vasodilators is indicated.

V. **HYPERTENSIVE CRISIS** is defined as severe hypertension characterized by a diastolic blood pressure of greater than 140 mm Hg. Blood pressure elevation to this degree can cause vascular damage, encephalopathy, retinal hemorrhages, renal damage, and death.

A. **Diagnosis.** A diastolic blood pressure of greater than 140 mm Hg, funduscopic findings of papilledema, changes in neurologic and mental status, and an abnormal renal sediment are the hallmarks of hypertensive crisis.

B. **Therapy.** Immediate lowering of the blood pressure is indicated.

1. Infusion of **sodium nitroprusside** is an effective treatment for hypertensive crisis.
   a. The patient's blood pressure should be monitored constantly so that the dose can be adjusted to maintain the blood pressure within the desired range . An excessive reduction in blood pressure can be reversed rapidly by reducing the dose of the infusion.
   b. Long-term administration of high-dose nitroprusside (7 μg /kg/min) can lead to cyanide intoxication. The likelihood of this complication increases in patients with renal dysfunction.

2. **Labetalol** is effective in treating this condition.

3. **Trimethaphan,** a ganglionic blocking agent, is useful in the treatment of hypertensive crisis.

DIRECTIONS: Each of the numbered items or incomplete statements in this section is followed by answers or by completions of the statement. Select the ONE lettered answer or completion that is BEST in each case.

1. A renal biopsy to determine the nature of glomerular disease in a patient with heavy proteinuria is absolutely contraindicated if the patient

(A) has a diastolic blood pressure of 120 mm Hg
(B) has a serum creatinine level of 2.5 mg/dl (normal = 0.8–1.4 mg/dl)
(C) is 65 years of age or older
(D) has nephrotic syndrome with no evidence of renal tubular casts
(E) has undergone a previous renal biopsy

2. A 71-year-old man is seen in the surgical intensive care unit for acute renal failure. The patient had an operation for removal of gallstones, after which he had a persistent drainage from his biliary catheter associated with spiking fevers to 102°F. The patient has been taking gentamicin (70 mg every 8 hours) and cephalothin (2 g four times a day) for the past 10 days. Over the last 4 days the serum creatinine level has increased at a rate of 1 mg/dl/day, but his urine output of 1.5 L/day has not diminished. He has had no history of hypotension at any time during this hospitalization. Physical examination shows normal blood pressure and vital signs. Results of laboratory studies show a creatinine level of 7.1 mg/dl, and renal ultrasonography reveals no evidence of obstruction. The most likely cause of this patient's acute renal failure is

(A) sepsis
(B) trauma to the ureter during surgery
(C) gentamicin nephrotoxicity
(D) acute glomerulonephritis
(E) cephalothin-induced acute renal failure

3. A 65-year-old man with long-standing hypertension well controlled with diuretics experiences two episodes of acute pulmonary edema that are successfully treated in the hospital. In the hospital, he is found to have a blood pressure of 210/120 mm Hg, despite continued use of his antihypertensive medication. A complete cardiac workup does not reveal any explanation for the pulmonary edema. His blood pressure is now 180/105 mm Hg despite the addition of a calcium channel blocker and a vasodilator to his antihypertensive regimen. Laboratory evaluation, including an evaluation for pheochromocytoma, is negative. What is the most likely cause of this patient's clinical condition?

(A) Progression of essential hypertension
(B) Renal artery stenosis
(C) Adrenal adenoma
(D) New-onset glomerulonephritis
(E) Renal vasculitis

4. A 39-year-old man comes to the emergency room experiencing labored breathing and mental obtundation. The physical examination is unremarkable. His laboratory studies show the following: serum sodium = 144 mEq/L, serum potassium = 3.7 mEq/L, serum chloride = 97 mEq/L, plasma bicarbonate concentration $[HCO_3^-]$ = 16 mEq/L, arterial pH = 7.38 and P_{CO_2} = 21 mEq/L. The acid–base disturbance is

(A) respiratory alkalosis
(B) metabolic acidosis
(C) metabolic acidosis and respiratory alkalosis
(D) metabolic acidosis and metabolic alkalosis

5. A 69-year-old woman has moderately severe renal failure: Tests were obtained during her most recent follow-up visit. Laboratory studies showed the following: serum sodium = 142 mEq/L, serum potassium = 5.1 mEq/L, serum chloride = 109 mEq/L, plasma bicarbonate concentration $[HCO_3^-]$ = 15 mEq/L, and creatinine = 4.2 mg/dl. The origin of metabolic acidosis in this patient is most likely due to

(A) bicarbonaturia
(B) impaired excretion of titratable acids
(C) decreased filtration of hydrogen ions (H^+)
(D) impaired ammonia excretion
(E) hypoaldosteronism

6. A 45-year-old man enters the hospital because of an episode of acute flank pain and red urine. The patient has been in good health until this episode, which began at night and awakened him. In the emergency room, he is found to have a normal physical examination, but also to have hematuria, with essentially normal laboratory studies. Radiography of the abdomen reveals a stone in the right kidney. An intravenous urogram shows the stone to be nonobstructing at that time. Further laboratory studies demonstrate normal serum calcium and phosphate, and a subsequent urine culture is negative. Which type of kidney stone is most likely to have caused this patient's condition?

(A) Calcium oxalate stone
(B) Uric acid stone
(C) Xanthine stone
(D) Struvite stone
(E) Cystine stone

7. A 70-year-old patient with long-standing hypertension develops, over a 6-month period, more severe hypertension—in spite of antihypertensive medication, his blood pressure has risen from 140/90 to 175/105 mm Hg. In addition, the patient developed an episode of "flash" pulmonary edema that led to his hospitalization for 1 week. He continued to take his antihypertensive medication faithfully but has developed some intermittent claudication in his left leg. He has a long history of smoking but has had no other medical problems. What is the most likely cause of this clinical disorder?

(A) Renal artery stenosis
(B) Pheochromocytoma
(C) Hyperaldosteronism
(D) Primary worsening of hypertension

8. A 58-year-old woman is admitted to the hospital for evaluation of polyuria. A water deprivation test is performed for 14 hours under strict medical observation.

Baseline	
Serum sodium	132 meq/L
Plasma osmolality	275 mOsm/kg
Urine osmolality	145 mOsm/kg

45 Minutes Following Vasopressin	
Serum sodium	130 mEq/L
Plasma osmolality	271 mOsm/kg
Urine osmolality	489 mOsm/kg

The most likely diagnosis is

(A) central diabetes insipidus
(B) nephrogenic diabetes insipidus
(C) electrolyte osmotic diuresis
(D) nonelectrolyte osmotic diuresis
(E) psychogenic polydipsia

9. A 78-year-old man enters the hospital because of abnormalities of urination. Today the patient is passing large amounts of urine; however, some days he passes no urine at all. On physical examination now, the patient has a blood pressure of 180/90 mm Hg but the rest of the physical examination is normal. Laboratory studies reveal a blood urea nitrogen (BUN) level of 120 mg/dl and a serum creatinine level of 4.2 mg/dl. Urinalysis reveals a specific gravity of 1.010; urine that is negative for protein, glucose, ketone bodies, and blood; and an occasional white blood cell per high-power field on microscopic examination. The most likely etiology of this patient's renal insufficiency is

(A) obstructive uropathy
(B) acute glomerulonephritis
(C) acute interstitial nephritis
(D) acute tubular necrosis (ATN)
(E) chronic renal failure of unspecified nature

10. A 47-year-old man enters the hospital with nephrotic syndrome. He reports that he initially experienced edema of his feet occurring in the morning, but this condition rapidly progressed until the edema extended to his midcalves and lasted throughout the day. He has been in good health all of his life and has not seen a physician in the last 5 years. His only complaints relate to the edema. Upon physical examination, his blood pressure is 155/100 mm Hg, his pulse is 88 bpm, his respiratory rate is 15, and his temperature is 98.6°F. Examination of the heart and lungs reveals no evidence of congestive heart failure. Examination of the abdomen reveals mild ascites with normal hepatic size. Examination of the extremities reveals +4 edema to the midcalf. Laboratory studies show a blood urea nitrogen (BUN) of 10 mg/dl and creatinine of 1.0 mg/dl. The rest of the laboratory studies are unrevealing. Urinalysis reveals 4+ protein and one red blood cell per high-power field. No red cell casts or other cellular elements are seen on urinalysis. The 24-hour urine contains 9.6 g of protein. Which disease is most likely to account for this patient's clinical condition?

(A) Membranous nephropathy
(B) Poststreptococcal glomerulonephritis
(C) Lupus nephritis
(D) Amyloidosis
(E) Diabetes mellitus

11. A 31-year-old man enters the hospital with acute onset of edema and hematuria. He had been well until 3 weeks before, when he had a sore throat and was treated with oral penicillin. Since that time he has felt generally in good health but has noted the onset of dark, tea-colored urine and swelling of his legs. He denies any other symptoms, including rash, joint pain, chest pain, and the use of any other medication but the penicillin. On physical examination, his blood pressure is 160/110 mm Hg, his pulse is 85 bpm, his respiratory rate is 15, and his temperature is 98.6°F. Findings on physical examination include only marked peripheral edema extending to midleg. Laboratory studies reveal a blood urea nitrogen (BUN) of 20 mg/dl, creatinine of 1.3 mg/dl, and normal electrolytes. The serum complement level, including CH_{50} and C_4, is reduced by 50%. The anti-deoxyribonuclease B antibody is increased, as is the antistreptolysin O titer. Anti-glomerular basement membrane (anti-GBM) antibody assay and antineutrophilic cytoplasmic antibody (ANCA) levels are within normal limits. Urinalysis reveals 4+ protein, 4+ blood, and no glucose. Microscopic examination reveals three to four red blood cell casts per high-power field as well as many red blood cells and white blood cells. No bacteria are visible. The most likely etiology of this patient's acute renal syndrome is

(A) poststreptococcal glomerulonephritis
(B) systemic lupus erythematosus (SLE)
(C) Goodpasture's syndrome
(D) immunoglobulin A (IgA) nephropathy
(E) allergic reaction to penicillin

12. A 64-year-old man enters the hospital because of renal insufficiency. The patient has been in good health until 6 months previously, when he developed persistent back pain. At that time, he was found to be severely anemic and his blood urea nitrogen (BUN) and creatinine levels were elevated to 42 and 4.6 mg/dl, respectively.

He now enters for further evaluation. He denies the use of any medications and any past history of renal injury. He denies any difficulty in voiding. He does complain of persistent weakness and easy fatigability, and his back pain has become more severe over the last 2 weeks. On physical examination, his blood pressure is 120/80 mm Hg, his pulse is 70 bpm, his respiratory rate is 15, and his temperature is 98.6°F. Major physical findings include severe pallor as well as clear evidence of muscle wasting. On urinalysis, there is 1+ protein on dipstick testing and 4+ on sulfosalicylic acid testing. Microscopic examination of the urine reveals an occasional broad and an occasional granular cast. Laboratory studies reveal the following: BUN = 61 mg/dl, creatinine = 5.1 mg/dl, serum sodium = 141 mEq/L, serum potassium = 5.6 mEq/L, serum chloride = 101 mEq/L, CO_2 = 14 mEq/L, serum calcium = 11.7 mg/dl, and serum phosphorus = 6.0 mg/dl. The most likely etiology of this patient's condition is

(A) renovascular disease
(B) thrombotic renal disease
(C) multiple myeloma
(D) systemic lupus erythematosus (SLE)

13. A 21-year-old woman enters the hospital because of severe anemia and acute renal failure. She had delivered a normal, full-term infant 3 weeks prior to admission and, following delivery, had felt extremely weak and fatigued. She sees her physician, who notes that she is extremely pale and performs a complete blood count (CBC), which reveals severe anemia as well as thrombocytopenia. Further laboratory screening reveals elevated blood urea nitrogen (BUN) and creatinine, and she is referred for admission. She denies any medication usage postpartum and any previous medical problems similar to this one. Her laboratory studies were normal at the time of her discharge from the hospital following delivery. On physical examination she has normal vital signs, and the only physical findings aside from her pallor are petechiae on her skin and multiple ecchymoses on her lower extremities. Laboratory studies reveal a hemoglobin of 6.3 mg/dl, a hematocrit of 18%, a platelet count of 23,000/μl, BUN of 94 mg/dl, and creatinine of 9.1 mg/dl. The serum antinuclear antibody (ANCA) level is normal, as are serum antineutrophilic cytoplasmic antibody (ACA) levels. A peripheral blood smear reveals multiple schistocytes. Urinalysis reveals many red blood cell casts. The most likely diagnosis is

(A) hemolytic–uremic syndrome
(B) Goodpasture's syndrome
(C) systemic lupus erythematosus (SLE)
(D) idiopathic thrombocytopenic purpura
(E) a drug reaction

14. A 69-year-old woman complains of easy fatigability, weight loss, and dizziness. Her medical history includes a remote history of tuberculosis. Physical examination reveals a blood pressure of 100/62 mm Hg and increased skin pigmentation. Laboratory studies reveal the following: serum sodium = 129 mEq/L, serum potassium = 6.1 mEq/L, serum chloride = 100 mEql/L, plasma bicarbonate concentration [HCO_3^-] = 21 mEq/L, glucose = 88 mg/dl, and blood urea nitrogen (BUN) = 30 mg/dl. The diagnosis that best fits these findings is

(A) adrenal insufficiency
(B) chronic renal failure
(C) adrenocorticotropic hormone (ACTH)–secreting tumor
(D) distal (type I) renal tubular acidosis

15. A 27-year-old man is referred for evaluation of hematuria. The patient has noted painless gross hematuria two to three times per year for the last 6 years, which has always remitted spontaneously within 1–2 days. On this occasion, bright-red blood has appeared in his urine for the past 8 days. He denies any trauma to his kidneys or any other recent illnesses. Although he has a younger brother with sickle cell anemia, the patient has been free from any symptoms of this abnormality, and there is no other known family history or evidence of any other renal disease, including kidney stones and infection. Urinalysis reveals red-to-pink urine, with numerous red blood cells per high-power field, and no proteinuria on orthotoluidine dipstick test. At this point, the most likely diagnosis is

(A) nephrolithiasis
(B) carcinoma of the kidney
(C) renal vein thrombosis
(D) prostatitis
(E) sickle cell trait

16. A 28-year-old architect is referred for evaluation of the cause of nephrolithiasis. The patient has had six kidney stones over the last 5 years, with the most recent one requiring surgical removal. He denies any history of urinary tract infections, but his father and paternal grandfather both had kidney stones. On physical examination, he is found to be normotensive; all other findings are normal. Laboratory studies reveal normal serum chemistries, including calcium, phosphorus, and magnesium determinations. Urinary determinations of calcium phosphate, uric acid, and protein also are normal. Urinalysis reveals a urine pH of 5 and occasional hexagonal crystals. What is the most likely etiology of this patient's nephrolithiasis?

(A) Calcium oxalate stones
(B) Uric acid stones
(C) Cystine stones
(D) Calcium phosphate stones
(E) Magnesium-ammonium-calcium-phosphate (struvite) stones

17. A 21-year-old man enters the hospital complaining that he has been passing dark reddish urine. The patient has recently recovered from a football-related knee injury that he incurred 3 months before, and the day before entering the hospital he engaged in vigorous physical activity for the first time since his knee injury. This morning he awoke with sore, painful muscles and the aforementioned change in the character of his urine. Physical examination of the patient is essentially normal except for the painful muscles. Findings on urinalysis include red–brown color, pH of 5.0, specific gravity of 1.02, 3 + dipstick test for blood, and no evidence of glucose, ketones, or bilirubin. Microscopic examination of the urine reveals occasional amorphous debris and three or four granular casts but no red blood cells. The most likely explanation for this urinalysis is

(A) myoglobinuria
(B) hemolyzed blood in the urine
(C) ingestion of foodstuffs containing red dye
(D) urinary tract infection
(E) renal trauma

18. A 37-year-old man enters the hospital with a history of recent onset of hemoptysis and acute renal failure. He had been in good health until 6 weeks ago when he noted the onset of a cough which, over the ensuing 3 days, produced streaky, blood-tinged sputum. His local physician ordered laboratory studies which revealed a serum creatinine of 1.2 mg/dl. A chest x-ray at that time revealed bilateral fluffy infiltrates. The patient was treated with antibiotics and followed over the next 3 weeks; during that time, the lung picture worsened and the serum creatinine rose to 2.5 mg/dl.

Now, the man appears ill and in moderate distress. His blood pressure is 120/80 mm Hg, his pulse is 110 bpm, his respiratory rate is 22, and his temperature is 99°F. Examination of the chest shows bilateral rales and a few scattered wheezes. Examination of the heart reveals tachycardia but is otherwise normal. Laboratory examination shows a blood urea nitrogen (BUN) of 65 mg/dl, a creatinine of 4.3 mg/dl, and electrolytes within normal limits. The hemoglobin level is 8.3 mg/dl, and the hematocrit is 28%. A chest x-ray reveals bilateral fluffy alveolar infiltrates. Examination of the sputum reveals blood. Urinalysis reveals many red blood cell casts. Serum antineutrophilic cytoplasmic antibody (ANCA) levels are negative, as are serum complement levels. The serum antiglomerular basement membrane (anti-GBM) antibody titer is elevated to 1:64. The most likely etiology of this disorder is

(A) Wegener's granulomatosis
(B) Goodpasture's syndrome
(C) systemic lupus erythematosus (SLE)
(D) microscopic polyarteritis nodosa
(E) idiopathic crescentic glomerulonephritis

19. A 60-year-old man enters the hospital complaining of nausea, weakness, and confusion of 1 week's duration. He has a long-standing history of hypertension and congestive heart failure that has been treated with increasing amounts of diuretics and digoxin without apparent benefit. Physical examination shows a blood pressure of 145/90 mm Hg (without orthostatic changes), jugular venous distention, bilateral basilar rales, and + 2 bilateral ankle edema. Laboratory studies show the following: serum sodium = 120 mEq/L, blood urea nitrogen (BUN) = 93 mg/dl, glucose = 135 mg/dl, plasma osmolality = 252 mOsm/kg, and urine osmolality = 690 mOsm/kg. Treatment of hyponatremia in this patient involves

(A) 3% sodium chloride infusion
(B) 0.9% sodium chloride infusion
(C) 50 mg hydrochlorothiazide daily
(D) salt and water restriction
(E) demeclocycline

DIRECTIONS: The set of matching questions in this section consists of a list of four to twenty-six lettered options (some of which may be in figures) followed by several numbered items. For each numbered item, select the ONE lettered option that is most closely associated with it. To avoid spending too much time on matching sets with large numbers of options, it is generally advisable to begin each set by reading the list of options. Then, for each item in the set, try to generate the correct answer and locate it in the option list, rather than evaluating each option individually. Each lettered option may be selected once, more than once, or not at all.

Questions 20–23
(A) Nodular glomerulosclerosis
(B) Positive fluorescent antinuclear antibody (ANA)
(C) Glomerular capillary endotheliosis
(D) Necrotizing granulomatous vasculitis
(E) Positive Congo red staining with amyloid

For each renal disorder listed, select the clinical feature with which it is most closely associated.

20. Lupus nephritis

21. Diabetic nephropathy

22. Toxemia of pregnancy

23. Wegener's granulomatosis

ANSWERS AND EXPLANATIONS

1. The answer is A [Part I: I D 2]. Hypertension is an absolute contraindication to performing a renal biopsy because the incidence of subclinical bleeding at the site is high (75%). In a hypertensive patient, this bleeding may lead to a major, life-threatening hemorrhage. Mild renal insufficiency (as evidenced by a small decrease in creatinine clearance), nephrotic syndrome without urinary casts, and moderately advanced age are not contraindications to performing a renal biopsy. Multiple renal biopsies may be performed in the same patient. A previous renal biopsy is not a contraindication for subsequent biopsies.

2. The answer is C [Table 6-1]. Approximately 5%–10% of patients treated with gentamicin develop a nonoliguric form of acute renal failure. Although the patient has received normal doses of gentamicin, its accumulation in the kidney has produced a late form of acute renal failure; the serum creatinine level then rises while an inappropriately high dosage is maintained. This rise exacerbates the renal insufficiency and prolongs the course of acute renal failure. The nonoliguric nature of this patient's clinical condition also is a typical finding in gentamicin nephrotoxicity. Although the patient could have obstructive uropathy, the negative results of ultrasonography strongly indicate otherwise. Cephalothin can produce an acute interstitial nephritis, but the patient's clinical course is much more compatible with the more common drug-induced disease of gentamicin nephrotoxicity. Acute glomerulonephritis usually is associated with hypertension and an active urinary sediment containing casts, protein, and red blood cells.

3. The answer is B [Part III: III A]. Hypertension that suddenly worsens in an older individual is a classic manifestation of the onset of atherosclerotic renal artery stenosis. These patients also typically manifest so-called "flash pulmonary edema" as a result of the acute elevations in sympathetic tone and in cardiac afterload that seem to characterize this condition. The decision to intervene is a difficult

one because surgery may be risky in patients with diffuse vascular disease. Newer treatments, such as angioplasty or stent placement, may improve the outcome of intervention but have not been fully studied. Essential hypertension could enter into a malignant phase but this is very uncommon in older patients who are under medical supervision. Adrenal adenoma is almost always associated with hypokalemia. Acute glomerulonephritis or renal vasculitis that produces hypertension tends to produce acute decrements in renal function. In this case, laboratory studies are reported to be normal, suggesting that these etiologies are not relevant in this case.

4. The answer is C [Part II: IV C, D]. Although the arterial pH is within the normal range, the patient is suffering from two separate acid–base disturbances (metabolic acidosis and respiratory alkalosis) which, together, tend to offset their effects on pH. The low P_{CO_2} in this case is much lower than would be expected if the patient had only respiratory compensation. Thus, if the patient has a single acid–base disturbance, namely metabolic acidosis, then the expected P_{CO_2} is calculated using Winters' formula:

$$\text{Expected } P_{CO_2} = 1.5 \times [HCO_3^-] + 8 \pm 2$$
$$= 1.5 \times 16 + 8 \pm 2$$
$$= 32 \pm 2$$

The measured P_{CO_2} of less than 32 indicates that the patient also has a primary respiratory disturbance, namely respiratory alkalosis.

5. The answer is D [Part II: IV D]. The most important factor that leads to metabolic acidosis in renal failure is the impaired synthesis and excretion of ammonia. This combination leads to impaired titration of hydrogen (H^+) ions that are secreted in the distal nephron. The net result is decreased net acid secretion.

6. The answer is A [Part I: VII A; Table 6-4]. The patient most likely has idiopathic calcium oxalate stones. This conclusion is based on the fact that it is the most common form of kidney stone, the stone is radiopaque, and many of the findings suggest that the other answers are wrong. First, uric acid stones are radiolucent, so a stone would not have been seen on the radiographic flat plate prior to the intravenous urogram. Second, xanthine stones are extremely rare and are also radiolucent. Third, struvite stones are found only in the setting of a urinary tract infection. The absence of a positive urine culture strongly suggests that struvite stones are not present. Fourth, while cystine stones could present in this fashion even though the patient is middle-aged, cystine stones typically present much earlier and represent less than 1% of the stones analyzed in large studies. Thus, on a purely statistical basis, the patient is unlikely to have cystine stones. However, all patients with kidney stone formation who have not had their stone crystallography analyzed should have a 24-hour cystine determination to be certain that cystinuria is not present.

7. The answer is A [Part III: III A]. Renal artery stenosis is a common complication in patients with long-standing hypertension and peripheral vascular disease. As many as 80% of patients with this combination of disorders have renal artery stenosis. It is typically atherosclerotic in nature and involves the ostia of the renal arteries. "Flash" pulmonary edema commonly accompanies this condition and probably represents acute changes in hemodynamic status induced by an increased sensitivity to the adrenergic nervous system. Other features of this disorder are worsening of hypertension as well as development of azotemia. This constellation of findings often necessitates intervention, with either percutaneous transluminal angioplasty (PCTA) or surgery.

8. The answer is E [Part II: I C 2 b (1), (2), (a), (b)]. Baseline urine osmolality is quite low, indicating a water diuresis and not an osmotic diuresis. To determine whether the patient has central versus nephrogenic diabetes insipidus (or alternatively, psychogenic polydipsia) requires testing with antidiuretic hormone (ADH). The substantial increase in urine osmolality after administration of vasopressin rules out nephrogenic diabetes insipidus. It is more likely that this patient has psychogenic polydipsia rather than central diabetes insipidus because baseline serum sodium is on the low side. This factor suggests that loss of water in the urine is actually caused by excess water intake, which would tend to decrease serum sodium concentration. In central diabetes insipidus, obligate urinary water losses would tend to raise serum sodium concentration above normal.

9. The answer is A [Part I: VIII A, C]. The incidence of prostatism in elderly men is so great that it must be considered the primary cause of renal insufficiency until proven otherwise. This patient's history is classic in that he had 1 or 2 days on which he seemed to pass no urine followed by days of high urine flow, a pattern that is caused by the gradual accumulation of large amounts of urine in the collecting system under pressure, which eventually may overcome some degree of obstruction. The high pressure is transmitted back to the kidney and results in renal insufficiency. Acute glomerulonephritis and acute interstitial nephritis are ruled out by the normal results of urinalysis. The possibility of acute tubular necrosis (ATN) should be considered, but no information in the history suggests recent surgery or nephrotoxic drug intake that would have produced ATN. The best way to screen for obstructive uropathy is renal ultrasonography, which would demonstrate dilated upper tract calyces.

10. The answer is A [Part I: X C; XII B 4]. This patient most likely has membranous nephropathy. The most common cause of nephrotic syndrome in patients of this age-group, it is characterized by an absence of evidence for a high degree of glomerular inflammation. Thus, the urinalysis, which reveals little in the way of cellular elements and heavy proteinuria, supports this diagnosis. Poststreptococcal glomerulonephritis and lupus glomerulonephritis are much more likely to demonstrate active urinary sediments with red cells and red cell casts. In addition, these conditions are often associated with systemic manifestations of the underlying disease; none are present in this patient. Amyloidosis could give a clinical picture similar to that described, but the vast majority of patients with systemic amyloidosis have systemic signs such as peripheral neuropathy, autonomic neuropathy, or cardiac disease at the time that they develop nephrotic syndrome. Diabetic nephropathy is unlikely because of the absence of history. Failure to find abnormal retinal findings on ophthalmoscopic examination would also make diabetic nephropathy an unlikely diagnosis.

11. The answer is A [Part I: X I]. The most likely etiology of this patient's acute renal syndrome is poststreptococcal glomerulonephritis. The finding of a reduced serum complement and elevated antistreptolysin O titer in the clinical setting of a streptococcal infection strongly suggests this cause. While systemic lupus erythematosus (SLE) may produce some aspects of the clinical picture, particularly the nephritic renal syndrome, the absence of other systemic signs of SLE makes this condition highly unlikely. However, an antinuclear antibody assay should be performed to fully exclude this diagnosis. Goodpasture's syndrome is unlikely in the absence of a history of pulmonary abnormalities or hemoptysis. Immunoglobulin A (IgA) nephropathy can present as a severe, acute nephritic picture but should not produce the other serologic abnormalities seen in this patient. A reaction to penicillin can result in an acute renal injury; however, like IgA nephropathy, it is not associated with the complement and antistreptococcal antibody titers that are seen. Furthermore, nephrotic syndrome would be an uncommon consequence of penicillin reaction, which much more typically presents as an acute interstitial injury to the kidney, with renal insufficiency, eosinophils and other white cell elements in the urine, and minimal proteinuria.

12. The answer is C [Part I: X P]. Multiple myeloma is the most likely etiology. The combination of hypercalcemia and acute renal failure raises the possibility of multiple myeloma as the bone breakdown secondary to tumor involvement releases large amounts of calcium to the extracellular fluid and hypercalcemia ensues. The renal failure in myeloma is primarily related to hypercalcemia combined with proteinaceous cast formation within the renal tubules, producing a form of intratubular obstruction as well as a tubular inflammatory lesion. The major diagnostic clue is the finding of a dipstick mildly positive urine with a sulfosalicylic acid strongly positive urine. Dipstick testing does not detect the negatively charged light-chain proteins, only the albumin. The sulfosalicylic acid test detects all forms of proteins. Renovascular lesions and thrombotic renal disease could present with this picture, although they should not be associated with hypercalcemia and severe back pain, and findings upon examination of the urine would not include proteins. Systemic lupus erythematosus (SLE) can, of course, be associated with severe anemia and joint manifestations, but hypercalcemia is not part of the picture.

13. The answer is A [Part I: XIV D 1 b]. The most likely cause of this condition is hemolytic–uremic syndrome. This syndrome is associated with platelet consumption as well as acute renal insufficiency. This condition may occur postpartum and can be diagnosed only by examining the entire clinical picture. Systemic lupus erythematosus (SLE) can present with thrombocytopenia and acute renal failure, but the negative antinuclear antibody (ANA) level in the absence of other systemic manifestations makes this answer unlikely. The finding of schistocytes on the peripheral smear also strongly supports the diagnosis of the microangiopathic picture, which explains to a greater extent the anemia seen. The only drug-associated cause of renal insufficiency which presents with severe thrombocytopenia of this degree as well as severe microangiopathic hemolytic anemia is cyclosporine or penicillamine treatment. Idiopathic thrombocytopenic purpura is not associated with concurrent renal disease. The correct therapy for this condition would be to perform plasma exchange, plasma infusions, or both, as the best way of limiting the injury associated with hemolytic–uremic syndrome. The etiology of this syndrome remains unclear, although it can be associated with bacterial infections, particularly when it occurs in epidemic form in children.

14. The answer is A [Part II: I B]. The findings of low blood pressure, increased skin pigmentation, hyperkalemia, and hyponatremia all point to the likely diagnosis of adrenal insufficiency. Adrenocorticotropic hormone (ACTH)–secreting tumors, while they may produce skin pigmentations, are usually associated with hypertension and hypokalemic alkalosis due to excess mineralocorticoid secretion. Hyperkalemia due to renal failure is seen when the glomerular filtration rate (GFR) is below 10–15 ml/min. The patient's blood urea nitrogen (BUN) of 30 mg/dl suggests only impaired renal function. Distal (type I) renal tubular acidosis is characterized by hypokalemia (although occasional cases of hyperkalemia have been described).

15. The answer is E [Part I: Table 6-3; XIV F2 b]. Sickle cell trait, nephrolithiasis, carcinoma of the kidney, renal vein thrombosis, and prostatitis all may be associated with hematuria. The finding of gross hematuria in a young man with a family history of sickle cell anemia, however, strongly suggests that, in the absence of other stigmata of sickle cell disease, he suffers from sickle cell trait. This abnormality commonly is associated with hematuria and is caused by sickling of red blood cells in the vessels on the surface of the renal pelvis and papilla, leading to small areas of infarction and bleeding. Renal tumor can produce bleeding, but it is rarely so persistent in the absence of other symptoms. Renal vein thrombosis can produce hematuria but usually in the setting of severe pain and proteinuria. Nephrolithiasis also may produce relatively silent hematuria if the stone has been present for a long period of time, but pain typically is associated with this condition. Urinary tract infection also can be associated with hematuria, but symptoms of infection (e.g., dysuria and fever) should be present.

16. The answer is C [Part I: Table 6-4]. The patient's clinical presentation is typical of any patient with kidney stone disease. In more than 90% of patients, nephrolithiasis is caused by calcium oxalate stone formation. In 50% of those individuals, hypercalciuria is present. In the absence of hypercalciuria and with the finding of hexagonal crystals in the urine, the physician must be highly suspicious that this patient has cystinuria. A urinalysis revealing cystine crystals is seen in approximately 40%–50% of patients; however, negative urinalysis should not deter the physician from measuring a 24-hour urinary cystine excretion. An initial presentation of cystinuria at age 25 or 30 is not unusual, but in some cases, patients are in their 70s and 80s before they present with cystinuria. The condition is an autosomal dominant trait, but a variety of phenotypic forms may be seen.

Treatment of cystine stones includes maintaining high urine flow rates (i.e., up to 4–5 L/day) and urine alkalinization if a urine pH value over 7.5 can be achieved by sodium bicarbonate administration. Cystine solubility is approximately 100 mg/L; therefore, if an individual excretes between 300 and 400 mg/24 hr, high fluid intake may prevent further stone formation. If, however, excretion is greater than 700 or 800 mg/24 hr, patients often may require D-penicillamine, a compound that forms mixed disulfides with cystine and renders cystine much more soluble in the urine.

If the patient in question has not had cystine demonstrated in his urine, the next critical test would have been an analysis of the kidney stone.

17. The answer is A [Part I: I A 1 b, 2 a, f; II C 3 a (5).] The finding of dark reddish urine

suggests a number of underlying conditions. However, the absence of red blood cells on microscopic examination of the urine combined with the positive dipstick test for blood strongly suggest the possibility of myoglobinuria. Myoglobin is a pigment that is detected by the orthotoluidine reagent on the dipstick. Although hemolyzed blood could be present in the urine, a few red blood cells should be noted, whereas none are seen in this patient's urine. Although foodstuffs do contain dyes that may color the urine, these dyes do not produce positive dipstick tests for blood. This clinical picture is most consistent with myoglobinuria caused by sudden, extreme physical exertion by an individual who is not well-conditioned. Such activity leads to muscle cell breakdown and the release of myoglobin into the circulation, with its ultimate filtration by the kidney and appearance in the urine.

18. The answer is B [Part I: X G]. The most likely etiology of this disorder is Goodpasture's syndrome. Wegener's granulomatosis can present with a pulmonary bleeding syndrome associated with acute glomerulonephritis, as seen in this patient and as evidenced by the hemoptysis as well as by the active urinary sediment. However, the negative antineutrophilic cytoplasmic antibody (ANCA) level and the absence of a destructive upper airway lesion on physical examination argue against Wegener's granulomatosis, and the finding of positive anti-glomerular basement membrane (anti-GBM) antibodies strongly points to Goodpasture's syndrome. Systemic lupus erythematosus (SLE) and microscopic vasculitis can present with pulmonary hemorrhage and renal insufficiency but neither is associated with the serologies seen in this patient. Idiopathic crescentic glomerulonephritis describes an entity similar to that seen in this patient, but the finding of positive serum anti-GBM antibody titers eliminates glomerulonephritis as an "idiopathic" entity.

19. The answer is D [Part II: I B 5]. Water restriction should help produce a negative water balance. Salt restriction is also needed because the patient has excess total sodium burden; this change should also optimize the response to diuretics. Hyponatremia in the setting of an expanded extracellular volume (e.g., congestive heart failure) develops because of diminished renal ability to excrete water in the face of continuing water ingestion. The renal diluting defect is the result of impaired delivery of tubular fluid to distal diluting nephron segments and is precipitated by enhanced proximal tubular reabsorption. The latter is caused by decreased renal perfusion as a result of impaired cardiac output. A decrease in effective arterial volume also stimulates antidiuretic hormone (ADH) release, which further impairs urinary dilution. Ideally, treatment should be directed at improving cardiac function. Digoxin and diuretics have been administered without significant benefit. The patient certainly cannot tolerate any saline infusions because this treatment would aggravate his congestive symptoms. Hydrochlorothiazide added to his regimen may not be potent enough to improve the refractory congestive symptoms; besides, hydrochlorothiazide itself impairs urinary dilution and may aggravate the hyponatremia. Demeclocycline for the treatment of hyponatremia is reserved for the chronic management of the syndrome of inappropriate antidiuretic hormone (ADH) (SIADH). Because of its potential nephrotoxicity, demeclocycline is contraindicated in all states of azotemia, as in this case.

20–23. The answers are: 20-B [Part I: X M 1 a (2)], **21-A** [Part I: X L 3], **22-C** [Part I: XV E 1, 2] **23-D** [Part I: X N 3]. The glomerular abnormalities of systemic lupus erythematosus (SLE) form a disease spectrum, with four associated major lesions: focal proliferative, diffuse proliferative, membranous, and mesangial forms of lupus nephritis. Serologic studies of the four lesions determine differing levels of anti-DNA antibodies and complement components, but common to all four are immunofluorescent findings for antinuclear antibody (ANA).

All lesions in the kidneys of individuals with diabetes mellitus are grouped under the term diabetic nephropathy. The foremost clinical feature of diabetic glomerular disease is an overt proteinuria, which develops after a prolonged course of diabetes mellitus. Although diffuse glomerulosclerosis is the most common lesion (found in 90% of all diabetic individuals) and is responsible for the proteinuria, the nephrosis, and the renal failure, it is neither specific nor diagnostic of diabetes. In contrast, the other major renal lesion associated with diabetes, nodular glomerulosclerosis (Kimmelstiel-Wilson syndrome), is both specific for and diagnostic of diabetes; however, it is not responsible for the nephrosis or the renal failure.

Preeclampsia is the toxemia of pregnancy; this syndrome includes hypertension, edema, and proteinuria. Eclampsia includes the preeclamptic spectrum of symptoms combined with associated maternal convulsions and coma. The primary pathologic renal feature is glomerular capillary endotheliosis.

Necrotizing granulomatous vasculitis (Wegener's granulomatosis) is characterized by upper or lower respiratory tract symptoms of necrotizing vasculitis and granulomatous inflammation. The kidneys are involved in approximately 50% of patients. Individually, the vasculitis and granulomatous inflammation are not specific for Wegener's granulomatosis; both must be histologically evident for diagnosis. The most recognizable presentation of the condition is the occurrence of necrotizing lesions.

A diagnosis of amyloidosis (i.e., systemic or focal accumulation of amyloid in tissue) is made by biopsy and positive Congo red staining of amyloid protein.

Chapter 7

Allergic and Immunologic Disorders

Donald P. Goldsmith

I. **OVERVIEW OF THE IMMUNE SYSTEM.** Immune responses are generated by natural and adaptive mechanisms that consist of both cellular and humoral components.

A. **Natural immunity** is nonspecific; that is, it is not influenced by previous antigen–antibody interactions.

1. **Phagocytic cells,** including **polymorphonuclear leukocytes** (**neutrophils** and **eosinophils**), **monocytes,** and **macrophages,** form the cellular component of the natural immune response. These cells ingest and destroy pathogenic organisms and other foreign material.

2. The **complement system,** a complex group of at least 15 serum proteins, mediates inflammatory reactions by attracting granulocytes and macrophages, promoting cell–cell interactions necessary for antigen processing, and stimulating the lysis of enveloped viruses and bacteria.

B. **Adaptive immunity** is characterized by direct responses to initial antigen presentation and **memory (anamnestic)** responses upon reexposure.

1. **Humoral immunity** involves the production of **immunoglobulins by B lymphocytes.**
    a. Immunoglobulins are divided into one of five classes, or **isotypes.**
        (1) **Immunoglobulin G (IgG),** the most prevalent serum immunoglobulin, is normally present at concentrations ranging from 800 to 1500 mg/dl. Four IgG subclasses—IgG1, IgG2, IgG3, and IgG4—have been identified.
        (2) **IgA** is the principal immunoglobulin in secretory fluids, with normal serum levels ranging from 80 to 350 mg/dl. It exists as a dimer linked to an associated secretory component by a J chain.
        (3) **IgM** exists in serum as a cluster of five monomeric units linked by a J chain and disulfide bonds. Normal serum levels of IgM range from 40 to 160 mg/dl.
        (4) **IgD** and **IgE** are monomeric proteins present in serum in trace amounts (i.e., approximately 3–5 mg/dl of IgD and 0.05 mg/dl of IgE).
    b. Antigen binding to membrane-bound immunoglobulin triggers the **differentiation of B cells into mature plasma cells** capable of secreting antigen-specific immunoglobulin (Figure 7-1).

2. **Cellular immunity** is mediated by **T lymphocytes.**
    a. **Subpopulations of T cells** have been defined on the basis of function and the presence of characteristic surface antigens.
        (1) **Cytotoxic T (Tc) cells** carry the CD8 surface antigen and are responsible for killing cells that express foreign antigens.
        (2) **Helper T (Th) cells** enhance the activity of B cells, macrophages, and other T cells. They bear the surface antigen CD4.
        (3) **Suppressor T (Ts) cells** are CD8 positive and inhibit the activity of other cells of the immune system.
    b. **Antigen interaction with T cells** stimulates the release of **lymphokines,** including interleukins, granulocyte–macrophage colony-stimulating factor (GM-CSF), tumor necrosis factor, and gamma interferon. These substances regulate various aspects of the immune response.

C. **Disorders of the immune system** result from immunopathologic expression of immune response mechanisms or deficiencies in the cellular and humoral components of these mechanisms.

II. **PATHOGENESIS OF THE IgE-MEDIATED ALLERGIC REACTION.** Antigen-stimulated release of chemical mediators from IgE-sensitized mast cells is characteristic of **IgE-mediated,** or **type I, hypersensitivity reactions.** These reactions figure prominently in many allergic disorders, including allergic rhinitis, urticaria, generalized anaphylaxis, insect sting sensitivity, and some drug reactions (see III–VII).

A. **The allergic response.** A hallmark of the allergic diathesis is the tendency to maintain a persistent IgE response after antigen presentation. Initial exposure to antigen stimulates the production of specific IgE molecules, which bind to high-affinity Fc receptors on the surface of mast cells. Upon reexposure, antigen cross-linking of these membrane-bound IgE molecules results in the release of vasoactive mediators and the subsequent clinical manifestations of pruritus, sneezing, and bronchospasm.

1. **Two types of IgE-binding Fc receptors** have been identified.
   a. **Type I receptors,** found on mast cells and basophils, bind avidly to IgE. Antigen bridging of any IgE bound to these receptors causes the membrane-bound enzyme **phospholipase C** to be activated. Enzyme activation triggers a cascade of reactions, culminating in the release of preformed mediators and the induction of additional, newly synthesized mediators.
   b. **Type II receptors** are found on certain kinds of monocytes, lymphocytes, eosinophils, and platelets. These receptors bind IgE less avidly than do type I receptors. Although the function of the type II receptor is not completely understood, its presence on alveolar macrophages suggests that it has a role in the pathogenesis of allergic asthma.

2. **Mediators**
   a. **Preformed mediators** are synthesized before antigen contact and stored in mast cells and basophils. Examples of such mediators include:
      (1) Histamine
      (2) Heparin
      (3) Serotonin
      (4) Eosinophil chemotactic factor of anaphylaxis (ECF-A)
      (5) Neutrophil chemotactic factor of anaphylaxis (NCF-A)
      (6) Proteases
   b. **Newly synthesized mediators** include:
      (1) Platelet-activating factor (PAF)
      (2) Slow-reacting substance of anaphylaxis (SRS-A)
      (3) Leukotrienes [e.g., leukotriene B4 (LTB4), leukotriene C4 (LTC4), and leukotriene D4 (LTD4)]
      (4) Prostaglandins and thromboxanes

B. **Clinical implications of IgE levels.** Increased levels of IgE have been implicated in the etiology of allergy.

1. Infants with elevated IgE levels during the first year of life are more likely to develop allergic symptoms later in childhood than are infants with normal levels.

2. Approximately 60% of adults with allergic disorders exhibit elevated IgE levels.

3. In patients with chronic rhinitis and bronchial asthma, the presence of antigen-specific IgE suggests that these symptoms are associated with allergy.

C. **Regulation of IgE synthesis** (see Figure 7-1)

1. **Differentiation of IgE-secreting B cells.** Bone marrow stem cells pass through a series of developmental steps to become mature B cells. **Induction of transcription** occurs during the last of these maturation phases, resulting in plasma cells capable of secreting the IgE isotype.

2. **T-cell involvement in IgE synthesis by B cells**
   a. **Th cells** enhance IgE synthesis, whereas **Ts cells** suppress synthesis. In normal

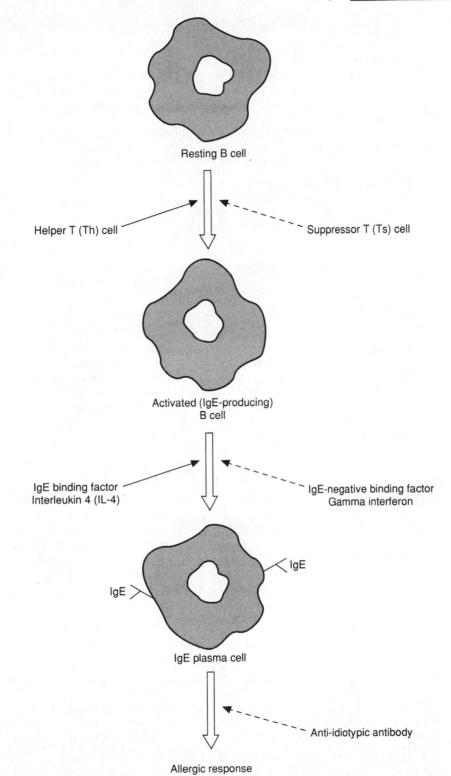

Figure 7-1. B-cell differentiation includes **immunoglobulin E (IgE) synthesis** and typically leads to allergic reaction. Each step (*open arrows*) can occur only if the stimulatory factors (*solid arrows*) at that step over-power the inhibitory factors (*dashed arrows*). In the last step, a sufficient amount of anti-idiotypic antibody can hamper IgE expression and thus prevent the allergic response.

individuals, the Ts cell population is typically dominant, blunting the IgE-mediated response.

- **(1)** Primary immunodeficiency disorders (see VIII) are sometimes accompanied by elevated levels of serum IgE.
- **(2)** In such cases, the number of Th cells is sufficient to induce IgE synthesis, and the number of Ts cells is inadequate to suppress synthesis.

  b. IgE synthesis is also regulated by T-cell–derived **IgE binding factors.** These factors may potentiate or suppress synthesis.

  c. The lymphokines **interleukin-4 (IL-4)** and **γ interferon,** derived from Th cells, enhance and block IgE synthesis, respectively. An imbalance between IL-4 and γ interferon may underlie elevated IgE levels in some patients.

3. **Anti-idiotypic antibodies** develop as a result of the heterogeneous composition of the variable domain of all immunoglobulins, including IgE. Because IgG anti-idiotypic antibodies inhibit certain antigen-specific IgE responses, a decrease in IgG antibodies leads to elevated IgE levels and an exaggerated IgE expression in some individuals.

D. **The late-phase reaction.** The IgE-mediated reaction may have a delayed, or late-phase, component, beginning 3–4 hours after the initial antigen challenge and resolving in 12–24 hours.

1. **Clinical implications.** This late-phase reaction may contribute to the chronicity of allergic rhinitis, atopic dermatitis, and asthma in some patients.

2. **Pathogenesis**
   a. Patients with severe and persistent allergic symptoms may have greater numbers of circulating mononuclear cells bearing type II Fc receptors, suggesting that these receptors have a role in the late-phase reaction.
   b. The release of a number of chemical mediators (i.e., chemotactic factors and histamine-releasing factors) is pivotal to the pathogenesis of the late phase reaction (Figure 7-2).

III. ALLERGIC RHINITIS

A. **Definition.** This inflammatory disorder of the nasal mucosa is characterized by nasal blockage, rhinorrhea, sneezing, and pruritus and is initiated by mast-cell mediators released during the IgE-mediated hypersensitivity reaction. There are two major classifications of allergic rhinitis.

1. **Seasonal allergic rhinitis** has periodic symptoms that occur only during the pollinating season of the antigen to which the patient is sensitive.

2. **Perennial allergic rhinitis** has continuous or intermittent symptoms that occur year round.

Figure 7-2. The **late-phase component of the immunoglobulin E (IgE)-mediated allergic reaction** is initiated by mediator release from mast cells and results in epithelial injury and inflammation of the airway and skin. The mediators released [i.e., eosinophil and neutrophil chemotactic factors of anaphylaxis (ECF-A and NCF-A), leukotriene B4 (LTB4), and monohydroxyeicosatetraenoic acids (HETE)] enhance infiltration by eosinophils and neutrophils. Eosinophils then produce major basic protein (MBP), a direct cause of airway epithelial injury, and platelet-activating factor (PAF), the trigger for platelets to secrete thromboxanes, which cause airway and cutaneous injury; both thromboxanes and PAF also are produced by neutrophils. Neutrophils and alveolar macrophages generate respiratory burst metabolites, another source of airway damage. The cycle is perpetuated by various stimulators of mast-cell mediator release, including thromboxanes, MBP, and the histamine-releasing factors produced by neutrophils, macrophages, and lymphocytes.

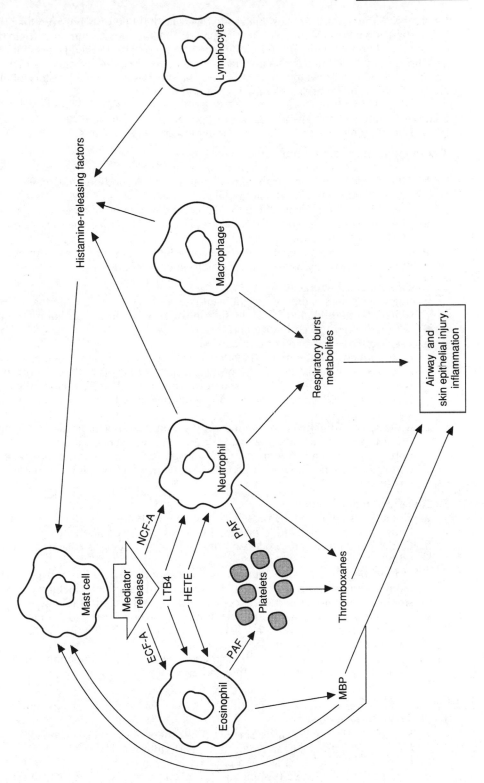

B. **Incidence.** Although accurate estimates are difficult to obtain, it is believed that 15%–20% of adults have allergic rhinitis, making this the most common chronic disorder of the respiratory tract. There is no apparent male or female predilection for allergic rhinitis, and no ethnic or racial patterns have been identified. Symptoms may begin at any age, but develop in most patients before age 20 years. A history of allergic disorders in the immediate family is common.

C. **Etiology.** Various aeroallergens (e.g., spores, pollens, and organic dusts) trigger the IgE-mediated hypersensitivity reaction that underlies allergic rhinitis.

1. **Common characteristics of aeroallergens**
   a. Aeroallergens usually are less than 50 μm in size.
   b. The allergens are lightweight and, therefore, easily wind-borne. (Heavier, insect-borne pollens do not cause allergic rhinitis.)
   c. The allergens are released into the environment in large numbers.
   d. The allergenic constituents usually are proteins with molecular weights of 10,000–40,000 daltons.
   e. Seasonal patterns for each pollen are consistent from year to year, but quantities of pollen vary depending on environmental conditions.

2. **Specific seasonal allergens**
   a. **Ragweed pollen** is the most significant cause of allergic rhinitis in the midwestern and eastern United States. Its season usually runs from late summer to early fall (mid-August to early October).
   b. **Tree pollens** elicit symptoms in early spring.
   c. **Grass pollens** are the major offenders in late spring and early summer. Because roses are fully blooming in late spring, sensitivity to grass pollen often is mistakenly called "rose fever." In the southeastern and southwestern United States, grass pollinates from early spring to late fall and may lead to nearly perennial symptoms.
   d. **Mold spores** initially appear in the early spring, reach peak levels in July and August, and subside after the first frost. In the United States, the clinically most important spores are *Alternaria* and *Cladosporium*. The highest mold spore counts occur when a windy period follows a few days of rainy and damp weather.

3. **Specific perennial allergens**
   a. **House dust.** Of the many diverse constituents of house dust, the common house mite is considered to be the primary antigenic component.
   b. **Epidermal antigens** are produced primarily by pets, such as cats, dogs, and rabbits.
   c. **Indoor molds** (i.e., spores found in homes) include *Aspergillus* and *Penicillium.*
   d. **Nonspecific irritants,** which probably are not true allergens, include cigarette smoke, air pollution, perfumes, cooking odors, and chemical fumes.
   e. **Occupational allergens** include platinum salts, wood dust, and laundry detergent enzymes, all of which are known to produce both allergic rhinitis and asthma in association with IgE antibodies.
   f. **Other.** Cockroach skin casts are also considered to be an important antigen, particularly in economically depressed areas.

D. **Clinical features**

1. **Chacteristic symptoms**
   a. **Sneezing**—often with paroxysms of 15–20 sneezes in quick succession—is characteristic and likely to occur in the early morning hours.
   b. **Pruritus** of the nose, palate, and pharynx is common and may lead to the "allergic salute" (repeated pushing up on the end of the nose), which, in turn, often results in a transverse nasal crease.
   c. **A thin, watery nasal discharge** usually is present and is associated with varying amounts of nasal obstruction and postnasal drainage. Mouth breathing is common.

    d. Excess lacrimation and ocular pruritus and soreness are common.

    e. Loss of olfaction and taste may result from chronic severe nasal congestion.

    f. Otitis media, resulting from impaired drainage of the eustachian tube, and **sinusitis,** resulting from impaired drainage of the paranasal sinuses, sometimes occur.

2. Characteristic physical findings usually are seen at the time of maximal exposure to the offending antigens (e.g., during the height of the pollen season).

    a. Nasal findings include the following.

        (1) The nasal cavity characteristically contains thin nasal secretions, and the mucosal surface is edematous, boggy, and usually pale or bluish in color.

        (2) Nasal polyps may be seen but are not common in allergic rhinitis. Their presence usually suggests cystic fibrosis in children and aspirin intolerance in adults.

        (3) Evidence of recent epistaxis in the anterior nasal vault may be seen if a patient's nasal congestion has led to frequent nose-rubbing.

    b. Conjunctival findings include injection and swelling, excess lacrimation, granularity, and, occasionally, chemosis. Infraorbital "shiners" (infraorbital venous congestion) may develop.

    c. Possible findings in children who have severe chronic nasal congestion include broadened bony dorsum of the nose, narrowed palatal arch, halitosis, retrognathic facies, excess gingival and pharyngeal lymphoid tissue, and dental abnormalities.

E. Diagnosis

1. Laboratory findings

    a. Accurately applied **skin tests** with potent and appropriate antigens are the best diagnostic procedures to identify the antigens causing IgE-mediated allergic rhinitis.

    b. An **increased IgE level** supports the diagnosis, but total IgE levels are increased in only 30%–40% of allergic rhinitis patients. The clinician must also consider other possible causes of elevated IgE levels, such as immunodeficiency disorders (see VIII).

    c. The **radioallergosorbent test (RAST)** is reserved for patients with extensive eczematoid dermatitis, significant dermatographism, or a complicated history without corroborative skin tests. IgG-blocking antibodies and high total IgE levels may interfere with the RAST.

    d. Peripheral eosinophilia may be seen, but is an **inconsistent** finding in patients with allergic rhinitis.

    e. A **stained smear of nasal secretions** at the time of clinically active disease often shows a higher number of eosinophils, but this finding also may be seen in patients with eosinophilic nonallergic rhinitis (see III E 2 d) or hyperplastic sinusitis, as well as in normal infants younger than 6 months of age.

    f. A **biopsy of the superficial nasal mucosa** (an office procedure now easily done using a disposable plastic curette) shows mast cells in the lamina propria and a mucosal basophilic infiltrate.

    g. Fiberoptic rhinoscopy may be indicated for unilateral nasal blockage, particularly when such blockage is unresponsive to usual medical therapy.

    h. Selected patients whose skin-test and RAST results are negative may benefit from **conjunctival and nasal mucosal challenges** with selected antigens, histamine, or methacholine. Experimental techniques are available to measure nasal mucosal blood flow and nasal air flow.

2. Differential diagnosis

    a. Nasal congestion with mild rhinorrhea sometimes is seen in **pregnant women** and in patients with **hypothyroidism.**

    b. Abuse of decongestant nasal spray and use of birth control pills, prazosin, thioridazine, perphenazine, propranolol, clonidine, and reserpine are associated with nasal blockage.

   c. Vasomotor rhinitis is a syndrome characterized by nasal blockage and rhinorrhea without evidence of immunologic or infectious nasal disease. Increased parasympathetic activity of the nasal mucosa is present. The condition is exacerbated by changes in body or environmental temperature, relatively high humidity, emotional stress, chemical fumes, tobacco smoke, and alteration of body position. Response to medical therapy often is poor.

   d. Symptoms of **eosinophilic nonallergic rhinitis** are similar to those of vasomotor rhinitis; however, in eosinophilic nonallergic rhinitis, nasal eosinophilia is present, nasal polyps are common, and symptoms usually respond to medical management.

   e. Infectious rhinitis often occurs in patients with underlying allergic rhinitis and usually is associated with reddened nasal mucosa, thick nasal secretions, sore throat, cervical adenopathy, and low-grade fever. Chronic infectious rhinitis may also occur with bronchiectasis and situs inversus as Kartagener syndrome [ciliary dysfunction syndrome (CDS)].

   f. A symptom complex known as the **aspirin triad** consists of nasal polyps, chronic sinus disease, and asthma, with exacerbation of symptoms after administration of aspirin or other nonsteroidal anti-inflammatory agents.

   g. Anatomic abnormalities, the most common of which is a partially deviated septum, may cause nasal obstruction. This should be recognizable during routine nasal examination, but, sometimes, fiberoptic rhinoscopy is needed. When unilateral discharge with a foul odor is present, obstruction by a foreign body should be suspected.

   h. Atrophic rhinitis is seen in older patients and is often secondary to trauma, specific infection, granuloma, or surgery. Mucosal secretions are minimal as a result of unciliated epithelial cells and a decrease in columnar epithelial cells. Anosmia, nasal crusting, and paradoxical symptoms of nasal blockage are characteristic.

F. **Therapy.** Management is stepwise and involves avoidance of any offending allergens and provocative substances, administration of selective pharmacologic agents, and, in some instances, initiation of immunotherapy.

   1. Avoidance. This aspect of management is most successful when a single antigen (e.g., animal dander) is responsible for symptoms. In patients with multiple sensitivities, sensible environmental precautions are recommended and appear to limit severe exacerbation of symptoms.

   2. Environmental measures. Nonspecific irritants, such as chalk dust, paint fumes, and tobacco smoke, may contribute to symptoms. Air conditioners reduce indoor mold and pollen counts, but must be properly maintained to avoid contamination by molds. Home air purifiers may also be helpful, but the benefits are unproven.

   3. Pharmacologic agents
     a. H_1-receptor antagonists (i.e., **antihistamines**) are useful in controlling rhinorrhea and pruritus. Many different agents are available, and, because of marked individual variation in efficacy and production of side effects, the clinician should be familiar with one or two preparations from each of the two major classes of H_1-receptor antagonists.
      (1) First-generation H_1-receptor antagonists
       (a) Ethanolamines (e.g., diphenhydramine) are effective, but often produce significant sedation and atropine-like side effects.
       (b) Ethylenediamines (e.g., pyrilamine) also are effective, produce less sedation than ethanolamines, and have minimal gastrointestinal side effects.
       (c) Alkylamines (e.g., chlorpheniramine) are effective and produce minimal to modest sedation.
      (2) Second-generation H_1-receptor antagonists
       (a) Terfenadine is administered twice daily and rarely produces sedation or anticholinergic or gastrointestinal side effects. Rare, but serious, adverse cardiovascular effects have been observed with concomitant ad-

ministration of ketoconazole and erythromycin and in association with significant hepatic dysfunction.

(b) **Astemizole** is administered once daily and has a clinical profile similar to that of terfenadine.

(c) **Loratadine,** also administered once daily, has not been associated with adverse cardiovascular effects.

b. **Adrenergic agonists** (also known as **sympathomimetic medications**)

(1) **Oral administration** of α-adrenergic agents (e.g., phenylpropanolamine and pseudoephedrine) is effective in reducing nasal congestion but not rhinorrhea. Central nervous system (CNS) stimulation may occur, but this effect often is negated when adrenergic agents are used in combination with a first-generation H_1-receptor antagonist. Short-term use is preferable (less than 10 days).

(2) **Topical application** of short-acting phenylephrine or long-acting oxymetazoline decreases nasal congestion, but regular administration for more than 3–4 days results in severe rebound nasal congestion (rhinitis medicamentosa).

c. **Cromolyn sodium.** A 4% solution of cromolyn sodium is available for topical nasal use. This medication must be administered frequently (3–6 times daily), but is effective in treating both seasonal and perennial allergic rhinitis. Side effects are minimal, and cromolyn sodium is preferred to corticosteroids.

d. **Corticosteroids**

(1) **Systemic** corticosteroids significantly improve symptoms during the height of a specific pollen season. This treatment is rarely indicated, however, and use of long-term oral corticosteroid therapy for perennial allergic rhinitis is ill-advised.

(2) **Topical.** Highly effective and rapidly metabolized topical steroid preparations (e.g., beclomethasone dipropionate and flunisolide acetate) are beneficial in the treatment of seasonal and perennial allergic rhinitis and also are useful during withdrawal of topical adrenergic agonists in patients with severe rhinitis medicamentosa. These preparations have minimal systemic side effects, and localized nasal mucosal abnormalities have not been identified with their long-term use.

4. **Immunotherapy** may be indicated if a patient continues to experience clinically significant symptoms after appropriate environmental, avoidance, and pharmacologic measures have been taken. Although double-blind studies have demonstrated the effectiveness of immunotherapy, the treatment is time consuming and does not provide complete relief for all patients.

IV. URTICARIA AND ANGIOEDEMA

A. Definitions

1. **Urticaria** (commonly known as **hives**) is a pruritic and transient skin eruption, with individual lesions presenting as erythematous circumscribed papules, or wheals, often with white edematous centers. Lesions are annular, round, figurate, or confluent. Repeated scratching often results in dermatographism (Table 7-1).

2. **Angioedema** may occur alone or jointly with urticaria. Compared with urticarial lesions, angioedema lesions are less pruritic, of longer duration, and found in deeper subcutaneous tissue—particularly in loose areas around the mouth, eyelids, and male genitalia. Angioedema in the submucosa of the upper respiratory or gastrointestinal tract may lead to laryngeal obstruction or abdominal pain with diarrhea, respectively.

B. Pathophysiology

1. **Histamine** is a primary mediator, causing dilatation of superficial cutaneous and mucosal venules, increased vascular permeability, and stimulation of cutaneous

TABLE 7-1. Physical Urticarias and Angioedemas

Type	Stimulus	Clinical Features	Diagnostic Test
Dermatographism	Stroking the skin	Exaggerated triple response of Lewis (wheal, flare, and edema), with occasional passive transfer to normal skin; possible immediate-pressure angioedema; may follow emotional stress or infection	Stroking the skin
Delayed pressure angioedema	Sustained heavy pressure	Deep, erythematous swelling typically affecting the hands or feet; disability secondary to discomfort	Application of pressure using inert weights
Cholinergic urticaria	Increase in core body temperature (e.g., fever, exercise, heat exposure, stress)	Intensely pruritic truncal 1- to 3-mm wheals, sometimes accompanied by excessive sweating, lacrimation, salivation, and abdominal cramping	Methacholine skin test; exercise challenge
Cold urticaria (idiopathic or inherited)	Sudden exposure to cold	Localized pruritus, erythema, and swelling in idiopathic form; papular lesions accompanied by chills, arthralgia, myalgia, and headache in inherited form; possible life-threatening edema of upper or lower respiratory tract	Ice cube challenge
Vibratory angioedema (hereditary or acquired)	Prolonged occupational exposure to vibration	Severe pruritus	Application of laboratory vortex to forearm
Solar urticaria (six types, based on wavelength triggering the reaction)	Exposure to sun or UV light	Progressive excoriation and lichenification of affected areas; possible presence of other metabolic or immunologic disorders (i.e., erythropoietic protoporphyria and SLE)	Exposure to specific UV wavelength
Aquagenic urticaria	Exposure to water	Pruritus sometimes accompanied by small wheals resembling those of cholinergic urticaria	Application of water compresses of varying temperatures

SLE = systemic lupus erythematosus; UV = ultraviolet.

type C sensory neurons that release neuropeptides such as **substance P.** The release of histamine from mast cells and basophils may be stimulated by IgE-related mechanisms, by direct cell activation, or by components of the complement cascade known as **anaphylatoxins** (e.g., C3a, C4a, and C5a). C5a also attracts mononuclear cells and neutrophils to the skin.

2. **PAF, prostaglandin D_2 (PGD_2), LTC4, and LTD4** evoke histamine-like vascular changes.

3. **Chemotactic factors affecting mononuclear cells, neutrophils, and platelets** are released by activated mast cells and basophils.

4. **GM-CSF and IL-3** stimulate basophil histamine release.

C. Clinical syndromes according to etiology

1. **Idiopathic urticaria.** In most cases of urticaria lasting several months, no specific cause can be identified. This type of urticaria thus is known as **chronic idiopathic urticaria;** it is most common in women 30–50 years of age.

   a. Histologic studies show perivascular infiltrates of the small blood vessels of the skin with no disturbance of vessel integrity. Neither immune complexes nor complement deposition is present, but the infiltrate contains large numbers of both mononuclear cells and hyperreleasable mast cells.

   b. The incidence of chronic idiopathic urticaria is not increased in individuals who have an underlying allergic disorder.

   c. Chronic urticaria also may be attributed to complement disorders, systemic illness, or physical stimuli (see IV C 3–5).

2. **IgE-mediated urticaria.** Most cases of **acute urticaria** can be attributed to an IgE-mediated reaction. The most common antigens eliciting this response are **nuts, shellfish, chocolate, penicillin,** and **hymenoptera venom.** Inhaled pollen may induce acute urticarial lesions in very sensitive individuals.

   a. Histologic studies of the initial reaction show **partial detachment of the collagen bundles** because of both fluid accumulation and dilatation of small blood vessels. In some individuals, a **late-phase response** characterized by a mixed cellular infiltrate occurs 48 hours after the initial response. This response can occur only if there has been a previous IgE-mediated response (see II A).

   b. The incidence of acute urticaria is increased in individuals with an underlying allergic disorder.

   c. Acute urticaria also may be brought on by a systemic illness or physical stimuli (see IV C 4–5).

3. **Complement-related disorders,** although rare, are well recognized. **Two major syndromes** exist.

   a. **Disorders associated with complement pathway activation.** Connective tissue disorders, such as systemic lupus erythematosus (SLE), hypocomplementemic vasculitis, and serum sickness caused by drugs or blood products, are sometimes associated with **chronic urticaria or angioedema.** In these disorders of the complement system, complement levels are often decreased but they also may be normal.

   b. **A deficiency in the inhibitor of the complement component C1 (C1-INH)** may be hereditary (e.g., in **hereditary angioedema**), idiopathic, or associated with underlying disorders, such as SLE or B-cell lymphomas.

      (1) **Genetics.** The inherited form is autosomal dominant, with 85% of patients exhibiting impaired synthesis of C1-INH and the remaining 15% exhibiting functionally inactive C1-INH.

      (2) **Diagnosis.** C1q levels are normal in hereditary C1-INH deficiency and decreased in the acquired forms. In both forms, a depressed C4 level during asymptomatic and symptomatic periods is characteristic, and the diagnosis usually is secured by documenting a quantitative or functional deficiency of C1-INH. Because this disorder is both life-threatening and treatable, recognition is vital.

4. **Systemic diseases.** Urticaria or angioedema sometimes may be the initial sign or a sequela of an underlying systemic illness.

   a. **Acute infectious diseases** in children, such as viral upper respiratory infection or streptococcal pharyngitis, may be associated with acute urticaria. Rare causes of chronic urticaria in adults are mycobacterial infection, chronic sinusitis, dental abscess, and helminthic infection.

   b. **Systemic inflammatory disorders,** such as SLE, inflammatory bowel disease, chronic hepatitis, and the early phase of either hepatitis A or infectious mononucleosis, may be associated with urticaria. Leukocytoclastic vasculitis of the skin may take the clinical form of urticaria with associated fever and arthralgia. In such cases, C1q-containing circulating immune complexes are present.

   c. **Thyroid disorders** (with or without hypothyroidism) are sometimes associated with persistent intractable urticaria. There is a marked female predilection for this condition, and antithyroid antibodies are commonly seen in affected patients.

5. **Physical urticarias and angioedemas** are induced by a physical stimulus, such as temperature, sunlight, or physical pressure. Although the pathogenic mechanism for most of these conditions is unknown, some are clearly IgE-dependent. Features of the physical urticarias and angioedemas are described in Table 7-1.

D. | **Therapy**

1. **Prevention of further episodes** involves avoidance of known evocative agents (e.g., foods, medications, and physical factors) and identification and management of underlying medical disorders.

2. **Treatment of existing episodes** usually is stepwise, depending on the presumed pathogenic mechanism.
   a. **H_1-receptor blockers** alone often are effective. Cyproheptadine appears to be useful in treating cold-induced urticaria, hydroxyzine in cholinergic urticaria, and diphenhydramine in solar urticaria. Cetirizine, a metabolite of hydroxyzine with strong H_1-blocker activity without sedative effects, is promising. Two newer, nonsedating H_1-receptor blockers, terfenadine and astemizole also are effective, particularly for delayed pressure urticaria.
   b. **Adding an H_2-receptor blocker,** such as cimetidine, may have a synergistic effect, because H_2 receptors make up approximately 15% of the histamine receptors in cutaneous blood vessels. Doxepin, which blocks both H_1 and H_2 receptors, is used to treat refractory urticaria.
   c. **Systemic steroids** are reserved for severe cases, with an alternate-day dosing regimen preferred.
   d. **Limited androgens,** such as danazol, are effective in treating C1-INH deficiency and some cases of steroid-responsive chronic idiopathic urticaria.
   e. **Ketotifen,** an experimental cromolyn-like drug, has potential either as standard early therapy or as a treatment for refractory urticaria.

V. **GENERALIZED ANAPHYLAXIS**

A. | **Definition.** Anaphylaxis is an acute life-threatening hypersensitivity syndrome. It affects multiple organ systems and results from the precipitous and massive release of mediators from both mast cells and basophils. Symptoms usually begin within minutes of exposure to the causative factor and peak within 1 hour.

B. | **Incidence.** Exact incidence rates are unknown. In Ontario, fatal anaphylaxis from any cause is estimated at 0.4 cases per 1 million population per year. One of every 2700 hospitalized patients in the United States experiences some anaphylactic symptoms.

C. | **Etiology.** A variety of mechanisms, summarized in Table 7-2, can initiate anaphylactic mediator release.

1. **IgE-mediated release.** The binding of IgE antibodies either to complete antigens (e.g., insulin) or to antigenic determinants on hapten-carrier complexes (e.g., the penicilloic acid moiety of penicillin coupled to serum albumin) often precipitates the release of mediators.

TABLE 7-2. Etiologic Mechanisms of Anaphylaxis

Mechanism	Typical Allergens

IgE-mediated mediator release	Drugs
	  Sulfonamides
	  Tetracyclines
	  Penicillins
	  Cephalosporins
	  Local anesthetics
	Insect venoms
	Allergen extracts
	Chymopapain
	Streptokinase
	Insulin
	Food
	  Shellfish
	  Nuts
	  Eggs
	  Milk

Direct mast cell mediator release	Drugs
	  Polymyxin B
	  Opiates
	  Vancomycin
	  Radiocontrast media

Anaphylatoxin-induced mediator release (via complement activation)	Human blood products
	  Plasma
	  Immunoglobulins
	  Cryoprecipitates

Other mechanisms	Nonsteroidal anti-inflammatory agents Sulfite additives Exercise Hormones

2. **Non–IgE-mediated release.** Certain substances (e.g., opiate analgesics and radio-contrast media) can stimulate degranulation of effector cells directly.

3. **Anaphylatoxin-mediated release.** Significant complement activation generates large amounts of the complement degradation products C3a and C5a. These fragments bind to mast-cell receptors, triggering mediator release.

4. **Other mechanisms**
   a. **Recurrent idiopathic anaphylaxis** has been linked to two recently described syndromes.
      (1) **Exercise-induced anaphylaxis.** Well-conditioned athletes are particularly susceptible to this condition, which is characterized by an unpredictable onset during mild, as well as strenuous, exercise. The patient often reports the ingestion of foods that provoke a positive skin reaction (e.g., shellfish or celery) shortly before exercise. In many cases, the combination of exercise and the ingestion of such foods triggers an anaphylactic reaction, whereas exercise or food intake alone does not.
      (2) **Hormonally related anaphylaxis.** In women of childbearing age, the recurrence of mild-to-severe anaphylactic episodes that increase in severity during menstruation suggests hormonal triggers. In such women, anaphylaxis may also be provoked by skin tests with progesterone or by infusions of releasing hormones, which induce ovarian secretion.
   b. In **other anaphylactic syndromes,** such as anaphylaxis induced by nonsteroidal anti-inflammatory agents, the etiologic and pathologic mechanisms are unknown.

TABLE 7-3. Signs and Symptoms of Anaphylaxis

Organ or Organ System Affected	Characteristic Signs and Symptoms
Skin	Pruritus Flushing Urticaria Angioedema
Eyes	Ocular pruritus Excess lacrimation Conjunctival injection
Respiratory system	Nasal congestion Rhinorrhea Cough Hoarseness Stridor Wheezing Laryngeal edema
Cardiovascular system	Weakness Palpitations Tachycardia Hypotension Arrhythmias Shock Cardiac arrest
Gastrointestinal system	Cramping Nausea Diarrhea Vomiting Abdominal distention Metallic taste

D. **Pathophysiology**

1. The **primary anaphylactic mediators** are:
   a. **Preformed substances** stored in secretory granules, such as histamine, mast-cell tryptase, and granulocyte chemotactic factors
   b. **Substances synthesized de novo from membrane lipids,** such as PAF, PGD_2, and sulfopeptide leukotrienes

2. **Physiologic sequelae** of mediator release include enhanced permeability of capillaries and postcapillary venules, decreased arteriolar tone, increased venous capacitance, and ventricular contractility.

E. **Clinical features.** The clinical presentation typically involves multiple organ systems, as summarized in Table 7-3. The severity of symptoms is increased in individuals who have undergone long-term administration of β-antagonists.

F. **Diagnosis** of anaphylaxis is based on clinical and laboratory findings characteristic of extensive mediator release.

1. **Essential diagnostic findings** include at least one of the following symptoms:
   a. Bronchial obstruction
   b. Upper airway obstruction
   c. Acute hypotension

2. **Additional findings** that support the diagnosis include:
   a. Characteristic allergic signs and symptoms involving organ systems other than those listed in Table 7-3
   b. Recent exposure to known allergens

    c. Absence of other medical disorders with similar clinical presentations, such as myocardial infarction (MI), vasovagal syncope, dysrhythmias, hypovolemic shock, pulmonary embolism, airway obstruction due to a foreign body, and panic disorder

    d. Elevated levels of plasma and urinary histamine and of mast-cell tryptase

3. Risk factors. Individuals with underlying bronchial asthma, ischemic heart disease, or congestive heart failure are more likely to suffer severe or fatal anaphylactic reactions.

G. **Therapy.** Effective management of the anaphylactic patient starts with knowing the duration of the present reaction, the existence of any underlying medical conditions, and the medication currently being taken by the patient.

1. Specific treatment measures include the following:

    a. Placement of the patient in a recumbent position, with legs elevated and neck extended

    b. If possible, elimination of the causative factor or delay of its absorption (e.g., removing an insect stinger or applying a tourniquet between the heart and the site of a precipitating drug injection)

    c. Maintenance of body temperature

    d. Administration of supplemental oxygen

    e. Use of an oropharyngeal airway, tracheal intubation, or cricothyrotomy if necessary to ensure maintenance of a patent airway

2. Pharmacologic therapy

    a. Aqueous epinephrine (0.3–0.5 ml administered subcutaneously) should be repeated every 20–30 minutes as needed. In addition, nebulized epinephrine can be used to assist in airway maintenance.

    b. Diphenhydramine (25–50 mg) can be administered intramuscularly or by slow intravenous infusion over 5 minutes.

    c. Cimetidine or **ranitidine** is administered by slow intravenous infusion over 5 minutes.

    d. Intravenous fluids, volume expanders, and **pressor agents** are used to maintain blood pressure.

    e. Persistent bronchospasm is usually treated with nebulized β_2**-adrenergic agonists** or intravenous aminophylline. Previous long-term administration of β-antagonists reduces the efficacy of the β-agonist therapy, but this effect may be countered by administration of intravenous glucagon.

    f. Prolonged or biphasic anaphylaxis may be treated by continued cautious administration of **subcutaneous epinephrine** or **intravenous hydrocortisone** every 6 hours.

VI. **INSECT STING SENSITIVITY.** Stings by insects of the Hymenoptera order (e.g., honeybee, yellow jacket, wasp, and white-faced and bald-faced hornet) may lead to sensitization and subsequent IgE-mediated hypersensitivity reactions.

A. **Incidence.** Population studies show that up to 25% of people with no history of a systemic reaction after a sting nonetheless may be sensitive, as judged by positive skin tests and the presence of venom-specific IgE antibodies. As many as 20% of these individuals may have a systemic allergic reaction if restung. It is estimated that 75–100 deaths occur in the United States each year from insect sting reactions, with most fatalities occurring in people older than age 40 years.

B. **Clinical features.** A nonallergic reaction to an insect sting consists of transient swelling, pain, and redness surrounding the injection site, all of which subside in 1–2 hours. Allergic reactions vary from scattered patches of urticaria to severe and fatal anaphylaxis.

1. **Local allergic reactions** extend a significant distance from the sting site (8 cm or more), peak in 24 hours, and often take 5–7 days to resolve.

2. **Anaphylactic reactions** may involve the skin (localized or generalized urticaria, angioedema, and generalized pruritus), the respiratory tract (laryngeal edema and bronchospasm), the vascular system (hypotension), and the gastrointestinal system (diarrhea, cramping pain, and nausea). The reaction pattern for repeat stings is often similar. Symptoms usually start within a few minutes of the sting.

3. **Rare reactions** include serum sickness, vasculitis, Guillain-Barré syndrome, and glomerulonephritis, all of which may or may not be associated with anaphylaxis.

C. Diagnosis

1. An accurate **history** of the symptoms and signs of a systemic allergic reaction after a sting is necessary. Vasovagal reactions often imitate allergic responses; thus, the physician must use all available resources to substantiate the clinical findings (e.g., records of the emergency room visit).

2. **Specific antivenom IgE antibodies** are detected by prick or intradermal tests. When skin test results are equivocal, a specific serum IgE–level RAST may be helpful.

D. Therapy

1. **Immediate therapeutic measures** are similar to those used in the treatment of anaphylaxis from any cause (see V G).

2. **Prophylactic therapy**
   a. When outside, at-risk individuals should observe **common sense measures,** such as wearing shoes, not wearing heavy perfumes or brightly colored clothes, and staying away from outdoor refuse containers.
   b. All at-risk individuals should own and know how to use an **epinephrine home injection kit.**
   c. Individuals who have had severe symptoms, such as hypotension, laryngeal edema, or bronchospasm, may need to undergo **specific venom immunotherapy.**
      (1) Maintenance dosage and intervals between doses are determined by measuring the patient's IgG antivenom antibodies.
      (2) Immunotherapy sometimes can be stopped without loss of protection after 3–5 years, even in the presence of declining IgG antivenom antibodies and persisting causative IgE antibodies. It is not known why some patients have loss of clinical reactivity after the therapy is stopped.

VII. DRUG REACTIONS

A. **Definitions.** Adverse drug reactions can be classified as **predictable** or **unpredictable,** with the former accounting for approximately 75% of all untoward effects. Unpredictable responses include **hypersensitivity,** or **allergic,** reactions, which constitute 7%–10% of all adverse reactions.

1. **Predictable responses** most often involve known pharmacologic actions, are dose-dependent, and occur in normal individuals. Examples include overdose, side effects, and secondary effects of a drug, as well as undesirable effects resulting from the interaction of two or more drugs (i.e., cross-reactions).

2. **Unpredictable responses** tend to occur in predisposed populations [e.g., on a hereditary basis, as in the association of the HLA-DR2 and DR3 loci with gold-induced nephritis], are not related to the expected pharmacologic action, and are most often independent of dose. Three types of responses have been characterized.

a. **Intolerance** refers to an adverse reaction that occurs at a subtherapeutic dose (e.g., vomiting at low doses of theophylline).

b. **Idiosyncrasy** is an unexpected and qualitatively abnormal response to a medication that is unrelated to the drug's known pharmacologic action (e.g., isoniazid-induced neuritis). Idiosyncratic reactions may occur on a hereditary basis (e.g., hemolytic anemia precipitated by quinolines in a patient with glucose-6-phosphate dehydrogenase deficiency).

c. **Hypersensitivity** results from an immunologic reaction that triggers an abnormal response unrelated to an expected pharmacologic action of the drug (e.g., penicillin-induced urticaria). Drug hypersensitivity reactions usually are categorized according to etiology, using the Gell and Coombs classification system.

   (1) **IgE-mediated reactions** occur when a pharmacologic agent or one of its metabolites binds with drug-specific IgE antibodies on mast-cell or basophil membranes. Subsequent exposure to the same drug promotes release of mediators such as histamines or leukotrienes, which contribute to the development of urticaria and angioedema, both of which occasionally progress to anaphylaxis.

   (2) **Cytotoxic reactions** result from complement-mediated damage to cell membranes precipitated by the binding of IgM or IgG antibodies to drug antigens on cell surfaces. These reactions usually involve blood cells (e.g., drug-induced thrombocytopenia and hemolytic anemia).

   (3) **Immune complex–mediated reactions** develop when soluble complexes of IgM or IgG antibodies and drug antigen are deposited in tissues. Complement activation occurs in the soluble phase or when the complex attaches to vessel walls, leading to inflammation and subsequent tissue injury. **Rash** (urticaria or palpable purpura) and **fever** are the most common clinical manifestations of immune complex–mediated reactions, followed by lymphadenopathy and arthralgia (as can be seen in serum sickness syndrome caused by heterologous serum, sulfonamides, penicillin, or hydantoin).

   (4) **Cell-mediated reactions** require sensitized T lymphocytes that recognize a drug or its metabolite. The antigen–T-cell interaction leads to a lymphokine-induced inflammatory response occurring 24–72 hours after drug administration. **Contact dermatitis** is the most common clinical example of a cell-mediated reaction. Drugs such as topical neomycin penetrate the skin, bind to carrier proteins, and migrate to regional lymph nodes. T cells become sensitized to the bound drug and migrate back to the skin. Subsequent reexposure to the inciting medication leads to T-cell–mediated inflammation. Another example of cell-mediated hypersensitivity is methicillin-induced interstitial nephritis.

B. **Clinical features.** Organ-specific syndromes resulting from drug allergy include the following.

1. **Hepatic syndromes** result primarily in hepatocellular changes or cholestasis. Hydantoin and halothane, for example, can cause hepatocellular damage, as can aspirin when administered to children with juvenile rheumatoid arthritis. Phenothiazines, azathioprine, and erythromycin estolate have been linked to cholestasis and painless jaundice.

2. **Renal involvement** most often takes the form of acute interstitial inflammation. Methicillin, sulfonamides, and cephalosporins have been implicated in this reaction. Fever, eosinophilia, macular rash, pyuria, hematuria, and proteinuria are characteristic.

3. **Pulmonary reactions** include pulmonary infiltration and bronchospasm.
   a. **Pulmonary infiltration** has been reported with use of nitrofurantoin, gold compounds, methotrexate, and, rarely, cromolyn sodium.
   b. **Drug-induced bronchospasm** may occur in asthmatic patients after administration of aspirin or other nonsteroidal anti-inflammatory agents. Excess leukotriene production, resulting from inhibition of the cyclooxygenase pathway, presumably is responsible for this reaction.

4. Dermatologic reactions are the most common manifestations of drug sensitivity.

    a. Urticaria, occasionally progressing to anaphylaxis, can be precipitated by a variety of medications; the most common offenders are penicillin, sulfonamides, cephalosporins, and allergen extracts. Most urticarial reactions are the result of IgE-mediated or direct histamine release.

    b. Fixed drug eruptions, which are most likely attributable to a cell-mediated reaction, may develop after ingestion of tetracycline, sulfonamides, and penicillin. In this reaction, discrete, nonpruritic lesions with a macular to bullous appearance occur at the same place each time the medication is taken.

    c. Photodermatitis is a characterized by a bright erythematous eruption or eczematoid lesions in areas exposed to ultraviolet light. Two presentations are recognized.

        (1) Phototoxicity as a result of ultraviolet light exposure occurs early in drug treatment. Drugs implicated in phototoxic reactions include doxycycline, coal tar derivatives, and psoralens.

        (2) Photoallergy occurs from 4–21 days after the ingestion of the causative agent. It appears to be a cell-mediated process in which ultraviolet light induces a chemical alteration of the drug, leading to tissue sensitization and subsequent injury. Phenothiazines, griseofulvin, and sulfonamides are common offenders.

    d. Contact dermatitis develops 48–72 hours after topical application of the implicated medication and is characterized by a vesicular T-cell–mediated inflammatory reaction. Common preparations causing these skin lesions are para-aminobenzoic acid (PABA), neomycin, and antihistamines.

    e. Febrile mucocutaneous reactions are uncommon, but may be severe. Cytotoxic, immune-complex, and cell-mediated reactions all contribute to the pathogenesis of these syndromes.

        (1) Stevens-Johnson syndrome, a severe form of erythema multiforme, may present as papular, urticarial, vesicular, or purpuric lesions involving two or more mucosal surfaces.

        (2) Lyell syndrome presents as epithelial bullae with subsequent desquamation **(toxic epidermal necrolysis).**

        (3) Drugs implicated in both syndromes include rifampin, phenobarbital, phenytoin, trimethoprim-sulfamethoxazole, and penicillins.

C. Diagnosis. Because there are so few specific diagnostic laboratory tests available to confirm drug allergy, obtaining an accurate history is essential. Drug allergy should be considered as the possible cause of almost any clinical symptom or sign because drug allergy reactions may mimic so many other clinical conditions.

    1. Clinical features suggesting drug hypersensitivity include:

        a. Prior exposure to the drug

        b. Onset of symptoms 7 or more days after initiating drug treatment (if there is no prior exposure)

        c. Administration of the drug at the recommended dose

        d. Symptoms and signs commonly associated with known allergic reactions

        e. Prompt disappearance of the symptoms following discontinuation of the implicated drug

    2. Specific diagnostic tests include:

        a. Immediate skin tests for IgE-mediated reactions (e.g., penicillin, insulin, and chymopapain)

        b. Delayed skin tests for cell-mediated reactions (e.g., PABA and nickel)

        c. RAST testing for specific IgE antibodies (e.g., penicillin)

        d. Coombs' antiglobulin test for cytotoxic reactions causing hemolytic anemia

D. Reactions to selected drugs and biologic agents

    1. Reactions to penicillin and its semisynthetic derivatives are among the most common adverse drug reactions. From 1% to 10% of patients receiving these drugs experience an allergic response. The newer monobactam group of β-lactams may be less allergenic than the β-lactam antibiotics previously available.

a. **Diagnosis.** When a β-lactam antibiotic is the only drug of choice for a patient with a history suggesting penicillin allergy, **skin testing** is recommended. Serial dilutions of benzylpenicilloyl polylysine (a **major determinant** of penicillin allergy that is associated with immediate or accelerated urticaria and anaphylaxis), aged penicillin G, and fresh penicillin G (both **minor determinants** of penicillin allergy that are associated with severe anaphylaxis) are applied via the prick method and then intradermally. If all three tests are negative, the likelihood of a reaction is estimated to be 1%–2%, and penicillin may be administered cautiously. Patients with a positive skin test should not receive penicillin or semisynthetic penicillins. Also, cephalosporins should be administered to such patients only cautiously, because 10%–20% of patients allergic to penicillin have a cross-reaction to cephalosporins.

b. **Therapy.** Desensitization to penicillin-related IgE-mediated reactions may be accomplished by administering penicillin in increments of increasing strength over 4–6 hours. This procedure should be carried out in a controlled setting with access to appropriate emergency treatment. The oral route has been found to be safer than the parenteral route and is preferred. Parenteral administration may be initiated after the completion of oral desensitization. The refractory, or desensitized, state may be maintained for weeks to months by administering the drug at least every 12 hours.

2. **Reactions to radiographic contrast dye** occur in 4%–8% of patients studied, with anaphylactoid responses occurring in as many as 1.7% of patients with reactions. Repeat anaphylactoid reactions may develop in up to 35% of patients. Because recently introduced **osmolarity contrast dyes** appear to be associated with a decreased risk of anaphylactoid reactions, they are now the agents of choice, particularly for those patients with a history of previous allergic reaction.

a. **Pathogenesis.** Anaphylactoid responses mimic IgE-mediated anaphylaxis and result from activation of the complement cascade and generation of anaphylatoxic complement components that precipitate mediator release from mast cells and basophils. Radiocontrast agents may also directly induce mediator release by disrupting cell membrane integrity.

b. **Clinical features** include symptoms of excess vagal stimulation, such as bradycardia, hypotension, nausea, or vomiting. These symptoms may be particularly severe, sometimes culminating in shock.

c. **Therapy** for an **existing** anaphylactoid reaction is identical to that for anaphylaxis from other causes (see V G). Vagal reactions can be treated with atropine. A pretreatment **prophylactic** regimen of prednisone and diphenhydramine significantly decreases the likelihood of a repeat anaphylactoid reaction. Some experts recommend the addition of ephedrine or an H_2-specific antihistamine.

3. **Insulin allergy and resistance**
   a. **Allergic reactions.** Because bovine insulin differs from human insulin by three amino acids and porcine insulin differs by only one amino acid, the bovine-based preparation is more allergenic. The newer human insulins, although less allergenic than the animal preparations, may still precipitate IgE-mediated hypersensitivity reactions. Certain histocompatibility antigens (HLA-DR2, HLA-DR3, and HLA-B7) may be associated with insulin allergic reactions, and as many as 50% of people exhibiting insulin allergy also have experienced allergic reactions to other drugs.
      (1) **Local allergic reactions** to insulin are characterized by pruritus, swelling, and mild erythema, usually occurring during the first few months of therapy. These reactions often subside completely after a few weeks; if not, antihistamines may be either administered systemically or mixed with the insulin. Dividing the dose among two or more injection sites or changing to a more purified insulin preparation also may be effective. Prolonged local reactions may result in lipoatrophy.

(2) Systemic allergic reactions are much less common than local reactions (i.e., they occur in less than 0.1% of patients) and are treated similarly to generalized anaphylaxis (see V G). If insulin therapy is reinstituted less than 24 hours after the systemic reaction, the next dose should be reduced from one third to one sixth, with slow incremental increases as needed to obtain metabolic control. A desensitization protocol must be implemented if the patient requires subcutaneous insulin and more than 24 hours have passed since the systemic reaction occurred.

b. Resistance

(1) Nonimmunologic causes of **insulin resistance** include infection, stress, pregnancy, obesity, Cushing's syndrome, acromegaly, pheochromocytoma, leprechaunism, and **type A insulin resistance syndrome** accompanied by acanthosis nigricans.

(2) Immunologic insulin resistance is mediated by IgG anti-insulin antibodies and is manifested by a need for increasing daily doses (up to 200 units/kg in adults and up to 2 units/kg in children). The presence of high-titer IgG antibodies to insulin or to the insulin receptor can be confirmed by a competitive binding assay.

(a) Although immunologic insulin resistance is rare, it occurs most often in people who have recently started insulin therapy or who have a history of allergic reactions. It often remits spontaneously in less than 6 months. Treatment, if required, involves first switching to a more purified insulin preparation and then, if symptoms have not improved, administering systemic corticosteroids. In rare cases, cyclophosphamide or 6-mercaptopurine may be required.

(b) Type B insulin resistance syndrome occurs most often in patients 60 years of age and older—elderly women are particularly susceptible. The syndrome is characterized by a lupus-like illness, acanthosis nigricans, and severe insulin resistance secondary to the production of anti-insulin receptor antibodies. Spontaneous improvement is rare, and immunosuppressive therapy may be required.

4. Vaccine reactions may occur after heterologous sera, tetanus toxoid, and egg-embryo–based viral vaccines are given.

a. Heterologous sera are used in the management of gas gangrene, botulism, and some snake and spider bites. Before treatment, skin tests are necessary to identify those patients in whom anaphylatic reactions are likely to develop. Skin tests, however, do not accurately predict the development of a serum sickness reaction.

b. Tetanus toxoid hypersensitivity usually occurs as fever accompanied by local swelling, tenderness, and erythema. Anaphylaxis is rare, and skin tests are rarely positive. Reactions are usually followed by high IgG-antibody titers and a hyperimmunized state. Antitoxin levels should be obtained if further immunization is deemed necessary.

c. Mumps, measles, influenza, yellow-fever, and **typhus vaccines** are grown on chick embryos, and anaphylaxis after vaccination in egg-sensitive individuals has been reported. Suspected sensitivity requires assessment by both prick and intradermal testing before vaccination. If a patient tests positive, the vaccine should be administered only according to a modified desensitization program.

5. Aspirin reactions usually present as urticaria or wheezing. Chronic rhinitis, sinusitis, and often intractable steroid-dependent asthma develop in a small, well-recognized subgroup of individuals between the ages of 30 and 60 years old. In these at-risk individuals, life-threatening severe bronchospasm may occur after aspirin ingestion. Those in whom chronic asthma develops cannot improve their asthma, however, by abstinence from aspirin or other nonsteroidal anti-inflammatory agents. Because there are no in vivo or in vitro tests for aspirin allergy, diagnosis can be made only from the patient's medical history and, in rare cases, by aspirin challenge. Oral desensitization has been successful in some individuals but must be done cautiously and under medically controlled circumstances.

E. Newly recognized drug allergy syndromes

1. **Sulfite-induced bronchospasm.** Sodium and potassium sulfite are commonly used as preservatives in foods, beverages, and medications. These products tend to liberate sulfur dioxide, a potent bronchoconstrictor for some individuals with underlying bronchial asthma. Reports of severe bronchospasm associated with sulfites used in fresh salad bars to prevent browning first brought this syndrome to medical attention in 1981.

   a. **Diagnosis.** Sulfite-induced asthma is characterized by the rapid onset of asthmatic symptoms (i.e., within 1–2 minutes) after ingestion of a sulfitic food, beverage, or medication. Bronchial challenge with an acidified sulfite solution confirms the diagnosis.

   b. **Therapy** is multifaceted and includes providing the patient with comprehensive dietary information, prophylactic medications, and a medical plan for treatment of an acute episode.

2. **Chymopapain anaphylaxis.** The proteolytic enzyme chymopapain is used to solubilize the nucleus pulposus and thus provide an alternative to diskectomy in the treatment of lumbar disk herniation. Up to 4% of patients undergoing this chymopapain procedure experience an IgE-mediated allergic reaction, and anaphylaxis develops in 1%. This high rate of sensitivity appears to result from people being repeatedly exposed to the enzyme, which is present in contact lens cleaning solutions, meat tenderizers, toothpastes, fruit juices, and debriding ointments.

   a. **Diagnosis of chymopapain sensitivity** is confirmed by standardized skin testing with a chymopapain test reagent and in vitro measurement of specific IgE anti-chymopapain antibodies.

   b. **Therapy.** Patients who demonstrate either in vivo or in vitro evidence of IgE-mediated sensitivity should not undergo the chymopapain procedure. Patients with a negative skin test should receive careful follow-up after surgery to determine whether chymopapain sensitivity developed during surgery.

3. **L-Tryptophan–related eosinophilia–myalgia syndrome.** L-Tryptophan, a dietary supplement, has been widely advertised to the general public as helpful for insomnia, premenstrual syndrome, and depression. In late 1989, an apparently new clinical entity associated with the ingestion of products containing L-tryptophan was recognized. The presence of peak "E," an unusual dimeric contaminant form of L-tryptophan, in certain lots of L-tryptophan from one manufacturer has been associated with the syndrome. Abnormal metabolism of tryptophan also occurs in some patients.

   a. **Clinical features.** The onset of symptoms, including intense myalgia and fatigue, is usually subacute, evolving over several weeks. Muscle weakness may be noted, as well as a transient maculopapular, urticarial, or vesicular skin rash. Hepatomegaly, extremity edema, early congestive heart failure, and arrhythmias may also occur. Interstitial lung infiltrates, accompanied by mild hypoxia and mild-to-moderate elevation of transaminases, C-reactive protein, and aldolase may be present. Absolute eosinophil counts are usually more than 2000 cells/μl, but values up to 30,000 cells/μl have been reported. Hyperplasia of bone-marrow eosinophil precursors can be seen, and muscle biopsies show a mononuclear infiltrate of lymphocytes and macrophages and variable eosinophil infiltrates in the fascia and perimysium.

   b. **Therapeutic recommendations** include cessation of all L-tryptophan–containing products, glucocorticoids for continuing symptoms, and nonsteroidal anti-inflammatory agents or narcotic analgesics for muscle pain. In severe cases, ancillary drugs such as methotrexate or cyclophosphamide have been tried with mixed success.

   c. **Prognosis.** Some patients improve rapidly after they stop taking L-tryptophan, but, in most patients, amelioration of symptoms is slow. Occasionally, the disorder continues to progress, and severe ascending polyneuropathy, scleroderma-like skin changes, pulmonary hypertension, recurrent muscle spasms, or cognitive dysfunction develop.

4. **Allergic reactions to latex** have recently emerged as a significant clinical problem. Natural latex is found in surgical gloves, catheters, balloons, condoms, and dental elastic adhesives.
   a. **Incidence.** Health care workers are particularly susceptible; up to 7.4% of surgeons and 5.6% of operating room nurses are allergic to latex. Children with spina bifida appear to have a high incidence of allergy.
   b. **Clinical features.** Urticaria on contact, rhinitis, conjunctivitis, and bronchospasm after inhalation are suggestive of latex allergy. Severe anaphylaxis may ensue during surgery, barium enema, or dental procedures.
   c. **Diagnosis.** Latex allergy is IgE-mediated, and the diagnosis is confirmed by prick skin testing or by RAST.
   d. **Prevention.** Nonlatex gloves and tubing are available and should be used during surgery in patients with known latex allergy. Premedication, antihistamines, and corticosteroids are also used to prevent severe reaction.

5. **Allergic reactions to streptokinase.** This enzymatic protein is commonly used as a thrombolytic agent.
   a. **Incidence.** The frequency of allergic reaction to streptokinase ranges from 1.7%–18.0%.
   b. **Clinical features.** Although not completely delineated, acute symptoms usually include urticaria, bronchospasm, and hypotension. Reexposure sensitivity is characterized by a delayed-onset serum sickness-like syndrome.
   c. **Diagnosis.** Streptokinase allergic reactions are IgE-mediated and corroborated by an immediate reaction to an intradermal test with 100 IU of streptokinase.
   d. **Prevention.** Substitute forms of thrombolytic therapy should be used in patients who demonstrate intradermal skin sensitivity or in those with known streptokinase allergy.

6. **Protamine sulfate sensitivity.** Protamine sulfate is a low–molecular-weight protein primarily used to neutralize heparin or to act as a complexing agent with insulin.
   a. **Clinical features.** Flushing, urticaria, hypotension or hypertension, ventricular fibrillation, wheezing, noncardiac pulmonary edema, thrombocytopenia, or neutropenia may develop. IgE-mediated anaphylactic and complement-mediated anaphylactoid mechanisms have been incriminated in patients with allergic reactions to protamine sulfate. Diabetic patients who have used protamine-containing insulins are at increased risk.
   b. **Diagnosis and therapy.** Skin testing is not reliable but pretreatment with antihistamines and corticosteroids may be helpful for patients suspected of being at high risk for allergic reactions.

F. **Prevention of drug reactions**

1. The concurrent administration of several medications should be avoided.

2. A detailed history of any previous drug reactions should be obtained for all patients, to guide the selection of a medication that is unlikely to cross-react.

3. Patients with documented allergic drug reactions should be instructed to carry identification (e.g., a medical alert bracelet). Medical records for such patients should be clearly marked.

4. Oral administration, when possible, is preferable to parenteral administration, because the incidence of reactions after oral administration is much lower.

5. Allergic reactions are unlikely to be discovered during premarketing trials, so particular vigilance is indicated when administering any new drug.

VIII. **IMMUNODEFICIENCY DISORDERS.** These disorders, which may be either **hereditary** or **acquired,** represent four distinct abnormalities of immune function.

A. **Complement system defects** may affect either the nine complement components or the associated regulatory proteins. The etiology, clinical features, and diagnosis of these syndromes are summarized in Table 7-4.

B. **Phagocyte disorders** (Table 7-5)

1. **Common clinical features** of these disorders include recurrent cutaneous and sino-pulmonary infections and chronic cutaneous and oral inflammation. Although the inflammatory response may be delayed, successive infections with *Staphylococcus aureus, Pseudomonas* species, *Haemophilus influenzae,* and *Aspergillus* are common and may be life-threatening.

2. **Therapy** consists primarily of the diagnosis, treatment, and prevention of pyogenic infections. However, such infections are often refractory to treatment, despite appropriate antibiotic therapy.
   a. A complete diagnostic workup is essential, including taking appropriate cultures and being especially vigilant for the development of superficial or visceral mycosis.
   b. Prompt surgical drainage is essential.
   c. Granulocyte transfusions are occasionally used when initial therapy is unsuccessful or complicated by visceral fungal infection.
   d. Bone marrow transplantation has been accomplished successfully with lasting amelioration of chronic granulomatous disease.
   e. **Future treatment modalities** may include administration of recombinant proteins (e.g., γ-interferon) to augment phagocyte function and genetic techniques for the detection and correction of the underlying defect.

3. **Genetic counseling** should be offered to families of affected individuals.

C. **Antibody deficiency syndromes** are characterized by an inability to produce antigen-specific antibody molecules. These disorders have a variety of causes, including abnormalities of the structural genes for the heavy chain of IgA, congenital infections, and medications. Table 7-6 lists the most common humoral immunodeficiency disorders.

1. **Common clinical features.** Most patients with these disorders present with recurrent infections caused by encapsulated bacteria, such as *Streptococcus pyogenes, Streptococcus pneumoniae,* and *H. influenzae.*

2. **Diagnosis** of the antibody deficiency syndromes is based on:
   a. Quantitative **determination of serum immunoglobulin levels**—principally, IgG, IgA, and IgM.
   b. **Functional immunoglobulin assays**
      (1) Determination of antibodies to **naturally occurring immunogens** (e.g., iso-hemagglutinins, anti-A, and anti-B IgM antibodies found in individuals with A, B, or O blood types)
      (2) Measurement of antibodies to **previously encountered antigens** (e.g., *Streptococcus* species, varicella virus, influenza virus, or Epstein-Barr virus)
      (3) Determination of **antibodies to prior immunizations** (e.g., IgG1 antibodies to tetanus and diphtheria toxins or IgG2 antibodies to the carbohydrate capsule of *H. influenzae*)
      (4) Assessment of **antibody production to newly introduced antigens** (e.g., magnitude of de novo response 3–4 weeks after administration of tetanus toxoid or pneumococcal vaccines)

3. **Therapy**
   a. The treatment of choice for most antibody deficiency syndromes is **replacement therapy** with intravenous immunoglobulin.

TABLE 7-4. Complement Deficiency Disorders

Defective Component	Inheritance	Phenotypic Expression	Clinical Features	Diagnosis
C1r, C1q, C2	Autosomal codominant trait involving null alleles	Impaired removal of immune complexes	Vasculitis syndrome; lupus-like syndrome; polymyositis; poikiloderma	Assessment of total hemolytic complement (CH_{50})*
C4	Autosomal codominant trait involving null alleles	Impaired removal of immune complexes	SLE and lupus-like syndrome; Sjögren's syndrome; Henoch-Schönlein syndrome	Assessment of total hemolytic complement (CH_{50})*
C3	Autosomal codominant trait involving null alleles	Impaired opsonization	Recurrent severe infections due to pyogenic or gram-negative organisms	Assessment of total hemolytic complement (CH_{50})*
C5–C9	Autosomal codominant trait involving null alleles	Impaired formation of the membrane attack complex, which mediates bacteriolysis	Recurrent meningococcal and gonococcal infections; increased susceptibility to some viruses; rheumatic disorders	Assessment of total hemolytic complement (CH_{50})*
Factors H, I (alternate pathway)	Autosomal codominant trait involving null alleles	Impaired opsonization	Recurrent infections due to pyogenic organisms	Rabbit RBC lysis in the absence of exogenous antibody

RBC = red blood cell; SLE = systemic lupus erythematosus.
* Followed by measurement of specific complement component levels.

TABLE 7-5. Disorders of Phagocyte Function

Disorder	Inheritance	Phenotypic Expression	Clinical Features	Diagnosis
Chronic granulomatous disease	Usually X-linked; may be inherited as autosomal recessive or autosomal dominant with incomplete penetrance	Abnormal NADPH oxidase function resulting in absence of respiratory burst	Onset of symptoms by age 1 year; granulomas (e.g., hepatosplenomegaly, lymphadenitis); aphthous stomatitis; seborrheic dermatitis	NBT test, confirmed by chemiluminescence
Chédiak-Higashi syndrome	Autosomal recessive	Impaired chemotaxis, intracellular bacteriolysis, and movement of neutrophils from bone marrow	Frequent viral and enteric bacterial infections; partial ocular and cutaneous albinism; neuropathy; nystagmus; mild neutropenia	Presence of giant lysosomal granules in granulocytes, melanocytes, and other granule-bearing cells
Leukocyte adhesion protein deficiency (surface glycoprotein)	Autosomal recessive, involving abnormal long arm on chromosome 21	Reduced neutrophil chemotaxis and spreading; reduced phagocytosis of iC3b-coated particles	Delayed umbilical cord separation, with subsequent omphalitis; cold skin abscesses; necrotizing deep soft tissue abscesses	Sustained granulocytosis; decreased surface-receptor iC3b activity
Job's syndrome (hyperimmunoglobulin E; recurrent infection)	Autosomal recessive	Reduced chemotaxis	Frequent sinopulmonary infections; cold skin abscesses; coarse facies; mucocutaneous candidiasis	Eosinophilia; markedly elevated serum IgE level

NADPH = the reduced form of nicotinamide–adenine dinucleotide phosphate; NBT = nitroblue tetrazolium.

TABLE 7-6. Humoral Immunodeficiency Disorders

Disorder	Inheritance	Phenotypic Expression	Clinical Features	Diagnosis
Bruton's agammaglobulinemia	X-linked	Pre–B-cell blocking factor	Recurrent severe infections due to pyogenic organisms, starting at 9–12 months of age; diarrhea caused by *Giardia lamblia*; chronic meningoencephalitis due to echovirus; autoimmune arthritis	Total immunoglobulin <100 mg/dl; severely reduced IgG, IgM, and IgA levels; marked decrease in B cells bearing surface immunoglobulin
Common variable immunodeficiency	Unknown pattern; equal sex distribution	Abnormal B-cell terminal differentiation	Less severe infections due to pyogenic organisms, starting between ages 20 and 40 years; giardiasis; sprue-like syndrome; nodular lymphoid hyperplasia; lymphoreticular malignancy; pernicious anemia; late development of autoimmune disorders	Reduced IgG, IgM, and IgA levels (total immunoglobulin may be <100 mg/dl); possible slight decrease in B cells bearing surface immunoglobulin
Selective IgA deficiency (inherited or sporadic)	Sporadic form affects 1 in 500 people (most common immunodeficiency disorder); inherited form involves genes on chromosome 14, which code for heavy chain of IgA	Arrested maturation of IgA-bearing cells	Recurrent respiratory or gastrointestinal bacterial infections; infections more severe in patients with IgA < 5 mg/dl; autoimmune and allergic disorders; no symptoms in 30% of cases; deficiency sometimes transient	Reduced serum IgA levels (below lower limit of age-normal values; may be <5 mg/dl); reduced IgG2 or IgG4 levels in 15% of cases; occasional mild abnormalities of T-cell function

TABLE 7-7. Cell Deficiency Disorders

Disorder	Inheritance	Phenotypic Expression	Clinical Features	Diagnosis	Therapy
DiGeorge syndrome	Unknown; few familial cases identified	Dysmorphogenesis of third and fourth pharyngeal pouches; hypoplastic thymus and parathyroid	Anomalies of the great vessels; neonatal tetany; hypoplastic mandible; hypertelorism; short upper-lip philtrum; low-grade or opportunistic infections (occasional or recurrent)	Total serum immunoglobulin usually normal; IgE levels possibly elevated; IgA levels possibly reduced; decrease in total T cells; hypocalcemia; mitogen-stimulated proliferation may be normal, decreased, or absent, depending on degree of thymic deficiency	Fetal thymus transplantation
Nezelof syndrome	Autosomal recessive; X-linked	Vestigial thymus; few thymocytes; Hassall's corpuscles absent	Failure to thrive; recurrent lung and skin infections; gram-negative sepsis; localized candidiasis; hyperplastic peripheral lymphoid tissue	Lymphopenia; possibly elevated serum immunoglobulin levels; marked decrease in total T cells; cutaneous anergy	Bone marrow transplantation

TABLE 7-8. Characteristics of Severe Combined Immunodeficiency (SCID)*

Inheritance	Phenotypic Expression	Clinical Features	Diagnosis	Therapy
Autosomal recessive in MHC deficiency (bare lymphocyte syndrome) and ADA deficiency; X-linked recessive	Absence of all adaptive immune mechanisms; vestigial thymus; few thymocytes or Hassall's corpuscles†	Skin infections, sepsis, pneumonia, and diarrhea, starting by age 3 months; marked failure to thrive; severe opportunistic infections (e.g., *Pneumocystis, Candida,* varicella); hypoplastic peripheral lymphoid tissue; chondrodysplasia;‡ possibility of death by age 2 years if untreated	Profound lymphophenia; cutaneous anergy; heterogeneous abnormalities of lymphocyte subpopulations; impaired in vitro lymphocyte proliferative response	Bone marrow transplantation; IV immunoglobulin replacement; experimental gene therapy trial in progress‡

ADA = adenosine deaminase; IV = intravenous; MHC = major histocompatibility complex.

* Includes ADA deficiency, which accounts for 40% of cases.

† Hassall's corpuscles may be present in ADA deficiency.

‡ Characteristic of ADA deficiency only.

TABLE 7-9. Partial Combined Immunodeficiency Disorders

Disorder	Inheritance	Phenotypic Expression	Clinical Features	Diagnosis	Therapy
Wiskott-Aldrich syndrome	X-linked recessive	Accelerated synthesis and catabolism of all Ig isotypes; intrinsic platelet abnormality	Eczema; thrombocytopenia; recurrent infections due to encapsulated pathogens, starting by age 1 year; *Pneumocystis* and herpesvirus infections, starting in late childhood; malignancy in 10%–12% of cases	Normal or slightly reduced IgG levels; elevated IgA levels; reduced IgM levels; impaired humoral response to polysaccharide antigens; mild-to-moderate depression of lymphocyte proliferative response	Bone marrow transplantation
Ataxia–telangiectasia	Autosomal recessive	Hypoplastic thymus; lack of Hassall's corpuscles; intrinsic Th- and B-cell defects	Progressive cerebellar ataxia; oculocutaneous telangiectasia; recurrent sinopulmonary infections; increased incidence of malignancy	Selective IgA deficiency (see Table 7-6) in 50%–80% of cases; low–molecular-weight IgM; mild depression of mitogen–stimulated proliferative response; decrease in Ts cells and T-cell total	None

Ig = immunoglobulins; Th cells = helper T cells; Ts cells = suppressor T cells.

b. Patients with selective IgA deficiency are treated as needed with **appropriate antibiotics** for bacterial infections. Immunoglobulin replacement therapy is limited to those individuals with accompanying IgG subclass deficiency.

D. **Cellular immunodeficiencies** include those limited to defects in T-cell function (Table 7-7), as well as combined disorders affecting both cellular and humoral immunity (Tables 7-8 and 7-9).

1. **Common clinical features.** T-cell deficiencies, whether partial or complete, typically result in recurrent infections of greater severity than those observed in the antibody deficiency syndromes.

2. **Diagnosis** of cellular immunodeficiency syndromes is based on a demonstrable decrease in the number or function of T cells. Specific T-cell assays include:
   a. **Quantitative assessment of circulating lymphocytes.** In normal individuals, 80%–85% of the circulating lymphocytes are T cells. Values below 1500 μl are considered abnormal.
      (1) The **total number** of T cells can be measured using the **E rosette test,** which counts the number of T lymphocytes binding sheep erythrocytes to form a rosette.
      (2) **Immunofluorescence labeling** with T-cell–specific monoclonal antibodies identifies T-cell subsets (e.g., anti-CD4 labels Th cells, and anti-CD8 labels Ts and Tc cell populations).
   b. **Delayed hypersensitivity skin tests to previously encountered common antigens** (e.g., *Candida albicans, Trichophyton,* streptokinase–streptodornase, mumps virus). Positive reactions to at least two antigens indicate intact cellular immunity.
   c. **Determination of in vitro responsiveness** of cultured T cells to **specific antigens, mitogens** (e.g., pokeweed, concanavalin A, or hemagglutinin), or **foreign cells**

E. The **human immunodeficiency virus (HIV)** selectively infects Th cells, leading to progressive deterioration of the immune system and, ultimately, **acquired immune deficiency syndrome (AIDS).** For a detailed discussion of AIDS, refer to Chapter 8. **Acquired immunodeficiency** may also be secondary to malnutrition, infection, malignancy, and drug or chemical exposure.

DIRECTIONS: Each of the numbered items or incomplete statements in this section is followed by answers or by completions of the statement. Select the **ONE** lettered answer or completion that is **BEST** in each case.

1. Which of the following components of the immune system is responsible for the secretion of lymphokines?

(A) B lymphocytes
(B) Eosinophils
(C) Macrophages
(D) Neutrophils
(E) T lymphocytes

2. Which of the following findings provides the best evidence of insect sting hypersensitivity?

(A) Positive prick or intradermal skin test
(B) Extensive local reaction lasting 5–7 days
(C) Documented evidence of a systemic allergic reaction
(D) Specific antivenom IgE antibodies
(E) Specific antivenom IgG antibodies

3. Which of the following tests is most useful in the diagnosis of allergic rhinitis?

(A) Radioallergosorbent test (RAST)
(B) Measurement of serum IgE levels
(C) Peripheral blood smear
(D) Immediate hypersensitivity skin test
(E) Stained nasal smear for eosinophils

4. Which of the following chemical mediators released during the late-phase reaction contributes to airway epithelial cell injury?

(A) Eosinophil chemotactic factor of anaphylaxis (ECF-A)
(B) Monohydroxyeicosatetraenoic acid (HETE)
(C) Histamine-releasing factors
(D) Respiratory burst metabolites
(E) Leukotriene B4 (LTB4)

5. Which one of the following immunodeficiency disorders is associated with normal IgG levels?

(A) Bruton's agammaglobulinemia
(B) DiGeorge syndrome
(C) Common variable immunodeficiency
(D) Selective IgA deficiency
(E) Wiskott-Aldrich syndrome

6. Urticarial lesions are best described as

(A) nonpruritic
(B) linear
(C) evanescent
(D) macular
(E) poorly circumscribed

7. Which one of the following drug reactions is mediated by IgG autoantibodies?

(A) Type B insulin resistance
(B) Chymopapain anaphylaxis
(C) Latex reaction
(D) Systemic reaction to an insect sting

8. In patients with acute anaphylaxis and drug-induced β-adrenergic blockade, which of the following therapeutic choices may be most useful in treating resistant hypotension?

(A) Subcutaneous aqueous epinephrine
(B) Intravenous pressor agents
(C) Intravenous glucagon
(D) Intravenous aminophylline

9. Which of the following clinical conditions is most commonly associated with latex allergy?

(A) Bronchial asthma
(B) Fibrosing alveolitis
(C) Diabetes mellitus
(D) Spina bifida
(E) Inflammatory bowel disease

DIRECTIONS: The set of matching questions in this section consists of a list of four to twenty-six lettered options (some of which may be in figures) followed by several numbered items. For each numbered item, select the ONE lettered option that is most closely associated with it. To avoid spending too much time on matching sets with large numbers of options, it is generally advisable to begin each set by reading the list of options. Then, for each item in the set, try to generate the correct answer and locate it in the option list, rather than evaluating each option individually. Each lettered option may be selected once, more than once, or not at all.

Questions 10–13 For each of the following patients with allergic rhinitis, select the most appropriate therapeutic intervention.

(A) Antigen avoidance
(B) Immunotherapy against known offending antigens
(C) Antihistamine–decongestant preparation
(D) Topical adrenergic agonist

10. A 34-year-old-woman with severe perennial allergic rhinitis loses 10–15 days of work each year as a result of secondary sinusitis. Immediate skin tests show significant positive reactions to house dust, *Cladosporium,* and grass and ragweed pollens. Various medications have been only partially successful in controlling symptoms.

11. A 20-year-old man has mild but persistent year-round symptoms of nasal congestion, rhinorrhea, and watery eyes. Immediate skin tests show positive reactions to house dust, *Alternaria,* and grass and ragweed pollens.

12. A 10-year-old girl has rhinorrhea and nasal pruritus after visiting a friend who has a kitten.

13. An 8-year-old boy regularly experiences moderately severe sneezing spells and watery eyes in May and June, September and October, and occasionally during January through March. Immediate skin tests show positive reactions to *Alternaria, Cladosporium,* house dust, and grass and ragweed pollens.

ANSWERS AND EXPLANATIONS

1. The answer is E [1 B 2 b]. Antigen interaction with T lymphocytes precipitates the release of lymphokines, substances that modulate other aspects of the immune response. Examples of lymphokines include the interleukins, granulocyte–monocyte colony-stimulating factor (GM-CSF), and γ-interferon. B lymphocytes secrete immunoglobulins, the humoral component of adaptive immunity. Eosinophils, neutrophils, and macrophages are phagocytic cells comprising the cellular component of the natural immune response.

2. The answer is C [VI C 1–2]. Clinical documentation of a systemic allergic reaction is essential to the accurate diagnosis of insect sting hypersensitivity. Typically, signs of anaphylaxis develop within minutes after the sting. Subsequent prick or intradermal skin testing, supplemented as necessary by antivenom IgE levels (determined by radioallergosorbent test [RAST]), provide confirming evidence of hypersensitivity. A large local reaction alone, whether of short or prolonged duration, does not provide sufficient evidence of IgE-mediated hypersensitivity. Antivenom IgG levels are used to chart the response to immunotherapy.

3. The answer is D [III E 1]. An accurately applied skin test is the most valuable tool for identifying the causative antigen in allergic rhinitis, yielding results in approximately 20–30 minutes. The radioallergosorbent test (RAST), albeit accurate, is more expensive and less discriminative than skin testing. Elevated immunoglobulin E (IgE) levels are observed in only 30%–40% of patients with allergic rhinitis and may be secondary to other unrelated disorders. Although eosinophils are usually identified in nasal secretions from patients with allergic rhinitis, they are also detected in eosinophilic nonallergic rhinitis and hyperplastic sinusitis. Peripheral eosinophilia seen in a peripheral blood smear is an inconsistent finding.

4. The answer is D [Figure 7-2]. Respiratory burst metabolites are released by activated neutrophils and alveolar macrophages during the late-phase reaction. Along with thrombox-

anes, platelet-activating factor (PAF), and major basic protein (MBP), these mediators contribute to the airway epithelial cell injury that is characteristic of the late-phase component of the IgE-mediated hypersensitivity reaction. Eosinophil chemotactic factor of anaphylaxis (ECF-A), leukotriene B4 (LTB4), and monohydroxyeicosatetraenoic acid (HETE) are chemotactic factors that enhance infiltration by eosinophils and neutrophils. Histamine-releasing factors may extend the late-phase reaction by prolonging mast-cell secretion.

5. The answer is B [Tables 7-6, 7-7, 7-9]. Although reduced levels of IgA or IgE may be seen in patients with DiGeorge syndrome (a T-cell deficiency disorder), the total serum immunoglobulin level usually is normal, and IgG levels are normal. In Bruton's agammaglobulinemia and common variable immunodeficiency, IgG, IgM, and IgA levels are all reduced, and the total immunoglobulin level is less than 100 mg/dl. Selective IgA deficiency is a humoral immunodeficiency in which IgA levels are extremely low; IgG4 and IgG2 are also reduced in 15% of patients with this disorder. Wiskott-Aldrich syndrome is a partial combined immunodeficiency disorder that is associated with eczema, thrombocytopenia, and recurrent infections early in life. Elevated IgA levels, depressed IgM levels, and normal or slightly reduced IgG levels are seen in patients with this disorder.

6. The answer is C [IV A 1]. Urticarial lesions are well circumscribed and intensely pruritic; dermatographism may result from prolonged scratching. Each lesion is transient, rarely lasting more than a few hours. Bouts of urticaria, however, may persist for several days or even years (as in chronic idiopathic urticaria). Individual lesions that last for longer than 48 hours and that are more painful than pruritic are likely to be due to small-vessel vasculitis, not urticaria.

7. The answer is A [VII D 3 b (2)]. Type B insulin resistance is caused by IgG autoantibodies that bind to insulin receptors, thereby inhibiting their function. This problem usually occurs in women with Sjögren's syndrome, systemic lupus erythematosus (SLE), or a less well-defined clinical syndrome also suggestive of autoimmunity. Chymopapain anaphylaxis, reactions to latex, and systemic reactions to insect stings are all IgE-mediated hypersensitivity responses.

8. The answer is C [V G 2]. Intravenous glucagon has a positive inotropic and chronotropic effect. In those patients taking β blocker medications, an even greater increase in blood pressure may occur. The other therapeutic agents are relatively ineffective in the face of β-adrenergic blockade.

9. The answer is D [VII E 4 a]. The highest prevalence of latex allergy occurs in children with spina bifida. This appears to be related to early surgical intervention with constant exposure to the natural latex in catheters and tubing. Surgeons and operating room nurses are at increased risk of developing latex allergy. Bronchial asthma, fibrosing alveolitis, diabetes mellitus, and inflammatory bowel disease are not commonly associated with the occurrence of latex allergy.

10–13. The answers are: 10-B [III F 4], **11-C** [III F 3 a–c], **12-A** [III F 1], **13-C** [III F 3 a–c]. Immunotherapy, which significantly ameliorates symptoms and is used when allergic rhinitis is severe, when medical complications or intolerance to medication occurs, and when various types of medications have been only partially successful, would be recommended for the 34-year-old woman.

Antihistamine–decongestant preparations remain the initial drugs of choice for the treatment of allergic rhinitis. These preparations usually control mild-to-moderate symptoms, such as those experienced by the 20-year-old man and the 8-year-old boy; however, some patients experience intolerable side effects, such as drowsiness. The second-generation antihistamines terfenadine and astemizole are less likely to cause such sedation.

Nasal cromolyn sodium, which in some cases is as effective as an antihistamine–decongestant in treating seasonal allergic rhinitis, could have been recommended for the 8-year-old boy with seasonal symptoms. Administration of nasal cromolyn sodium, however, requires the patient to carry a nasal pump and administer the treatment approximately four times daily before expected antigen exposure, making it inconvenient for some patients. Patients who cannot tolerate oral medications may respond to cromolyn sodium, however. It is somewhat effective for perennial allergic rhinitis, but is more often used to alleviate acute seasonal symptoms.

Topical adrenergic preparations are used for no longer than 2–3 days to treat acute nasal congestion that could lead to sinusitis. They are used sometimes before air travel by individuals who are susceptible to barotitis media.

Antigen avoidance is most successful when a single antigen can be identified as the causative agent. Because the 10-year-old girl developed symptoms only after being exposed to her friend's kitten, it is likely that avoiding cats will alleviate her symptoms. Antigen avoidance is not feasible for all patients, however. For example, while a patient may be able to avoid animal dander indoors, the avoidance of multiple outdoor antigens is likely to prove difficult, if not impossible. Nonetheless, sensible environmental precautions help to limit exacerbation of symptoms.

Chapter 8

Infectious Diseases

Thomas Fekete

I. **GENERAL PRINCIPLES OF HUMAN–MICROBE INTERACTION.** The normal human body harbors a complex microbial ecosystem. Generally, these **commensal** organisms (referred to as the **indigenous flora**) are considered to be nonpathogenic. Infection and disease may result, however, when the body is challenged by a known pathogen or when the body's defense system is disturbed, allowing uncontrolled growth or invasion by the indigenous flora.

A. **Normal human–microbe ecology.** Microorganisms can interact with humans in the following ways:

1. **Most indigenous organisms seldom cause disease.** Many of the organisms normally found on the skin and mucous membranes (e.g., *Staphylococcus epidermidis* and *Corynebacterium* species) are ubiquitous but may cause disease in unusual settings (e.g., when host defenses are significantly impaired or when artificial material, such as a catheter or a prosthetic joint, is present).

2. **Some indigenous organisms may cause disease in other body sites.** Many bacteria that normally exist in one body site may cause morbidity elsewhere. For example, α-hemolytic (viridans) streptococci are commensals in the oropharynx but can cause endocarditis if they are inoculated into the blood and settle on a previously damaged heart valve. Also, enteric aerobes and anaerobes, which normally exist in high density in the colon, can cause peritonitis and abscess formation if the colon is perforated and these bacteria spill into the abdominal cavity.

3. **Transient organisms may cause disease.** The body's normal flora may allow the temporary growth of certain microbes, which disappear spontaneously but may cause disease while present. For example, patients with invasive meningococcal disease first have pharyngeal carriage of *Neisseria meningitidis,* but only a tiny fraction of individuals with meningococci in the pharynx ever develop systemic disease.

4. **Pathogenic organisms usually cause disease.** Most viruses, as well as *Chlamydia* and *Rickettsia,* rarely are isolated from humans except during or following an acute illness. Some pathogenic bacteria include *Brucella* and *Salmonella* species, *Neisseria gonorrhoeae,* and *Mycobacterium tuberculosis.*

B. **Host defense mechanisms.** The human body has many ways of defending itself from potentially pathogenic microorganisms.

1. **Anatomic barriers** are integral in preventing infection. These include physical barriers, such as intact skin and mucous membranes, and functional barriers, such as the muscular protection of the glottis and bladder neck.
   a. **Herpetic whitlow** occurs when broken skin comes into contact with herpes simplex virus.
   b. Similarly, nonsterile intravenous injection of drugs may allow skin flora to enter the bloodstream and lead to the development of **endocarditis.**
   c. Mechanical devices, such as indwelling bladder catheters and endotracheal tubes, allow **bacterial colonization** of normally sterile sites; this colonization may lead to infection.

TABLE 8-1. The Human Immune System

Component	Source	Function	Causes of Diminished Function	Opportunistic Organisms
Cellular immunity				

Neutrophil	Bone marrow	Phagocytosis; acute inflammation	Genetic disorders
			  Chronic granulomatous disease
			  Myeloperoxidase deficiency
			Acquired causes
			  Cytotoxic therapy
			  Leukemia
			  Aplastic anemia
			  Drug reaction
				Endogenous flora; enteric bacilli; *Pseudomonas aeruginosa*; *Candida* species; *Aspergillus* species

Eosinophil	Bone marrow	Modulate hypersensitivity reactions to multicellular parasites	Idiopathic; corticosteriod therapy	None known
Monocyte/ macrophage	Bone marrow	Release cytokines; interact with lymphocytes; phagocytosis	Cytotoxic therapy; lymphoreticular malignancy	
T lympho- cyte	Thymus; bone marrow	Modulate activity of B lymphocytes, macrophages, and T lymphocytes	Genetic disorders; autoimmune disease; lymphoreticular malignancy; AIDS; organ transplantation; corticosteroid therapy	*Mycobacterium* species; fungi; *Listeria* species; *Nocardia* species
Humoral immunity				
Antibody	Plasma cells	Facilitate phagocytosis; inactivate toxins	Genetic disorders; multiple myeloma; splenectomy	Viruses; pyogenic bacteria
Complement	Liver	Enhance phagocytosis; direct cell destruction	Genetic disorders; severe liver disease	*Neisseria* species (especially with deficiency of complement components (C5–C9)

AIDS = acquired immune deficiency syndrome.

2. **Cellular immunity.** The cellular arm of the immune system has several components (Table 8-1).
   a. **Neutrophils** (polymorphonuclear leukocytes) are phagocytic cells that are impor- tant for ingesting and killing microorganisms that breach normal body defenses.
      (1) When neutrophils are reduced substantially in number (a condition termed

neutropenia), pyogenic bacteria and fungi that are commensals of the skin or gut, such as *Escherichia coli* and *Candida albicans,* can cause serious infections.

(2) Functional abnormalities of neutrophils may result in syndromes of varying type and severity.

  (a) For example, patients with **chronic granulomatous disease,** which is due to a deficiency of nicotinamide adenine dinucleotide phosphate (NADPH) oxidase, are prone to infections by catalase-producing organisms such as *Staphylococcus aureus,* many gram-negative bacilli, and fungi. These infections start early in life and tend to be severe and recurrent.

  (b) Conversely, patients with **lazy leukocyte syndrome** tend to have mild, easily treatable infections associated with the upper respiratory tract.

b. **Monocytes** and their tissue forms, **macrophages,** also are important for the ingestion of pathogenic microbes as well as for the production of cytokines, interleukins, and other modulators of the immune system. Some microorganisms are resistant to macrophage killing. After phagocytosis, these bacteria may be protected from those antibiotics that do not penetrate macrophages. Examples of these bacteria are *Salmonella, Legionella,* and *Mycobacterium* species.

c. **Lymphocytes** are the third component of the cellular immune system. **T lymphocytes,** or **T cells,** have many roles in modulating the activities of other T cells, monocytes, and **B lymphocytes,** or **B cells** (see Chapter 7 I B 2).

  (1) Antigen-specific T cells are responsible for delayed hypersensitivity and for controlling infections caused by a variety of agents, including species of *Mycobacterium, Pneumocystis,* and *Cryptococcus.*

  (2) T cells are broadly divided into **helper T (Th) cells** and **suppressor T (Ts) cells** based on their effect on the immune system in terms of augmenting or diminishing the immune response. Th cells (e.g., CD4 cells) tend to up-regulate the immune response; Ts cells (e.g., CD8 cells) tend to down-regulate the immune response.

  (3) T cells also seem to have a pivotal role in the manifestations of autoimmune diseases.

3. **Humoral immunity** (see Table 8-1)

a. **Antibody-mediated immunity** involves the production of antibody by activated B cells, which are stimulated by exposure to the proper antigen and to Th cells to differentiate into **plasma cells.** Plasma cells essentially are factories for the production of immunoglobulins, which they excrete into their environment. Immunoglobulins facilitate phagocytosis and activate complement and, thus, lead to a more rapid clearance of the antigen. The absence or profound deficiency of immunoglobulins leads to recurrent infections caused primarily by encapsulated bacteria (e.g., *Haemophilus influenzae* and *Streptococcus pneumoniae*).

b. Another host defense is provided by the **complement system**—a cascading series of glycoproteins that either tag foreign material to promote phagocytosis or directly damage or destroy infective organisms. Severe complement deficiencies can predispose a person to infections. For example, the reduced production of one or more of the late complement components (i.e., C5–C9) permits overwhelming neisserial infections.

C. **Thermal regulation.** One of the most recognized features of infectious diseases, regardless of body site of infection is the elevation of body temperature.

1. **Normal regulation of body temperature.** The normal core body temperature is approximately 37° (± 1°) C. Monocytes secrete a polypeptide called **interleukin-1 (IL-1),** which stimulates the hypothalamus to raise the body's temperature **set point.** The rise in set point causes alterations in circulation, metabolism, and perspiration, which ultimately lead to a rise in body temperature. Body temperature usually is measured by placing a thermometer in the mouth or the rectum, or it is measured directly from the tympanic membrane or the superior vena cava. (Mouth breathing or the recent ingestion of very hot or cold beverages may reduce the ac-

curacy of orally measured temperature readings, which tend to be 0.5°C–1.0°C lower than rectal temperatures). Temperature readings above 38.3°C are considered abnormal. **Hypothermia** (body temperature below 36°C) is sometimes a response to overwhelming infection, especially in neonates and the elderly.

2. **Conditions associated with fever.** Almost any infectious process may be accompanied by fever, although the absence of fever should not exclude the consideration of an infection. Fever may also occur with myocardial infarction, pulmonary embolism, drug reactions, autoimmune disease [e.g., systemic lupus erythematosus (SLE), rheumatoid arthritis, and temporal arteritis], or tumor (e.g., lymphoma and renal cell carcinoma). The actual pattern of fever rarely helps to narrow the range of etiologic factors that may be causing the fever.

3. **Fever management. Antipyretic drugs** (e.g., aspirin, acetaminophen, and nonsteroidal anti-inflammatory agents) can modify a fever, but seldom completely suppress a fever caused by infection. When fever is extreme (i.e., > 42°C) or when the tachycardia and circulatory changes accompanying fever are poorly tolerated, it is wise to try to reduce body temperature. In most settings, however, fever is merely uncomfortable, and the attempt to eliminate it may be comparatively more unpleasant because of the shaking and sweating that are sometimes associated with fever lysis.

4. **Beneficial effects of fever.** Fever does play a role in host defense because many infective microbes prefer lower temperatures; however, the clinical significance of this protection is unknown. In addition, some elements of the immune system are more efficient at higher temperatures whereas others are less efficient. The net effect on recovery from infection is not known.

D. **Microbial virulence factors** are important in determining the likelihood of infection. To infect a host, microorganisms or their products must adhere to host tissue.

1. **Some microbes invade host cells or breach barriers** to reach the susceptible body sites and, along the way, avoid or overcome host defenses. In some situations (e.g., chickenpox or measles), microbes can easily infect an otherwise healthy individual who has normal host defenses but no prior exposure to the microbe.

2. **Some microbes cause disease at the contact site with the host.** An example is *Giardia lamblia,* which is confined to the lumen of the small bowel and causes abdominal cramping and diarrhea.

3. **Some microbes have a special ability to produce a toxin or virulence factor** to cause disease. For example, a toxin elaborated by some strains of *S. aureus* [toxic shock syndrome toxin 1 (TSST-1)] is responsible for **toxic shock syndrome** (TSS; see VII D 1 a).

4. **In some situations, microbes work in groups to cause disease** when an individual organism lacks an essential virulence or survival quality to act alone. An example is **delta hepatitis,** which can occur only in the presence of ongoing hepatitis B infection.

5. Because of the selective pressures induced by using antimicrobial agents to treat or prevent infections in man and animals, **microorganisms that are resistant to antibiotics may have a propensity for causing infections.** This is especially true where antibiotic use is widespread, such as in hospitals and nursing homes.

E. **Epidemiologic considerations.** In addition to host and microbial characteristics, environmental circumstances also help determine the nature and severity of an infection.

1. **Contagious diseases** are spread from person to person through direct physical contact (e.g., syphilis) or by infectious aerosols (e.g., tuberculosis). Smallpox was eradicated successfully in part because preventive measures could be directed to potential contacts of documented cases.

2. **Vectors and fomites**
   a. When an animal is a host or carrier of a disease without becoming ill itself, that animal is a **vector** of infection. Most vectors are insects or arthropods. In gen-

eral, infections that are related to animals or their products (e.g., meat, milk, or eggs) are called **zoonoses.**

   b. Fomites are inanimate objects capable of spreading infection. Fomites are most commonly identified in hospitals where enhanced patient susceptibility and a high concentration of virulent organisms coexist.

3. Geography. Some diseases occur exclusively or at substantially greater frequency in certain areas. For example, malaria no longer is transmitted by mosquito bites in the United States. When considering such a disease in a diagnosis, a history of travel to or residence in an appropriate area is important. Duration of exposure can also be important, such as in filariasis, which leads to elephantiasis only after repeated exposure to the mosquito vector over a period of months to years.

4. Season. Many infections occur more commonly during a particular time of the year. This may be due to certain activities that might expose an individual to risk and that are seasonal in nature (e.g., hunting and fishing) or to environmental factors that favor the growth of the microbe or its insect vector.

   a. Influenza infections occur most commonly in the winter.

   b. Enterovirus meningitis tends to occur in the summer.

II. USE OF ANTI-INFECTIVE THERAPY

A. General principles. Because the use of antibiotics can be life-saving, it is important to recognize when to initiate treatment. However, any type of medical intervention presents potential hazards, and the indiscriminate use of antibiotics is no exception. In general, there are three circumstances that prompt antimicrobial therapy.

1. Organism-based treatment

   a. When cultures or stains from a patient demonstrate a credible microorganism, appropriate antibiotic treatment is initiated.

   (1) For example, a urethral exudate with gram-negative intracellular diplococci is presumptive evidence for gonorrheal urethritis, and chemotherapy is warranted on the basis of this test alone.

   (2) Blood cultures positive for *Streptococcus sanguis* in a patient with a history of mitral valve disease and a fever call for prompt therapy for bacterial endocarditis.

   b. Techniques for recognizing specific antigens of microorganisms also may be used to help initiate therapy. An example is the finding of cryptococcal antigens in the cerebrospinal fluid (CSF) in a patient with chronic meningitis.

   c. Isolation of an organism allows in vitro testing of antibiotic susceptibility, but, for many microbes, resistance patterns are predictable enough to permit treatment without these further tests.

2. Syndrome-based treatment. Syndrome-based treatment is initiated when all three of the following conditions pertain:

   a. The clinical picture strongly suggests specific organ disease.

   b. The tests needed to make a microbiologic diagnosis are not available or practical.

   c. The most likely causative organisms all respond to the same treatment.

   (1) For example, if gram-negative diplococci are not found on the Gram stain of a urethral exudate, therapy for nongonococcal urethritis may be initiated.

   (2) Several organisms cause nongonococcal urethritis, and distinguishing among them is unnecessary because they all respond to tetracycline. Patients with recurrent or unresponsive disease, however, may require further diagnostic evaluation.

3. Empiric therapy is given when the diagnosis is uncertain but clinical experience suggests that the patient outcome in a particular setting is improved with antimicrobial therapy.

a. Generally, empiric therapy is initiated while awaiting the results of diagnostic tests to identify a specific causative organism.

b. Fever often develops as the first sign of infection in patients with severe neutropenia from cancer therapy. These patients may succumb to their infection before final reports are received from the laboratory. Thus, antimicrobial therapy should begin at the first sign of fever.

c. **Prophylaxis** is used when a specific infection or complication is to be avoided. Generally, this form of empiric therapy is restricted to a fixed and brief period during which there is a risk of infection. Examples include the use of penicillin before dental procedures in patients with heart valve disease and the use of perioperative antibiotics in surgery.

B. **Dosage and route.** When considering the use of antibiotics, the appropriate dosage and route of administration must be established.

1. **Dosage**
   a. Dosing usually is based on pharmacologic and clinical data related to the size and age of the patient, the desired level of the drug in the target tissue, the drug's rate of elimination (often estimated by examining kidney and liver function), and the expected penetration of the drug into the infected tissue.
   b. Guidelines for proper dosing usually are provided with the drug itself and are widely available in publications. Occasionally, blood or tissue levels of the drug must be measured to ensure safe and effective concentrations.

2. **Route.** In general, parenterally administered (i.e., intravenous or intramuscular) drugs are more reliably absorbed than orally administered drugs and are used:
   a. In patients who cannot tolerate orally administered drugs
   b. In patients in whom institution of therapy is urgent
   c. When no oral form of the drug exists

C. **Cost** of antibiotic treatment has become more important with the proliferation and availability of similar drugs and increased attention to cost containment. When all other factors are equal, cost may influence which drug is prescribed. With intravenously given drugs, there is a cost of diluents and of labor involved in preparing and infusing the drugs. The cost of administration is lower with intramuscularly given drugs and is lowest with oral agents.

D. **Specific antibiotic spectrum.** The range, or **spectrum,** of microorganisms inhibited or killed by an antibiotic is an important consideration in deciding which drug to use. The results of in vitro testing are helpful in selecting an antibiotic that is most likely to be effective against an infective organism. Even when the particular organism has not been tested, it may be assumed—on the basis of either local patterns of antibiotic susceptibility or general experience in treating certain syndromes—that a given drug is likely to be effective in that setting. However, susceptibility patterns merit close scrutiny because they may change over time.

E. **Toxicity and side effects.** Although life-threatening toxicity rarely occurs with antibiotic treatment, the specific risks of each drug administered should be familiar to the physician so that side effects can be anticipated and minimized.

1. **Allergic reactions**—sometimes fatal—can occur with almost any pharmaceutical agent but are more common with the β-**lactam antibiotics** and sulfonamides than with other antimicrobials.

2. **Chloramphenicol,** which is seldom used, is associated with **bone marrow suppression,** including irreversible aplastic anemia.

3. Many drugs can cause **renal dysfunction,** the most prominent being the **aminoglycosides.** This toxicity is reversible and usually of minor clinical significance, but recovery may take weeks or months. In rare instances, dialysis may be needed.

4. **Abnormalities in blood coagulation** (e.g., changes in the levels of clotting factors or in the number or function of platelets) have been associated with several β-**lactam antibiotics** and sometimes result in clinically significant bleeding.

5. **Ototoxicity** is an infrequent but potentially debilitating side effect of **aminoglyco-sides** and **vancomycin.** Either auditory or vestibular impairment can occur; often, it is irreversible.

F. **Adult immunization**

1. It is important for adults to have immunity to **all of the childhood diseases except pertussis.** (Although pertussis may occur in adults, it usually is mild, and the available vaccines are not well tolerated when administered to adults.)

   a. If there has been no previous vaccination, a series of tetanus and diphtheria vaccines should be administered. Booster doses of tetanus should be given every 10 years to all adults. Toxoid may be given earlier if an individual has a tetanus-prone wound and the previous dose of toxoid was given more than 5 years earlier. Passive immunization with tetanus immunoglobulin is indicated if a wound has been extensively contaminated with dirt. Diphtheria toxoid is usually coadministered with tetanus.

   b. Killed poliovirus vaccine should be given to adults who are not already immune—especially those with children who are due to receive live poliovirus vaccine.

   c. Because rubella in a pregnant woman can result in a devastating infection of the fetus, all women of childbearing age should be immune to rubella. Serum tests for antibody to rubella are widely available to help identify adults who need vaccination.

   d. If there is no history of mumps or measles illness or vaccination, the appropriate live virus vaccines for these illnesses should be given.

2. Special vaccination issue pertain to the **elderly** and to **chronically ill** patients, especially those with cardiac or pulmonary disease. All such patients should receive **pneumococcal vaccination** once and, in the appropriate season, should have annual **influenza vaccination.**

3. **Travelers** to countries where **yellow fever** is endemic (most of tropical Africa and South America) should receive this vaccine. Cholera and typhoid immunizations may be recommended for certain travelers. Hepatitis A vaccine is recommended for travelers who expect to encounter poor sanitary facilities, especially those resulting in human fecal contamination of food or water.

4. Universal immunity to **hepatitis B** and **varicella** are current public health goals. Both vaccines can be given safely to people who are already immune by virtue of prior infection or vaccination. Both vaccines are less effective in people with impaired immune status. Because varicella vaccine is a live virus vaccine, it should be used cautiously or not at all in patients with known advanced immunodeficiency.

   a. Adults who have durable immunity to varicella-zoster virus from a clinical bout of chickenpox in childhood do not need vaccination.

   b. Adults with no history of chickenpox or no serologic evidence of immunity should receive two doses of vaccine.

   c. Adults without a history of hepatitis B or vaccination for it should receive three doses of vaccine.

5. **Asplenic individuals** should have **pneumococcal** and **meningococcal vaccinations,** even though protection from these infections is incomplete. In preparation for elective splenectomy, immunizations should be performed before surgery.

III. **EFFECTIVE USE OF THE MICROBIOLOGY LABORATORY.** To maximize the usefulness of any microbiology laboratory, it is necessary to be familiar with its specific capabilities and procedures. The following are general guidelines.

A. **Obtaining and handling specimens**

1. **Fresh specimens are superior to old ones.** This is especially true when quantitative results are important (e.g., colony counts of urine cultures) or when the target organism is fragile (e.g., protozoal trophozoites in stools). If immediate delivery of a specimen is not possible, proper maintenance of the specimen should be ensured until it can be processed.

    a. Some bacteria (e.g., *N. gonorrhoeae*) are sensitive to cold and should not be refrigerated.

    b. Specimens to be cultured for anaerobes should be maintained in a prereduced, oxygen-free environment or in a syringe without any air and without a needle. They should be transported to the laboratory for immediate plating.

2. **Large specimens are better than small ones.** In most cases it is preferable to have adequate material to culture than to have only a swab—the laboratory technologist should have the final choice as to which portion to use. Sometimes, multiple specimens are needed to identify microorganisms (e.g., *M. tuberculosis*) that are shed infrequently or in small numbers.

3. **Biological hazards should be labeled and handled properly.** Laboratories have instituted **universal precautions** and treat all specimens as potentially infectious. Some bacteria and fungi may be especially hazardous in pure culture (e.g., *Brucella, Francisella,* and *Coccidiodes*), and the laboratory should be notified if these organisms are suspected clinically so that appropriate care can be taken.

B. **Interpreting negative and positive cultures.** When a diagnosis rests on identifying an organism obtained from a clinical specimen, it is crucial to recognize what represents simple contamination by other body flora or inanimate sources. Laboratory results are more credible when a specimen has been stained and shown to contain the appropriate cell type (e.g., neutrophil or alveolar macrophage in sputum) and lacks evidence of contamination (e.g., squamous epithelial cells in sputum or urine). When care and attention have been lavished on a good specimen, almost any positive result is significant.

1. If antibiotics have been administered, the potential for positive cultures is reduced, and the predictive value of negative cultures also is diminished.

2. When cultures are truly negative, the use of special media and growth conditions should be considered. Supplementary nutrients or suppression of other organisms may be necessary to permit growth and identification.

3. Cultures that are repeatedly positive for a given organism may be more convincing than a single positive specimen. This is especially true for blood cultures. Specimens taken from normally sterile sites such as CSF and joint and pleural fluids usually are reliable when obtained aseptically. However, if they are culture-positive for skin or mucous membrane commensals, repeat cultures can be helpful.

4. Corroborative tests such as antigen detection, specific nucleic acid probes, and seroconversion (i.e., the development of antibodies to a pathogen) can establish the significance of a single culture-positive specimen or establish a diagnosis when cultures have not been obtained or are negative.

C. **Interpreting antimicrobial susceptibility tests.** In vitro testing of antimicrobial susceptibility can provide useful information about the specific microbe causing an infection. For many bacteria, these tests can be accomplished rapidly, with results sometimes available in hours. However, **the conditions used in susceptibility testing do not necessarily simulate conditions in the patient.**

1. The results of susceptibility testing may show the microorganism to be susceptible, intermediately susceptible, or resistant to the drug being tested. This information presupposes that the drug concentration at the site of infection will be similar to what usually is found in serum. It also assumes that the organism will be inhibited or killed at the infection site if it is exposed to such a drug concentration.

2. Another way to assess susceptibility is to determine the actual concentration of antibiotic needed to inhibit the microorganism. This usually is done by exposing the microbe to varying concentrations of the drug and observing which is the lowest one to inhibit growth (called the **minimum inhibitory concentration,** or **MIC**). The lower the MIC, the more susceptible the organism. In some instances, however, clinical experience shows that a drug is ineffective despite in vitro data that suggest it would work. For example, cephalosporins are not useful in treating infections caused by methicillin-resistant *S. aureus,* although blood and tissue levels in excess of the MIC are easily achievable.

3. Direct measurement of serum or tissue levels of the drug being used may be desirable so that the dosage can be adjusted to avoid toxicity and to maximize therapeutic benefit. This is especially true for patients who may have less predictable blood or tissue levels of antibiotic due to altered drug metabolism or excretion secondary to renal or hepatic dysfunction.

IV. RISK FACTORS FOR INFECTION.
Sometimes it is possible to identify patient characteristics that modify the likelihood or severity of an infection. Although some of these risk assignments have been accepted without adequate validation, there is sound evidence that a substantially increased risk of infection exists among certain groups of individuals. In general, the intensity or frequency of exposure and the degree of susceptibility correlate with potential hazard of infection.

A. Diabetes. In general, diabetic patients are not known to have infections more frequently than individuals without glucose intolerance. However, there are a few significant differences.

1. Diabetic patients tend to have more **foot and lower leg ulcers,** which may become infected. When such soft tissue infections occur, they are more likely to involve gram-negative rods, and they are more difficult to cure than those occurring in nondiabetic individuals.

2. Diabetic patients have more **genital infections** with *Candida* species—especially vulvovaginal candidiasis. Urinary tract infections may be more common and more severe in diabetic patients, and the increased morbidity probably is related to bladder dysfunction in those patients with diabetic neuropathy. It is often recommended that urinary tract infections be more vigorously treated in diabetic patients.

3. Some **rare diseases** occur almost exclusively in diabetic patients.
   a. **Malignant otitis externa** is a painful, rapidly progressive, and locally destructive disease of the external auditory canal and may extend to the temporal bone and the brain. *Pseudomonas aeruginosa* is the causative agent (see V B 1 a.)
   b. **Rhinocerebral mucormycosis** is a fungal infection that starts in the nose or paranasal sinuses and is locally destructive. It is found in patients with severe metabolic acidosis, such as diabetic patients with ketoacidosis.
   c. **Synergistic gangrene** is a soft tissue infection, which often is due to streptococci and obligate anaerobes. It may involve the skin or the underlying fascial structures and tends to progress relentlessly unless treated with extensive surgical debridement.

B. Alcoholism. Acute and chronic alcohol use can impair neurologic function and decrease the efficacy of neutrophils. In addition, chronic alcohol use can result in severe organ damage, especially to the liver.

1. Alcoholics have a greater incidence of pneumococcal, aspiration, and gram-negative bacillary **pneumonias** than the general population. Tuberculosis, anaerobic lung abscess, and empyema also are more common.

2. When ascites is present, alcoholics may develop **spontaneous bacterial peritonitis,** a bacterial infection of ascitic fluid that occurs in the absence of bowel perforation. This infection, usually caused by gram-negative aerobic bacilli or enterococci, also occurs in nonalcoholic patients with ascites.

C. **Injection drug use.** Several infections are more common in injection drug users than in comparable individuals who do not use such substances. **Fever** in an injection drug user must be evaluated carefully because pyogenic bacterial infections can progress rapidly if treatment is delayed.

1. **Infections related to unsterile techniques.** Injection drug users are prone to a variety of suppurative complications because, in most cases, the preparation of the drug is not aseptic, the equipment is not sterile, and skin cleansing is inadequate.
   a. The most serious infection is **bacterial endocarditis,** which often occurs on the tricuspid valve (a valve rarely infected in other populations). Usually, the bacterium responsible is *Staphylococcus aureus.*
   b. **Superficial skin infections** are common, and infectious arthritis—usually caused by *P. aeruginosa* or *S. aureus*—is seen frequently.
   c. **Tetanus,** although rare, occurs more frequently in injection drug users because they are more likely to have improperly cleaned wounds and low levels of immunity.

2. **Infections related to sharing needles.** Some contagious diseases can be transmitted efficiently via the small amount of blood in used needles and syringes. For example, the incidence of hepatitis B and human immunodeficiency virus (HIV) infection is increased in injection drug user populations. Hepatitis C and delta hepatitis are also more common.

D. **Homosexuality**

1. **Homosexual men.** The increased risk of infections in sexually active homosexual men was first recognized in the mid-1970s. The etiologic agents include *Shigella* species, *N. gonorrhoeae, G. lamblia, Chlamydia trachomatis, Entamoeba histolytica, Treponema pallidum,* hepatitis A virus, and human papillomavirus (HPV). HIV, hepatitis B virus, and non-A, non-B hepatitis virus have been recognized as being hyperendemic among American homosexual men, especially those living in urban communities. The incidence of many of these infections has declined recently as sexual practices have changed in response to the HIV epidemic.

2. **Homosexual women.** The incidence of infectious diseases is not known to be increased among homosexual women.

E. **Occupation** may predispose workers to certain infections by permitting exposure to various infective agents.

1. In some cases, the risk of occupation-related infection is unpredictable, as in the outbreaks of **Pontiac fever,** which were related to the aerosolization of *Legionella pneumophila*–contaminated water via air-conditioning ducts throughout an office building.

2. In other cases, the risk of infection is influenced by factors outside the immediate work environment. For example, the risk of brucellosis among slaughterhouse workers is determined largely by the number of livestock infected and to a lesser extent by the degree of the worker's exposure to the blood of infected livestock.

3. When an increased risk is predictable, certain preventive measures can be instituted, such as the immunization of veterinarians against rabies.

F. **Internal prostheses.** The advances in modern surgery have made it possible to replace malfunctioning body parts, most notably joints and heart valves. When a prosthesis (or any foreign material) is inserted into the body, there is a possibility that an infection will develop at the site of insertion. Because of the human body's reaction to foreign material, a prosthetic organ is susceptible to infection by a greater number and variety of organisms than is the native, damaged organ. In addition, the clinical presentation of these infections may be atypical, and the time interval between surgery and any manifestation of sepsis may be long (e.g., many years). *S. epidermidis* is involved in many of these infections. In most cases, bacteria are inoculated at the time of surgery, although secondary hematogenous or percutaneous spread is possible.

1. **Diagnosis** of these infections depends on recognition of the characteristic clinical presentation. Infected joints almost always cause local pain and may be accompanied by erythema, loosening of the prosthesis, tenderness, and fever. Infected heart valves are almost always associated with fever and may be associated with valve dysfunction. These infections resemble native valve endocarditis.

2. **Therapy** is most successful when it includes the removal or replacement of the prosthetic device as well as systemic antibiotic treatment.

G. **Indwelling catheters**

1. Like internal prostheses, catheters such as intravenous or intra-arterial lines, bladder catheters, and endotracheal tubes offer sites of diminished host responsiveness. Furthermore, they provide communication between the external environment and the ordinarily sterile internal environment of the body.

2. In addition to intrinsic host factors, two important factors determine the likelihood of catheter-related infection: the duration of catheterization and the degree of asepsis maintained during catheterization. The duration of catheterization is the important factor in tracheal and urethral catheterization. Both factors are important for vascular catheterization.

   a. For long-term intravenous access with a surgically implanted catheter such as a Hickman silastic catheter, the risk of infection can be reduced, although not eliminated by meticulous attention to sterile technique during insertion and by avoiding site such as the groin that are prone to microbial contamination. These catheters are usually used for intravenous hyperalimentation or for venous access in seriously ill patients who may already be at high risk for infection.

   b. For the patient who needs intravenous access for a short or intermediate period of time and has catheters placed in the arms, the sites should be changed every 48–72 hours. When a catheter is placed in a central vein for temporary intravenous access, the maximal duration of the catheterization at a given site is not absolute; however, there is a substantial risk of infection after a few days, and catheters should be removed as soon as possible or at the first sign of sepsis.

   c. Vascular catheters generally are maintained with a high degree of care to avoid infection (e.g., aseptic dressing changes and the application of antibiotic-containing ointments to the insertion site); however, the importance of these measures in preventing infection is unknown.

   d. Despite the high risk of infection with the use of catheters, there is no indication for systemic antibiotic prophylaxis before or during catheterization.

H. **Granulocytopenia.** A specific risk that has been identified and carefully studied is related to the absence of adequate numbers of circulating neutrophils, or **granulocytopenia.** The risk of infection is inversely related to the duration and degree of granulocytopenia. Neutrophil counts greater than 500/μl are adequate protection from most opportunistic infection.

1. In most granulocytopenic patients, the underlying disease is a hematologic malignancy, although reduced neutrophil levels can be seen in association with aplastic anemia, drug-induced agranulocytosis, and cytotoxic chemotherapy.

2. The indigenous flora of granulocytopenic patients is likely to be altered during hospitalization and with the administration of antibiotics. The microflora most commonly associated with infections in granulocytopenic patients is derived from their indigenous flora. Bacteria such as *E. coli* and *P. aeruginosa* and fungi such as *C. albicans* are most commonly found.

3. Molds such as *Aspergillus* species may cause serious, often fatal, infections in granulocytopenic patients. Spores are inhaled from the environment.

4. Persistent **fever** is the hallmark of infection in the neutropenic patient. Because uncontrolled infection can result in rapid clinical deterioration in these patients, antimicrobials are given immediately after appropriate culture specimens are obtained.

5. Granulocytes released into the circulation after the use of colony-stimulating factors such as filgrastim are fully fuctional. Thus, granulocytopenia following chemotherapy of solid tumors is often brief and unaccompanied by serious infection.

I. **Corticosteroids** are used to treat a variety of medical problems. Although steroids typically cause an increase in the number of circulating white blood cells (WBCs), they have an immunosuppressive effect that is strongly dose related.

   1. The expression of this immunodeficiency is seen mostly in the increased incidence of infection usually controlled by cellular immunity (e.g., mycobacterial, fungal, nocardial, and cytomegaloviral infections). Steroids also alter some diagnostic tests, most notably the expression of delayed hypersensitivity.

   2. Steroids are used widely in transplantation procedures involving the kidney, heart, lung, liver, and bone marrow. In part, the infections experienced by these patients are related to corticosteroids and the other drugs (i.e., cyclosporine, tacrolimus, and azathioprine) used to prevent organ rejection.

J. **Neurologic deficits.** Neurologic dysfunction may predispose the patient to infection if such deficits cause body defenses to be more easily breached. The following are examples.

   1. Elimination of the gag reflex, whether by stroke or coma, may predispose the patient to aspiration of oral or gastric contents.

   2. A hypoesthetic limb may become secondarily infected; for example, diabetic neuropathy can result in skin ulceration and infection.

   3. When neuromuscular control of the bladder is lost, long-term catheterization (with its attendant complications) may be necessary.

K. **Age.** The likelihood of acquiring certain infections varies considerably with age. In general, the maturation of the immune system is responsible for the changing pattern of infections in early childhood, and the presence of other medical illnesses accounts for most of the changes in late adulthood. Diminished immune response in the elderly may predispose them slightly to infection. For example, there are lower titers of antibody to influenza virus after immunization in the elderly than in younger adults.

L. **Nosocomial infection.** Infections acquired after 2 or more days in the hospital are called nosocomial infections. Although they can involve any body site, they have some important common characteristics.

   1. Etiology and pathogenesis
      a. Residence in the hospital predisposes patients to skin and mucosal colonization by microbial flora different from that found in ambulatory patients. Specifically, enteric gram-negative rods (e.g., *E. coli, Klebsiella*) or *P. aeruginosa* are found in the alimentary tract and may spill over onto the skin or into the respiratory tree. The degree of illness influences the likelihood and rapidity of acquiring hospital flora.
      b. Antimicrobials given to prevent or treat infection may predispose patients to colonization and subsequent infection by hospital flora.
      c. Instrumentation in the hospital (e.g., endotracheal tubes, intravenous catheters) may bypass some of the natural host defenses.
      d. Failure to observe appropriate infection control measures may permit the dissemination of hospital flora. The most important route for such dissemination is on the hands of health care workers.

   2. Prevention
      a. Proper technique upon insertion of devices such as endotracheal tubes and in-

travenous catheters is essential. Prompt discontinuation when they are no longer needed may reduce the burden of nosocomial infections.

b. Hands must be washed or gloves changed between patient contacts.

c. Universal precautions have been instituted in health care facilities to reduce the risk of transmission of many potentially hazardous microbes, including blood-borne viruses such as HIV type 1 (HIV-1) and hepatitis B virus. It is extremely important to be familiar with the institutional policy of each health care facility in which one works. The essential principles of universal precautions are to treat each clinical specimen as potentially infective, to reduce sharp (e.g., needlestick) exposures, to avoid splashes of body fluids onto mucous membranes, and to dispose of potentially hazardous substances safely.

d. For some diseases, especially tuberculosis, **reduction of exposure of health care workers** and **other patients** to aerosol droplets exhaled by an infected patient is important. In the setting of documented or suspected infection by such organisms, a private room with appropriate ventilation is required. Reduction of time spent in the room and fastidious use of masks by the patient and health care workers can reduce risk of transmission in this setting

e. Protective isolation is intended to protect the patient from exogenous sources of colonization or infection. This measure is usually applied to patients with extensive burns or with extreme neutropenia. There are many different practices of protective isolation, but careful hand washing and use of gloves are probably most important.

3. Treatment. The use of empiric antibiotics to treat suspected infections is influenced by the duration of hospitalization and the likelihood that the infection was acquired nosocomially. Knowledge of the antimicrobial susceptibility patterns of nosocomial microbes can be especially useful.

V. SPECIFIC INFECTIONS ACCORDING TO BODY SITE

A. **Central nervous system (CNS) infections** are classified according to their location. They include meningitis, encephalitis, and intracranial abscess.

1. Meningitis

a. Acute meningitis is an inflammatory disease involving the arachnoid layer of the meninges and the fluid that circulates in the ventricles and the subarachnoid space—the **cerebrospinal fluid (CSF).**

(1) Classification. There are two major classifications of meningitis—**bacterial** and **aseptic.** In both forms, there is fever, headache, and stiff neck.

(a) In bacterial meningitis, the CSF has a pyogenic nature, with an elevated WBC, an increased fraction of neutrophils, an elevated protein level, and a normal or lowered glucose level.

(b) In aseptic meningitis, the CSF is characterized by a mildly elevated WBC, a normal or mildly elevated protein level, and a normal glucose level (i.e., greater than two thirds of the serum level).

(2) Etiology. The etiologic agents of meningitis can be divided into those causing bacterial meningitis and those causing aseptic meningitis.

(a) The **causes of bacterial meningitis vary with the age of the patient**—*E. coli* and *Streptococcus agalactiae* occur most frequently in infants, *H. influenzae* predominates in young children (aged 2 months to 6 years), *N. meningitidis* is most common in adolescents and young adults, and *S. pneumoniae* is most common in adults older than 25 years. *Listeria monocytogenes* is found most commonly in cancer patients and immunosuppressed individuals.

(b) **Aseptic meningitis** usually is a **viral disease** or may reflect an **inflammatory process adjacent to the meninges** (e.g., cerebritis, brain abscess, sinusitis, or otitis) The CSF in partially treated bacterial meningitis usually has a pyogenic nature, although antibiotics may modify the disease in such a way as to create an aseptic pattern. Drug hypersensitivity also may cause an aseptic meningitis (usually with a predominance of neutrophils in the WBC) and may occur rarely with ibuprofen or a variety of other agents.

(3) Clinical features. When bacteria cause meningitis, this manifestation usually is part of a **systemic, bacteremic infection.** An exception occurs when bacteria gain access to the meninges after trauma or surgery or via a bony defect (usually in the temporal area or the cribriform plate).

(a) With disease due to *H. influenzae* or *S. pneumoniae,* focal infection such as **pneumonia** or **otitis** also may be apparent.

(b) With disease due to *N. meningitidis,* there may be a characteristic systemic infection consisting of a **petechial** or **purpuric skin rash and hypotension,** which can develop rapidly.

(c) With aseptic meningitis due to echoviruses or coxsackieviruses, there may be a characteristic **rash resembling rubella** or a **vesicular** or **petechial rash.**

(4) Therapy

(a) Antibiotics have a significant impact on the outcome of bacterial meningitis. Without treatment, death is almost certain; with treatment, however, the mortality rate is reduced to approximately 20% of those patients who are not moribund at the time of diagnosis. Bactericidal antibiotics should be given in dosages that permit the drug to achieve killing levels in the CSF. Because there is a barrier to virtually all drugs, reducing drug penetration from the blood into the CSF, maximum tolerated systemic dosages should be given even at the end of the course (usually a total of 2 weeks).

(i) In adults, penicillin or ampicillin is effective against almost all of the common agents of bacterial meningitis.

(ii) If resistant organisms are found, one of the most broad-spectrum cephalosporins (e.g., cefotaxime or ceftriaxone) should be used. Often, treatment is initiated with one of these agents when the most likely etiologic factor is not apparent on Gram stain.

(iii) *S. pneumoniae* organisms resistant to penicillin (and sometimes cephalosporins) are being isolated more frequently. In the critically ill patient with suspected or established pneumococcal meningitis, vancomycin should be added to the regimen until susceptibility information is available.

(b) There is **no specific chemotherapy for aseptic meningitis.** Any underlying disease should be treated. If drug hypersensitivity is suspected, the offending agent should be stopped.

b. Chronic meningitis

(1) Etiology. The most common causes of chronic meningitis are tuberculosis, cryptococcal disease, malignancy, and sarcoidosis.

(2) Clinical features. Chronic meningitis may have an indolent presentation, with symptoms similar to acute meningitis or with altered mentation with or without fever. CSF abnormalities may progress with time if the underlying disease is untreated. In many of these diseases, the CSF glucose level is low. Chronic meningitis should be considered when a low CSF glucose level is noted in a patient who is found not to have acute bacterial meningitis.

(3) Therapy is directed at the underlying disease.

(a) Tuberculosis is treatable if there is not already extensive neurologic deterioration. Most **antituberculous drugs** (e.g., isoniazid and rifampin) achieve high levels in the CSF and are useful in the treatment of tuberculous meningitis.

(b) Cryptococcal meningitis may be difficult to treat and has a high relapse rate, especially when it occurs as a complication of HIV infection. Treatment usually begins with **amphotericin B alone or in combination**

with flucytosine, but there is a high rate of failure and relapse. **Triazole drugs** such as fluconazole are useful in the prevention of relapse and may be appropriate as first-line therapy as well.

  (c) **Malignancy** involving the meninges is difficult to treat and may require **neural radiotherapy** or **intrathecal chemotherapy.**

  (d) **Sarcoidosis** usually is treated with **corticosteroids.**

2. **Encephalitis** is an inflammatory process involving the brain.
   a. **Etiology.** Most encephalitides are caused by viruses, several of which are transmitted by the bites of infective mosquitoes.
   b. **Clinical features.** Encephalitis usually presents with altered mentation, seizures, or both. The CSF may be normal or have an aseptic pattern.
   c. **Diagnosis** is made by measuring rising titers of antibody to one of the encephalitis viruses in a patient with a compatible clinical syndrome. When **herpes simplex encephelitis** is suspected, brain biopsy and culture or empiric antiviral treatment is recommended. Successful treatment of herpes encephalitis depends on initiation of medications before there is extensive neurologic deterioration.
   d. **Differential diagnosis**
      (1) *Toxoplasma gondii* can cause encephalitis in a patient with diminished T-cell function e.g., due to acquired immune deficiency syndrome (AIDS) or post-transplant immunosuppressive therapy.
      (2) Some intoxications and immune diseases (e.g., systemic lupus erythematosus) may have a presentation indistinguishable from encephalitis.
      (3) Endocarditis also should be considered.
   e. **Therapy.** With the exception of herpes simplex encephalitis, the treatment of viral encephalitis is **supportive.** Toxoplasmosis, drug intoxication, endocarditis, and immune diseases are treatable, and associated encephalitis usually responds.

3. **Intracranial abscess.** Suppurative infections can involve the contents of the calvarium, usually by direct spread from an infected sinus or ear.
   a. **Etiology.** The bacteriology of intracranial infections reflects the types of organisms that cause disease in more superficial contiguous structures, such as streptococci and anaerobic bacteria. Abscesses can be localized to the extradural (also called epidural) or subdural spaces or in the brain parenchyma. Rarely, hematogenous spread of bacteria can give rise to intracranial abscesses. Less common agents are *Toxoplasma, Nocardia,* and *Cryptococcus* species, which usually are seen in immunocompromised patients.
   b. **Diagnosis. Computed tomography (CT)** or **magnetic resonance imaging (MRI)** of the brain is helpful in making the diagnosis. Early scans may be equivocal, but studies repeated within a few days are almost always positive, especially with the use of contrast.
   c. **Therapy.** Bacterial abscesses are treated with appropriate **antibiotics** that penetrate brain tissue well. These might include penicillin, chloramphenicol, and metronidazole. The usual treatment is given for infection by *Toxoplasma* (i.e., pyrimethamine and sulfadiazine), *Cryptococcus* (i.e., amphotericin B and flucytosine), or *Nocardia* (i.e., a sulfa drug with or without trimethoprim). Surgical excision or decompression is not always needed, but some patients, especially those with large lesions or slow response to treatment, require **serial aspirations** or more aggressive surgical debridement.

B. **Head and neck infections**

1. **Otitis.** Infections of the ear can involve any of the ear's three major anatomic areas—the outer, middle, or inner ear.
   a. **Outer ear infections** tend to be minor irritations of the external auditory canal. Topical antibiotic treatment is used for external otitis. An exception is **malignant otitis externa**—a destructive process most commonly found in diabetic patients (see IV A 3 a). Malignant otitis externa requires antibiotics that are effective against *Pseudomonas* infection plus surgical debridement and drainage.

b. Middle ear infection, or **otitis media,** typically is a disease of children and presents as ear pain and reduced auditory acuity. Otoscopy shows a dull, poorly mobile tympanic membrane with or without pus behind it. The most common causes are pneumococci, *Streptococcus pyogenes, Moraxella catarrhalis* and *H. influenzae.* In chronic cases, especially if multiple courses of antibiotics have been given, enteric gram-negative rods and anaerobes may be involved. Therapy for acute otitis media is amoxicillin, amoxicillin with clavulanic acid, trimethoprim with sulfamethoxazole, or an oral cephalosporin. Cultures and appropriate therapy are suggested for chronic otitis media.

c. Inner ear infections rarely are caused by bacteria. However, several viruses may be associated with a syndrome of **vertigo** with or without **tinnitus.** No treatment is helpful.

2. **Sinusitis.** The paranasal sinuses have continuous exposure to the external environment via the ostia in the nose. Under normal conditions, there are host defenses that maintain the sterile environment of the sinuses. However, when mucociliary clearance is interruped because of structural or functional abnormalities, infection can supervene. In addition, patients with mid- to late-stage HIV infection are prone to recurrent or chronic sinusitis.

   a. Etiology. As in middle ear infections, **virulent bacteria** such as pneumococci and *H. influenzae* are most likely to cause acute disease, and anaerobic or enteric organisms are associated with more chronic infections. Bacterial sinusitis may follow and mimic viral upper respiratory infections; however, only the bacterial infections go on to develop suppurative complications of the CNS.

   b. Diagnosis. Sinus radiography shows mucosal thickening or opacification or air–fluid levels in sinusitis. Tenderness and edema help to localize disease to the sinuses but are not present in all patients.

   c. Therapy
   (1) In mild cases, **antibiotics** (e.g., penicillin, cephalosporins, macrolides, or sulfa drugs) alone or in combination with decongestants are adequate.
   (2) Functional **endoscopic sinus surgery** can be useful in patients with repeated or persistent infection.

3. **Odontogenic infections,** the most common infections occurring in the oral cavity, usually are local and respond to simple measures such as draining abscesses, restoring carious teeth, and maintaining good oral hygiene. Sometimes, however, soft tissue infections in the mouth can dissect through tissue planes and involve deeper structures of the face or neck. Examples are **Ludwig's angina,** which is an infection extending to the floor of the mouth, and **retropharyngeal abscess,** which can track down to the mediastinum. The involved bacteria are streptococci and indigenous oral anaerobes.

4. **Eye infections.** Normally, the eyes also are resistant to infections.
   a. Conjunctivitis. Superficial infections of the conjunctiva usually are bacterial or viral and resolve spontaneously. An exception is **gonorrheal conjunctivitis**—a rare adult disease that must be treated vigorously.

   b. Keratitis is an infection of the cornea. Because the transparency of the cornea is crucial for vision, diagnostic tests such as bacterial and viral smears and cultures are warranted. Initial therapy is guided by the clinical picture, because a variety of organisms can cause keratitis, including *S. aureus, P. aeruginosa,* streptococci, numerous fungi, and herpes simplex virus. It is important to recognize keratitis caused by herpes simplex virus so that appropriate antiviral therapy can be instituted to prevent blindness.

   c. Endophthalmitis is an infection of the internal structures of the eye. It is most commonly caused by bacteria and may follow eye surgery or distant infection. Systemic and topical antibiotics, selected on the basis of clinical findings and Gram stain of ocular material, are administered to prevent irreversible destruction of the eye. However, the prognosis for normal visual acuity after endophthalmitis is poor.

C. **Respiratory tract infections**

1. **Upper respiratory infections.** Infections involving the nose, throat, larynx, airways, and adjacent structures are the most common causes of morbidity in the United States.

   a. **Etiology.** Upper respiratory infections almost invariably are viral; rarely is a specific cause sought or found.

   b. **Clinical features.** These "colds" and "flus" involve rhinorrhea, coryza, cough, a slight fever, and, sometimes, sore throat. During seasons when influenza is epidemic in a community, headache, cough, myalgia, and a more marked temperature elevation may suggest this diagnosis.

   c. **Therapy** for colds is symptomatic although influenza A virus infections may resolve more quickly when amantadine or rimantadine is administered.

   d. **Prevention** of most upper respiratory disease is difficult due to the ubiquity and extreme infectivity of most epidemic viruses. Influenza is preventable in many cases by timely administration of vaccine developed against the epidemic strains that exist during a particular season. Immunization should be directed at individuals who are at greatest risk for complications of upper respiratory infection, such as elderly or chronically ill individuals. Yearly immunization has a favorable impact on influenza morbidity and mortality.

2. **Pharyngitis** is common.

   a. **Etiology.** The major etiologic agents of pharyngitis are viruses, *Mycoplasma pneumoniae, Chlamydia pneumoniae,* and *S. pyogenes* (group A streptococci).

   b. **Clinical features** include **sore throat** that occurs with or without objective findings of erythema or exudate on the oropharynx or tonsils.

   c. **Therapy**

   (1) Although treatment for group A streptococcal pharyngitis may accelerate healing and reduce symptoms, the major purpose of treating this disorder is **prevention of subsequent rheumatic fever,** a rare sequela of streptococcal pharyngitis.

   (2) Viral pharyngitis does not improve with any known chemotherapy.

   (3) It is not known whether treatment of mycoplasmal or chlamydial pharyngitis is beneficial.

3. **Tracheobronchitis** is an infection of the airways.

   a. **Etiology.** Most cases of tracheobronchitis are associated with infection by mycoplasma or by **viruses,** such as influenza or parainfluenza virus (in adults) or respiratory syncytial virus (in young children). Bacteria may play a role, however, in patients with chronic obstructive pulmonary disease (COPD). *H. influenzae, S. aureus,* and *P. aeruginosa* are believed to be pathogenic in those with cystic fibrosis.

   b. **Clinical features and laboratory findings.** Cough with abundant, thick sputum is characteristic of tracheobronchitis. Fever, chest pain, and wheezing also may occur. If rales or consolidation is found, pneumonia is suggested. The WBC and chest x-ray are unchanged from baseline in uncomplicated tracheobronchitis.

   c. **Therapy.** Simple supportive measures usually suffice. Antibiotics usually are given to patients with COPD, although the benefit of such therapy is not clearly documented. Cystic fibrosis patients undergo chest physical therapy and receive antimicrobial agents according to sputum bacteriology.

4. **Pneumonia** is an infection of the alveoli, pulmonary interstitium, or both.

   a. **Etiology.** The causes of pneumonia are innumerable and include bacteria, viruses, fungi, and parasites. Identification of the specific cause of pneumonia, therefore, is necessary for effective treatment.

   b. **Clinical features and diagnosis**

   (1) **Patient history** may reveal an underlying condition. For example, the incidence of bacterial pneumonia is increased in association with COPD or alcoholism. Fever is usually, but not invariably, present. Evidence of extra fluid in the lungs is noted as rales or consolidation on physical examination and infiltrate on chest radiograph. In addition to information gained from

the patient's history, physical examination, and chest radiograph, the appearance of the sputum can be useful for making the appropriate diagnosis.

(2) Because of the **vast differential diagnosis,** it is helpful to consider pneumonia in two ways:

    (a) Whether it developed at home (**community-acquired**) or in a hospital or institution (**hospital-acquired** or **nosocomial**)

    (b) Whether it had a rapid onset with chills, fever, and cough (**classical**) or a more indolent onset (**atypical**)

c. Pneumonia syndromes

  (1) Classical community-acquired pneumonia

    (a) **Etiology.** This syndrome most frequently is caused by *S. pneumoniae.* However, *H. influenzae, M. catarrhalis,* and enteric gram-negative bacilli also can cause this clinical picture.

    (b) **Diagnosis.** Gram staining of expectorated sputum shows large numbers of neutrophils (i.e., > 25 per low-power field) and few squamous cells (< 10 per low-power field). The bacterial flora may be mixed, but often there is a predominance of one morphologic type such as the lancet-shaped gram-positive cocci, which appear in pairs in pneumococcal pneumonia.

    (c) **Therapy**

      (i) When the presentation is truly classic—with a single shaking chill, rust-colored sputum, and a moderate fever accompanied by a Gram stain suggesting pneumococci—penicillin is the drug of choice. The decision whether to give oral or parenteral therapy is influenced by the severity of the illness and the need for hospitalization.

      (ii) Erythromycin is used in penicillin-allergic patients when symptoms blend into those seen in the atypical form or when the Gram stain is inconclusive.

      (iii) If the Gram stain reveals gram-negative rods, therapy appropriate for *Haemophilus* or enteric gram-negative bacilli is given, usually in the hospital.

      (iv) If gram-negative cocci appear singly or in pairs, treatment should be directed toward *M. catarrhalis.*

  (2) Atypical community-acquired pneumonia

    (a) **Etiology.** This syndrome usually is caused by *M. pneumoniae* or *C. pneumoniae* although a variety of viruses may be responsible, including adenovirus, parainfluenza virus, and respiratory syncytial virus.

    (b) **Diagnosis.** Atypical community-acquired pneumonia is less severe than the classical form, with a less diagnostic sputum. Systemic symptoms (e.g., myalgia, arthralgia, and skin rash) are more prominent, and chest complaints (e.g., pleuritic pain and productive cough) are less marked in atypical pneumonia than in classical pneumonia. Gram stain shows some neutrophils and a variety of bacterial forms. Cultures seldom are diagnostic. Chest radiographs usually show patchy, bilateral infiltrates and little or no pleural effusion.

    (c) **Differential diagnosis**

      (i) Pulmonary aspiration of oral secretions can lead to an **aspiration pneumonia,** especially in a setting of diminished protection of the airways (e.g., following unconsciousness, a seizure, or vocal cord paralysis).

      (ii) Tuberculosis is another consideration in a case of a slowly evolving pulmonary infection. However, there usually is other evidence of tuberculosis (e.g., radiographic findings, an exposure history, or a positive acid-fast smear of the sputum).

      (iii) Legionnaires' disease also may occur in this way.

    (d) **Therapy**

      (i) When aspiration is suspected, an antibiotic with good activity against oral anaerobes and streptococci (e.g., penicillin or clindamycin) is suggested.

      (ii) Tuberculosis always is treated with combinations of antibiotics (see VII C 2).

      (iii) Legionnaires' disease usually responds to erythromycin, although some patients may require hospitalization for the intravenous administration of large doses.

(3) Classical (acute) hospital-acquired pneumonia.

    (a) Etiology. This syndrome can be caused by a variety of bacteria. Patients often are granulocytopenic, postoperative, or intubated. Because these patients usually have pharyngeal colonization by enteric gram-negative aerobes, the pneumonia is likely to involve these organisms. All risk factors should be taken into consideration when assessing these patients.

    (b) Diagnosis. Gram stain and culture of sputum are important in determining the organisms involved in this infection. Sometimes, more invasive tests such as bronchoscopy and lung biopsy are needed to confirm the diagnosis.

    (c) Therapy. When the Gram stain suggests inflammation and shows abundant gram-negative rods, recommended treatment is a β-lactam antibiotic with activity against a wide variety of enteric gram-negative organisms, with or without an aminoglycoside. Knowledge of susceptibility patterns in the hospital can help in choosing empiric therapy. When culture results are available, more specific therapy can be given. In neutropenic patients, broad coverage (including activity against *P. aeruginosa*) is used. If *Legionella* is seriously considered, erythromycin should be added.

5. Lung abscess

  a. Etiology. This infection may be the result of a pyogenic pneumonia caused by pathogens such as *S. aureus* or *S. pyogenes*. More commonly, however, lung abscess occurs as a late stage in the evolution of an untreated anaerobic or mixed flora pneumonia, such as occurs when oral or gastric contents enter the airway. Neurologic impairment of normal glottal reflexes predisposes patients to aspiration and lung abscess.

  b. Clinical features. Approximately half of the patients are afebrile, and some have long-standing constitutional complaints such as weight loss. A foul smelling sputum is highly suggestive of anaerobic infection.

  c. Therapy. Most lung abscesses drain into the tracheobronchial tree and can be cured with appropriate antimicrobial therapy, although the duration of therapy often is long.

6. Thoracic empyema

  a. Etiology. This infection also is related to underlying pneumonia. Any pyogenic pneumonia may give rise to a pleural effusion, which may become infected. Rarely, anaerobic empyema is the only manifestation of thoracic infection; presumably, this occurs as a sequela to an anaerobic pneumonia or lung abscess, which may not be apparent at the time of the empyema.

  b. Therapy

    (1) Noninfected parapneumonic effusions with a relatively low WBC and a pH above 7.2 usually resolve with systemic antimicrobial therapy.

    (2) Infected effusions, or those with a very low pH or a high WBC, usually require thoracostomy drainage.

D. | **Gastrointestinal infections**

1. Food poisoning syndromes represent a diverse collection of intoxications or infections associated with ingestion of food or beverage that has been contaminated with pathogenic organisms, toxins, or chemicals. Disregarding the purely chemical entities such as heavy metal poisoning, mushroom poisoning (see Chapter 5 IV D 5 b), and polychlorinated biphenyl (PCB) poisoning, food poisoning syndromes can be divided into those causing **gastrointestinal symptoms** and those causing **neurologic symptoms.**

a. **Gastrointestinal food poisoning** is the most familiar type of food poisoning (see also Chapter 5 IV D 4 and Table 5-1). Diarrhea, nausea, vomiting, and abdominal pain are the most common manifestations.

   (1) **Clinical categories** usually are based on the incubation period, the food vehicle, and the nature of the gastrointestinal complaint.

      (a) Preformed toxins give rise to the shortest onset syndromes. For example, the enterotoxin-mediated syndromes caused by staphylococci, *Bacillus cereus,* and *Clostridium perfringens* manifest within a few hours after ingestion of the contaminated food.

      (b) Diseases that depend on the growth of bacteria require a period of hours to days to manifest, and it may be difficult to relate the illness to a specific exposure. Cultures of various leftovers sometimes are helpful; in other cases, a careful recall of foods consumed by the patient is diagnostic.

   (2) **Therapy.** Almost all forms of gastrointestinal food poisoning are self-limited and remit spontaneously within 1 or 2 days.

b. **Neurologic food poisoning** syndromes are rare. However, it is usually critical to establish the diagnosis so that appropriate therapy can be instituted immediately.

   (1) **Botulism** is an intoxication caused by a preformed toxin of *Clostridium botulinum.* Although the toxin is destroyed by heating, the duration or degree of heating may be inadequate to do so. Often, a gastrointestinal prodrome occurs before the classic flaccid paralysis sets in.

   (2) **Fish poisoning.** The other major category of neurologic intoxications is related to seafood (see also Chapter 5 IV D 5 a).

      (a) Consumption of **contaminated shellfish** can result in two types of poisoning—paralytic and neurotoxic.

         (i) **Paralytic shellfish poisoning** results from contamination by neurotoxin-producing dinoflagellates of the genus *Gonyaulax.* This syndrome includes paresthesias followed by muscle weakness.

         (ii) **Neurotoxic shellfish poisoning** results from shellfish contamination by dinoflagellates of the genus *Gymnodinium.* This syndrome is characterized by paresthesias without muscle weakness. Consumption of fleshy fish can give rise to a similar neurologic syndrome called **ciguatera** [see Chapter 5 IV D 5 a (1)].

      (b) Consumption of certain **contaminated fish,** such as tuna and bonito, can result in an illness resembling a histamine reaction. This syndrome is called **scombroid.**

   (3) **Monosodium glutamate intoxication** (sometimes called **Chinese restaurant syndrome**) is characterized by a burning and tightness in the upper body accompanied by systemic symptoms such as flushing, diaphoresis, cramps, and nausea.

   (4) **Therapy.** Neurologic food poisoning syndromes usually resolve completely but require patient reassurance and supportive medical care during the intoxication. Identifying the vehicle is crucial to prevent further cases. Specific antitoxin therapy is available for botulism and should be administered as soon as possible after the diagnosis is established. Supportive measures may include tracheal intubation for patients with botulism or paralytic shellfish poisoning.

2. **Infectious diarrhea**

   a. **Introduction.** Acute diarrhea often can be attributed to microorganisms including bacteria viruses, and protozoa. The occurrence of any infectious diarrhea suggests a break in optimal hygienic measures. The disease is transmitted either through fecal contamination of food or water or from human to human via fomites or by sexual contact.

   b. **Etiology.** Determining the specific etiologic agent of infectious diarrhea can be laborious and is often unsuccessful. It may be useful to distinguish invasive from noninvasive processes.

c. Pathogenesis

(1) Invasive process. Certain agents of acute diarrhea invade the terminal ileum and colon where they destroy mucosal cells and cause inflammation. The most common invasive agents are *Shigella, Salmonella, Entamoeba,* and *Campylobacter* species.

(2) Noninvasive process. Other agents of acute diarrhea are enterotoxigenic and adhere to mucosal cells in the small intestine where they produce diarrheal toxins. The most common noninvasive agents are enterotoxigenic *E. coli, Vibrio cholerae* (rarely found in the United States), *Cryptosporidium, G. lamblia,* and rotavirus.

d. Clinical features vary with respect to the presence of abdominal pain, cramps, and blood or mucus in the stool and to the frequency and nature of the bowel movements.

(1) Diarrhea due to invasive agents generally is associated with rectal bleeding, fever, and systemic symptoms such as headache.

(2) Diarrhea due to noninvasive agents usually occurs without fever and is associated with fewer systemic complaints. However, there can be substantial fluid loss from watery diarrhea in these patients.

e. Diagnosis. It is important to distinguish among the various infectious diarrheal diseases because their therapies are different.

(1) Microscopic examination

(a) Fecal leukocytes. A useful test is to examine the stool for WBCs using Gram stain or preparations stained with methylene blue.

(i) Invasive agents may secrete cytotoxin or penetrate the mucosal wall of the bowel. Either mechanism may lead to the presence of leukocytes in the stool. [The diarrhea associated with *Clostridium difficile,* sometimes called **pseudo-membranous colitis** (see Chapter 5 V H), also is associated with pus in the stool as are several of the sexually transmitted proctitides and **inflammatory bowel diseases** (i.e., ulcerative colitis and regional enteritis, or Crohn's disease).]

(ii) Noninvasive agents do not cause the migration of leukocytes into the bowel wall and the stool. However, special techniques are needed to identify *Microsporidium or Cryptosporidium* in the stool, and the laboratory may not perform these tests routinely.

(b) Trophozoites or cysts in the stool suggest the presence of protozoa such as *E. histolytica* or *G. lamblia.*

(2) Stool culture

(a) The presence of fever or the identification of fecal leukocytes suggests an invasive pathogen. When the clinical severity or the epidemiologic setting of the illness makes the precise diagnosis important, the stool can be cultured for the most common of these pathogens (i.e., *Shigella, Salmonella,* and *Campylobacter*).

(b) Evaluation of the stool for protozoa (i.e., the **ova and parasite test**) also is recommended.

(c) *C. difficile* produces an enterotoxin leading to diarrhea, fever, and stool leukocytosis. (In severe cases, a pseudomembrane may be present in the rectum or colon.) Disease occurs during or shortly after the administration of antibacterial agents and is especially common in nosocomial diarrhea. Culture and toxin assays are available to diagnose *C. difficile* infection.

(3) Proctosigmoidoscopy or colonoscopy may aid in the differential diagnosis of inflammation-related diarrhea, especially to distinguish infectious from noninfectious causes.

(4) Biopsy. In cases of persistent diarrhea in which less invasive techniques have failed to provide a diagnosis, biopsy of the large bowel (for *E. histolytica*) or the small bowel (for *G. lamblia* or *Cryptosporidium*) may be diagnostic.

f. Therapy

(1) Fluid and electrolyte replacement is paramount, regardless of the agent of the diarrhea, and should be adjusted according to the patient's degree of depletion.

(2) Specific **antimicrobial therapy** may be necessary.

(a) Among the bacterial causes of acute diarrhea, only *Shigella* infections are routinely treated. The inherent delay in diagnosis makes it unnecessary to treat most *Campylobacter, Salmonella,* and *E. coli* infections except in severely ill patients or those with impaired immunity. Most cases in previously healthy people resolve without incident within a few days to 1 week. When treatment is indicated, fluoroquinolones are usually effective.

(b) Antimicrobial agents usually are indicated for giardiasis and amebiasis.

g. Prognosis. The prospect for complete recovery from infectious diarrhea is excellent for all patients except those who are severely immunocompromised. In most cases, a cause is not established or even investigated. All of the bacterial causes of infectious diarrhea can be followed by asymptomatic excretion for days to weeks after clinical resolution.

E. Intra-abdominal infections

1. Peritonitis is an inflammation of the lining of the abdominal cavity and may result from bacterial infection or chemical irritation. It is characterized by sharp abdominal pain often with tenderness and rebound tenderness. Bowel sounds are often diminished or absent because of the secondary ileus associated with peritonitis. Bacterial peritonitis that occurs without other abdominal disease is described as **primary** (spontaneous) **peritonitis;** when it occurs after rupture or perforation of a hollow organ, it is said to be **secondary peritonitis.** It is crucial to distinguish between primary and secondary peritonitis because a ruptured viscus requires surgical repair.

a. Primary peritonitis

(1) Etiology. Primary peritonitis is almost always preceded by ascites, usually secondary to hepatic cirrhosis. The causative organism most often is an enteric pathogen, usually *E. coli.* Other gram-negative rods, enterococci, and pneumococci are also seen.

(a) In children, primary peritonitis historically has been seen most often in association with **nephrotic syndrome** and ascites. The causative organisms usually are streptococci, pneumococci, and enteric gram-negative bacteria.

(b) In adults, primary peritonitis usually develops in the setting of **hepatic cirrhosis** and ascites. The causative organism most often is an enteric pathogen, usually *E. coli* or an enterococcus.

(2) Clinical features include abdominal pain and distention, rebound tenderness, nausea, vomiting, fever, and hypotension.

(3) Diagnosis. Paracentesis of peritoneal fluid, with smear and culture for appropriate bacteria, is needed for the diagnosis. Cultures may be somewhat insensitive and may need to be repeated. WBCs greater than $250/\mu l$ in peritoneal fluid suggest bacterial infection. Abdominal free air is not seen on abdominal x-ray. In some cases, exploratory laparotomy is required to rule out secondary peritonitis.

(4) Therapy. Systemic antibiotics are necessary for the treatment of primary peritonitis. If the Gram stain does not show a characteristic organism, empiric therapy for *E. coli, Klebsiella pneumoniae,* and pneumococci should be started. Because patients with advanced liver disease may be fragile, the mortality rate, even in appropriately treated patients, may be 20%.

b. Secondary peritonitis

(1) Etiology. The causes of secondary peritonitis are many, but the process is the same in most cases. Usually, enteric pathogens gain access to the abdominal cavity through a tear or necrotic defect of an abdominal organ.

Common examples include ruptured appendix and perforated peptic ulcer. In most cases, the infection is polymicrobial and the causative agents are endogenous organisms.

   (2) Clinical features. The early symptoms of secondary peritonitis are similar to those of spontaneous peritonitis. Abdominal pain, nausea, vomiting, and fever are common complaints. Tachycardia and shock may develop.

   (3) Diagnosis
    (a) Diagnosis may be difficult in patients without the usual clinical features. For example, corticosteroid therapy may mask the pain and tenderness that usually characterize peritonitis, but septic complications continue to develop.
    (b) The most important laboratory finding in secondary peritonitis is the presence of **free air in the abdomen,** as determined by chest or abdominal x-ray. Careful and repeated observation and consultation with a general surgeon help to distinguish surgically remediable disease from mimicking conditions.

   (4) Therapy. In most cases, **surgical repair** of the damaged viscus and **drainage of abdominal pus** are the cornerstones of therapy. Antibiotics with activity against enteric gram-negative bacilli and anaerobes (especially *Bacteroides fragilis*) also are important. The need for coverage for enterococci is controversial.

  c. Peritonitis and peritoneal dialysis. Peritonitis is a frequent complication of peritoneal dialysis, whether it is performed acutely or on a continuous basis. Ordinarily, the dialysis need not be interrupted, and systemic or peritoneally administered antibiotics can be used for treatment. Skin flora are often implicated, but gram-negative rods and fungus are sometimes seen.

2. Postoperative intra-abdominal abscesses often are difficult to diagnose.
 a. Etiology and pathogenesis
  (1) Postoperative abscesses develop most frequently when the bowel has been breached in the operative procedure; however, they may occur when nonviable tissue or accumulations of blood, serum, urine, or bile are present in the abdominal cavity.
  (2) Traditionally, these infections occur within several days of the operative procedure, but they may be delayed by weeks or months. They tend to develop near the anatomic site of the surgery, although the contour of the abdomen may allow infected fluid to move to other locations.
 b. Diagnosis. CT and ultrasonography are the most commonly used techniques for locating these abscesses. Most importantly, there must be a high index of suspicion for patients who have prolonged fever, abdominal pain, or both after surgery.
 c. Therapy. Once intra-abdominal abscesses have been identified, **they should be evacuated,** either by repeat surgery or via a temporary flexible drainage catheter. **Antimicrobial therapy** should be administered based on the results of Gram stain and cultures. Anaerobes play a major role in intra-abdominal abscesses and should be suspected when the fluid is foul-smelling or shows polymicrobial morphology on Gram stain. In selecting antimicrobial treatment, the onus is to prove that anaerobes are *not* present.

3. Hepatic and splenic abscesses
 a. Etiology and pathogenesis. Although liver and spleen are relatively protected from infection, bacterial (pyogenic) abscesses may develop. They may be single or multiple and often are multibacterial. Hepatic abscesses are usually associated with biliary disease or portal vein bacteremia. Splenic abscesses are associated with systemic bacteremia, hemoglobinopathy, trauma, endocarditis or intravenous drug use.
 b. Clinical features. Patients with these abscesses commonly have fever, chills, and pain near the affected organ. However, clinical findings may be subtle, making localization and diagnosis difficult.

    c. Diagnosis is usually made by cross-sectional anatomic imaging such as CT scanning, MRI, or ultrasonography. Occasionally, nuclear medicine studies such as liver–spleen or gallium scans are helpful. Blood cultures should always be done.

    d. Therapy is primarily surgical, with excision of abscesses from the liver or splenectomy. Catheter drainage is another option for selected patients. **Systemic antimicrobial therapy is mandatory.**

4. Cholecystitis and cholangitis are inflammatory diseases of the gallbladder and biliary tree, respectively.

    a. Cholecystitis (see Chapter 5 VIII B and C) is a common medical problem.

        (1) Etiology and pathogenesis. Infection need not be present nor be prominent feature of cholecystitis. In most cases, obstruction of the gallbladder is found, and the bile, which is normally sterile, may be colonized by bacteria such as *E. coli, K. pneumoniae,* or enterococci.

        (2) Clinical features include right upper abdominal pain, anorexia, nausea, vomiting, and low-grade fever with chills.

        (3) Diagnosis is made on the basis of the clinical presentation and evidence of gallstones or gallbladder dysfunction as demonstrated by ultrasonography or cholecystography.

        (4) Therapy. Cholecystitis usually is treated adequately with **conservative** measures. Cholecystectomy is recommended for recurrent disease, rupture, or empyema of the gallbladder. Chemical dissolution of gallstones with bile acids or lithotripsy may be useful in selected patients. Antibiotics are seldom needed in patients who do not require surgery.

    b. Cholangitis (see also Chapter 5 VIII G) is a more serious problem than cholecystitis.

        (1) Etiology and pathogenesis. Cholangitis tends to occur with obstruction of the intrahepatic or common bile duct (usually by gallstones or malignancy). Bacterial colonization (most often with *E. coli*) in this setting usually leads to infection.

        (2) Clinical features are similar to but more severe than those for cholecystitis and include right upper abdominal pain, high fever with shaking chills, and jaundice **(Charcot's triad),** often in the setting of gallbladder disease.

        (3) Diagnosis is based on the characteristic presentation of Charcot's triad and the finding of moderate to severe leukocytosis with elevated serum bilirubin and alkaline phosphatase. Bacteremia is also commonly found. Patients with recent biliary surgery or cancer in the liver or pancreas have an especially high risk for developing cholangitis.

        (4) Therapy usually consists of **antimicrobial agents** that are active against enteric organisms, accompanied by **decompressive surgery. Endoscopic sphincterotomy** or **percutaneous transhepatic drainage** may be used in lieu of or in preparation for open surgical drainage.

F.   **Urinary tract infections** (see Chapter 6, Part I: IX)

1. Incidence. These are the most common bacterial infections encountered in clinical practice. Outside the geriatric population, urinary tract infections occur much more frequently in women than in men. It is estimated that 20% of women have at least one of these infections in their lifetime.

2. Etiology. Most urinary tract infections are caused by gram-negative bacteria, including *E. coli* (most commonly), *Klebsiella* species, and *Proteus* species. Less common causes include gram-positive cocci, such as *Staphylococcus* species (especially *Staphylococcus saprophyticus*) and enterococci.

3. Clinical features

    a. In general, symptomatic urinary tract infections are characterized by the irritative symptoms of urinary frequency, urgency, and pain. Flank pain and fever suggest upper tract involvement.

b. The composition of the urinary sediment in urinary infections is characterized by a large number of neutrophils and a variable number of red cells. White cell casts may be observed in kidney infections.

c. Quantitative urine cultures do not distinguish between upper and lower tract infections.

4. Clinical syndromes

a. There is standard agreement that a bacterial count exceeding 10^5 organisms per milliliter of urine combined with irritative voiding symptoms and pyuria indicate significant disease, not simple contamination. However, there are two clinically important situations that are not covered by this definition of urinary tract infections.

    (1) The first category includes patients with symptoms of true urinary tract infection but with fewer than 10^5 bacteria per milliliter of urine.

    (2) The second category termed **asymptomatic bacteriuria,** includes patients with no symptoms of urinary tract infection but a urine bacterial count exceeding 10^5/ml. This condition is not rare and occurs most often in women and in older patients.

b. Catheter-related infections. Bacteriuria is an inevitable concomitant complication of prolonged bladder catheterization. It can be delayed by careful aseptic insertion and strict closed drainage; however, after 1 or 2 weeks some degree of colonization is common and ultimately, bacterial counts exceeding 10^5/ml of urine are reached.

c. Prostatitis is a complication of many urinary tract infections in men. Acute prostatitis is characterized by perineal pain and irritative voiding symptoms.

d. Urethritis is often a symptom of a sexually transmitted disease (e.g., gonorrhea or chlamydial infection). Copious urethral discharge is diagnostic of urethritis, but mildly symptomatic urethritis can mimic a urinary tract infection.

5. Diagnosis

a. Diagnostic tests seldom are needed to make a decision to treat a patient with symptoms of urinary infection, dipstick evidence of bacteriuria or pyuria, and an abnormal urinary sediment. In patients with previous infections or other risk factors, urine culture is helpful.

b. There is controversy concerning when to examine a patient for anatomic abnormalities as an explanation for urinary tract infections. Most evidence suggests that cystoscopy and urography seldom reveal treatable causes of infection and should be reserved for patients with frequent recurrences and jeopardized kidney function.

c. When blood cultures are positive in the context of a urinary tract infection, involvement of the kidneys or prostate gland is implied. Fever also suggests renal involvement.

d. Rectal examination may reveal enlargement or tenderness of the prostate, and purulent discharge may be expressed from the urethra after prostatic examination.

6. Therapy usually is directed at the agent most likely to be responsible for the infection.

a. E. coli has a propensity for causing infections in otherwise healthy individuals. Thus, in the absence of cultures, antibiotics effective against *E. coli* should be given. Many oral agents can be used, including trimethoprim and sulfamethoxazole used alone or together, quinolones, tetracyclines, and some penicillin preparations such as amoxicillin with clavulanic acid. Used alone, ampicillin is likely to be ineffective because there is a large number of ampicillin-resistant *E. coli.* Cephalosporins are widely used to treat uncomplicated urinary tract infections, but they possess no special qualities for this indication and are often expensive.

    (1) A 3-day course of therapy is adequate to cure most infections (especially cystitis) where urine drug levels seem to be the most important determinant of effectiveness.

(2) Failure to cure infections rapidly does not alter the efficacy of future therapy. In rare instances, refractory infection may require a long course of therapy—sometimes up to several months—although briefer courses (i.e., 2 weeks) often are successful.

b. The therapeutic approach to **asymptomatic bacteriuria** is debated; however, treatment is indicated for patients with a known structural or functional abnormality of the kidneys and for pregnant patients.

c. **Catheter-related bacteriuria** is more likely to be caused by antibiotic-resistant bacteria or yeast. The use of frequent bladder catheterizations (several times daily) rather than an indwelling catheter may lessen the risk of these infections. This approach has been most effective in paraplegic patients who otherwise would require prolonged bladder drainage through an indwelling catheter.

d. **Prostate infections** are difficult to treat. Fluoroquinolones, which enter the prostate gland, are the best therapeutic agents for prostatitis.

G. **Skin and soft tissue infections.** Bacterial, fungal, and viral infections of the skin and related structures (e.g., hair follicles and sweat glands) are common.

1. **Bacterial skin infections** usually start in areas of trauma or previous disease.

   a. **Etiology.** In otherwise healthy individuals, gram-positive cocci such as *S. pyogenes* and *S. aureus* cause most skin infections. Immunocompromised individuals are subject to a wider variety of pathogens, including enteric gram-negative bacilli and *P. aeruginosa*.

   b. **Clinical features.** There are three major forms of bacterial skin infection—**cellulitis, abscess,** and **ulcer.**

   (1) **Cellulitis** is characterized by redness, warmth, and tenderness of the skin. It may involve a limited area or may spread widely and rapidly. Any part of the body can be affected. Fever and leukocytosis are common. In some patients, a rapidly progressive cutaneous infection caused by group A streptococci and characterized by significant systemic features can cause severe skin damage and even death.

   (2) **Abscesses** represent deeper, circumscribed infections, which often start in accessory structures such as hair follicles. They may be warm or of normal skin temperature and frequently contain pus. Fever is most likely to be present in cases of large, multiple, or deep abscesses.

   (3) **Ulcers** are not usually the result of bacterial infection alone but reflect tissue damage from ischemia or trauma. Invariably, ulcers are colonized by bacteria and may lead to deep soft tissue or bone infection. They usually occur in dependent areas (e.g., the sacrum) or in areas of poor blood flow (such as may occur in the foot of a diabetic patient).

   c. **Therapy**

   (1) **Cellulitis requires antibiotic management.** Agents active against streptococci and staphylococci usually are effective, including semisynthetic penicillins (e.g., nafcillin), cephalosporins, vancomycin, and clindamycin.

   (2) **Abscesses should be drained,** although some rupture spontaneously. Antibiotics are seldom needed unless there is accompanying cellulitis.

   (3) **Skin ulcers** usually are managed by **debridement and antibiotic therapy** with agents active against enteric gram-negative rods and anaerobes. Skin grafting may be beneficial.

2. **Fungal skin infections** usually are acquired by exposure of the skin to pathogenic fungi. Exceptions are cutaneous manifestations of blastomycosis or of candidal fungemia.

   a. **Clinical features.** Fungal infections that start in the skin fall into three groups.

   (1) **Dermatophytosis** is a superficial infection of the epidermis due to dermatophytic fungi (e.g., *Trichophyton, Microsporum,* and *Epidermophyton* species). Athlete's foot and ringworm are examples. The skin usually is flaky and may be slightly discolored but is not frankly painful.

   (2) **Candidiasis** is a red, tender edematous rash occurring in moist body parts and caused by *C. albicans.* Intertrigo in the axillary or inframammary area is an example.

(3) **Mixed bacterial flora and fungi** (usually *Candida* species) can be involved in superficial infection. This may be evident during or after administration of antibacterial therapy.

b. **Diagnosis** of all fungal infections rests on potassium hydroxide preparations (or Gram stains) and on fungal cultures.

c. **Therapy**

(1) Dermatophytosis is treated with topical therapy for limited disease or with oral therapy for extensive infection. **Azoles** (e.g., ketoconazole, fluconazole) are most commonly used.

(2) Candidiasis is treated topically, but special attention should be given to keeping the affected area clean and dry. Rarely, systemic therapy is required.

(3) Mixed bacterial and fungal infections usually do not require specific antifungal therapy.

3. **Viral skin infections** may be cutaneously inoculated, as in the case of herpes simplex, but more commonly are a manifestation of systemic viral infection or an immune response to infection. An example of this is **varicella (chickenpox),** in which the virus is acquired via the respiratory tract and spreads to the skin following a viremia.

4. **Deep soft tissue infections** are rare but serious infections usually caused by streptococci, anaerobes, and gram-negative rods. There may be comparatively little abnormality of the skin in some of these infections (e.g., **fasciitis**). Combinations of medical and surgical therapy usually are used, but even so, many patients succumb to these infections.

a. **Gangrene** is an infection of the skin and soft tissues caused by a mixed anaerobic and aerobic bacterial flora that usually includes C. perfringens. It is characterized by cellulitis and gas in the soft tissues. Therapy is surgical debridement and antibiotic therapy (e.g., with penicillin).

b. **Fasciitis** is a rare infection of subdermal tissue planes. It usually occurs postoperatively, after rupture of an abdominal viscus, or in diabetic patients. The bacteriology is one of mixed anaerobes, streptococci, and, occasionally, gram-negative bacilli.

H. **Osteomyelitis.** Bone infections can be classified according to their pathogenesis. In general, bone infections develop in three ways: by extension from a contiguous infection, by direct inoculation during surgery or as a result of trauma, and by hematogenous spread.

1. **Osteomyelitis due to contiguous infection or inoculation.** Bone infection should be suspected in a patient with a history of **trauma** or **surgery** or with obvious **soft tissue infection** overlying bone, although the bone involvement may be difficult to prove.

a. **Etiology.** Almost any bacterium can be responsible including *S. aureus, P. aeruginosa,* or anaerobes.

b. **Clinical features** may simply be those of the adjacent infection. Pain is common, and fever is variable.

c. **Diagnosis** may be difficult. Radiographic evidence of osteomyelitis lags behind the symptoms and pathologic changes by approximately 7–10 days. Although bone scanning is sensitive for osteomyelitis, it cannot distinguish bone infection from more superficial soft tissue infection. The definitive diagnosis rests on bone biopsy and bacterial culture.

d. **Clinical course and therapy.** The clinical course guides the length of treatment, but, generally, **long courses of antibiotics** are needed. Devitalized bone, poor blood supply, and adjacent infection may be reasons for extended (months) therapy.

2. **Hematogenous osteomyelitis** should be suspected in a febrile patient who experiences pain and swelling over a bone but has no obvious source of infection.

a. **Etiology.** The bacteriology of this disease is largely *S. aureus.* However, *Salmonella* species seem to be more important in patients with sickle cell disease. Vertebral osteomyelitis also is somewhat different in that gram-negative bacilli may be introduced from the urinary tract via venous channels.

b. **Diagnosis.** Radiography and bone scanning are helpful. The erythrocyte sedimentation rate usually is elevated. Bone aspiration and culture are recommended for microbiologic diagnosis. Blood cultures also should be obtained.

c. **Therapy.** The treatment is a prolonged course of **antibiotics.** Nonviable bone may need to be removed surgically because it provides a site for potential relapse.

I. **Intravascular infections and endocarditis.** Intravascular infections manifest as **viremia, bacteremia, fungemia,** or **parasitemia,** depending on the type of infective organism demonstrated in the blood. Such infections may reflect **invasion or failure of containment at a localized site** (e.g., the bowel or lung) or a **primary infection of the blood vessels or the heart** (e.g., endocarditis).

1. **Local infections** lead to positive blood cultures with a frequency dependent on the site and severity of the infection and on the organism or organisms responsible for the infection.

   a. For example, among hospitalized patients with pneumococcal pneumonia, 10%–25% have bacteremia. The prognosis for these patients is worse than for those without bacteremia because the bacteremic patients tend to have more diffuse lung involvement and more virulent organisms.

   b. Even when blood cultures do not demonstrate a particular organism, metastatic infection or dissemination (e.g., cryptococcal meningitis or miliary tuberculosis) strongly suggests blood-borne spread.

2. **Septic shock** is a commonly recognized clinical entity defined as a systemic infection accompanied by hypotension that is not attributed to hypovolemia or intrinsic cardiac disease. In most cases, blood cultures are positive during these episodes.

   a. Septic shock sometimes is called **gram-negative sepsis** based on the observation that the bacteria most frequently responsible are gram-negative enteric bacilli. It has been postulated that **endotoxin** (the lipopolysaccharide coat of gram-negative organisms) is the cause. However, an indistinguishable clinical disease can be caused by gram-positive bacteria, viruses, and yeast.

   b. Antibiotic therapy is critical for patient recovery. High-dose corticosteroid therapy to supplement usual supportive measures is controversial but is not thought to improve survival.

3. **Catheter-related infections** are serious problems associated with hospitalization. Infection seldom is caused by the infusion of contaminated fluid. Rather, these infections most commonly occur at the **site of cannulation.**

   a. **Diagnosis** is made by demonstrating either local skin infection at the cannulation site or positive blood cultures and the presence of the same bacteria in significant numbers on a semiquantitative culture of the catheter.

   b. **Therapy** requires removing the catheter when local infection is present. When vascular access is crucial and the catheter has been aseptically inserted into the vena cava (e.g., a **Hickman catheter**—a wide-bore silastic catheter used for chemotherapy, hyperalimentation, or drawing blood), conservative therapy with antibiotics alone may cure the infection. Fungal infections usually cannot be cured without removal of the catheter.

4. **Vascular graft infection** is one of the most serious consequences of vascular surgery. Although native blood vessels may become infected in atherosclerotic processes or in pyogenic processes involving the arterial wall itself (**mycotic aneurysm**), these events are rare. When arteries are bypassed because of arterial insufficiency or for hemodialysis vascular access, the surgical site can become infected.

   a. **Diagnosis** rests on finding consistently positive blood cultures in a patient with such a graft. In chronic infections, immunologic disease may manifest as an elevated erythrocyte sedimentation rate, abnormal urinary sediment, and positive blood tests for circulating immune complexes.

    b. Therapy. The best chance of cure is with removal of the entire prosthetic device. When this is not possible, revascularization—circumventing the site of infection—can be tried. Antibiotic therapy alone cannot ensure a positive outcome and must be carried out for usually 6 weeks or more.

5. Endocarditis usually results from infection of the cusp of a heart valve, although any part of the endocardium or any prosthetic material inserted into the heart may be involved.

    a. Etiology. A variety of organisms may cause endocarditis, although bacteria account for almost all cases. The specific agent of endocarditis depends on which cardiac structures are affected.

        (1) Infection of normal valves is rare and usually associated with intravenous drug use. *S. aureus* is the most common pathogen.

        (2) Infection of previously damaged valves usually is due to viridans streptococci. The other agents of endocarditis in this setting are enterococci, *S. aureus,* and various small gram-negative rods comprising part of the normal oral flora.

        (3) Infection of prosthetic valves. Staphylococci (both coagulase positive and coagulase negative) are the most common agents of early-onset disease (occurring < 2 months postoperatively), and streptococci are the most common agents of late-onset disease (occurring > 2 months postoperatively).

    b. Clinical features vary widely.

        (1) Common findings include **fever,** which is almost universal, and a **heart murmur.** Endocarditis is one of the most common causes of fever of unknown origin.

        (2) Less commonly, there is evidence of **embolic disease,** such as stroke or splenic artery embolism and infarction. Most emboli are small and may give rise to uncommon but diagnostically helpful physical findings including **Roth's spots, Osler's nodes, Janeway lesions,** and **conjunctival hemorrhage.**

        (3) There may be a variety of constitutional symptoms such as myalgia, back pain, confusion, or fatigue.

        (4) Moderate anemia is associated with endocarditis that has been present for more than 2 weeks.

    c. Laboratory diagnosis

        (1) Blood cultures are critical and are positive in more than 90% of cases of endocarditis. (Previous use of antibiotics may lower this figure.) Because of the continuous bacteremia of endocarditis, virtually all cultures are positive and it is rarely necessary to obtain more than three or four cultures.

        (2) For patients with culture-negative endocarditis, there is little incremental value in collecting several additional blood samples for culture. Sometimes, the microbiology laboratory can enhance isolation by using **special culture techniques.**

        (3) Immune complexes may cause a **glomerulonephritis,** which is manifest by elevated serum creatinine, hematuria, and casts in the urine. The role of immune complexes in other aspects of endocarditis is not well understood.

    d. Therapy for endocarditis has been carefully studied. When untreated, this infection is almost uniformly fatal. In general, prosthetic valve disease is more difficult to treat medically or surgically.

        (1) Antibiotic therapy alone provides an excellent chance of cure for streptococcal disease on a native valve and for staphylococcal disease on the tricuspid valve. The key is to provide an adequate dosage for a long enough period of time, usually 2–6 weeks, depending on the organism.

        (2) In medical failures, **valve replacement** may be a necessary adjunct to antibiotic therapy. Other indications for valve surgery include:

            (a) Fungal endocarditis (an absolute indication)

            (b) Congestive heart failure

   (c) Recurrent major emboli
   (d) Inability to provide a full course of antibiotic therapy
   (e) Inability to sterilize the blood after 10–14 days

VI.   SEXUALLY TRANSMITTED DISEASES

A.   **Modes of transmission.** Sexually transmitted diseases (STDs) usually affect healthy adults. Multiple STDs can be present at once. There are three ways microorganisms may be transmitted during intimate sexual relations.

 1. Cutaneous inoculation is the most common route for the five "classical" STDs (i.e., syphilis, gonorrhea, chancroid, lymphogranuloma venereum, and granuloma inguinale) as well as for herpes simplex. Apposition of an infected site to a susceptible site in a partner results in a physical transfer of microorganisms. Abrasion or trauma may facilitate the infection of skin.

 2. Blood-borne infection can be transmitted by sexual activity. Hepatitis B, cytomegalovirus (CMV), and HIV are all transmitted by inoculation of microscopic amounts of blood or serum.

 3. Enterically acquired infection may occur with sexual activity because the anal area is close to the genitals or is also used for sexual interaction. *Shigella, Entamoeba,* and hepatitis A are examples of sexually transmissible enteric diseases.

B.   **Urethritis**

 1. Etiology. Urethritis is classified as **gonococcal** or **nongonococcal.**
  a. Gonococcal urethritis is caused by *N. gonorrhoeae.* In almost all cases of gonococcal urethritis, Gram stain of the urethral discharge shows gram-negative intracellular diplococci.
  b. Nongonococcal urethritis is caused by *C. trachomatis, Ureaplasma urealyticum,* or some other, yet unidentified, agent. (In 25% of cases of gonococcal urethritis, one of these organisms also is present and patients may have recurrent symptoms after therapy for gonorrhea.)

 2. Clinical features
  a. Dysuria is observed in most cases of urethritis, whether gonococcal or nongonococcal.
  b. Urethral discharge is observed more frequently in men than women and may be purulent (usually in gonococcal disease) or cloudy and mucoid (usually in nongonococcal disease).

 3. Therapy
  a. A variety of **antibiotic regimens** can be used to treat gonorrhea. However, resistance patterns change and up-to-date recommendations should be sought.
  b. Many clinicians recommend that treatment with a tetracycline or macrolide follow gonococcal therapy to eliminate possible simultaneous nongonococcal urethritis. A 7-day course of a tetracycline or erythromycin or a single dose of azithromycin is usually sufficient, although some patients experience a relapse within a few weeks. These patients usually respond to another course of antibiotics.

C.   **Pelvic inflammatory disease (PID)** refers to a complex of infections involving the uterus, fallopian tubes, or ligaments of the uterus.

 1. Etiology
  a. *N. gonorrhoeae, C. trachomatis,* or a mixture of pelvic anaerobes may be involved, although it is difficult to determine which of these is responsible when instituting therapy.
  b. The presence of an intrauterine device (IUD) may predispose patients to PID.

2. **Clinical features and laboratory findings.** The symptoms may be contemporaneous with menstruation and usually consist of lower abdominal or pelvic pain and tenderness on palpation of the cervix, uterus, or adnexa; fever is not necessarily a significant feature. A cervical discharge or pelvic mass may be present, and the WBC may be normal or elevated.

3. **Diagnosis**
   a. It is important to obtain cultures for *N. gonorrhoeae.* If there is fluid in the retro-uterine cul-de-sac, culdocentesis can be performed and may help to sort out the possible causes.
   b. Ultrasonography of the pelvis may demonstrate an adnexal mass or abscess, which should be followed up carefully.

4. **Therapy.** No simple therapy is effective in all cases of PID. Hospitalization is suggested when pain is incapacitating or when parenteral therapy is given. Combinations of antibiotics are usually needed to cover the three major categories of possible pathogens.

5. **Complications.** The most serious long-term complications of PID are infertility, ectopic pregnancy, and the need for hysterectomy.

D. **Infectious proctitis** is an inflammation of the rectal mucosa.

1. **Etiology.** Infectious proctitis can be caused by a variety of microorganisms. When anal sex is practiced, gonorrhea, syphilis, chlamydial infection, and herpes should be considered. When there is no history of anal sex, shigellosis and amebiasis are more likely causes.

2. **Clinical features and diagnosis.** Proctalgia, a change in bowel habits, and a mucoid or bloody anal discharge between bowel movements suggest infectious proctitis. A sexual history should be obtained to aid in the diagnosis, and appropriate diagnostic studies (e.g., sigmoidoscopy, culture and Gram stain of the discharge, and biopsy) should be performed.

3. **Therapy.** When specific agents of infectious proctitis can be identified, appropriate antibiotic treatment should be administered. In general, the same regimens used to treat these pathogens in other body sites are effective in proctitis. For gonorrheal proctitis, however, cure rates are lower than for gonorrheal urethritis, and post-therapy cultures should be obtained.

E. **Syndromes of genital ulcers and lymphadenopathy**

1. **Incidence.** Ulcerative lesions of the genitalia are common outpatient problems. Men are more commonly affected by these entities than women.

2. **Etiology.** There are many causes, which vary in different parts of the world. In the United States, **genital herpes** is the most common cause of genital ulcers, followed by **syphilis.** Other causes include **lymphogranuloma venereum, chancroid,** and **granuloma inguinale (donovanosis)**—all of which are uncommon in the United States. (Gonorrhea is one STD that does not cause genital ulcer syndromes.)

3. **Clinical features** (Table 8-2)
   a. Genital herpes initially presents as itching and soreness followed by the appearance of erythema and, eventually, the development of herpetic vesicles. In immunocompromised patients (e.g., transplant recipients, patients with HIV), vesicles may be confluent and lead to large ulcers.
   b. Syphilis, in its primary form, presents as a painless, often solitary, chancre (ulcer) with a hard, indurated base. Oral and vulvar lesions may be subtle.
   c. Lymphogranuloma venereum presents as nodes that are disproportionately large compared to the ulcers. There often is a depression between the inguinal and femoral nodes (the **groove sign**).
   d. Chancroid is characterized by multiple, painful ulcers with ragged, undermined edges and suppurative inguinal nodes.

TABLE 8-2. Syndromes of Genital Ulcers and Lymphadenopathy

Disease	Causative Organism	Diagnostic Tests	Clinical Findings	Therapy
Genital herpes	Herpes simplex virus	Direct immunofluoresence; culture	Lesion—multiple, vesiculopustular; painful	None; acyclovir
Syphilis	*Treponema pallidum*	Darkfield microscopy; RPR test	Lesion—usually solitary; indurated; painless	Penicillin; tetracycline
			Nodes—rubbery; not fluctuant	
Lymphogranuloma venereum	*Chlamydia trachomatis*	Culture; serologic examination	Lesion—small papule or vesicle	Tetracycline; erythromycin
			Nodes—large; suppurative; both sides of inguinal ligament affected (groove sign)	
Chancroid	*Haemophilus ducreyi*	Gram stain; culture (special media needed)	Lesion—ragged; soft; dirty looking	Erythromycin; ceftriaxone; trimethoprim–sulfamethoxazole; fluoroquinolone
			Nodes—tender; suppurative	
Granuloma inguinale	*Calymmatobacterium granulomatis*	Biopsy with Giemsa or Wright's stain	Lesion—large; slowly advancing; rolled edges; not indurated	Tetracycline; trimethoprim–sulfamethoxazole
			Nodes—not prominent	

RPR = rapid plasma reagin.

    e. Granuloma inguinale is a more indolent infection characterized by a painless, beefy-red lesion with ragged edges and less prominent adenopathy. It is rare in the United States. The clinical characteristics and course of illness are more like genital cancer than other STDs.

4. Diagnosis
    a. When a **genital ulcer** is noted, a **smear** for herpes and a **darkfield examination** for spirochetes can help make a quick diagnosis. Darkfield examinations, however, can be technically difficult. In all cases, serologic testing for syphilis should be done.
    b. Confirmation of **lymphogranuloma venereum** is difficult and may be done by culturing *C. trachomatis* from a lesion or a node or by showing a serologic reaction to this organism.
    c. **Chancroid** is diagnosed by eliminating other causes of genital ulcers and isolating *Haemophilus ducreyi* from the ulcers or suppurative nodes. However, *H. ducreyi* can be difficult to grow in culture, even under optimal conditions. In most patients, a clinical suspicion of chancroid and negative tests for syphilis and herpes simplex are enough to initiate treatment.
    d. The diagnosis of **granuloma inguinale** is confirmed by demonstration of Donovan bodies in edge scrapings prepared with Giemsa or Wright's stain. An experienced cytopathologist may be needed to make the identification. Granuloma inguinale is very rare in the United States.

5. Therapy. Identification and treatment of sexual contacts is always desirable.
    a. Herpes infections are self-limited but recurrent. Acyclovir may shorten the course and reduce symptoms, but it does not affect the natural history of these infections.
    b. Syphilis is treated with varying schedules of penicillin, depending on the stage. Ceftriaxone or tetracycline may be useful for patients with penicillin intolerance or other special requirements.
    c. Lymphogranuloma venereum is treated with a tetracycline or macrolide.
    d. Chancroid is treated with erythromycin, ceftriaxone, fluoroquinolones, or tri-

methoprim–sulfamethoxazole. However, resistance patterns of *H. ducreyi* are variable, and up-to-date recommendations should be acquired.

  e. Granuloma inguinale is treated with a tetracycline or trimethoprim–sulfamethoxazole.

6. Late complications

  a. Herpes simplex recurrences tend to be most common early after acquisition but may continue to occur for many years and may become severe in immunocompromised patients. Herpes can also complicate parturition and cause devastating infection of neonates.

  b. Syphilitic chancres heal spontaneously after 1–2 weeks. However, in the secondary phase, syphilis can present as a multisystem disease including, but not limited to, lymphadenopathy, rash (especially on the palms and soles), fever, pharyngitis, and meningitis. The multisystem disease resolves spontaneously, and a latent, noninfective phase ensues. Most patients remain seropositive. Approximately 10% of patients develop serious late complications of the aorta or the CNS. The neurologic lesions are varied but include pupillary disturbances, posterior spinal column problems, and major cognitive impairment. In tertiary syphilis, treatment may halt progression but is unlikely to reverse damage.

  c. Lymphogranuloma venereum may rarely lead to genital or rectal scarring.

  d. Chancroid and granuloma inguinale tend to cause only local problems.

VII. OTHER INFECTIOUS DISEASES AND SYNDROMES

A. Infections associated with adenopathy and splenomegaly. Syndromes of adenopathy (both local and general), splenomegaly, and fever are common medical problems. The differential diagnosis should include tumors, rheumatic diseases, and vasculitis as well as specific infectious processes.

1. Generalized lymphadenopathy and fatigue are the classic signs of **infectious mononucleosis.**

  a. Mononucleosis most commonly is caused by the **Epstein-Barr virus** and is associated with splenomegaly, pharyngitis, and an atypical lymphocytosis.

  b. CMV causes a mononucleosis syndrome that is virtually indistinguishable from Epstein-Barr virus–induced mononucleosis.

  c. Both infections tend to occur in adolescents and young adults and may be subclinical.

  (1) They are distinguished by serologic tests such as the **Monospot test,** which usually demonstrates the presence of heterophile antibody in Epstein-Barr virus infection and the absence of heterophile antibody in CMV infection.

  (2) Specific antibody testing for the two viruses can confirm the diagnosis in equivocal cases.

  (3) Both viruses can be transmitted by intimate contact including, but not limited to, sexual intercourse.

  d. Some cases of mononucleosis are caused by *T. gondii,* but this infection usually is subclinical or presents as a mild "viral-type syndrome" in healthy adults.

2. Secondary syphilis and **early HIV infection** can manifest as fever, adenopathy, and fatigue.

3. Splenomegaly out of proportion to adenopathy

  a. This clinical presentation is characteristic of only a few infections, such as malaria, schistosomiasis, and kala-azar (visceral leishmaniasis)

  b. This syndrome also should suggest a **malignancy** such as lymphoma or Hodgkin's disease, an **infiltrative disease** such as Gaucher's disease, a **congestive disease** such as hepatic cirrhosis, or a **connective tissue disease** such as systemic lupus erythematosus (SLE).

  c. Local infections, such as splenic abscess and left-sided subphrenic abscess, may manifest as a palpable spleen.

4. Localized adenopathy helps to pinpoint a potential **infection** or **tumor.**

    a. A few small (<8 mm) lymph nodes in the inguinal axillary or cervical region may be present in most healthy adults. If the nodes are nontender and firm but not rock hard and do not change over a period of weeks to months, they usually do not demand attention.

    b. Lymphadenopathy in other areas is unusual without an obvious infection in the region drained by those nodes.

    c. Cutaneous inoculation with an infective agent may result in a local lesion and regional adenopathy. Examples are sporotrichosis (from exposure to *Sporothrix schenckii,* a plant-associated fungus) and cat-scratch disease (*Bartonella henselae* infection following cat bite or scratch).

    d. Lymphadenopathy alone or with a variety of constitutional problems occurs in mid to late stages of HIV infection.

B. **Infections associated with eosinophilia.** Eosinophils are granulocytes that have limited ability to phagocytose bacteria but are prominent in hypersensitivity reactions and in infections by multicellular parasites that have an invasive phase.

1. The finding of eosinophilia (i.e., an increase in the number of circulating eosinophils above 500/μl) should stimulate the search for an infection.

    a. Eosinophilia is seen most often with infection by helminths that are not limited to the lumen of the bowel, such as the **schistosome** (blood fluke), which belongs to the group called **trematodes. Pinworm** (from the helminth group called **nematodes**) does not tend to stimulate eosinophilia because it has no tissue phase.

    b. *Strongyloides stercoralis* is the most important helminth associated with eosinophilia in the United States. Strongyloidiasis should be suspected in persons who live or have lived in tropical areas (or in the southeastern United States) and who have persistent eosinophilia with or without cutaneous or gastrointestinal complaints. Because the *Strongyloides* larvae can cross the bowel wall, they may be associated with episodes of polymicrobial bacteremia involving typical bowel flora. Untreated disease can last for decades and worsen during periods of immunosuppression.

    c. Protozoa (e.g., *Entamoeba* and *Giardia*) seldom elicit eosinophilia.

    d. Most bacterial infections cause eosinopenia because of the effect of endogenous steroid production. Medically prescribed corticosteroids reduce eosinophilia of any origin.

2. Many noninfectious diseases may stimulate eosinophil production, release, or both. The most frequently encountered are **atopic** or **allergic diseases.**

3. When a drug such as an antibiotic is the allergen or hapten, eosinophilia acts as a marker for an allergic reaction to the drug. The eosinophilia tends to resolve quickly after the offending drug has been withdrawn.

C. **Tuberculosis** remains a major medical problem in certain immigrant and underprivileged groups in the United States as well as a widespread disease throughout the world. The diagnosis is based on identification of acid-fast bacilli—specifically, *M. tuberculosis*—on special stain or culture. The diagnosis may be difficult to establish, however, because many patients have too few bacteria to be seen on direct stain, and it takes several weeks of incubation for specimens to grow.

1. Clinical syndromes

    a. Pulmonary tuberculosis is the most common form and, in most adults, is characterized by an increased cough (possibly with altered sputum), weight loss, hemoptysis, and fatigue. The chest x-ray usually is abnormal and shows signs of a prior exposure to *M. tuberculosis* (e.g., calcified or enlarged intrathoracic lymph nodes and infiltrates in the posterior segment of the upper lobes). Most cases of pulmonary tuberculosis are believed to be a reactivation of *M. tuberculosis* acquired months to years earlier rather than reinfection or initial infection by this bacterium. Primary disease may resemble bacterial pneumonia and should be suspected especially when a close contact has recently been discovered to have active tuberculosis.

b. **Extrapulmonary tuberculosis** can develop in any organ, but the most seriously affected are the kidneys, bones, and meninges. Again, the diagnosis rests on finding *M. tuberculosis* in body fluid or tissue. Only approximately 40% of patients with extrapulmonary tuberculosis have clinical or radiographic evidence of lung involvement.

2. **Therapy** is aimed at curing the patient who has a definite diagnosis of tuberculosis. To be effective, the treatment must include **at least two antimicrobial agents;** single-agent treatment has a high risk of failure due to the selection of drug-resistant strains of the infecting tubercle bacillus.

   a. Because of their potency and reliability, **isoniazid** and **rifampin** are the drugs of choice for tuberculosis. Other first-line drugs include ethambutol, pyrazinamide, and streptomycin. Most authorities recommend starting three or four drugs in the initial treatment of tuberculosis to provide adequate coverage even in the unexpected circumstance of isoniazid or rifampin resistance.

   b. Second-line drugs are are used mainly for patients who are intolerant of the first-line agents or who have drug-resistant disease. These drugs include ethionamide, kanamycin, and cycloserine.

   c. The usual duration of therapy is 6–12 months, depending on the patient and the regimen.

3. **Prevention**

   a. **Skin testing.** The **tuberculin skin test** is used widely to screen certain high-risk populations, particularly those who have been exposed to an infectious individual. The test involves an intradermal injection of the **purified protein derivative (PPD)** of tuberculin. After 48–72 hours, the injection site is examined for visible and palpable induration. Because of a possible cross-reaction following exposure to other mycobacteria, a single tuberculin skin test to determine sensitization to *M. tuberculosis* is considered positive only if the induration at the skin test site measures at least 1 cm in diameter in immunocompetent people and 0.5 cm in immunosuppressed individuals.

   b. **Chemoprophylaxis.** Certain individuals are at extremely high risk for the development of significant symptomatic tuberculosis. In many cases, disease can be prevented by administering isoniazid alone for 9–12 months, at a dosage of 300 mg/day. Pyridoxine is usually coadministered with isoniazid to prevent the development of peripheral neuropathy. The high-risk groups include:

      (1) Individuals younger than 30 years of age who have positive skin tests for tuberculosis

      (2) Individuals of any age who previously had negative skin tests but recently had positive skin tests for tuberculosis

      (3) Individuals with positive skin tests who receive chronic corticosteroid therapy

      (4) Individuals who live in the same house or come in close contact with an infected and contagious patient

   c. **Immunization** of children and adults with Bacille Calmette-Guérin (BCG) has been reported to reduce the risk of acquiring tuberculosis. BCG is a live bacterial vaccine and should not be used when there is known immunodeficiency. The PPD skin test can become positive after BCG administration. This vaccine is seldom used in the United States, but is widely used in other countries.

   d. **Isolation.** Because of the **potential hazard of transmission** of tuberculosis in the hospital, it is important to identify potentially infective patients and to ensure adequate containment of their infectious aerosols.

      (1) Waiting for a positive acid-fast bacillus smear may introduce an excessive delay, so any patient suspected of having highly contagious tuberculosis should be housed in a priviate room with air pressure less than that in the hallway. Visitors and staff should wear masks.

      (2) Smears are useful in confirming the diagnosis. Finding three consecutive negative smears may be enough to discontinue isolation, but in some clini-

cal settings, it may still be appropriate to continue treatment until the final cultures are available weeks later.

D. Infections associated with diffuse rash and fever

1. **Toxin-associated diseases**
   a. **Toxic shock syndrome** (TSS) occurs when a susceptible individual is colonized or infected by a strain of *S. aureus* that produces a toxin (TSST-1). Most adults have antibody to this toxin and are thus immune. Many cases have been associated with tampon use in young women, but current tampons seem to be safer and menstrual TSS is considerably less common than in the early 1980s.
      (1) **Clinical features**
         (a) TSS is characterized by fever, hypotension, diarrhea, mucous membrane changes, and a diffuse erythematous rash with desquamation on the hands and feet. Multisystem involvement is the rule with gastrointestinal, renal, hepatic, hematopoietic, and musculoskeletal organs affected.
         (b) TSS varies from a mild illness to a life-threatening disease. Hypotension from fluid loss and lack of vascular tone is the most ominous prognostic sign. There may be recurrences unless protective antibody is formed.
      (2) **Therapy.** The treatment for acute illness is **supportive,** consisting of fluids and pressors, and antistaphylococcal therapy is given to prevent recurrence.
   b. **Scarlet fever** is an illness caused by infection with toxigenic *S. pyogenes* (group A streptococcus). It is characterized by fever, rough erythematous diffuse rash, mucous membrane erythema (including strawberry tongue), and local streptococcal infection (usually involving the skin). It is less severe than TSS and usually responds to supportive measures and antistreptococcal therapy.
   c. **Streptococcal shock** is a more fulminant condition that resembles TSS clinically.

2. **Non–toxin-mediated illness with fever and rash**
   a. **Kawasaki disease** usually affects young children. It is characterized by prolonged fever, digital swelling, conjunctivitis, mucous membrane erythema, lymphadenopathy, and thrombocytosis. The major late sequela is vasculitis, especially coronary artery aneurysm. Treatment is with aspirin and gamma globulin.
   b. **Adverse reactions to medications** include combinations of fever, rash, and eosinophilia. Reaction severity ranges from trivial to life-threatening.
      (1) The most common offending agents include anticonvulsants, oral hypoglycemics, and antibiotics (especially β-lactams and sulfa drugs). Unlike acute hypersensitivity reactions, which occur within minutes to hours of administration, the rash or fever of drug-induced reactions usually appears after a variable interval of uneventful therapy.
      (2) The most serious reaction, toxic epidermal necrolysis **(Stevens-Johnson syndrome),** is characterized by diffuse macular eruption and extensive involvement of the mucous membranes. If the affected skin sloughs, fatality may occur due to fluid derangement and sepsis.
   c. A number of **viral exanthems** (skin rashes) and **enanthems** (mucous membrane rashes) are well described. Most usually affect children and unvaccinated individuals and are mild, each having a characteristic appearance and course. Measles (rubeola), erythema infectiosum, and coxsackievirus are among the best known.
   d. **Spotted fevers** are caused by *Rickettsia* species. In the United States, the most well known is **Rocky Mountain spotted fever (RMSF),** caused by *Rickettsia rickettsii* and most often found in the southeastern part of the country. RMSF is transmitted by the bite of the dog tick (*Dermacentor* species). After a delay of several days, there is headache, fever, and a rash, which starts peripherally and moves centrally. Infection involves the vascular endothelium and may be fatal for 15%–20% of untreated patients. Usually, tetracycline or chloramphenicol is effective if given early enough. A similar syndrome, usually without rash, can be caused by *Ehrlichia chaffeensis,* another tick-borne rickettsial pathogen.

E. Legionnaires' disease

1. Etiology

a. Legionnaires' disease is a pneumonia caused by *L. pneumophila,* a gram-negative bacterium that dwells in warm aquatic environments.

b. Several legionella-like organisms have been discovered, which produce similar but distinct disease patterns

2. Epidemiology

a. Infection occurs when contaminated water is aerosolized and then inhaled (e.g., during nebulizer treatments). Some outbreaks of legionnaires' disease have been connected to the airborne spread of contaminated fluid from air-conditioning cooling towers or from potable water.

b. Individuals who are particularly vulnerable to infection include cigarette smokers, people with underlying lung disease, and immunosuppressed individuals (e.g., those receiving steroid therapy).

3. Clinical features

a. Fever occurs in almost all cases, is abrupt, and usually is associated with shaking chills. A sudden headache may precede the rapid increase in temperature.

b. Cough is a common symptom, which initially is nonproductive but progresses to a productive cough that may be associated with slight hemoptysis.

c. Less common symptoms include diarrhea, nausea, vomiting, and pleuritic pain.

4. Diagnosis. The diagnosis is made by **culturing the bacterium** from infected body sites (e.g., lung tissue, pleural fluid, or sputum) or by demonstrating the bacterium by immunofluorescent, nucleic acid hybridization, or antigen detection techniques. When *L. pneumophila* infection cannot be confirmed by these methods, increasing titers of antibodies from the acute phase to convalescence can be diagnostic.

5. Therapy. The preferred therapy for all *Legionella* infections is **erythromycin.** Alternative treatments include erythromycin combined with rifampin or possibly a quinolone (or another macrolide).

F. Lyme disease

1. Etiology. Lyme disease is a multisystem infection caused by a spirochete, *Borrelia burgdorferi,* which is transmitted by tick bite.

2. Epidemiology. The incidence of Lyme disease is related to the presence of its vector (usually *Ixodes* ticks) and infected wild mammals, such as deer and mice. In the United States, endemic foci have expanded from initial small areas in New England to include areas as far south as Georgia as well as areas in the midwest and the Pacific states. Lyme disease is the most common tick-borne illness in the United States.

3. Clinical features. Lyme disease is divided into three phases. The phases may follow each other closely or be separated by periods without symptoms.

a. The **first phase** is characterized by an enlarging erythematous rash **(erythema migrans)** at the site of the original tick bite. There may be central clearing or a few satellite lesions. The patient is often constitutionally ill with malaise, headache, and mild fever.

b. The **second phase** involves the heart (conduction abnormalities, arrhythmias) or the nervous system (cranial or peripheral neuropathies or aseptic meningitis). **New onset of Bell's palsy** (paralysis of cranial nerve VII) should suggest the possibility of Lyme disease.

c. The **third phase** consists of an oligoarticular arthritis or some persistent, mild neuropsychiatric disturbances and only affects a few patients.

4. Diagnosis is difficult. In early illness, the production of antibody to *B. burgdorferi* may not be detectable. Conversely, people living in endemic areas may have antibody without any clinical illness. The organism may be demonstrated rarely in skin biopsies and can sometimes be cultured by special research laboratories. High levels of immunoglobulin M (IgM) antibody and increasing levels of IgG antibody to one or more *B. burgdorferi* antigens corroborate clinical suspicions of Lyme borreliosis.

5. **Therapy.** Early **antibiotic therapy** seems to prevent disease progression for most patients. Tetracyclines are preferred for adolescents and adults; penicillin is an alternative. For later-stage disease, high dosages of penicillin, tetracycline (especially doxycycline), and ceftriaxone have been shown to relieve symptoms. Some oral cephalosporins and azithromycin have also been shown to be useful.

VIII. RETROVIRUS INFECTION OF HUMANS

A. **Introduction.** Retroviruses are single-stranded RNA viruses characterized by the presence of **reverse transcriptase,** an enzyme that uses the viral RNA as a template to make a copy of complementary DNA for integration into the host cell. Many animals can be infected with species-specific retroviruses.

1. Retroviruses known to cause disease in man are the **human T-cell lymphotropic viruses**—HTLV-I, HTLV-II—and HIV.

2. HIV comprises two types—type 1 (HIV-1) and type 2 (HIV-2).

B. **Epidemiology.** All of these agents can be transmitted from person to person via sexual activity or mingling of blood (as occurs via blood transfusion or sharing of blood-contaminated needles) and from mother to child in utero.

1. **HTLV-I** is found most commonly in the Caribbean basin and in southern Japan. Up to 10% of the population in certain villages may be infected.

2. **HTLV-II** is not known to have such marked geographic clusters and incidence seems to be low worldwide.

3. **HIV**
   a. **HIV-1** is found worldwide. Because of a long latent period and the possibility of one person infecting many others via sexual activity or needle sharing, an explosive spread of this virus has led to a striking change in its distribution since 1981, when it was first identified. Male homosexual activity was the predominant mode of transmission in North America and Europe through the 1980s. Intravenous drug use and heterosexual transmission account for an increasing share of new infections, especially among women—one of the fastest growing groups to be infected. In Africa, heterosexual activity is the predominant mode of transmission.
   b. **HIV-2** is found primarily in west Africa.

C. **Clinical features**

1. **HTLV-I** is the causative agent of adult T-cell leukemia–lymphoma. This unusual malignancy, which is associated with skin involvement and hypercalcemia, is difficult to treat. However, **most people** infected with HTLV-1 **have no clinical illness** even after years or decades of infection.

2. **HTLV-II** has not been categorically associated with any illness, although it has been reported in patients with hairy cell leukemia.

3. **HIV**
   a. **HIV-1** infection can be arbitrarily divided into three general stages, which may overlap.
      (1) **Early illness** (seroconversion stage). Within a few weeks or months after exposure to HIV, living virus and viral antigens can be found in the blood. Although most patients are totally asymptomatic, approximately 40% of patients have a brief illness marked by headache, fever, skin rash, or lymphadenopathy, which resolves spontaneously wuthin a few weeks. Most

people who become infected with HIV-1 develop antibody within 3–6 months of exposure.

    (2) Almost all HIV-1 infected patients have a clinical **latent period,** during which there is no clinical illness but virus can be detected and is replicating. During this phase of infection, viral turnover is high because the host is able to contain the infection. With time, the virus alters the host immune response, the earliest indications of which may be declining numbers of Th cells (CD4), normal to increased numbers of Ts cells (CD8), and a dramatic change in the ratio of Th to Ts cells from the normal ratio of 2:1. Some patients have minor viral infections or other symptoms; for example, more frequent than usual recurrences of oral or genital herpes simplex, herpes zoster, oral hairy leukoplakia, mild fever, sweats, weight loss, and diarrhea. Common bacterial infections (e.g., pneumonia and tuberculosis) may occur with increased frequency at any point in HIV-1 infection, including the early stage of disease. These complications tend to become more common as the duration of HIV-1 infection increases.

    (3) Advanced symptomatic HIV-1 infection is manifested as AIDS. Previous case definitions of AIDS depended heavily on the documentation of specific opportunistic infections or malignancies. The current definition still includes these criteria but also subsumes most of them with two fairly simple laboratory tests: evidence for HIV-1 infection and fewer than 200 CD4 cells per microliter of blood. Lesser degrees of symptomatic immune depression used to be called AIDS-related complex (ARC), but HIV infection is best thought of as a continuum, with evidence of progressive immune depletion correlating with increased probability of specific infection or malignancy; nonspecific localized or generalized complaints such as fever, fatigue, or night sweats; or organ dysfunction such as renal failure or dementia.

  b. HIV-2 infection follows the same general pattern as HIV-1, but much less is known. The clinical course is usually milder or slower. Several well-described cases of AIDS have been associated with HIV-2 in the absence of HIV-1. It will probably be shown that determinants of immunosuppression are the most significant predictors of whether opportunistic infection or malignancy will occur.

D. Therapy

1. HTLV-1. Therapy for HTLV-1 related malignancies with conventional cancer chemotherapy has been disappointing; however, the use of zidovudine and interferon has resulted in some durable remissions. There is no need for treatment of asymptomatic HTLV-1 infections.

2. HTLV-II. There is no need to treat HTLV-II infection at any stage.

3. HIV

  a. HIV-1. The progression of HIV-1 infection can be influenced by chemotherapy.

    (1) After acquisition of HIV, careful evaluation and timely **retroviral therapy** may delay the development of significant complications. Because recommendations change quickly, the decision of which kind of single or combination therapy to use should be based on current studies.

    (2) A variety of **reverse transcriptase inhibitors** [e.g., zidovudine, azidothymidine or (AZT)] can alter disease course when administered before symptoms develop. However, this alteration may not be sustained after a period of 1 or 2 years, and an equivalent outcome may be achieved by watching for changes in symptoms before beginning drug therapy.

    (3) In later-stage infection, **antiretroviral therapy** can partly reverse the immunologic depredations of HIV-1, but survival benefits are often measured in months rather than years. Viral resistance to each agent is relatively easily demonstrated in vitro and by observation and may limit the benefits of antiretroviral chemotherapy.

    (4) Newer agents and combinations of agents are constantly being tested, and recommendations are constantly changed.

b. HIV-2. Treatment for HIV-2 infection tends to mirror that of HIV-1 and is much less extensively studied.

E. **Prognosis.** Although there are a number of interventions available to alter the course of HIV-1 infection and treat the complicating infections and malignancies, there have been no cures. The median length of survival after acquisition of HIV-1 is approximately 10–15 years, but the length of survival after the diagnosis of AIDS is usually 4 years or less. Patients with Kaposi's sarcoma and relatively normal CD4 numbers have the best prognosis among AIDS patients.

F. **Prevention**
  a. Screening. There is **no systematic screening program** for retroviral infections. Applicants to the military are screened for HIV-1 infection, and blood donors are screened for HTLV-1 and HIV-1. Most testing is done on a voluntary basis, and many states require an informed consent or some equivalent document for HIV-1 testing. Because, most HTLV-I–and -II–infected patients never develop clinical disease, there is little call for screening for these agents. The HIV-1 screening tests are very sensitive, specific, and widely available for HIV-1 infection, but they may not detect the antibody response to HIV-2.
  b. Controlling spread of infection. Preventive measures for controlling the spread of HIV include **education** about risk factors, **sexual abstinence,** use of **barrier precautions** (condoms), **avoidance of childbirth** in women known to be HIV-1 infected, **needle exchange programs,** and **universal testing blood products.** Treatment of HIV-1–infected pregnant women with zidovudine substantially decreases prenatal and peripartum transmission of HIV.

G. **Complications of HIV-1 infection** can result from direct damage caused by the virus or from the opportunistic infections or malignancies that accompany the decline of the immune system in late-stage HIV-1 infection. In general, direct effects of HIV-1 include fevers, night sweats, weight loss, decreased libido, and muscle wasting.

  1. Types of complications
    a. Skin lesions
      (1) Some lesions are rare in patients without HIV infection but are relatively common with HIV-1 infection.
        (a) Kaposi's sarcoma
        (b) Eosinophilic folliculitis
        (c) Disseminated molluscum contagiosum
        (d) Bacillary angiomatosis
        (e) Thrush
      (2) The following common disorders are more severe in people with HIV-1 infection:
        (a) Psoriasis (including psoriatic arthritis)
        (b) Seborrheic dermatitis
        (c) Alopecia
        (d) Onychomycosis (fungal infections of the nail beds)
        (e) Severe or recurrent genital candidal infection
        (f) Carcinoma of the uterine cervix
    b. Lymphatic system. Lymph nodes are often enlarged, although usually this is not reflective of a specific infection or tumor. The enlarged nodes are characterized on biopsy as having reactive hyperplasia.
      (1) Lymphomas in HIV-1–infected patients often occur as extranodal disease but may cause nodal enlargement later.
      (2) Several **infectious agents** can cause lymph node enlargement including *T. pallidum, M. tuberculosis,* and *Histoplasma capsulatum.* Node aspirate or biopsy is useful in distinguishing among these organisms.
      (3) Kaposi's sarcoma may be found in lymph nodes.
    c. Nervous system involvement can be diffuse or focal. Some cognitive or motor dysfunction is common and tends to become more severe. Usually, there is evi-

dence of cerebral atrophy, and no opportunistic agent can be found to explain the dementia.

    (1) Meningitis is caused most frequently by *Cryptococcus neoformans,* a ubiquitous yeast. Headache and neck stiffness range from mild or transient to severe, and the CSF is often normal or near normal with regard to cell count, protein level, glucose concentration, and general appearance. Cryptococci are seen on India ink preparations, and cryptococcal antigen can be demonstrated in serum and CSF.

      (a) Aseptic meningitis with headache, nuchal rigidity, and lymphocytic pleocytosis often occurs in the early stage of HIV-1 infection and occasionally in later stages.

      (b) Other forms of meningitis, although relatively uncommon, occur more often than in the general population.

    (2) Neuropathy may be a part of HIV-1 infection, an opportunistic infection, or a side effect of treatment. For example, vincristine, which may be used for some AIDS-related malignancies, induces dose-related peripheral neuropathy as do certain reverse transcriptase inhibitors such as zalcitabine (ddC) and didanosine (ddI).

    (3) Space-occupying lesions of the CNS are found with some frequency in HIV-1 infection. The presentation is usually one of focal neurologic abnormality (often accompanied by seizures) and an abnormal CT or MRI scan.

      (a) *T. gondii,* a protozoan parasite found worldwide, is the most common cause of **brain abscess** in AIDS patients.

      (b) Lymphomas located in deep brain structures and **progressive multifocal leukoencephalopathy** (caused by the JC virus) are also disproportionately common.

  d. Eye. HIV-1 may be associated with some direct toxicity for the eye and optic nerve, but CMV retinitis is the most common and serious ocular complication of AIDS. The lesions are predominantly retinal and spare the choroid. They usually progress over weeks and can lead to blindness. Involvement of both eyes is the rule, and CMV retinitis is often part of a systemic illness including predominantly the gastrointestinal tract. Treatment for CMV disease is effective but must be continued for life to prevent recurrence.

  e. Upper alimentary tract

    (1) The upper gastrointestinal tract is most frequently affected by **local candidal or herpes simplex infections,** which can extend into the esophagus, or by **Kaposi's sarcoma,** which can be found throughout the intestine. Endoscopic esophageal brushings or biopsy can distinguish between the two most common opportunists.

    (2) Visual examination of the oral cavity is sufficient for identifying **oral hairy leukoplakia,** an Epstein-Barr virus–related infection that predominantly involves the lateral tongue but may extend to other parts of the oral cavity.

    (3) Aphthous ulcers of the mouth and esophagus are common, and esophageal ulcers can be large and painful.

  f. Liver

    (1) In the late stage of HIV-1 infection, the liver often is the site of **opportunistic infections** such as histoplasmosis, mycobacteriosis [due to *M. tuberculosis* and *Mycobacterium avium-intracellulare* (MAI)], cryptococcosis, and CMV. Hepatic candidiasis, which is sometimes seen in leukemia as part of systemic fungal disease, is not seen in AIDS.

    (2) The same populations who are at risk for HIV-1 infection are also at risk for blood-borne **hepatitis, hepatitis B, hepatitis C, delta hepatitis,** and **non-A, non-B hepatitis.** Peliosis hepatis is a treatable liver infection caused by *B. henselae,* the agent of cat-scratch disease.

  g. Gastrointestinal tract distal to the esophagus

    (1) HIV-1 can cause an **enteropathy** distinct from the infectious diarrheas.

    (2) In addition, *Cryptosporidium* species, *Microsporidium, Cyclospora, Isospora,* and *G. lamblia* are potentially causes of **watery diarrhea** and **diffuse abdominal pain** in HIV-1–infected patients.

(3) The stomach and small bowel may also be sites of origin of **extranodal lymphoma.**

(4) **CMV colitis** can be the cause of severe abdominal pain, diarrhea, and fever, and it occasionally can lead to perforation or megacolon.

h. Lungs. The lungs are the most common target organ for symptomatic disease in AIDS.

(1) **Pneumocystis carinii pneumonia (PCP)** develops in the majority of patients who do not receive prophylaxis. In HIV–infected patients, PCP has a subacute presentation that delays diagnosis. By the time patients come to medical attention, there is fever, dry cough, and hypoxemia. Chest radiographs may be normal or have interstitial markings or fluffy infiltrates. Usually, diagnosis is made by examining bronchoalveolar lavage fluid, bronchial washings or brushings, or sputum. Even after initiation of treatment, the disease may progress temporarily but ultimately yields to effective therapy in 90% of patients.

(2) **Bacterial pneumonias** also occur more commonly in HIV-1–infected patients than in otherwise healthy people. Although these pneumonias may be more severe than in immunocompetent patients, they usually respond to routine antimicrobial therapy. Pneumococcus is the most common cause of bacterial pneumonia in adult HIV-1–infected patients. Bacterial pneumonia can occur simultaneously with PCP.

(3) **Fungal pneumonia** is less common and is usually a part of systemic cryptococcal, *Coccidioides,* or *Histoplasma* infection. Awareness of exposure to the agents of endemic mycoses (e.g., *Coccidioides* or *Histoplasma*) is crucial to make the diagnosis and to initiate appropriate therapy.

(4) **Viral pneumonia** can be severe in HIV-1–infected patients. CMV, a herpesvirus known to cause severe lung disease in other patients with Th-cell deficiencies (especially bone marrow transplant recipients), may cause a fatal pneumonia alone or with PCP in HIV-1–infected patients.

(5) **Mycobacterial disease** is common.

(a) Infection with **M. tuberculosis** may appear relatively early in HIV-1 infection. It has a higher propensity to disseminate in patients who have Th-cell (CD4) depletion but usually responds to antimycobacterial therapy. Recently, there has been an increase in the incidence of multiply resistant (to isoniazid and rifampin) *M. tuberculosis.* These strains are difficult to treat; in immunologically competent patients the clinical response may only be 60%, whereas it is considerably lower in HIV-infected patients.

(b) **Nontuberculous mycobacteria,** usually MAI, may be found in sputum. In HIV-1–infected patients, the lungs are a fairly minor target organ for this agent, which usually infects the liver, spleen, blood, and bone marrow.

(6) A **noninfectious pneumonitis** characterized by lymphocytic infiltration of the lungs has been seen frequently in children with HIV-1 infection and is being recognized more commonly in adults.

i. Cardiovascular system. Cardiomyopathy may be found in HIV-1–infected patients, presumably as a direct consequence of the retrovirus.

j. The **musculoskeletal system** is frequently involved in all stages of HIV-1 infection. Manifestations are seldom life threatening, but do cause substantial morbidity. Except for AIDS-associated arthritis, most of these manifestations are clinically similar to entities in patients without HIV-1 infection. However, the incidence and severity of these manifestations are greater in HIV-1–infected patients and tend to be worse in the late stage of HIV-1 infection.

(1) **Articular manifestations**

(a) **Arthralgias** occur in up to one third of HIV-1–infected individuals. The pain is intermittent and usually affects the large joints.

(b) **Reiter's syndrome** has been reported to affect approximately 5% of HIV-1–infected homosexual men, although it seems to be rarer in people who acquire HIV-1 through needle sharing or heterosexual activity.

(c) Although uncommon, **psoriatic arthritis** may occur at a higher rate in HIV-1–infected patients who have psoriasis than in HIV-seronegative patients with psoriasis.

(d) **AIDS-associated arthritis** is severe and debilitating. It affects the large joints and produces only a mild synovitis. Intra-articular steroids may give considerable relief.

(2) Muscular diseases

(a) **Myalgias** are common in HIV-1 infection, especially in the early mononucleosis-like illness associated with seroconversion.

(b) **Polymyositis** with proximal muscle weakness and elevated serum levels of muscle enzymes (e.g., creatine kinase) occurs in approximately 2% of HIV-1–infected people. It may also occur as a side effect of zidovudine therapy.

(3) **Bone and joint infections** are fairly uncommon in HIV-1 infection, except among injection drug users. The causative agents are a mixture of common organisms (see V H) and opportunistic agents, such as mycobacteria and fungi.

(4) Various forms of **vasculitis and connective tissue disease** (e.g., Sjögren's syndrome) seem to occur with higher than expected frequency.

k. Hematopoietic abnormalities are common in HIV-1 infection.

(1) **Immune thrombocytopenia** may occur in mid to late HIV-1 infection and resembles idiopathic thrombocytopenic purpura or thrombotic thrombocytopenic purpura.

(2) **Anemia** is common in late HIV-1 infection. The pattern is usually one of chronic disease with normochromic, normocytic indices. Some antiretroviral therapies and antimetabolites used to prevent infections may induce macrocytic anemia. Serum levels of vitamin B_{12} are often low, but vitamin B_{12} therapy does not improve hematologic parameters. Many patients with low levels of erythropoietin respond to erythropoietin replacement therapy.

(3) **Neutropenia.** In addition to the expected depletion of lymphocytes, HIV-1 infection may be accompanied by neutropenia. This may be a sign of disseminated bacterial or opportunistic infection, and blood and bone marrow culture (including mycobacterial cultures) can be helpful. Antiretroviral and antimetabolite therapies may contribute to neutropenia.

(4) **Immunoglobulin disorders** are common. The most frequently described is a polyclonal increase in gamma globulin with an inability to produce novel immunoglobulins. Thus, patients with advanced HIV-I infection may respond poorly to vaccination and may not demonstrate good serologic responses to acute infections, especially when challenged during the late stage of HIV infection.

l. Endocrine system. A variety of endocrine abnormalities, including thyroid and adrenal insufficiencies, have been reported in HIV-1 infection.

2. Treatment of infections associated with HIV infection. Treatment regimens may be the same or more intensive than those for the same infection in immunocompetent people or patients with other causes of immune depression. Many of the infections associated with HIV are potentially chronic; lifelong secondary prophylaxis and close vigilance are necessary to control recurrences. Recommendations for treatment of these infections are revised constantly, and current information should always be sought.

3. Prevention of complications

a. Tuberculosis

(1) **Screening.** Early skin testing is most useful for identifying people at risk for recrudescence of previously acquired infection, because many patients become anergic in the later stages of HIV infection. Aggressive contact tracing of people who are known to be infectious with tuberculosis can also identify people at risk before they become ill with recently acquired tuberculosis.

(2) Prophylactic isoniazid reduces the risk of recurrent tuberculosis when administered for 6–12 months to patients who have had positive PPD skin tests.

b. **MAI infection. Rifabutin prophylaxis** is advocated by some caregivers for patients with fewer than 100 CD4 cells/mm^3. Although rifabutin does delay or prevent the development of MAI infection, it may not prolong life because MAI is the principal cause of death in a small minority of people with AIDS.

c. **PCP.** Every person who has already experienced PCP should receive secondary prophylaxis. Because PCP is a common complication of mid- to late-stage HIV infection, and because preventive therapy is safe and effective, it has become general practice to offer PCP prevention to every HIV-infected person when the CD4 count declines to below 300/mm^3. First-line prophylaxis for PCP is trimethoprim—sulfamethoxazole. For patients intolerant of this medication, dapsone, clindamycin/primaquine, or pentamidine would be considered. Therapy is life-long.

d. **Syphilis** can recrudesce in HIV-infected persons. **Standard treatments** are usually effective, but careful follow-up is indicated. When there is a question of whether a cure has been achieved, a more intensive regimen (e.g., that for the treatment of neurosyphilis) is recommended.

e. **Cryptococcal disease** can be prevented or delayed by the use of **fluconazole** in patients with late-stage HIV-infection. Although fluconazole is safe and prevents or delays the occurrence of thrush, controlled studies show no survival benefit to this regimen as compared to with waiting for and treating fungal infections as they occur.

f. **Toxoplasmosis.** Many prophylactic regimens for PCP also can prevent clinical toxoplasmosis from occurring. However, it is not usually advisable to add anti-toxoplasma medications to the preventive regimen of a person who is intolerant to the kind of PCP prophylaxis that also prevents toxoplasmosis.

g. **Bacterial pneumonia.** Early administration of **pneumococcal vaccine** is recommended for every HIV-infected person. A single dose should be adequate for a lifetime.

h. **Hepatitis. Hepatitis B vaccine** is recommended for universal use. Because the vaccine is safe and the route of transmission of hepatitis B is similar to that of HIV, vaccination of HIV-infected persons is logical.

i. **Enteritis.** Because many meats and animal products such as milk and eggs can be contaminated with bacteria that cause enteric infection, HIV-infected persons should be advised to consume only pasteurized milk and to eat well-cooked eggs and meats.

j. **Cryptosporidial infection.** The discovery of *Cryptosporidium* in municipal water supplies is worrisome for the person with advanced HIV-infection. It is not clear whether the use of water filters and bottled water can substantially reduce the risk of this infection.

STUDY QUESTIONS

DIRECTIONS: Each of the numbered items or incomplete statements in this section is followed by answers or by completions of the statement. Select the ONE lettered answer or completion that is BEST in each case.

1. A 70-year-old man is admitted to the hospital for elective liposuction. The night before surgery, a nurse reports a rectal temperature of 38.1°C. After a careful examination shows no obvious source of infection, a single blood sample is sent for culture. The surgery is uneventful, but 3 days later, *Corynebacterium* is identified on blood culture. Which of the following best explains this finding?

(A) The patient has bacterial endocarditis caused by *Corynebacterium*.
(B) While taking the rectal temperature, the nurse inadvertently caused *Corynebacterium* bacteremia.
(C) Toothbrushing just before the blood collection resulted in transient *Corynebacterium* bacteremia.
(D) Inadequate skin preparation or careless handling resulted in contamination of the blood culture.

2. A 19-year-old man with acute nonlymphocytic leukemia is admitted to the hospital 2 weeks after his first round of chemotherapy. His temperature is 39.2°C, and physical examination shows no localized abnormalities. Chest radiograph shows a Hickman catheter with its tip in the right atrium. The white blood cell count (WBC) is 300/μl with no polymorphonuclear or band cells in the differential count. Blood cultures are obtained. The next step is to

(A) initiate antistaphylococcal treatment for the possibility of Hickman catheter–related bacteremia
(B) administer broad-spectrum antibiotics with excellent activity for enteric gram-negative rods and *Pseudomonas aeruginosa*
(C) await results of blood cultures and other diagnostic tests because infection could be caused by almost any microorganism
(D) initiate oral prophylaxis to prevent bacterial and fungal infections
(E) administer parenteral antifungal therapy

3. A 20-year-old woman with a history of seizures for which she has taken phenytoin for 4 months has a fever of 38.7°C; she has felt febrile for 2 weeks. She has no respiratory or urinary symptoms. Physical examination findings are normal except for elevated body temperature. Chest radiograph, urinalysis, and complete blood count findings are normal. Which would be the best next step?

(A) Admit the patient for toxic shock syndrome (TSS)
(B) Administer acetaminophen
(C) Treat occult urinary tract infection with antibiotics
(D) Discontinue phenytoin and prescribe another anticonvulsant

4. A sexually active 24-year-old woman known to be HIV-1–infected has had a fever for 2 days and has a productive cough. Chest radiographs show an infiltrate in the right lung. Two weeks earlier, her helper T (Th) cell (CD4) count was 510/μl. Gram stain of sputum shows many white blood cells and squamous epithelial cells with a mixed bacterial flora. Testing for nontreponemal antigen (rapid plasma reagin) is positive at 2 dilutions, and treponemal antigen testing is positive also. Which is the most likely cause of the pneumonia?

(A) *Streptococcus pneumoniae*
(B) *Pneumocystis carinii*
(C) Cytomegalovirus (CMV)
(D) *Mycobacterium avium-intracellulare* (MAI)
(E) Syphilis

5. A 62-year-old man has right upper quadrant abdominal pain, nausea, and vomiting. Physical examination shows only guarding over the liver. Ultrasound examination confirms the diagnosis of gallstones without dilated bile ducts. The patient is allergic to penicillin (a rash developed after penicillin therapy for a sore throat). In addition to dietary changes, which of the following treatments would be best?

(A) No antibiotics
(B) Erythromycin
(C) Oral quinolone
(D) Trimethoprim–sulfamethoxazole
(E) Amoxicillin

6. Two weeks after emergency surgery for a perforated duodenal ulcer, a 39-year-old woman complains of fever and vague abdominal pain. Her only medication is ranitidine. On physical examination, she appears a little pale, has a temperature of 38°C, and has a slight fullness in the epigastrium. Computed tomography (CT) scan of the abdomen shows an area of fluid collection measuring 3 × 3 × 8 cm in the left paracolic gutter. The most effective next step would be

(A) antibiotic therapy with an agent highly effective against aerobic gram-negative rods (e.g., aztreonam)
(B) antibiotic therapy effective against abdominal anaerobes (e.g., clindamycin)
(C) catheter drainage of the fluid collection and antibiotics appropriate for culture results
(D) no therapy unless blood cultures are positive or the collection changes in size

7. Which of the following features points to a community-acquired bacterial (nonmycoplasma, nonchlamydial) pneumonia?

(A) Pleuritic chest pain
(B) Nonproductive cough
(C) Myalgias and headaches
(D) Bilateral infiltrates on chest radiograph
(E) Prolonged cough and fever (>14 days)

8. Generalized lymphadenopathy rarely is found in cases of

(A) human immunodeficiency virus type 1 (HIV-1)
(B) infectious mononucleosis
(C) malaria
(D) syphilis

9. A 14-year-old girl from Pennsylvania goes to Wisconsin for a 2-week camping trip. Two weeks after she returns, she notices a solitary circular rash on her left calf just above the area normally covered by her socks. Overall, she feels well, and there is gradual progression of the rash over the next week. Which of the following diseases endemic in Wisconsin or Pennsylvania did she most likely acquire?

(A) Blastomycosis
(B) Lyme disease
(C) California encephalitis
(D) Rocky Mountain spotted fever (RMSF)

10. Which of the following is the strongest indication to consider valve replacement surgery in a patient with infective endocarditis?

(A) Hematuria
(B) Positive cultures for *Staphylococcus aureus* on the second day of therapy
(C) Splinter hemorrhages and Osler's nodes
(D) Progressive congestive heart failure

11. An 18-year-old woman takes a summer job working in a day care center. A month after starting, she develops a rash over her whole body. The lesions are small vesicles on a slightly erythematous base. Except for a slight cough and fever of 38°C, she feels well. She has proof of having received her childhood immunizations. Which of the following statements is most correct?

(A) The patient probably has an elevated total white blood cell (WBC) count and a differential with an abundance of neutrophils and band forms.
(B) Within 1 week, the patient will recover totally with lifelong immunity and no further sequelae.
(C) The patient probably missed a routine childhood immunization.
(D) The patient may be infectious to other family members.

12. Which of the following statements about intracranial abscess is true?

(A) Magnetic resonance imaging (MRI) scans are usually not helpful.
(B) The source of infection is usually cardiac.
(C) Antimicrobials active against *Pseudomonas aeruginosa* are usually a part of the treatment.
(D) Surgical excision is not usually needed.

13. A 12-year-old boy has had fever and bloody diarrhea for 1 week and has lost 4 pounds of body weight. A single stool specimen yields no enteric pathogens on culture, and no ova or mature parasites are observed on direct examination. Which of the following is the best reason for his illness?

(A) Regional enteritis
(B) Giardiasis
(C) Travelers' diarrhea caused by enterotoxigenic *Escherichia coli*
(D) Cryptosporidiosis

14. Which of the following features of the cerebrospinal fluid (CSF) is typical for bacterial meningitis but rare in viral meningitis?

(A) headache and stiff neck
(B) leukocyte pleocytosis
(C) increased cerebrospinal fluid (CSF) protein
(D) decreased CSF glucose (i.e., to less than half of the serum level)

15. A 70-year-old man with chronic lung disease should receive annual immunization for

(A) influenza
(B) tetanus
(C) pneumococcal pneumonia
(D) pertussis

16. Which of the following diseases causes dysuria in men?

(A) *Chlamydia trachomatis* infection
(B) syphilis
(C) trichomoniasis
(D) granuloma inguinale

17. Most upper respiratory infections

(A) are caused by bacteria
(B) can be prevented by immunization
(C) are treatable with amantadine or rimantidine
(D) involve the nose, sinuses, throat, larynx, or ears

18. When a patient needs a peripheral intravenous catheter for approximately 1 week, the most important feature (among the ones listed below) in preventing catheter-related infections is

(A) Using a powerful antimicrobial ointment at the junction of the hub and the skin
(B) Changing the catheter site every 48–72 hours
(C) Giving systemic antibiotics for the entire duration of catheter placement
(D) Shaving the skin before cleansing it

ANSWERS AND EXPLANATIONS

1. The answer is D [III B]. Inadequate skin preparation or careless handling resulted in contamination of the blood culture. Even though all the answers are possible, the most likely one is simple contamination—2%–5% of blood cultures are contaminated by skin flora from the patient or the phlebotomist. *Corynebacterium* makes up a small fraction of oral and rectal flora and is less likely to enter the blood from these sites. Endocarditis caused by *Corynebacterium* is rare and almost never involves native valves.

2. The answer is B [II A 3]. The next step is to administer broad-spectrum antibiotics with activity against enteric gram-negative rods and *Pseudomonas aeruginosa.* The heightened susceptibility of neutropenic patients to die quickly of overwhelming sepsis makes early intervention obligatory. Even though many clinicians include antibiotic coverage for staphylococci, the most common bacteria encountered are gram-negative rods. Antifungal treatment is used if antibacterial therapy fails to control the fever or if a specific fungal infection is found. Prophylaxis is started before having evidence of active infection.

3. The answer is D [VII D 2 b]. The next best step is to discontinue the phenytoin and prescribe another anticonvulsant. Of the many drugs that cause fever as an unwanted side effect, anticonvulsant agents lead the list. Prolonged fever can have many causes other than medication reactions and may be difficult to diagnose. In ambulatory patients, common bacterial infections are fairly well excluded by normal findings on chest radiograph, urine, and blood tests. TSS is a multisystem illness in which fever is only one component. Although juvenile rheumatoid arthritis affects patients in this age group, aspirin would be more appropriate than acetaminophen.

4. The answer is A [V C 4 b, c (1); VIII E 9]. The most likely cause of the pneumonia is *S. pneumoniae.* Although *P. carinii* is the most common single infection in patients with HIV-1 infection, the productive cough, localized infiltrate, and brief duration argue against *P.*

carinii pneumonia (PCP). In addition, the Th cell (CD4) count of more than 500 suggests that serious opportunistic infections such as PCP, CMV, or MAI are unlikely for some time. Syphilis, which may have been present, almost never involves the lungs.

5. The answer is A [V E 4 a]. Uncomplicated cholecystitis with obstruction of the biliary ducts or empyema of the gallbladder is best managed conservatively. Although some bacteria may be found in the bile at the time of cholecystectomy, there is rarely progression to infection. Erythromycin essentially has no activity for any of the agents associated with cholecystitis or cholangitis. Amoxicillin is contraindicated for patients who are allergic to penicillin. Severely ill patients should be hospitalized to manage the possibility of serious complications.

6. The answer is C [V E 2]. Catheter drainage of the fluid collection and antibiotics appropriate for culture results would be the most effective step to take next. The most likely explanation for the clinical findings and the CT abnormality is a postoperative intra-abdominal abscess. These rarely heal without drainage. Surgical drainage is effective, but a lesion that can be reached safely with a catheter may be drained equally effectively and more safely. Antibiotics are usually used as adjunctive therapy. The flora of these abscesses is usually mixed with enteric aerobes and anaerobes. Good cultures can be useful in refining the exact therapeutic regimen.

7. The answer is A [V C 4 c (2)]. Symptoms and signs of acute, focal pneumonia—such as rapid onset, local consolidation, pleuritis, and purulent sputum—all suggest bacterial pneumonia. So-called atypical pneumonia, caused by *Mycoplasma pneumoniae,* has a subacute presentation characterized by a more indolent course and constitutional findings such as rash, myalgias, and headache. Chest radiographs are useful in sorting out the classes of pneumonia. Atypical pneumonia rarely has significant pleural effusion but often more extensive abnormalities than suspected on clinical evaluation, whereas bacterial pneumonia is usually focal and unilateral and may have substantial pleural effusion.

8. The answer is C [VII A 1, 2]. Malaria is characterized by **lack** of lymphadenopathy, although splenomegaly and fever are characteristic. Although generalized enlargement of lymph nodes is a nonspecific finding, it often can lead to the diagnosis of a clinical entity. When the lymphadenopathy is coupled with fatigue and an atypical lymphocytosis, infectious mononucleosis is suggested. This syndrome most often is caused by Epstein-Barr virus, but a similar clinical picture is produced by cytomegalovirus infection. The infections can be distinguished using serologic tests (e.g., the Monospot test) or specific antibodies. Secondary syphilis also should be considered in patients with a short duration of adenopathy and can be confirmed on the basis of serologic tests and the finding of an appropriate rash. Reactive, hyperplastic lymph nodes are common in HIV-1 infection.

9. The answer is B [VII F]. Only Lyme disease and RMSF occur with a rash as a common feature. California encephalitis (which is spread by mosquito) has few, if any, skin manifestations but does cause a syndrome of progressive neurologic deterioration that resolves spontaneously in most cases. Blastomycosis, a disease that enters the body through the respiratory tract and may metastasize to other organs, almost never generates a circular rash. RMSF has a rash that usually begins peripherally but is rarely solitary. The course of disease is usually fairly rapid in contrast to this indolent but progressive lesion that is typical of erythema migrans.

10. The answer is D [V I 5 d]. Although all the answers reflect aspects of endocarditis, the only absolute indications for valve replacement are fungal endocarditis, congestive heart failure, valve ring abscess, and failure to clear infection after a long course of antimicrobial therapy. Some authorities recommend valve replacement after multiple significant emboli. Minor emboli and immunologic phenomena are not cause for valve replacement.

11. The answer is D [II F 4]. Although a varicella vaccine does exist, its implementation has not bee universal. Thus, many children and adults are still susceptible to varicella. Sequelae of varicella infection are rare and include pneumonia, meningitis, and hepatitis as well as herpes zoster (shingles). The WBC is normal or slightly depressed in most of the childhood exanthems.

12. The answer is D [V A 3]. Cross-sectional imaging studies (such as computed tomography scans and MRIs) are critical to the diagnosis and management of intracranial abscess. Surgery is often undertaken to obtain a specimen for culture or to decompress the abscess. Total surgical excision is rarely required in the patient who is responding well to medical therapy. Although occasional patients do have cardiopulmonary sources for infection, most patients have contiguous infection of the middle ear or sinuses.

13. The answer is A [V D]. Regional enteritis, ulcerative colitis, and a variety of invasive infectious pathogens can cause bloody diarrhea. A single stool specimen may miss any of these agents. *Giardia lamblia* and cryptosporidium usually cause an upper small bowel lesion that leads to watery diarrhea without fever. Travelers' diarrhea is a toxin-mediated infection that also leads to minimal inflammatory changes in the bowel.

14. The answer is D [V A 1 a (1)]. Acute meningitis is an inflammatory process involving the arachnoid layer of the meninges and the CSF. Two major forms of acute meningitis are recognized—bacterial and aseptic. Because the two forms have a similar clinical presentation of fever, headache, and stiff neck, the interpretation of CSF findings is important in the management of acute meningitis. Aside from a diagnostic Gram stain, lowered CSF glucose (i.e., to less than half of the simultaneous serum level) and the presence of a neutrophil pleocytosis are the most characteristic findings in bacterial meningitis. An increased CSF protein level also is a consistent finding in bacterial meningitis; however, CSF protein may be mildly elevated in the aseptic form as well. The pleocytosis in aseptic meningitis is modest (usually <100 cells/μl) and is characterized by a preponderance of lymphocytes.

15. The answer is A [II F 2]. Immunity to pertussis is not essential for adults of any age, and a periodic booster for tetanus is all that is required. A single vaccination for pneumococcal infection should be given to all persons with chronic cardiopulmonary disease and to all adults older than age 60 years. Reimmunizations may not be needed at all, and certainly no more than once every 5–7 years. However, the immunity conferred by influenza vaccine is short-lived and strain specific. Yearly immunizations for influenza are strongly recommended for the elderly and those with chronic cardiopulmonary diseases.

16. The answer is A [VI B 1,2]. Chlamydial infection is one of the most common causes of urethritis and frequently manifests with dysuria. Syphilis and granuloma inguinale do affect the external genitals but tend to spare the urethral mucosa. Trichomonas is sometimes found in the male genitals, but it is almost always without symptoms.

17. The answer is D [V C 1]. Most upper respiratory infections are caused by viruses that are seldom cultured (e.g., rhinovirus, coronavirus). Influenza, a viral infection that can be prevented by vaccination or treated with amantadine or rimantidine, is an important cause of upper respiratory infections during epidemics. However, on a yearly basis, influenza accounts for a small minority of all such infections. Bacterial complications such as sinusitis and otitis affect a small percentage of those who have upper respiratory infections.

18. The answer is B [IV G]. Assuming that all catheters are placed under the best possible conditions, keeping them clean and dry is all the daily care they need. Short plastic catheters are prone to infection over time, so routine replacement is recommended. This rule does not apply to central catheters (placed directly into a central vein or threaded up along the arm). There is no benefit to shaving the skin except to provide a better surface for the adhesive tape used to secure the catheter.

Chapter 9

Endocrine and Metabolic Diseases

E. Victor Adlin

I. **DISORDERS OF THE PITUITARY GLAND**

A. **Anterior pituitary disease** results from insufficient production of pituitary hormones (hypopituitarism), excessive production of pituitary hormones (acromegaly, Cushing's disease, or hyperprolactinemia), or the local effects of pituitary tumors.

1. **Pituitary tumors** make up 10% of intracranial tumors. Most are benign, but their continued slow growth in the confined sellar and suprasellar areas may cause serious neurologic damage.

   a. **Types**

      (1) **Pituitary adenomas** are classified by cell type, based on electron microscopy and immunohistochemical staining.

         (a) **Somatotroph tumors** produce growth hormone (GH), **corticotroph tumors** produce adrenocorticotropic hormone (ACTH), and **lactotroph tumors** produce prolactin.

         (b) An older classification system, based on light microscopy, categorizes these tumors as eosinophilic, basophilic, or chromophobic adenomas.

      (2) **Craniopharyngiomas,** the most common tumors of the hypothalamic–pituitary area in children, arise from remnants of cells from Rathke's pouch.

         (a) These tumors usually are located above the sella turcica, but they may produce changes within the sella itself.

         (b) They may be solid or cystic, may contain cholesterol-rich fluid, and often contain areas of calcification.

      (3) **Meningiomas** and **metastatic tumors** may involve the hypothalamic–pituitary area.

   b. **Clinical features**

      (1) **Excess hormone production** by pituitary adenomas may lead to **acromegaly** (see I A 3), **Cushing's disease** (see V B 1 a), or **hyperprolactinemia** (see I A 4).

         (a) In rare cases, these tumors may produce excess thyroid-stimulating hormone (TSH), causing hyperthyroidism.

         (b) Follicle-stimulating hormone (FSH) and luteinizing hormone (LH) are frequently produced in excess by pituitary tumors, but this usually does not result in a clear-cut clinical syndrome.

      (2) **Insufficient hormone production,** due to compression and destruction of pituitary and hypothalamic cells, produces the syndrome of **hypopituitarism** (see I A 2).

      (3) **Neurologic effects**

         (a) **Optic nerve compression.** Pituitary tumors may press upward on the inferior surface of the optic chiasm. Vision loss tends to occur first in the superior temporal quadrants, with bitemporal hemianopia in more advanced cases.

         (b) **Headache** is common.

         (c) Other neurologic manifestations such as mental status changes, cranial nerve abnormalities, vomiting, and papilledema are less common.

      (4) **Microadenomas.** Sensitive imaging techniques [e.g., magnetic resonance imaging (MRI)] can reveal pituitary microadenomas (tumors less than 10 mm in diameter) in 10%–20% of apparently normal women. If hyperprolactinemia or other hormone abnormalities are not present and if follow-up study shows no progressive enlargement, these should be regarded as incidental findings of no clinical significance.

(5) Multiple endocrine neoplasia, type I (MEN I, Wermer syndrome) is a syndrome consisting of tumors, often functioning, of the pituitary, parathyroids, and pancreatic islets.

c. Diagnosis

(1) Diagnostic imaging

(a) Skull x-rays may show enlargement or distortion of the sella when tumors are 10 mm or more in diameter (**macroadenomas**). Suprasellar calcification suggests the presence of a craniopharyngioma.

(b) Microadenomas may be visualized with more sensitive procedures such as **MRI with gadolinium enhancement** or **computed tomography (CT).**

(2) Hormone studies. Pituitary adenomas that secrete excess GH, ACTH, or prolactin can be diagnosed by measuring hormone levels, even if the adenoma is too small to be visualized by diagnostic imaging.

d. Therapy

(1) Surgery is indicated for pituitary adenomas that produce neurologic symptoms and for some tumors that cause syndromes associated with hormone overproduction.

(a) Transsphenoidal pituitary microsurgery is used for intrasellar tumors that have minimal or no suprasellar extension. Small adenomas often can be removed without damage to normal pituitary tissue.

(b) Transfrontal resection may be necessary for large tumors that extend far outside the sella turcica or compress the optic chiasm.

(2) Radiotherapy, used alone or in conjunction with surgery, may decrease the size of pituitary tumors and decrease hormone production.

(3) Medical therapy

(a) Hormone replacement is required if hypopituitarism is present.

(b) Bromocriptine may decrease the size and hormone production of prolactin-secreting adenomas.

2. Hypopituitarism

a. Etiology

(1) Pituitary tumors, most commonly chromophobic adenomas and craniopharyngiomas, may destroy normal hypothalamic–pituitary tissue.

(2) Sheehan's syndrome is hypopituitarism caused by infarction of the anterior pituitary gland during childbirth. The pituitary gland doubles in size during pregnancy, largely because of hyperplasia of the lactotropes. The blood supply does not keep pace with the enlargement, however, and hypotensive episodes during a complicated delivery may lead to infarction.

(3) Surgery for the removal of pituitary or other brain tumors may cause damage to the hypothalamus, the pituitary gland, or both.

(4) Less common causes of pituitary or hypothalamic destruction include **sarcoidosis, hemochromatosis, Hand-Schüller-Christian disease, tuberculosis, syphilis,** and **fungal infections.**

b. Clinical features

(1) GH deficiency causes **growth failure in children.** GH deficiency has been thought to have no important clinical effects in adults, but recent studies have suggested that it increases adipose tissue and decreases lean body mass, leading to reduced strength and exercise capacity.

(2) Gonadotropin (LH and FSH) deficiency causes **amenorrhea** and **genital atrophy in women** and **loss of potency and libido in men.** If adrenal androgens are deficient as well, because of concomitant ACTH deficiency, pubic and axillary hair may be lost, especially in women.

(3) TSH deficiency results in the symptoms and physical changes of **hypothyroidism** (see II B 2 a–b).

(4) ACTH deficiency leads to **adrenal insufficiency** (see V C). Secondary adrenal insufficiency (caused by pituitary disease) differs in several clinical manifestations from primary adrenal insufficiency (caused by adrenal disease).

(a) Hyperpigmentation of the skin and mucous membranes is characteristic of primary adrenal disease.

(i) It is caused by the elevated ACTH levels that result, by negative feedback, from low plasma cortisol levels. [ACTH and melanocyte-stimulating hormone (MSH) are derived from the same large precursor molecule (proopiomelanocortin), so when ACTH is increased, MSH is increased as well. MSH stimulates melanocytes and causes pigmentation].

(ii) ACTH (and therefore, MSH) levels are low in secondary adrenal insufficiency; consequently, hyperpigmentation is not characteristic of this condition.

(b) Electrolyte changes (i.e., decreased serum sodium and increased serum potassium levels) are minimal in secondary adrenal insufficiency, since aldosterone production by the adrenal cortex (which promotes sodium retention) depends mainly on renin and angiotensin (which are undisturbed) rather than on ACTH.

(5) Prolactin deficiency may be responsible for the postpartum failure of lactation in Sheehan's syndrome but otherwise produces no clinical manifestations.

(6) With slow, progressive destruction of pituitary tissue, **failure of GH and gonadotropin secretion** occurs early. With continuing loss of tissue, TSH and finally ACTH and prolactin fall below normal levels.

(7) Deficiency of individual pituitary hormones may occur. Isolated GH deficiency and isolated gonadotropin deficiency are not uncommon, especially in children. Isolated deficiencies of TSH and ACTH are very uncommon.

c. Diagnosis

(1) Evaluation of target organ function is often the first step in the diagnosis of hypopituitarism; this condition is often suspected because of failure of more than one target organ (i.e., the thyroid, the adrenal glands, or the gonads). Tests of thyroid, adrenal, ovarian, and testicular function are described in sections II, V, VI, and VII, respectively.

(2) Measurement of pituitary hormones

(a) GH levels may be undetectable under basal conditions in normal individuals; therefore, provocative maneuvers are needed to prove inadequacy of hormone production.

(i) Insulin-induced hypoglycemia is the most consistently effective test stimulus for GH. Regular insulin, in a dose of 0.1–0.15 U/kg, is given as an intravenous bolus, and GH levels are measured after 30, 60, and 90 minutes have passed. The fall in the serum glucose level, usually maximal at 30 minutes, is followed by a rise in GH to a level greater than 8–10 ng/ml in normal individuals. The patient must be observed closely during the test; central nervous system (CNS) symptoms of hypoglycemia require immediate intravenous administration of glucose.

(ii) Levodopa (L-dopa) is almost as consistently effective as insulin, and administration is considerably more convenient. L-Dopa is given orally in a dose of 0.5 g, and GH levels are measured at 30, 60, and 90 minutes.

(iii) Administration of **arginine or glucagon with propranolol** and **exercise** are also methods of stimulating GH production.

(b) Levels of other pituitary hormones can be measured by radioimmunoassay, but since low values cannot be distinguished reliably from normal values, the evaluation is useful only in special situations.

(i) If thyroid function is subnormal [e.g., a low thyroxine (T_4) and low triiodothyronine (T_3) uptake], the TSH level should be elevated if the disorder originates in the thyroid; a low (or low-normal) TSH value strongly suggests hypopituitarism.

(ii) If adrenal insufficiency is present (e.g., if levels of serum cortisol are low), the ACTH level should be elevated if the disorder originates in the adrenal gland; a low (or low-normal) ACTH level strongly suggests hypopituitarism.

        (iii) In postmenopausal women, or in men with inadequate testicular function (i.e., a low testosterone level), LH and FSH levels should be high; low (or low-normal) values suggest hypopituitarism.

   (3) Other provocative tests

      (a) Insulin-induced hypoglycemia stimulates cortisol production as well as GH production. Cortisol levels can be measured in the same blood samples in which GH is measured. An increase in serum cortisol of at least 10 μg/dl to a level of 20 μg/dl or higher indicates normal function of the entire hypothalamic–pituitary–adrenal axis.

      (b) The **metyrapone test** evaluates ACTH reserve function.

         (i) Metyrapone inhibits 11β-hydroxylation, the enzymatic step that produces cortisol from its precursor, 11-desoxycortisol. Oral metyrapone administration causes a fall in cortisol production, which stimulates ACTH output by the pituitary gland. The increased ACTH stimulates production of 11-desoxycortisol.

         (ii) If the serum level of 11-desoxycortisol increases as expected after metyrapone administration, it indicates that both pituitary ACTH reserve and adrenal response to ACTH are normal.

  d. Therapy

   (1) The **underlying cause** of the patient's pituitary insufficiency (e.g., enlarging pituitary tumors, granulomatous diseases) should be sought and treated, if possible.

   (2) Hormone replacement

      (a) GH administration can stimulate growth and increase the ultimate height in children with isolated GH deficiency or panhypopituitarism. Synthetic human growth hormone of recombinant DNA origin is available, but must be given by injection and is expensive. GH replacement in adults with GH deficiency is being given experimentally but is not standard practice.

      (b) Thyroid hormone is given in usual replacement doses (see II B 4).

      (c) Cortisol is given in usual replacement doses (see V C 4).

      (d) Estrogen–progesterone combinations may be given to women to restore menstrual function, and **testosterone** may be given to men to restore libido and potency.

      (e) Fertility is considerably more difficult to achieve because it depends on the precisely controlled administration of **gonadotropins** or **gonadotropin-releasing hormone (GnRH).**

         (i) GnRH has been successful in restoring ovulation in women and sperm production in men, but only in cases in which hypothalamic production of GnRH is impaired but the pituitary retains its ability to secrete LH and FSH in response to GnRH.

         (ii) GnRH stimulates LH and FSH production only if it is administered in a way that mimics normal physiologic secretion; that is, it must be given by regular pulsatile injection every 90–120 minutes. (Constant, rather than pulsatile, administration of GnRH has the opposite effect. It decreases pituitary LH and FSH production).

3. Acromegaly

  a. Etiology. Acromegaly is caused by a pituitary adenoma that produces GH.

   (1) In many cases, the adenoma is large enough to distort the sella turcica and can be seen on lateral skull x-ray; in other cases, CT scan or MRI is needed to visualize the tumor; in a few cases, no tumor can be visualized.

   (2) Pathologically, the tumors are eosinophilic or chromophobic adenomas. Immunohistochemical staining reveals that these adenomas are composed of somatotroph cells.

  b. Clinical features. Excess GH secretion may cause changes in bone, soft tissues, and metabolic processes.

Table 9-1. Skeletal and Soft Tissue Manifestations of Acromegaly

Enlargement of hands (especially fingertips) and feet
  Increased ring, glove, and shoe sizes
Coarsening of facial features
  Thick skin folds
    Brows and nasolabial creases
  Enlargement of nose
  Enlargement of mandible
    Prognathism
    Spreading of teeth
Enlargement of internal organs
  Heart, lungs, liver, spleen, and kidneys
Skin thickening and interstitial edema, with swelling and firmness of soft tissues
Osteoarthritis
Entrapment neuropathies (especially carpal tunnel syndrome)
X-ray changes
  Enlargement of sinuses
  Tufting of distal phalanges, cortical thickening

(1) Bone and soft tissue changes

(a) In children, excess GH secretion may cause increased linear growth of long bones, resulting in **gigantism.** After closure of the epiphyses at puberty, these changes cannot occur.

(b) In adults, soft tissue growth and bone enlargement, especially in the acral areas of the skeleton, lead to **diverse manifestations,** many of **which affect the patient's appearance** (Table 9-1). These changes are gradual and may not be obvious to the patient or the patient's family until the present appearance is compared with that on old photographs.

(2) Metabolic changes

(a) Decreased glucose tolerance, a result of the anti-insulin actions of GH, is common, although overt diabetes occurs in only 10% of acromegalic patients.

(b) A tendency to develop **hyperphosphatemia** is caused by the increased tubular reabsorption of phosphate that is induced by GH.

c. Diagnosis of acromegaly depends on the clinical manifestations. Abnormalities in the blood levels of GH, insulin-like growth factor I (IGF-I, formerly called somatomedin C), or both, confirm the diagnosis.

(1) GH levels should be measured in the morning under basal conditions, if possible before the patient arises from bed, because exercise or stress can raise GH levels, especially in women.

(a) A level higher than 10 ng/ml favors the diagnosis of acromegaly.

(b) In acromegalic patients, GH levels measured 1–2 hours after ingestion of 100 g of glucose are not suppressed to less than 2 ng/ml as they are in normal individuals. Acromegalic patients may even show a paradoxical increase in GH after glucose administration, whereas the level falls in normal individuals. [If the basal level of GH is greatly increased (e.g., greater than 30–50 ng/ml), as is common in acromegaly, demonstration of nonsuppressibility of GH by glucose is not necessary.]

(2) IGF-I is a growth factor produced by the liver under the stimulation of GH. IGF-I levels may be elevated in acromegalic patients whose GH level is normal or equivocal. Elevated levels of IGF-I provide an additional index of GH activity and further evidence of the diagnosis.

d. Therapy

(1) Transsphenoidal pituitary adenomectomy causes prompt normalization of GH levels in the majority of patients; permanent cure is common when the adenoma is small but uncommon when the tumor is large and extends beyond the sella turcica.

    (2) Conventional radiotherapy lowers GH levels slowly; normal levels may not be reached until 3–10 years after treatment, if at all.

    (3) Octreotide is an analogue of somatostatin that can be given by subcutaneous injection. It lowers GH levels in many patients with acromegaly, and may be useful in patients in whom surgery and radiotherapy have been unsuccessful.

4. Hyperprolactinemia. As many as 50% of all pituitary adenomas have been found to secrete prolactin.

  a. Etiology

    (1) Prolactin-secreting pituitary adenomas (prolactinomas) are more common in women than in men, usually appearing during the reproductive years and causing menstrual abnormalities and galactorrhea (the galactorrhea-amenorrhea syndrome). Men tend to have larger tumors at the time of diagnosis, which usually are suspected because of neurologic impairment and hypogonadism.

    (2) Damage to the hypothalamus or pituitary stalk by tumors, granulomas, and other processes may prevent the normal regulatory effect of hypothalamic dopamine on lactotrope activity, resulting in hypersecretion of prolactin.

    (3) Drugs that can inhibit dopamine activity and, thus, interfere with its regulation of prolactin secretion include psychotropic agents (e.g., phenothiazines, butyrophenones, tricyclic antidepressants), antihypertensives (e.g., methyldopa, reserpine), metoclopramide, cimetidine, and others.

  b. Clinical features

    (1) Amenorrhea or menstrual irregularity is due to the inhibition of hypothalamic GnRH production by prolactin as well as the direct effects of the prolactin on the ovaries.

    (2) Galactorrhea is a direct result of prolactin excess.

    (3) Loss of potency and libido, with low testosterone levels, is the common endocrine manifestation in men.

  c. Diagnosis

    (1) Prolactin levels are elevated. A serum prolactin level greater than 300 ng/ml strongly suggests the presence of a prolactinoma. Functional causes of hyperprolactinemia, such as drugs, seldom elevate the level above 100–200 ng/ml.

    (2) CT scanning and **MRI** are used to visualize an adenoma.

  d. Therapy for prolactinoma depends on the size of the tumor and its manifestations. A small, nonenlarging tumor in a woman with insignificant galactorrhea who does not desire pregnancy may not require treatment. If pregnancy is desired, if the galactorrhea or amenorrhea is unacceptable, or if the tumor is enlarging or causing local symptoms, therapeutic options include **surgery, administration of bromocriptine,** and **radiotherapy.**

    (1) Transsphenoidal surgery cures most patients with small prolactinomas. Large tumors with suprasellar extension, however, usually are not cured by surgery.

    (2) Bromocriptine is remarkably effective in decreasing prolactin levels, usually to normal, which promptly relieves the galactorrhea and restores normal menses and fertility; it frequently reduces tumor size as well. However, many patients may not tolerate bromocriptine; its side effects include nausea, headache, dizziness, and fatigue.

      (a) Initial dosages of 1.25 mg once or twice daily may need to be increased to 10–20 mg daily for full effect.

      (b) Because of the poor surgical results in patients with large tumors, many physicians recommend initial treatment with bromocriptine. If the tumor shrinks, there is a greater chance for successful surgery.

(3) **Radiotherapy** may be used in conjunction with surgery and bromocriptine to further reduce tumor size and function.

B. **Posterior pituitary disease. Arginine vasopressin [antidiuretic hormone (ADH)]** is produced by cells in the supraoptic and paraventricular nuclei of the hypothalamus, travels down the pituitary stalk in the axons of these cells, and is stored in the nerve endings in the posterior lobe of the pituitary gland (i.e., in the neurohypophysis). Inadequate ADH production may follow damage to the hypothalamus, the pituitary stalk, and, less commonly, the posterior pituitary gland, and it results in **diabetes insipidus.** Excessive ADH production produces the **syndrome of inappropriate secretion of ADH (SIADH).**

1. **Diabetes insipidus** that is due to ADH insufficiency is termed **central** diabetes insipidus and that due to renal unresponsiveness to ADH is termed **nephrogenic** diabetes insipidus.
   a. **Etiology**
      (1) Approximately 50% of the cases of diabetes insipidus are **idiopathic.**
      (2) **Injury to the hypothalamic–pituitary area** may result from head trauma, brain tumors, and neurosurgical procedures.
      (3) **Less common causes** of diabetes insipidus include **sarcoidosis, syphilis, Hand-Schüller-Christian disease,** and **encephalitis.**
   b. **Clinical features**
      (1) **Polyuria,** with urine volumes of 3–15 L daily, results from the inability to reabsorb free water and to concentrate urine in the absence of adequate ADH.
      (2) **Thirst** results, which leads to **increased fluid intake.** A conscious patient with a normal thirst mechanism and free access to water will maintain hydration; the disease in such a patient is an inconvenience rather than a threat to life. However, rapid and life-threatening dehydration may occur in an infant or in an unconscious patient.
      (3) Laboratory abnormalities include a **dilute urine** (with osmolality < 200 mOsm/kg and specific gravity < 1.005) and a high-normal or slightly **elevated plasma osmolality.**
   c. **Diagnosis**
      (1) **Measurement of plasma osmolality** in the untreated patient helps to distinguish the causes of polyuria. In diabetes insipidus, the loss of free water is primary and plasma osmolality tends to be high (280–310 mOsm/kg). In psychogenic polydipsia, excessive fluid intake is primary and plasma osmolality tends to be low (255–280 mOsm/kg).
      (2) **Water deprivation.** Fluid intake is withheld until urine osmolality reaches a plateau (i.e., an hourly increase of < 30 mOsm/kg for 3 consecutive hours). When urine osmolality is stable, plasma osmolality is measured. Five units of aqueous vasopressin or 2 μg of desmopressin is then injected subcutaneously, and urine osmolality is measured again 1 hour later.
         (a) The responses typical of normal individuals and of patients with partial, complete, and nephrogenic diabetes insipidus are shown in Table 9-2.

Table 9-2. Response to Water Deprivation Test

Diagnosis	Increase in Urine Osmolality above 280 mOsm/kg with Dehydration	Further Increase in Urine Osmolality in Response to ADH
Normal	+	−
Complete central diabetes insipidus	−	+
Partial central diabetes insipidus	+	+
Nephrogenic diabetes insipidus	−	−

ADH = antidiuretic hormone.

(b) Patients with partial diabetes insipidus show an increase in urine osmolality with dehydration, but the incompleteness of their response is demonstrated by a further increase after ADH is injected.

(3) Infusion of hypertonic saline solution (2.5% sodium chloride administered intravenously for 45 minutes at 0.25 ml/kg/min) after a water load (20 ml/kg in 30–60 minutes) causes a sharp decrease in urine flow in normal subjects because of stimulation of ADH secretion. Patients with diabetes insipidus cannot respond to this stimulus.

(4) Differential diagnosis. In a patient with polyuria and dilute urine, central diabetes insipidus must be differentiated from nephrogenic diabetes insipidus and compulsive water drinking.

(a) Nephrogenic diabetes insipidus is a condition in which the renal tubules fail to respond to normal circulating levels of ADH.

(i) The condition may be familial, starting in infancy, or it may occur later in life in association with hypokalemia, hypercalcemia, chronic renal disease, sickle cell anemia, amyloidosis, or the use of certain drugs (e.g., lithium, demeclocycline, methoxyflurane).

(ii) The clinical features are the same as those caused by ADH deficiency. The difference is seen in the failure of nephrogenic diabetes insipidus to respond to administration of ADH.

(b) Compulsive water drinking (psychogenic polydipsia) is a primary psychiatric abnormality that leads to polyuria and dilute urine. Differentiation from diabetes insipidus may be difficult. It is most common in young or middle-aged women who often have a history of psychiatric disorders.

d. Therapy

(1) Desmopressin (dDAVP) is a synthetic analogue of vasopressin that can be administered topically; 0.05–0.2 ml is applied to the upper respiratory mucous membranes twice daily by nasal cannula or nasal spray. A parenteral preparation is available for use in acutely ill or postoperative patients.

(2) Chlorpropamide. A side effect of this oral hypoglycemic agent is the potentiation of the action, the secretion, or both, of endogenous ADH.

(a) Patients who have at least partial ADH production often become asymptomatic when 250–500 mg of chlorpropamide is taken daily.

(b) The physician and patient must watch for hypoglycemia, a possible side effect of chlorpropamide.

(3) Thiazide diuretics have the paradoxical effect of decreasing urine output in patients with diabetes insipidus.

(a) The volume depletion induced by the diuretic increases sodium and water reabsorption in the proximal tubule, thus blunting the effect of the defective water absorption in the distal and collecting tubules.

(b) Thiazides are only partially effective, decreasing urine volume by 30%–50%. However, they are the only drugs useful for treating nephrogenic diabetes insipidus, because their action does not depend on distal tubular response to ADH.

2. SIADH

a. Etiology

(1) ADH production by **malignant tumors,** particularly oat cell carcinoma of the lung and carcinoma of the pancreas, was the originally recognized cause of SIADH.

(2) More commonly, excess ADH production is caused by other disease processes through unknown mechanisms via the hypothalamic–neurohypophyseal axis or by diseased tissue. These disease processes include **pulmonary diseases** (e.g., pneumonia, tuberculosis) and **central nervous system (CNS) disorders** (e.g., stroke, head injury, encephalitis).

(3) Drugs (e.g., chlorpropamide, carbamazepine, vincristine, clofibrate) may stimulate hypothalamic–neurohypophyseal ADH production.

b. Pathophysiology. ADH excess causes water retention and extracellular fluid volume expansion, which is then compensated for by increased urinary sodium excretion. Clinically, significant volume expansion (i.e., edema or hypertension) is not present, because of the natriuresis. However, the water retention and the sodium loss both contribute to **hyponatremia, which is the hallmark of SIADH.** If water intake is minimized, this sequence of events does not occur and serum sodium levels do not fall.

   c. **Clinical features. Hyponatremia** refers to a serum sodium level less than 135 mEq/L.

     (1) Symptoms of lethargy, confusion, agitation, headache, nausea and vomiting, and focal neurologic abnormalities are common when the sodium level declines rapidly or when it reaches a level less than approximately 125 mEq/L.

     (2) Seizures and coma may occur with more severe hyponatremia.

   d. **Diagnosis** of SIADH is based on the following conditions.

     (1) **Hyponatremia** is present, with low serum osmolality.

     (2) **Daily urinary sodium excretion exceeds 20 mEq/L,** despite the low serum sodium levels, and urine osmolality is higher than serum osmolality. (Other causes of hyponatremia, such as sodium depletion, cause renal retention of sodium, with less than 20 mEq/L excreted daily.)

     (3) Conditions that might appropriately stimulate ADH secretion because of volume depletion must be excluded. These include adrenal insufficiency, fluid loss, edematous states (e.g., heart failure, nephrosis, cirrhosis), and renal failure.

   e. **Therapy.** The cause of SIADH should be treated when possible.

     (1) **Fluid restriction** to 500–1000 ml daily is effective in increasing the serum sodium level and is the mainstay of treatment. The limiting factor is patient compliance.

     (2) If hyponatremia is severe, hypertonic (3%) saline should be administered to elevate the serum sodium level above 120 mEq/L.

       (a) Serum sodium should not be increased rapidly to a level exceeding 125 mEq/L, or CNS damage may result (see Chapter 11 XI B 1).

       (b) Salt loading is of only temporary value because the additional sodium is soon excreted in the urine.

     (3) If fluid restriction cannot be enforced, 300 mg of **demeclocycline** can be administered 3 or 4 times daily. Demeclocycline is an antibiotic with the useful side effect of inhibiting renal tubular response to ADH.

II. **DISORDERS OF THE THYROID GLAND.** The thyroid may produce too little or too much hormone; it may undergo chronic enlargement and inflammation (**chronic thyroiditis**); and it is a common site for benign and malignant tumors. Thyroid disease is suggested by symptoms of hypothyroidism (i.e., insufficient thyroid hormone effect) or **hyperthyroidism** (i.e., excess thyroid hormone effect) or by localized or diffuse thyroid enlargement (**goiter**). Initially, thyroid disease usually is evaluated by thyroid function tests, which estimate hormone production. Information on the physical characteristics and function of separate areas of the thyroid may then be obtained, if necessary, by isotope scans and other imaging techniques.

A. **Thyroid function studies**

   1. **Serum T_4 determination** measures the total bound (99.95%) and free (0.05%) T_4 in the circulation. The serum T_4 concentration is elevated in hyperthyroidism and decreased in hypothyroidism.

     a. The proteins that bind T_4, mainly thyroxine-binding globulin (TBG), are elevated by estrogen treatment, pregnancy, congenital TBG excess, and sometimes by liver disease.

       (1) If the binding proteins are elevated, the total T_4 concentration in the blood is high but the concentration of free T_4 (the active form of the hormone at

the tissue level) remains normal because it is regulated by the normally functioning T_4-TSH feedback mechanism.

(2) If the concentration of free T_4 is normal, the patient is euthyroid, and the elevated level of total T_4 is misleading.

b. The converse is also true. TBG levels may be lowered by androgen treatment, congenital TBG deficiency, the nephrotic syndrome, or cirrhosis. In this case, the concentration of total T_4 is low, but the patient maintains a normal level of free T_4 and is euthyroid.

c. Therefore, the T_4 concentration alone is not an adequate test to evaluate thyroid function. Either the T_4 concentration must be measured in conjunction with a test that evaluates protein binding (i.e., the T_3 uptake test), or free T_4 itself must be measured.

2. **Serum T_3 determination** measures the concentration of the total bound and free T_3 in the circulation. The total T_3 measurement may give the same misleading results as the total T_4 measurement if there is an abnormality in binding proteins.

3. **T_3 uptake test**

a. This test is performed by combining in a tube the patient's serum, a known amount of radiolabeled T_3, and an insoluble binder of T_3, such as a small piece of resin. The binding proteins from the patient's serum and the resin compete for the labeled T_3.

(1) If the binding proteins are increased, less T_3 binds to the resin, and if the proteins are decreased, more T_3 binds to the resin.

(2) The result, which is expressed as a percent of labeled T_3 bound to the resin, is a measure of the unoccupied binding sites on the patient's thyroid hormone–binding proteins.

b. **Interpretation**

(1) The T_3 resin uptake is elevated in hyperthyroidism. Thyroid hormone is increased in the blood; therefore, the hormone bound to protein is also increased, leaving fewer unoccupied binding sites. Consequently, there is increased labeled T_3 binding to resin. Conversely, the T_3 resin uptake is decreased in hypothyroidism.

(2) In both instances, the T_3 resin uptake varies directly with changes in the total T_4 and total T_3 concentrations and confirms the diagnosis suggested by the total T_4 and total T_3 levels.

(3) However, if the levels of total T_4, total T_3, or both are increased or decreased because of abnormalities of the binding proteins, rather than hypothyroidism or hyperthyroidism, the T_3 resin uptake changes in the opposite direction (i.e., when binding protein is increased, there is an increase in total T_4 concentration; when there is increased binding protein, there is an increase in unoccupied binding sites and, therefore, decreased T_3 resin uptake).

4. **Free T_4 index**

a. If the total T_4 level and T_3 resin uptake are known, an index can be calculated that estimates the free T_4 level.

(1) The patient's T_3 resin uptake is divided by the average normal T_3 resin uptake, and the total T_4 is multiplied by this fraction.

(2) The result, which is called the free T_4 index, has approximately the same normal range as the total concentration of T_4. This process considers the effects of abnormalities of thyroid hormone-binding proteins on the total T_4 measurement.

b. **Example.** A patient has a total of T_4 of 15.0 μg/dl (normal = 4.5–12.5 μg/dl). If the T_4 resin uptake is 45%, the free T_4 index equals 45% divided by 30% (which is the average normal uptake) multiplied by 15.0 or 22.5. This result suggests a diagnosis of hyperthyroidism. If the T_3 resin uptake is 15%, the free T_4 index is 7.5 (15/30 × 15.0), suggesting that the patient is euthyroid but has an increased level of T_4-binding proteins.

5. Serum TSH measurement

a. In primary **hypothyroidism,** measuring the serum TSH concentration is a very sensitive test, because it usually becomes elevated even before thyroid hormone levels (total T_4 or total T_3) decline below normal. TSH elevation is caused by the negative feedback effects of low thyroid hormone levels.

b. In **hyperthyroidism,** the elevated thyroid hormone concentrations lead to suppression of serum TSH to levels below normal; this can be detected if a sufficiently sensitive assay is used. This finding is a very sensitive indication of hyperthyroidism, because TSH may be suppressed even when thyroid hormone levels are not elevated above the normal range.

6. Radioactive iodine uptake by the thyroid gland 24 hours after administration of the isotope is increased in hyperthyroidism and decreased in hypothyroidism. This test is especially useful in detecting forms of hyperthyroidism in which the thyroid gland itself is not synthesizing excess hormone; that is, the hyperthyroidism associated with exogenous thyroid hormone administration, subacute thyroiditis, and ectopic hormone production (e.g., caused by struma ovarii). In these situations, blood hormone levels are high, but the radioactive iodine uptake is low.

B. Hypothyroidism

1. Etiology

a. Chronic thyroiditis (see II D 2) is the most common cause of spontaneous hypothyroidism in the United States.

b. Idiopathic atrophy of the thyroid is also common. Antithyroid antibodies frequently are present. This may represent an atrophic form of chronic thyroiditis.

c. Hypothyroidism frequently develops following the treatment of Graves' disease, and the prevalence may approach 50% in patients treated with radioactive iodine. However, hypothyroidism also may occur after Graves' disease is treated by subtotal thyroidectomy or antithyroid drugs.

d. Secondary hypothyroidism is caused by any of the conditions that may affect the hypothalamic–pituitary axis and cause hypopituitarism (see I A 2 a).

e. Less common causes of hypothyroidism include congenital athyreosis, congenital biochemical defects that prevent thyroid hormone production, and insensitivity of the tissues to thyroid hormone. Iodine deficiency is an uncommon cause of hypothyroidism in most highly developed countries, but it is common in some areas of the world.

2. Clinical features

a. Symptoms (Table 9-3)

(1) As metabolism slows because of the lessened effects of thyroid hormone on tissues, the patient may experience **weakness, lethargy, sleepiness and fatigue, and slowness of speech and thought.**

(2) A puffy appearance, constipation, and a **constant feeling of cold** are common.

(3) Slight to moderate **weight gain** reflects the decreased metabolism, but massive weight gain does not occur because appetite tends to be diminished.

Table 9-3. Symptoms of Hypothyroidism

Weakness, lethargy, and fatigue ("slowing down")
Dry skin and coarse hair
Puffy eyelids, face, and hands; swollen legs
Cold intolerance
Constipation
Weight gain
Hoarseness
Menorrhagia
Hearing loss

Table 9-4. Physical Findings in Hypothyroidism

Thickened, puffy features
Yellowish, dry skin
Nonpitting edema
Hypothermia
Bradycardia
Slow return of deep tendon reflexes
Loss of lateral portion of eyebrows

  (4) Edema of the larynx and middle ear may cause **voice changes and hearing loss** in severe cases.
  (5) Excess and **irregular menstrual bleeding** may be associated with anovulatory cycles.
 b. Physical findings (Table 9-4)
  (1) Puffiness and **nonpitting edema** are caused by the accumulation of mucinous mucopolysaccharide-rich material in the tissues. The term **myxedema** describes this phenomenon and is sometimes used synonymously with severe hypothyroidism.
  (2) The characteristic puffy, dull appearance and the **slow return phase** of the Achilles and other **deep tendon reflexes** are perhaps the most helpful physical findings in suggesting hypothyroidism.
 c. Effects on organ systems. All organ systems are affected; some of the most important changes are listed in Table 9-5.
 d. Cretinism is severe **hypothyroidism beginning in infancy.** Cretinism is marked by mental retardation and impairment of physical growth and development.
  (1) Short limbs and a large head, with a broad, flat nose, widely set eyes, and a large tongue characterize this form of dwarfism.
  (2) Epiphyseal dysgenesis, with abnormalities of the ossification centers, affects the femoral and humeral heads and other parts of the skeleton.
  (3) Early recognition and treatment prevent the otherwise irreversible mental and physical impairment.
 e. Myxedema coma may result if severe hypothyroidism goes untreated. This serious condition may occur gradually (over years) or more acutely in response to precipitating factors (e.g., infection, exposure to cold).
  (1) Hypothermia, hypoglycemia, shock, hypoventilation, and ileus may be present in myxedema coma in addition to the severely depressed state of consciousness.
  (2) The mortality rate is 50%–75%.

Table 9-5. Effects of Hypothyroidism on Organ Systems

Cardiovascular system
 Decrease in cardiac output
 Pericardial effusion
Respiratory system
 Hypoventilation
 Pleural effusion
Gastrointestinal tract
 Constipation
Nervous system
 Decreased mental function
 Psychiatric changes (e.g., psychosis, depression)
Blood
 Normochromic normocytic anemia

3. **Diagnosis**
   a. **Overt hypothyroidism** is suggested in severe cases by the characteristic symptoms and physical findings; however, mild cases may escape detection unless laboratory tests are performed. Routine laboratory screening is especially recommended for newborns and elderly individuals with nonspecific complaints.
      (1) Serum T_4 and T_3 levels are decreased, and T_3 uptake is depressed.
      (2) An increased serum concentration of TSH is the earliest and most sensitive indicator of primary hypothyroidism. If the TSH level is elevated, the diagnosis may be confirmed by the finding of a decreased serum free T_4 or free T_4 index.
   b. **Subclinical hypothyroidism** is a common condition in which serum TSH is elevated but serum free T_4 or the free T_4 index is normal rather than decreased. Many of these patients progress to overt hypothyroidism. The decision to treat patients with subclinical hypothyroidism must be made on a case-by-case basis. A greater degree of TSH elevation and the presence of symptoms that might be caused by hypothyroidism are factors favoring a decision to treat.

4. **Therapy**
   a. **Thyroid hormone preparations.** Thyroid extract derived from animal sources and synthetic preparations containing both T_4 and T_3 have been used in the past and are still available. However, synthetic L-thyroxine sodium is the agent of choice.
      (1) The administered T_4 is slowly converted to T_3, and the proportions of circulating T_4 and T_3 approximate those of euthyroid individuals.
      (2) The peaks and valleys of blood T_3 levels, which are seen when exogenous T_3 is given, are avoided.
   b. **Initiation of treatment**
      (1) Patients with severe hypothyroidism, older patients, and patients with cardiovascular disease may have an increased sensitivity to thyroid hormone and are at risk for acute cardiovascular and other complications if the hypothyroidism is corrected too quickly. Therefore, these patients should be given a very small dose of thyroid hormone initially (i.e., 25 μg of L-thyroxine), which is increased to a full maintenance dose during a 6- to 12-week period.
      (2) Younger patients and patients with less severe hypothyroidism may be started on a slightly higher dose (50 μg of L-thyroxine) and advanced to a full replacement dose more quickly (e.g., the dose may be raised to 100 μg in 2 weeks and to 125 μg or 150 μg in another 2 weeks).
   c. **Maintenance therapy.** Most patients require 75–150 μg of L-thyroxine daily. When this dose is tolerated and symptoms of hypothyroidism have resolved, the dose should be further adjusted so that serum TSH and thyroid hormone levels are maintained in the normal range.
   d. **Myxedema coma** has a high mortality rate **and must be treated rapidly,** despite the risk associated with sudden hormone replacement.
      (1) L-thyroxine is given intravenously as 500-μg bolus injection, followed by daily maintenance doses.
      (2) Ancillary treatment includes the temporary use of adrenal corticosteroids and respiratory support.

C. **Hyperthyroidism**

1. **Etiology**
   a. **Graves' disease (diffuse toxic goiter) is the most common cause of hyperthyroidism.** It is an autoimmune disorder in which an abnormal immunoglobulin G (thyroid-stimulating immunoglobulin) binds to receptors for TSH on the thyroid follicular cells, causing diffuse enlargement of the gland and stimulation of thyroid hormone production. Graves' disease is most common in women between the ages of 20 and 50 years, although others may be affected.
   b. **Plummer's disease (nodular toxic goiter)** is less common than Graves' disease and usually affects older individuals.

      (1) Discrete areas of the thyroid function autonomously, for unknown reasons, secreting excessive amounts of thyroid hormone.

      (2) The pathognomonic feature is the presence of unaffected thyroid tissue, the function of which is suppressed by the high thyroid hormone levels and consequent TSH suppression but which can be shown to concentrate radio-active iodine after TSH injection.

    c. Subacute thyroiditis (see II D 1) may cause transient hyperthyroidism.

    d. Factitious hyperthyroidism may be caused by surreptitious ingestion of thyroid hormone by patients. Inadvertent administration of excessive doses of the hormone by physicians may have the same result.

    e. Rare causes of hyperthyroidism include excess TSH production by **pituitary tumors, teratomas of the ovary** that produce thyroid hormone (**struma ovarii**), and overproduction of hormone by the thyroid gland following iodine ingestion, which is called jodbasedow.

2. Clinical features. Thyroid hormone increases oxygen consumption by tissues, raising heat production and energy metabolism. It interacts with the sympathetic nervous system in a way that seems to increase tissue sensitivity to catecholamines and adrenergic stimuli. It affects protein, fat, carbohydrate, and vitamin metabolism. These and other actions lead to profound changes in many organ systems when thyroid hormone is in excess.

    a. Metabolic changes include an **elevated basal metabolic rate** and **weight loss,** despite increased appetite and food intake. **Sweating** and **heat intolerance** reflect the increased heat production.

    b. Cardiovascular effects

      (1) The heart rate is increased; **sinus tachycardia** is common, with rates of 120 bpm or higher in severe cases.

      (2) Systolic blood pressure tends to be elevated and diastolic blood pressure decreased, with a **wide pulse pressure.**

      (3) Myocardial excitability is increased, and arrhythmias (e.g., **atrial fibrillation, premature ventricular contractions**) may occur.

    c. Gastrointestinal symptoms of loose stools or **diarrhea** are common.

    d. Skin and hair changes. The **skin is warm and moist** because of peripheral vasodilation and increased sweating. **Fine, silky hair** is characteristic.

    e. CNS effects include **emotional lability, restlessness,** and **fine tremor.**

    f. Muscle weakness and **fatigue** are common.

    g. Ophthalmopathy

      (1) Stare and **lid lag** (i.e., slow closing of the upper lid when the eye moves downward, revealing sclera between the lid and cornea) may occur in any form of hyperthyroidism.

      (2) True **thyroid exophthalmos,** however, is seen only in Graves' disease, occurring in approximately 50% of cases. The eye is pushed forward because of mucinous and cellular **infiltration of the extraocular muscles.** There is **inflammation of the conjunctiva** and surrounding tissues. The patient may complain of **tearing, eye irritation, pain,** and **double vision.** In severe cases, vision may be threatened.

    h. Thyroid storm is a sudden exacerbation of the signs and symptoms of hyperthyroidism.

      (1) Thyroid storm may be precipitated by intercurrent illness, trauma, surgery, or childbirth.

      (2) Marked fever, tachycardia, and agitation are present and may progress to stupor and coma, with vascular collapse.

      (3) The mortality rate is 50%–75%.

3. Diagnosis

    a. Presenting symptoms of weight loss, nervousness, palpitations, muscle weakness, and diarrhea are characteristic of hyperthyroidism.

    b. Family history of thyroid disease is common.

    c. Physical examination often reveals a fidgety, hyperkinetic patient with warm, moist skin; fine, silky hair; and a fine tremor of the hands.

(1) The eyes may be prominent, with retraction of the upper lid and a staring appearance.

(2) The thyroid is enlarged in most cases. In Graves' disease, the enlargement is uniform, and a bruit may be heard over the gland; in Plummer's disease, one or more nodular areas are usually felt.

(3) The heart rate often exceeds 100 bpm.

(4) The return phase of the deep tendon reflexes is brisk.

d. Laboratory studies show an increase in the serum concentration of total T_4, the serum concentration of total T_3, and the T_3 resin uptake. The radioactive iodine uptake is high. Serum TSH levels are low.

4. **Therapy.** The **adrenergic manifestations of hyperthyroidism** (e.g., sweating, tachycardia, tremor) may be diminished by **β-blockers.** These drugs do not affect thyroid function but provide symptomatic relief until thyroid hormone levels can be lowered to normal.

   a. Treatment of Graves' disease. The most common methods for treatment of Graves' disease are **antithyroid drugs, subtotal thyroidectomy,** and **radioactive iodine.**

   (1) Antithyroid drugs

   (a) Mechanism of action. Methimazole and **propylthiouracil (PTU)** inhibit the oxidation of iodide and the coupling of iodotyrosines, thus decreasing the synthesis of thyroid hormone. PTU, in addition, decreases the conversion of T_4 to T_3 in peripheral tissues.

   (b) Medical treatment of Graves' disease. Full doses (i.e., 30–40 mg of methimazole or 300–400 mg of PTU) are given daily until the patient is euthyroid.

   (i) Although blockade of hormone synthesis is rapid, clinical improvement occurs only after a few weeks or months, because a large pool of stored hormone continues to be released from the thyroid.

   (ii) After clinical improvement, the dose is tapered to the lowest dose that maintains euthyroidism, and the drug is continued for $1-1\frac{1}{2}$ years. Treatment is then discontinued in the hope that a lasting or permanent remission has occurred.

   (c) Drug toxicity

   (i) Skin rash or joint pain occurs in 3%–5% of patients, necessitating a switch to the alternative drug.

   (ii) Agranulocytosis occurs in fewer than 0.5% of patients but is life threatening. For early detection of agranulocytosis, patients should be instructed to stop the drug immediately if fever, sore throat, mouth ulcers, or other unexplained symptoms occur. Treatment should be resumed only after examination shows a normal white blood cell count.

   (d) Advantages of antithyroid drugs

   (i) Hospitalization, surgery, and anesthesia are avoided.

   (ii) There is less likelihood of the occurrence of post-treatment hypothyroidism than in patients treated with radioactive iodine.

   (e) Disadvantages of antithyroid drugs

   (i) Permanent remission occurs in fewer than 50% of patients treated.

   (ii) Successful treatment depends on patient compliance, which is less of a problem when treatment is by surgery or radioactive iodine.

   (2) Subtotal thyroidectomy

   (a) Preparation for surgery. Operation on a thyrotoxic patient produces the risk of thyroid storm; therefore, treatment should be initiated with antithyroid drugs long enough in advance for the patient to return to a euthyroid state before surgery.

   (b) Advantages of surgery

   (i) Cure of hyperthyroidism is rapid.

   (ii) The success rate is high; most patients are cured, and fewer become hypothyroid after surgery than after treatment with radioactive iodine.

    (iii) Patient compliance is required for a shorter period than it is in prolonged antithyroid drug treatment.

  (c) Disadvantages of surgery

    (i) The patient must be hospitalized, and surgical and anesthetic risks are incurred.

    (ii) Surgical complications include hypoparathyroidism and recurrent laryngeal nerve paralysis.

(3) Radioactive iodine

  (a) Method of treatment. A single dose of iodine 131 (^{131}I) causes a decrease in function and size of the thyroid gland in 6–12 weeks. Approximately 75% of patients with Graves' disease are made euthyroid by a single dose; those who are still thyrotoxic after 12 weeks are given a second dose. Additional doses can be given if needed. Eventually, almost all patients are cured in this way.

  (b) Advantages of radioactive iodine

    (i) Hospitalization, surgery, and anesthesia are avoided.

    (ii) The rate of cure approaches 100%.

    (iii) Little patient compliance is required.

  (c) Disadvantages of radioactive iodine

    (i) Multiple treatments may be needed.

    (ii) Hypothyroidism, the treatment of which requires long-term patient compliance, occurs in approximately 10% of patients after 1 year and continues to develop at a rate of 2%–3% each year. After 10–15 years, as many as 50% of patients are hypothyroid. This complication is easily treated, however, with a single daily dose of L-thyroxine sodium.

    (iii) There is a slight risk of genetic effects (comparable in magnitude to the effects of a barium enema or intravenous urogram) in future offspring. No increase in the risk for leukemia, thyroid cancer, or other malignancies has been found in patients treated with radioactive iodine, however.

(4) Choice of therapy

  (a) Radioactive iodine is the treatment of choice for most patients older than 30–40 years.

  (b) In younger patients, the choice is more difficult. In patients with mild clinical manifestations, slightly to moderately elevated thyroid hormone levels, and an only moderately enlarged thyroid, a trial of antithyroid drugs is reasonable, because patients with mild disease have a better chance for a lasting remission.

  (c) Surgery may be a better choice for patients with large goiters and severe disease and for patients who are unwilling to take antithyroid drugs for a prolonged period.

  (d) Radioactive iodine treatment may be considered even in young patients (i.e., those younger than 30 years of age), if there are reasons to avoid surgery or drugs.

b. Treatment of Plummer's disease. Because antithyroid drug therapy does not lead to permanent remission in patients with Plummer's disease, the options for treatment are surgery and radioactive iodine.

  (1) Thyroidectomy or removal of a hyperfunctioning nodule rapidly cures the hyperthyroidism and relieves symptoms of pressure or tracheal or esophageal obstruction that may be caused by a large goiter.

  (2) Radioactive iodine treatment requires much larger doses in patients with Plummer's disease than in patients with Graves' disease because the affected thyroid cells are relatively radioresistant. However, because the unaffected thyroid cells are functionally suppressed, they do not trap ^{131}I and are spared the effects of radiation; therefore, hypothyroidism following radioactive iodine treatment is less common in patients with Plummer's disease.

c. Treatment of thyroid storm

(1) The mainstay of treatment is iodine, which acts within 24 hours by inhibiting the release of thyroid hormone. Sodium iodide is given in an intravenous dose of 1–2 g over 24 hours, or potassium iodide may be given orally.

(2) Antithyroid drugs are administered, but because they block hormone synthesis without inhibiting the release of release of preformed hormone, their effect is less rapid.

(3) β-Blockers and adrenal corticosteroids also are used.

D. Thyroiditis

1. **Subacute thyroiditis** (also called granulomatous thyroiditis and de Quervain's thyroiditis)

   a. Etiology. The cause of subacute thyroiditis generally is considered to be viral. Mumps and coxsackievirus, among others, have been suspected.

   b. Clinical features

   (1) **Early symptoms** may include a prodrome of malaise, upper respiratory symptoms, and fever that lasts 1 or 2 weeks. Then, the thyroid gland becomes enlarged, film, and tender, with pain radiating to the ears, neck, or arms.

   (2) **Hyperthyroidism** may occur, due to thyroid hormone leaking from damaged follicles into the circulation.

   (3) **Disease course.** The thyroid pain and hyperthyroidism subside in a few weeks or months. The gland usually returns to normal size; if enlargement persists, chronic thyroiditis should be suspected.

   c. Diagnosis is suspected when the thyroid becomes acutely swollen, tender, and painful, especially if symptoms of hyperthyroidism are present. Diagnosis is confirmed by a **very low radioactive iodine uptake in the face of high serum T_4 and T_3 levels.** The radioactive iodine uptake is low because the follicular cells are injured and unable to trap iodine and because the high levels of circulating thyroid hormone suppress TSH.

   d. Therapy is symptomatic, because the disease is self-limited.

   (1) Aspirin, nonsteroidal anti-inflammatory drugs (NSAIDs), and adrenal corticosteroids (in severe cases) relieve the pain and tenderness.

   (2) β-Blocking drugs can be used to relieve symptoms of hyperthyroidism.

2. **Chronic thyroiditis (Hashimoto's thyroiditis)**

   a. Etiology. Chronic thyroiditis is a common autoimmune disorder that mainly affects women. Antithyroid antibodies are present in most patients.

   b. Clinical features

   (1) **Thyroid gland enlargement,** the main clinical manifestation, is the result of autoimmune damage that leads to lymphocytic infiltration, fibrosis, and a weakened ability of the thyroid to produce hormone.

   (2) **Hypothyroidism** is present in approximately 20% of patients when the disease is first diagnosed, but it may develop later in some patients.

   (3) **Pain and tenderness of the gland** sometimes occur, as in subacute thyroiditis.

   c. Diagnosis is suspected in any patient with a firm, nontoxic goiter; a high titer of antithyroglobulin antibodies, antimicrosomal antibodies, or both is confirmatory. Thyroid function tests usually are normal unless the patient has hypothyroidism.

   d. Therapy with L-thyroxine sodium often decreases the size of the goiter and, therefore, is useful even in patients with normal thyroid function. The presence of hypothyroidism makes this treatment necessary.

3. **Painless thyroiditis** (also called silent thyroiditis and lymphocytic thyroiditis with spontaneously resolving hyperthyroidism) is a syndrome that resembles subacute thyroiditis in some ways and chronic thyroiditis in others.

a. Like subacute thyroiditis, painless thyroiditis is associated with transient, self-limited hyperthyroidism, often with thyroid gland enlargement, and a low radioactive iodine uptake. Thyroid pain and tenderness are absent, however.

(1) Recognition of this cause of self-limited hyperthyroidism is important, because, in the absence of thyroid pain to suggest thyroiditis, the syndrome could easily be mistaken for Graves' disease and be treated inappropriately.

(2) The low radioactive iodine uptake is the most useful finding for distinguishing painless thyroiditis from Graves' disease.

b. Like chronic thyroiditis, painless thyroiditis involves lymphocytic infiltration of the thyroid. However, although antithyroid antibodies may be present, the titers are lower than in chronic thyroiditis.

4. **Rare forms of thyroiditis**
   a. **Suppurative thyroiditis** is caused by pyogenic bacterial infection. It is treated with antibiotics and surgical drainage, if necessary.
   b. In **Riedel's struma** (fibrous thyroiditis), fibrous connective tissue replaces normal thyroid tissue and infiltrates surrounding structures. Surgery is indicated to exclude cancer and to relieve tracheal compression.

E. **Thyroid cancer**

1. **Epidemiology**
   a. Thyroid cancer is common; it is found at autopsy in approximately 5% of patients with no known thyroid disease. However, death due to thyroid cancer is uncommon—approximately 1200 individuals die of it each year in the United States.
   b. These contradictory observations are explained best by the behavior of thyroid cancer. It is usually indolent and tends to remain localized to the thyroid for many years, which is the reason for the low mortality rate.

2. **Etiology**
   a. **Radiation exposure.** Incidence of thyroid cancer is increased in atomic bomb survivors and in individuals who received x-ray therapy to the neck (e.g., for enlarged thymus or enlarged tonsils) in childhood.
   b. **Genetic factors.** One form of thyroid cancer, medullary carcinoma, may be familial.
   c. **TSH** can induce thyroid cancer in animals, and the growth of many human thyroid cancers is stimulated by TSH.

3. **Types.** Thyroid cancer may present as a solitary thyroid nodule or, less commonly, as multiple nodules or a mass in the neck. These tumors occasionally cause hoarseness, symptoms of tracheal or esophageal compression (e.g., dyspnea, dysphagia), or pain.
   a. **Papillary carcinoma,** which accounts for 60% of all thyroid cancer, affects the youngest age group—50% of patients are younger than 40 years of age.
   (1) The neoplasm consists of columnar cells in folds (the papillae). It tends to grow slowly, often remaining localized to the thyroid for years, and eventually spreads via the lymphatic system to other parts of the thyroid and to regional nodes.
   (2) There are few recurrences after treatment, especially in young patients with small primary tumors.
   b. **Follicular carcinoma,** which comprises 25% of all thyroid cancer, histologically may resemble normal thyroid tissue.
   (1) It often functions like normal thyroid tissue, trapping iodine in a TSH-dependent fashion.
   (2) Follicular carcinoma is more malignant than papillary cancer and often spreads to bone, the lungs, and the liver. The 10-year survival rate is 50%.
   c. **Medullary carcinoma,** which accounts for 5% of all thyroid cancer, arises from the parafollicular cells (or C cells) of the thyroid. It has a hyalin stroma, which may stain for amyloid.
   (1) Approximately 20% of these carcinomas are familial and may be a compo-

nent of **MEN type II** (Sipple's syndrome), a syndrome of medullary thyroid carcinoma and pheochromocytoma.

(2) This tumor often produces calcitonin and occasionally produces other hormones.

(3) It is more malignant than follicular carcinoma, with both local lymphatic and distant hematogenous spread.

d. **Anaplastic carcinoma,** which accounts for 10% of thyroid cancer, usually affects patients older than 50 years of age and is highly malignant. It invades rapidly, metastasizes widely, and usually causes death within a few months.

4. **Therapy.** Papillary, follicular, and medullary carcinoma usually are treated with a combination of surgery, suppression with thyroid hormone, and radioactive iodine. Anaplastic carcinoma generally is treated palliatively. It may require surgery to relieve obstruction; chemotherapy may delay death.

a. **Surgery**

(1) Papillary carcinoma, when small and limited to a single area of the thyroid, often is treated by removal of the involved lobe and the isthmus.

(2) Follicular carcinoma and more extensive papillary tumors usually are treated by near-total thyroidectomy; just enough tissue is left in association with the posterior capsule to spare the parathyroid glands. This more extensive procedure is more likely to be complicated by hypoparathyroidism, but it is followed by less tumor recurrence.

b. **Suppression therapy.** Because many thyroid cancers grow more rapidly with TSH stimulation, TSH should be suppressed with the highest dose of L-thyroxine that does not cause hyperthyroidism. This treatment is continued indefinitely.

c. **Radioactive iodine therapy.** Follicular cancers often accumulate radioactive iodine, and many papillary cancers contain some follicular elements.

(1) A radioactive iodine scan in a patient whose normal thyroid tissue has been removed surgically may show functioning metastases that can be ablated with ^{131}I.

(2) In addition, radioactive iodine can be used to ablate any normal thyroid tissue that remains after near-total thyroidectomy, allowing subsequent scans to indicate metastatic tumor.

F. **Thyroid nodules** are present in 1% of individuals in their 20s and in 5% of individuals in their 60s; cancer is found in 10%–20% of the nodules that are investigated.

1. **Pathology.** Thyroid nodules may be true adenomas, cysts, localized areas of chronic thyroiditis, colloid nodules, hemorrhagic necrotic tissue, or carcinoma.

2. **Diagnosis**

a. **Risk assessment**

(1) **X-ray treatment** of the head or neck in childhood is associated with an increased prevalence of thyroid nodules and thyroid cancer in adult life.

(2) **Sex.** A higher percentage of nodules are malignant in men than in women (although nodules are much more common in women).

(3) **Age.** A higher percentage of nodules are malignant in younger individuals (although nodules are much more common in older individuals). In children, 50% of nodules are malignant.

(4) **Disease course.** Malignancy is suggested by recent growth of the nodule or by continuing growth despite suppressive therapy with L-thyroxine. Malignancy is less likely if the nodule disappears after aspiration of cyst fluid, if the nodule is visible as a "warm" or "hot" spot on scintiscan (i.e., as demonstrated by its uptake of radioactive iodine), or if the nodule shrinks with suppressive therapy.

(5) **Physical examination**

(a) Malignancy is suggested when the nodule is fixed in place and no movement occurs on swallowing.

(b) It also is suggested by an unusually firm consistency or irregularity of the nodule or by regional lymph node enlargement.

Table 9-6. Results of Fine-Needle Aspiration Biopsy of Thyroid Nodules

Cytologic Findings	% of Nodules	% Positive for Cancer
Benign	61	2.5
Equivocal	24	15
Malignant	15	97

Adapted with permission from Ashcraft MW, Solomon DH: The thyroid nodule. *Ann Intern Med* 96:221–232, 1982.

  (c) Malignancy is less likely if there are multiple nodules or if the nodule is less than 1 cm in diameter.
 b. **Laboratory evaluation**
  (1) **Radioactive iodine thyroid scintiscanning** identifies the nodule as "hot," "warm," or "cold."
   (a) Because most cancers appear on scan as cold areas, only cold nodules are considered to have a significant risk of malignancy.
   (b) Of all nodules, 70%–90% are cold, and most of these are benign. Therefore, scanning may indicate a greatly reduced risk of malignancy in a nodule that is warm or hot, but it does not yield much additional information on the risk of malignancy in a nodule that is cold.
  (2) **Fine-needle aspiration biopsy** is safe, and easily performed in an office setting. Cells, not sections of tissue, are obtained and must be evaluated by a skilled cytopathologist. The overall results and predictive values are shown in Table 9-6.

3. **Therapy.** The goal of management is surgical removal of the nodules with a high probability of malignancy and careful observation of the others, usually with attempted suppression by ʟ-thyroxine.
 a. **Surgical removal** of the nodule is indicated if one of the following occurs.
  (1) The history and physical examination raise a suspicion of cancer.
  (2) The cytologic findings are equivocal or malignant.
  (3) The nodule grows despite suppressive therapy with ʟ-thyroxine.
 b. **Careful long-term observation** of the nodule, with suppressive ʟ-thyroxine therapy, is indicated if there are no suspicious findings in the history or on physical examination and the cytologic findings are benign. Finding the nodule to be functioning (i.e., "warm" or "hot" on scintiscan) further supports a decision for conservative management.

III. DISORDERS OF THE PARATHYROID GLANDS

A. **Primary hyperparathyroidism and hypercalcemia.** Primary hyperparathyroidism is the result of oversecretion of parathyroid hormone (PTH), which in turn causes hypercalcemia. When primary hyperparathyroidism was first recognized in the early 1920s, patients exhibited severe bone disease, recurrent urinary calculi, and systemic illness caused by marked hypercalcemia. Now the disease is diagnosed much earlier, and, as a result, most cases are less severe.

1. **Epidemiology.** Primary hyperparathyroidism is common, affecting approximately 1 individual in every 1000 who are screened. The disease is especially common in middle-aged and elderly women.

2. **Etiology**
 a. A single **parathyroid adenoma** causes 80%–90% of cases, and **hyperplasia** of all four glands causes 10%–20% of cases of primary hyperparathyroidism. Parathyroid carcinoma is a rare cause.

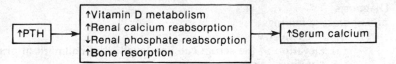

FIGURE 9–1. Actions of parathyroid hormone (PTH) in maintaining normal calcium homeostasis.

b. Predisposing factors
   (1) Although most cases seem to arise without a known cause, a history of **radiation to the neck** is present in 10% or more of patients.
   (2) Familial occurrence of parathyroid hyperplasia and of the MEN syndrome, which often involves parathyroid adenomas or hyperplasia, indicates that **genetic factors** may be important.

3. Pathophysiology. PTH is important in maintaining normal calcium homeostasis (Figure 9-1).
   a. PTH raises the serum calcium level by stimulating vitamin D production (which is important for gastrointestinal absorption of calcium), by increasing renal tubular reabsorption of calcium, by decreasing renal tubular reabsorption of phosphate, and by promoting movement of calcium from the bone.
   b. Decreased circulating levels of ionized calcium stimulate PTH production, causing calcium levels to return to normal; conversely, increased circulating levels of ionized calcium inhibit PTH production. However, a parathyroid adenoma may function autonomously, producing excessive PTH despite high serum calcium levels and causing the abnormalities of primary hyperparathyroidism.

4. Clinical features. The routine measurement of serum calcium levels in multichannel screening tests has led to early diagnosis of primary hyperparathyroidism. The disease commonly presents as mild asymptomatic hypercalcemia, although occasionally patients are seen with the classic findings of advanced kidney and bone disease. Patients with serum calcium levels greater than 11 or 12 mg/dl often have gastrointestinal symptoms, neurologic symptoms, or both.
   a. Renal manifestations
      (1) Although PTH increases renal calcium reabsorption, the hypercalcemia and resulting increased glomerular filtration of calcium commonly lead to **hypercalciuria,** which may cause the formation of **urinary calculi.**
      (2) Chronic hypercalcemia may cause deposition of calcium within the renal parenchyma (nephrocalcinosis) and eventual **renal failure.**
   b. Skeletal manifestations. PTH excess increases the rate of osteoclastic bone resorption and can lead to the disorder of bone metabolism called **osteitis fibrosa cystica.**
      (1) Symptoms include bone pain, fractures, and areas of swelling and deformity localized to involved bones.
      (2) There are areas of **demineralization** in the skeleton. In severe cases, there may be **bone cysts** and "**brown tumors,**" which are localized lesions consisting of proliferating osteoclasts, osteoblasts, and fibrous tissue.
      (3) Radiographs may show **generalized osteopenia,** with demineralization of the skull and other areas. **Subperiosteal resorption** of bone occurs in the phalanges and distal portions of the clavicles. Loss of the lamina dura around the teeth is characteristic.
   c. Gastrointestinal manifestations related to the hypercalcemia of hyperparathyroidism include anorexia, weight loss, constipation, nausea and vomiting, and abdominal pain. Patients with hyperparathyroidism may have an increased incidence of peptic ulcer disease and pancreatitis.
   d. Neurologic manifestations also are related to the hypercalcemia of hyperparathyroidism. Emotional changes and abnormal mentation may occur. Fatigue and muscle weakness are common.

5. **Diagnosis**
   a. **Laboratory findings**
      (1) **Blood chemistry**
         (a) **Elevation of the serum calcium level is the hallmark of primary hyperparathyroidism.**
         (b) The serum phosphate level is lowered in many, but not all, cases.
         (c) Because the serum chloride level tends to be increased (because of PTH-induced bicarbonaturia), the serum chloride to phosphate ratio usually is elevated (> 33); this finding is more consistent than that of hypophosphatemia.
         (d) The serum alkaline phosphatase level is elevated only in patients with significant bone disease.
      (2) **Urine chemistry. Hypercalciuria** is common, but, because of the calcium-reabsorbing action of PTH, approximately one third of patients have normal urine calcium levels.
   b. **PTH assay.** An elevated blood PTH level in the presence of hypercalcemia is strong evidence for primary hyperparathyroidism because other causes of calcium elevation tend to suppress PTH levels. The **immunoradiometric assay** for intact PTH is more sensitive and specific than previously used assays.
   c. **Diagnostic imaging**
      (1) Noninvasive techniques, such as **ultrasonography, CT scanning, MRI,** and **isotope scans** may demonstrate parathyroid adenomas in 60%–80% of cases.
      (2) A much more difficult procedure is **selective venous catheterization,** in which blood samples are taken from veins draining various areas of the neck and mediastinum. A marked increase in PTH concentration suggests the location of the adenoma. This procedure is done in patients facing a second operation after an unsuccessful neck exploration.

6. **Differential diagnosis.** Hypercalcemia may be caused by entities other than primary hyperparathyroidism (Table 9-7).
   a. **Tumors**
      (1) **Malignant tumors with bone metastases** may cause hypercalcemia through an increase in bone resorption due to local effects and sometimes through locally acting humoral substances (e.g., osteoclast activating factor) produced by the metastatic tumor.
      (2) **Tumors that cause hypercalcemia in the absence of bone metastases** do so by producing **PTH-related peptide (PTHrP),** a humoral factor that acts like PTH and binds to PTH receptors but is not measured by the PTH radioimmunoassay. PTHrP may produce biochemical effects like those of PTH, including hypophosphatemia and increased urinary nephrogenous cyclic

Table 9-7. Causes of Hypercalcemia

Primary hyperparathyroidism

Malignancy
  With bone metastases (e.g., breast cancer, myeloma, lymphoma)
  Without bone metastases (e.g., hypernephroma; pancreatic cancer; squamous cell carcinoma of the lung, cervix, and esophagus; head and neck tumors)

Sarcoidosis

Familial hypocalciuric hypercalcemia

Hypervitaminosis D

Milk–alkali syndrome

Hyperthyroidism

Thiazide therapy

Immobilization

adenosine 3′, 5′-monophosphate (cAMP). Humoral hypercalcemia of malignancy may be differentiated from primary hyperparathyroidism by finding an elevated level of PTHrP and a normal or low level of PTH.

b. Sarcoidosis may cause hypercalcemia because of production of 1,25-dihydroxyvitamin D_3 by granulomatous tissue. If no other findings indicate the presence of sarcoidosis and the PTH concentration is not elevated, a therapeutic trial may be helpful. Serum calcium levels decline within 1 week of the start of glucocorticoid administration (e.g., 40 mg prednisone daily) in most cases of sarcoidosis but are unaffected in most cases of primary hyperparathyroidism.

c. Familial hypocalciuric hypercalcemia is a poorly understood autosomal dominant disorder in which mild to moderate hypercalcemia is present, but complications such as urinary calculi and renal failure rarely occur.

  (1) PTH levels are normal or mildly elevated, and the parathyroid glands may be hyperplastic, but subtotal parathyroidectomy does not cure the hypercalcemia.

  (2) Diagnostic clues are the familial occurrence and the low (rather than high) urinary calcium excretion.

  (3) Because surgical treatment is not beneficial and is not recommended, this condition should be ruled out in patients with apparent primary hyperparathyroidiism.

d. Vitamin D intoxication, which is usually seen in patients receiving pharmacologic doses of the vitamin for the treatment of hypoparathyroidism, results in hypercalcemia.

  (1) The diagnosis should be apparent from the patient's history.

  (2) If a sufficiently rapid fall in serum calcium levels does not result when vitamin D ingestion is stopped, glucocorticoids should be given. Glucocorticoids inhibit the action of vitamin D on intestinal calcium absorption and rapidly lower serum calcium levels.

e. Milk-alkali syndrome is caused by the ingestion of large quantities of calcium and absorbable alkali, and it is characterized by hypercalcemia, systemic alkalosis, and renal damage due to nephrocalcinosis. The ingestion of more than 5 g of calcium carbonate (or 2 g of elemental calcium) daily, which is approximately double the dose usually recommended for the prevention or treatment of osteoporosis, is necessary before there is risk of this syndrome developing.

f. Other causes of hypercalcemia

  (1) Hyperthyroidism may cause hypercalcemia due to increased bone turnover. The diagnosis is usually evident because the hyperthyroidism, not the hypercalcemia, is the presenting complaint.

  (2) Thiazide diuretics decrease urinary calcium excretion but rarely cause hypercalcemia; they should be avoided, however, in patients with hyperparathyroidism.

  (3) Prolonged immobilization may lead to hypercalcemia because of continuing bone resorption in the absence of normal postural stimuli for bone formation. This problem is particularly common in children who are confined to bed for long periods (e.g., in a total body cast for treatment of multiple traumatic fractures).

  (4) Paget's disease. Increased bone turnover and localized bone tumors due to defective regulation of bone metabolism in this condition may produce hypercalcemia, especially during periods of immobilization.

  (5) Recovery from acute renal failure. A syndrome of hypercalcemia may develop during the recovery period following rhabdomyolysis and acute renal failure. During the first 2–3 days after muscle injury, the initial muscle damage leads to local calcium and phosphate deposition. When renal function returns to normal, calcium and phosphate exit from sites of muscle damage and enter the circulation to produce hypercalcemia. This defect typically occurs 2–3 weeks after the acute muscle injury.

7. Therapy. Asymptomatic patients older than age 50 years with serum calcium levels no greater than 11.4–12.0 mg/dl often have no progression of their disease during periods of 10 years or more. Such patients should be followed closely and operated on only if the calcium level rises or if the patient develops renal or skeletal symptoms or other manifestations of severer disease.

a. Surgery

   (1) Initial surgical exploration. When the diagnosis of primary hyperparathyroidism is made with confidence, surgical exploration of the neck usually is undertaken.

      (a) In most cases, a **single adenoma** is found and removed.

      (b) If **parathyroid hyperplasia** is found, the surgeon may remove three glands and part of the fourth, or the surgeon may remove all parathyroid tissue and transplant a portion to the muscles of the forearm, from which the removal of additional parathyroid tissue may easily be accomplished if necessary.

   (2) Repeat surgical exploration. Approximately 10% of initial neck explorations fail to reveal abnormal parathyroid tissue or cure the disease. The patient is then reevaluated, and additional invasive and noninvasive localizing procedures are considered before a second operation is performed.

   (3) Postoperative course. Transient hypocalcemia is common after the removal of a parathyroid adenoma because the remaining normal glands are likely to have been suppressed by long-standing hypercalcemia.

      (a) Patients usually recover within a few weeks.

      (b) In the occasional patient with severe bone disease, marked intractable hypocalcemia may persist for several months, because, when the excess PTH stimulus is suddenly removed, the demineralized bone becomes avid for calcium (the ''hungry bones'' syndrome).

b. Medical therapy is used if surgery is contraindicated by other illnesses, if the patient refuses surgery, or if surgery is unsuccessful.

   (1) Increased fluid intake and activity help to minimize hypercalcemia.

   (2) Oral phosphate in doses of 1–2 g daily often lowers the serum calcium level. The main complication, extraskeletal calcification, is uncommon if this dose is not exceeded.

   (3) Estrogen may lower mildly elevated serum calcium levels to normal, apparently by decreasing bone resorption. This treatment often is useful, because two-thirds of cases of primary hyperparathyroidism occur in postmenopausal women, in whom estrogen administration may be considered to be physiologic hormone replacement.

c. Emergency treatment of hypercalcemia is necessary if the calcium level increase above 13–15 mg/dl before the adenoma can be removed or if surgical treatment is refused or is unsuccessful. Hypercalcemia caused by diseases other than hyperparathyroidism (e.g., hypercalcemia due to malignancy) also may be treated by the following methods.

   (1) Hydration, sodium diuresis. Four to six L or more of intravenous saline daily, with large doses of furosemide, increase renal calcium excretion and reduce serum calcium levels.

   (2) Bisphosphonates, such as **pamidronate** and **etidronate,** bind to hydroxyapatite in bone and block dissolution of this mineral; they also inhibit osteoclast activity. The resulting inhibition of bone resorption produces a decline in serum calcium levels over 1–7 days. Pamidronate (60–90 mg) is given intravenously in a single dose over 24 hours; this can be repeated in 7 days if necessary. Etidronate (7.5 mg/kg) is given intravenously over 4 hours once daily for 3–7 days, depending on the response.

   (3) Plicamycin (formerly called mithramycin) is an antineoplastic agent that lowers serum calcium levels by inhibiting osteoclastic bone resorption. A single intravenous dose of 25 μg/kg administered over 4–6 hours may lower the serum calcium levels for several days. This drug is commonly used in treating hypercalcemia due to malignancy.

   (4) Gallium nitrate is a potent inhibitor of bone resorption. It is given in a dose of 200 mg/square meter of body surface area/day by continuous infusion for 5 days. Potential nephrotoxicity limits its use to patients without renal failure.

(5) Calcitonin lowers serum calcium levels by inhibiting osteoclastic bone resorption. It is the fastest acting hypocalcemic agent and is very safe, but it is less potent than plicamycin, gallium nitrate, or pamidronate, and its effect tends to decrease after several days. Salmon calcitonin, 4 U/kg, is given intramuscularly or subcutaneously every 12 hours.

(6) Glucocorticoids lower serum calcium levels in patients with sarcoidosis and vitamin D intoxication, and sometimes in patients with myeloma and hematologic malignancy. However, glucocorticoids do not lower serum calcium levels in patients with hyperparathyroidism.

B. Hypoparathyroidism and hypocalcemia

1. **Etiology**
   a. **Surgical removal of the parathyroid glands** is the common cause of hypoparathyroidism.
      (1) This may be an unavoidable result of radical neck dissection for cancer or a rare complication of subtotal thyroidectomy.
      (2) **Temporary hypoparathyroidism** following neck surgery is not uncommon and may be due to ischemic injury to the glands; however, recovery usually occurs in a few weeks or months.
   b. **Idiopathic hypoparathyroidism** is much less common. It usually is diagnosed in childhood, may be familial, and sometimes is associated with adrenal insufficiency and mucocutaneous candidiasis. It is probably of autoimmune etiology.

2. **Pathophysiology. PTH deficiency leads to hypocalcemia, the hallmark of hypoparathyroidism,** through the same mechanisms by which increased secretion of PTH causes hypercalcemia (see III A 3). In addition, the decreased renal phosphate clearance leads to **hyperphosphatemia,** which is present in most cases of hypoparathyroidism.

3. **Clinical features and diagnosis.** Hypocalcemia produces acute symptoms related to increased neuromuscular irritability. In addition, long-term changes may occur as a result of effects on ectodermal tissues and ectopic calcium deposition.
   a. **Symptoms and signs**
      (1) **Latent tetany**
         (a) Mild hypocalcemia may cause **muscular fatigue and weakness** as well as **numbness** and tingling around the mouth and in the hands and feet.
         (b) **Chvostek's sign** may be positive (i.e., a tap over the facial nerve in front of the ear elicits a contraction of the facial muscles and upper lip). However, Chvostek's sign may be positive in 10% of normal individuals.
         (c) **Trousseau's sign** may be positive; that is, inflation of a blood pressure cuff on the arm to a pressure higher than the patient's systolic pressure for 3 minutes elicits carpal spasm (flexion of the metacarpophalangeal joints and extension of the interphalangeal joints, with drawing together of the fingers and adduction of the thumb).
      (2) **Overt tetany.** Severe hypocalcemia causes **twitching and cramps of the muscles with carpopedal spasm. Laryngeal stridor** and **seizures** may occur in severe cases.
      (3) **Long-term effects of hypocalcemia**
         (a) **Ectodermal changes** include atrophy, brittleness, and ridging of the nails; dryness and scaling of the skin; and enamel defects and hypoplasia of the teeth.
         (b) **Calcification of the basal ganglia** may occur and is occasionally associated with parkinsonian signs and symptoms.
         (c) **Calcification of the optic lens may lead to cataract formation.**
   b. **Laboratory abnormalities. Hypocalcemia** and **hyperphosphatemia** are consistently present in hypoparathyroidism. PTH levels, of course, are low, but clini-

cal assays may not be sensitive enough to distinguish between low and normal levels.

4. **Differential diagnosis**
    a. **Pseudohypoparathyroidism**
        (1) Pseudohypoparathyroidism is a hereditary disease with two distinct areas of clinical expression.
            (a) **Calcium metabolism is abnormal** because of end-organ resistance to the action of PTH; that is, the kidney and bone cannot respond to PTH, even though its concentration in the serum is normal or increased. The result is hypocalcemia and hyperphosphatemia, as are seen in true hypoparathyroidism.
            (b) **Developmental and skeletal abnormalities (Albright's hereditary osteodystrophy)** are present.
                (i) The most common abnormalities are short stature, shortening of the metacarpal and metatarsal bones, and mental deficiency.
                (ii) The skeletal abnormalities sometimes occur in the absence of any disorder of calcium metabolism; this has been called "pseudopseudohypoparathyroidism."
        (2) If Albright's hereditary osteodystrophy is not present and if hypocalcemia is not clearly postsurgical in its onset, the differentiation between true hypoparathyroidism and pseudohypoparathyroidism may depend on laboratory tests.
            (a) PTH levels may be sufficiently elevated in pseudohypoparathyroidism to distinguish the syndrome clearly from hypoparathyroidism.
            (b) Injection of PTH is followed promptly by increased urine concentrations of phosphate and cAMP and, within 1 or 2 days, by an increase in serum calcium in patients with hypoparathyroidism. No response occurs in patients with pseudohypoparathyroidism.
    b. **Hypoalbuminemia** causes a decrease in the fraction of serum calcium that is bound to protein and, therefore, a decrease in total serum calcium; because the ionized fraction of serum calcium remains normal, however, there are no clinical manifestations of calcium deficiency. This should not be considered a form of true hypocalcemia. For each decrement in serum albumin of 1 g/L, the serum calcium is expected to decline about 0.8 mg/dl.
    c. **Renal failure.** Hypocalcemia in renal failure is caused by many factors. These include renal phosphate retention (with resultant hyperphosphatemia), reduced production of 1,25-dihydroxyvitamin D_3 by the diseased kidneys, and bone resistance to the calcemic action of PTH.
    d. **Malabsorption** associated with gastrointestinal disease may lead to inadequate calcium absorption and consequent hypocalcemia.
    e. **Vitamin D deficiency** or resistance to the actions of vitamin D may cause hypocalcemia through decreased gastrointestinal absorption of calcium.
    f. **Acute pancreatitis** may lead to intra-abdominal precipitation of calcium soaps in areas of fat necrosis. Whether this explains why hypocalcemia is sometimes seen in patients with acute pancreatitis is uncertain.
    g. **Osteoblastic metastasis** of prostate, breast, or lung cancer may produce hypocalcemia, presumably due to rapid bone uptake of calcium.
    h. **Hypomagnesemia** decreases production of PTH and inhibits the actions of PTH and vitamin D on bone, leading to hypocalcemia.

5. **Therapy**
    a. **Hypoparathyroidism.** PTH is neither practical nor available for long-term therapy. Instead, treatment with **supplemental calcium,** combined with **vitamin D** to enhance its absorption, is effective in correcting the hypocalcemia and hyperphosphatemia of hypoparathyroidism, even in cases caused by end-organ unresponsiveness to PTH (e.g., pseudohypoparathyroidism).
        (1) **Calcium supplementation.** Usually 1–2 g of elemental calcium are given daily.
            (a) Commonly used preparations include calcium gluconate (each 1-g tab-

let contains 90 mg of elemental calcium), calcium carbonate (each tablet of Os-Cal 500 contains 500 mg of calcium), and calcium glubionate (each tablespoon of Neo-Calglucon contains 345 mg of calcium).

   (b) The calcium is given in three or four divided doses. The dose can easily be raised or lowered to regulate serum calcium levels.

(2) Vitamin D

   (a) Calciferol. Vitamin D$_2$ (ergocalciferol) has been used for years in the treatment of hypoparathyroidism.

   (i) Because vitamin D$_2$ must be converted to 1,25-dihydroxyvitamin D$_3$ to be fully effective (a conversion that is greatly inhibited in the absence of PTH), large doses are necessary. The average daily dose is 50,000 U, with a range of 25,000–150,000 U, although the recommended dietary allowance in normal person is only 200–400 U.

   (ii) The onset of action is slow (1–2 weeks), but the effect may persist for months after administration is stopped.

   (b) Calcitriol (1,25-dihydroxyvitamin D$_3$) has largely replaced calciferol in the treatment of hypoparathyroidism. The main advantage of calcitriol over vitamin D$_2$ is the faster onset and cessation of action, which may lead to more precise control of blood calcium levels. Calcitriol is given in doses of 0.25–2.0 μg/day.

   b. Treatment of acute hypocalcemia, which may occur shortly after parathyroid resection and may cause severe tetanic symptoms, consists of intravenous administration of calcium. Calcium gluconate (10%) in a dose of 1–2 g is given intravenously in approximately 10 minutes followed by slow infusion of one g of calcium gluconate over the next 6–8 hours.

IV. DISORDERS OF GLUCOSE HOMEOSTASIS

A. **Diabetes mellitus is characterized by hyperglycemia** and other metabolic derangements that are **caused by inadequate action of insulin** on body tissues, because of either reduced circulating levels of insulin or resistance of target tissues to its actions. Because of the prevalence and importance of certain complications, diabetes may be considered to be a syndrome consisting of metabolic abnormalities, microvascular disease (i.e., retinopathy and nephropathy), large vessel disease (i.e., accelerated atherosclerosis), and peripheral and autonomic neuropathy.

1. Classification (Table 9-8). In general, diabetes mellitus is divided into two categories—**type I or insulin-dependent diabetes** (formerly called juvenile-onset diabetes) and **type II or noninsulin-dependent diabetes** (formerly called maturity-onset diabetes). Syndromes that overlap these two categories and are related to the stage or severity of the disease are impaired glucose tolerance, gestational diabetes, previous abnormality of glucose tolerance, potential abnormality of glucose tolerance, and diabetes associated with certain other diseases.

   a. Type I diabetes affects approximately 10% of diabetic patients.

   (1) "Dependence" on insulin means not only that insulin is needed for optimal control of blood glucose, which also may be true for patients with type II disease, but that, **without exogenous insulin, the patient is prone to the development of ketoacidosis.** This is thought to reflect a complete or almost complete absence of insulin in these patients, in contrast to the partial lack of insulin or the resistance to insulin characteristic of patients with type II diabetes.

   (2) Other key features of type I diabetes are its occurrence in children and young adults and its occurrence in individuals who are lean rather than obese.

   b. Type II diabetes commonly affects overweight individuals older than 40 years of age.

Table 9-8. Major Types of Primary Diabetes Mellitus

	Type I Diabetes Mellitus	Type II Diabetes Mellitus
Prevalence	0.2%–0.5%; men = women	2%–4%; women > men
Age at onset	Usually < 25 years	Usually > 40 years
Genetics	<10% of first-degree relatives affected; 50% concordance in identical twins	>20% of first-degree relatives affected; 90%–100% concordance in identical twins
HLA	Associated with HLA-DR3, HLA-DR4, HLA-DQ	None
Autoimmunity	Increased prevalence of autoantibodies to islet cells and other tissues	None
Body build	Usually lean	Usually obese—80% are >15% above ideal body weight
Metabolism	Ketosis prone; insulin production absent	Ketosis-resistant; insulin levels may be high, normal, or low
Treatment	Insulin	Weight loss; possibly an oral agent (e.g., a sulfonylurea) or insulin

HLA = human leukocyte antigen.

       (1) Because some insulin is produced by these patients, **ketoacidosis does not occur.**
       (2) Insulin therapy may be necessary, however, to prevent severe hyperglycemia.
     c. Related syndromes
       (1) Impaired glucose tolerance. This is a disorder of glucose metabolism in which blood glucose levels are higher than those of normal individuals and lower than those of diabetic patients.
          (a) Impaired glucose tolerance increases the patient's risk for the macrovascular complications of diabetes (i.e., atherosclerosis) but not for the microvascular complications.
          (b) Although affected individuals have an increased risk of development of diabetes, the disease does not develop in most.
       (2) Gestational diabetes. Diabetes or impaired glucose tolerance develops in 2%–3% of pregnant, previously nondiabetic women, most often in the last trimester of pregnancy.
          (a) β-Cell reserve is apparently inadequate for the increased insulin requirements of pregnancy.
          (b) Careful screening for gestational diabetes and intensive treatment are essential because of an increased risk of neonatal morbidity.
          (c) The glucose tolerance of most patients returns to normal within a few weeks after delivery, although diabetes develops in many patients as many as 5–15 years later.
       (3) Previous abnormality of glucose tolerance. This term refers to individuals with normal glucose levels who formerly were glucose intolerant or diabetic because of pregnancy, illness, obesity, or medications.
       (4) Potential abnormality of glucose tolerance. This syndrome occurs in individuals with an increased risk of future diabetes because of a history of having had large babies (greater than 9 pounds), the presence of diabetes in an identical twin, or similar factors.
       (5) Diabetes or impaired glucose tolerance **may occur secondary** to certain diseases that affect the production or action of insulin, such as **chronic pancreatitis, Cushing's syndrome, acromegaly, insulin receptor abnormalities,** and others.

2. **Etiology.** The cause of diabetes mellitus is unknown. Many etiologic factors are suspected, with major differences between those factors that are etiologic for type I and type II diabetes.
   a. **Type I diabetes**
      (1) **Etiologic factors**
         (a) **Genetic factors**
            (i) Fifty percent of identical twins of patients with type I diabetes are diabetic.
            (ii) There is a strong association between type I diabetes and certain human leukocyte antigens (HLAs) (see Table 9-8).
         (b) **Autoimmune factors**
            (i) Antibodies to islet-cell antigens are commonly present in diabetic patients shortly after the disease is diagnosed, although they usually disappear within a few years.
            (ii) Antibodies against other tissues, such as antithyroid antibodies, also are increased.
         (c) **Environmental factors** are suggested because the concordance rate for diabetes in identical twins is 50% rather than 100%, which would be the rate predicted if the disease were totally genetic. Also, seasonal occurrence has been observed, with an increased diagnosis of new cases in the fall and winter.
      (2) How these factors interact to cause diabetes is speculative. For example, a viral infection may trigger β-cell destruction in an individual with genetically determined susceptibility to such an infection and to autoimmune reactivity to islet-cell antigens.
   b. **Type II diabetes**
      (1) **Genetic factors** are even more important etiologically in type II than in type I diabetes. There is a 90%–100% concordance rate for diabetes in identical twins.
      (2) **Obesity** is a significant factor—80% of patients with type II diabetes are more than 15% above their ideal weight. Obesity is associated with resistance to the action of insulin both in diabetic and nondiabetic individuals; this resistance may be caused partly by decreased numbers of insulin receptors and partly by abnormal insulin action beyond the receptor.
      (3) Genetically susceptible individuals may be unable to sustain the increased insulin production needed to maintain carbohydrate homeostasis in the face of insulin resistance, with resulting diabetes.

3. **Pathophysiology**
   a. **Levels of insulin**
      (1) In **type I diabetes,** some insulin may be produced for a few years after the disease is diagnosed, but insulin production eventually ceases totally.
      (2) In **type II diabetes,** insulin levels vary and often are similar to the levels is nondiabetic individuals of similar weight. However, these insulin levels are not normal but are low, when considered in relation to the elevated blood glucose concentrations of the diabetic patient, and they reflect a decrease in β-cell sensitivity to glucose.
   b. **Consequences of impaired insulin action.** Impaired insulin action may be caused by inadequate insulin secretion, by target-tissue resistance to the action of insulin, or both.
      (1) **Hyperglycemia.** Insulin increases the synthesis of glycogen in the liver and in muscle and increases the uptake of glucose in muscle and adipose tissue. In the absence of adequate insulin action, hepatic glucose production increases (with increased glycogenolysis and increased gluconeogenesis) and peripheral glucose use decreases. The result is hyperglycemia.
      (2) **Other metabolic derangements**
         (a) Insulin normally acts as an anabolic, storage-promoting agent. It stimulates fatty acid formation from glucose and esterification of fatty acids to form triglycerides, and it stimulates amino acid storage as protein.

(b) Inadequate insulin action on target tissues causes inadequate disposal of ingested nutrients and excessive consumption of endogenous metabolic fuels. Blood fatty acids and lipids are increased because of decreased lipogenesis and increased lipolysis; blood amino acids are increased because of decreased protein synthesis and increased catabolism of muscle protein.

c. Levels of other hormones
   (1) Glucagon levels are often elevated in diabetic patients. This may contribute to hyperglycemia through glucagon's action in stimulating glycogenolysis and the resulting increase in glucose levels.
   (2) Epinephrine, cortisol, and GH levels may be increased during periods of stress or poor diabetic control. This may contribute to hyperglycemia through the anti-insulin effect and diabetogenic action of these hormones.

4. Clinical features
   a. Polyuria and polydipsia. The most common symptom of hyperglycemia is increased urine volume, which is caused by glucose-induced osmotic diuresis. Increased fluid intake is a response to the resulting dehydration and thirst.
   b. Weight loss results from the loss of glucose in urine and the catabolic effects of the decrease in insulin action, despite increased food intake. Generalized weakness also reflects the metabolic derangements.
   c. Infections of the skin, vulva, and **urinary tract** are especially common in uncontrolled diabetes because hyperglycemia decreases resistance to infection.
   d. Blurring of vision is caused by changes in the shape and refractive qualities of the optic lens that result from hyperglycemia-induced osmotic alterations.

5. Diagnosis. Diabetes mellitus is often suspected because of typical clinical manifestations, such as polyuria and unexplained weight loss; however, a definitive diagnosis is based on **elevated glucose levels.**
   a. Fasting serum glucose levels that are persistently higher than 140 mg/dl are diagnostic of diabetes.
   b. Postprandial glucose levels may be measured 2 hours after a standard meal or after a 75-g glucose load.
   (1) Values of 140 mg/dl or higher are diagnostic of impaired glucose tolerance, and values of 200 mg/dl or higher indicate diabetes.
   (2) This measurement is more sensitive than a measurement of fasting glucose levels because the ability to return blood glucose to normal 2 hours after a meal is usually lost earlier than the ability to maintain a normal fasting glucose level.
   c. A glucose tolerance test is seldom needed to diagnose diabetes if fasting serum or postprandial glucose levels have been evaluated. However, the glucose tolerance test is the diagnostic standard in questionable cases.
   (1) After at least 3 days of a normal diet, which includes a minimum of 150 g of carbohydrate, the patient ingests a 75-g glucose load. Serum glucose levels are measured at 0, 30, 60, 90, and 120 minutes.
   (2) The criteria for the diagnosis of impaired glucose tolerance and diabetes mellitus are listed in Table 9-9.

Table 9-9. Glucose Tolerance Test

Diagnosis	Fasting Glucose Level (mg/dl)	Maximum Level at 30, 60, or 90 Minutes (mg/dl)	Level at 120 Minutes (mg/dl)
Normal	<115	<200	<140
Impaired glucose tolerance	115–139	≥200	140–199
Diabetes mellitus	≥140	≥200	≥200

d. Urine glucose levels. Glucose appears in the urine only when the renal threshold of approximately 180 mg/dl is exceeded.

   (1) This threshold varies widely and tends to increase with age; therefore, urine glucose measurement is an insensitive and unreliable test for diabetes.

   (2) However, it can be a rough guide to the presence or absence of marked hyperglycemia and occasionally may be of use in the day-to-day management of diabetes.

6. Acute complications of diabetes. Diabetic ketoacidosis, hyperosmolar nonketotic coma, and hypoglycemic coma are acute, life-threatening complications of diabetes mellitus; they cause rapid mental and physical deterioration and require prompt treatment. Because each of these complications may present with an alteration in mental status that often progresses to coma, and because each of these conditions requires different treatment, accurate diagnosis is essential.

a. Diabetic ketoacidosis occurs in an insulin-dependent diabetic patient whose circulating insulin is insufficient to allow glucose use by peripheral tissue and to inhibit glucose production and tissue catabolism. Increased levels of glucagon and hormones that increase in response to stress (i.e., epinephrine, norepinephrine, cortisol, and GH) contribute to the metabolic derangements.

   (1) Precipitating factors. Ketoacidosis may occur after several days of worsening diabetic control or may appear suddenly within a few hours.

   (a) Precipitating factors include any event that decreases insulin availability or causes stress that increases the need for insulin.

   (b) Common factors are the omission of insulin doses, infections, injuries, emotional stress, excessive alcohol ingestion, and intercurrent illness.

   (2) Pathophysiology

   (a) Hyperglycemia. Insufficient insulin reduces peripheral glucose use and, together with glucagon excess, increases hepatic production of glucose through the stimulation of gluconeogenesis and glycogenolysis and the inhibition of glycolysis. Protein breakdown in peripheral tissues provides a flow of amino acids to the liver as substrate for gluconeogenesis. Hyperglycemia is the result.

   (b) Osmotic diuresis results from the elevated serum glucose (and ketone) levels and produces **hypovolemia, dehydration,** and **loss of sodium, potassium, phosphate, and other substances in the urine.** Volume depletion stimulates catecholamine release, which further opposes insulin action in the liver and contributes to lipolysis.

   (c) Ketogenesis. The lipolysis that results from insulin lack and catecholamine excess mobilizes free fatty acids from their stores in adipose tissue. Instead of reesterifying the incoming fatty acids to form triglycerides, the liver shifts its metabolic pathways toward the production of ketone bodies.

   (i) Glucagon increases the hepatic level of carnitine, which enables fatty acids to enter the mitochondria, where they undergo β-oxidation to ketone bodies.

   (ii) Glucagon decreases the hepatic content of malonyl coenzyme A, an inhibitor of fatty acid oxidation.

   (d) Acidosis. The increased hepatic production of ketone bodies (acetoacetate and β-hydroxybutyrate) exceeds the body's ability to metabolize or excrete them.

   (i) The ketone bodies' hydrogen ions are buffered by bicarbonate, leading to a decrease in serum bicarbonate and pH.

   (ii) Arterial carbon dioxide tension (Pa_{CO_2}) also decreases because of ventilatory compensation.

   (iii) The anion gap increases because of the elevated plasma levels of acetoacetate and β-hydroxybutyrate.

   (iv) The result is metabolic acidosis that is associated with an increased anion gap.

(3) Clinical features and diagnosis
    (a) Physical findings
        (i) Patients with diabetic ketoacidosis exhibit **rapid, deep breathing (Kussmaul's respiration),** which occurs as the body tries to compensate for metabolic acidosis by increasing carbon dioxide excretion.
        (ii) An **odor of acetone** is often detected on the breath.
        (iii) Marked dehydration is common, with **dry skin and mucous membranes** and **poor skin turgor. Orthostatic hypotension** may be present due to intravascular volume depletion.
        (iv) Clouding of consciousness is present in most cases, and approximately 10% of patients are **comatose.**
    (b) Laboratory abnormalities
        (i) Hyperglycemia. Serum glucose levels in ketoacidosis may be only slightly increased, but more often they are markedly elevated, averaging approximately 500 mg/dl. Renal function affects the degree of hyperglycemia—glucose levels are greatly elevated only when urinary excretion of glucose is limited by volume depletion or renal abnormalities.
        (ii) Hyperketonemia. Serum levels of acetoacetate, acetone, and β-hydroxy butyrate are greatly increased. The agent nitroprusside, in the form of tablets or reagent strips, is commonly used to measure serum and urine ketone bodies. It reacts only with acetoacetate. If the other ketone bodies are increased to a much greater or much lesser extent than acetoacetate, the results of the test may be misleading.
        (iii) Metabolic acidosis is indicated by a **low serum bicarbonate level** (usually below 10 mEq/L) and **a low blood pH.** The anion gap is increased.
        (iv) Urinary levels of glucose and ketone bodies are increased. The diagnosis of diabetic ketoacidosis can be made rapidly if marked **glycosuria** and **ketonuria** are present.
        (v) Other laboratory findings. Serum potassium concentration may be increased initially because of potassium ion movement from the intracellular to the extracellular space in metabolic acidosis. Later, the serum potassium level is low because of both renal losses and the movement of potassium ions back into cells as the acidosis is corrected. **Serum sodium concentration** tends to be low, mainly because of dilution as the osmotic effect of the hyperglycemia increases extracellular water. **Serum osmolality** is high, usually greater than 300 mOsm/kg.
(4) Therapy. The treatment of diabetic ketoacidosis has four main components.
    (a) Insulin is administered to increase glucose use in the tissues, to inhibit the flow of fatty acids and amino acids from the periphery, and to counter the effects of glucagon on the liver.
        (i) Route of administration. If volume depletion and vascular collapse are present, poor tissue perfusion may impair the absorption of intramuscular or subcutaneous insulin, in which case the insulin should be administered intravenously.
        (ii) Dosage. A priming dose of 0.1 U/kg of regular insulin is given intravenously and is followed by the infusion of 0.1 U/kg/hr or approximately 5–10 U/hr. Similar doses may be given intramuscularly when blood pressure is normal and tissue perfusion seems adequate. Much higher doses were used in the past, and many physicians still advocate their use. If the serum glucose level does not decrease (75–100 mg/dl/hr), the serum level of ketone bodies does not fall, and serum pH does not increase in few hours, then larger doses of insulin (50–100 U/1–2 hr) must be given.

      (iii) After the acidosis and hyperglycemia have resolved and the urine has become free of ketone bodies, treatment with intermediate-acting insulin is resumed.

   (b) **Fluid replacement** corrects the dehydration caused by glucose-induced osmotic diuresis. The fluid deficit in patients with diabetic ketoacidosis averages 3–5 L, which must be promptly replaced.

      (i) Approximately 1 L of normal saline (0.9% NaCl) is given each hour for the first 2 hours, and then half-normal saline (0.45% NaCl) is given at a slower rate. When the serum glucose level falls to 200–300 mg/dl, 5% or 10% glucose is infused to prevent hypoglycemia.

      (ii) Fluid replacement lowers serum glucose levels, even without insulin, by increasing urine flow (and hence, glycosuria) and by decreasing the levels of catecholamines and cortisol, which were increased by the stimulus of volume depletion.

   (c) **Minerals and electrolytes must be replaced** because they are lost via osmotic diuresis.

      (i) **Potassium.** Body stores of potassium are low and must be replaced. If initial serum potassium levels are elevated (due to severe acidosis), replacement is delayed; when the levels become normal or low, after therapy has been initiated, potassium chloride is infused at a rate of 20–40 mmol/hr. This can be given as potassium phosphate or potassium chloride, depending on the blood levels of calcium and phosphorus; too much phosphate replacement may cause hypocalcemia.

      (ii) **Phosphate** must also be replaced. Approximately 10–20 mmol/hr may be given as potassium phosphate, for a total of 40–60 mmol.

      (iii) **Bicarbonate** is given only when the arterial pH declines below 7.1 in order to maintain the pH above that level. Because diabetic ketoacidosis is corrected by fluids and insulin, excessive administration of bicarbonate may result in rebound alkalosis. Some physicians recommend bicarbonate administration only when the pH decreases below 6.9.

   (d) **Treatment of precipitating factors and complications**

      (i) Urinary tract infections as well as other infections must be investigated and treated.

      (ii) Meningitis, stroke, and myocardial infarction may escape detection in a patient whose sensorium is clouded by ketoacidosis.

      (iii) Nasogastric aspiration should be performed if the patient is unconscious and has been vomiting or has gastric dilatation.

      (iv) Blood or plasma expanders should be given if hypotension persists despite fluid replacement.

b. **Hyperosmolar nonketotic coma** is much less common than ketoacidosis, but it has a much higher mortality rate. It occurs mainly in elderly patients with type II diabetes, often previously undiagnosed.

 (1) **Pathophysiology.** Often a precipitating factor (e.g., infection, increased glucose ingestion, omission of insulin, or intercurrent illness) causes increasing hyperglycemia within a few days or weeks. Osmotic diuresis, without adequate fluid intake, causes dehydration and progressive decline in mental status. Ketoacidosis is mild or absent, presumably because enough insulin is present to inhibit hepatic ketogenesis.

 (2) **Clinical features.**

   (a) The **hyperglycemia** tends to be more marked than it is in ketoacidosis, with plasma glucose concentrations typically approximately 1000 mg/dl.

   (b) In the absence of ketoacidosis, the osmotic diuresis continues for a longer time before the diagnosis is made and therefore produces more severe **dehydration.**

    (c) **Serum osmolality** is very high, averaging approximately 360 mOsm/kg. The dehydration and hyperosmolality may cause **mental obtundation, seizures,** and **focal neurologic signs.**

    (d) Lactic acidosis may be present because of the hypovolemia and indicates a worse prognosis.

  (3) **Therapy** is similar to that for diabetic ketoacidosis. Fluid replacement and reversal of the hyperglycemia with insulin are the main goals. Fluid replacement in elderly patients with cardiovascular disease requires care to avoid volume expansion, which might precipitate heart failure.

c. **Hypoglycemic coma** must be rapidly differentiated from diabetic ketoacidosis and hyperosomolar nonketotic coma, because therapy is obviously quite different.

  (1) **Etiology**

    (a) Hypoglycemia in insulin-treated diabetic patients ("insulin shock") may be caused by **excessive insulin dosage, delay in the ingestion of a meal, and excessive physical activity.** Sulfonylureas may cause hypoglycemic reactions, but much less often than does insulin.

    (b) Insulin-dependent diabetic patients may be susceptible to hypoglycemia because of **insufficient levels of the counterregulatory hormones** that normally prevent a fall in serum glucose. The response of glucagon to hypoglycemia is frequently impaired in these patients, and epinephrine production may become impaired if autonomic neuropathy develops. (Epinephrine prevents severe hypoglycemia both by stimulating glucose production and by producing symptoms that alert the patient to hypoglycemia, prompting rapid glucose ingestion.)

  (2) **Clinical features.** Hypoglycemia produces symptoms through the following two mechanisms:

    (a) A fall in the serum glucose concentration stimulates catecholamine production and sympathetic nervous system outflow. **Adrenergic stimulation** then causes sweating, tachycardia, palpitations, tremulousness, and muscular weakness.

    (b) Prolonged hypoglycemia deprives the CNS of its main source of fuel, glucose. **CNS symptoms** of hypoglycemia usually occur later than the adrenergic symptoms, and they are potentially more serious. Mental changes may progress from **somnolence** and confusion to coma. Headache, slurred speech, focal neurologic signs, and seizures may occur.

  (3) The **diagnosis** of hypoglycemia is obvious if symptoms of sweating, palpitation, and tremulousness occur at the time of peak action of a recent insulin dose. Patients learn to recognize this reaction and treat it by drinking orange juice or eating candy. Less obvious is the cause of coma in a diabetic patient brought to the emergency room. Clues that suggest hypoglycemia rather than ketoacidosis are the history of a missed meal or unusually vigorous exercise, the finding of profuse sweating rather than dehydration, and the absence of Kussmaul's respiration. A fingerstick blood glucose determination is useful for rapid confirmation of hypoglycemia.

  (4) **Therapy**

    (a) A patient who is unable to take glucose orally is given **50 ml of 50% glucose intravenously** over 3–5 minutes, followed by a constant infusion of 5% or 10% glucose.

      (i) Some patients regain consciousness immediately, others more slowly.

      (ii) Glucose infusion may have to be maintained during the expected duration of action of the insulin or oral agent responsible for the hypoglycemia. If the hypoglycemia is caused by **chlorpropamide,** this may be several days.

    (b) An intramuscular injection of 1 mg of **glucagon** may increase the serum glucose level rapidly, allowing the patient to regain consciousness and take oral glucose. Teaching a patient's family members to inject glucagon may decrease the frequency of emergency room visits.

(c) Following an episode of insulin-induced hypoglycemia, the insulin dosage, diet, or both should be readjusted to prevent subsequent attacks.

7. **Chronic complications of diabetes.** Patients with diabetes frequently develop microvascular disorders involving the small blood vessels of the eye, kidney, and muscle; macrovascular disease (i.e., atherosclerotic disease of the medium and large vessels), and diabetic neuropathy (i.e., abnormalities of the peripheral and autonomic nervous system).

   a. **Pathogenesis**

      (1) **Microvascular complications and neuropathy.** The Diabetes Control and Complications Trial, a 10-year randomized controlled trial in 1441 patients with type I diabetes, has shown conclusively that better control of serum glucose levels reduces the incidence of retinopathy, nephropathy, and neuropathy. Several mechanisms have been proposed by which elevated glucose levels may cause these complications:

         (a) Nonenzymatic glycosylation of proteins in capillary basement membranes and other tissues, similar to the process that produces glycosylated hemoglobin, may produce damage to these tissues that is related to the blood glucose levels.

         (b) When glucose levels are elevated, the enzyme aldose reductase converts glucose to sorbitol, which may cause damage in nerve cells, the retina, and renal tissue.

      (2) **Macrovascular complications.** Atherosclerosis, leading to coronary, cerebrovascular, or peripheral vascular disease, is associated with diabetes mellitus. Unlike the microvascular complications, however, it is also associated with the lesser degree of glucose elevation known as decreased glucose tolerance. Increased insulin levels, as a result of insulin therapy (in type I diabetes) or insulin resistance (in type II diabetes), are suspected of contributing to atherosclerosis.

   b. **Diabetic retinopathy** is directly related to the duration and severity of diabetes. Prevalence increases from 3% at the time that diabetes is diagnosed to 20%–45% after 10 years. Of new cases of blindness in adults, 20% are caused by diabetes.

      (1) **Types**

         (a) **Background (simple, nonproliferative) retinopathy** makes up 90%–95% of all cases. Increased capillary permeability, vascular occlusion, and weakness of supporting structures lead to the findings on funduscopic examination of venous dilatation, exudates, hemorrhages, and microaneurysms.

         (b) **Proliferative retinopathy** makes up 5%–10% of all cases. In response to vascular occlusion and ischemia, new vessels form on the surface of the retina (neovascularization) and may grow into the vitreous body of the eye.

            (i) Preretinal or vitreous hemorrhage may lead to clot retraction and scar formation, with retinal detachment.

            (ii) Vitreous hemorrhage may cause sudden blindness.

      (2) **Therapy**

         (a) Background retinopathy is less likely to progress if diabetic control is good. Annual screening for retinopathy is recommended, because blindness may be prevented by early treatment.

         (b) Proliferative retinopathy may be treated with **laser-beam photocoagulation,** which is effective in obliterating new vessels. **Vitrectomy** is beneficial in selected cases.

   c. **Diabetic nephropathy.** The renal lesion that is specific for diabetes is **intercapillary glomerulosclerosis (Kimmelstiel-Wilson syndrome).** Other renal diseases associated with diabetes are papillary necrosis, chronic interstitial nephritis, and arteriosclerotic disease.

      (1) **Incidence.** Significant renal disease develops in approximately 40% of patients with type I diabetes and 20% of patients with type II diabetes. Nearly

all patients with severe glomerulosclerosis also have retinopathy. Almost 33% of new cases of end-stage renal disease are caused by diabetes.

(2) Pathogenesis. Hyperglycemia may cause increased intraglomerular pressure, leading to damage to the basement membrane, deposition of protein in the mesangium, glomerulosclerosis, and renal failure. **Pathologic features** of diabetic glomerulosclerosis include an increase in the mesangial matrix and increased width of the glomerular basement membrane, hyaline arteriosclerosis of the afferent and efferent arterioles, and IgG and albumin deposits lining the tubular and glomerular basement membranes. Diabetic kidneys tend to be large, even when end-stage renal disease is present.

(3) Clinical features

    (a) The first manifestation is usually **proteinuria,** which often progresses to the **nephrotic syndrome.**

        (i) Microalbuminuria, which can be detected by special tests, predicts the later occurrence of renal failure.

        (ii) The presence of **hypertension** is also associated with an increased risk of renal failure in diabetic patients.

    (b) When renal failure occurs, the progression to **end-stage renal disease** is rapid; transplantation or dialysis usually becomes necessary within 3 years.

(4) Prevention. Progression of diabetic nephropathy can be prevented or delayed by intensive glycemic control and by control of coexisting hypertension. Angiotensin-converting enzyme (ACE) inhibitors slow the progression of renal disease by their antihypertensive effect and probably by an action independent of blood pressure control. A low-protein diet (0.6–0.89 g of protein/kg body weight) may also slow the progression of renal disease.

d. Diabetic neuropathy is common. Older patients with a relatively long history of diabetes and severe hyperglycemia have an increased incidence of this complication. Accumulation of sorbitol in Schwann cells, with subsequent cell damage, may play a causative role. Slowing of nerve conduction velocity occurs, with changes in Schwann-cell function and eventual segmental demyelination and axonal degeneration.

(1) Types

    (a) Peripheral polyneuropathy is the most common syndrome.

        (i) Distal, bilateral sensory changes predominate. Weakness and upper extremity involvement are less frequent.

        (ii) Symptoms include paresthesias and pain of the feet, and examination may show decreased reflexes, loss of vibratory sense, and loss of pain sensation.

        (iii) Neuropathic ulcers of the feet are a common manifestation of diabetic neuropathy and are more common than ischemic ulcers.

    (b) Autonomic neuropathy is less common than peripheral polyneuropathy, but usually it is seen in patients who have peripheral polyneuropathy. **Postural hypotension** is the chief manifestation. Other clinically important problems are sexual impotence in diabetic men and urinary retention with abnormal bladder function. Abnormal gastrointestinal motility may result in delayed gastric emptying (diabetic gastroparesis), constipation, and diarrhea. The adrenergic symptoms of hypoglycemia may be decreased or absent, leading to delayed recognition and treatment of insulin reactions.

    (c) Less common forms of diabetic neuropathy are **radiculopathy,** causing lancinating pain in a single dermatome, and **mononeuropathy,** involving cranial nerves or proximal motor nerves.

(2) Therapy

    (a) Improved diabetic control may lessen the symptoms of peripheral polyneuropathy. Symptomatic treatment of painful neuropathy may be attempted with amitripyline, phenytoin, carbamazepine, and topical capsaicin.

(b) Several drugs that inhibit aldose reductase, thus decreasing sorbitol formation, have been tried; none is yet approved for use in the United States.

e. Atherosclerosis. The incidence of atherosclerosis is considerably increased in diabetic patients; that is, diabetes, like hypertension, smoking, hyperlipidemia, obesity, and a positive family history, is a major risk factor for the development of atherosclerosis.

(1) Coronary artery disease is twice as common in diabetic patients compared with nondiabetic patients. Small-vessel disease may contribute to myocardial ischemia.

(2) Peripheral vascular disease, which is common in diabetic patients, is most likely to affect the legs and feet. Small-vessel disease may play a major role—ischemic changes in a foot with a normal pedal pulse on examination is typical of diabetes. Foot infections, poorly healing ulcers, and eventual gangrene, resulting in amputation, are frequent complications.

8. Treatment of diabetes

a. Goals of treatment

(1) Control of symptoms. The polyuria, weight loss, increased incidence of infections, blurring of vision, and other symptoms of diabetes are related to the hyperglycemia. Return of serum glucose levels to normal brings relief of these symptoms.

(2) Prevention of acute complications. Diabetic ketoacidosis and nonketotic hyperglycemic coma are prevented by careful management of diabetes.

(3) Prevention of long-term complications. The Diabetes Control and Complications Trial clearly showed that intensive therapy, with lowering of blood glucose below the levels needed to control symptoms and prevent ketoacidosis, delays or prevents the onset of retinopathy, nephropathy, and neuropathy.

b. Diet. Before insulin was available, severe restriction of carbohydrate intake was necessary to prolong life in type I diabetic patients. In patients receiving insulin, the **regularity and timing of carbohydrate intake** may be more important than the quantity. Many physicians believe it is equally important to **avoid excessive fat intake,** which increases the risk of atherosclerosis. In seeking to balance these considerations, physicians recommend that caloric intake be comprised of 12%–20% protein, 50%–60% carbohydrate, and 20%–30% fat.

(1) Specific objectives

(a) Type I diabetes. The chief goals of dietary treatment are to provide adequate calories for growth and exercise and to ensure day-to-day regularity of food intake so that the availability of insulin is coordinated with carbohydrate intake.

(b) Type II diabetes. The chief goal in most cases is to attain the patient's ideal weight by means of caloric restriction and regular exercise. Because many patients will become normoglycemic with diet alone if significant weight loss is achieved, initial treatment should emphasize the importance of diet. Most patients, however, are not able to lose enough weight to control glucose levels through diet alone.

(2) Diet calculation

(a) The ideal body weight should be estimated.

(i) For men, the allowance is 106 pounds for the first 5 feet in height, and 6 pounds for each additional inch.

(ii) For women, the allowance is 100 pounds for the first 5 feet in height, and 5 pounds for each additional inch.

(iii) For heavy-framed individuals, 5–15 pounds may be added.

(b) The total daily caloric requirement should be determined. The ideal body weight should be converted to kilograms by dividing the number of pounds by 2.2. The data in Table 9-10 can then be used to determine the daily caloric need, which varies with the patient's activity level and need to gain or lose weight.

Table 9-10. Daily Caloric Requirement*

| | Activity Level | | |
Body Build	Sedentary	Moderately Active	Very Active
Obese	20–25	30	35
Normal	30	35	40
Underweight	35	40	45–50

* Calories (kcal) required per kilogram of ideal body weight per day. These estimates are intended to produce weight loss in the obese, weight gain in the underweight, and maintenance of weight in normal individuals.

(c) The protein, carbohydrate, and fat intake should be determined by calculating 20% of the total calories as protein (4 kcal/g), 50% as carbohydrate (4 kcal/g), and the remaining 30% as fat (9 kcal/g).

(d) The total food intake should be divided into meals. For the average person, two sevenths of the total should be eaten at breakfast, at lunch, and at dinner, and one seventh should be eaten at bedtime. Food exchange lists are available to aid in apportioning the food components to each meal.

(3) Additional suggestions

(a) Increased intake of polyunsaturated fats and reduced intake of saturated fats are desirable. Cholesterol intake should not exceed 300–500 mg/day.

(b) For a balanced amino acid content, 50% of protein should be derived from the meat exchange list.

(c) Increased fiber intake, in the form of unprocessed bran, cereals, fruits, and vegetables, may lower blood glucose levels and decrease the need for insulin.

c. Oral hypoglycemic agents

(1) Sulfonylurea derivatives (Table 9-11) reduce serum glucose levels in patients with type II diabetes. They are often used in patients with mild to moderate diabetes whose glucose levels are not controlled by diet alone.

(a) Mode of action

(i) The acute effect of these agents is to increase insulin output by the β-cells.

(ii) With long-term use, they may also have a minor effect in increasing the action of insulin on peripheral tissues.

(b) Clinical use

(i) The patients most likely to respond to oral agents are those with type II diabetes of recent onset, who have not required insulin in the past or who have needed less than 20 U daily.

(ii) After it is evident that therapy via diet alone will not be sufficient, an oral agent may be prescribed. A low dose is given initially and

Table 9-11. Sufonylurea Derivatives: Their Dosages and Duration of Action

Drug	Usual Starting Dose (mg)	Daily Dose Range (mg)	Duration of Action (hr)
Tolbutamide	1000–2000 in 1 or 2 doses	500–3000	6–12
Tolazamide	100–250 in 1 dose	100–1000	12–24
Acetohexamide	250 in 1 dose	250–2000	12–24
Chlorpropamide	250 in 1 dose	100–750	60–90
Glyburide	2.5–5 in 1 dose	1.25–20	24
Glipizide	5 in 1 dose	2.5–40	24

is increased at intervals of approximately 1 week until good glucose control is achieved or maximal recommended dosage is reached.

   (iii) If oral agents are not effective (primary failure), insulin therapy must be initiated. Oral agents may produce satisfactory glycemic control for months or years, with secondary failure eventually occurring for unknown reasons.

(c) **Side effects**

   (i) **Hypoglycemia** may result from excessive dosage, interaction with drugs that potentiate the action of sulfonylureas, renal or hepatic disease, or inadequate food intake. Prolonged duration of the hypoglycemia, which is associated especially with chlorpropamide, may necessitate hospitalization and continuous intravenous glucose infusion for several days.

   (ii) **Sensitivity to alcohol,** with reactions similar to those seen with disulfiram, may occur, especially in association with chlorpropamide.

   (iii) **Hyponatremia** may result from the action of chlorpropamide (and, less commonly, other agents) potentiating the effect of ADH on the renal tubules.

   (iv) **Skin reactions, gastrointestinal symptoms,** and **bone marrow depression** occur rarely.

(d) **Choice of agent.** Glipizide and glyburide, which are newer, do not cause the alcohol intolerance and hyponatremia that are occasionally associated with older drugs. For the most part, however, none of the sulfonylureas has any definite advantage over the others.

(2) Metformin

(a) **Mode of action.** Unlike the sulfonylureas, metformin **potentiates the action of insulin** but does not increase its secretion. It increases glucose uptake and use.

(b) **Clinical use.** Because its mechanism of action is different from that of the sulfonylureas, metformin may be used along with a sulfonylurea. It may also be used with insulin or as a single agent.

(c) **Side effects**

   (i) **Gastrointestinal symptoms** (e.g., metallic taste, anorexia, nausea and vomiting, diarrhea) may occur.

   (ii) **Lactic acidosis** is a serious but rare potential complication, unless the patient has a predisposing condition such as renal failure, liver disease, alcoholism, or any condition that may cause tissue hypoxia (e.g., heart failure, pulmonary disease). These conditions are strong contraindications to the use of metformin.

(d) **Dose.** The starting dose is 500 mg with supper; this can be raised gradually to a maximum of 2500 mg daily in divided doses.

d. Insulin

(1) Indications

(a) Patients with type I diabetes are, by definition, dependent on insulin treatment.

(b) Insulin is indicated in type II patients in whom satisfactory control of blood glucose levels is not obtained with diet and oral hypoglycemic drugs. Patients whose diabetes is usually well controlled with oral agents may require insulin temporarily during stress or illness or after surgery.

(c) Gestational diabetes that is not controlled by diet should be treated with insulin.

(2) Insulin preparations

(a) Insulin produced from the pancreatic tissue of pigs and cattle is rapidly being replaced by human insulin prepared by recombinant DNA technology.

Table 9-12. Insulin Preparations and Their Onset, Peak, and Approximate Duration of Action

Types	Onset of Action (hr)	Peak Effect (hr)	Duration of Action (hr)
Fast-acting			
Regular human insulin	$\frac{1}{2}$	$2\frac{1}{2}$–5	8
Intermediate-acting			
NPH human insulin	$1\frac{1}{2}$	4–12	24
Lente insulin (beef)	$2\frac{1}{2}$	7–15	24
70% NPH human, 30% regular human insulin	$\frac{1}{2}$	2–12	24
Long-acting			
Ultralente insulin (beef)	4	10–30	36

NPH = isophane insulin suspension.

(b) Insulin preparations are available with rapid (regular insulin), intermediate, and long durations of action (Table 9-12). A mixture of 70% isophane insulin suspension (NPH) and 30% regular insulin combines early onset of action with 24-hour duration of action.

(3) **Evaluation of glucose control**
  (a) Patients treated with insulin may have blood sugar determinations every week or every several weeks if their glucose control is stable, or determinations may be made several times daily if glucose levels are unstable or if the insulin dose is being adjusted. In hospitalized patients and in patients who learn to measure their blood sugar levels at home, glucose levels are commonly measured before breakfast and at one or more additional times daily (e.g., at 4 P.M., at bedtime, or before each meal). Home monitoring is done using test strips (e.g., Dextrostix) with or without a meter (e.g., Glucometer).
  (b) Fasting serum glucose levels less than 140 mg/dl and 2-hour postprandial glucose levels below 200 mg/dl are considered to be satisfactory in most patients.
    (i) Lower glucose levels are essential in pregnant women and are desirable in patients who are well motivated to achieve optimal control.
    (ii) In patients with **"brittle" diabetes** (i.e., diabetes characterized by widely fluctuating glucose levels and frequent hypoglycemia) and, often, in insulin-resistant patients, higher glucose levels may have to be tolerated.
  (c) **Glycosylated hemoglobin measurements**
    (i) The free amino acid groups of hemoglobin and other body proteins combine with glucose to form a reversible compound (Schiff base), which can then become a stable glycosylated protein (Amadori rearrangement). The extent of this nonenzymatic glycosylation is dependent on the concentration of glucose in blood; that is, the percent of hemoglobin that is glycosylated depends on the blood glucose levels that were present during the life span of the currently circulating red blood cells.
    (ii) The glycosylated hemoglobin level, therefore, reflects the degree of hyperglycemia during the preceding 6–12 weeks, and it may be useful in estimating the average control of serum glucose levels during this time.

(4) **Insulin regimens**
  (a) **Single dose of intermediate-acting insulin.** The simplest regimen, and the most commonly used, is a single dose of an intermediate-acting insulin daily before breakfast. An initial dose of 10–20 U of NPH or 70% NPH, 30% regular insulin is given, and its effect on blood and urine

glucose levels is observed. The dose can be raised by 4–10 U every few days.

(b) Split dose of intermediate-acting insulin. If a single morning dose of intermediate-acting NPH or Lente insulin produces a good afternoon glucose level but fails to maintain control until the next morning, an evening dose can be added. Approximately two thirds of the daily dose is given before breakfast, and one third is given before dinner. The morning dose is adjusted according to the afternoon glucose level, and evening dose is adjusted according to the morning fasting glucose level.

(c) Intensive insulin therapy

    (i) Multiple injections. In patients with unstable diabetes, the increase in blood sugar levels after meals may best be controlled by a dose of regular insulin before each meal. Basal insulin requirements may be supplied by a single dose of intermediate- or long-acting insulin each morning. Frequent home glucose measurements allow the adjustment of each dose and the addition of extra doses when necessary.

    (ii) Portable infusion pump. The closest control of serum glucose levels is achieved by the constant infusion of regular insulin through a needle placed subcutaneously in the abdominal wall or thigh. A basal rate of approximately 12.5–15 mU/kg/hr is supplemented with pulse doses 15–30 minutes before each meal. The benefit of tighter glucose control with intensive therapy must be balanced against the increased risk of hypoglycemia and the inconvenience of the portable pump.

(5) Factors affecting insulin requirements

(a) Intercurrent illness or other stress may increase insulin needs, perhaps because of increased levels of catecholamines. A temporary increase in the dosage of intermediate-acting insulin or supplementary doses of regular insulin may be needed.

(b) Exercise increases glucose use and may cause hypoglycemia unless the insulin dose is reduced or extra carbohydrate is ingested.

(c) Somogyi effect. Insulin-induced hypoglycemia causes release of counterregulatory hormones such as epinephrine and glucagon; this may then cause rebound hyperglycemia. If the cause for this hyperglycemia is not recognized, the insulin dose may be increased, leading to even more severe hypoglycemia. Hypoglycemia during the hours of sleep may be an unrecognized cause of increased morning fasting glucose levels; if this is the case, a decrease in the insulin dose may correct the morning hyperglycemia.

(6) Complications of insulin therapy

(a) Local allergy. Red, itchy lumps may form at the injection site minutes or hours after an insulin dose. This reaction tends to occur within a few weeks of initial insulin treatment and usually resolves in a few weeks or months.

(b) Systemic allergy. Generalized urticaria, angioedema, and anaphylaxis are rare but life-threatening reactions to insulin. Because a ketosis-prone patient cannot survive without insulin, that patient must be hospitalized and insulin desensitization must be performed. An initial intradermal dose of 1/10,000 U of insulin is given and is increased every 30 minutes.

(c) Antibody-mediated insulin resistance is caused by IgG insulin-binding antibodies in the serum.

    (i) Insulin resistance is often defined as a need for more than 200 U daily, and it is more common in patients who have been exposed to insulin intermittently.

    (ii) Antibody-mediated resistance is often self-limited, resolving within 6 months.

(iii) Treatment consists of switching to human insulin (if not already in use) and cautious use of glucocorticoids if necessary (the excessively sudden release of antibody-bound insulin in response to steroid therapy may cause hypoglycemia).

(d) Lipodystrophy

(i) Lipohypertrophy. Local swellings, composed of fibrous and fatty tissue, may occur at insulin injection sites, perhaps because of a local lipogenic effect of insulin on the fat cells. The swellings may regress if human insulin is used and the site of lipohypertrophy is avoided.

(ii) Lipoatrophy. Pits may form at injection sites due to the disappearance of subcutaneous fat. These may slowly disappear if human insulin is injected into the perimeter of the atrophic area.

B. **Hypoglycemia.** There is no simple definition of hypoglycemia. Glucose levels less than 45 or 55 mg/dl may be associated with hypoglycemic symptoms, but some normal individuals have glucose levels lower than this without symptoms after several days of fasting or several hours after a glucose load, with resultant excessive secretion of insulin. If the diagnosis is in doubt, **Whipple's triad** (i.e., symptoms of hypoglycemia, low serum glucose levels, and relief of the symptoms when normoglycemia is restored) may be used as a criterion.

1. **Insulinomas** are rare tumors that arise from the β-cells of the islets of Langerhans. Most are single, benign adenomas, but approximately 10% of these tumors are multiple, and 10% are malignant. They occur with equal frequency in the head, the body, and the tail of the pancreas. β-Cell hyperplasia may occasionally produce a similar syndrome.

   a. **Clinical features.** Insulinomas produce excessive quantities of insulin, leading to **fasting hypoglycemia** (i.e., a category of hypoglycemia in which the lowest levels of serum glucose and the severest symptoms occur after prolonged periods without food intake).

      (1) Symptoms are most likely to occur in the early morning or late afternoon or after fasting or exercise.

      (2) The symptoms of hypoglycemia are the same as those that result from insulin overdose in diabetic patients [see IV A 6 c (2)].

      (3) Patients may gain weight before the diagnosis is made because they learn to relieve or avoid hypoglycemic symptoms by frequent snacking on carbohydrates.

   b. **Diagnosis**

      (1) **An elevated serum insulin concentration** when the glucose level is low is strong evidence for the presence of an insulinoma, if an exogenous insulin source is excluded.

         (a) In normal individuals, insulin levels fall as glucose levels fall, and insulin levels become undetectable at glucose levels less than 30 mg/dl.

         (b) If the serum glucose concentration is less than 45 mg/dl, an insulin level higher than 10 mU/ml is abnormal.

      (2) **A prolonged fast,** extending for 24–72 hours, may be necessary to demonstrate fasting hypoglycemia with inappropriately high insulin levels.

      (3) **C-peptide suppression test.** If prolonged fasting does not produce hypoglycemia but an insulinoma is still suspected, hypoglycemia can be induced with the administration of exogenous regular insulin (0.1 U/kg intravenously over 1 hour).

         (a) The induced hypoglycemia suppresses endogenous insulin production in a normal individual but fails to suppress the autonomous insulin production by an insulinoma.

         (b) Serum insulin measurement cannot be used to evaluate endogenous insulin production because the injected insulin would be measured as well. However, C peptide, which is separated from the proinsulin molecule when the latter is cleaved to form insulin, can be measured. Because C peptide is not present in injected insulin, its concentration in serum reflects endogenous insulin production. A level of C peptide that is greater than 1.2 mg/ml after an insulin infusion suggests the autonomous insulin production of an insulinoma.

(4) Proinsulin, the large precursor molecule of insulin, is produced in increased amounts by insulinomas. Proinsulin normally makes up 5%–20% of the total insulin in blood that is measured by radioimmunoassay; in patients with an insulinoma, proinsulin usually exceeds 25%.

(5) Diagnostic imaging. MRI, CT, ultrasonography (including intraoperative ultrasound), and selective arteriography may be used to identify and localize an insulinoma. These tumors may be small, however, averaging 1–2 cm, and they often cannot be visualized.

c. Therapy

(1) Surgical removal of an adenoma or partial pancreatectomy for multiple adenomas or β-cell hyperplasia is the treatment of choice.

(2) Medical therapy is reserved for patients whose tumors cannot be completely removed because of metastatic disease, because previous surgical attempts have failed, or because illness or patient refusal makes surgery infeasible.

(a) Diazoxide inhibits the release of insulin from β-cells. A dose of 200 mg daily, which can be raised as high as 800 mg if necessary, can prevent hypoglycemia in patients with an inoperable insulinoma.

(b) Streptozocin is an antibiotic that specifically destroys β-cells. It is used to treat malignant β-cell tumors.

2. Factitious hypoglycemia is caused by the surreptitious self-administration of insulin or an oral hypoglycemic drug, most often by an individual who is familiar with health care, such as a nurse or medical technologist, or by a diabetic or relative of a diabetic. Differentiation from hypoglycemia caused by an insulinoma may depend on special studies.

a. Serum C-peptide measurement indicates the source of insulin secretion [see IV B 1 b (3)]. The low glucose and high insulin levels that are pathognomonic of an insulinoma should be accompanied by increased C-peptide levels; if the latter are low, indicating an exogenous source of the high insulin concentration, the disease is factitious.

b. Ingestion of a sulfonylurea, however, stimulates endogenous insulin production and the C-peptide level is high; therefore, **screening of blood or urine for sulfonylureas** is also necessary to rule out factitious disease.

3. Extrapancreatic tumors may cause hypoglycemia. These usually are large, intra-abdominal tumors, most often of mesenchymal origin (e.g., fibrosarcoma), although they may be hepatic carcinomas or other tumors. The mechanism of hypoglycemia is poorly understood; increased use of glucose by some tumors and production by others of an insulin-like substance have been observed.

4. Ethanol-induced hypoglycemia occurs in patients whose glycogen stores are depleted because of inadequate recent food intake, usually 12–24 hours after a bout of heavy drinking.

a. The oxidation of ethanol to acetaldehyde and acetate generates NADH and decreases the availability of nicotinamide-adenine dinucleotide (NAD), which is needed for gluconeogenesis, and generates NADH. When neither glycogenolysis nor gluconeogenesis is available to maintain hepatic glucose production in the fasting state, hypoglycemia results.

b. Prompt recognition with glucose administration is essential because the mortality rate is higher than 10%.

5. Liver disease may result in impairment of glycogenolysis and gluconeogenesis sufficient to cause fasting hypoglycemia. This is seen in fulminant viral hepatitis or acute toxic liver disease but not in the usual, less severe cases of cirrhosis or hepatitis.

6. **Other causes of fasting hypoglycemia** include cortisol deficiency, GH deficiency, or both, which may occur in **adrenal insufficiency** or **hypopituitarism.** Hypoglycemia may occur in patients with **renal failure** and **heart failure;** however, the causes are poorly understood.

7. **Reactive hypoglycemia.** Insulinoma and the other conditions discussed previously produce hypoglycemia most commonly in the fasting state. Another, smaller group of disorders causes hypoglycemia a few hours after the ingestion of carbohydrates, thus the term "reactive hypoglycemia."
   a. **Alimentary hypoglycemia** occurs in patients who have had a gastrectomy or other surgical procedure that leads to abnormally rapid movement of food into the small bowel. Rapid absorption of carbohydrate stimulates excessive insulin secretion, causing hypoglycemia several hours after a meal.
   b. **Reactive hypoglycemia of diabetes.** Patients with early diabetes occasionally have a late but excessive release of insulin after a carbohydrate-containing meal. The glucose level is elevated after 2 hours but then decreases to hypoglycemic levels 3–5 hours following the meal.
   c. **"Functional" hypoglycemia,** although commonly diagnosed in patients with chronic fatigue and anxiety, is probably a rare condition. Hypoglycemia is not a cause of chronic fatigue, depression, and lack of energy.
      (1) **Clinical features.** Hypoglycemia, with adrenergic symptoms such as sweating and palpitations, occurs 2–5 hours after a carbohydrate-rich meal, presumably because of increased insulin production or insulin sensitivity.
      (2) **Diagnosis**
         (a) The overdiagnosis of functional hypoglycemia stems in part from misinterpretation of the 5-hour glucose tolerance test. One in four normal individuals has a serum glucose level less than 50 mg/dl 3–5 hours after the nonphysiologic stimulus of 75–100 g of glucose, and some normal individuals have levels less than 35 mg/dl, without symptoms. These responses do not prove functional hypoglycemia.
         (b) The diagnosis depends on finding hypoglycemia that coincides with the patient's typical symptoms and on finding relief of symptoms by carbohydrate ingestion.
      (3) **Therapy** consists of eating four to six small meals daily that are low in carbohydrate and high in protein.

V. DISORDERS OF THE ADRENAL GLAND

A. **General considerations**
   1. Diseases of the **adrenal cortex** are caused by the excessive production of cortisol (**Cushing's syndrome**), aldosterone (**primary aldosteronism**), and adrenal androgens (**congenital adrenal hyperplasia**) and by inadequate production of cortisol and aldosterone (**Addison's disease**).
   2. Loss of the **adrenal medulla** does not cause illness, but **catecholamine overproduction by a pheochromocytoma** (a tumor of the adrenal medulla) causes a characteristic hypertensive syndrome.

B. **Cushing's syndrome** is caused by excessive concentrations of cortisol or other glucocorticoid hormones in the circulation.
   1. **Etiology**
      a. The most common cause of spontaneous Cushing's syndrome is **bilateral adrenal hyperplasia** (also known as **Cushing's disease**).* Bilateral adrenal hyperplasia is caused by increased creased pituitary secretion of ACTH.

* Excess production of ACTH by the pituitary gland is Cushing's disease. Cushing's syndrome is a nonspecific designation that is associated with increased glucocorticoid levels from any origin.

(1) Whether the primary defect originates in the hypothalamus (through elaboration of excessive corticotropin releasing factor) or in the pituitary gland is uncertain.

(2) Pituitary tumors that are large enough to be seen on skull radiograph, which are usually chromophobic adenomas, are present in approximately 10% of these patients, and smaller basophilic adenomas are found in more than 50%.

b. Adrenal adenomas and adrenal carcinomas may cause Cushing's syndrome.

c. Ectopic ACTH production by tumors, such as oat cell carcinoma of the lung, carcinoma of the pancreas, bronchial carcinoid tumors, and others, causes adrenal hyperplasia and Cushing's syndrome.

d. Iatrogenic Cushing's syndrome is seen more often than the spontaneously occurring syndrome. It is an expected complication in patients receiving long-term glucocorticoid treatment for asthma, arthritis, and other conditions.

2. Clinical features

a. Central obesity is caused by the effect of excess cortisol secretion on fat distribution. Fat accumulates in the face, neck, and trunk, while the limbs remain thin. The **"moon face," "buffalo hump"** (cervical fat pad), and **supraclavicular fat pads** contribute to the cushingoid appearance of affected individuals.

b. Hypertension results from the vascular effects of cortisol as well as other actions of the hormone, including sodium retention.

c. Decreased glucose tolerance is common; 20% of patients have overt diabetes. This is a result of the increased hepatic gluconeogenesis and decreased peripheral glucose utilization caused by elevated levels of cortisol.

d. Symptoms of androgen excess (e.g., oligomenorrhea, hirsutism, and acne) may occur in women with Cushing's disease because of stimulation by ACTH of adrenal androgen production.

e. Purple striae are linear marks on the abdomen, where the thin, wasted skin is stretched by underlying fat.

f. Muscle wasting and weakness reflect the catabolic effects of cortisol on muscle protein.

g. Osteoporosis is a frequent result of cortisol excess. It is caused by increased bone catabolism and perhaps by the inhibitory effects of cortisol on collagen synthesis and calcium absorption.

h. Susceptibility to bruising is probably caused by enhanced capillary fragility.

i. Psychiatric disturbances, especially depression, are frequent results of cortisol excess.

j. Growth retardation in children may be severe.

3. Diagnosis. Although serum and urine cortisol levels are elevated in Cushing's disease and Cushing's syndrome, overlap with normal values is fairly common, and elevated levels are seen in normal persons at times of stress. Therefore, tests of the suppressibility of cortisol are usually necessary.

a. The **overnight dexamethasone suppression test** is recommended as an initial screening procedure for any patient suspected of having Cushing's syndrome. The patient takes 1 mg of dexamethasone orally at 11 P.M., and the serum cortisol level is measured at 8 A.M the following morning.

(1) The serum cortisol level is less than $5 \mu g/dl$ in most individuals, indicating normal suppression of ACTH and cortisol by the dexamethasone. Because this test is very sensitive, the diagnosis need not be considered further in these cases.

(2) Patients with Cushing's syndrome will have cortisol levels greater than 5 $\mu g/dl$ and usually greater than 10 $\mu g/dl$. This result indicates that further study is needed. (The test is not very specific; mental or physical stress may produce a false-positive result.)

b. The **standard dexamethasone suppression test** is the most relied upon biochemical test for Cushing's syndrome, although false-positive and false-negative results occur in approximately 10–20% of cases. The suppressibility of the hypothalamic–pituitary–adrenal axis is tested by the administration of dexameth-

Table 9-13. Standard Dexamethasone Suppression Test

Method		
Day	Dosage (Dexamethasone)	Measurements
1	None (baseline)	24-hour urinary 17-hydroxycorticosteroid and 4 P.M. serum cortisol levels
2, 3	Low-dose (0.5 mg every 6 hours)	Repeat measurements on day 3
4, 5	High-dose (2.0 mg every 6 hours)	Repeat measurements on day 5

Response		
Diagnosis	Suppression with Low Dose*	Suppression with High Dose†
Normal	Yes	Yes
Cushing's disease	No	Yes
Adrenal tumor or ectopic ACTH production	No	No

ACTH = aderenocorticotropic hormone.
* 17-hydroxycorticosteroid excretion <3 mg/24 hr; serum cortisol level <5 μg/dl.
† >50% fall in 17-hydroxycorticosteroid baseline levels; serum cortisol level <10 μg/dl.

asone in both low and high doses, each for 2 days, with measurement of the serum cortisol concentration and the urinary 17-hydroxy corticosteroid level on the second day of each dose level (Table 9-13).

(1) The pattern of response helps to distinguish normal individuals from those with Cushing's syndrome and to separate patients with Cushing's disease from those with adrenal tumors or ectopic ACTH production.

(2) Patients with Cushing's disease behave as though their feedback response to glucocorticoids is intact but set at a higher than normal level; they respond to high but not to low doses of dexamethasone. Patients with adrenal tumors and ectopic ACTH secretion produce corticoids autonomously, without suppression even by high doses of dexamethasone.

c. **ACTH measurement** may help to differentiate the causes of Cushing's syndrome.

(1) ACTH levels are usually high-normal or slightly elevated in patients with Cushing's disease and may be markedly elevated in patients with ectopic ACTH production.

(2) When an autonomously functioning adrenal tumor is the source of excess cortisol secretion, pituitary secretion of ACTH is suppressed due to the excessive cortisol production, and the ACTH level is extremely low or undetectable.

d. Several **newer tests** may prove to be useful.

(1) The **overnight high-dose dexamethasone suppression test** is more convenient to perform than the standard test. Serum cortisol is measured at 8 A.M. on two consecutive days; 8 mg of dexamethasone is taken at 11 P.M. on the first day. A decrease in the serum cortisol level of less than 50% on the second day indicates failure of suppression and has the same significance as failure of suppression with high-dose dexamethasone in the standard test.

(2) **Corticotropin-releasing hormone (CRH) stimulation test.** CRH is injected and the response of ACTH and cortisol is measured. The response tends to be normal or exaggerated in pituitary Cushing's disease but absent in ectopic and adrenal Cushing's syndrome.

(3) **Inferior petrosal sinus sampling.** ACTH concentrations are measured in venous blood obtained by catheterization of the inferior petrosal sinuses. A high concentration, compared to that in peripheral blood, indicates that a pituitary adenoma is the cause of ACTH excess; if one superior petrosal sinus has a high ACTH concentration while the other has a concentration

similar to peripheral blood, the adenoma is likely to be on the side of the pituitary corresponding to the high concentration.

e. Other laboratory findings

   (1) The **serum cortisol** level in normal individuals is highest in early morning and decreases throughout the day, reaching a low point at about midnight. Although the morning level may be increased in patients with Cushing's syndrome, a loss of the normal diurnal variation and an increase in the evening level are more consistent findings.

   (2) The **24-hour urinary free cortisol excretion rate** is increased in most patients with Cushing's syndrome. This test and the overnight dexamethasone suppression test are the most useful screening tests for Cushing's syndrome.

   (3) **Nonspecific laboratory abnormalities** include leukocytosis, with a relatively low percentage of lymphocytes and eosinophils, and an elevation in the serum glucose level.

f. Radiographic findings

   (1) **Skull radiographs** reveal enlargement of the sella turcica in the 10% of patients with Cushing's syndrome who have **macroadenomas** but they do not reveal most of these tumors, which are **microadenomas** averaging 5–6 mm in diameter.

   (2) **CT scans with injection of contrast medium** detect approximately 50% of the pituitary adenomas that cause Cushing's disease. **MRI with gadolinium contrast,** however, reveals approximately 75% of these tumors and is the method of choice.

   (3) **CT scans of the adrenal gland** reveal most adrenal tumors. Uniform enlargement of both adrenal glands suggests an ACTH-dependent form of Cushing's syndrome, either Cushing's disease or the ectopic ACTH syndrome.

4. Therapy

a. Adrenal adenomas can usually be resected completely, with cure of the disease. Cortisol replacement may be needed for several months to a year postoperatively, until the remaining normal adrenal tissue, suppressed by the previous high cortisol levels, regains its ability to produce cortisol.

b. Adrenal carcinoma is often inoperable when first diagnosed due to metastases, usually to the liver and the lungs. Mitotane, metyrapone, and aminoglutethimide are drugs that block adrenal steroid production, and they may relieve the manifestations of excess cortisol production in patients with inoperable adrenal carcinoma. Prolonged survival of these patients is uncommon.

c. The ectopic ACTH syndrome can be cured by removal of the tumor, but this is not possible in most cases. The tumor causing the syndrome is usually the main problem rather than the Cushing's syndrome itself.

d. Cushing's disease may be treated in several ways.

   (1) **Pituitary irradiation** is effective in many children, but it cures fewer than one third of adult patients; the reason for the difference in response between children and adults is unclear.

   (2) **Bilateral adrenalectomy** cures Cushing's disease but leaves the patient with **Addison's disease** and the need for lifelong steroid replacement. Additionally, adrenalectomy is sometimes followed by the development of **Nelson's syndrome,** in which a pituitary adenoma undergoes rapid growth, perhaps because it is no longer inhibited by above normal levels of cortisol.

   (3) **Transsphenoidal pituitary surgery is the treatment of choice.** Even when tumors cannot be seen on CT scan or MRI, transsphenoidal exploration may disclose a microadenoma. Surgery is successful in 50%–95% of cases and is followed by normal pituitary and adrenal function as well as cure of Cushing's disease.

C. **Adrenal insufficiency (Addison's disease)**

1. Etiology

a. Primary adrenal insufficiency

   (1) **Idiopathic atrophy of the adrenal cortex,** due to an autoimmune process, is the most common cause of adrenal insufficiency.

     (2) Tuberculosis may involve the adrenal glands, with destruction of both cortices and medullae.

     (3) Iatrogenic causes

        (a) Bilateral adrenalectomy for Cushing's disease results in adrenal insufficiency.

        (b) Adrenal suppression following prolonged steroid therapy may persist for up to 1 year or longer.

     (4) Less common causes of adrenal destruction include **amyloidosis, fungal infections, syphilis, bilateral adrenal hemorrhage** (especially in patients receiving anticoagulants), and **metastatic malignancy. Acquired immune deficiency syndrome (AIDS)** sometimes leads to adrenal insufficiency through cytomegalovirus and other infections of the adrenal glands.

  b. Secondary adrenal insufficiency is due to pituitary disease and results from any of the causes of hypopituitarism (see I A 2 a).

2. Clinical features. The symptoms of adrenal insufficiency are caused by both cortisol and aldosterone deficiencies.

  a. Cortisol deficiency

     (1) Hyperpigmentation of the skin is caused by increased melanocyte-stimulating hormone (MSH) activity that accompanies the increased pituitary secretion of ACTH. The latter is a feedback response to the cortisol deficiency.

        (a) Hyperpigmentation is most noticeable over exposed areas, on mucous membranes, and in skin creases and scars.

        (b) In secondary adrenal insufficiency (which is caused by pituitary disease), ACTH levels are low rather than elevated and hyperpigmentation is absent.

     (2) Hypotension, often orthostatic, is caused by the absence of the pressor effect of cortisol on vascular tone and by a decrease in cardiac output.

     (3) Gastrointestinal symptoms include anorexia, nausea and vomiting, and weight loss.

     (4) Hypoglycemia is related to decreased cortisol-induced gluconeogenesis.

     (5) Mental symptoms may include lethargy and confusion. Psychotic manifestations occur on occasion.

     (6) Intolerance to stress. Patients who cannot increase their cortisol output in response to severe stress risk an acute exacerbation of the symptoms discussed above, with life-threatening vascular collapse.

  b. Aldosterone deficiency*

     (1) Sodium loss results from reduced aldosterone-mediated reabsorption of sodium in the distal renal tubules. **Hypovolemia, decreased cardiac output,** and **decreased renal blood flow with azotemia** as well as weakness, hypotension, and weight loss may be related to sodium depletion.

     (2) Potassium retention caused by aldosterone deficiency may lead to **hyperkalemia** and **cardiac arrhythmias.**

3. Diagnosis

  a. ACTH testing is needed for a definitive diagnosis. The normal adrenal gland sharply increases its output of cortisol in response to ACTH; absence of this response proves adrenal insufficiency.

     (1) Short ACTH test. The serum level of cortisol is measured before and 1 hour after an intravenous or intramuscular injection of 0.25 mg (25 U) of cosyntropin, a synthetic form of ACTH. The serum cortisol level should increase at least 7 μg/dl and should reach a level of 18 μg/dl or higher. Although this test is useful as an office procedure, it is less reliable than the standard ACTH test.

---

* The renin–angiotensin system is not affected by secondary adrenal insufficiency, and because it, rather than ACTH, has primary control of aldosterone production, there is usually no deficiency of aldosterone in secondary adrenal insufficiency.

(2) Standard ACTH test

  (a) ACTH in a dose of 25–40 U is given intravenously for 8 hours. The 24-hour urinary excretion rate of free cortisol or the 17-hydroxycorticosteroid excretion rate is measured the day before the infusion and on the day of the infusion. In addition, serum cortisol levels are measured before the infusion is started and 6–8 hours after the infusion is started. Dexamethasone in 0.5-mg doses every 6 hours may be given during the test to protect the patient against adrenal insufficiency.

  (b) A normal response is a threefold to fivefold increase in urinary corticoid excretion and a 15–40 μg/dl increase in serum cortisol level.

  (c) If hypopituitarism is suspected, the ACTH infusion should be given daily for 4 or 5 days. A lack of response on the first or second day, followed by a stepwise increase and eventual normal response by the fourth or fifth day, is typical of secondary adrenal insufficiency; the adrenal tissue is suppressed by long-term ACTH deficiency, but it can be "primed" by daily stimulation.

  (d) Alternatively, ACTH can be administered intravenously continually for 48 hours. Urinary 17-hydroxycorticosteroid excretion of less than 27 mg in the first 24 hours indicates adrenal insufficiency. In the second 24 hours, patients with primary adrenal insufficiency excrete less than 4 mg, whereas those with secondary disease excrete more than 10 mg.

b. Laboratory findings

  (1) Nonspecific laboratory abnormalities may include **hyponatremia, hyperkalemia, hypoglycemia,** and an **increased eosinophil count** (glucocorticoids lower the eosinophil count). Chest radiography may reveal a **small heart.**

  (2) Plasma cortisol, urinary free cortisol, and urinary 17-hydroxycorticosteroid levels are low. Baseline levels, however, may overlap with the values in normal individuals, which is why ACTH testing is necessary for a definitive diagnosis.

4. Therapy

  a. Glucocorticoid replacement is needed in all patients. The usual dose of cortisol is 20 mg orally each morning and 10 mg each evening. The dose must be increased during times of stress. Typical doses would be 40–60 mg daily during minor stress (e.g., common cold or dental extraction), 100 mg during moderate stress (e.g., influenza or minor surgery), and "stress doses" of 300 mg or more during severe stress (e.g., major surgery or a serious infection or injury).

  b. Mineralocorticoid replacement is not required by all patients. Persistence of low blood pressure, weakness, and low serum sodium and high serum potassium levels indicate a need for mineralocorticoid treatment in addition to cortisol. **Fludrocortisone** is given in a daily dose of 0.05–0.2 mg.

5. Adrenal crisis (addisonian crisis) is an acute, life-threatening complication of Addison's disease in which the manifestations of adrenal insufficiency are greatly exaggerated.

  a. Clinical features. Fever, vomiting, abdominal pain, altered mental status, and **vascular collapse** may occur if Addison's disease remains untreated or in a treated patient following acute stress if additional glucocorticoid replacement is not provided.

  b. Therapy. Immediate intravenous administration of 100 mg of cortisol over 5–10 minutes should be followed by an additional 300 mg in the next 24 hours. Intravenous saline is also needed, and mineralocorticoid replacement should be provided if hypotension and volume depletion persist.

D. **Primary aldosteronism**

1. Etiology. Excessive adrenal production of aldosterone is usually caused by a single **small** (0.5–3.0 cm) **adrenal adenoma.** Less often (i.e., in 20%–40% of cases), there is bilateral hyperplasia of the adrenal cortex.

2. Clinical features. Aldosterone increases the reabsorption of sodium and the excretion of potassium and hydrogen ions in the distal renal tubules.

    a. Sodium retention causes blood pressure elevation, which is the chief clinical manifestation of this syndrome.

      (1) The amount of sodium and water that are retained is limited by compensatory mechanisms that increase renal sodium excretion in response to extracellular fluid volume expansion; sodium balance is restored after 1–2 kg of fluid have accumulated.

      (2) Although this amount of volume expansion does not cause edema, the long-term increase in cardiac output and, perhaps, other effects of mineralocorticoid excess lead to hypertension.

    b. Potassium loss causes hypokalemia, which may produce **muscle weakness, paresthesias,** and **tetany** in severe cases.

      (1) Hypokalemic nephropathy may cause polyuria.

      (2) Metabolic alkalosis is a result of the renal loss of potassium and hydrogen ions.

3. Diagnosis

    a. Laboratory diagnosis of primary aldosteronism

      (1) Hypokalemia in a hypertensive patient is often the clue that triggers the search for primary aldosteronism, although not all patients with aldosteronism have a low serum level of potassium.

      (2) Aldosterone must be measured under standardized conditions because it is affected by sodium balance, diuretics, and other factors.

        (a) Diuretics and vasodilators must be discontinued at least 2 weeks before studies of aldosterone (and renin) are undertaken.

        (b) Random aldosterone measurements in patients with primary aldosteronism may overlap those of normal individuals; sodium loading may be necessary to differentiate the aldosterone levels in patients with primary aldosteronism (which are not suppressed by a sodium load) from the levels in normal individuals (which are suppressed by a sodium load). Two of the many ways that this procedure can be performed are as follows.

          (i) The **24-hour urinary aldosterone excretion rate** can be measured after the patient has ingested more than 150 mEq of sodium for at least 3 days. (This can be ensured by giving sodium chloride tablets.) Sodium loading may further lower serum levels of potassium; therefore, caution is necessary if the patient is hypokalemic. An elevated aldosterone level in a 24-hour urine sample that contains more than 150 mEq of sodium suggests primary aldosteronism.

          (ii) Plasma levels of aldosterone can be measured after 2000 ml of normal saline have been infused over 4 hours. Normally, the values are less than 8–10 ng/dl. Severe hypertension or congestive heart failure are contraindications to saline infusion.

      (3) Plasma renin activity is the most useful indicator of whether elevated aldosterone production is primary or secondary.

        (a) Secondary aldosteronism is caused by conditions that originate outside the adrenal gland and that reduce the effective arterial blood volume, thus diminishing the pressure or tension sensed by the juxtaglomerular cells.

          (i) Such conditions include heart failure, nephrosis, cirrhosis, volume depletion caused by diuretics, and renovascular disease.

          (ii) Decreased pressure on the juxtaglomerular cells stimulates renin release, which increases angiotensin II and, in turn, aldosterone. Thus, **the high aldosterone level is accompanied by increased renin activity.**

        (b) In **primary aldosteronism,** the enhanced aldosterone production is caused by an adrenal abnormality, not by increased renin activity; the resulting volume expansion suppresses renin production. This combination of **increased aldosterone production and reduced renin activity**

can be caused only by primary aldosteronism, and it is a reliable indicator of this diagnosis.

(c) Suppression of renin activity is diagnosed with certainty only if levels remain low following manipulations that are known to stimulate renin in normal individuals, such as dietary sodium restriction, several hours of upright posture, or furosemide administration.

b. Adenoma versus hyperplasia. Aldosteronism that is due to an adenoma must be distinguished from aldosteronism that is due to hyperplasia because the distinction affects treatment, which is usually surgical in cases of adrenal adenoma and medical in bilateral hyperplasia.

(1) The biochemical changes of aldosteronism—the hypokalemia, the increased aldosterone level, and the low renin activity—are more pronounced in cases caused by a unilateral adenoma than in cases caused by hyperplasia.

(2) The plasma aldosterone concentration may be measured at 8 A.M., after 8 hours of recumbency, and again at noon, after 4 hours of ambulation.

    (a) Levels are higher after ambulation in normal subjects and in patients with bilateral hyperplasia, because renin and angiotensin are stimulated by the upright posture and sympathetic outflow.

    (b) However, patients with unilateral adrenal adenomas have a paradoxical fall in plasma aldosterone levels, presumably because when renin is profoundly suppressed, aldosterone is influenced mainly by the diurnal fall in ACTH.

(3) **Adrenal vein aldosterone concentrations** may be measured in blood samples obtained by selective catheterization. A very high level on one side indicates an adenoma; high levels on both sides indicate bilateral hyperplasia.

(4) **CT scans** and **MRI** sometimes reveal aldosterone-producing adenomas, but these tumors may be small and often cannot be visualized.

4. Therapy

a. Surgery

(1) Removal of a unilateral adenoma results in cure of the hypertension in approximately 60% of cases and improvement in another 25%.

(2) In contrast, only 20%–50% of patients with bilateral hyperplasia are improved by surgery, even if bilateral adrenalectomy is performed. Medical therapy is preferable.

b. Medical therapy. Spironolactone inhibits the effects of aldosterone on the renal tubule. A dose of 200–400 mg daily corrects the hypokalemia and often corrects the hypertension.

E. **Congenital adrenal hyperplasia**

1. Etiology and pathophysiology. Congenital adrenal hyperplasia is caused by a defect in one of the enzymes that are necessary for the synthesis of cortisol. Cortisol deficiency stimulates ACTH, which causes hyperplasia of the adrenal cortex and overproduction of whatever ACTH-dependent steroids are not affected by the enzyme deficiency (mainly adrenal androgens).

2. Clinical features

a. Androgen excess is caused by increased adrenal production of dehydroepiandrosterone, androstenedione, and testosterone.

(1) If present during fetal development, this disorder may cause **ambiguous genitalia** in female infants. If androgen excess is manifested in the postnatal period, it may cause **virilization** in prepubertal girls or in young women.

(2) In male infants, the consequence of androgen excess during fetal development is macrogenitosomia. In the postnatal period, the consequence is **precocious puberty.**

b. The cortisol deficit usually does not cause major clinical manifestations because the ACTH stimulation and adrenal hyperplasia maintain cortisol levels in the low-normal range, despite the enzyme deficiency.

    c. Other manifestations occasionally occur, depending on the specific enzyme affected.

      (1) 21-Hydroxylase deficiency accounts for 95% of cases of adrenal hyperplasia.

        (a) In the mild (simple virilizing) form, only the androgen-excess symptoms are of importance.

        (b) In the severe (salt-losing) form, the production of aldosterone is impaired as well as that of cortisol; mineralocorticoid deficiency leads to hyponatremia, hyperkalemia, dehydration, and hypotension.

      (2) In **11-hydroxylase deficiency,** deoxycorticosterone, a mineralocorticoid, as well as adrenal androgens are overproduced. This causes hypertension through mechanisms that are similar to those causing hypertension in primary aldosteronism.

      (3) In **17-hydroxylase deficiency,** deoxycorticosterone is overproduced, resulting in hypertension. However, because 17-hydroxylase is necessary for sex steroid synthesis, there is androgen deficiency as well as estrogen deficiency. This causes the development of ambiguous genitalia in male infants and primary amenorrhea in women.

3. Diagnosis. Concentrations of adrenal androgens and precursors of cortisol are increased in blood and urine. The most useful measurements are of **blood testosterone, androstenedione, dehydroepiandrosterone,** and **17-hydroxyprogesterone** (a cortisol precursor) as well as **urinary 17-ketosteroids** and **pregnanetriol** (a metabolite of 17-hydroxyprogesterone).

4. Therapy

    a. Medical therapy. Cortisol administration suppresses the overproduction of ACTH and adrenal androgens. In the salt-losing syndrome, mineralocorticoid replacement with fludrocortisone may be necessary.

    b. Surgery. Reconstructive surgery of the external genitalia in female infants is done in the first few years of life.

F. **Pheochromocytoma** is a tumor of **chromaffin cells,** the cells that synthesize and store catecholamines. Chromaffin cells are located mainly in the adrenal medulla, but they also are located in sympathetic ganglia and elsewhere. The cells in the adrenal medulla produce epinephrine and norepinephrine; the extra-adrenal chromaffin cells make only norepinephrine.

1. Epidemiology

    a. Incidence. Pheochromocytoma is found in approximately 0.5% of patients with severe hypertension and in less than 0.05% of all hypertensive patients. However, because it may cause a dramatic and debilitating syndrome, often with fatal complications if undetected, diagnostic efforts and awareness are required out of proportion to the frequency of occurrence.

    b. Familial occurrence. Pheochromocytomas may occur sporadically or may occur as part of one of several familial syndromes.

      (1) MEN type II (Sipple's syndrome) is characterized by multiple pheochromocytomas and medullary carcinoma of the thyroid; hyperparathyroidism is often present.

      (2) Neurofibromatosis and von Hippel-Lindau disease may be associated with pheochromocytoma.

2. Pathology. Most pheochromocytomas are single tumors of the adrenal medulla. However, 10%–20% are located outside of the adrenal gland, and 1%–3% are in the chest or neck. Approximately 20% are multiple and 10% are malignant.

3. Clinical features. The manifestations of pheochromocytoma (Table 9-14) are caused by increased levels of circulating catecholamines.

    a. Hypertension is paroxysmal in approximately 50% of cases and is sustained in the rest. The diagnosis is often suggested by the **paroxysmal nature of the symptoms,** caused by variations in the function of the tumor. Attacks typically last less than 1 hour and may be precipitated by exercise, induction of anesthesia,

Table 9-14. Manifestations of Pheochromocytoma

Hypertension
Headache
Sweating
Palpitations
Nervousness and tremor
Weight loss

urination (suggesting a pheochromocytoma of the bladder), or palpation of the abdomen.

b. **Other features** that suggest the presence of a pheochromocytoma are **hyperglycemia, hypermetabolism,** and **postural hypotension** in a hypertensive patient.

4. **Diagnosis.** Pheochromocytoma is suspected far more often than it is diagnosed. Many patients with symptoms of catecholamine excess prove to have normal hormone levels.

   a. The levels of **urine catecholamines** and their metabolites are elevated in most confirmed cases.

      (1) The **24-hour urinary metanephrine excretion rate** may be the most useful screening test, but tests of **urinary free catecholamine** (i.e., epinephrine and norepinephrine) and **vanillylmandelic acid** concentrations are also of value.

      (2) Stressful illness can raise catecholamine levels twofold; greater than twofold elevations are more suggestive of pheochromocytoma.

   b. **Serum catecholamine levels** are variable and are more difficult to interpret than the 24-hour urine measurements.

   c. The **clonidine suppression test** is useful in patients with mild catecholamine elevation. Three hours after an oral dose of 0.3 mg of clonidine, the plasma level of norepinephrine is lowered into the normal range in most normal individuals but it remains elevated in patients with pheochromocytoma.

   d. **CT scans** or **MRI** of the abdomen detect as many as 90% of these tumors because they usually are greater than 1 cm in diameter.

   e. **Adrenal scanning** with ^{131}I iodobenzylguanidine is especially useful for localizing extra-adrenal tumors, but this procedure is not widely available.

5. **Therapy**

   a. **Medical therapy**

      (1) The α- and β-adrenergic blocking agents are useful for inoperable tumors and for preparation for surgery.

         (a) α-**Adrenergic blocking agents** relieve the hypertension and adrenergic symptoms.

            (i) **Phenoxybenzamine** is given orally, starting with 10 mg twice daily and increasing to 40 mg twice daily, if necessary.

            (ii) **Phentolamine** can be given intravenously to treat acute severe elevations in blood pressure.

            (iii) **Prazosin, terazosin,** or **doxazosin** can also be given to produce sustained α-adrenergic blockade.

         (b) **Beta-adrenergic blocking agents** should not be used alone, because unopposed α-adrenergic stimulation may lead to exacerbation of the hypertension. β-Blockers are sometimes useful in conjunction with α-blockers.

      (2) **Metyrosine,** which is an inhibitor of tyrosine hydroxylase, blocks the formation of norepinephrine and epinephrine and is an alternative agent for the relief of the symptoms of pheochromocytoma. It may be used when patients are intolerant of the adrenergic-blocking agents.

    b. Surgery. Surgical removal of the pheochromocytoma is the treatment of choice. Careful exploration of the adrenal gland and the periaortic sympathetic chain should be performed.

      (1) Complications that frequently occur during and after surgery are extreme swings in blood pressure, cardiac arrhythmias, and shock. These are caused by the sudden removal of the source of the source of excess catecholamine production and by the low blood volume that results from long-term constriction of the vascular compartment.

      (2) To prevent vascular instability during removal of a pheochromocytoma, patients are treated with α-blockers to maintain normal blood pressure for at least 1 week before surgery. β-Blockers may be added for a few days before surgery, especially if tachycardia or another arrhythmia is present.

VI.   **FEMALE REPRODUCTIVE DISORDERS.** Endocrine disorders that affect the female reproductive system usually cause menstrual abnormalities and include those disorders in which menarche does not occur **(primary amenorrhea)** and those disorders that cause cessation of menstrual periods after menarche **(secondary amenorrhea).** Androgen-excess syndromes are a common cause of reproductive abnormalities that also are considered in this section.

  A.   **Primary amenorrhea** (Table 9-15)

    1. Gonadal dysgenesis (Turner's syndrome) occurs in 1 in 2500–10,000 live female births.

      a. Etiology and pathophysiology. Gonadal dysgenesis is caused by a **chromosomal abnormality** that is not familial and is not related to the mother's age. Patients have a chromatin-negative buccal smear and a 45,X karyotype.

      b. Clinical features

        (1) Ovaries fail to develop; only bilateral streaks of connective tissue are present, without germ cells. Estrogen deficiency, caused by the absence of ovarian tissue, results in **sexual infantilism,** with absence of breast development and other secondary sexual characteristics, and increased levels of LH and FSH.

        (2) Somatic abnormalities are associated with gonadal dysgenesis.

          (a) Most patients are short, between 48 and 58 inches in height.

          (b) Other features, present in varying numbers of patients, include a short, webbed neck, epicanthal folds, low-set ears, a shield-like chest with widely spaced nipples, cubitus valgus (wide carrying angle), and renal and cardiac abnormalities.

      c. Therapy

        (1) Estrogen therapy induces the development of secondary sexual characteristics. If estrogen is given cyclically with progesterone, regular menstrual bleeding will occur, but fertility is not possible.

Table 9-15. Causes of Primary Amenorrhea

Gonadal causes
Gonadal dysgenesis (Turner's syndrome)
Testicular feminization syndrome
Resistant ovary syndrome
Extragonadal causes
Hypopituitarism
Hypogonadotropic hypogonadism
Delayed menarche
Congenital adrenal hyperplasia
Abnormalities of the uterus or vagina

(2) Removal of streak gonads. Gonadal dysgenesis may occur in patients with sex chromosome mosaicism in which one or more cell lines bear a Y chromosome. The frequency of gonadoblastoma and other gonadal tumors is increased in patients with these gonads, and their prophylactic removal is recommended.

2. **Testicular feminization syndrome.** Patients with this syndrome are genetic males with a 46,XY karyotype, but they have normal female external genitalia and are raised as girls.
   a. **Pathogenesis.** The basic defect is resistance of target tissues to the action of androgens. The fetal testes produce testosterone, but because the wolffian ducts and genital tissues cannot respond to testosterone, female differentiation of the external genitalia takes place. The fetal testes also produce müllerian duct inhibiting factor, which has its normal effect in inhibiting the müllerian anlage, and so the fallopian tubes, uterus, and upper vagina do not develop.
   b. **Clinical features.** The result is a phenotypic woman with a vagina that ends in a blind pouch, hypoplastic male ducts instead of the fallopian tubes and uterus, and testes located in the abdomen, inguinal canal, or labia majora. Endogenous estrogen stimulates normal breast development at puberty. The condition is suspected when menarche fails to occur or when a testis is felt as an abdominal mass, which is explored.
   c. **Therapy.** The testes are prone to malignant degeneration and should be removed. Estrogen treatment is then given to maintain secondary sexual characteristics.

3. **Resistant ovary syndrome.** Inability of the ovaries to respond to normal or increased stimulation by gonadotropins may be a result of autoimmune destruction of the ovaries or other conditions.

4. **Hypogonadotropic hypogonadism**
   a. **Panhypopituitarism** due to destructive lesions of the hypothalamic–pituitary area (see I A 2 a) causes primary or secondary amenorrhea, depending on whether the problem is prepubertal or postpubertal in onset.
   b. **Isolated gonadotropin deficiency** is most often caused by defective hypothalamic production of GnRH, usually of unknown etiology. In **Kallmann's syndrome,** this defect is associated with anosmia.

5. **Delayed menarche** should be considered when menstrual periods have not begun by 16 years of age.
   a. A diagnosis of delayed menarche, as opposed to that of primary amenorrhea, can only be made in retrospect, after spontaneous menstrual periods have begun. A family history of late pubertal development suggests that spontaneous menarche may yet be expected.
   b. If severe psychological stress is caused by the absence of sexual development, it may be necessary to give one or more 6-month courses of estrogen therapy, with long treatment-free periods to observe whether spontaneous puberty will occur.

B. **Secondary amenorrhea** (Table 9-16)

1. **Hypothalamic** (also called **"psychogenic," "functional,"** and **"idiopathic"**) **amenorrhea is** the **most common form of nonphysiologic secondary amenorrhea.** Obvious psychological stress may or may not be present. LH and FSH levels are low in some cases and normal in others. If the hypothalamic releasing hormone GnRH is infused in physiologic fashion (pulse doses every 90–120 minutes), all abnormalities may be corrected—ovarian follicles mature, ovulation takes place, a corpus luteum develops and functions, and pregnancy may occur. This supports the clinical impression that most cases of functional or idiopathic amenorrhea are caused by abnormal hypothalamic GnRH production.

2. **Malnutrition.** Menarche seems to occur when a critical body weight is reached, and menstruation often ceases when the weight of a woman whose menstrual

Table 9-16. Causes of Secondary Amenorrhea

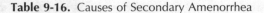

> Pregnancy
> Menopause
> Uterine causes
>   Intrauterine synechiae (Asherman's syndrome)
>   Hysterectomy
> Hypothalamic–pituitary causes
>   Hypopituitarism
>   Hypothalamic ("psychogenic") amenorrhea
>   Malnutrition, chronic illness
>   Exercise
>   Discontinuation of oral contraceptives
> Ovarian causes
>   Primary ovarian failure ("premature menopause")
>   Oophorectomy
>   Radiotherapy, chemotherapy
> Estrogen excess
>   Ovarian tumors
> Prolactin excess
>   Pituitary tumors
> Androgen excess
>   Polycystic ovary syndrome
>   Overproduction of adrenal androgen
>   Ovarian tumors

cycle was previously normal falls below this critical weight, whether because of food deprivation, chronic illness, excessive dieting, or anorexia nervosa.

3. **Exercise.** Amenorrhea is present in up to 50% of female ballet dancers, runners, and athletes. Exercise-related weight loss is at least partially responsible; the risk of amenorrhea is much higher in women who have lost more than 10%–15% of their body weight. Levels of LH, FSH, and estrogen tend to be low, suggesting a hypothalamic abnormality.

4. **"Post-pill amenorrhea"** refers to a delay of more than 6 months in the return of menses after the discontinuation of oral contraceptive use. It occurs in fewer than 1% of oral contraceptive users. Other causes of amenorrhea must be excluded before contraceptive use is blamed.

5. **Primary ovarian failure ("premature menopause")** is similar to normal menopause; that is, ovarian function declines, estrogen levels decrease and gonadotropin levels increase. However, primary ovarian failure occurs before 40 years of age. Autoantibodies against ovarian antigens have been found in some cases.

6. **Ovarian tumors** (e.g., granulosa–theca cell tumors) may inhibit normal menstrual cycling by producing excessive quantities of estrogen.

7. **Prolactin excess** is a common cause of secondary amenorrhea (see I A 4 b).

C. **Androgen excess syndromes**

1. **Polycystic ovary syndrome** (also called the Stein-Leventhal syndrome), a disorder of unknown etiology, is characterized by a chronic lack of ovulation, associated with symptoms of androgen excess and often with obesity. It is present in 3%–7% of reproductive-age women.
   a. **Pathophysiolosy** (Figure 9-2)
      (1) The ovary produces excess androgenic steroids, especially **androstenedione.** The androstenedione is converted to estrone, an estrogen, in fat and other peripheral tissues. The increased circulating and intraovarian levels of

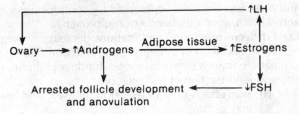

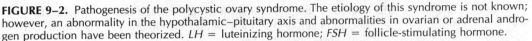

FIGURE 9–2. Pathogenesis of the polycystic ovary syndrome. The etiology of this syndrome is not known; however, an abnormality in the hypothalamic–pituitary axis and abnormalities in ovarian or adrenal androgen production have been theorized. *LH* = luteinizing hormone; *FSH* = follicle-stimulating hormone.

androstenedione and other androgens prevent the maturation of graafian follicles, causing **anovulation.**

(2) The increased circulating level of estrone has a positive feedback effect on pituitary production of LH and a negative effect on production of FSH. The **increased LH level** causes hyperplasia of ovarian thecal cells and stroma and increased androgen production. The **decreased FSH level** contributes to the lack of follicle maturation.

(3) **Obesity** may enhance the elevated levels of sex steroids by decreasing sex-hormone–binding globulin, thus increasing the level of free testosterone, and by increasing the peripheral conversion of androstenedione to estrone.

(4) As a result of the **arrested follicle development,** the ovaries are enlarged, with thickened capsules and many small follicular cysts. Stromal and thecal hyperplasia are seen on microscopic examination.

(5) The initiating event in this cycle is uncertain, and it may not be the same in all cases. Some authorities believe that the basic abnormality is in the hypothalamic–pituitary axis, with constant (rather than cyclic) overproduction of LH; others believe that excess ovarian secretion of androgen is the primary event. Abnormalities of adrenal androgen production have been found in these patients, and some investigators believe that this may initiate the cycle; there are reports of disappearance of the polycystic ovary syndrome following the removal of an androgen-secreting adrenal adenoma.

b. **Clinical features**

(1) **Infertility and menstrual abnormalities** are the result of chronic anovulation. Most patients have amenorrhea or oligomenorrhea. The prolonged, noncyclic, unopposed estrogenic stimulation of the endometrium may cause functional bleeding and an increased risk of endometrial carcinoma.

(2) **Androgen excess** causes oiliness of the skin, acne, and hirsutism in the majority of women with this syndrome. Signs of true virilization (e.g., deepening of the voice, enlargement of the clitoris) are rare.

(3) **Obesity** is present in approximately 40% of patients.

c. **Laboratory findings**

(1) An **increased LH-to-FSH ratio** ($\geq$ 2) is a useful diagnostic finding. The LH level is usually elevated, and the FSH level is in the low-normal range.

(2) **Serum testosterone and androstenedione levels** are usually elevated. Increased levels of the androgens of predominantly adrenal origin (i.e., dehydroepiandrosterone and dehydroepiandrosterone sulfate) are found less often.

(3) **Serum estrone levels** are usually high, and estradiol levels are normal.

d. **Therapy.** The two **main goals of treatment are the relief of symptoms of androgen excess and the induction of ovulation and fertility.** Treatment of the former (e.g., with birth control pills) may preclude treatment of the latter; a clear view of therapeutic goals in each case is, therefore, essential.

(1) **Androgen excess.** Oral contraceptives, glucocorticoids, and spironolactone are used to treat the hirsutism and other symptoms associated with androgen excess. Some authorities advocate initial testing to determine whether

androgen levels can be suppressed by contraceptives or by glucocorticoids, and others prefer a trial and error approach.

   (a) **Estrogen–progestin combinations** decrease androgen levels by feedback inhibition of pituitary LH production and by stimulation of hepatic synthesis of sex-hormone–binding globulin, which decreases the unbound fraction of testosterone.

      (i) Side effects of fluid retention, nausea, and break-through bleeding may occur.

      (ii) Potential complications, which are related to the estrogen dose and to cigarette use, include thrombophlebitis, myocardial infarction, and hypertension.

   (b) **Glucocorticoids** decrease adrenal androgen production by suppressing ACTH; they may also lower ovarian androgen secretion, although the mechanism is unknown.

      (i) Because ACTH production peaks in early morning, a bedtime dose of 0.5 mg of dexamethasone is recommended.

      (ii) Potential undesired side effects are weight gain, depression, and suppression of the hypothalamic–pituitary–adrenal response to stress.

   (c) **Spironolactone,** an aldosterone antagonist that is used mainly for its diuretic and antihypertensive properties, has additional actions that make it useful in the treatment of hirsutism.

      (i) Spironolactone decreases ovarian and adrenal synthesis of androgens and inhibits androgen binding to receptors in hair follicles and other target tissues.

      (ii) A dose of 100 mg once or twice daily is often effective.

   (d) The effects of hormone therapy in diminishing the growth of unwanted facial and body hair are seldom dramatic and usually take place over a period of 3–6 months. Mechanical methods of hair removal are usually needed as well (e.g., shaving, electrolysis, bleaching, chemical depilatories, and wax treatments).

(2) Infertility

   (a) **Clomiphene citrate** blocks the binding of estrogen to receptors in target tissues. By blocking estrogen's negative feedback effects on the hypothalamus and pituitary gland, it stimulates LH and FSH production.

      (i) If given on the fifth day through the ninth day following a menstrual period induced by progesterone, clomiphene citrate often stimulates follicle maturation and ovulation.

      (ii) Ovulation can be induced with clomiphene citrate in approximately 80% of patients.

   (b) **Human menopausal gonadotropin** has both FSH and LH bioactivity.

      (i) It is injected daily until increasing serum estrogen levels and ultrasonography of the ovary indicate that follicle maturation has occurred.

      (ii) Then human chorionic gonadotropin (hCG), which has mainly LH activity, is injected to induce ovulation. Because the risk of ovarian hyperstimulation and of multiple gestation is high, this therapy should be reserved for resistant cases of infertility.

   (c) **GnRH,** when given intravenously or subcutaneously in pulse doses every 90–120 minutes, may induce ovulation without causing ovarian hyperstimulation. This is a promising new form of treatment.

(3) Chronic anovulation and abnormal menstrual bleeding. Unopposed noncyclic stimulation of the endometrium by estrogen may cause functional bleeding and may increase the risk of endometrial cancer. Persistent endometrial proliferation can be interrupted either with progestin treatment (e.g., 10 mg daily of medroxyprogesterone acetate for 10 days every 1–3 months) or with cyclic estrogen–progestin therapy.

2. **Androgen-producing ovarian tumors** are rare. Arrhenoblastoma, the most common of these tumors, makes up less than 1% of solid ovarian tumors; others are hilar cell tumors, adrenal rest tumors, and granulosa cell tumors.
   a. Testosterone levels tend to be higher than those in the polycystic ovary syndrome, and virilization occurs more frequently.
   b. Androgen levels are not suppressed by treatment with glucocorticoids or estrogen–progestin combinations, as they often are in the polycystic ovary syndrome.
   c. Diagnosis depends on detection of the tumor by pelvic examination (the majority are palpable) and on diagnostic imaging techniques.

3. **Hyperthecosis** of the ovary is probably a severe form of the polycystic ovary syndrome, but the androgen excess is more evident.
   a. The **diagnosis** depends on the histologic finding of luteinized thecal and stromal cells.
   b. **Medical therapy** is not effective, and oophorectomy may be necessary.

4. **Adrenal tumors,** either adenomas or carcinomas, may produce excess androgens with or without excess cortisol. High levels of adrenal androgens (urinary 17-ketosteroids, serum dehydroepiandrosterone) that cannot be suppressed by dexamethasone suggest this diagnosis; 24-hour urinary 17-ketosteroid levels greater than 50–100 mg strongly suggest adrenal carcinoma.

5. **Congenital adrenal hyperplasia** is discussed in the section on disorders of the adrenal gland (see V E).

6. **Idiopathic hirsutism,** or idiopathic androgen excess syndrome, is a poorly understood but common condition in which mild hirsutism and sometimes acne and menstrual irregularities occur in the absence of marked hormone abnormalities.
   a. Testosterone levels may be high-normal or slightly elevated, or there may be elevations in testosterone (with decreased sex-hormone–binding globulin) and adrenal androgens.
   b. Polycystic ovaries and LH and FSH abnormalities are absent. Whether the ovary or adrenal gland is the source of mild androgen excess is unclear.
   c. Estrogen–progestin combinations, glucocorticoids, and spironolactone (see VI C 1 d) sometimes decrease the androgen levels and the symptoms. Because of its effectiveness and minimal side effects, spironolactone is usually the treatment of choice.

VII. MALE REPRODUCTIVE DISORDERS AND GYNECOMASTIA

A. **Hypogonadism** in men affects two separate functions—the production of spermatozoa by the seminiferous tubules and the secretion of testosterone by the Leydig cells. The seminiferous tubule defect causes infertility; the testosterone deficiency leads to inadequate development and maintenance of secondary sexual characteristics.

1. **Physical and developmental effects**
   a. **Before puberty,** testicular failure prevents normal sexual development.
      (1) The penis and testes remain small, and spermatozoa are absent.
      (2) Facial and body hair are sparse.
      (3) The voice remains high-pitched, and muscle mass and strength are diminished.
      (4) Increased growth of long bones (because of delayed epiphyseal closure) produces the "eunuchoidal habitus," in which the arm span is more than 2 inches greater than the height, and the floor-to-pubic symphysis distance is more than 2 inches greater than the symphysis-to-crown distance.
   b. **After puberty,** loss of libido and sexual potency may be the first symptoms of testicular failure. Partial regression of secondary sex characteristics may occur gradually, with slowing of facial and body hair growth and decreased muscle mass.

Table 9-17. Causes of Hypogonadism in Men

Hypogonadotropic syndromes
   Hypopituitarism
   Hypogonadotropic eunuchoidism
     Kallmann's syndrome
   Delayed puberty
Hypergonadotropic syndromes
   Klinefelter's syndrome
   Testicular agenesis
   Testicular injury
     Mumps orchitis
     Other infections (e.g., gonorrhea)
     Trauma
     Surgery
     Radiotherapy
     Cancer chemotherapy
     Cryptorchidism
     Myotonic dystrophy

2. **Clinical syndromes**
  a. **Hypogonadotropic syndromes** (Table 9-17). The causes of hypogonadism are divided into **disorders of the hypothalamic–pituitary axis (hypogonadotropic hypogonadism) and disorders that originate with testicular damage,** with consequent feedback stimulation of LH and FSH **(hypergonadotropic hypogonadism).**
    (1) **Hypogonadotropic (secondary) hypogonadism** is characterized by deficiency of LH and FSH, with resulting testosterone deficiency and eunuchoidism. **Kallmann's syndrome** is a form of hypogonadotropic hypogonadism that is associated with midline defects such as agenesis of the olfactory lobes, anosmia, and cleft palate. It is more common in men than in women. The basic hormonal defect is in the hypothalamus, rather than in the pituitary gland; this has been demonstrated by LH and FSH response to GnRH administration.
    (2) **Delayed puberty** is a retrospective diagnosis. Puberty may occur spontaneously up to about 20 years of age; until this age, true hypogonadotropic hypogonadism cannot be diagnosed with certainty unless associated abnormalities such as anosmia are present. The diagnosis of delayed puberty is suggested by a family history of late maturation.
      (a) If delayed puberty is suspected, a course of therapy with low doses of testosterone can be initiated to induce pubertal changes; true puberty may be induced by this treatment.
      (b) Testosterone should be given for no more than 6 months at a time, with 6 months between courses, to avoid causing epiphyseal closure and limitation of ultimate height and to allow recognition of the onset of spontaneous puberty, if it should occur.
  b. **Hypergonadotropic syndromes (primary hypogonadism)**
    (1) **Klinefelter's syndrome,** in which the presence of two or more X chromosomes causes congenital testicular damage, occurs in approximately 1 in 400 male births.
      (a) Approximately 80% of patients have a **47,XXY karyotype.**
        (i) The testes are small (less than 2 cm in length).
        (ii) There is hyalinization of the seminiferous tubules and **azoospermia.**
        (iii) Leydig cell function is variable. Testosterone levels are deficient and **eunuchoidism** is present in many, but not all, cases.

      (iv) Gynecomastia is present, and LH and FSH levels are elevated, even (for unknown reasons) in patients without testosterone deficiency.

      (v) Mental deficiency is an associated finding in 25% of all patients.

    (b) The only available treatment is testosterone replacement in those patients who require it.

  (2) Testicular agenesis is recognized by failure of pubertal development and absence of testes in the scrotum or in the inguinal canals. Loss of the testes occurs after 7–14 weeks' gestation, because absence of testicular hormones before this stage would result in a female phenotype.

  (3) Mumps orchitis affects mainly germinal cells; if the disease is bilateral, infertility may result, although this is uncommon. Testosterone production is usually unimpaired.

  (4) Cryptorchidism, especially if it is bilateral, may be associated with hypogonadism because the undescended testes are damaged by trauma or torsion.

    (a) An association between hypogonadism and cryptorchidism may exist because the cryptorchidism is sometimes a consequence of an intrinsic abnormality in the testes.

    (b) Treatment with hCG or GnRH may induce testicular descent in some cases.

  (5) Myotonic dystrophy is a syndrome consisting of myotonia, cataracts, and testicular atrophy.

3. Therapy

  a. Testosterone deficiency. Although oral androgenic steroids are available, they do not provide fully virilizing blood levels of male hormones. The usual treatment of male hypogonadism is the injection of 200–300 mg of a long-acting testosterone preparation (e.g., Delatestryl or DEPO-Testosterone) every 2–3 weeks. A transdermal system for administration of testosterone through the scrotal skin (Testoderm) is also available.

  b. Infertility. Sperm production and fertility cannot be induced in individuals with primary testicular injury. In hypogonadotropic hypogonadism, spermatogenesis can sometimes be brought about by providing the testes with adequate gonadotropic stimulation.

    (1) This can be done either by injections three times per week of hCG (which has LH activity) and human menopausal gonadotropin (which has FSH activity) or by administration via portable infusion pump of pulse doses of GnRH every 90–120 minutes.

    (2) Both of these methods are expensive and impractical for long-term use, but they have been used successfully in some highly motivated men for the several months that are necessary to induce spermatogenesis.

B. **Gynecomastia** is enlargement of the male breast. In true gynecomastia, firm, sometimes tender, glandular tissue is present. The disorders that cause gynecomastia are usually associated with increased levels of estrogens, decreased levels of androgens, or both.

1. Pubertal gynecomastia. At 12–15 years of age, approximately two thirds of normal boys have some degree of gynecomastia, usually a small, firm subareolar nodule that disappears in most cases within 1–2 years.

  a. In the occasional boy with persistent breast enlargement, medical treatment with **danazol,** a weak synthetic androgen that inhibits gonadotropin, or with the antiestrogen **tamoxifen,** may be tried.

  b. If this is ineffective, however, **reduction mammoplasty** must be considered if psychological stress is severe.

2. Hypogonadism, either primary (hypergonadotropic) or secondary (hypogonadotropic), may be associated with gynecomastia.

3. Refeeding after a period of starvation often leads to transient gynecomastia, which may last for several months. Renewed secretion of previously inhibited gonadotropins and sex steroids and decreased hormone inactivation by the starved liver may be contributing factors.

4. **Liver disease,** especially alcoholic cirrhosis, is a common cause of gynecomastia.
   a. Estrogen levels are increased because of accelerated conversion of androgenic precursors by peripheral tissues.
   b. Also, alcohol inhibits the testicular production of testosterone and the pituitary production of gonadotropins and increases hepatic metabolism of testosterone.

5. **Chronic renal failure** is associated with gynecomastia, especially after the start of hemodialysis. The refeeding phenomenon may play a role, as may an increase in the ratio of estrogens to androgens in chronic renal failure.

6. **Drugs**
   a. **Estrogens,** commonly used to treat prostatic carcinoma, stimulate the breast directly.
   b. **Spironolactone, cimetidine,** and **digitalis** also produce gynecomastia. They are believed to inhibit androgen action by displacing dihydrotestosterone from its intracellular receptor.
   c. **Marijuana** binds to estrogen receptors and may cause gynecomastia through a direct estrogenic action.
   d. Other drugs that may cause this problem include **phenothiazines, tricyclic antidepressants, methyldopa, reserpine,** and **isoniazid.**

7. **Tumors** may cause gynecomastia.
   a. **Adrenal** and **testicular tumors** may cause gynecomastia through the production of estrogen.
   b. **Testicular choriocarcinomas** may cause gynecomastia through the secretion of hCG, which stimulates testicular estrogen production.
   c. Other malignant tumors may cause the condition through the ectopic production of gonadotropins.

8. **Hyperthyroidism** increases the conversion of androgens to estrogens in the peripheral tissues and increases the circulating level of sex-hormone–binding globulin, which raises the estrogen to androgen ratio. These hormonal changes may cause gynecomastia in men with hyperthyroidism.

VIII. METABOLIC BONE DISEASE. The metabolic bone diseases are commonly classified into three main categories: osteomalacia, osteoporosis, and osteitis fibrosa cystica. Osteitis fibrosa cystica is discussed briefly in the section on hyperparathyroidism (see III A 4 b).

A. **Osteomalacia**

1. **Definition.** Osteomalacia is a **skeletal abnormality** in which there is **inadequate mineralization of bone matrix.** In children, this usually takes the form of rickets, caused by vitamin D deficiency. In adults, osteomalacia may be caused by many specific abnormalities of calcium, phosphorus, and vitamin D metabolism.

2. **Etiology**
   a. **Vitamin D deficiency**
      (1) Deficiency of vitamin D causes osteomalacia because its most active metabolite, 1,25-dihydroxyvitamin D_3 is essential for the absorption of calcium and phosphate from the gastrointestinal tract.
      (2) Deficiency of vitamin D is uncommon in the United States; most Americans obtain the recommended dietary allowance of 200–400 U of vitamin D from fortified foods, especially dairy products. However, dietary deficiency may still occur because of poverty, food faddism, eating disorders such as anorexia nervosa, or lack of sun exposure in elderly, debilitated patients.

(3) Exposure to sunlight converts 7 dehydrocholesterol in the skin to vitamin D_3 and this is an important source of the vitamin. Absence of sunlight may contribute to vitamin D deficiency.

b. Abnormal metabolism of, or response to, vitamin D

(1) Liver disease, when far advanced, may cause osteomalacia by interfering with the normal hepatic conversion of vitamin D to 25-hydroxyvitamin D_3.

(2) Anticonvulsant drugs, such as phenobarbital and phenytoin, if taken over a long period, may alter the metabolism of vitamin D by inducing hepatic microsomal enzymes. Osteomalacia and decreased serum levels of 25-hydroxyvitamin D_3 have been described in patients receiving long-term treatment with anticonvulsants.

(3) Vitamin D-dependent rickets type I is an autosomal recessive disorder caused by impaired activity of renal 1-α-hydroxylase, leading to inadequate conversion of 25-hydroxyvitamin D_3 to 1,25-dihydroxyvitamin D_3 (calcitriol). It is treated with small, physiologic doses (0.5–1.0 μg) of calcitriol.

(4) Vitamin D-dependent rickets type II, also autosomal recessive, is caused by resistance to the action of vitamin D due to altered structure or function of the calcitriol receptors. To overcome this resistance, large, supraphysiologic doses of calcitriol, along with calcium supplementation, must be used.

c. Renal abnormalities

(1) Renal osteodystrophy may occur in patients with chronic renal failure of any cause. Both osteomalacia, caused by impaired renal production of 1,25-dihydroxyvitamin D_3, and osteitis fibrosa cystica, caused by the secondary hyperparathyroidism of renal failure, are present in varying degrees.

(2) X-linked hypophosphatemic rickets is an X-linked dominant disorder in which the primary abnormality is renal loss of phosphate. This is caused by decreased proximal tubular reabsorption of phosphate and relative deficiency of calcitriol production. Supraphysiologic doses of calcitriol, together with phosphate, may raise the serum phosphate level, decrease the bony abnormalities of rickets, and increase growth.

(3) In **Fanconi's syndrome,** renal tubular defects may lead to the loss of phosphate as well as calcium, glucose, and amino acids, with resulting osteomalacia.

d. Gastrointestinal disorders. Any disease or surgical procedure that leads to malabsorption and steatorrhea may reduce the absorption of calcium, phosphate, and vitamin D, and osteomalacia may result.

e. Tumors, such as hemangiopericytomas and giant cell tumors of bone, may produce a humoral substance that causes phosphaturia and osteomalacia; the syndrome (**"oncogenic osteomalacia"**) is cured by removal of the tumor.

3. Pathophysiology

a. The **common defect** in the various diseases associated with osteomalacia is the **lack of calcium and phosphorus for mineralization of bone matrix.**

(1) Circulating phosphate levels are usually low, either because of decreased gastrointestinal absorption or excessive renal excretion.

(2) Calcium levels may be low, but they are often normal because of compensatory parathyroid hyperactivity.

b. Rickets is caused by defective mineralization of bone before closure of the cartilagenous growth plates. Deformity occurs because of pressure on weakened growth plates and on the abnormally soft shafts of the long bones. After closure of the growth plates, only osteomalacia can occur, with defective mineralization of mature lamellar bone.

c. Histologically, bone biopsy shows an excess of unmineralized bone matrix, which is seen as an increase in the volume and thickness of osteoid seams covering the bone surfaces.

4. Clinical features

a. Pain and tenderness are common in affected areas of the skeleton, especially the spine, ribs, pelvis, and lower extremities.

    b. Muscle weakness is common, affecting particularly the proximal muscles of the legs.

    c. Skeletal deformities and fractures occur in severe cases.

        (1) The long bones may bow because of the softening of the skeleton.

        (2) Rickets in children is associated with widening of the epiphyses; swelling of the wrists, knees, ankles, and costochondral joints; bowlegs; and disturbances in growth.

5. Laboratory findings

    a. X-rays may show **decreased bone density** and coarsening of the trabecular pattern. **Looser's zones** are radiolucent bands that are perpendicular to the periosteal surface, caused by pseudofractures.

    b. Although laboratory abnormalities depend on the cause and the severity of the osteomalacia, they often include **low serum phosphate, low or normal serum calcium, and increased serum alkaline phosphatase levels.**

6. Therapy

    a. Treatment of the primary disorder is sometimes possible (e.g., correction of a bowel disorder causing malabsorption or removal of a tumor causing osteomalacia).

    b. Vitamin D is usually the mainstay of treatment.

        (1) In simple vitamin D deficiency, a physiologic dose of 400 U of vitamin D daily may be all that is needed.

        (2) Large doses of calcitriol, which does not require biochemical transformation to achieve full activity, may be needed in the uncommon syndromes caused by altered metabolism or action of vitamin D or renal wasting of phosphate.

B. **Osteoporosis**

1. Definition. Osteoporosis is a decrease in total bone volume or, simply, too little bone. The bone that is present is normal. The decrease in bone mass leads to an increased susceptibility to fractures. Both increased bone resorption and decreased bone formation have been observed.

2. Etiology

    a. Decreased bone mass at maturity

        (1) After reaching its peak in an individual of approximately 30–35 years of age, bone mass declines throughout the remaining years of life. A low total bone mass at maturity, a relatively rapid rate of bone loss, or both contribute to the development of "involutional" osteoporosis.

        (2) Genetic factors affect the bone mass at maturity.

            (a) Men and blacks have greater peak bone mass and less osteoporosis; women and individuals of northern European ancestry have less bone mass at maturity and more osteoporosis.

            (b) A familial tendency toward osteoporosis has been observed.

    b. Calcium deficiency. Evidence suggests that calcium intake in American women is less than is needed to maintain calcium balance.

        (1) More than 75% of women older than 35 years of age fail to ingest the recommended daily allowance of 1000 mg of calcium. Also, calcium absorption decreases in later life.

        (2) The need to maintain normal serum levels of calcium may lead to increased bone resorption, through the action of PTH. (The effect of PTH on bone is to increase the rate of calcium and phosphate resorption, and when serum calcium levels are low, the secretion of PTH increases.)

    c. Hormone changes. When estrogen levels decrease, whether because of ovarian disease, oophorectomy, or normal menopause, the rate of bone loss is accelerated.

        (1) Estrogen deficiency may result in less stimulation of osteoblastic activity and may increase the sensitivity of bone to the action of PTH.

        (2) The increased rate of bone loss persists for 5–10 years after menopause.

3. **Classification**
   a. **Two types** of osteoporosis have been described.
      (1) **Postmenopausal osteoporosis** primarily affects women within 15 years of menopause. The loss of trabecular bone is accelerated, and fractures of the vertebrae, which consist mainly of trabecular bone, are common.
      (2) **Senile osteoporosis** affects men and women older than 75 years of age, causing loss of both cortical and trabecular bone. Fractures of the hip, which is largely cortical bone, occur as do vertebral fractures.
   b. **Secondary osteoporosis** may be associated with glucocorticoid therapy or spontaneous Cushing's syndrome, malabsorption syndromes or malnutrition, multiple myeloma, and prolonged immobilization, among other things.

4. **Clinical features**
   a. **Fractures**
      (1) **Vertebral compression fractures** typically affect T8 to L3 and occur more commonly in women. They may cause acute back pain that persists for several months or may occur gradually and painlessly.
      (2) **Hip fractures,** characteristically in the neck and intertrochanteric regions of the femur, are common in both men and women older than 65 years of age. Loss of function frequently results, and, because of complications, mortality rates may be as high as 20% within 1 year.
      (3) The **distal radius** and other areas also may be the site of fractures.
   b. **Pain and deformity.** Back pain may persist long after an episode of vertebral fracture because of spinal deformity and alteration of spinal mechanics. Several inches may be lost from height, and severe kyphosis may be the result of multiple vertebral fractures.

5. **Diagnosis**
   a. **Radiography of the spine** may reveal a decrease in bone density, with accentuation of the cortical outlines and prominence of the trabeculae.
      (1) However, approximately 30% of bone tissue must be lost before these abnormalities appear on plain radiographs.
      (2) Wedge-shaped deformities and compression fractures on spinal radiographs also suggest the diagnosis of osteoporosis.
   b. **Dual energy absorptiometry (DXA),** the best method for evaluating bone mineral density, is the reference standard for the diagnosis of osteoporosis.

6. **Therapy.** Prevention of osteoporosis is easier than treatment. Therapeutic agents can slow the rate of bone loss but are less effective in restoring bone mass that has been lost.
   a. **Estrogen.** An important means of preventing osteoporosis is the administration of estrogen after menopause. Estrogen decreases the accelerated rate of bone loss that occurs following menopause. Obese women have higher estrogen levels after menopause, which decreases their risk for osteoporosis.
      (1) The decision to use postmenopausal estrogen replacement should be based on the benefits and risks of estrogen use in each patient.
         (a) There is a greater risk for osteoporosis and, therefore, greater **potential benefit of estrogen** use in an individual who:
            (i) Has a small stature and slender build
            (ii) Has a family history of osteoporosis
            (iii) Is white and of northern European ancestry
            (iv) Experienced early menopause
            (v) Smokes
         (b) The **adverse effects of estrogen,** which must be balanced against its benefits, are:
            (i) Possible symptoms of nausea, breast tenderness, and fluid retention
            (ii) A fourfold to eightfold increase in the risk for endometrial cancer (if estrogen is taken without progesterone)
            (iii) Increased risk that unscheduled uterine bleeding may occur and require gynecologic investigation

                (iv) Increased risk for gallbladder disease and hypertension

                (v) A possible small increase in the risk of breast cancer

        (c) Other benefits of estrogen therapy, such as the relief of menopausal symptoms, must be considered. The most important benefit of estrogen may be its favorable effects on the blood lipoprotein pattern (i.e., it decreases low-density lipoprotein (LDL) levels and increases high-density lipoprotein (HDL) levels, thereby reducing the risk of atherosclerosis and cardiovascular disease). These benefits may outweigh the other risks and benefits associated with estrogen therapy.

    (2) Treatment of osteoporosis

        (a) Once a patient is known to have osteoporosis, the benefit of estrogen treatment clearly outweighs the risk, provided that there are no major contraindications to estrogen use, such as breast cancer.

        (b) Estrogen has been shown to reduce the rate of vertebral, hip, and wrist fractures, even when started years after menopause.

    (3) Mode of administration

        (a) Estrogen can be given in relatively low doses, such as 0.625 mg of conjugated estrogens or 20 μg of ethinyl estradiol daily.

        (b) The cyclic administration of estrogen for 25 days each month, with the addition of a progestin (e.g., medroxyprogesterone acetate in a dose of 5–10 mg daily) for the final 10–14 days, reduces the risk of uterine cancer. The use of progestins is being questioned, however, because these may lessen the favorable effect of estrogens on blood lipid patterns.

        (c) Alternatively, 0.625 mg of conjugated estrogens and 2.5 mg of medroxyprogesterone acetate can be given every day. In a majority women, this leads to endometrial atrophy. The periodic bleeding that makes cyclic estrogen–progestin therapy unacceptable to many women often stops within 1 year.

        (d) In women who have had a hysterectomy, estrogen can be given daily without cycling and without progesterone, because there is no risk of endometrial cancer.

  b. Calcium

    (1) Patients with osteoporosis should ingest at least 1500 mg of elemental calcium daily.

        (a) Because the average American takes in only about 500 mg of calcium in food, calcium supplements should be given. Calcium carbonate tablets (e.g., 500 mg of Os-Cal two or three times daily) are usually well tolerated.

        (b) Exogenous calcium may reduce the rate of bone loss and the fracture rate in patients with osteoporosis whose usual calcium intake is inadequate.

    (2) Because of the safety of calcium supplementation and the prevalence of inadequate calcium intake, many authorities recommend calcium supplementation for all susceptible women, starting before menopause.

  c. Calcitonin, a hormone secreted by the parafollicular cells of the thyroid, inhibits osteoclast activity and decreases the rate of bone loss and fractures in osteoporosis. It is given by injection, and may be given by nasal spray (Miacalcin), which is more acceptable to many patients. The nasal spray delivers 200 units of calcitonin, the daily dose, in one puff; the patient alternates nostrils each day because of possible nasal irritation.

  d. Bisphosphonates are agents that bind to hydroxyapatite in bone and decrease osteoclastic bone resorption.

    (1) Etidronate (Didronel) has been used to treat osteoporosis, but unlike calcitonin and alendronate it has not been approved for this indication by the Food and Drug Administration. It must be given intermittently because daily administration may interfere with mineralization of bone.

    (2) Alendronate (Fosamax) does not inhibit bone mineralization, and is given daily. Its effectiveness in increasing bone mineral density and in decreasing the fracture rate has been greater than that of calcitonin or etidronate.

(a) The dose is 10 mg once daily.

(b) The main side effects of alendronate are gastrointestinal symptoms, especially esophageal irritation and in a few cases esophageal erosion. To prevent these complications and to maximize drug absorption the patient must take alendronate with a full glass of water on arising in the morning, 30 minutes before the first meal, beverage, or other medication, and must not lie down for 30 minutes after the pill is swallowed.

e. **Sodium fluoride** has been found effective in the treatment of osteoporosis in some studies but not in others. Its role in therapy is not yet defined.

f. **Vitamin D** in pharmacologic doses (more than 1000 units daily) has not been proved to be effective in the treatment of osteoporosis. But physiologic doses, 400–800 units daily, have decreased the fracture rate in populations of elderly persons who may be deficient in vitamin D because of poor nutrition and lack of exposure to sunlight. Vitamin D supplementation of 400–800 units daily should be recommended in such individuals, and perhaps in patients with osteoporosis.

STUDY QUESTIONS

DIRECTIONS: Each of the numbered items or incomplete statements in this section is followed by answers or by completions of the statement. Select the ONE lettered answer or completion that is BEST in each case.

1. A 23-year-old man with gynecomastia is found to have a 47,XXY karyotype. This patient probably also has which one of the following conditions?

(A) Abnormal liver function tests
(B) Low blood levels of luteinizing hormone (LH) and follicle-stimulating hormone (FSH)
(C) High blood levels of estrogen
(D) Azoospermia
(E) Enlargement of the testes

2. An 18-year-old woman is evaluated because she has never had a menstrual period. Pelvic examination is normal except that the vagina ends in a blind pouch. A karyotype is reported to be 46,XY. Which one of the following diagnoses is most likely?

(A) Congenital adrenal hyperplasia
(B) Turner's syndrome
(C) Kallmann's syndrome
(D) Testicular feminization syndrome
(E) Polycystic ovary syndrome

3. A 55-year-old woman has been treated for type II diabetes with isophane insulin suspension (NPH), 35 U once daily before breakfast. Home glucose measurements on a typical day are 7 A.M. (fasting), 238 mg/dl; 11 A.M., 155 mg/dl; 4 P.M., 128 mg/dl; 8 P.M., 125 mg/dl. Which of the following changes in insulin therapy would be reasonable?

(A) Raising the dose of insulin
(B) Adding regular insulin to the dose of NPH
(C) Giving the dose in the evening instead of the morning
(D) Adding a dose of regular insulin before supper
(E) Adding a second dose of NPH insulin before supper

4. Which of the following tests is the most sensitive for the diagnosis of a pituitary microadenoma?

(A) Serum prolactin measurement
(B) Visual field examination
(C) Computed tomography (CT) scan with contrast injection
(D) Magnetic resonance imaging (MRI) with gadolinium injection
(E) Insulin-tolerance test

5. Primary hyperparathyroidism is successfully treated with the removal of a single parathyroid adenoma in a 60-year-old woman. Following surgery, she has a prolonged period of hypocalcemia, which requires continuous treatment with large doses of vitamin D and calcium. After 2–3 months, the need for vitamin D and calcium subsides and she remains normocalcemic without treatment. This patient probably had which one of the following conditions?

(A) Accidental destruction of the other three parathyroid glands
(B) Removal of the wrong parathyroid gland
(C) Severe pancreatitis caused by her hyperparathyroidism
(D) Unrecognized pseudohypoparathyroidism
(E) Severe bone disease

6. A patient with polycystic ovary syndrome is most likely to have which of the following findings?

(A) Deepening of the voice, enlargement of the clitoris, and a high testosterone level
(B) Oligomenorrhea, obesity, a high luteinizing hormone (LH) level, and a low follicle-stimulating hormone (FSH) level
(C) Amenorrhea, acne, a low LH level, and a low FSH level
(D) Facial hirsutism, acne, and increased urinary pregnanetriol, and 17-ketosteroids
(E) Facial hirsutism, normal menstrual periods, and normal levels of FSH, LH, and testosterone

7. Hypothyroidism should be treated with daily administration of which one of the following thyroid hormone preparations?

(A) Thyroid extract
(B) Thyroglobulin
(C) Thyroxine (T$_4$)
(D) Triiodothyronine (T$_3$)
(E) T$_4$ and T$_3$

8. Which one of the following is the most common complication of radioiodine treatment of Graves' disease?

(A) Thyroid storm
(B) Subacute thyroiditis
(C) Thyroid cancer
(D) Hypothyroidism
(E) Leukemia

9. Which one of the following hormones is most commonly found to be elevated in patients with pituitary adenomas?

(A) Growth hormone (GH)
(B) Adrenocorticotropic hormone (ACTH)
(C) Prolactin
(D) Thyroid-stimulating hormone (TSH)
(E) Somatomedin C

10. The syndrome of painless thyroiditis can best be distinguished from Graves' disease by which one of the following findings?

(A) Thyroid enlargement
(B) Low blood thyroid-stimulating hormone (TSH) levels
(C) Elevated blood thyroxine (T$_4$) levels
(D) Low radioactive iodine uptake
(E) Tenderness and pain involving the thyroid gland

11. A 23-year-old man is evaluated because of a diagnosis of hypogonadism. Which one of the following findings would suggest primary testicular disease rather than hypothalamic or pituitary disease?

(A) Anosmia
(B) Increased levels of follicle-stimulating hormone (FSH) and luteinizing hormone (LH)
(C) Eunuchoidal habitus
(D) Loss of libido and sexual potency
(E) Decreased sperm number and motility

12. Osteomalacia caused by excessive urinary loss of phosphate is associated with which one of the following?

(A) Vitamin D deficiency
(B) Vitamin D-dependent rickets type I
(C) X-linked hypophosphatemic rickets
(D) Treatment with anticonvulsant drugs
(E) Severe liver disease

13. Excessive production of aldosterone results in which one of the following clinical features?

(A) Sodium depletion
(B) Acidosis
(C) Hypotension
(D) Potassium retention
(E) Plasma renin activity suppression

DIRECTIONS: Each set of matching questions in this section consists of a list of four to twenty-six lettered options (some of which may be in figures) followed by several numbered items. For each numbered item, select the ONE lettered option that is most closely associated with it. To avoid spending too much time on matching sets with large numbers of options, it is generally advisable to begin each set by reading the list of options. Then, for each item in the set, try to generate the correct answer and locate it in the option list, rather than evaluating each option individually. Each lettered option may be selected once, more than once, or not at all.

Items 14–16

(A) Graves' disease
(B) Hypothyroidism
(C) Pregnancy
(D) Subacute thyroiditis
(E) Nontoxic goiter

For each result of thyroid function tests, select the clinical condition with which it is most likely to be associated.

14. Elevated serum thyroxine (T_4), low radioactive iodine uptake

15. Elevated serum T_4, low triiodothyronine (T_3) resin uptake

16. Elevated serum T_4, elevated radioactive iodine uptake

Items 17–21

(A) Graves' disease
(B) Testicular feminization syndrome
(C) Addison's disease
(D) Hypopituitarism
(E) Acromegaly

For each primary pathological process, select the disease it is most likely to cause.

17. Excessive production of hormone by an endocrine tumor

18. Destruction of an endocrine gland by tumor, trauma, or infarction

19. Stimulation of an endocrine gland by autoimmune mechanisms

20. Destruction of an endocrine gland by autoimmune mechanisms

21. Impaired sensitivity of peripheral tissues to normal circulating levels of a hormone

ANSWERS AND EXPLANATIONS

1. The answer is D [VII A 2 b (1) (a)]. The 47, XXY karyotype indicates Klinefelter's syndrome. Elevation of gonadotropin levels, small testes, and gynecomastia also are common findings in Klinefelter's syndrome.

2. The answer is D [VI A 1 a, 2 b, C 1 b; VII A 2 a (1)]. Patients with the testicular feminization syndrome have a normal male karyotype, and testes (located In the abdomen or groin) that produce testosterone. But because there is resistance of the tissues to the effects of testosterone, the external genitalia develop as female during fetal life. Turner's syndrome (gonadal dysgenesis) is characterized by a 45,X karyotype. Kallmann's syndrome is more common in men than in women and is often accompanied by anosmia and cleft palate. Polycystic ovary syndrome usually causes secondary, not primary, amenorrhea, and this patient has none of the other typical clinical features (e.g., oily skin, obesity, or hirsutism). Congenital adrenal hyperplasia is not associated with a short vagina and blind pouch, both of which are typical of testicular feminization.

3. The answer is E [IV A 8 d (3) (b), (4) (b)]. The pattern of glucose levels suggests that the dose of isophane insulin suspension (NPH) is effective during the day, but does not retain its effect until the next morning. Giving more insulin in the morning or adding regular insulin would risk causing hypoglycemia in the afternoon and evening when glucose levels are already at a satisfactory level. A second dose of NPH before supper, however, would be expected to have its maximal action in the early morning, which is the time that an increased glucose-lowering effect is desired.

4. The answer if D [I A 1 b (3) (a), (4), c (1) (b)]. Magnetic resonance imaging (MRI) with gadolinium is the most sensitive test for the detection of microadenomas, revealing them in 10%–20% of normal women. Overscretion of prolactin is present in only 30%–50% of patients with pituitary adenomas. Impaired growth hormone (GH) response to insulin-induced hypoglycemia or visual field changes

function or to compress the optic chiasm. Computed tomography (CT) scans reveal very small adenomas, but MRI with gadolinium is even more sensitive.

5. The answer is E [III A 7 a (3)]. When primary hyperparathyroidism causes osteitis fibrosa cystica, the sudden correction of the primary hyperparathyroidism and consequent removal of the source of excessive parathyroid hormone (PTH) allows the skeleton to undergo rapid repair and remineralization, which creates a marked but self-limiting demand for calcium and phosphate. If the patient had hypoparathyroidism after surgery, the hypocalcemia would probably have been permanent and the need for treatment would not have resolved.

6. The answer is B [VI C 1]. Polycystic ovary syndrome is characterized by a chronic lack of ovulation associated with symptoms of androgen excess and often with obesity. Severe virilization and marked testosterone elevation are more likely to be caused by an ovarian tumor or hyperthecosis than by the polycystic ovary syndrome. A low luteinizing hormone (LH) level and an increased urinary pregnanetriol concentration are not characteristic of the polycystic ovary syndrome. Hirsutism without other clinical or laboratory abnormalities usually is diagnosed as "idiopathic hirsutism."

7. The answer is C [II B 4 a]. Thyroxine (T_4) is the agent of choice. Thyroid extract and thyroglobulin contain varying proportions of the two thyroid hormones, thyroxine (T_4), and triiodothyronine (T_3), making it difficult to interpret blood T_4 and T_3 levels and to adjust the dosage precisely. Preparations containing T_3 must be given several times daily to maintain a normal blood level of T_3 because T_3 has a short half-life. T_4, however, has a long half-life and is converted to T_3 in the liver and elsewhere; hypothyroid patients taking the correct optimal dose of T_4 once daily have normal, stable blood levels of both T_4 and T_3.

8. The answer is D [II C 4 a (3) (c) (ii)–(iii)]. Hypothyroidism occurs in approximately 50% of patients treated with radioiodine 10–15 years after treatment. Thyroid storm and subacute thyroiditis are rare complications. No increased incidence of thyroid cancer, leukemia, or other malignancies has been attributed to radioiodine therapy.

9. The answer is C [I A 1 a (1), b (1), 4] As many as 50% of all pituitary adenomas have been found to secrete prolactin, and blood prolactin levels should be measured in a patient suspected of having a pituitary tumor. Acromegaly due to growth hormone (GH) excess and Cushing's disease due to adrenocorticotropic hormone (ACTH) excess are considerably less common, and overproduction of thyroid-stimulating hormone (TSH) is rare. Somatomedin C (insulin-like growth factor I) is increased in acromegaly but is not elevated in most patients with pituitary tumors.

10. The answer is D [II D 3 a (2)] Low radioactive iodine uptake is the most useful finding for distinguishing painless thyroiditis from Graves' disease. Inflammation and injury to thyroid cells, as well as a lack of thyroid-stimulating hormone (TSH), inhibit radioactive iodine uptake in painless thyroiditis, whereas the uninjured and immunoglobulin-stimulated thyroid cells in Graves' disease concentrate radioactive iodine at an increased rate. Enlargement of the thyroid gland and increased blood levels of thyroid hormone, with suppression of TSH, may occur in both Graves' disease and painless thyroiditis. The gland is not tender or painful in either condition.

11. The answer is B [VII A 1, 2]. Increased gonadotropin production indicates primary testicular failure with negative-feedback stimulation of the hypothalamic–pituitary axis. Hypogonadism, whether caused by hypothalamic–pituitary disease or testicular disease, is associated with loss of libido and potency and abnormalities of sperm production. A eunuchoidal habitus results from continued growth of long bones due to delay in testosterone-induced epiphyseal closure; therefore, eunuchoidal habitus can result from either primary testicular failure or hypothalmic–pituitary disease. Anosmia is sometimes associated with hypothalamic failure to secrete gonadotropin-releasing hormone (GnRH).

12. The answer is C [VIII A 2 a, b, c (2)]. X-linked hypophosphatemic rickets is characterized by excessive excretion of phosphate in the urine caused by decreased proximal tubular reabsorption of phosphate and a relative deficiency of 1,25-dihydroxyvitamin D_3 production. Vitamin D deficiency prevents normal gastrointestinal absorption of calcium and phosphorus. Liver disease and anticonvulsant drugs may impair the hepatic conversion of vitamin D to 25-hydroxyvitamin D_3. In vitamin D-dependent rickets type I, conversion of 25-hydroxyvitamin D_3 to 1,25-dihydroxyvitamin D_3 is impaired.

13. The answer is E [V D 2, 3 a (3) (b)]. Plasma renin activity suppression is a clinical feature of primary aldosteronism. Excess circulating levels of aldosterone increase the reabsorption of sodium, in exchange for potassium and hydrogen ions, in the distal tubules. The resulting expansion of extracellular fluid volume causes suppression of plasma renin activity and eventually causes hypertension. The loss of potassium and hydrogen ions causes a tendency toward metabolic alkalosis.

14–16. The answers are: 14-D [II D 1 c], **15-c** [II A 1 a], **16-A** [II C 3 d]. In subacute thyroiditis, injured thyroid follicular cells release thyroid hormone, raising the blood level of thyroxine (T_4). Radioactive iodine uptake is low, however, because the injured follicular cells are unable to trap iodine normally. Also, thyroid-stimulating hormone (TSH) is suppressed by the increased level of circulating thyroid hormone, and this further reduces the radioactive iodine uptake.

The high estrogen levels in pregnancy cause increased production of T_4-binding globulin. This raises the serum level of total T_4 and lowers the triiodothyronine (T_3) resin uptake. The patient remains euthyroid, however, because the serum free T_4 level remains normal.

In Graves' disease, the follicular cells trap increased amounts of iodine and produce increased amounts of thyroid hormone. Therefore, both the radioactive iodine uptake and the serum T_4 level are elevated. This combination of findings indicates hyperthyroidism, caused either by Graves disease or by Plummer's disease.

17–21. The answers are: 17-E [I A 3 a], **18-D** [I A 2 a], **19-A** [II C 1 a], 20-C [V C 1 a (1)], **21-B** [VI A 2 a]. The usual cause of acromegaly is a growth hormone (GH)-secreting pituitary adenoma. Whether these adenomas arise de novo or are caused by excessive hypothalamic production of GH-releasing hormone is not known. Rarely, GH-releasing hormone production by an islet-cell adenoma may cause acromegaly.

Pituitary tumors may compress normal tissue, impairing its function. Surgical removal of the tumor may further damage the hypothalamus and pituitary gland. Ischemic infarction at childbirth (Sheehan's syndrome) and various destructive, infectious, and granulomatous lesions also cause hypopituitarism.

Graves' disease is caused by abnormal stimulation of the thyroid gland by thyroid-stimulating immunoglobulin. This immunoglobulin G (IgG) antibody binds to receptors for thyroid-stimulating hormone (TSH). It then stimulates growth and hormone production by the thyroid follicular cells.

Addison's disease is most commonly caused by atrophy of the adrenal cortex. Anti-adrenal antibodies are often present. Other evidence of autoimmunity, such as antibodies against other tissues and the presence of other autoimmune diseases, also are common findings. Hemorrhage into the adrenals and infectious agents (e.g., tuberculosis) are less common causes of Addison's disease.

The testicular feminization syndrome results from the inability of tissue to respond to testosterone and other androgens. If not stimulated by androgens, the fetal external genitalia develop as female organs. Therefore, a genetic male infant with testes and normal male testosterone levels is born with female external genitalia and is considered to be a normal female.

Chapter 10

Rheumatic Diseases

Douglas C. Conaway

I. OSTEOARTHRITIS

A. **Definition.** Osteoarthritis is a common age-related deterioration of articular cartilage and underlying bone.

B. **Etiology.** Osteoarthritis has no single known cause. The factors listed below are believed to interact to cause varying degrees of articular damage in individual patients.

1. **Wear and tear.** Repetitive microtrauma in subchondral bone may cause changes that impair its ability to absorb the longitudinal forces of joint impact loading, leading to cartilage degeneration.

2. **Aging**
   a. **Decreased proteoglycan aggregation.** Although the number and function of chondrocytes are preserved in aging cartilage, proteoglycan aggregation may be diminished. This proteoglycan abnormality may impair the ability of articular cartilage to dissipate loading forces.
   b. **Loosening of type II collagen.** Separation of the collagen network may occur with repetitive mechanical stress. Defects in type IX (cross-linking) collagen may contribute to loosening in the type II collagen backbone.

3. **Genetic factors**
   a. **Erosive osteoarthritis.** Genetic factors appear to be particularly important in the development of erosive osteoarthritis of the distal and proximal interphalangeal (DIP and PIP) joints. This variant is 10 times more common in women because it is autosomal dominant in women and recessive in men.
   b. **Type II collagen gene defect.** A defect has been discovered in the gene coding for type II collagen synthesis that allows early degeneration of the type II collagen. A type of premature polyarticular osteoarthritis associated with mild epiphyseal dysplasia is associated with the presence of this abnormal type II gene in several families.

4. **Inflammation.** Immunoglobulin and complement deposits have been found in superficial articular cartilage in patients with osteoarthritis, suggesting that antigenic components of exposed cartilage can elicit a mild inflammatory response in osteoarthritis.

5. **Obesity** increases loading stress on weight-bearing joints, especially the knees.

6. **Neuropathy.** Muscle tone around a joint modulates the forces of joint impact loading. If proprioceptive input to the joint is impaired, abnormal muscle tone may result in osteoarthritis by transferring abnormal forces to the joint.

7. **Deposition diseases** (e.g., hemochromatosis, ochronosis, Wilson's disease, crystal deposition diseases) cause deposition of substances in the cartilage matrix, which can result in direct chondrocyte injury or can impair the ability of the matrix to dissipate loading forces.

C. **Pathogenesis.** Osteoarthritis is a metabolically active condition, not a degenerative one. Repair and synthetic processes counteract the destructive processes, until the repair processes are overwhelmed late in the disease course.

1. **Initial insult.** Damage to chondrocytes leads to release of neutral proteases and collagenases and to degradation of the matrix. The cytokines **interleukin-1 (IL-1)** and **tumor necrosis factor-α (TNF-α)** are the principal mediators of these catabolic effects.

523

2. Repair. Damage also leads to stimulation of chondrocyte replication and increased proteoglycan synthesis. **Transforming growth factor-β (TGF-β)** and **fibroblast growth factor (FGF)** are the major mediators of these anabolic effects, and metalloproteinase inhibitors also are released by chondrocytes at the time of injury to protect against enzyme-mediated cartilage breakdown.

3. Progressive damage. Eventually, repair processes are overwhelmed and collagen is progressively altered. The cartilage swells, and proteoglycan concentration diminishes.

4. Mechanical factors
  a. Proteoglycan loss leads to impaired cartilage elasticity and transmission of increasingly abnormal forces to the chondrocytes.
  b. Subchondral bone sclerosis also causes transmission of increased joint loading forces to chondrocytes.

D. Pathology

1. Cartilage changes
  a. Early in osteoarthritis, cartilage changes in **color** from blue to yellow due to loss of proteoglycan.
  b. Localized areas of **softening** are the earliest pathologic changes in osteoarthritis.
  c. Superficial **chipping and flaking** of cartilage signify more advanced disease.
  d. Vertical **fibrillations** in the cartilage indicate further progression.
  e. Focal and later confluent **erosions** eventually progress to full-thickness cartilage loss if healing forces are overwhelmed by destructive forces.

2. Bone changes
  a. New bone formation can occur under the cartilage (seen as eburnation on x-ray) or at the joint margin (seen as osteophytic spurs on x-ray).
  b. Subchondral cysts. Large pseudocystic areas can form in the juxta-articular bone due to transmission of increased mechanical forces to bone; presumably, these cysts fail to heal because of impaired perfusion from subchondral microfractures.

E. Classification (Table 10-1)

1. Primary osteoarthritis has no underlying cause for joint damage. It typically involves the DIP and PIP joints and the first carpometacarpal (CMC) joints. Knees, hips, and first metatarsophalangeal (MTP) joints often are involved as well as cervical and lumbar spine facet joints. The joint involvement may be **generalized** or it may occur in an isolated, **sporadic** fashion. **Erosive** osteoarthritis is a unique subset that occurs predominantly in middle-aged women and has autosomal dominant, sex-influenced characteristics. Episodic erythema, swelling, and tenderness occur in involved joints, especially the DIP and PIP joints of the hands. Characteristic radiographic abnormalities include bone erosions and ankylosis, which are unusual in typical osteoarthritis. **Diffuse idiopathic skeletal hyperostosis** is noninflammatory axial and peripheral enthesis hyperostosis manifested by radiographic "whiskering" at tendon or ligament insertion and flowing osteophytes adjacent to vertebral disks.

2. Secondary osteoarthritis exhibits an underlying cause for degenerative joint disease and may involve joints not typically affected by primary osteoarthritis (e.g., elbow, wrist). A primary metabolic, inflammatory, or mechanical process leads secondarily to osteoarthritis (see Table 10-1).

F. Clinical features

1. Symptoms of osteoarthritis vary with the joint involved and the severity of the disease.
  a. Pain. Most patients experience the gradual onset of a deep, aching pain, which worsens with activity and is relieved by rest. With more severe disease, pain can occur even at rest and interfere with sleep.

TABLE 10-1. Classification of Osteoarthritis

Primary osteoarthritis (multiple sites)
Heberden's nodes
Generalized osteoarthritis
"Erosive" osteoarthritis
Diffuse idiopathic skeletal hyperostosis

Primary osteoarthritis (local)
Cervical spine
Hip
First carpometacarpal joint
Distal interphalangeal joints
Lumbar spine
Knee
First metatarsophalangeal joint
Proximal interphalangeal joints

Secondary osteoarthritis
Congenital (e.g., hip dysplasia)
Deposition disease
   Ochronosis
   Wilson's disease
   Hemochromatosis
   Gout
   Calcium pyrophosphate deposition disease
Neuropathic joint (e.g., diabetes mellitus, syphilis)
Endocrine/metabolic (e.g., acromegaly)
Osteonecrosis (especially hips, knees)
Infection (tuberculosis)
Inflammation (rheumatoid arthritis)

   b. Morning stiffness in osteoarthritis is brief (less than 30 minutes) in contrast to that occurring in inflammatory rheumatic conditions, which may last much longer.

   c. Gelling phenomenon refers to the sensation of renewed stiffness in osteoarthritic joints after prolonged inactivity.

2. Signs

   a. Tenderness. Mild or moderate tenderness can be present in involved joints.

   b. Painful range of motion in large joints (e.g., knees, hips) is the equivalent of tenderness in small joints.

   c. Crepitus (i.e., a grinding sound or sensation) can be felt and sometimes heard when a joint is put through a full range of motion. Crepitus is caused by surface incongruities in the joint.

   d. Warmth. Involved joints usually are cool but can feel warm with flare-ups of disease activity.

   e. Joint enlargement. Soft tissue swelling may occur if an effusion is present, More commonly, bone enlargement occurs in the form of osteophytes.

   f. Deformity. Varus (medial) or **valgus** (lateral) **angulation** of joints can occur late in the disease. Gross bone enlargement and joint subluxation also can occur in severe disease.

      (1) Heberden's nodes specifically refer to enlargement of the DIP joints of the hand.

      (2) Bouchard's nodes specifically refer to enlargement of the PIP joints of the hand.

G. **Diagnosis** of osteoarthritis is made on the basis of the patient history combined with physical, laboratory, and radiographic findings.

1. Joint involvement
    a. Joint distribution. The particular joints involved should suggest whether the osteoarthritis is primary or related to an underlying disorder (see I E 1–2).
    b. Joint swelling is typically **bony,** sometimes with superimposed **fluid.**

2. Laboratory findings
    a. Hematologic findings generally are normal, including the erythrocyte sedimentation rate.
    b. Synovial fluid findings. Typical osteoarthritic synovial fluid is slightly turbid, contains no crystals, and has a white cell count that is only mildly inflammatory (i.e., < 2000 cells/μl and < 25% neutrophils).

3. Radiographic findings are common after age 40 in joints typically affected by osteoarthritis, and they often are asymptomatic.
    a. Findings typically present include:
        (1) Joint space narrowing (due to loss of cartilage)
        (2) Subchondral sclerosis (increased subchondral bone density)
        (3) Marginal osteophytes
        (4) Subchondral cysts
    b. Findings typically absent include:
        (1) Periarticular osteopenia
        (2) Marginal erosions (except in the distal DIP and PIP joints in the erosive osteoarthritis variant)
    c. Clinical correlates
        (1) Comparison views. Obtaining x-rays of the contralateral joint can be helpful.
        (2) Standing views best demonstrate the amount of cartilage loss in knees.

4. Differential diagnosis
    a. Monoarticular problems
        (1) Periarticular abnormality. Patients may complain of pain in a joint yet have involvement of a periarticular structure such as a tendon, ligament, or bursa as the real cause of symptoms.
        (2) Other causes. Bacterial infections and crystal-mediated problems must always be considered if only one joint is involved. Trauma, hemorrhage, and monoarticular presentations of inflammatory diseases also can be confused with osteoarthritis.
    b. Polyarticular problems
        (1) Inflammatory rheumatic disease. Systemic complaints (e.g., anorexia, weight loss, fatigue, fever), prominent morning stiffness, and findings of inflammatory rheumatic diseases should be sought.
        (2) Soft tissue syndromes. Disorders associated with regional aching (regional myofascial pain) or generalized aching [e.g., fibromyalgia, polymyalgia rheumatica (PMR)] also should be considered in polyarticular presentations.

H. Therapy

1. Nonpharmacologic therapy
    a. General advice to patients. Joint overuse or repetitive trauma must be avoided. **Weight loss** may be beneficial in arthritis of weight-bearing joints such as the knees. Osteoarthritis pain improves with rest, so **joint rest** is particularly important when pain is prominent.
    b. Supports
        (1) A **knee cage or brace** sometimes is used when knee ligamentous instability coexists with osteoarthritis.
        (2) A **soft cervical collar** may be used for symptomatic flare-ups of cervical spine osteoarthritis.
        (3) A **lumbar corset** (back brace) sometimes is used to buttress sagging abdominal or back muscles in patients with low back pain.
        (4) A **cane** may be helpful in supporting a patient with unilateral hip or knee osteoarthritis.

    (5) Arch supports (orthotics) or cushioned shoes may decrease the transmission of weight-bearing forces to the hips and knees.

  c. Exercise. Isometric strengthening of supporting muscles around joints may be helpful (e.g., quadriceps-setting exercises in knee arthritis). Swimming is the best form of **aerobic exercise** for a patient with osteoarthritis of the hips or knees; running should be avoided by these patients.

  d. Heat/cold modalities. Application of moist heat or heating pads, or even ice, often can temporarily lessen the pain of osteoarthritis.

2. Pharmacologic therapy

  a. Analgesics

    (1) Topical. Direct application of **capsaicin** (substance P inhibitor) or a **nonsteroidal anti-inflammatory drug (NSAID)** to the skin overlying a painful joint can relieve pain.

    (2) Systemic. Pain-relieving medications such as **acetaminophen** often are effective in moderate to high doses for mild to moderate osteoarthritis. Narcotics should be avoided, although **propoxyphene** may be useful in severe cases for management of pain associated with flare-ups of disease activity.

  b. NSAIDs. Pain relief with low to moderate doses of aspirin or other NSAIDs may be useful. Elderly patients have more gastrointestinal and renal side effects from these drugs and, thus, should be carefully monitored when receiving such treatment.

  c. Corticosteroids. Oral steroids have no place in the management of osteoarthritis. Occasional **intra-articular** injections of corticosteroids may be of temporary benefit in flare-ups, but repeated use of steroids carries the risk of possible acceleration of the disease process.

3. Surgery. In advanced disease of the knee or hip, **total joint replacement** can be dramatically effective in alleviating pain and restoring function. **Angulation osteotomy** is still performed in osteoarthritis of the knee to treat unicompartmental disease.

II. CRYSTAL-RELATED JOINT DISEASES

A. Gout

1. Definition. Gout is the name given to a group of disorders of purine metabolism that are characterized by **serum uric acid elevation** (hyperuricemia) and **urate deposition** in articular or extra-articular tissues. Elevation of serum uric acid alone is not sufficient for the diagnosis of gout; in fact, only 10% of patients with hyperuricemia develop gout. Some unknown factor predisposes some patients to urate deposition and articular inflammation in the setting of sustained hyperuricemia.

2. Etiologic classification of hyperuricemia. All gouty syndromes are characterized by either episodic or constant **elevation of serum uric acid** concentration **above 7 mg/dl.** Patients with elevated serum uric acid can be classified as **overproducers** or **underexcreters** of uric acid, depending on the amount of uric acid excreted during a 24-hour period. Excessive dietary intake of purines can contribute to hyperuricemia in both types of patient.

  a. Overproducers, who comprise approximately 10% of the gout population, excrete **more than 750–1000 mg** of uric acid per day on an unrestricted diet. These patients synthesize greater than normal amounts of uric acid de novo from intermediates or via breakdown of purine bases from nucleic acids. The defect causing uric acid overproduction can be **primary** (associated with purine pathway enzymatic defects) or **secondary** (increased cell turnover associated with alcohol use, hematologic malignancies, chronic hemolysis, or cancer chemotherapy).

  b. Underexcreters, who comprise approximately 90% of the gout population, excrete **less than 700 mg** of uric acid per day.

(1) This group includes patients with combined defects, because overproducers of uric acid also may be underexcreters. The decreased renal excretion of uric acid is the basis for hyperuricemia in these patients.

(2) The most common causes of decreased uric acid excretion are **drug effects** (diuretic, alcohol, and low-dose aspirin interference with tubular handling of urate) and **renal disease** (chronic renal failure, lead nephropathy). Subtle renal tubular defects in urate handling may also be **inherited** and predispose to underexcretion.

3. Associated conditions. The following conditions occur more commonly in patients with gout but are not known to be causal.

a. Obesity. Serum uric acid level rises with body weight. Gout is significantly more common in individuals who are more than 15% overweight, partly because of decreases in urate excretion.

b. Diabetes mellitus. Impaired glucose tolerance is common in gout and may be a function of obesity.

c. Hypertension is common in patients with gout, but no independent correlation exists between blood pressure and serum uric acid level. Obesity probably is responsible for a high rate of hypertension in patients with gout.

d. Hyperlipidemias (types II and IV) are common in gout; however, diet, alcohol intake, and body weight seem to be more important associations in these patients.

e. Atherosclerosis. Death in patients with gout is commonly attributable to cardiovascular or cerebrovascular diseases. However, the above-mentioned risk factors that commonly occur in gout patients seem to explain the tendency for accelerated atherogenesis.

4. Clinical stages of gout

a. Asymptomatic hyperuricemia is characterized by an increased serum uric acid level in the absence of clinical evidence of deposition disease (i.e., arthritis, tophi, nephropathy, or uric acid stones).

(1) Hyperuricemia. The risk of acute gouty arthritis or nephrolithiasis increases as the serum uric acid concentration increases. However, most patients do not develop either of these conditions.

(2) Hyperuricosuria. The risk of uric acid stone formation in patients with hyperuricemia is most closely related to a urinary uric acid excretion exceeding 1000 mg/day. These patients also are at risk for **acute obstructive uropathy,** a form of acute renal failure occurring most often following combination chemotherapy for cancer. Large purine loads lead to sudden increases in serum uric acid levels, with subsequent precipitation of uric acid crystals in the collecting tubules and ureters.

b. Acute gouty arthritis—the second stage and primary manifestation of gout—is an extremely painful, acute-onset arthritis.

(1) Typical patient. Most patients (80%–90%) are middle-aged or elderly men who have had sustained asymptomatic hyperuricemia for 20–30 years before the first attack. Women seem to be spared until menopause, perhaps via an estrogen effect on uric acid clearance. Onset of acute gouty arthritis in the teens or twenties is unusual and most often associated with a primary or secondary cause of uric acid overproduction.

(2) Typical attack

(a) Presentation. A monoarticular, lower extremity presentation is most common with 50% of patients experiencing their first attack in the first MTP joint (called **podagra**). Many attacks occur suddenly at night, with rapid evolution of joint erythema, swelling, tenderness, and warmth. intense joint inflammation can extend into the soft tissues and mimic cellulitis or phlebitis. Fever can occur in severe attacks.

(b) Course. Attacks usually resolve in a few days, although some can extend over several weeks. The joint usually returns to normal between attacks. Polyarticular involvement can occur in some cases, and a typical progression from monoarticular to polyarticular involvement occurs by extension to adjacent joints.

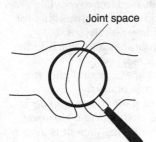

Joint space

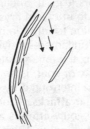

Joint space

Crystal either is shed
or forms spontaneously

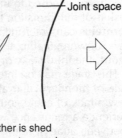

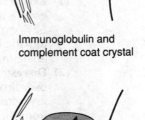

Immunoglobulin and
complement coat crystal

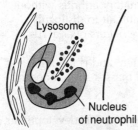

Lysosome

Nucleus
of neutrophil

Neutrophil chemotaxis
and ingestion of crystal

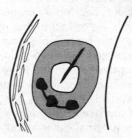

Fusion of the lysosome
and crystal

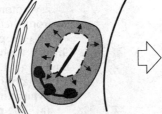

Undigested crystal ruptures
lysosome, releasing enzyme

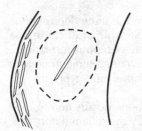

Lysosomal enzyme release
kills cell; inflammation
is increased

Increased synovial permeability
leads to lipoprotein coating,
downregulates inflammation

FIGURE 10-1. Postulated pathogenesis of crystal-induced joint inflammation. *Ig* = immunoglobulin; *C3* and *C4* = complement components C3 and C4; *LP* = lipoprotein.

(3) Pathogenesis of acute attacks (Figure 10-1).
  (a) Sustained hyperuricemia leads to the development of **microtophi** (i.e., small crystal aggregates) in the synovial membrane and cartilage.
  (b) Through several mechanisms, microtophi are disrupted and crystals are released into the joint space. Spontaneous urate crystallization can also occur in conditions of urate supersaturation of joint fluid. (Trauma, joint temperature changes, and fluctuations in serum or synovial fluid uric acid concentration are potential initiators of these processes.)
  (c) Urate crystals are coated by **immunoglobulins** and **complement components.** These adherent proteins enhance phagocytosis by neutrophils.
  (d) Phagosomes in the crystal-containing neutrophils fuse with lysosomes, and the lysosomal enzymes digest the protein coating of the crystals. The naked crystals then apparently disrupt the phagosomal membranes.
  (e) Neutrophils are damaged by the crystals, and lysosomal enzymes are released into synovial fluid, potentiating inflammation.

  (f) Inflammatory mediators (e.g., IL-6) can be released from synovial macrophages exposed to uric acid crystals and may be responsible for extension of inflammation to other joints and into soft tissues.

  (g) Lipoproteins can enter inflamed synovial membranes and attach to the crystals, downregulating the inflammatory process.

 c. Intercritical gout, the third stage of gout, is an asymptomatic period after the initial attack. This stage may be interrupted by new acute attacks.

  (1) Recurrence of monoarticular attacks. About 7% of patients never experience a new attack of acute gouty arthritis after the first episode. However, 62% experience a recurrence within 1 year. Typically; the patient is asymptomatic between attacks, but attacks eventually become more frequent and abate more gradually if urate deposition remains untreated over time.

  (2) Disease progression. Attacks tend to become polyarticular and more severe over time. Some patients develop a chronic inflammatory arthritis without asymptomatic intervals—a condition that may be difficult to distinguish from rheumatoid arthritis. Tophaceous gout typically occurs over a 10- to 20-year period of untreated urate deposition.

 d. Chronic tophaceous gout develops in the untreated patient and is the final stage of gout. The tophus is a collection of urate crystal masses surrounded by inflammatory cells and variable fibrosis.

  (1) Typical locations of tophaceous deposits

   (a) The pinna of the external ear is a potential site of tophus development, although deposition here is uncommon.

   (b) Other common locations are the surfaces of chronically involved joints and subchondral bone as well as extensor surfaces of the forearms, olecranon bursae, and the infrapatellar and Achilles tendons.

  (2) Pathogenesis of tophaceous gout

   (a) Although microtophi may form in joints early in the urate deposition phase, aggregates that are large enough to be palpable or to cause anatomic deformities take years to develop. The rate of tophus formation is directly related to the severity and duration of hyperuricemia in gout patients. Tophi do not occur in patients with asymptomatic hyperuricemia.

   (b) Erosion of cartilage and adjacent subchondral bone occurs due to displacement of normal tissue by the tophus and by the inflammatory reaction to it.

 e. Renal complications may arise at any stage of gout, but nephrolithiasis is the only common clinical presentation of renal involvement. Proteinuria and impaired ability to concentrate urine related to urate deposition in the renal interstitium have been described in gout patients (see Chapter 6, Part I: XI B 3).

 5. Diagnosis

  a. Acute gouty arthritis

   (1) Laboratory findings

    (a) Serum findings. The serum uric acid value often is not helpful in the clinical diagnosis of acute gout. Serum uric acid concentration is normal in at least 10% of patients at the time of an acute attack, and an elevated serum uric acid level is not specific for acute gout.

    (b) Synovial fluid findings. The demonstration of **urate crystals,** especially intracellular crystals, in synovial fluid is diagnostic. These **crystals characteristically are needle-shaped and negatively birefringent** in red-compensated, polarized light, and they may be present in neutrophils during an acute attack. Synovial fluid white cell counts of 10,000–60,000/μl (predominantly neutrophils) also are common in acute attacks.

   (2) Colchicine trial. In a typical clinical setting (i.e., a middle-aged man with an acute attack of podagra), a good clinical response to colchicine treatment is reasonably specific for acute gout. Other forms of acute arthritis (e.g., sarcoid arthropathy, pseudogout) can respond to colchicine; therefore, this trial may not be as specific in less typical presentations.

b. Chronic tophaceous gout

(1) **Physical appearance.** Tophi are firm, movable, and cream-colored or yellowish in appearance if superficially located. If they ulcerate, a chalky material is extruded.

(2) **Radiographic findings.** Tophaceous deposits appear as well-defined, large erosions (punched-out erosions) of the subchondral bone. These erosions are most common at the first MTP joint and at the bases and heads of phalanges; however, any articulation can be affected. Typical gouty erosions have an **overhanging edge** of subchondral new bone formation. Periarticular osteopenia is absent.

(3) **Aspiration.** Tophi can be aspirated and crystals demonstrated by polarized microscopy.

6. Therapy. In all stages of gout, secondary causes of hyperuricemia (e.g., medications, obesity, excess dietary purine intake, alcohol intake, other disease) should be altered if possible.

a. Asymptomatic hyperuricemia. In general, patients without evidence of urate deposition do not require treatment other than correction of underlying causes. Patients with uric acid elevations that chronically exceed 10 mg/dl have a greater than 90% chance of developing acute gout at some time, but most physicians wait for an acute attack to begin treatment.

b. Acute gouty arthritis. Drug treatment of the acute attack is most effective when started very early after symptoms begin. As with any inflammatory arthritis, rest or immobilization of the involved joint is an important adjunct to treatment.

(1) **Colchicine** inhibits neutrophil chemotaxis and inflammatory mediator release by suppressing phospholipase A_2; it can be used intravenously to treat acute attacks. Caution is necessary in elderly patients and in those with renal or hepatic impairment due to increased bone marrow toxicity. Colchicine can be used orally for acute attacks, but nausea, vomiting, and diarrhea often appear before therapy is successful.

(2) **NSAIDs** often are used in high but quickly tapered doses to treat acute attacks. Any of these agents can be used, although drugs that affect uric acid clearance (e.g., salicylates, diflunisal) should be avoided, because any fluctuation in serum urate can prolong acute attacks. Caution is warranted when using NSAIDs in the presence of gastrointestinal, hepatic, or renal disease.

(3) **Corticosteroids.** Intra-articular injections of corticosteroids can be used to treat acute gout of a single joint, particularly when the use of other agents is contraindicated.

(4) **Drugs that alter serum uric acid concentrations** (e.g., **allopurinol, probenecid**) should be avoided during acute attacks because raising or lowering serum uric acid can prolong attacks. In patients already taking such drugs, the dosage should not be altered.

c. Intercritical gout. Prophylactic treatment with small doses of colchicine (0.6 mg once or twice daily) or small doses of an NSAID can be used to forestall new attacks.

d. Chronic or tophaceous gout. Therapy for chronic gout centers on control of hyperuricemia. Drugs that increase renal uric acid excretion (uricosuric drugs) or that decrease uric acid production (xanthine oxidase inhibitors) are available. The aim of this treatment is to reduce serum urate below 6 mg/dl, to allow reduction in serum supersaturation by urate and mobilization of tissue uric acid deposits. Patients who have had a recent acute attack should receive low-dose colchicine or an NSAID to prevent new attacks caused by fluctuation in serum urate.

(1) **Uricosuric drugs** (e.g., **probenecid,** sulfinpyrazone) can be used in patients who excrete less than 700 mg of uric acid daily, who have normal renal function, and who have no history of urinary stones.

      (2) Xanthine oxidase inhibitors include **allopurinol,** which is an analog of hypoxanthine. This drug inhibits de novo uric acid synthesis and competitively inhibits xanthine oxidase via enzymatic conversion to oxypurinol. Inhibition of uric acid synthesis with xanthine oxidase inhibitors is preferred in patients with urate excretion greater than 1000 mg/day, creatinine clearance less than 30 ml/min, tophaceous gout, or a history of nephrolithiasis. Dosages are reduced in the presence of renal failure to avoid toxicity.

B. Calcium pyrophosphate dihydrate (CPPD) deposition disease

1. **Definition.** Deposition of CPPD crystals in cartilage and periarticular connective tissues can cause a gamut of articular manifestations, ranging from asymptomatic deposition to acute and chronic inflammatory arthritis. The acute form of CPPD deposition disease is commonly called **pseudogout.**

2. **Etiologic classification**
   a. **Hereditary CPPD disease.** A high prevalence of CPPD disease has been noted in many families, with autosomal dominant transmission the typical pattern. Secondary metabolic associations with CPPD disease typically are not present in these families.
   b. **Osteoarthritis.** Chondrocalcinosis and CPPD crystals can occur as a result of severe osteoarthritis. CPPD disease can also cause osteoarthritis by damaging cartilage.
   c. **CPPD disease associated with metabolic disorders.** Correction of underlying metabolic disorders, if possible, does not seem to alter the progression of CPPD disease.
      (1) **Probable associations.** CPPD disease occurs at a higher than expected frequency in association with certain diseases and conditions. Potential abnormalities of calcium, phosphorus, or cartilage metabolism can explain the associations, which include:
          (a) Hyperparathyroidism
          (b) Hemochromatosis
          (c) Hypothyroidism
          (d) Hypophosphatasia
          (e) Hypomagnesemia
          (f) Wilson's disease
      (2) **Possible associations.** CPPD disease may or may not occur at a higher than expected frequency in association with:
          (a) Gout
          (b) Diabetes mellitus
          (c) Ochronosis

3. **Pathogenesis** (see Figure 10-1)
   a. **Crystal deposition**
      (1) **Site.** The initial site of CPPD deposition appears to be articular cartilage surrounding lacunae in the midzone. Later, deposition occurs in clefts of degenerated cartilage and in scattered foci in the cartilage matrix and synovial membrane, eventually forming large crystalline masses.
      (2) **Process.** An alteration of cartilage ground substance, the ionic composition of the matrix (i.e., calcium and pyrophosphate), or a combination of both is required for crystallization. Possibly, an altered condition of the matrix (e.g., removal of an inhibiting agent or addition of a nucleating agent) allows crystals to form in the microenvironment around the chondrocyte as pyrophosphate is released from the cell. A cell surface ectoenzyme, nucleoside triphosphate pyrophosphohydrolase (NTP-PPH), generates pyrophosphate in the process of scavenging extracellular adenosine triphosphate (ATP); the increased energy requirement of greater proteoglycan synthesis in osteoarthritis thus may lead to CPPD production.
   b. **Crystal-mediated joint damage.** CPPD deposits stiffen the cartilage, impairing its weight-bearing properties and accelerating osteoarthritic change. The acute

arthritic attacks are believed to be induced by the release of crystals from the cartilage into the joint space.

(1) **Factors mediating crystal release**

    (a) **Matrix loosening.** CPPD crystals in cartilage exist in equilibrium with synovial fluid calcium and pyrophosphate concentrations. Decreases in serum calcium concentration can lead to decreases in synovial fluid pyrophosphate levels and solubilization of joint CPPD crystals as equilibrium is restored. Loss of marginal CPPD deposits may cause the entire deposit to loosen in the matrix, with subsequent release of abundant CPPD crystals into the joint space. Thus, fluctuations of serum calcium concentration in the setting of acute medical illness or during the perioperative period may initiate acute crystal release.

    (b) **Loss of matrix.** Enzymatic erosion of cartilage due to an associated inflammatory arthritis (e.g., gout, infectious arthritis) also may cause crystal release.

    (c) **Biomechanical forces.** Impaired dissipation of weight-bearing forces on cartilage also may lead to crystal loosening and release into the joint space.

(2) **Factors affecting acute attacks**

    (a) **Inflammatory response.** Neutrophils are attracted to crystals coated with IgG, complement, fibronectin, fibrinogen, or kininogen. Crystals are ingested, causing the release of inflammatory mediators such as prostaglandins and collagenase.

    (b) **Degree of response.** CPPD crystals are somewhat less inflammatory than urate crystals. Generally, fewer are released in the acute attack, the crystals adsorb inflammatory proteins less well, and CPPD crystals are not membranolytic.

4. **Clinical syndromes**

  a. **Pseudogout** accounts for 25% of cases of CPPD disease. Acute swelling, pain, stiffness, and erythema develop in previously asymptomatic joints. The knee is most commonly involved (50% of cases), but almost any synovial joint can be involved, including the first MTP joint. Spread to adjacent joints can occur, and precipitation of attacks by acute medical or surgical illness is common, occurring in 10%–20% of cases. Systemic findings such as fever and leukocytosis can occur, especially in elderly patients. Joints typically return to normal between attacks, which may last days to weeks.

  b. **Pseudo-rheumatoid arthritis** accounts for 5% of cases of CPPD disease. In some patients, a smoldering chronic arthropathy can occur. Subacute episodes of pain and swelling in one or more joints can be superimposed on a more chronic picture of prolonged morning stiffness, fatigue, synovial thickening, and progressive deformities.

  c. **Pseudo-osteoarthritis** accounts for 50% of cases of CPPD disease. These patients present with a clinical and radiographic picture similar to that of degenerative joint disease, although about half have superimposed acute attacks of pseudogout. Flexion contractures are more common than in typical osteoarthritis, and bilateral knee varus deformities or isolated patellofemoral arthritis may occur more commonly than in osteoarthritis. A small percentage of these patients may have such severe joint destruction (e.g., of the shoulders or knees) that the clinical and radiographic appearance is that of a **neuropathic joint disorder,** even in the absence of underlying neurologic disease or apparent proprioceptive deficit.

  d. **Asymptomatic CPPD** disease occurs in 20% of cases. These patients do not have joint pain; the disease typically is uncovered by the finding of asymptomatic chondrocalcinosis on radiography. The prevalence of this finding—and of the other, clinically evident, forms of CPPD disease—increases with age and is seen in as many as 7% of elderly people screened.

5. **Diagnosis.** The finding of typical crystals on synovial fluid analysis is diagnostic of pseudogout. Chondrocalcinosis seen on radiography is evidence for a diagnosis of

CPPD deposition. However, chondrocalcinosis may be present in patients who never develop acute pseudogout.

a. **Synovial fluid findings.** Chunky, rhomboid **crystals that exhibit weakly positive birefringence** in red-compensated, polarized light are the hallmark of the acute arthritis syndromes associated with CPPD disease. These may be intracellular (in neutrophils) or extracellular, but they usually are much less prevalent than in a typical gout-involved joint. Synovial fluid leukocytosis of 10,000–20,000 cells/μl (mostly neutrophils) is typical.

b. **Radiographic findings**
   (1) **Chondrocalcinosis.** Calcification of articular hyaline cartilage, fibrocartilage (most commonly in the knee menisci, intervertebral disk annuli, symphysis pubis, and wrist triangular fibrocartilage), synovial membrane, tendons, and bursae can occur, usually in a stippled, linear fashion.
   (2) **Osteoarthritis.** Osteoarthritic changes in atypical joints [e.g., the wrist, elbow, and shoulder and the metacarpophalangeal (MCP) joints] suggest CPPD disease. Subchondral bone cysts may be more extensive in x-rays of joints affected by CPPD disease, and hook-shaped osteophytes characteristically are present with MCP involvement.
   (3) **Pseudoneuropathic joint.** Radiographic findings typical of neuropathic joint disorders, including extreme joint disorganization and bone fragments, can be found in severe cases of CPPD disease.

c. **Clinical diagnostic distinctions**
   (1) **Clinical or radiographic evidence of osteoarthritis** in joints not usually involved by osteoarthritis should suggest CPPD disease as an alternative diagnosis.
   (2) **Attacks of acute inflammatory arthritis** in a setting of apparent osteoarthritis should suggest CPPD disease.
   (3) **Acute arthritis occurring shortly after a medical illness or surgical procedure** should suggest a crystal-mediated arthritis, such as gout or pseudogout.
   (4) **Radiographic changes more typical of osteoarthritis** in a patient thought to have rheumatoid arthritis should suggest CPPD disease as an alternative diagnosis.
   (5) **The presence of diseases commonly associated with CPPD disease** (e.g., hyperparathyroidism, hemochromatosis) should suggest CPPD disease as a possible cause of any joint manifestations. In people younger than 55 years of age or in those with recurrent, polyarticular disease, an associated metabolic disease is more likely. In these patients, determinations of calcium, magnesium, alkaline phosphatase, copper, and ferritin levels as well as liver and thyroid function tests should be considered.
   (6) **Neuropathic joint presentations** should prompt investigation for CPPD disease as well as potentially associated neurologic disorders.

6. **Therapy**
   a. **Acute attacks.** Typical treatment involves aspiration of inflammatory joint fluid, intra-articular injection of corticosteroid, and use of NSAIDs.
   b. **Prophylaxis.** Similar to gout, some evidence suggests that recurrent acute attacks can be minimized by the chronic use of small oral doses of colchicine (0.6 mg once or twice daily).

C. **Hydroxyapatite arthritis.** Hydroxyapatite crystals, the typical complexed form of calcium in bone, also can cause several rheumatic syndromes.

1. **Clinical syndromes**
   a. **Crystal deposition in osteoarthritis.** Mineral formation in cartilage may be a result of abnormal cartilage metabolism in more severe forms of osteoarthritis. Joint effusions in these patients contain crystals of hydroxyapatite as often as they contain CPPD crystals.
   b. **Calcific periarthritis.** Hydroxyapatite deposition in bursae and tendon sheaths can cause episodes of acute inflammation (i.e., periarthritis and peritendinitis),

with acute attacks of pain, swelling, and erythema. Discrete clumped deposits can be found radiographically around the shoulders, greater trochanters, wrists, elbows, and digits and in other periarticular areas. These deposits can be shown to disintegrate gradually on radiographs taken several weeks after the acute periarthritis.

   c. **Destructive arthritis.** Hydroxyapatite crystals can be associated with a chronic destructive arthropathy, which is characterized by erosive radiographic changes, large (usually noninflammatory) effusions, proliferative synovitis, synovial mineral deposition, and periarticular ligamentous instability. This syndrome occurs most often in the knee and shoulder **("Milwaukee shoulder")** of elderly patients. Synovial fluid analysis shows few white cells ($500–1000/\mu l$), with monocytes predominating. High concentrations of neutral proteases and collagenases sometimes are present.

2. **Diagnosis.** Light microscopic examination of synovial fluid occasionally reveals brownish globules that are large clumps of hydroxyapatite crystals. Isolated crystals are too small to be seen with ordinary light or polarized light microscopy. A calcium stain, **alizarin red S,** can be used as a screening test for the presence of hydroxyapatite or CPPD crystals in effusions. Aspirates from bursae or tendon sheaths may yield milky or pasty material that contains high concentrations of these hydroxyapatite crystals.

3. **Associated conditions.** Disorders of calcium and phosphorus metabolism should be sought if multiple deposits are found.

4. **Therapy.** Mechanical splinting and NSAIDs are used to treat acute episodes of periarthritis. NSAIDs often are used in the chronic hydroxyapatite arthropathy as well. Periodic aspiration of the large synovial effusions that occur in the Milwaukee shoulder may help to preserve ligamentous integrity and remove destructive enzymes. Corticosteroid injections may help to treat acutely symptomatic joints.

III. RHEUMATOID ARTHRITIS

A. **Definition.** Rheumatoid arthritis is a chronic inflammatory disorder of unknown cause that typified by polyarticular, symmetrical joint involvement as well as characteristic extra-articular involvement. **Rheumatoid factor** (see III D 3) frequently is present in the serum of affected individuals.

B. **Epidemiology**

1. **Prevalence and sex distribution.** As many as 1% of adults may have rheumatoid arthritis, depending on the criteria used to make the diagnosis. Clinically meaningful forms of disease are less common—0.5% of women and 0.1% of men have forms of the illness that require ongoing treatment.

2. **Human leukocyte antigen (HLA) associations.** There is an increased prevalence of the B cell alloantigen HLA-DR4 in patients with rheumatoid arthritis. Evidence also suggests that similar amino acid sequences coded by the third hypervariable region of the DR β chain may explain disease association with HLA-DR4, -DR1, -Dw4, and -Dw14. HLA-DR4 positivity also is a marker for more severe rheumatoid arthritis.

3. **Seropositivity for rheumatoid factor.** Patients who have rheumatoid factor in their serum appear to have a different illness from patients who are seronegative. Seropositive patients tend to have more severe disease, more erosions, and more extra-articular features.

C. **Etiology.** No single factor or agent is known to cause rheumatoid arthritis. Presumably, an initial insult (possibly infectious) interacting with the host's genetically established immune responses determines whether an initial synovitis is suppressed or perpetuated.

1. **Extra-articular agent.** The earliest inflammatory changes in the rheumatoid joint involve inflammation and occlusion of small subsynovial vessels, suggesting that the agent is carried in the circulation to the joint.

2. **Infectious agent.** An infectious etiology is suggested because virus-like particles often are present in synovial biopsies early in the disease course and because polyarthritis occurs in association with several human and animal bacterial or viral illnesses. However, no direct evidence of infection has been discovered. Symmetrical inflammatory arthritis can occur in patients who have parvovirus or rubella virus infections, although the joint findings are not typically persistent.

3. **Genetic factors.** A genetic susceptibility to altered immune responses probably is important in rheumatoid arthritis. There is no known association of HLA-A or HLA-B haplotypes with the disease, but a significant association exists between rheumatoid arthritis and the presence of HLA-DR4 and related alloantigens of the major histocompatibility complex (MHC). The presence of these and other genetically coded immune response alloantigens may be important in modulating the host's cellular and humoral immune responses to potential etiologic agents.

4. **Effects of Epstein-Barr virus on the immune response.** Rheumatoid arthritis patients have a defect in their ability to regulate B cells infected with Epstein-Barr virus. The virus may act as a polyclonal activator of B-cell autoantibody production in rheumatoid arthritis and, as such, may have a role in perpetuating (not initiating) the disease.

D. **Pathogenesis.** An unknown etiologic agent (an exogenous one or an "altered" endogenous one) initiates a nonspecific immune response. The joint lesion in rheumatoid arthritis begins as an inflammatory lesion in the synovial membrane that can progress to a proliferative one (**the pannus**), which can deform by destroying adjacent cartilage and bone. Alternatively, the inflammatory or proliferative lesions can regress, either spontaneously or with disease-altering therapies. Immune-response genes may also be important in determining the type, intensity, and chronicity of the immune response.

1. **Synovial cell interactions** are important for maintenance of articular inflammation. Intercellular messages are transmitted by **cytokines** (small proteins that can amplify and perpetuate inflammation in the rheumatoid joint). In general, cytokines produced by macrophages and fibroblasts [IL-1, IL-6, granulocyte–macrophage colony-stimulating factor (GM-CSF), TNF-α] are present at high concentrations in the rheumatoid synovium. **Lymphokines** produced by T cells (IL-2, IL-3, IL-4, interferon gamma) are present at relatively low concentrations, apparently suppressed by substances secreted by macrophages.

   a. **Macrophage–T cell.** Macrophage and helper T-cell (CD4$^+$ T-cell) interrelationships are central to the amplification of the immune response. Macrophages process antigen and present it (in association with class II MHC molecules) to the CD4$^+$ T cells, which then become activated by the interaction. Certain bacterial toxins or retroviral proteins can function as **superantigens,** binding to HLA molecules or T-cell receptors directly, potentially amplifying the inflammatory response.

   b. **Th cell–B cell.** Activated CD4$^+$ T cells stimulate B cell proliferation and differentiation into antibody-producing cells. These B cells are factories for the production of **rheumatoid factor.**

   c. **CD4$^+$ T cell–synovial cell.** CD4$^+$ T cells produce soluble mediators (lymphokines) that can modulate the function of synovial lining cells, both macrophage-like and fibroblast-like. The fibroblast-like lining cell produces collagenase and prostaglandins, and stimulates the growth of connective tissue; all of these effects may be important in the destructive effects of the synovial pannus.

   d. **Macrophage–endothelial cell.** The ingrowth of capillaries is important to the propagation of synovitis and the later growth of the pannus. Macrophages signal capillary endothelial cells to migrate and replicate by heparin-binding growth factors.

2. **Synovial fluid phase**
   a. In contrast to the mononuclear response in the synovium, the **neutrophil** is the predominant cell in rheumatoid synovial fluid inflammation. Numerous factors chemotactic for neutrophils are present in the inflamed joint [e.g., complement fragments, leukotriene B4 (LTB4), immune complexes with rheumatoid factor]. These neutrophils release oxygen-free radicals and hydrolytic enzymes that can destroy cartilage.
   b. Bacterial, mycobacterial, and human **heat shock proteins** share many antigenic sequences and may cross-react with collagen or proteoglycan molecules; therefore, an infection could generate autoimmunity or localize an inflammatory response to a joint.

3. **Rheumatoid factor.** Eighty percent of patients with rheumatoid arthritis have antibodies to the Fc portion of immunoglobulin, called **rheumatoid factor.** The synovium produces immunoglobulin, most of which consists of IgM and IgG rheumatoid factors. These immunoglobulins form complexes in synovial fluid, which activate complement. Rheumatoid factor aggregates also are ingested by macrophages (which secrete cytokines) and neutrophils (which release digestive enzymes); both actions amplify inflammation.

4. **Chronic proliferative lesion.** A mass of fibroblastic, vascular, and inflammatory cells (i.e., the **pannus**) accumulates at the margin of the synovial membrane–cartilage border, driven by platelet-derived growth factor (PDGF) and other locally produced growth factors. The mass can cause local erosions of cartilage and bone; cytokines (e.g., IL-1) drive the synovial lining cells to secrete prostaglandins and proteolytic enzymes, thus degrading collagen and proteoglycans in the cartilage. IL-1 and prostaglandins also can stimulate bone resorption in periarticular areas.

5. **Joint destruction.** Destructive change is unpredictable, and counteracting anti-inflammatory cytokines (e.g., TGF-β) can down-regulate the effects of IL-1 and TNF-α, leading to cartilage repair and immunosuppression. Native IL-1 inhibitors perform similar functions. These compensatory mechanisms often are overwhelmed, and unimpeded synovial inflammation and proliferation lead to loss of cartilage and bone as well as anatomic distortion. Secondary degenerative joint disease results from the continued inflammation and alterations in biomechanical joint loading forces.

E. Clinical features

1. **Synovitis**
   a. **Articular involvement.** Fairly symmetrical, bilateral joint involvement is typical, often sparing the DIP joints of the hands. MCP, PIP, and wrist joint involvement is so common as to be part of the American Rheumatism Association revised criteria for disease diagnosis (Table 10-2).
   b. **Tendon and ligament involvement.** Synovial linings outside joints can be involved as well.
      (1) **Palmar flexor tendinitis** can cause carpal tunnel syndrome.
      (2) **Rotator cuff tendinitis** can cause shoulder pain and limitation of motion.
      (3) **Atlantoaxial ligament involvement** in the cervical spine can lead to instability between the C1 and C2 vertebrae and potential neurologic complaints.

2. **Extra-articular features** (Table 10-3) more often exist in patients who are seropositive for rheumatoid factor and patients who have more severe and established disease.
   a. **Rheumatoid nodules** are the most common features of extra-articular disease and are found in 20%–25% of patients. These firm, subcutaneous masses typically are found in areas of repetitive trauma (e.g., the extensor surfaces of the forearm), although they also can appear in the viscera (e.g., lungs).
   b. **Eye involvement** also is common. **Keratoconjunctivitis sicca** is seen in 10%–15% of rheumatoid arthritis patients who have a secondary form of Sjö-

TABLE 10-2. The 1987 American Rheumatism Association Revised Criteria for the Classification of Rheumatoid Arthritis

Criterion	Definition
1. Morning stiffness	Morning stiffness in and around the joints, lasting at least 1 hour before maximal improvement
2. Arthritis of three or more joint areas	At least three joint areas simultaneously have had soft tissue swelling or fluid (not bony overgrowth alone) observed by a physician; the fourteen possible areas are right or left PIP, MCP, wrist, elbow, knee, ankle, and MTP joints
3. Arthritis of hand joints	At least one area swollen (as defined above) in a wrist, MCP, or PIP joint
4. Symmetrical arthritis	Simultaneous involvement of the same joint areas (as defined in 2) on both sides of the body (bilateral involvement of PIPs, MCPs, or MTPs is acceptable without absolute symmetry)
5. Rheumatoid nodules	Subcutaneous nodules over bony prominences, or extensor surfaces, or in juxta-articular regions, observed by a physician
6. Serum rheumatoid factor	Demonstration of abnormal amounts of serum rheumatoid factor by any method for which the result has been positive in < 5% of normal control subjects
7. Radiographic changes	Radiographic changes typical of rheumatoid arthritis on posteroanterior hand and wrist radiographs, which must include erosions or unequivocal bony decalcification localized in or most marked adjacent to the involved joints (osteoarthritis changes alone do not qualify)

For classification purposes, a patient is said to have rheumatoid arthritis if he or she has satisfied at least four of these seven criteria. Criteria 1 through 4 must have been present for at least 6 weeks. Patients with two clinical diagnoses are not excluded. Designation as classic, definite, or probable rheumatoid arthritis is **not** to be made. PIP = proximal interphalangeal; MCP = metacarpophalangeal; MTP = metatarsophalangeal. (Reprinted from Arnett FC, Edworth SM, Bloch DA, et al: American Rheumatism Association 1987 revised criteria for the classification of rheumatoid arthritis. *Arthritis Rheum* 31:315, 1988.)

TABLE 10-3. Extra-articular Features of Rheumatoid Arthritis

Skin	**Nerve**
Nodules (20%–25% of patients)	Entrapment (carpal tunnel syndrome)
Vasculitis (purpura)	Vasculitis
Eye	Distal sensory neuropathy
Sicca complex (10%–15% of patients)	Mononeuritis
Episcleritis	**Blood**
Scleritis	Anemia of chronic disease
Heart	Thrombocytosis
Pericarditis	Felty's syndrome
Myocarditis (rare)	**Metabolism**
Valve dysfunction (rare)	Amyloidosis
Lung	**Vessels**
Pleural effusion	Vasculitis
Interstitial fibrosis	Skin
Nodules	Nerve
	Viscera (rare)

gren's syndrome (see X). The often subtle inflammation of scleritis or episcleritis occurs less commonly.

c. **Other organ involvement** is noted in Table 10-3.

F. **Diagnosis.** Rheumatoid arthritis is a sustained, inflammatory polyarthritis that typically is fairly symmetrical. It is a diagnosis of exclusion of other forms of polyarthritis, which it may imitate. The patient must have arthritis for at least 6 weeks to eliminate viral syndromes or other causes of nonsustained polyarthritis. Finding rheumatoid factor in the serum is useful in patients who have other features of inflammatory polyarthritis, but as many as 40% of patients with rheumatoid arthritis will not have this marker initially.

1. **History.** Patients with rheumatoid arthritis often have **prolonged** (longer than 1 hour) **morning stiffness. Constitutional complaints** (weight loss, anorexia, fatigue) are common. Patients with rheumatoid arthritis have **pain in involved joints,** which typically is worse in the morning.

2. **Physical examination.** Classically involved joints are the wrists and the **MCP and PIP joints of the hand;** DIP joints are typically spared, as is the axial skeleton except for the cervical spine. **Soft tissue swelling,** rather than bony enlargement, is typical around involved joints, unless secondary degenerative changes have occured; limitation of joint motion and warmth may be noted. **Rheumatoid nodules** often are present in highly expressed disease; they can be found over extensor prominences, especially near the olecranon.

3. **Laboratory findings.** The complete blood count may reveal a **normocytic, normochromic anemia** of chronic disease, leukocytosis, and thrombocytosis. These findings along with an increased erythrocyte **sedimentation rate** reflect chronic inflammation. **Rheumatoid factor** typically is present in 60% of patients in the first year of disease and in 80% of patients with sustained disease. Thirty percent of patients seronegative for rheumatoid factor have antibodies to **keratinized** epithelium (AKA), a fairly specific but insensitive diagnostic test that may become more widely available. Synovial fluid findings reflect mild to moderate inflammation; leukocyte counts are 5000–25,000 and consist mainly of neutrophils.

4. **Radiographic findings.** Early characteristics include **soft-tissue swelling** and loss of bone in periarticular areas **(periarticular osteopenia).** Signs of sustained inflammation include loss of bone at joint margins **(erosions)** and **joint space narrowing** as a result of cartilage loss.

5. **Differential diagnosis** (Figure 10-2). Because rheumatoid arthritis is one of many illnesses characterized by chronic polyarticular inflammation, diagnosis relies on excluding other such illnesses and searching for symmetrical periarticular soft tissue swelling and inflammatory characteristics of rheumatoid arthritis.

a. **Nonarticular disorders.** Fibromyalgia is a syndrome of generalized aching and tenderness in specific soft tissue areas, without joint involvement or inflammation. Tendon, neurologic, and vascular complaints also may mimic joint pain.

b. **Noninflammatory disorders**

(1) **Osteoarthritis** usually causes bony rather than soft tissue swelling, and the involved joints typically are the DIP and PIP joints of the hand, the hips, and the knees. The lumbar and cervical spine can be involved as well. Constitutional and inflammatory complaints are absent, and synovial fluid leukocyte counts are less than 2000/mm^3.

(2) **Metabolic disorders** (e.g., CPPD, hemochromatosis, Wilson's disease) cause bony degenerative change in atypical joints (e.g., MCP joints).

c. **Axial joint inflammation.** Inflammation of the axial spine (especially the sacroiliac joints) is characteristic of the spondylarthropathies, and inflammatory back pain due to **sacroiliitis** should be sought. Inflammatory back pain is insidious, day-after-day pain starting in the sacroiliac area and typically associated with prolonged morning stiffness. It is worsened with rest and improved by exercise, the opposite of mechanical low-back pain. The absence of sacroiliac joint in-

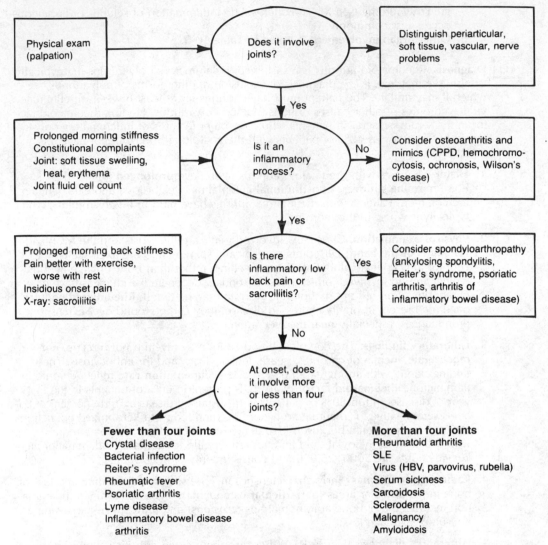

FIGURE 10-2. Flowchart for the diagnosis of polyarthritis. Rheumatoid arthritis is a diagnosis of exclusion. The evaluation of chronic polyarthritis requires a careful history and physical examination for identification of organ changes typical of other illnesses that can cause arthritis. Selected laboratory and radiographic testing also can be helpful in reaching a diagnosis. *HBV* = hepatitis B virus; *CPPD* = calcium pyrophosphate dihydrate; *SLE* = systemic lupus erythematosus.

volvement does not rule out these disorders, but its presence makes spondylarthropathy likely.

d. **Oligoarticular presentations.** Certain illnesses must be considered more strongly when the initial inflammatory presentation involves four or fewer joints and is asymmetrical. These disorders include crystal diseases, infectious arthritis (e.g., Lyme disease, gonococcemia, endocarditis), reactive arthritis (e.g., rheumatic fever), and spondylarthropathies (e.g., Reiter's syndrome, psoriatic arthritis).

e. **Polyarticular presentations.** It also is important to consider inflammatory disorders that initially involve four or more joints and are fairly symmetrical. Although rheumatoid arthritis is the prototype, many other illnesses must be distinguished, based on clinical features or organ involvement not typical of rheumatoid arthritis. Detailed history and physical examination with basic laboratory data are critical in distinguishing among disorders that feature polyarthritis.

(1) **Other rheumatic diseases** (e.g., lupus, scleroderma, polymyositis/dermatomyositis, polymyalgia rheumatica, vasculitis) are distinguished by the features of the primary illness.

(2) **Viral disorders** (e.g., rubella, hepatitis B, parvovirus infection) are distinguished by a typical rash, serologic markers, or organ involvement.

(3) **Malignancies** may present as long bone pain, digital clubbing, and periostitis mimicking polyarthritis (hypertrophic osteoarthropathy) or as paraneoplastic polyarthritis.

(4) **Sarcoidosis** exhibits mediastinal adenopathy on chest x-ray and usually erythema nodosum when it includes a polyarthritis.

(5) **Amyloidosis** is associated with Congo red–positive deposits in typical organs, subcutaneous tissue, and joints.

G. **Therapy.** In all patients with rheumatoid arthritis, an attempt is made to control pain and reduce inflammation without causing undesirable side effects. Preservation of joint function and the ability to maintain life-style are important long-term goals.

1. **Nonpharmacologic therapy**
   a. **Patient education.** Educating the patient about the disease process is particularly important in chronic diseases such as rheumatoid arthritis, in which a patient's compliance with instructions and drug treatment is critical to the outcome.
      (1) **Description of the illness.** The various disease courses of rheumatoid arthritis must be described, emphasizing the fact that most patients do well if they are appropriately treated. The chronicity and intermittency of symptoms must be discussed so that the patient understands that spontaneous fluctuations in an extended disease course are normal. The patient must be educated about the systemic nature of the disease process, so that both patient and family will understand the fatigue, malaise, and weight loss that often accompany this illness.
      (2) **Rest and exercise.** Patients should be advised to rest or splint acutely involved joints to reduce inflammation. Brief periods of bed rest may be useful in patients with severe polyarticular exacerbations, and regular naps may help patients deal with the fatigue of rheumatoid arthritis. Conversely, exercises to strengthen muscles surrounding involved joints should be encouraged when the arthritis is under good control. All joints should be put through a full range of motion once daily to prevent contractures.
   b. **Physical medicine**
      (1) All patients with rheumatoid arthritis benefit from coordination of their nonpharmacologic treatment by a **physiatrist.**
      (2) **Physical therapists** can help patients strengthen weakened muscle groups to protect damaged joints. They can show patients range-of-motion exercises that prevent joint contractures.
      (3) **Occupational therapists** can help patients obtain devices to assist them, can construct splints for involved joints, and can aid in rehabilitating patients for activities of daily living and employment.

2. **Pharmacologic therapy.** Several categories of drugs are available for treatment of rheumatoid arthritis. NSAIDs typically are the first-line drug therapy for the disease. Slower-acting, or second-line, drugs are added for more sustained disease not satisfactorily controlled by NSAIDs. Corticosteroids are not thought of as first- or second-line therapies but often are used intra-articularly for disease flare-ups or orally to help a patient who is waiting for a second-line drug to work.
   a. **NSAIDs.** Aspirin is the prototypic drug of this class. Nonacetylated salicylates also have been developed, which cause less suppression of prostaglandin synthesis. Numerous other agents (e.g., ibuprofen, diclofenac, naproxen, piroxicam) also have been developed; these agents have similar potency to aspirin, cause fewer side effects, and require fewer pills.

(1) **Use.** NSAIDs are used to control pain and inflammation acutely by suppression of prostaglandin synthesis or inhibition of leukocyte function, or both. Some patients with rheumatoid arthritis need only NSAIDs to control their illness, but most use them in combination with other drugs.

(2) **Toxicity.** Typical toxicities include dyspepsia, peptic ulcers (primarily of the stomach), hypertension, and renal dysfunction. Clinical hepatitis and bone marrow toxicity are very rare.

b. **Corticosteroids** have potent anti-inflammatory effects, but they have equally potent and predictable toxicities. These drugs are used most commonly in rheumatoid arthritis to control serious extra-articular manifestations (e.g., vasculitis).

(1) **Systemic administration.** In rare situations, such as severe progressive active disease, prednisone doses no higher than 5–10 mg once daily in the morning may be used to allow continued functioning. Continual attempts to taper the dosage of these drugs should be made.

(2) **Local instillation.** Injectable corticosteroid preparations can be instilled into one or two joints inflamed "out of phase" with other involved joints. These injections should be performed only occasionally, because cartilage loss may result from frequent injections into the same joint.

c. **Second-line agents** are drugs that have no analgesic effect and generally require weeks to months before anti-inflammatory effects are evident. Examples include sulfasalazine, low-dose methotrexate, antimalarial agents, gold, and D-penicillamine.

(1) **Use.** Second-line agents may be useful for patients with rheumatoid arthritis that is not controlled by NSAIDs (with or without corticosteroids). Most rheumatologists now use them within the first few weeks of disease onset when patients have sustained synovitis, certainly with extra-articular disease features, and preferably before bone erosions develop.

(a) These drugs are most often employed singly, but are used in combination in patients with a bad prognosis or refractory disease. Methotrexate in combinations with hydroxychloroquine, sulfasalazine, or cyclosporine is often used in severe disease.

(b) When employed, second-line agents usually must be given for periods of several months before being abandoned as ineffective.

(2) **Toxicity.** Differences exist between agents. Gold and D-penicillamine typically cause skin rash, cytopenias, and membranous glomerulonephritis. Antimalarial agents cause dyspepsia and, occasionally, serious ocular toxicity. Methotrexate can cause hepatic fibrosis and acute interstitial pneumonitis, but it more often causes reversible mucosal ulcers, dyspepsia, or cytopenia as a result of folate depletion. Sulfasalazine most often causes gastrointestinal distress but can cause hematologic cytopenias or hepatic dysfunction.

d. **Assessment of response.** One judges the effectiveness of drug therapy by measuring reduction in morning stiffness, constitutional complaints, number of swollen and tender joints, and erythrocyte sedimentation rate. Sometimes, improvement in anemia of chronic disease and resolution of thrombocytosis occurs. Indices that measure a patient's ability to perform activities of daily living (health assessment questionnaires) also are used.

3. **Surgery** may be necessary early as well as late in the course of rheumatoid arthritis. Synovectomies may decrease the inflammatory process in joints or tendon sheaths that remain inflamed despite drug therapy that has been effective in other joints. Later, arthroplasties or total joint replacements may be appropriate to relieve pain or help restore function in structurally damaged joints.

H. Prognosis

1. **Prognostic factors** (Table 10-4). Inability to control disease activity and the presence of several of these indicators suggests a poor prognosis and the need for more aggressive therapy, perhaps including combinations of second-line agents and low-dose oral glucocorticoids.

TABLE 10-4. Indicators of Poor Prognosis in Patients with Rheumatoid Arthritis

Many persistently inflamed joints
Poor functional status (ascertained from health-assessment questionnaires)
Low formal education level
Rheumatoid factor positivity
HLA-DR4 positivity
Extra-articular disease
Persistently elevated acute phase reactants (e.g., erythrocyte sedimentation rate)
Radiographic evidence of erosions

HLA = human leukocyte antigen.

    2. Mortality. Many patients with rheumatoid arthritis have a reasonably good prognosis if they respond well to treatment. Adequate early response to the use of NSAIDs or antimalarials, with or without corticosteroids, is a favorable prognostic sign. However, recent epidemiologic studies suggest that patients with severe and persistent disease have increased mortality rates; in those with the most highly expressed forms of rheumatoid arthritis, mortality rates approach those found in stage IV congestive heart failure or stage IV Hodgkin's disease. The increase in mortality appears to be the result of organ compromise caused by extra-articular features (e.g., interstitial lung disease, cardiac complications, vasculitis), complications of drug therapy, and infection.

IV. SPONDYLARTHROPATHIES

A. **Unifying characteristics** (Table 10-5). The spondylarthropathies are a group of inflammatory arthritides that are distinct from rheumatoid arthritis. Typical distinguishing features include the following.

    1. Clinical features
        a. Skeletal
            (1) Axial. As a group, the spondylarthropathies prominently involve the axial skeleton, particularly the **sacroiliac joints.** With the exception of the cervical spine, the axial skeleton is not commonly involved in rheumatoid arthritis.
            (2) Appendicular. Inflammatory arthritis of the appendicular skeleton also occurs in these disorders, but the involvement tends to be oligoarticular and asymmetrical. In contrast, rheumatoid arthritis usually is polyarticular and symmetrical.

TABLE 10-5. Distinguishing Characteristics
of Spondylarthropathies

Axial skeleton inflammation
Enthesis inflammation, often asymmetric
Characteristic extraskeletal features
   Uveitis or conjunctivitis
   Urethritis
   Inflammatory bowel lesions
   Psoriasis-like rashes
Association with HLA-B27
Absence of rheumatoid factor

HLA = human leukocyte antigen.

       (3) **Enthesis.** In both the axial and appendicular skeletons, inflammation of tendon and ligament sites of attachment to bone is common (e.g., costochondritis, Achilles tendinitis, plantar fasciitis). Tendon inflammation is less prominent in rheumatoid arthritis.

    b. Extraskeletal

       (1) **Nodules.** Rheumatoid nodules are not found in the spondylarthropathies.

       (2) **Internal organ involvement.** The typical eye involvement in the spondylarthropathies (conjunctivitis and anterior uveitis), cardiac involvement (aortitis), and genitourinary involvement (urethritis and prostatitis) are much different from the usual extra-articular features of rheumatoid arthritis.

    c. Laboratory findings. Several cardinal laboratory features of chronic inflammation (i.e., anemia, thrombocytosis, and elevated gamma globulin levels) are not commonly present in the spondylarthropathies as they are in rheumatoid arthritis. Erythrocyte sedimentation rate may be increased but is not a good measure of disease activity. Rheumatoid factor typically is absent.

    d. Radiographic findings. The characteristic changes seen radiographically are those of periosteal new bone formation at the site of the enthesopathic lesions (see IV A 3), both at axial locations (in the form of **syndesmophytes**) and appendicular locations. Although erosive changes can occur, they occur most typically in the axial skeleton (in the hips, sacroiliac joints, and shoulders).

    e. Therapeutic response. Several second-line agents commonly employed in treating rheumatoid arthritis (gold, D-penicillamine, or hydroxychloroquine) have no proven role in the treatment of spondylarthropathy, with the exception of psoriatic peripheral arthropathy. Sulfasalazine and methotrexate are used for both rheumatoid arthritis and the appendicular arthritis of the spondylarthropathies, but NSAIDs alone typically are sufficient to treat the spondylarthropathies.

2. Genetic factors. The strong association of the histocompatibility antigen **HLA-B27** with clinical expression of the spondylarthropathies provides evidence for genetic transmission of these disorders.

    a. This relationship also is a major reason for grouping these disorders. The independent correlation of HLA-B27 with specific features of spondylarthropathies (e.g., sacroiliitis, aortitis, anterior uveitis) explains both the clinical overlap among these diseases and their familial clustering.

    b. The role of the antigen in disease causation is not understood. However, transgenic rats can express HLA-B27 on cell surfaces and develop clinical features of spondylarthropathies, so this gene product is clearly involved in disease causation or perpetuation.

    c. Disease susceptibility is also associated with other unknown genes, perhaps T-cell receptor genes, accounting for the tenfold increase in risk associated with HLA-B27 positivity in spondylitis families.

3. Pathology

    a. The basic pathologic lesion in the spondylarthropathies is an **enthesopathy**—an inflammation occurring at the site where ligaments and tendons attach to bone. This type of inflammation explains the frequency of sacroiliitis, ascending spinal lesions, and peripheral tendon lesions (e.g., Achilles tendinitis) in patients with these diseases.

    b. Although inflammatory synovitis that is indistinguishable from rheumatoid synovitis can be seen in these illnesses, it is not typically as widespread, chronically active, and potentially destructive as it is in rheumatoid arthritis (psoriatic arthritis mutilans is a notable exception).

4. HIV-related spondylarthropathic disease. Some HIV-positive patients have spondylarthropathic illness often with features of **Reiter's syndrome** or **psoriatic arthritis.** Most commonly, however, they have skin, joint, and tendon features that prevent easy classification into one illness or the other, suggesting that these spondylarthropathic illnesses have a common pathogenesis.

B. **Specific disorders**

1. **Ankylosing spondylitis**

   a. **Definition.** Ankylosing spondylitis is the spondylarthropathy that is most closely associated with inflammation of the axial skeleton. **Back pain** and **limited spinal mobility** caused by **sacroiliitis** and variable ascent of the inflammation up the spine dominate the clinical expression of this disease.

   b. **Epidemiology**

      (1) **Prevalence.** Ankylosing spondylitis may be as common as 1 in 1000 white individuals, because the frequency of disease parallels the prevalence of the HLA-B27 antigen in the population (1%–2% of the 6% of whites with HLA-B27 antigen may have ankylosing spondylitis). The frequency of ankylosing spondylitis is lower in black and Asian populations, paralleling the prevalence of the antigen in these groups.

      (2) **Gender distribution.** Ankylosing spondylitis may be as prevalent in women as in men if x-ray findings of sacroiliitis are considered to be diagnostic of the disease. However, women tend to have somewhat milder disease with more peripheral joint manifestations.

      (3) **Familial aggregation.** The risk of ankylosing spondylitis in an HLA-B27–positive family member of an affected proband is 20%, as compared to 1%–2% for the general population of those with HLA-B27.

   c. **Etiology**

      (1) The major histocompatibility antigen HLA-B27 occurs in 90%–95% of white patients with ankylosing spondylitis, but the association is less marked in nonwhite populations (40%–50% of blacks with ankylosing spondylitis have HLA-B27).

      (2) Because the gene coding for the expression of HLA-B27 resides on chromosome 6, autosomal transmission occurs. Thus, children of a proband who is heterozygous for the gene controlling HLA-B27 production have a 50% probability of eventual expression of the antigen on cell surfaces.

      (3) **The presence of HLA-B27 on cell membranes** is thought to be important in the causation of ankylosing spondylitis. The disease is somehow caused or perpetuated by the presence of a short amino acid sequence in the peptide-binding cleft of the HLA-B27 molecule that is able to bind a unique arthritis-causing peptide.

         (a) **Receptor theory** (Figure 10-3A). One current theory is that this marker is a receptor for an environmental factor (e.g., bacterial peptide antigen, virus), which then can cause disease. The **athritogenic peptide theory** is a variation in which an immune response to a bacterial peptide is increased because the peptide (after intracellular processing) is particularly well-presented by HLA-B27.

         (b) **Molecular mimicry theory** (Figure 10-3B). A bacterial or other environmental antigen presented on the cell surface with a different HLA molecule might share similar sequences with the HLA-B27 molecule. If this class I complex (non–HLA-B27 plus peptide) is recognized by the cytotoxic $CD8^+$ T cell as HLA-B27, an immune response can be mounted against HLA-B27 (**autoimmunity**) or suppressed against the disease-causing peptide (**tolerance**). Either condition could lead to clinical disease expression.

         (c) **Thymic selection theory.** HLA-B27 may function at the level of the thymus by allowing selection of **arthritogenic T cells.**

   d. **Clinical features**

      (1) **Disease onset** usually occurs in the second or third decade of life (see V E 3 b for discussion of childhood disease).

      (2) **Disease course.** The disease begins with the gradual onset of chronic sacral backache, which is associated with prolonged morning stiffness and which improves with exercise. Most patients have prolonged, unremitting low back pain for years. The disease may be mild and cause minimal interference with function, or it may be severe and deforming.

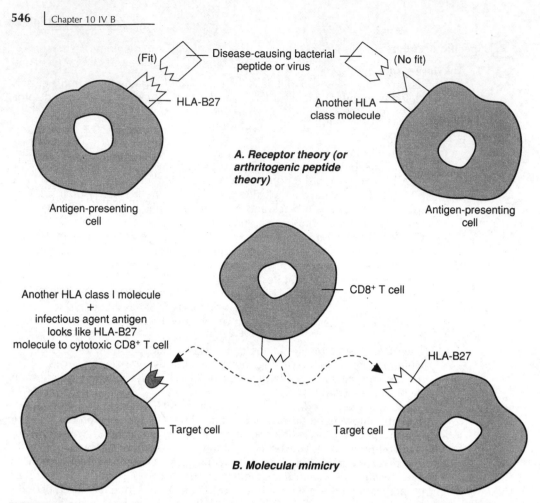

FIGURE 10-3. Human leukocyte antigen B27 (*HLA-B27*) as the cause of ankylosing spondylitis. (*A*) Receptor theory. A bacterial peptide or virus forms a complex externally with HLA-B27. The arthritogenic peptide theory, a variation of the receptor theory, maintains that the bacterial or viral peptide is processed intracellularly and only presented on the cell surface in association with the HLA-B27 molecule. (*B*) Molecular mimicry theory. An immune response is mounted against HLA-B27 (autoimmunity) or suppressed against the disease-causing peptide (tolerance) because the immune system cannot distinguish between their similar amino acid sequences.

    (3) Manifestations of disease
        (a) Axial skeletal involvement. Symmetrical inflammation of the sacroiliac joints (sacroiliitis) is the most common presentation. Inflammation and consequent calcification of the spinal ligaments and the intervertebral zygoapophyseal joints can cause limited spinal mobility, and intercostal ligament enthesopathy can cause limitation of chest wall expansion.
        (b) Peripheral joint involvement typically is a feature of more severe ankylosing spondylitis. Erosive hip and shoulder involvement is not uncommon and may be severe. More distal synovitis is less common, although 35% of patients with ankylosing spondylitis have some evidence of peripheral joint disease.
        (c) Extraskeletal features. Constitutional complaints, fatigue, and weight loss are not as common in ankylosing spondylitis as in rheumatoid arthritis, but may occur. Anterior uveitis occurs in 25% of patients with ankylosing spondylitis, and sometimes occurs as an isolated clinical association of HLA-B27. Aortic root inflammation can occur, usually in patients with long-standing disease; this process can lead to aortic

valve insufficiency or, if it extends into the conduction system, complete heart block. Upper lobe pulmonary fibrosis and chronic prostatitis are other uncommon extraskeletal features.

e. **Diagnosis** of ankylosing spondylitis is made by blending historical, physical, and radiographic evidence as well as by excluding mechanical low back pain, other spondylarthropathies, and other inflammatory arthritides.

(1) **Historical information**

(a) **Inflammatory low back pain** can be distinguished from mechanical low back pain. Inflammatory sacroiliitis has a gradual onset, in early adulthood, and is persistent for more than 3 months; the pain is associated with prolonged morning back stiffness and is relieved by exercise and worsened by rest. In contrast, the onset of mechanical low back pain usually occurs later in life, with sudden, self-limited episodes that are worsened by exercise and improved by bed rest.

(b) **Familial association.** Patients with ankylosing spondylitis often have other affected family members.

(c) **Associated complaints.** Evidence of prior inflammatory eye symptoms, recurrent oligoarthritis, and inflammatory tendinitis should be sought.

(2) **Physical findings**

(a) **Musculoskeletal examination.** Each sacroiliac joint should be evaluated for tenderness, lumbar spinal mobility should be assessed in all directions, and chest expansion should be evaluated to assess severity of chest wall enthesopathic lesions.

(b) **General physical examination.** Evidence of associated abnormalities should be sought, including ocular erythema, aortic insufficiency murmurs, and peripheral arthritis and tendinitis.

(3) **Laboratory findings.** The only characteristic laboratory abnormality in ankylosing spondylitis is the variable presence of HLA-B27 in different population groups, and, in general, testing for this antigen is not necessary for the diagnosis.

(4) **Radiographic findings.** Sacroiliac involvement is best seen on an anteroposterior x-ray of the pelvis. Blurred joint margins, periarticular sclerosis, erosions, and joint space widening are characteristic, but total joint obliteration is typical of long-standing disease. If the illness is more severe or longstanding, ascending spinal involvement can occur, with flowing calcifications that bridge the intervertebral disk, culminating in a **bamboo-spine** appearance on x-ray.

(5) **Differential diagnosis**

(a) **Mechanical low back pain,** as previously mentioned, must be differentiated from inflammatory low back pain.

(b) **Other disorders.** Sacroiliitis is highly unusual in nonspondylitic diseases. Characteristic skin lesions may suggest that a patient with sacroiliitis has psoriasis or Reiter's syndrome. Prominent urethritis may also suggest Reiter's syndrome, and prominent bowel complaints may suggest inflammatory bowel disease when a patient also has sacroiliitis.

f. **Therapy.** Patient education and multidisciplinary treatment are important therapeutic components in ankylosing spondylitis, as they are in rheumatoid arthritis.

(1) **Goals.** Short-term goals involve control of pain and reduction of inflammation without causing drug toxicity. Prevention of postural deformity and retention of employment are long-term goals.

(2) **Education**

(a) **Cigarette smoking.** Individuals with enthesopathic chest wall restriction or fibrotic lung disease should be discouraged from smoking.

(b) **Genetic counseling.** Patients should be made aware of the familial incidence of the illness so that it can be diagnosed early in children and treatment of spondylitic symptoms begun.

(c) **Protection of brittle spine.** Patients with extensive spinal involvement must understand that minimal trauma can cause a spinal fracture. Wearing a hard or soft collar should be recommended for automobile driving.

(3) **Exercise.** Spinal extension exercises and correct posture are important for prevention of deformity. Hard mattresses and small cervical pillows help to prevent excessive spinal flexion during sleep.

(4) **Drug therapy.** In contrast to rheumatoid arthritis, NSAIDs are the mainstay of treatment. Second-line agents useful in rheumatoid arthritis are not thought to be effective in ankylosing spondylitis, although methotrexate and sulfasalazine are being used for prominent peripheral joint arthritis with variable success. Local joint or peritendinous instillation of a corticosteroid sometimes is beneficial in patients with prominent peripheral disease manifestations not controlled by NSAIDs.

g. **Prognosis.** Most patients with ankylosing spondylitis remain employable and continue to function well in society. The progression to severe, deforming disease cannot be predicted on the basis of HLA-B27 status or other criteria. Patients with severe spondylitis tend to have brittle spines, more cardiopulmonary disease, and other extraspinal complications; these patients may have shortened life spans.

2. **Reiter's syndrome**

a. **Definition.** Reiter's syndrome is another spondylarthropathy that is strongly associated with HLA-B27. Reiter's syndrome is an eponym for **seronegative reactive arthritis** that is associated with characteristic extra-articular findings. It is a predominantly lower extremity oligoarthritis triggered by **urethritis, cervicitis,** or **dysenteric infection.** The variable features of the typical syndrome include **mucocutaneous lesions, inflammatory eye lesions,** and **sacroiliitis.**

b. **Epidemiology**

(1) **Incidence.** Reiter's syndrome occurs in 1%–3% of patients after nonspecific urethritis and 0.2% of patients after dysentery outbreaks caused by *Shigella flexneri.* HLA-B27 is present in 75%–80% of cases. Patients with the marker who develop nonspecific urethritis or *S. flexneri* dysentery have a 20%–25% chance of developing Reiter's syndrome.

(2) **Gender distribution.** Reiter's syndrome is diagnosed in men much more commonly than in women, in part because cervicitis is less symptomatic than urethritis. However, the arthritis tends to be less severe in women as well.

c. **Etiology and pathogenesis.** Specific infections trigger the clinical expression of arthritis in susceptible patients, including chlamydial and mycoplasmal urethritis as well as dysenteric infections caused by certain serotypes of *Shigella, Salmonella,* and *Yersinia.* The presence of the organism may not be necessary for later exacerbations or chronic activity of the disease, although some polymerase chain reaction and electron microscopic studies of inflamed synovium suggest the persistence of chlamydial organisms or fragments in Reiter's syndrome. The unusual severity of Reiter's syndrome in patients with AIDS suggests that functioning CD4$^+$ cells are not necessary in the inflammatory response.

(1) **Exaggerated immune response.** Conceivably, infectious antigens cross-react with self antigens such as HLA-B27 and stimulate an exaggerated immune response that can include a noninfectious arthritis.

(2) **Suppressed immune response.** It is also conceivable that this molecular mimicry between HLA-B27 and bacterial peptides prevents the host immune system from recognizing the pathogen, thus allowing dissemination and production of disease at widely varied sites. This theory is supported by evidence that suggests persistence of organisms or fragments at sites of chronic inflammation.

(3) **Protected site of infection.** Persistent subclinical genitourinary or gastrointestinal infections (e.g., *Chlamydia, Shigella*) could cause recurrent shedding of organisms or bacterial antigens to joints. Persistent specific IgA responses to causative organisms and improvement with surgical removal of the urethra in venereal onset of Reiter's syndrome supports this theory.

d. Clinical features

    (1) Disease onset. Reiter's syndrome begins most often in young adulthood. One to three weeks after an episode of urethritis or dysentery, any of the typical clinical features of the syndrome can occur. The disease often is misdiagnosed because these features tend to occur serially rather than simultaneously.

    (2) Manifestations of disease

        (a) Musculoskeletal

            (i) Arthritis. A lower extremity oligoarthritis is the most common joint presentation. The arthritis may be acute and self-limited, but it is more commonly relapsing or chronic.

            (ii) Enthesopathy. Inflammation of the tendons and ligaments are as much a part of Reiter's syndrome as they are of ankylosing spondylitis. Plantar fasciitis and Achilles tendinitis are most typical. **Dactylitis** (sausage toe), a lesion involving both joint and tendon inflammation in the same digit, also is a common feature of Reiter's syndrome.

            (iii) Sacroiliitis. Asymmetrical involvement of sacroiliac joints occurs in approximately 20% of patients with Reiter's syndrome. Less frequently, asymmetrical ascending spinal disease occurs. The consequent back pain has typical inflammatory characteristics, but only rarely does the ascending spinal disease limit thoracic or cervical spinal mobility.

        (b) Genitourinary. Symptomatic or asymptomatic **urethritis** is extremely common in patients with Reiter's disease. Chronic **prostatitis** also is common, affecting as many as 80% of patients in some series.

        (c) Ocular. Both **conjunctivitis** and **anterior uveitis** are common features. The conjunctival inflammation is an acute, usually self-limited manifestation, which may be recurrent. Anterior uveitis occurs in more established forms of disease; it may be chronic and require topical or systemic corticosteroids to prevent visual deterioration.

        (d) Mucocutaneous. Fleeting and painless oral ulcers are the typical mucous membrane features of Reiter's syndrome. **Keratoderma blennorrhagica** is the characteristic scaling, plaque-like lesion found anywhere on the body, including the palms and soles. This lesion resembles pustular psoriasis clinically and pathologically. **Circinate balanitis** is a painless, erythematous erosion of the glans penis that may expand to surround the urethral orifice. Each of these skin lesions occurs in approximately 20%–30% of patients with Reiter's syndrome, although circinate balanitis is the most common.

        (e) Cardiovascular. Early cardiovascular changes in Reiter's syndrome include transient **pericardial rubs** or **first-degree heart block.** In more severe, long-standing disease, an **aortitis** identical to that seen in ankylosing spondylitis can cause valvular insufficiency or conduction system lesions.

e. Diagnosis

    (1) General considerations. Reiter's syndrome can be difficult to diagnose when the onset of various clinical features is widely separated over time, but it is quite easy if **arthritis, dysentery** or **urethritis, conjunctivitis,** and **mucocutaneous lesions** appear simultaneously. A tentative diagnosis can be made when a seronegative asymmetrical oligoarthritis is associated with any of these extra-articular features. Because Reiter's syndrome is, strictly speaking, a reactive arthritis, the temporal appearance of arthritis after urethritis or a dysenteric illness is especially convincing. Because the mucocutaneous lesions, urethritis, and cervicitis often are asymptomatic, they must be sought specifically while taking the patient history and during the physical examination.

    (2) Laboratory findings. Eighty percent of whites with Reiter's syndrome have HLA-B27. The synovial fluid typically is mildly to moderately inflammatory, with neutrophil predominance and no important distinguishing characteristics.

(3) Radiographic findings. Asymmetrical, oligoarticular erosions, joint space narrowing, and periarticular osteopenia can be seen radiographically in established disease. Periosteal new bone formation is a characteristic feature of Reiter's syndrome, especially adjacent to the insertions of the Achilles tendon and plantar fascia. Sacroiliitis, if it occurs, typically is asymmetrical, and the occasional patient with spondylarthropathy has asymmetrical, large syndesmophytes at scattered vertebral levels.

(4) Differential diagnosis

    (a) Diseases most likely to mimic acute Reiter's syndrome are gonococcal arthritis and other infectious arthropathies, even Lyme disease. Thus, appropriate tissues should be cultured and serologies obtained. Crystal-mediated arthritis (i.e., gout and pseudogout) and the arthritis of rheumatic fever should be excluded.

    (b) Diseases most likely to mimic chronic recurring Reiter's syndrome include other spondylarthropathies, especially psoriatic arthritis or ankylosing spondylitis. Close attention to the symmetry and severity of sacroiliac and spinal involvement, to extraskeletal features, and to the presence or absence of infectious triggers may help to differentiate these illnesses. Many cases of so-called **seronegative rheumatoid arthritis** may actually be cases of Reiter's syndrome. Typical clinical features as well as radiographic evidence of sacroiliac joint and periostitic involvement should be sought. The presence or absence of HLA-B27 may be helpful in diagnosing particularly difficult cases.

f. Therapy

(1) Goals of treatment are essentially the same as in ankylosing spondylitis [see IV B 1 f (1)].

(2) Exercise. Patients should be advised to rest to lessen inflammation and to perform appropriate exercises that will allow preservation of joint function and prevention of contractures.

(3) Drug therapy

    (a) NSAIDs are the mainstay of treatment of Reiter's syndrome. Aspirin, however, is relatively ineffective in this illness.

    (b) Corticosteroids. Occasional intra-articular instillation may be useful in the management of particular joints that do not respond to treatment with NSAIDs.

    (c) Second-line agents. Both azathioprine and methotrexate have been used to control particularly severe and chronic disease, and sulfasalazine is used for arthritis unresponsive to NSAIDs. The effects of these medications on disease course are not yet known. HIV testing should be considered for patients with Reiter's syndrome severe enough to require immunosuppressive medications.

    (d) Antibiotics. Trials of tetracycline-like drugs, used for 3-month periods early in Reiter's syndrome associated with urethritis, suggest that antibiotic treatment may lessen the severity and chronicity of arthritis.

g. Prognosis. Chronic or recurrent disease appears to be common. In 60%–80% of patients with Reiter's syndrome, skeletal or extraskeletal complaints, or both, recur or become chronic. Neither gender nor HLA-B27 status appears to affect outcome. Perhaps as many as 25% of patients with Reiter's syndrome are functionally disabled by their illness. Long-term problems with aortic regurgitation and conduction disturbances are unusual but increase with the duration of the disease. Patients who have HLA-B27 antigen have more sacroiliitis and are more likely to have recurrent or chronic disease.

3. Psoriatic arthritis

a. Definition. Any form of inflammatory arthritis associated with psoriasis is called psoriatic arthritis. Rheumatoid factor generally is absent.

b. Epidemiology

(1) Psoriatic arthritis occurs much more commonly in patients who have a first-degree relative with the disorder.

(2) Psoriasis occurs two to three times more commonly in patients with arthritis than in the normal population. Conversely, as many as 10%–20% of patients with psoriasis may have an inflammatory arthritis.

c. **Etiology.** Although a hereditary etiology is apparent in psoriatic arthritis, its characteristics are not fully understood. HLA-B27 is highly associated with sacroiliitis in psoriasis, and HLA-B27, -B13, and -DR7 are independently associated with arthritis and psoriasis at an increased frequency. Unknown environmental factors also may be important in disease expression.

d. **Clinical features**

   (1) **Disease onset.** Most patients with psoriatic arthritis develop the disease in their late thirties to early forties. Most patients develop skin lesions before the arthritis, but as many as 16% develop inflammatory arthritis before the psoriasis.

   (2) **Patterns of arthritis.** Five patterns of psoriatic arthropathy have been distinguished, although the typical patient often has the skeletal manifestations of several of these patterns. Peripheral joint and tendon involvement may be more severe in the upper than in the lower extremities.

   (a) **DIP arthritis** is the classic form of psoriatic arthritis. It is strongly associated with typical fingernail abnormalities as well as DIP joint redness, soft tissue swelling, and erosive changes seen radiographically in a clinical picture resembling primary erosive osteoarthritis.

   (b) **Asymmetrical oligoarthritis.** Large and small joint oligoarthritis is another clinical form of psoriatic arthritis. **Sausage digits** are common in this form as a manifestation of joint and enthesis involvement of a single phalanx.

   (c) **Symmetrical polyarthropathy.** A fairly symmetrical polyarthropathy can occur in conjunction with psoriasis, and it can be difficult to distinguish from rheumatoid arthritis. As many as 25% of these patients may be seropositive for rheumatoid factor.

   (d) **Arthritis mutilans** is an unusually destructive form of psoriatic arthritis because of the severe periarticular bone resorption that occurs in the small finger joints. "Telescoping digits" characterize the end stage of this uncommon form of arthritis. Widespread joint ankylosis also can occur.

   (e) **Sacroiliitis.** As many as 20% of patients with psoriatic arthritis can have clinical or radiographic evidence of sacroiliitis, usually asymmetrical. Ascending spinal syndesmophytes occur in an asymmetrical and patchy fashion.

   (3) **Extra-articular features**

   (a) **Skin.** Arthritis is more likely to occur in patients with severe skin involvement than in those with mild psoriasis, although it can occur in the presence of localized cutaneous lesions. Skin and joint flares of disease can occur in association with each other or independently in individual patients.

   (b) **Nails.** Nail abnormalities most commonly occur in conjunction with DIP joint lesions; however, nail changes are noted more frequently in all of the peripheral forms of psoriatic arthritis in comparison to psoriasis uncomplicated by arthritis. Multiple **pitting,** transverse depressions, and **onycholysis** are the characteristic abnormalities found.

   (c) **Ocular.** The only other extra-articular features that occur commonly in patients with psoriatic arthritis are conjunctivitis (in 20% of cases) and anterior uveitis (in 10% of cases).

e. **Diagnosis**

   (1) **Clinical considerations.** An association should be made between the typical skin and nail lesions and the joint and spinal involvement to diagnose psoriatic arthritis. The skin manifestations may be subtle, so particular care must be taken to check the elbows, scalp, groin, navel, and buttock cleft.

   (2) **Laboratory findings.** Laboratory indicators of chronic disease (e.g., anemia, thrombocytosis) typically are absent. Patients usually are seronegative for rheumatoid factor, although 25% of patients with symmetrical polyarthritis are seropositive.

    (3) **Radiographic findings**
        (a) **DIP joint erosions** can lead to joint space widening, and proximal phalangeal bone resorption can lead to a "pencil-in-cup" abnormality seen in arthritis mutilans. This severe destruction also can occur in more proximal joints.
        (b) **Spinal involvement.** Asymmetrical sacroiliitis and asymmetrical patchy syndesmophytes are seen and are similar to those seen in Reiter's syndrome.
        (c) **Enthesopathy.** Calcifications at tendon and ligament insertions occur.
    (4) **Differential diagnosis**
        (a) **Reiter's syndrome** is distinguished from psoriatic arthritis by its characteristic extra-articular features and its tendency to involve the lower extremities more than the upper extremities. In psoriatic arthritis, upper extremity peripheral joint involvement is more common.
        (b) **Rheumatoid arthritis.** A presentation of symmetrical polyarthritis, seropositivity for rheumatoid factor, and rheumatoid nodules in a patient with psoriasis may be diagnosed as rheumatoid arthritis. Other overlapping presentations of the two diseases may be difficult to diagnose as being one or the other.

  f. Therapy. Drug treatment for psoriatic arthritis is similar to that for the other spondylarthropathies in that NSAIDs are the cornerstone of therapy; an importance difference is that gold can be administered intramuscularly to treat sustained manifestations of peripheral arthritis. Sulfasalazine also is effective. Methotrexate is often the first agent used if NSAIDs are not sufficient; it has been particularly successful in controlling both the skin disease and refractory arthritis. Other cytotoxic drugs (e.g., azathioprine) also have been used in treatment of severe skin and joint disease.

  g. Prognosis. Most patients with psoriatic arthritis can avoid significant deformity and remain employed. The 5% or so who develop arthritis mutilans obviously are exceptions.

4. Enteropathic arthropathies
  a. Definition. Inflammatory arthritis associated with either Crohn's disease or ulcerative colitis is typified by a seronegative, migratory polyarticular involvement that waxes and wanes with the activity of the bowel disease. Sacroiliitis and spondylitis can also occur in affected individuals.

  b. Clinical syndromes
    (1) **Peripheral arthritis.** In 10%–20% of patients with severe ulcerative colitis or Crohn's disease—usually those with other extra-intestinal manifestations—a predominantly lower extremity arthritis or tendinitis occurs in association with flare-ups of bowel disease. The arthritis often occurs abruptly and usually remits completely within weeks. There is no association with HLA-B27 in this peripheral arthritis. Treatment is directed at control of the bowel disease, although NSAIDs or local or systemic corticosteroids may help to control the articular complaints.
    (2) **Spondylitis.** The spondylitis of inflammatory bowel disease is associated with HLA-B27 in about 50% of patients. The radiographic findings are typical of those found in primary ankylosing spondylitis (i.e., symmetrical sacroiliac joint changes and, less commonly, ascending symmetrical spondylitis without skin lesions). Approximately 5% of patients with inflammatory bowel disease develop sacroiliitis or spondylitis, but the activity of these lesions and that of the bowel disease are independent of one another. NSAIDs usually are effective in controlling symptoms but can cause increased bowel complaints; sometimes only nonacetylated salicylates can be tolerated by these patients.

  c. Differential diagnosis. Whipple's disease can be confused with enteropathic arthropathies, because most patients manifest prominent bowel and joint complaints. In fact, sacroiliitis occurs in about 20% of cases. However, Whipple's disease is quite rare and most commonly presents in middle-aged men with weight loss, skin hyperpigmentation, lymphadenopathy, fever, and symptoms of malabsorption.

V. JUVENILE RHEUMATOID ARTHRITIS (JUVENILE CHRONIC ARTHRITIS)

A. **Definition.** Juvenile rheumatoid arthritis is a **chronic inflammatory arthritis** that begins before age 18 years. Prior to considering a diagnosis of juvenile rheumatoid arthritis, arthritis should be present in one or more joints for more than 6 weeks, and other rheumatic diseases should be excluded.

B. **Epidemiology.** The annual incidence of juvenile rheumatoid arthritis may be as high as 0.01%. Although the apparent HLA associations would suggest that the altered immune responses are genetically transferable, familial aggregation of cases is uncommon.

C. **Etiology and pathogenesis.** The same factors important in the development of adult rheumatoid arthritis also apply to juvenile rheumatoid arthritis (see III C–D). Etiologic factors are unknown but may include infectious agents. **Immune system dysfunction** is apparent in the prolongation and maintenance of synovitis. A subset of patients with juvenile rheumatoid arthritis have an immunodeficiency state (IgA deficiency), which may be important In disease pathogenesis.

D. **Pathology.** The **synovial lesions** cannot be distinguished histologically from those in adult rheumatoid arthritis. The **inflammatory lesion** can involve the growing epiphysis, however, and can result in involved bones that are longer or shorter than normal. Chronically involved joints exhibit **fibrous ankylosis** more often than in adult rheumatoid arthritis. **Pannus formation** can occur, although typically later in the disease course than in adults with rheumatoid arthritis. As a consequence, destructive joint disease also is much less common in juvenile rheumatoid arthritis.

E. **Classification.** Three primary subtypes of juvenile rheumatoid arthritis (i.e., systemic-onset juvenile rheumatoid arthritis, pauciarticular arthritis, and polyarticular arthritis) can be distinguished in the first 6 months of illness. Making distinctions between subtypes of illness appears to be important prognostically and therapeutically. Important classification features are the **presence or absence of prominent systemic features** and the **total number of involved joints.** The cervical spine, wrist, and ankle articulations are counted as one joint each for classification purposes; all other joints are counted separately.

1. **Systemic-onset juvenile rheumatoid arthritis,** also called **Still's disease,** occurs in approximately 10%–20% of patients and is characterized by an early pattern of **prominent systemic complaints** and **extra-articular involvement.** Boys are affected as commonly as girls, and a peak age of incidence is not evident.
    a. **Clinical features**
        (1) **Typical features of the early disease course** are **high spiking fevers** and marked **constitutional complaints.** Overt arthritis may not be part of the early course but develops within weeks to months of the onset of illness. A characteristic **nonpruritic, fleeting, maculopapular rash** occurs in 90% of patients and may be most apparent with fever spikes.
        (2) **Common features of active disease** include lymphadenopathy, hepatosplenomegaly, and pleuropericarditis.
        (3) **The most serious manifestation of systemic-onset juvenile rheumatoid arthritis is pericarditis,** sometimes associated with a large pericardial effusion requiring pericardiocentesis. Accompanying myocarditis is rare.
    b. **Laboratory findings**
        (1) **Hematologic findings** include a strikingly elevated erythrocyte sedimentation rate, prominent leukocytosis and thrombocytosis, and moderate to se-

vere anemia of chronic disease, although there often is striking micro-cytosis.

(2) **Serologic findings** only rarely include rheumatoid factor and antinuclear antibodies (ANAs). Early reports show association with HLA-B8, -B35, -DR4, and -Dw7.

c. **Disease course.** Disease flare-ups are punctuated by relatively symptom-free intervals. Polyarticular arthritis becomes evident at some point in the first 6 months of illness, although some children may have only myalgia and arthralgia at disease onset.

(1) Approximately 50% of patients may begin to develop symptoms of disease that resemble the polyarticular arthritis subset, with progressive joint involvement determining disease outcome and systemic features becoming less evident over time.

(2) The remaining 50% of patients eventually recover completely.

2. **Polyarticular arthritis** occurs in approximately 30%–40% of patients and **involves five or more joints** in the first 6 months of illness. **Systemic features usually do not dominate** the early course of disease. Girls are affected much more often than boys. Polyarticular arthritis can be further separated into **rheumatoid factor–positive or–negative subsets.** Patients who are seropositive for rheumatoid factor present most often in late childhood; a peak age of incidence is not evident for patients who are seronegative for rheumatoid factor.

a. **Clinical features**

(1) Typically, inflammatory polyarticular arthritis may have an acute or a gradual onset similar to the presentation of adult rheumatoid arthritis. Symmetrical large and small joint involvement also is typical. Prominent features may include cervical spine, sacroiliac joint, and temporomandibular joint disease.

(2) Rarely, patients have symptoms and signs of anterior uveitis typical of that seen in spondylarthropathies.

(3) Patients who are seropositive for rheumatoid factor can have subcutaneous nodules as in adult-onset rheumatoid arthritis.

b. **Laboratory findings**

(1) **Hematologic findings** frequently include moderate elevation of erythrocyte sedimentation rate, leukocyte count, and platelet count. Patients usually develop a mild normochromic, normocytic anemia of chronic disease.

(2) **Serologic findings** include rheumatoid factor in 10%–20% and ANAs in 20%–40% of patients.

c. **Disease course.** Polyarticular arthritis can be chronic and persistent or can pursue a more intermittent, relapsing course.

(1) Patients with polyarticular arthritis who are seropositive for rheumatoid factor are at greatest risk for chronic, erosive, and severe arthritis and significant disability. These patients have disease that is very similar to adult-onset rheumatoid arthritis.

(2) Patients who are seronegative for rheumatoid factor less often have severe disease or disease that lasts into adulthood.

3. **Pauciarticular arthritis** occurs in approximately 50% of patients and involves **four or fewer joints** in the first 6 months of illness. This patient group is composed of three subsets.

a. **Oligoarthritis and anterior uveitis** affect girls more often than boys, and peak incidence is in early childhood.

(1) **Clinical features**

(a) Typically, the arthritis is asymmetrical, mild, and involves the knee. Other peripheral joints also can be involved, but the axial skeleton usually is spared.

(b) Systemic symptoms and signs are mild or absent.

(c) Potentially serious **anterior uveitis** unrelated to arthritis activity can develop in 20%–40% of patients. This usually chronic eye lesion can be asymptomatic and can lead to **blindness** if unrecognized or inadequately treated.

    (2) Laboratory findings

        (a) Hematologic findings usually do not include anemia, thrombocytosis, and leukocytosis. The erythrocyte sedimentation rate is normal or only minimally elevated.

        (b) Serologic findings include ANA positivity in 60% of patients, which identifies those at higher risk for chronic uveitis. Rheumatoid factor typically is not present. Associations with HLA-DR5, -DRw8, and -DPw2 may be important in this subset.

    (3) Disease course. Most patients have pauciarticular involvement that is manageable and not disabling. In approximately one-third of patients, the disease evolves into a more polyarticular form.

  b. Axial skeleton oligoarthritis predominantly affects boys, with disease onset usually beginning in late childhood.

    (1) Clinical features. The sacroiliac joints most often are involved, but asymmetrical hip or knee arthritis also can occur. Acute anterior uveitis can occur as in adult spondylarthropathies, but this feature is not the chronic and sight-threatening form seen in the other pauciarticular subset.

    (2) Laboratory findings

        (a) Hematologic findings are not distinct in this subset.

        (b) Serologic findings indicate that 50% of these patients have HLA-B27, but few have rheumatoid factor.

    (3) Disease course. Most of these patients develop features of ankylosing spondylitis, psoriatic arthritis, or Reiter's syndrome in later life.

  c. Oligoarthritis with prominent dactylitis is a third presentation seen most frequently in girls of any age. **Psoriasis** commonly affects these patients and their families.

F. Diagnosis

  1. Difficulties in diagnosis. Diagnosing arthritis in a child may be difficult. Children may avoid using an involved joint instead of complaining of pain. Irritability, regressive behavior, or emotional withdrawal may be the child's response to the pain of an inflamed joint. Once joint involvement has been discovered, disease should be present for at least 6 weeks before a diagnosis of juvenile rheumatoid arthritis is seriously considered. Within the first 6 months, an attempt should be made to classify the patient into a clinical subset.

    a. Synovial fluid findings. In juvenile rheumatoid arthritis, the synovial fluid usually is mildly inflammatory (i.e., a white cell count of 10,000–20,000/mm^3); however, the number of white cells present may not parallel disease activity. Joint fluid culture and analysis are especially important in pauciarticular forms to exclude infection (bacterial or mycobacterial) or hemorrhage (e.g., due to trauma or hemophilia).

    b. Radiographic findings are nonspecific.

      (1) Early findings may include only soft tissue swelling, periarticular demineralization, or periosteal bone proliferation.

      (2) Late findings include epiphyseal changes (either premature closure or overgrowth, depending on epiphyseal activity at the time of involvement) and articular erosion or joint space narrowing.

      (3) Distinctive long bone periosteal elevation in leukemia may allow differentiation from juvenile rheumatoid arthritis, and localized joint abnormalities (e.g., osteonecrosis, osteochondritis) may have distinct radiographic presentations.

      (4) Cervical spine involvement, particularly with ankylosis at C2–C3, is common in juvenile rheumatoid arthritis.

  2. Differential diagnosis

    a. A variety of **genetic or inborn metabolic disorders** as well as nonrheumatic conditions can superficially resemble juvenile rheumatoid arthritis. It is specifically important to rule out **infectious etiologies** (e.g., Lyme disease, tuberculosis) and **malignancies** (e.g., leukemia) as causes of childhood arthritis.

b. **Other rheumatic diseases** [e.g., rheumatic fever, systemic lupus erythematosus (SLE), spondylarthropathies] may require a period of observation for characteristic extra-articular features to evolve.

G. **Therapeutic approach**

1. **Education of patients and parents** about inflammatory arthritis is important, and the generally favorable course of juvenile rheumatoid arthritis should be emphasized. Long-term goals of suppression of disease activity and prevention of deformity should be instituted, and the child's psychological and emotional development should not be neglected.

2. **Therapy.** The use of appropriate therapy is important in relieving pain and maintaining function. Parents should be urged to perform active roles in giving physical therapy and medications, encouraging school attendance, and maintaining the child's ability to be self-sufficient.

   a. **Pharmacologic therapy**

      (1) **Salicylates** are no longer the primary drug used in treating juvenile rheumatoid arthritis because of concerns about the potential precipitation of Reye's syndrome by aspirin.

      (2) **Other NSAIDs.** Currently, tolmetin and naproxen are most often prescribed as initial treatment. Indomethacin, although not formally approved for children, also may be effective.

      (3) **Gold compounds.** Patients with chronically active, progressive disease that is not responsive to NSAIDs may need a second-line agent such as gold. Many of these patients have a polyarticular syndrome and are seropositive for rheumatoid factor. Gold is potentially dangerous in systemic-onset juvenile rheumatoid arthritis because it presents a high risk of cholestatic jaundice and disseminated intravascular coagulation (DIC).

      (4) **Corticosteroids**

         (a) In **patients with systemic complaints who have life-threatening manifestations** (e.g., pericarditis), moderate- to high-dose systemic corticosteroids may be required.

         (b) In **nonambulatory children with polyarticular disease,** a small every-other-day dose of corticosteroids may promote weight bearing. The consequences of being nonambulatory in childhood outweigh possible corticosteroid complications in this clinical situation.

         (c) Local corticosteroid injections often are effective in managing **pauciarticular disease** or more **severely involved joints in polyarticular disease.**

         (d) In the treatment of **chronic uveitis,** systemic corticosteroids may be needed if initial treatment with topical or local corticosteroids and dilating agents is not effective. Patients at high risk for chronic uveitis (oligoarticular subgroup) should be evaluated every 3 months to determine treatment effectiveness.

      (5) **Other second-line agents** (e.g., hydroxychloroquine, D-penicillamine) also are used in the treatment of juvenile rheumatoid arthritis, but with limited success. Recent experience with methotrexate is more encouraging, and sulfasalazine is becoming more popular because it has rapid onset of effect (less than 2 months), infrequent serious toxicity, and moderate efficacy.

      (6) **Intravenous infusions of gamma globulin** have been used to control severe systemic-onset or polyarticular disease.

   b. **Surgery.** Patients sometimes may benefit from early synovectomy. Correction of deformities and total joint replacements may be needed in chronic, severe disease. Jaw implants have been used for micrognathia.

   c. **Physical and occupational therapy** are especially important in treating patients with juvenile rheumatoid arthritis. Children must learn and practice exercises that will maintain muscle tone and prevent joint contractures. Night splints may

chondral bone. Closed-needle aspiration usually is appropriate, because open surgical drainage prolongs immobilization and delays return of effective function.

    b. Open surgical drainage. Hip infections, especially in children, are best handled by immediate open drainage. Joints that do not respond to needle drainage are treated either by open drainage or by arthroscopy.

    c. Arthroscopic drainage. Arthroscopy is an attractive alternative to open drainage, because lysis of adhesions and removal of inflamed synovium can often be accomplished without the prolonged immobilization of open drainage.

3. Other ancillary measures

    a. Continuous passive motion early in treatment is somewhat more effective than complete immobilization at preventing loss of cartilage and subchondral bone. The avascular cartilage depends on joint motion for nutrition.

    b. Ambulation. Weight bearing and ambulation of involved joints should be avoided until effusions are gone; otherwise, **postinfectious inflammatory arthritis** can delay recovery.

4. Response to treatment

    a. Trends in the following clinical and laboratory parameters allow clinicians to assess therapeutic progress:

        (1) Resolution of fever

        (2) Resolution of synovial effusion

        (3) Improvement in joint pain, tenderness, and range of motion

        (4) Resolution of leukocytosis (blood, synovial fluid)

        (5) Sterility of synovial fluid cultures

    b. Failure of improvement should lead to reconsideration of diagnosis, reconsideration of choice or dosage of antibiotic, and consideration of open or arthroscopic drainage.

VII. SYSTEMIC LUPUS ERYTHEMATOSUS

A. **Definition.** SLE is a chronic immune disorder characterized by multisystem involvement and clinical exacerbations and remissions. **Circulating immune complexes** and **autoantibodies** cause tissue damage and organ dysfunction. Manifestations involving the skin, serosal surfaces, central nervous system (CNS), kidneys, and blood cells are particularly characteristic. Evidence for the autoimmune nature of this disorder lies in the laboratory finding of ANAs, the demonstration of immune complexes in tissues, and the utilization of complement.

B. **Epidemiology**

    1. The overall **prevalence** of SLE is approximately 15–50 cases per 100,000 population. The prevalence in young women of childbearing age is approximately eight to ten times that in men. Black women are affected approximately three times as often as white women.

    2. The frequency of occurrence of lupus is higher in the relatives of affected individuals than in the general population, and the disease concordance rate in identical twins approaches 50%.

C. **Etiology.** No single cause of lupus has been discovered. Complex interrelationships among environmental factors, genetically determined host immune responses, and hormonal influences probably are critical in the initiation as well as the expression of the disease.

    1. Environmental factors. Viruses and drugs or toxins have been pursued as causative agents, but neither has been shown to cause idiopathic SLE. Microbial toxins and viral (particularly retroviral) products can function as **superantigens,** binding to the helper T-cell receptors and MHC class II molecule complexes nonspecifically. Binding to B cell MHC class II molecules might activate helper T cells to generate **autoimmune responses.**

2. **Genetic factors.** Twin and family studies suggest a genetic predisposition to SLE. The disease occurs commonly in families with hereditary deficiencies of early complement components. Histocompatibility antigens HLA-DR2 and HLA-DR3 are present much more commonly in SLE patients than in controls. Some of the HLA-DR3 association may be due to linkage with a deletion for a C4a gene. Specific combinations of histocompatibility antigens may be associated with the production of specific autoantibodies (e.g., HLA-DR or HLA-DQ associations with Ro and La antibodies).

3. **Autoimmunity.** Loss of tolerance to autoantigens is central to the pathogenesis of SLE, and genetic tendencies toward the development of autoantibodies, B-cell hyperactivity, and T-cell dysfunction are evident in patients with the disease. The tendency to develop autoimmunity in SLE is not MHC-linked but may be caused by genes outside the histocompatibility loci.

4. **Apoptosis.** Programmed cell death, or apoptosis, leads to the orderly replacement of old cells in all organs, including the B and T lymphocytes of the immune system. Defects in apoptosis genes have been discovered in lupus mouse kindreds, resulting in the development of autoimmunity, perhaps related to failure to delete autoreactive T cells or autoantibody-producing B cells.

5. **Hormonal influences.** Lupus is predominantly a disease of women of childbearing age, but hormonal factors probably are more important in modulation of the expression of disease than in causation. Estrogen may be a permissive factor in polyclonal B cell activation.

D. **Pathogenesis.** All of the clinical features of SLE are manifestations of cellular and humoral immune dysfunction; however, **atherosclerosis** can be a secondary effect of vascular damage that leads to further organ ischemia.

1. **Immune complexes.** Circulating antigen–antibody (immune) complexes are deposited in blood vessels and the renal glomerulus, initiating a pathologic response that damages these tissues. These complexes are characteristic features of active disease, and their size, solubility, concentration, and complement-fixing properties as well as vessel hydrostatic forces are important in determining tissue deposition.

2. **Reticuloendothelial dysfunction.** The chronic circulation of immune complexes seems to be important in their pathogenicity, as occurs in a chronic serum sickness reaction. At times, the ability of the reticuloendothelial system to remove immune complexes from the circulation may be overwhelmed. Patients with C4a gene deletions more commonly have SLE, perhaps as a result of impaired immune complex clearance.

3. **Autoantibodies** are produced either in the setting of specific, antigen-driven, induction of autoreactive lymphocyte clones or polyclonal activation of different B cell lineages. These autoantibodies can cause:
   a. **Tissue damage.** Antibodies to red cells, white cells, or platelets can cause immune cytopenias.
   b. **Cellular dysfunction.** Antibodies to lymphocytes can impair lymphocyte function and intercellular signalling; antineuronal antibodies crossing a breached blood–brain barrier can impair neuron function.
   c. **Immune complex formation.** Complexes of antibodies and double-stranded DNA are important in mediation of autoimmune renal disease.

4. **Lymphocyte dysfunction.** B cell hyperactivity, impaired CD8$^+$ cell function, and augmented CD4$^+$ cell activity are present in various combinations in lupus patients, leading to autoantibody production and increased generation of immune complexes.

E. **Pathology**

1. **Characteristic microscopic changes**
   a. **Hematoxylin bodies.** Amorphous masses of nuclear material bound with immunoglobulin can be found in connective tissue lesions that become purple–blue when stained with hematoxylin. Neutrophils that ingest these bodies in vitro are called **LE cells.**
   b. **Fibrinoid necrosis.** In SLE, immune complexes of DNA, antibody to DNA, and complement may stain with eosin (which can stain immune complexes as well as fibrin) in vessel walls and connective tissue, demonstrating so-called "fibrinoid necrosis."
   c. **Onion-skin lesions.** Lesions characteristic of SLE in splenic arteries are called onion-skin lesions because of the concentric deposition of collagen around them, presumably formed as vasculitic lesions heal.

2. **Tissue changes**
   a. **Skin.** Although some of the milder skin lesions in SLE have only nonspecific lymphocytic infiltration in perivascular locations in the dermis, more typical lupus lesions show **dermal–epidermal junction deposits of immunoglobulins** and complement as well as necrosis. Classic discoid lesions show follicular plugging, hyperkeratosis, and the loss of skin appendages. Frank vasculitic lesions also can occur in small dermal vessels.
   b. **Kidney.** Immune complex deposition in the kidney can lead to various histologic pictures of inflammation. A cardinal characteristic of renal pathology in SLE is the tendency of these pathologic pictures to change over time, based either on changes in disease activity or therapy. Biopsy specimens are graded with regard to activity (active inflammation) and chronicity (glomerular sclerosis and fibrotic interstitial change); the most treatable lesions have high activity and low chronicity.
      (1) **Mesangial disease** refers to **mesangial hypercellularity** caused by the presence of immunoglobulin deposits and is the most common renal pathologic lesion in SLE.
      (2) **Focal proliferative nephritis** involves cellular proliferative change only in **segments of glomeruli** and in **less than 50% of glomeruli.**
      (3) **Diffuse proliferative nephritis** involves cellular proliferation in **most of the segments** of the glomerulus and in **more than 50% of glomeruli.**
      (4) **Pure membranous nephritis** consists of **subepithelial** glomerular basement membrane immunoglobulin deposits without glomerular hypercellularity (called **wire looping** on light microscopy), although patients may have overlapping combinations of proliferative and membranous forms on biopsy.
      (5) **Interstitial inflammation** can also occur in all of the above pathologic pictures.
   c. **CNS.** Large vessel vasculitic lesions can occur (although they are uncommon) in focal presentations of the disease, but focal areas of perivascular small vessel inflammation, microinfarction, or microhemorrhages are more typical and do not correlate well with abnormalities found on imaging studies [computed tomography (CT) or magnetic resonance imaging (MRI) scans] or the neurologic examination. The **phospholipid antibody syndrome** may be associated with the small vessel occlusive lesions.
   d. **Vasculitis.** Inflammatory lesions of capillaries, venules, and arterioles, caused by immune complex deposition and variable cellular infiltration, are responsible for much of the tissue destruction and damage seen in SLE.
   e. **Other tissue lesions.** Nonspecific mild synovitis and lymphocytic infiltration of muscles occur frequently. Nonbacterial endocarditis often is present but typically is asymptomatic.

F. **Clinical features and laboratory findings**

1. **Manifestations of disease.** Fatigue, weight loss, and fever are prominent **systemic complaints** in this disease.

a. **Skin.** The **butterfly rash** (i.e., facial erythema over the cheeks and nose) and the chronic, potentially scarring, **discoid lesions** (i.e., coin-shaped lesions with hyperemic margins, central atrophy, and depigmentation) are the most classic. Less commonly, bullous and maculopapular eruptions can occur. Nonscarring, psoriasiform lesions **(subacute cutaneous lupus)** have recently been described. Recurrent mucous membrane ulceration, generalized or focal alopecia, digital vasculitis, and photosensitivity also are potential dermatologic features of SLE.

b. **Nerve**

   (1) **CNS.** Focal or diffuse neurologic disorders occur in approximately 50% of patients. **Generalized manifestations** include severe headache, reactive depressions, psychoses, cognitive disturbances, and seizures. Psychosis in some lupus patients correlates with the presence of antibody to ribosomal P protein. **Focal seizures** also have been described, and hemiparesis, cranial nerve deficits, transverse myelitis, and movement disorders may pinpoint discrete areas of involvement. Lumbar puncture, electroencephalography (EEG), and CT scan often are unrevealing, although MRI scanning reveals CNS lesions in many patients, especially those with focal presentations.

   (2) **Peripheral nervous system.** Some patients have sensory or sensorimotor neuropathies, and those with vasculitis of the vasonervorum may manifest mononeuritis multiplex.

c. **Heart.** Symptomatic **pericarditis** occurs in aproximately 20% of SLE patients and pericardial effusions on echocardiography in as many as 50%, but tamponade is uncommon. **Myocarditis** (conduction abnormalities, arrhythmias, and congestive heart failure) is less common and may be reversible if treated promptly with corticosteroids. Although **coronary vessel vasculitis** can occur in fulminant cases, premature atherosclerosis in steroid-treated patients is a more common cause of myocardial infarction in lupus patients. **Nonbacterial endocardial lesions** (Libman-Sacks endocarditis) can be associated with embolic CNS events, valvular dysfunction, or infective endocarditis.

d. **Lung.** At some time in the disease course, approximately 30% of SLE patients have symptomatic **pleuritis** and fewer have friction rubs or actual effusions apparent on ultrasonography. Diaphragmatic fibrosis or diaphragm dysfunction may present as **"shrinking lung syndrome,"** with a restrictive picture on pulmonary function testing. Parenchymal involvement **(lupus pneumonitis)** can be difficult to distinguish from acute infections; lupus infiltrates may be unilateral or bilateral, tend to be fleeting, occur with active disease, and lack purulent sputum. **Hemoptysis** occurs as a feature of pulmonary vasculitis and may herald an **adult respiratory distress syndrome** picture. **Diffuse interstitial lung disease** is recognized, albeit uncommonly. **Pulmonary hypertension** as a result of isolated pulmonary vascular involvement also occurs.

e. **Gastrointestinal tract.** Although symptoms of nausea, vomiting, and abdominal pain are common, diagnostic testing often is unrevealing. Overt **intestinal vasculitis** can lead to bowel infarction, perforation, and hemorrhage. Lupus- or corticosteroid-related **pancreatitis** and reversible gastric damage or hepatitis induced by NSAIDs as occur as well.

f. **Kidney.** Most lupus patients have some clinical and pathologic evidence of renal involvement. Active disease often is announced by abnormalities in the urinary sediment (i.e., red blood cells, white blood cells, or cellular casts formed in the absence of acute bacterial infection). Other clinical laboratory features typically associated with active renal disease are elevations in serum creatinine and blood urea nitrogen (BUN) levels (chronic elevations can be caused by scarring from old disease); decreased levels of serum complement components or increased titers of antibodies against double-stranded DNA are immunologic features that parallel renal disease activity in many, but not all, patients. The renal biopsy often can aid in treatment decisions and the determination of prognosis, although the biopsy pathology may change with disease course or therapy.

   (1) **Mesangial disease** is the most common and mildest form of renal involve-

ment and may be asymptomatic. Many patients have mild proteinuria or red or white cells in the urinalysis. Treatment usually is not required.

(2) **Focal proliferative nephritis** often has a good prognosis as well and typically requires treatment with corticosteroids alone; however, its more severe presentations blend with diffuse proliferative nephritis clinically and prognostically.

(3) **Diffuse proliferative nephritis** is the most severe pathologic lesion and usually is associated with hypertension, severe proteinuria, and some degree of renal insufficiency. The most severe cases can be associated with **crescents** and the rapid development of severe renal insufficiency. Corticosteroids and cytotoxic agents typically are required for preservation of renal function.

(4) **Membranous glomerulopathy** classically presents as large amounts of protein in the urine and nephrotic syndrome, usually with relatively few cells in the urine. Corticosteroid therapy may help control the protein loss. Slowly progressive renal insufficiency may develop over time; it is not clear whether the addition of cytotoxic agents retards this progression.

g. **Muscle and bone. Arthralgia** and **symmetrical arthritis** often are features of acute SLE, but the rare joint deformities (**Jaccoud's arthropathy**) that occur are a function of tendon or ligament laxity rather than erosive joint disease. Inflammatory muscle involvement usually is subclinical, but clinical inflammatory myopathy can occur.

h. **Other.** Photosensitivity can trigger systemic symptoms as well as skin manifestations. Raynaud's phenomenon and secondary Sjögren's syndrome each occur in approximately 25% of patients.

2. **Laboratory findings**

a. **Hematologic findings.** Anemia is common during active disease and more often is the anemia of chronic disease than hemolytic anemia. Antibodies to leukocytes also occur, with autoimmune lymphopenia a common feature of active disease; neutropenia is less common. Antibodies to platelets can cause chronic immune thrombocytopenia or more acute falls in the platelet count with active disease. Elevation of the erythrocyte sedimentation rate is common and in some patients correlates with disease activity.

b. **Coagulation parameters.** Antibodies to the phospholipid components of individual clotting factors can interfere with coagulation testing, causing prolongation of the partial thromboplastin time (PTT) not correctable by the addition of normal plasma. Paradoxically, patients with the PTT prolongation (the **"lupus anticoagulant"**) have a higher frequency of thrombosis than bleeding.

c. **Serologic findings.** Phospholipid antibodies also can cause false-positive test results for syphilis, more often by interference with reagin [e.g., rapid plasma reagin (RPR) or Venereal Disease Research Laboratories (VDRL)] testing than with antitreponemal [e.g., fluorescent treponemal antibody absorption (FTA-ABS)] testing.

d. **Immunologic findings.** Lupus patients commonly have **low complement component (C3 and C4) levels** as a result of immune complex activation; in many patients, falls in serum complement levels parallel disease flare-ups if complement synthesis is unchanged. **Hypergammaglobulinemia** reflects B cell hyperactivity. By far the most significant immunologic findings in SLE patients are **autoantibodies.**

(1) **ANAs.** Approximately 99% of patients with SLE have ANAs. These antibodies are detectable by an immunofluorescence technique that involves human epithelial cell lines (e.g., HEp-2 cells). When the test serum is applied to the epithelial cells that have been frozen and cut to expose nuclear components, the patient's ANAs interact with the nuclear material, and this interaction can be detected by fluorescence microscopy. A **diffuse** or **homogeneous** immunofluorescent staining **pattern** is most common in SLE, although **speckled, nucleolar,** and **rim patterns** also can be seen.

(a) **Antibodies** to **double-stranded DNA** are found in over 65% of SLE patients with active disease; they are found less often or at lower titer in patients with inactive disease. When present, they are fairly specific for a diagnosis of SLE. Some of these antibodies give a **rim pattern** of ANA nuclear fluorescence.

(b) **Antibodies** to **histones.** Patients either with SLE or the drug-induced lupus syndrome can have antibodies to the structural proteins of DNA. These antibodies often yield **homogeneous** or **diffuse pattern** ANAs.

(c) **Antibodies** to **small nuclear ribonucleoproteins (SnRNPs)** frequently are present in SLE.

   (i) Two of these, **antibody** to **Smith (Sm) antigen** and **antibody** to **U$_1$RNP,** commonly give **speckled patterns** of immunofluorescence on ANA substrates. The Sm antigen includes the U$_1$RNP epitope as well as several other uridine-rich RNPs (uRNPs), so lupus patients with antibody to Sm often have antibodies to U$_1$RNP, but the converse is not true. Antibody to Sm is relatively specific for SLE; isolated antibody to U$_1$RNP is seen in **mixed connective tissue disease.**

   (ii) Antibodies to another snRNP, the **Ro particle,** are typically found by precipitin testing rather than immunofluorescence, although patients with antibody to Ro may have positive ANAs when tested against the new HEp-2 cell lines. Antibody to Ro typically is associated with forms of SLE that have prominent dermatologic and photosensitive components and also is a marker for Sjögren's syndrome. It is present in most cases of **ANA-negative SLE.**

   (iii) Patients with SLE and Sjögren's syndrome also may have antibodies to a related snRNP, **La,** which are almost always found in patients who also have antibody to Ro.

(2) **Antibodies** to **membrane** and **cytoplasmic components.** Antibodies to transfer RNA (tRNA) and ribosomal nucleoproteins can be found in SLE. Other cytoplasmic autoantibodies possibly are made to cell membrane constituents (e.g., phospholipids) and are responsible for the tissue specificity of some autoantibodies (e.g., antibodies to gastric parietal cells, thyroid epithelial cells, and blood cellular elements).

G. **Diagnosis** of SLE involves careful consideration of historical and physical findings that suggest this multisystem disease. A common presentation would be a systemically ill patient with characteristic rash, polyarthritis, and serositis, but the possibility of lupus should be entertained even when patients present with seemingly isolated hematologic cytopenias, CNS disease, or glomerulonephritis. In suspicious settings, the physician seeks laboratory evidence of autoimmunity and attempts to exclude other illnesses.

1. **Diagnostic criteria** (Table 10-8). The 1982 American Rheumatism Association revised criteria for the diagnosis of SLE are useful when the disease is suspected, and the presence over time of any four of the eleven criteria strongly suggests the diagnosis. Although findings such as alopecia, periungual vasculitis, and low serum complement levels are not part of the criteria, they may be supportive evidence in individual patients.

2. **Differential diagnosis.** The physician must be careful to exclude other chronic rheumatic diseases, especially rheumatoid arthritis, overlap syndromes (inflammatory myopathies or scleroderma overlapping with SLE), and vasculitic syndromes, in arriving at the diagnosis of SLE. The following syndromes also should be considered in the setting of possible SLE.

   a. **Mixed connective tissue disease** is a term used to describe patients with clinical features of several connective tissue diseases and high titers of antibody to U$_1$RNP. Patients with this disease may have cutaneous features of SLE, dermatomyositis, or scleroderma; inflammatory muscle disease; and a destructive form of arthritis more typical of rheumatoid arthritis. Furthermore, the severe renal and CNS manifestations of SLE usually are not present. When followed for pro-

TABLE 10-8. The 1982 American Rheumatism Association Revised Criteria for Classification of Systemic Lupus Erythematosus

Criterion	Definition
Malar rash	Fixed erythema, flat or raised, over the malar eminences, tending to spare the nasolabial folds
Discoid rash	Erythematous raised patches with adherent keratotic scaling and follicular plugging; atrophic scarring may occur in older lesions
Photosensitivity	Skin rash as a result of unusual reaction to sunlight—documented by patient history or observed by a physician
Oral ulcers	Oral or nasopharyngeal uleration, usually painless—observed by a physician
Arthritis	Nonerosive arthritis involving two or more peripheral joints, characterized by tenderness, swelling, or effusion
Serositis	Pleuritis—convincing history of pleuritic pain or friction rub heard by a physician or evidence of pleural effusion **or** Pericarditis—documented by ECG or friction rub or evidence of pericardial effusion
Renal disorder	Persistent proteinuria exceeding 0.5 g/day or greater than 3+ if quantitation not performed **or** Cellular casts—may be red cell, hemoglobin, granular, tubular, or mixed
Neurologic disorder	Seizures—in the absence of offending drugs or known metabolic derangements (e.g., uremia, ketoacidosis, electrolyte imbalance) **or** Psychosis—in the absence of offending drugs or known metabolic derangements (e.g., uremia, ketoacidosis, electrolyte imbalance)
Hematologic disorder	Hemolytic anemia—with reticulocytosis **or** Leukopenia—less than 4000/μl total on two or more occasions **or** Lymphopenia—less than 1500/μl on two or more occasions **or** Thrombocytopenia—less than 100,000/μl in the absence of offending drugs
Immunologic disorder	Positive LE cell preparation **or** Antibody to native DNA in abnormal titer **or** Antibody to Smith nuclear antigen **or** False-positive serologic test for syphilis known to be positive for at least 6 months and confirmed by *Treponema pallidum* immobilization or fluorescent treponemal antibody absorption (FTA-ABS) test
Antinuclear antibody	An abnormal titer of antinuclear antibody by immunofluorescence or an equivalent assay at any point in time and in the absence of drugs known to be associated with drug-induced lupus syndrome

Reprinted from Tan EM, Cohen AS, Fries JF, et al American Rheumatism Association: 1982 revised criteria for the classification of systemic lupus erythematosus (SLE). *Arthritis Rheum* 25:1271–1277, 1982.

longed periods of time, most patients with this disease more closely resemble patients with scleroderma or SLE.

b. **Drug-induced lupus.** Chronic ingestion of several drugs can precipitate a syndrome of **polyserositis, arthritis,** and **antihistone ANAs.** The drugs most commonly associated include hydralazine, procainamide, penicillamine, isoniazid, and phenytoin. Renal disease is rare in this syndrome, and dermal and CNS features are less common than in idiopathic SLE. Drug-induced SLE typically resolves upon discontinuation of the drug. Hepatic acetylation of drugs such as hydralazine, isoniazid, and procainamide is apparently slow in patients who develop this syndrome, although these drugs typically are tolerated well by patients with SLE.

c. **Discoid lupus.** Patients can have typical skin manifestations of SLE without systemic disease. Fifteen percent of these patients have positive ANAs. These patients should be considered to have SLE when other disease features are present.

3. **Associated syndromes**

a. **Neonatal lupus syndrome** can develop in infants of mothers who have high-titer **IgG antibodies** to **Ro.** In this syndrome, the maternal antibodies apparently cross the placenta, bind to fetal tissue, and cause immunologic injury. The most typical features include evanescent lupus skin lesions, but transient thrombocytopenia or hemolytic anemia can occur. The most serious clinical presentation occurs when the antibody to Ro binds to fetal cardiac tissue and causes congenital heart block, which can require permanent pacing. Most mothers of affected infants develop a mild version of some autoimmune disease over time, often SLE.

b. **Phospholipid antibody** syndrome can occur as a mimic of SLE or as part of the disease. One-third to half of lupus patients exhibit phospholipid antibody if tested, although the associated clinical syndrome occurs less commonly.

(1) Antibodies to phospholipid can be detected by finding that patients exhibit **prolonged PTTs** (associated with the presence of lupus anticoagulant when tested), **false-positive syphilis serologies** (RPR or VDRL), or **anticardiolipin (antiphospholipid) tests** when assayed. Patients may have positive results on one or all of these tests and still have the clinical syndrome, which paradoxically involves **hypercoagulability** rather than the tendency to hemorrhage expected by a prolonged PTT.

(2) Manifestations most commonly include **venous or arterial thromboses,** sometimes of large vessels, and can also include **episodic thrombocytopenia. Pregnant patients may experience fetal death** after the first trimester or premature birth, and these problems may recur in successive pregnancies. Some of these patients exhibit placental thrombosis, infarction, or insufficiency, but the cause of fetal death is not always clear.

(3) **Management** primarily involves **chronic anticoagulation therapy,** typically with warfarin, after the first episode of clinical thrombosis.

H. **Therapy** for SLE must be individualized to the features that a particular patient exhibits, and it need not always include corticosteroids. Patients must understand that the prognosis in this chronic disease generally is better than they fear and that their compliance with medication regimens and avoidance of disease precipitants (e.g., ultraviolet light, emotional stress) often can favorably affect the disease course. Physicians must be alert to disease flares related to surgery, antecedent infections, or the postpartum period. Sulfonamides and oral contraceptives may precipitate flare-up of disease in some patients.

1. **Sunscreens.** Topical sunscreens containing para-aminobenzoic acid (PABA) or benzophenones are effective in protecting the one-third of lupus patients who are photosensitive.

2. **NSAIDs** are used in full anti-inflammatory doses for fever, joint complaints, and serositis. Mild elevation in transaminase levels often develops in SLE patients on

these drugs, and aseptic meningitis has been reported in lupus patients on ibuprofen, tolmetin, and sulindac.

3. **Antimalarial drugs** (e.g., hydroxychloroquine, choloroquine) often are used to treat fatigue, skin disease, and arthritis in patients with SLE. Retinal pigmentary deposition leading to blindness is a rare complication of antimalarial treatment since hydroxychloroquine replaced chloroquine, but patients should be screened by an ophthalmologist at 6-month intervals.

4. **Corticosteroids**
   a. **Topical preparations.** Some of the skin manifestations are improved by treatment with topical glucocorticoids two to three times daily, although discoid lesions usually require additional treatment with antimalarial agents.
   b. **Systemic corticosteroids**
      (1) **Glucocorticoids** in varying doses are often required to control severe manifestations of SLE and less severe symptoms when they are persistent and disabling. These drugs should be used cautiously, because long-term treatment usually is needed and typical side effects ensue. **Chronic arthritis** and **serositis** may require glucocorticoids if NSAIDs are not sufficient. Severe **hemolysis,** life-threatening **thrombocytopenia, pneumonitis, CNS** or **peripheral nervous system disease,** clinically evident **cardiac** or **skeletal muscle disease, renal disease,** and **vasculitis** are typical indications for systemic glucocorticoids. Usually the drug dosage selected is proportionate to the severity of the illness; the dosage is tapered as manifestations subside. Alternate-day therapy is ideal for patients with only nephritis, but patients who are systemically ill typically require daily doses.
      (2) **"Pulse" corticosteroids.** Large doses of corticosteroids sometimes are administered intravenously for particularly severe cases of SLE. Serious **renal** and **CNS manifestations** have been the typical indications for pulse treatment, but dangerous **cardiopulmonary** and **hematologic involvement** also might warrant this aggressive treatment.

5. **Cytotoxic agents** (e.g., azathioprine, cyclophosphamide) sometimes are employed to treat severe, refractory features of lupus, particularly **renal disease.** Intravenous "pulse" use of cyclophosphamide has become popular for the treatment of diffuse proliferative glomerulonephritis and acute severe manifestations of lupus refractory to corticosteroids.

6. **Intravenous immunoglobulin.** Large doses of immunoglobulin have been given intravenously to treat refractory manifestations of lupus, particularly **immune-mediated thrombocytopenia** or **hemolytic anemia.** Typical doses are 400 mg/kg, administered daily for 5 days. This therapy is expensive, often must be given monthly, and **cannot be given to IgA deficient patients** because of the risk of anaphylaxis.

7. **Plasma exchange.** Removal of antibodies by **plasmapheresis** and replacement of globulin fractions with albumin or fresh frozen plasma can temporarily remove pathologic antibodies in patients with lupus but is associated with a quick rebound in antibody levels if immunosuppression is not also used. Although this therapy is not of major effect in lupus, it may have a place in life-threatening lupus manifestations. When cytotoxic therapy is used with plasmapheresis, plasma exchange precedes intravenous cyclophosphamide "pulses" in the hope that antibody-secreting cells stimulated by the antibody removal phase will then be more susceptible to destruction by the alkylating agent.

8. **Ancillary drugs** are important in managing particular features of the disease. Phenytoin and phenobarbital are useful in the control of seizure disorders, and antipsychotic agents with or without corticosteroids help treat acute or chronic psychoses.

I. **Prognosis** clearly is better today than in the presteroid era; milder forms of disease are recognized and, presumably, appropriate drug treatment improves morbidity and mortality rates. **Renal disease** and **infectious complications** are still major causes of death, and prominent **CNS disease** can lead to severe disability. The mortality rate is higher in patients of lower socioeconomic status and educational attainment, a characteristic common to many chronic illnesses. Steroid-related complications can be crippling (e.g., avascular necrosis of the femoral head and osteoporotic vertebral fractures) or fatal (e.g., premature coronary atherosclerosis).

VIII. SCLERODERMA

A. Definition. Scleroderma (systemic sclerosis) is a connective tissue disease characterized by widespread **small vessel obliterative disease** and **fibrosis of the skin** (especially distal, digital skin) and **multiple internal organs,** including the heart, lungs, kidneys, and gastrointestinal tract. The description best fits the diffuse form, but localized forms also exist. These latter forms involve patches of skin and subcutaneous tissues but do not include digital skin involvement, Raynaud's phenomenon, or internal organ changes.

B. Epidemiology. Scleroderma is a relatively rare disease; familial clustering is uncommon. The disease is three to four times more common in women than in men. Coal miners are at a higher risk for the disease, possibly as a result of exposure to silica dust.

C. Etiology. The etiology of scleroderma is unknown. In some cases it seems likely that an environmental agent (e.g., toxin, virus) causes vascular endothelial injury, with later immunologic responses leading to continued endothelial damage and tissue fibrosis. Supportive evidence includes the initiation of a fibrosing syndrome in patients with polyvinyl chloride exposure, Spanish "toxic oil" syndrome, and L-tryptophan–related eosinophilia myalgia syndrome (EMS).

D. Pathogenesis. Whether the initiating event is environmental or immunologic, the early lesion seems to be one of **vascular endothelial damage,** especially in small vessels. Unregulated immunologic processes appear to be responsible for continuing vascular damage and widespread **dermal** and **internal organ fibrosis.**

1. **Vascular endothelial damage. Intimal hyperplasia** of small vessels in skin and internal organs occurs at the earliest stage of disease. **Luminal narrowing** from this endothelial fibrotic process can lead to tissue ischemia; this process is enhanced by release of the potent vasoconstrictor endothelin from damaged vessels. **Physiologic vasoconstrictive stimuli** (e.g., cold, emotion, platelet-derived thromboxane A_2, serotonin) can result in further narrowing and symptomatic **Raynaud's phenomenon** in skin or internal organs. Local release of the physiologic vasodilators nitric acid and endothelium-derived relaxation factor (EDRF) is diminished in damaged vessels. In patients with renal vascular involvement, increased renin–angiotensin production can cause a vicious circle of vasoconstriction, which is the presumed mechanism for **renal crisis** in this illness.

2. **Tissue fibrosis** may be caused by the healing of ischemic lesions from small vessel injury and from immune processes causing increased fibroblastic activity. **Cytokines** and **growth factors** secreted by lymphocytes, monocytes, and platelets (e.g., PDGF, TGF-β) lead to increased secretion of collagen and ground substance by fibroblasts with the consequent development of fibrotic lesions. Mast cells are present in increased amounts in scleroderma skin and may interact with lymphocytes in cytokine-driven fibroblast activation.

3. **Autoantibodies.** Scleroderma patients often demonstrate ANAs; their relationship in scleroderma patients to disease pathogenesis is unknown, but these antibodies may help to distinguish subsets of the illness (see VIII E 2).

E. Clinicopathologic features

1. **Organ involvement.** The degree of skin change and the type and progression of internal organ involvement are different in the **limited form** as compared to the **diffuse form** of scleroderma. Also, spontaneous fluctuations in disease activity can occur.

   a. **Skin involvement** occurs in **95% of patients** with scleroderma. An early **edematous phase** of small vessel endothelial injury and increased permeability may progress through an **indurative phase** as increasing amounts of collagen are produced in the subcutaneous tissue. Epidermal and skin appendage atrophy may occur in late forms of the disease **(atrophic phase)** as the skin becomes progressively bound to underlying tissue.

      (1) **Distribution.** Changes most often begin in the fingers and hands and may spread to involve more proximal tissues including the trunk and face. The lower extremities often are less severely involved.

      (2) **Associated features**

         (a) **Raynaud's phenomenon** occurs in **95% of patients** with scleroderma. Episodic vasospasm of the damaged small vessels in the digits results in a **triphasic color change** of the involved area as blood flow ceases (white), returns sluggishly (blue), and exhibits reactive hyperemia (red).

         (b) **Telangiectasias** can occur in involved areas as well as on mucous membranes.

         (c) **Subcutaneous calcifications** can occur, especially in finger tips.

         (d) **Salt-and-pepper changes.** The skin can become taut, shiny, and immobile, and hyperpigmented areas can alternate with depigmented areas.

         (e) **Microcapillary abnormalities.** The distal nail bed proliferates and the capillary bed becomes visibly abnormal, with dilatation, tortuosity, and loss of vessels. These abnormalities can be seen in patients by examining the proximal nail beds with wide-field microscopy.

         (f) **Skin ulcers.** Distal digital ulcers and finger tapering occur due to distal infarctions and consequent loss of digital pulp, sometimes resulting in infection.

   b. **Gastrointestinal tract**

      (1) **Esophageal dysfunction** is the most common manifestation of internal organ involvement. **Esophageal motility dysfunction** and **reflux** develop as collagen replaces smooth muscle in the lower two-thirds of the esophagus; striated muscle in the upper one-third of the esophagus is relatively unaffected. **Esophageal strictures** can result from the constant reflux, and **ulceration** can occur at the gastroesophageal junction. Barium swallow and esophageal manometry may be helpful in documenting disease extent.

      (2) **Similar small bowel involvement** leads to intestinal hypomotility and intermittent cramping, diarrhea, and **bacterial overgrowth malabsorption syndrome. Wide-mouth diverticuli** can be seen in the transverse and descending colon in areas of patchy muscularis involvement. Lower gastrointestinal contrast radiographic studies or malabsorption testing may demonstrate small bowel or colonic involvement.

   c. **Lung.** Widespread small pulmonary arterial narrowing and fibrotic change eventually can lead to **isolated pulmonary hypertension.** More commonly, a fibrotic proliferation in the peribronchial and perialveolar tissues leads to progressive **interstitial lung disease.** Patients with interstitial lung disease present with symptoms of progressive dyspnea on exertion and demonstrate a restrictive pattern on pulmonary function testing, a better disease indicator than chest x-ray changes. Pleuritis is uncommon in scleroderma as compared to other rheumatic diseases (e.g., rheumatoid arthritis, SLE).

   d. **Heart.** Clinical cardiac involvement can take several forms. Clinically, acute and chronic pericarditis are unusual, but effusions often can be seen on ultrasonography and are associated with myocardial involvement. If interstitial myocardial disease is extensive, frank **cardiomyopathy** can result, producing congestive heart failure, arrhythmias, and conduction disturbances. Angina can be a result of fibrotic involvement of small myocardial vessels. Ambulatory electro-cardiogram (ECG) monitoring or exercise stress testing can help to uncover dangerous arrhythmias or subtle ischemia in need of treatment.

e. **Kidney.** Sudden renal failure **(scleroderma renal crisis)** can occur often as a combination of interlobular artery fibrotic damage and some vasoconstrictive stimulus (e.g., diuresis, blood loss, surgery). Massive renin–angiotensin release in response to decreased renal perfusion worsens the vasoconstriction, and acute renal failure can occur. **Malignant hypertension** and **microangiopathic hemolytic anemia** often accompany these renal events. **Chronic renal failure** and **death** occur unless emergent treatment restores renal perfusion. Some but not all patients demonstrate new hypertension, urinary protein, or elevated serum creatinine testing before acute renal decompensation, so these features should be monitored periodically.

f. **Muscle.** In many patients, a mild indolent myopathy manifested by minor enzyme elevations and perhaps mild weakness occurs but does not require treatment. In some patients, an overt **inflammatory myopathy** identical to polymyositis can occur **("overlap" presentation).**

g. **Joint and tendon.** More than 50% of patients with scleroderma develop swelling, stiffness, and pain in finger, wrist, and knee joints. Mild, self-limited inflammatory arthritis can occur early in the disease, but typical joint involvement is limited to synovial fibrosis and impaired range of motion due to the generalized restriction of the fibrotic process. Tendon sheath involvement is not unusual; carpal tunnel syndrome can result from extensive tendon sheath fibrosis in the wrist.

h. **Nerve.** Neurologic involvement typically is limited to fibrotic **entrapment neuropathies** of the median and trigeminal nerves.

2. **Clinical syndromes.** Classification of the disease into **limited** and **diffuse forms** is important because of differences in organ involvement and, thus, prognosis. In general, the more widespread visceral involvement of the diffuse form gives it a poorer prognosis than the limited variant. Scleroderma can also exist in **overlap forms,** the most distinct of which is called **mixed connective tissue disease.**

a. **Diffuse scleroderma** is typified by **proximal skin involvement** (skin proximal to the MCP joints or forearms in various definitions) and the presence of **Scl-70 antibodies** or **antinucleolar ANAs.** Visceral organ involvement in this form typically occurs earlier than in the limited variant. Renal involvement is much more common than in the limited form, and pulmonary fibrosis occurs earlier and more quickly.

b. **Limited scleroderma** typically has skin involvement limited to the distal extremities and face, and also is known as the **CREST variant** (involving the coexistence of subcutaneous **calcinosis, Raynaud's phenomenon, esophageal motility dysfunction, sclerodactyly,** and **telangiectasia). Anticentromere antibody** is most closely associated with this form, and visceral involvement is usually more slowly progressive than in the diffuse form. One exception is the early development of **pulmonary vascular hypertension** in this form due to obliterative changes in pulmonary arterioles. The pulmonary fibrosis so typical of the diffuse variant occurs more slowly in this form but can become severe after several decades of disease.

c. **Mixed connective tissue disease** is a rheumatic syndrome that can include clinical features of scleroderma, SLE, and polymyositis in association with the presence of high titers of **antibody** to **U_1RNP.** Most cases evolve into more typical scleroderma or SLE over time.

F. Diagnosis

1. **Clinical approach.** A diagnosis of scleroderma should be entertained in the presence of symptoms of **Raynaud's phenomenon, distal skin thickening,** and **visceral organ involvement.** In addition to physical evidence of internal organ change, the physician should evaluate distal nail beds for the suggestive capillary abnormality and attempt to document the location and extent of the skin thickening to differen-

tiate local from generalized forms. Characteristic ANA test results may also be useful in classifying patients.

a. Raynaud's phenomenon. The abnormal vascular response to cold or emotional stimuli is present in most patients with the diffuse or limited form of scleroderma, but most patients with Raynaud's phenomenon do not have scleroderma or another form of connective tissue disease. As many as 5%–10% of nonsmoking individuals in population surveys may have Raynaud's phenomenon; typical screening procedures for scleroderma would include examination for finger edema, fingernail-fold capillary abnormalities, and ANAs. Patients with none of these features are unlikely to develop scleroderma. Because patients can have Raynaud's phenomenon in association with other connective tissue diseases (SLE, polymyositis), a clinical search for these illnesses should be made as well.

b. Distal skin thickening is a diagnostic feature of both the diffuse and limited forms of scleroderma. Patients with diffuse scleroderma also have more proximal involvement, typically of the upper arms, upper legs, or trunk. Fewer than 5% of patients may have visceral involvement typical of scleroderma without skin thickening (**scleroderma sine scleroderma**).

c. Laboratory findings. Differences in ANA testing may discriminate between diffuse and limited forms of scleroderma. Patients with the diffuse form often have **Scl-70 antibodies** or **antinucleolar ANAs.** Patients with the more limited forms often have **anticentromere antibodies.**

d. Visceral involvement. Typical internal organ involvement (see VIII E 1) will lend further support for scleroderma diagnosis and help discriminate between diffuse and limited forms.

2. **Differential diagnosis.** Skin thickening can be seen in other illnesses besides scleroderma. Typically, Raynaud's phenomenon, the characteristic distal hand involvement, and visceral organ changes of scleroderma are absent.

a. Local scleroderma. Two forms of purely local disease, **morphea** and **linear scleroderma,** have similar clinical and pathologic appearance to sclerodermatous skin. These forms present as localized fibrotic plaques (morphea) or as longitudinal bands (linear scleroderma).

    (1) Morphea may present at any age (it is more common in childhood) as a disease characterized by small circumscribed skin lesions (**guttate morphea**) or larger patches (**morphea en plaque**). Some patients with chronic Lyme disease have very similar atrophic skin lesions, so an appropriate clinical syndrome should be sought and Lyme serology obtained in these patients.

    (2) Linear scleroderma occurs most commonly in children and young adults. Facial involvement (**coup de sabre**) can be extremely disfiguring. The principal impact of linear scleroderma can be interference with function or growth of underlying muscle or bone leading to extremity wasting or contractures.

b. Eosinophilic fasciitis. Pain, swelling, and tenderness develop in one or more extremities, sometimes after an episode of vigorous exercise. Induration of involved skin and subcutaneous tissue develops, but without Raynaud's phenomenon or sclerodactyly. Patients often have marked peripheral blood eosinophilia, and a full-thickness skin biopsy (including underlying fascia and muscle) is required to demonstrate the deep fascial eosinophils and chronic inflammatory cell infiltrate.

c. Eosinophilia–myalgia syndrome. A new clinical syndrome related to the ingestion of ʟ-**tryptophan dietary supplements** can be confused with scleroderma (due to the skin thickening in some cases) and may be responsible for some cases of eosinophilic fasciitis. Patients who take ʟ-tryptophan likely have ingested a toxic contaminant generated by the synthetic process, although some may metabolize ʟ-tryptophan abnormally. The cornerstones of diagnosis are **eosinophilia (> 1000/μl) and severe myalgia** found in the absence of other possible causes. Variable features include skin rashes and induration, interstitial pulmonary infiltrates, and polyneuropathy. Elevation of muscle enzymes [aldolase, not creatine kinase (CK)] and hepatic enzymes also can occur.

G. **Therapy**

1. **General.** No therapy is of proven value in scleroderma. Trials of D-**penicillamine** suggest possible effectiveness in slowing skin and internal organ involvement.

2. **Specific disease features**

a. **Skin involvement.** D-Penicillamine appears to be effective in slowing or reversing skin involvement in the diffuse form, particularly when used early in disease. **Nitroglycerin ointment** applied directly to fingertip ulcerations may help heal them. **Colchicine** helps to prevent painful inflammatory episodes related to subcutaneous calcinosis. **Interferon gamma** may inhibit fibroblast proliferation and collagen production; it has helped improve skin thickening in non-blinded trials.

b. **Raynaud's phenomenon.** Patients should understand the need to cover their head, hands, and trunk in cold weather to minimize reflex vasoconstriction, and smoking should be discouraged. **Calcium channel blocking agents** are the most useful vasodilating agents in the treatment of scleroderma. **Intravenous prostaglandin infusions** have been used with success for treating refractory vasospastic episodes and for healing skin ulcerations. **Ketanserin,** a serotonin antagonist, has helped heal digital skin ulcers.

c. **Esophageal involvement** should be managed by the usual antireflux measures. **Mucosal protective agents** (e.g., sucralfate) and **histamine (H_2)-receptor blockers** (e.g., cimetidine) may be added to antacids for symptomatic reflux esophagitis, and **omeprazole** (a proton pump inhibitor) can he used for refractory esophagitis symptoms. **Cisapride,** a prokinetic agent, may help treat reflux and motility disorders.

d. **Interstitial pulmonary involvement** may be treated with **corticosteroids** or D-**penicillamine,** but neither treatment is clearly efficacious. A 6-month regimen of daily **oral cyclophosphamide with prednisone** may be the most effective therapy for progressive pulmonary fibrosis. Tobacco smoking may be synergistic in pulmonary injury. No treatment is known to be effective for the primary pulmonary hypertension-like syndrome, although **vasodilators** and **intravenous prostaglandins** are often used.

e. **Lower gastrointestinal involvement.** Bacterial overgrowth malabsorption may be improved by treatment with **broad-spectrum antibiotics** (e.g., tetracycline). **Prokinetic agents** (e.g., octreotide, cisapride) help constipation and bloating related to lower gastrointestinal motility dysfunction.

f. **Muscle involvement.** When inflammatory myositis occurs in overlap syndromes, **corticosteroids** are used, as in polymyositis. **NSAIDs** (e.g., aspirin) should be used in treating articular symptoms.

g. **Renal involvement** is best managed by aggressive control of hypertension. The **angiotensin-converting enzyme (ACE) inhibitors** (e.g., captopril, enalapril) are major advances in controlling blood pressure in patients with scleroderma and may help to reverse the angiotensin-dependent vasoconstrictive state of scleroderma renal crisis. The avoidance of hypovolemia in diuresis and in the perioperative state is important.

h. **Cardiac involvement.** Medications useful for control of angina, congestive heart failure, and arrhythmias are employed when these complications occur.

IX. **INFLAMMATORY MYOPATHIES (POLYMYOSITIS AND DERMATOMYOSITIS)**

A. **Definition. Polymyositis** is an idiopathic inflammatory muscle disease associated with prominent proximal muscle weakness, muscle enzyme elevations, characteristic myopathic electromyogram (EMG) patterns, and inflammatory infiltrates on muscle biopsy. When this complex is accompanied by a characteristic rash it is called **dermatomyositis.** Dermatomyositis is much more common than polymyositis in children.

B. **Epidemiology.** Polymyositis is a rare disease, occurring in approximately 1 in 200,000 individuals, with a peak incidence in childhood and in late adulthood. It is twice as common in females as in males and may be associated with malignancy in the adult-onset form.

C. **Etiology and pathogenesis.** The basic cause of polymyositis is unknown. However, it is believed that an initiating viral infection and altered immune responses are potentially important in causation and pathogenesis. Lymphocyte-mediated muscle cell damage is thought to be the central pathogenetic factor in this disease, although small vessel damage is also an important factor in dermatomyositis.

1. **Infections** can cause acute myositis.
   a. **Elevated titers of antibodies to picornaviruses** (e.g., coxsackievirus B) have been found in some juvenile dermatomyositis patients, and high titers of antibodies to *Toxoplasma gondii* have been found in some adult polymyositis patients.
   b. Isolation of these organisms from muscle of patients with polymyositis or dermatomyositis has not been accomplished, and antibiotic treatment for toxoplasmosis has not improved myositis in patients with high titers of antibody to *T. gondii.*

2. **Autoimmunity**
   a. **Humoral.** Most patients with inflammatory myopathies demonstrate autoantibodies when human tumor cell lines [i.e., human epithelial cells **(HEp-2)**] are used as testing substrate, but it is not known whether these antibodies interfere with the normal physiologic function of their antigens. **Molecular mimicry** may be important in polymyositis/dermatomyositis, because autoantibodies directed against tRNA synthetases are found in some patients, perhaps resulting from mimicry between a virus and an epitope on the intracellular enzyme. Vascular deposits of immune complexes and complement are associated with endothelial cell injury and small vessel obstruction in dermatomyositis, especially in juvenile dermatomyositis.
   b. **Cellular**
      (1) **Polymositis.** Peripheral blood lymphocytes from polymyositis patients produce a lymphotoxin that is cytotoxic to muscle cells. In addition, cytotoxic CD8$^+$ T cells are the predominant cell type found in the inflammatory infiltrate in muscle, apparently attacking muscle cells expressing increased numbers of class I MHC-restricted markers.
      (2) **Dermatomyositis.** Some studies suggest that CD4$^+$ T cells and B cells are predominant in dermatomyositis infiltrates, in contrast to the predominantly CD8$^+$ T-cell infiltrates in polymyositis. Perhaps humoral mechanisms are relatively more important in dermatomyositis than in polymyositis.

D. **Pathology.** The major sites of inflammation are skeletal muscle and, less commonly, cardiac muscle. Skin involvement is a minor pathologic feature.

1. **Inflammatory infiltrate.** Lymphocytes and plasma cells are the predominant inflammatory cells, although macrophages, eosinophils, and neutrophils also can be seen in muscle tissue. CD8$^+$ cells infiltrate muscle fibers in polymyositis. In dermatomyositis, CD4$^+$ cells and B cells often are clustered around small blood vessels within the muscle.

2. **Muscle fiber damage.** Spotty muscle fiber necrosis and degeneration occur, with loss of cross striations and variation in the size of surviving fibers. Increased numbers of muscle nuclei and enhanced basophilic staining of fibers indicate regeneration in the midst of cell death. Interstitial fibrotic infiltrates occur in chronic cases.

E. **Clinical features.** Inflammatory myopathies are clinically grouped into specific syndromes, depending on specific organ manifestations and laboratory findings.

1. **Organ involvement**
   a. **Skin.** The rash of dermatomyositis consists of erythematous patches, which sometimes are scaling or atrophic and are distributed over the face, neck, upper chest, and extensor surfaces. Only scattered inflammatory infiltrates in the dermis are evident on biopsy.
      (1) Pathognomonic skin findings include **heliotrope lids** (a violet discoloration and swelling of the eyelids) and **Gottron's sign** (heaped-up erythematous papules over the MCP or PIP joints).
      (2) Other significant findings include **mechanic's hands** (roughened erythematous skin and hypertrophic changes of the palms and fingers) as well as the erythematous **V sign** (anterior chest) and **shawl sign** (neck and upper back).
   b. **Lung.** Chronic interstitial lung disease can occur, especially in association with synthetase antibodies. Aspiration pneumonitis and ventilatory insufficiency also can occur.
   c. **Joint.** A mild, symmetrical inflammatory arthritis occurs uncommonly and rarely is destructive; it is seen most often in patients with the synthetase antibodies [see IX E 2 b (2)(a)].
   d. **Muscle.** Most patients have gradual but steady progression of muscle weakness; however, some patients have such fulminant courses that **acute respiratory failure** or **myoglobinuric renal failure** can ensue.
      (1) **Skeletal muscle weakness** is the primary manifestation of polymyositis.
         (a) **Symmetrical, proximal, upper and lower extremity weakness** occurs, causing difficulty with rising from a chair, sitting up in bed, or combing hair.
         (b) **Pharyngeal muscle involvement** can lead to swallowing difficulties and aspiration, and respiratory muscle dysfunction can lead to respiratory failure.
      (2) **Cardiac muscle involvement** is not as common, but when it occurs it presents as cardiomyopathy with congestive heart failure, arrhythmias, and conduction disturbances.

2. **Laboratory findings**
   a. **Muscle enzymes.** An increased concentration of enzymes typically present in skeletal muscle is prominent in polymyositis. **CK** and **aldolase** are routinely measured, and CK fractionation may suggest myocardial involvement if the **MB fraction** (i.e., the CK isoenzyme found mainly in myocardium but also in regenerating skeletal muscle) is increased. However, in most patients, CK elevation is caused by the **MM band** (i.e., the fraction most prevalent in skeletal muscle). Serum **myoglobin** levels are also elevated in most patients and may be more sensitive than CK levels in some myositis patients. Enzyme elevations usually correlate with activity of the muscle disease and are used as a parameter to evaluate treatment response.
   b. **Autoantibodies.** Most patients with polymyositis/dermatomyositis (80%–90%) have antibodies to nuclear or cytoplasmic antigens. Routine ANA testing is done against HEp-2 cells; other myositis-specific antibodies require specialized testing (e.g., immunoprecipitation).
      (1) **Nonspecific autoantibodies.** ANAs, particularly **speckled-pattern ANAs,** are the most common autoantibodies in the inflammatory myopathies, occurring in more than 50% of patients. Other antibodies also can be seen, including **Ro antibodies, La antibodies, PM/Scl antibodies,** and **Ku antibodies.**
      (2) **Specific autoantibodies.** Several autoantibodies are formed only in inflammatory myopathies; they target cytoplasmic or nuclear constituents of myocytes.
         (a) **Synthetase antibodies (anti-aminoacyl–tRNA synthetases)** are directed against cytoplasmic enzymes involved in specific amino acid attachment to tRNA. **Jo-1 antibody,** found in 20% of myositis patients, is the most common, directed against histidyl–tRNA synthetase.

      (b) **Signal recognition particle antibodies (SRP antibodies)** recognize one of the components of the SRP, a cytoplasmic protein complex involved in polypeptide transfer across the endoplasmic reticulum.

      (c) **Mi-2 antibodies** target a nuclear protein of unknown function, in contrast to the cytoplasmic proteins of the other myositis-specific antigens (MSA).

3. **Clinical syndromes**

   a. **Polymyositis** is characterized by upper and lower extremity proximal muscular weakness and elevated muscle enzymes. All organ manifestations listed in IX E 1 can occur, except the skin findings. Patients with polymyositis tend to have disease that is less responsive than dermatomyositis to therapy, particularly those patients with **SRP antibodies.** These patients tend to have treatment-resistant, acutely severe disease often associated with cardiac muscle involvement. Patients with polymyositis who have **PM/Scl antibodies** tend to do relatively well.

   b. **Dermatomyositis** is characterized by the muscle weakness, elevated muscle enzymes, and organ manifestations seen in polymyositis, but the distinct feature of this syndrome is the presence of **skin involvement.** In general, dermatomyositis patients respond reasonably well to therapy. Two distinct subsets have different features and prognoses.

      (1) **Synthetase antibodies subset.** These patients typically present with **mechanic's hands, interstitial lung disease,** and **symmetrical polyarthritis.** They also may have fever and prominent Raynaud's syndrome. Patients in this subset may respond well to initial therapy but experience flare-ups with steroid tapering; the pulmonary disease often is severe and may be fatal.

      (2) **Mi-2 antibodies subset.** These 5%–10% of myositis patients have **heliotrope lids, Gottron's sign,** the **shawl sign,** and the **V sign.** They respond well to therapy and typically have a good prognosis.

   c. **Polymyositis or dermatomyositis associated with malignancy.** Visceral malignancies occur in approximately 10%–25% of cases, especially in elderly individuals with late-onset inflammatory myopathy. The incidence of malignancy is thought to be higher in patients with dermatomyositis than in those with polymyositis. The most common malignancies are those that are typical in middle-aged or elderly individuals (i.e., cancers of the lung, gastrointestinal tract, breast, uterus, and ovaries). Removal of the malignancy occasionally results in remission of the muscle disease, but the prognosis in general for these patients is poor; they die of their malignancy or uncontrollable muscle disease.

   d. **Juvenile dermatomyositis.** Most children have dermatomyositis rather than polymyositis. Late in the disease course, young patients may develop muscle contractures from calcific deposits in the chronically damaged muscle. A widespread small artery and capillary vasculitis may lead to skin, muscle, and bowel ischemic lesions. Otherwise, prognosis is similar to that in adult forms of inflammatory myopathy.

   e. **Overlap syndromes.** Muscle disease that is identical to polymyositis can occur in SLE, rheumatoid arthritis, systemic sclerosis, and Sjören's syndrome. These patients often have milder muscle disease that is responsive to therapy, and prognosis is determined by the features of the underlying disease more than the muscle findings.

   f. **Inclusion body myositis.** This syndrome is considered a subset of inflammatory myopathies because of the associated CD8^{+}-cell cytotoxicity directed against muscle fibers. The syndrome tends to affect **older males** and has a gradual disease onset and progression. Although patients have muscle weakness, CK elevations, and myopathic EMGs, they are distinguished from typical polymyositis patients by having **distal as well as proximal weakness,** typical **absence of autoantibodies,** and a **characteristic muscle biopsy** showing vacuolar changes and distinctive electron microscopic findings. The clinical features often are poorly responsive to immunosuppressive therapy, but patients have an excellent 5-year survival rate because of the slow progression of the disease.

F. **Diagnosis**

1. **Approach to the diagnosis**
   a. **Distinctive muscle findings.** A clinical diagnosis of inflammatory myopathy typically is considered when patients present with **proximal muscle weakness or increased muscle enzymes** (e.g., CK, aldolase). True proximal muscle weakness must be distinguished from generalized fatigue, distal weakness more typical of neuropathy, and pain-related weakness (i.e., joint or tendon pain that prevents full muscle contraction). Patients with true proximal muscle weakness complain of being unable to comb their hair or to rise from a squatting or sitting position. If true proximal weakness appears likely from the history and physical examination, CK testing is performed and EMG and biopsy of symptomatic deltoid or quadriceps muscle should be considered. Gallium scanning, indium-labelled lymphocyte scanning, and magnetic resonance imaging may show that inflammation is spotty. In addition, these tests may help localize the best biopsy sites and measure disease activity. The diagnosis of polymyositis is likely if a patient has three of the following muscle criteria:
      (1) Characteristic proximal muscle weakness
      (2) Inflammatory cell infiltrate and myofibril degeneration on muscle biopsy
      (3) Increased muscle enzyme levels
      (4) Myopathic EMG changes
   b. **Supportive findings**
      (1) The **characteristic skin findings** are supportive evidence if found and sometimes precede clinical evidence of muscle involvement.
      (2) Because 90% of polymyositis patients have autoantibodies when their serum is tested against HEp-Z cells, the presence of a positive test for autoantibodies also is supportive evidence for the disease, particularly if a **myositis-specific antibody** is found.

2. **Consideration of malignancy.** A search for a malignancy is warranted in middle-aged or elderly polymyositis or dermatomyositis patients. Thorough physical examination, chest x-ray, and routine hematologic and biochemical testing as well as urinalysis and stool testing for occult blood should be performed. Abnormalities found should be pursued through additional testing.

3. **Differential diagnosis.** Other entities should be considered in making a diagnosis of inflammatory myopathy, especially when the presentation is somewhat atypical. Some disorders can be eliminated on clinical grounds; others require laboratory testing, EMG, or muscle biopsy.
   a. **Endocrine disorders**
      (1) **Hypothyroidism** can present as proximal muscle aching, weakness, and mild-to-moderate CK elevation.
      (2) **Hyperthyroidism** can present as diffuse weakness; CK levels typically are normal.
      (3) **Cushing syndrome** patients may have lower more than upper extremity proximal muscle weakness; muscle enzymes are normal.
   b. **Drugs.** Numerous drugs and toxins can cause muscle weakness and sometimes CK elevation; these effects usually resolve when the agent is removed. Some of the most common of these agents include alcohol, cholesterol-lowering drugs (e.g., clofibrate, gemfibrozil, lovastatin), colchicine, chloroquine, corticosteroids, D-penicillamine, and zidovudine.
   c. **Muscle diseases.** Muscular dystrophies and metabolic muscle diseases can be distinguished by careful family history, distinguishing patterns of weakness, and lack of inflammation on muscle biopsy. Some require exercise testing with venous lactate determinations or electron microscopic examination of muscle.
   d. **Neurologic diseases.** Early in the disease course, illnesses such as myasthenia gravis or amyotrophic lateral sclerosis (ALS) can mimic inflammatory myopathy. The presence of ocular muscle involvement or characteristic EMG or nerve conduction velocity (NCV) findings can help in diagnosing these diseases.
   e. **Infections**
      (1) **Bacterial.** Some cases of Lyme disease are associated with myopathy.

(2) Viral. Acute and convalescent serologies can distinguish viral illness. Common causes include coxsackievirus, echovirus, influenza virus, and HIV.

(3) Parasitic. Serologic testing can help distinguish toxoplasmosis or trichinosis from polymyositis.

f. Sarcoidosis may exhibit inflammatory muscle involvement, which can be distinguished by characteristic organ involvement and finding noncaseating granulomas on muscle biopsy.

G. Therapy

1. **Corticosteroids.** Large doses of corticosteroids appear to be effective in controlling the muscle disease in most patients. Prednisone usually is begun at a dose of 60 mg/day and is reduced gradually over several months as muscle strength improves and CK level falls. Alternate-day regimens can be used to prevent steroid toxicity but only after the normalization of CK level and return of muscle strength.

2. **Immunosuppressive agents.** Patients who do not respond to the above-mentioned corticosteroid schedules within 3 months are considered to be nonresponders to treatment. Frequently, the addition of methotrexate or azathioprine allows control of the muscle disease and gradual tapering of the steroids. The $CD4^+$ cell-specific drug cyclosporine also has been effective in some patients who do not respond to general immunosuppression.

3. **Physical therapy.** When the disease process has been clinically controlled (i.e., CK levels normalized and muscle strength improved), muscle strengthening exercise and aerobic training can be initiated. Mild exercise and passive stretching to prevent contractures should be used in active disease.

4. **Hydroxychloroquine** may help the rash of dermatomyositis.

5. **Intravenous immunoglobulin** has been helpful in some steroid-resistant patients.

6. **Plasmapheresis** has been shown not to be effective in the idiopathic inflammatory myopathies.

X. SJÖGREN'S SYNDROME

A.
Definition. Sjögren's syndrome (also called **sicca syndrome**) is an idiopathic, autoimmune disorder characterized by dry mouth (**xerostomia**) and dry eyes (**keratoconjunctivitis sicca**). Variable **lacrimal** or **salivary gland enlargement** can occur (related to lymphocytic infiltration of lacrimal and salivary glands).

B.
Classification. Sjögren's syndrome is divided into primary and secondary forms. The two forms can be distinguished on the basis of clinical features and HLA associations.

1. **Primary Sjögren's syndrome** has characteristic organ and exocrine glandular features and a significantly increased association with **HLA-DR3.** Patients can present with a variety of clinical manifestations that are uncommon in the secondary form, mainly due to a wider attack on exocrine glands in the primary form. Specific organ involvement is as follows:
   a. **Skin:** Dry skin and vagina, Raynaud's phenomenon, and purpura (vasculitis)
   b. **Lung:** Recurrent infections and interstitial fibrosis
   c. **Gastrointestinal tract:** Angular cheilitis, oral candidiasis, beefy red tongue, recurrent parotitis, dysphagia, atrophic gastritis, chronic active hepatitis, biliary cirrhosis, and pancreatitis
   d. **Kidney:** Renal tubular acidosis and interstitial nephritis
   e. **Muscle:** Indolent myositis
   f. **Nerve:** CNS involvement (possibly vasculitis, with clinical manifestations similar to CNS lupus) and peripheral neuropathy

   g. Hematologic system: Splenomegaly with neutropenia, lymphomas, and pseudo-lymphomas

   h. Joint: Arthralgias or mild inflammatory arthritis

   i. Endocrine system: Chronic thyroiditis [increased thyroid-stimulating hormone (TSH) levels and antithyroid antibodies, perhaps in as many as 50% of patients]

   j. Vasculitis (polyarteritis-like)

2. **Secondary Sjögren's syndrome** occurs in the setting of another rheumatic disease (e.g., rheumatoid arthritis, SLE, scleroderma) and has an increased association with **HLA-DR4.** Patients usually have symptoms that are limited to lacrimal and salivary gland abnormalities, although they also have typical features of a primary rheumatic disease.

C. Diagnosis

1. **Clinical approach.** Patients are most commonly evaluated for Sjögren's syndrome when they have complaints of **dry eyes, dry mouth,** or **salivary gland enlargement.** Primary Sjögren's syndrome also should be considered in the setting of **cutaneous vasculitis** (purpura), **CNS dysfunction** similar to that which occurs in SLE (either focal neurologic abnormalities or diffuse features such as depression, psychosis, or cognitive dysfunction), or the conspicuous presence of other clinical features listed in X B 1.

   a. Complaints of **gritty eyes and dry mouth** can be investigated as follows.

   (1) Ophthalmologic slit-lamp examination with fluorescein or rose bengal staining can be used to examine for the punctate staining of keratoconjunctivitis. The **Schirmer test,** which measures the degree of tear wetting on filter paper, is a supportive test; limited wetting suggests that keratoconjunctivitis found on staining is sicca-related.

   (2) Lip biopsy. The lower lip mucosa can be biopsied to search for characteristic lymphocytic infiltration of the minor salivary glands in that location.

   b. Salivary gland enlargement. MRI of the parotid gland may show a nonhomogenous density, which can be distinguished from parotitis, tumor, and normal glandular tissue.

   c. Salivary flow rate tests (sialometry) and **radiographic studies (sialography)** are sensitive but nonspecific tests and are not often used.

   d. Laboratory findings. Many laboratory abnormalities occur and may offer suggestive evidence; however, no specific laboratory test is diagnostic.

   (1) Tests suggesting chronic inflammation. Anemia of chronic disease, elevated erythrocyte sedimentation rate, hypergammaglobulinemia, and rheumatoid factor often are found in Sjögren's syndrome, whether primary or secondary.

   (2) Autoantibody findings. ANAs are seen frequently in Sjögren's syndrome; antibodies to the small RNA protein **Ro** are found in **70%** of patients and antibodies to the protein **La** are found in **40%** of patients. La antibodies rarely are found without Ro antibodies, and the presence of both is relatively specific for Sjögren's syndrome. Salivary duct antibodies are common only in the secondary form.

2. **Differential diagnosis**

   a. Salivary gland enlargement also may be caused by a lymphoid or parotid gland neoplasm, granulomatous infiltration (sarcoidosis), alcohol use, cirrhosis, diabetes, amyloidosis, graft-versus-host disease, hyperlipidemias, or infection (e.g., bacterial mumps, HIV).

   b. Dry mouth may be caused by the use of certain drugs, including tricyclic antidepressants, phenothiazines, and antihistamines.

   c. Dry mouth and dry eyes are common in the geriatric population, and they often are present without any other features of Sjögren's syndrome.

D. Therapy

1. **General considerations**

   a. Scrupulous oral hygiene is important to prevent rampant dental caries.

    b. Patients with primary Sjögren's syndrome who demonstrate salivary gland or lymphoid tissue enlargement must be considered **at risk for lymphoma,** because non-Hodgkin's lympomas occur at 40 times the normal rate in these patients.

2. Symptomatic treatment

    a. Xerostomia. Avoidance of drugs that dry out the mouth and frequent drinks of water or other liquids to keep the mouth wet are the usual symptomatic measures for this condition. Artificial salivas are now commercially available, which may help with mouth wetting and dental caries prevention, and electrical stimulation may help some patients increase salivary flow.

    b. Keratoconjunctivitis sicca. Artificial tears (methyl cellulose) are used as often as needed to keep the eyes lubricated.

    c. Features of severe disease. Progressive pneumonitis, vasculitis, neuropathy, and **CNS involvement** may require anti-inflammatory treatment with corticosteroids and immunosuppressive drugs.

E. **Prognosis** for patients with primary Sjögren's syndrome depends on the severity of involvement of organs other than the salivary glands, particularly the CNS. Also, the risk of lymphoma is higher in more severe cases. Features of the primary rheumatic disease determine the prognosis for patients with secondary Sjögren's syndrome.

XI. VASCULITIS

A. **Definition.** Vasculitic syndromes are a group of clinically disparate disorders characterized by **necrosis and inflammation of blood vessel walls.** Vasculitis can exist as the primary feature of an idiopathic condition or as a secondary manifestation of infectious, malignant, or rheumatic disease.

B. **Etiology.** Most of the vasculitic syndromes are idiopathic. Hepatitis B surface antigen (HBsAg) and hepatitis C virus have been found in immune complexes of several different syndromes, including some cases of polyarteritis nodosa and essential mixed cryoglobulinemia. HIV, parvovirus, and CMV have been associated with vasculitis diseases, particularly polyarteritis. Methamphetamine abuse also has been implicated in the causation of vessel lesions in some cases of polyarteritis.

C. **Pathogenesis.** Individual syndromes often demonstrate features of disordered humoral and cellular immunity.

1. Disordered humoral immune response. In some vasculitic syndromes (e.g., leukocytoclastic vasculitis perhaps polyarteritis nodosa), soluble immune complexes form and deposit in vessel walls, fix complement, and attract inflammatory cells, which cause damage. Antibodies may also react directly with neutrophils or endothelial cells to cause vessel damage [e.g., Wegener's granulomatosis and antineutrophil cytoplasmic antibodies (ANCA)]. The site and degree of damage are determined by many variables, including:

    a. Physical and biochemical characteristics of the immune complexes

    b. Variations in blood pressure (hydrostatic forces)

    c. Changes in blood vessel size and permeability

    d. Endothelial cell adhesive properties

    e. Effectiveness of reticuloendothelial system removal of immune complexes

    f. Degree of turbulence in vessels (e.g., immune complexes deposit at branch points)

    g. Degree of persistence or recurrence of antigen exposure (e.g., toxin versus hepatitis B)

    h. Variations in host immune response [e.g., antineutrophil cytoplasmic antibody (ANCA) in patients with Wegener's granulomatosis]. An inhaled antigen or other immune system challenge may activate neutrophils, which in the presence of ANCA degranulate, recruit T cells and monocytes, and damage vessel walls.

2. **Disordered cellular immune response.** Disorders involving granuloma formation are the best examples of the contributions of the cellular immune response to vasculitic processes. Interactions between macrophages and CD4$^+$ T cells in response to unknown antigens lead to granuloma formation in and around vessel walls. In giant cell arteritis, age-related vessel degeneration in large arteries may expose antigens typically hidden to the immune system, which then elicit a cellular immune response; there may also be an HLA-DR4 association with this disease and proliferation of specific T cell clones in vessel lesions.

D. **Classification.** The current systems for classifying vasculitic syndromes use clinical features, size of the involved vessel, and type of cellular infiltrate to separate the syndromes (Table 10-9). Nonspecific hematologic and immunologic abnormalities (e.g., anemia, leukocytosis, elevated erythrocyte sedimentation rate, hypocomplementemia) often exist in many of these syndromes, but these are not noted in Table 10-9 unless they are specifically important for the diagnosis of a particular syndrome. It is important to understand that these syndromes often blur and overlap in actual patients.

E. **Vasculitic syndromes**

1. **Hypersensitivity vasculitis**
   a. **Typical hypersensitivity vasculitis syndrome.** Hypersensitivity vasculitis (also called **leukocytoclastic vasculitis** or **cutaneous vasculitis**) is immune-complex-mediated inflammation of small vessels (arterioles, capillaries, venules). The cause often is unclear. In many cases, hypersensitivity vasculitis seems to occur as an exaggerated immune response to a **drug** (e.g., penicillin) or **infection** (viral or bacterial antigen), causing a self-limited immune complex vasculitis. The skin almost always is involved, with palpable purpura, petechiae, urticariae, ulcers, or other lesions. Polyarticular arthritis is common. Distinct organ involvement may allow further classification.
   b. **Distinctive subsets**
      (1) **Henoch-Schönlein purpura** is a systemic, small-vessel vasculitis that occurs primarily in children, often following a streptococcal pharyngitis.
          (a) **Clinical features** typically include palpable purpura, polyarticular arthralgias or inflammatory arthritis, abdominal pain or gastrointestinal bleeding due to mesenteric vessel involvement, and immune complex-mediated glomerulonephritis. A distinctive feature is **IgA deposition** in the vascular lesions.
          (b) **Course.** Most cases of Henoch-Schönlein purpura resolve spontaneously over a period of days to weeks. Patients with severe renal or gastrointestinal involvement may require steroids.
      (2) **Serum sickness** is an immune complex vasculitis that often follows a drug (e.g., penicillin, sulfonamide) or foreign protein exposure by 7–10 days. Antilymphocyte globulin now is one of the most common causes. Hepatitis B arthritis–dermatitis syndrome is a serum sickness–like response to HbsAg.
          (a) **Clinical features.** Urticaria, purpura, arthritis, and arthralgias are characteristic, and lymphadenopathy and immune complex glomerulonephritis are common.
          (b) **Course.** Resolution is typical following removal of the inciting agent.
      (3) **Hypocomplementemic urticarial vasculitis**
          (a) **Clinical features.** Patients with this form of vasculitis exhibit urticaria, typically lasting longer than 24 hours and, sometimes, arthritis, glomerulonephritis, or gastrointestinal involvement. **Hypocomplementemia** is a consistent feature, apparently related to antibodies directed against C1q; the degree of complement depression typically parallels disease activity.
          (b) **Course.** The disease follows a relapsing, remitting course and may require corticosteroids for the more disabling manifestations.

TABLE 10-9. Major Vasculitic Syndromes: Clinicopathologic Distinctions

Syndrome	Clinical Features	Pathology		Diagnosis	Therapy
		Vessel Size	Cellular Infiltrate		
Hypersensitivity vasculitis (serum sickness; drug reactions; Henoch-Schönlein purpura; mixed essential cryoglobulinemia)	Skin involvement predominant Visceral involvement typically minimal and self-limited	Small (capillaries; venules; arterioles)	Leukocytoclastic vasculitis with all lesions at the same developmental stage	Skin biopsy	Supportive Corticosteroids for serious vessel involvement
Polyarteritis nodosa	Multisystem illness Major arterial ischemic lesions that spare lungs and spleen Nodose skin lesions uncommon	Small and medium-sized arteries	Necrotizing arteritis at vessel branch points Simultaneous lesions at various stages	Biopsy of involved organ Visceral angiography	Corticosteroids; cytotoxic agents added if no response
Allergic angitis (Churg-Strauss disease)	Prominent allergic, asthmatic history Lung involvement Blood eosinophilia common	Varying (capillaries; venules; small arteries)	Granulomatous infiltrates with eosinophils	Biopsy of involved organ, typically lung	Corticosteroids; cytotoxic agents added if no response
Wegener's granulomatosis	Upper and lower respiratory tract involvement Prominent renal abnormalities	Small (arteries; veins)	Necrotizing granulomas in upper and lower airways Focal necrotizing arteritis in lungs Necrotizing glomerulonephritis in kidneys	Lung biopsy (sinus biopsy usually non-diagnostic); c-ANCA	Cyclophosphamide; corticosteroids added if disease is fulminant; switch to methotrexate may lessen cyclophosphamide toxicity after induction
Giant cell arteritis (temporal arteritis)	Polymyalgia rheumatica in 50% Occurs in patients older than 50 Signs and symptoms of cranial artery involvement High erythrocyte sedimentation rate	Large arteries (especially temporal artery)	Giant cell and chronic mononuclear infiltrates in vessel walls	Temporal artery biopsy	Corticosteroids
Takayasu's arteritis	Large vessel claudication Occurs in young (often Asian) women	Large arteries (aortic arch)	Giant cell and chronic mononuclear infiltrates in vessel walls	Angiography Chest MRI Neck ultrasonography	Corticosteroids Large vessel reconstructive surgery

ANCA = antineutrophil cytoplasmic antibody; c-ANCA = cytoplasmic ANCA; MRI = magnetic resonance imaging.

(4) Mixed essential cryoglobulinemia is an idiopathic disorder caused by cold-precipitated immunoglobulin (cryoglobulin) complexes, which produce a vaso-occlusive or inflammatory injury. The syndrome typically occurs in patients who have type II (mixed) cryoglobulin. Many patients have been found to have hepatitis C or less often, hepatitis B, in the immune complexes.

  (a) Clinical features include recurrent attacks of palpable purpura, Raynaud's phenomenon, arthralgia, and immune complex glomerulonephritis. Gastrointestinal, hepatic, and pulmonary dysfunction are occasional features.

  (b) Course. Severe renal involvement is the most common reason for treatment, which may include corticosteroids, cytotoxic agents, or removal of the cryoglobulin by apheresis. Interferon alpha may help when the disease is associated with hepatitis B or C.

2. **Polyarteritis nodosa** is a necrotizing vasculitis of small and medium-sized arteries, which presents as a multisystem illness. Ischemic arterial lesions are caused by vessel wall inflammation, in some cases associated with immune complex deposition.

  a. **Clinical features. Constitutional complaints** (e.g., fever, weight loss, anorexia) are common, and **multiorgan ischemic dysfunction** is the rule; the lung and spleen typically are spared.

  (1) Renal involvement is most common and presents as severe hypertension, proteinuria and active sediment from glomerulonephritis, or renal insufficiency.

  (2) Other common features include arthralgias, myalgias, peripheral nervous system abnormalities (sensory polyneuropathies, mononeuritis multiplex), and skin lesions (infarctions, nodose lesions). Insidious congestive heart failure, diffuse or focal CNS dysfunction, and gastrointestinal involvement also can occur, depending on the size of the ischemic lesions.

  (3) Microscopic polyarteritis is a clinical variant typified by prominent lung involvement and segmental glomerulonephritis, sometimes rapidly progressive. The vessels involved tend to be smaller (capillaries, arterioles, and small arteries). **Perinuclear ANCA (p-ANCA)** is commonly found (50%–80% of patients) and abdominal angiography is typically negative (because the smaller vessels are involved).

  b. **Course.** Treatment with corticosteroids, cytotoxic agents, or both is necessary, the illness typically is fatal if untreated. Interferon alpha may help in hepatitis B- or C-associated cases.

3. **Allergic angiitis (Churg-Strauss disease)** is a granulomatous vasculitis that typically occurs in patients with asthma.

  a. **Clinical features.** Allergic angiitis is typically a triphasic disease. **Asthma** occurs first, often associated with **blood eosinophilia. Tissue infiltrates,** especially **pulmonary** ones, occur next; eosinophils are often present in these lesions, sometimes in granulomas. **Vasculitis** of small or medium-sized vessels occurs last, commonly involving skin, nerve, or muscle lesions.

  b. **Course.** The farther apart in time the three phases of illness occur, the milder the disease; the closer together, the more explosive. Catastrophic lung, gastrointestinal tract, cardiac, or nerve lesions may mandate aggressive intravenous corticosteroid and cytotoxic therapy, but more indolent forms are often easily controlled with moderate corticosteroid doses.

4. **Wegener's granulomatosis** is a granulomatous, small-vessel vasculitis that typically involves the upper and lower respiratory tract and kidney.

  a. **Clinical features**

  (1) Respiratory tract. Pulmonary features typically include upper airway complaints (e.g., sinusitis, rhinitis) as well as lower airway symptoms (e.g., cough, shortness of breath, hemoptysis). Cavitary or multiple infiltrates may be seen on chest x-ray.

  (2) Kidney. Renal involvement is characterized by abnormal sediment or renal functional impairment.

(3) Organs. Other, less classical features include skin lesions (palpable purpura), arthritis, ocular or orbital inflammation (typically with proptosis), cardiac lesions, and CNS or peripheral nervous system involvement.

(4) Presence of cytoplasmic ANCA (c-ANCA). c-ANCA is often found in patients with active, multi-organ disease. In these patients, the presence of c-ANCA may be a relatively specific diagnostic test.

b. Course. Although corticosteroids may be used initially, cytotoxic agents such as cyclophosphamide are uniformly required to prevent death. Methotrexate may have a role in maintaining disease remission.

5. **Takayasu's arteritis** is a granulomatous inflammation of the vessels of the aortic arch that is characterized pathologically by a panarteritis containing mononuclear and giant cells. Young, often Asian, women are at highest risk for this disorder.

   a. Clinical features

     (1) Generalized aching similar to polymyalgia rheumatica often occurs early in the illness. Features of **large artery ischemia** develop weeks to months later and may include upper extremity claudication, angina, and congestive heart failure from cardiac or aortic involvement. Pulmonary and mesenteric vessels also can be involved.

     (2) Findings on physical examination include arterial bruits, pulse deficits, and blood pressure differences between extremities.

   b. Course. Patients may require steroids early in the course of the illness; later, vascular reconstruction may be required for occlusive lesions. Cytotoxic agents are typically added if steroids do not control inflammatory disease.

6. **Giant cell (temporal) arteritis** usually is a granulomatous inflammation of the carotid artery and its branches, but it sometimes can involve the vertebral artery or other aortic branches. The pathology is indistinguishable from that of Takayasu's arteritis.

   a. Clinical features. The disease rarely occurs in patients younger than age 50.

     (1) Approximately 50% of patients have **polymyalgia rheumatica** (i.e., aching and stiffness of shoulder and hip girdles associated with an erythrocyte sedimentation rate exceeding 50 mm/hr, age greater than 50 years, and constitutional complaints such as fever, malaise, and weight loss), and most patients have features related to ischemia in the carotid artery region (i.e., headache, visual symptoms, jaw claudication, scalp tenderness, neurologic complaints).

     (2) Superficial temporal artery involvement is common but often is clinically silent. Potential clinical features include tenderness, nodules, or erythema. Even when the artery is clinically normal, temporal artery biopsy typically reveals pathology.

   b. Course. Patients require steroids early and in high doses to prevent **blindness,** the most serious complication of this illness.

7. **Other vasculitic syndromes** do not fit into the major categories of vasculitis due to distinct clinical features or overlapping pathologic ones.

   a. Vasculitis as a secondary feature of a primary disease. Certain diseases can exhibit vasculitic inflammation as a secondary feature. The vasculitis typically is small-vessel, cutaneous vasculitis but sometimes can overlap with polyarteritis-like vessel involvement, especially in **rheumatoid arthritis** and **lupus.** Dermal and CNS vasculitic lesions are recently recognized secondary features of **Sjögren's syndrome. Hematologic malignancies** and bacterial and viral **infections** also can include vasculitic features, usually with the skin the predominant organ involved.

   b. Behçet syndrome is defined by the presence of recurrent oral and genital ulcers. Patients also may have eye inflammation, **pathergic skin lesions** (lesions occurring at sites of skin injury), and vasculitis of the CNS or other organs.

   c. Kawasaki disease (mucocutaneous lymph node syndrome) is a febrile illness of infants and young children characterized by conjunctival injection; diffuse maculopapular rash with associated edema, erythema, and eventual desquamation of the hands and feet; cracked lips; "strawberry tongue"; and cervical adenopathy. A coronary vasculitis can develop in 25% of patients and lead to aneurysm, myocardial infarction, and sudden death. The incidence of this vasculitis has greatly decreased, however, since the advent of intravenous immunoglobulin therapy, which, along with aspirin, is the treatment of choice in this disease.

   d. Isolated CNS vasculitis is a granulomatous inflammation of small or medium-sized arteries of the brain. Typically, patients do not have clinical or laboratory evidence of inflammation elsewhere. Presenting features often are combinations of diffuse CNS complaints (headache, altered mental status, poor memory) and more focal ones (cranial nerve defects, hemiparesis). A chronic meningitis picture typically is found on lumbar puncture in these patients, and enhanced MRI scan of the brain is a sensitive but nonspecific indication of possible involvement.

F. **Diagnosis**

   1. Recognizing a possible vasculitis. Combinations of clinical features will suggest the possibility of a vasculitis.

     a. Specific clinical data. The history and physical examination should be performed with attention to signs of organ ischemia or vessel abnormalities. Laboratory data may suggest a general inflammatory process or point to a specific syndrome (Table 10-10).

     b. Syndrome recognition. The diagnostic investigation should aim to identify patterns of organ involvement or distinct clinical features that suggest a vasculitic process. Overlap between vasculitic categories may blur the diagnosis.

   2. Confirming the diagnosis. If the clinical evaluation suggests a reasonable chance of vasculitis, the appropriate approach to making a diagnosis usually lies in biopsy of involved tissue or visceral angiography; ANCA testing may be helpful when microscopic polyarteritis or Wegener's granulomatosis are suspected.

     a. Biopsy of a fresh lesion from clinically involved tissues is the preferred method of diagnosing vasculitis; if involved, the skin often is the easiest tissue to obtain.

       (1) Diagnosis of **Wegener's granulomatosis** often relies on open lung biopsy demonstration of granulomatous vasculitis, as paranasal sinus tissue typically shows nonspecific inflammation and renal tissue shows only glomerulonephritis.

       (2) Diagnosis of **temporal arteritis** requires examination of a 3- to 5-cm segment of the superficial temporal artery in multiple sections; biopsy of the contralateral side may be needed if the first biopsy is negative and clinical suspicion remains high.

       (3) Biopsy of leptomeninges and clinically involved brain tissue may be needed when **isolated CNS vasculitis** is strongly suspected.

     b. Visceral angiography. When polyarteritis is suspected and appropriate tissue cannot be obtained for biopsy or when the biopsy is unrevealing, abdominal three-vessel angiography may show aneurysms or arteriopathy (discrete narrowing) suggestive of small to medium-sized artery vasculitis. Aortic arch and large vessel angiograms, carotid ultrasonography, and MRI studies of the chest are useful in Takayasu's arteritis, because the involved vessels often cannot be safely biopsied. CNS angiograms may be warranted when isolated CNS vasculitis is suspected.

     c. Presence of ANCA. ANCA are typically IgG antibodies directed against cytoplasmic components of neutrophils and monocytes.

       (1) c-ANCA is directed against **proteinase-3** and is a fairly specific diagnostic feature of **Wegener's granulomatosis.** Its presence is a fairly sensitive indicator when the disease is active and multiple organs are involved, but it is less often present in limited forms or inactive disease.

       (2) p-ANCA is directed against **myeloperoxidase** (or other neutrophil antigens) and is often present in cases of **microscopic polyarteritis;** it is not a specific indicator because p-ANCA can be seen in other vasculitides, inflammatory bowel disease, various forms of glomerulonephritis, and other rheumatic diseases such as SLE.

TABLE 10-10. Clinical Data Suggesting Vasculitis

History	Physical Examination	Laboratory Studies
Constitutional complaints Malaise Anorexia Fever Weight loss **Drug exposure** (prescribed or illicit) **Infection** Human immunodeficiency virus (HIV) Hepatitis B or C virus **Organ ischemic complaints** Angina Extremity or jaw claudication Visual complaints Transient ischemic attacks	**Vessel findings** Blood pressure/pulse deficits Hypertension (sudden onset) Vessel tenderness, nodules, bruits **Skin findings** Palpable purpura Infarctions Ulcers **Muscle findings** Tenderness, cramping **Nerve findings** Sensory/motor neuropathies Focal/diffuse CNS dysfunction **Testis** Tenderness Erythema	**Nonspecific tests** (chronic inflammation) Anemia (chronic disease) Thrombocytosis Increased erythrocyte sedimentation rate Increased gamma globulins **Test indicating potential ischemia** Abnormal renal function (↑ creatinine, BUN) Abnormal muscle/liver enzymes (↑ CK, AST, ALT) Electrocardiogram **Tests pointing toward specific diagnoses** HIV (several syndromes) HBsAg (20%-30% of polyarteritis patients) Hepatitis C RNA ANA (SLE more likely) c-ANCA (Wegener's granulomatosis) p-ANCA (microscopic polyarteritis) Cryoglobulins (mixed essential cryoglobulinemia) Anti-Ro (Sjögren's syndrome, SLE)

ALT = alanine aminotransferase; ANA = antinuclear antibody; ANCA = antineutrophil cytoplasmic antibody; c-ANCA = cytoplasmic ANCA; p-ANCA = perinuclear ANCA; AST = aspartate aminotransferase; BUN = blood urea nitrogen; CNS = central nervous system; CK = creatine kinase; HBsAg = hepatitis B surface antigen; SLE = systemic lupus erythematosus.

3. **Differential diagnosis.** Numerous conditions should be considered in the differential diagnosis of vasculitis. Important disorders and the tests used to eliminate them include:
   a. **Bacterial endocarditis** (blood culture)
   b. **Left atrial myxoma** (two-dimensional or transesophageal echocardiogram)
   c. **Cholesterol embolism** syndrome (biopsy showing refractile crystals)
   d. **Thrombotic diseases,** such as **antiphospholipid syndrome** (antiphospholipid antibody) and **DIC** or **thrombotic thrombocytopenic purpura** (PT, PTT, platelet count, fibrinogen, fibrin split products)

G. **Therapy.** The management of patients with vasculitis is complex. In all patients with known vasculitic disease, it is important to record the extent of disease initially and to monitor organ involvement (in terms of clinical, biopsy, and angiographic evidence). The tempo of disease progression also should be gauged to determine the best treatment.

1. **Antigen removal.** Drugs that may be causing vasculitic processes should be stopped; plasmapheresis has been used in attempt to remove known antigens (HBsAg, hepatitis C) and unknown antigens (cryoglobulin).

2. **Treatment of primary disease.** Control of any primary rheumatologic, infectious, or malignant process generally is the most effective way to control vasculitis that is a secondary feature.

3. **Immunosuppressive treatment.** Vasculitis syndromes that are not related to a removable antigen or treatable primary disorder often should be controlled with immunosuppressive agents—either **corticosteroids, cytotoxic drugs,** or a combination of both. **Cyclosporine,** working specifically on activated CD4 + T cells, has been used in some vasculitis diseases, particularly to counteract eye involvement in Behçet's and some cases of refractory small vessel vasculitis.

   a. **Corticosteroids** alone should be attempted as first-line pharmacologic treatment in all patients except those with Wegener's granulomatosis. Daily dosing usually is required, although alternate-day dosing may be sufficient once systemic features of the illness are controlled. **Low-dose aspirin therapy** is often added to treatment of vasculitis disorders to counteract the potential **vasoocclusive** effects of glucocorticoids.

   b. **Cytotoxic drugs** (e.g., cyclophosphamide)

      (1) **Wegener's granulomatosis** almost always is fatal without cytotoxic therapy; thus, patients should be started on a combination of one of these agents and corticosteroids.

      (2) **Polyarteritis nodosa and allergic angiitis** also often require cytotoxic drugs in addition to steroids for control of disease manifestations, although recent prospective studies have shown benefit in decreasing disease recurrences but not in preventing mortality.

      (3) In other disorders, cytotoxic drugs typically are added to corticosteroid therapy if the steroid doses cannot be easily lowered without the disease flaring.

4. **Other drugs.** Agents such as dapsone, colchicine, NSAIDs, hydroxychloroquine, and H_1- or H_2-blocking antihistaminic agents have been used, particularly in refractory small-vessel vasculitis.

5. **Plasmapheresis,** which removes antibodies and immune complexes from plasma, has not been shown to improve outcome in systemic necrotizing vasculitis (e.g., polyarteritis, allergic angiitis). In **mixed cryoglobulinemia,** whether or not it is related to hepatitis B or C infection, plasmapheresis may improve disease features, at least temporarily.

STUDY QUESTIONS

DIRECTIONS: Each of the numbered items or incomplete statements in this section is followed by answers or by completions of the statement. Select the ONE lettered answer or completion that is BEST in each case.

1. Which of the following joint findings is most suggestive of an inflammatory, rather than an osteoarthritic, cause of joint pain?

(A) Painful range of motion
(B) Crepitus
(C) Bony articular enlargement
(D) Swelling and warmth
(E) Instability

2. A 68-year-old man presents with an acutely red and swollen right great toe without history of trauma. Which of the following findings is most useful for making a diagnosis of gout in this patient?

(A) Persistent elevation of serum uric acid
(B) Good response to colchicine trial
(C) Radiograph showing marginal joint erosion in the first metatarsophalangeal (MTP) joint
(D) An associated right ankle effusion
(E) A painless elbow nodule

3. Which of the following forms of juvenile rheumatoid arthritis is most likely to be associated with serious eye complications?

(A) Polyarticular arthritis that is seropositive for rheumatoid factor
(B) Polyarticular arthritis that is seronegative for rheumatoid factor
(C) Oligoarticular arthritis without axial spine involvement
(D) Oligoarticular arthritis with axial spine involvement
(E) Systemic-onset juvenile rheumatoid arthritis

Questions 4–5

An 18-year-old woman comes to an emergency room complaining of severe right knee, right wrist, and left ankle pain. She has several skin lesions on her arms and legs; some are petechial and others are vesiculopustular. Physical examination also reveals tenderness and swelling of tendons around the involved joints but no actual joint swelling.

4. Which of the following tests is most likely to yield the diagnosis?

(A) Pelvic examination and cervical culture
(B) Joint fluid aspiration
(C) Antinuclear antibody (ANA) testing
(D) Rheumatoid factor testing
(E) Streptococcal enzyme testing

5. While awaiting results of laboratory testing, this patient should receive which of the following treatments?

(A) Corticosteroids
(B) Nonsteroidal anti-inflammatory drugs (NSAIDs)
(C) Antibiotics
(D) Local care of skin lesions
(E) Splinting of painful joints

6. A 50-year-old woman complains of a 2-month history of her hands becoming painful and turning white or blue in the cold; progressive skin tightness and thickening of fingers, hands, and forearms; shortness of breath on exertion; and a sensation of lower chest burning and food sticking upon swallowing. Antibody testing shows the presence of antinuclear antibody (ANA) and elevated titers of antibody to Scl-70. Which of the following pathogenetic explanations best fits this patient's illness?

(A) Infiltration of mucopolysaccarides into underlying subepithelial tissues
(B) Unregulated fibroblastic collagen synthesis
(C) Raynaud's phenomenon leading first to ischemia and later to tissue fibrosis
(D) Vascular endothelial damage and immunologically mediated tissue fibrosis
(E) Carcinomatous paraneoplastic process

7. Which of the following manifestations is more likely to be found in the diffuse form of systemic sclerosis than in the CREST form?

(A) Esophageal motility dysfunction
(B) Pulmonary involvement
(C) Distal skin thickening
(D) Renal disease
(E) Telangiectasias

8. Which of the following therapies is essential for treating polymyositis?

(A) Antimalarial drugs
(B) Nonsteroidal anti-inflammatory drugs (NSAIDs)
(C) Corticosteroids
(D) Bed rest
(E) Aerobic exercise

9. Which one of the following clinical features is typical of all of the spondylarthropathies?

(A) Enthesopathic inflammation
(B) Urethritis
(C) Skin lesions
(D) Bowel inflammation
(E) Oral ulcers

Questions 10–12

A 57-year-old previously well man has been ill for 2 more with fatigue, malaise, dyspnea on exertion, abdominal pain, and progressive numbness in his feet. He has lost 20 pounds over the same time period. Recently, he developed mild inflammatory polyarthritis of the hands and has physical signs suggesting a mononeuritis in the right median nerve distribution. Chest x-ray shows cardiomegaly and findings of early pulmonary edema.

10. What is the most likely diagnosis?

(A) Hypersensitivity vasculitis
(B) Rheumatoid arthritis
(C) Systemic lupus erythematosus (SLE)
(D) Polyarteritis nodosa
(E) Churg-Strauss syndrome

11. Which test will most likely yield the correct, diagnosis?

(A) Serum rheumatoid factor
(B) Sural nerve biopsy
(C) Skin biopsy
(D) Serum hepatitis B surface antigen (HBsAg)
(E) Right arm arteriography

12. The best initial therapy would be

(A) nonsteroidal anti-inflammatory drugs (NSAIDs)
(B) antibiotics
(C) cyclophosphamide and corticosteroids
(D) antimalarial agents
(E) cyclosporine

DIRECTIONS: Each set of matching questions in this section consists of a list of four to twenty-six lettered options (some of which may be in figures) followed by several numbered items. For each numbered item, select the ONE lettered option that is most closely associated with it. To avoid spending too much time on matching sets with large numbers of options, it is generally advisable to begin each set by reading the list of options. Then, for each item in the set, try to generate the correct answer, and locate it in the option list, rather than evaluating each option individually. Each lettered option may be selected once, more than once, or not at all.

Questions 13–15

(A) Rheumatoid arthritis
(B) Lyme disease
(C) Gonococcal arthritis
(D) Systemic lupus erythematosus (SLE)
(E) Polymyositis
(F) Sjögren's syndrome
(G) Polymyalgia rheumatica
(H) Reiter's syndrome
(I) Pseudogout

For each of the following case descriptions, select the most appropriate diagnosis.

13. A 20-year-old woman complains of 2 weeks of fever, pleuritic chest pain, stiffness and swelling in wrists and metacarpophalangeal (MCP) and proximal interphalangeal (PIP) joints, an erythematous rash over both cheeks, and bilateral pre-tibial edema.

14. A 50-year-old man complains of a gritty sensation in his eyes and dry mouth, which he has experienced for several months. He has vague arthralgias in his hands and knees but only bulge signs (small amount of synovial fluid) in the knees on physical examination. He has scattered purpuric lesions over both calves and ankles.

15. An 80-year-old man complains of right knee pain and swelling. He has bony enlargement of the second and third MCP joints bilaterally as well as wrist, PIP, and distal interphalangeal (DIP) joints. His knee is swollen, and range of motion is moderately limited by pain. An x-ray shows only flecks of calcium in the meniscal cartilage of the knee.

ANSWERS AND EXPLANATIONS

1. The answer is D [I F; III F 1–2]. A swollen and warm joint is more likely to be affected by an inflammatory arthritis than by osteoarthritis. The presence of synovial fluid is more commonly associated with inflammatory arthritis than osteoarthritis, and warmth suggests some degree of inflammation. Osteoarthritis typically is associated with bony joint enlargement in response to cartilage and subchondral bone injury. Painful joint range of motion, joint crepitus, and joint instability could occur in either an inflammatory or osteoarthritic joint problem.

2. The answer is B [II A 5 a (1)–(2)]. The most specific way to make a diagnosis of acute gout is to aspirate the involved joint and to identify negatively birefringent, needle-shaped crystals under red-compensated polarized light. The next best way to make a diagnosis of gout is to give oral colchicine hourly until the patient develops significant improvement in joint inflammation or gastrointestinal side effects that prevent further colchicine use. Rarely do patients with other diagnoses [e.g., sarcoid arthritis, calcium pyrophosphate deposition (CPPD) disease] respond to colchicine trial. The other tests are too nonspecific to be of diagnostic use.

3. The answer is C [V E 3 a (1) (c)]. Patients with oligoarticular arthritis without axial spine involvement are most likely to develop chronic and potentially severe anterior uveitis, which can be clinically quite subtle even as it leads to progressive visual loss. About 20%–40% of patients in this subset develop anterior uveitis, and the group that is antinuclear antibody (ANA)-positive appears to be at highest risk. Patients with axial spine involvement can also develop anterior uveitis, but this tends to be acute, self-limited, and easily treatable.

4–5. The answers are: 4-A [VI D 1 a, E 1 a], **5-C** [VI F 1]. This patient has clinical features suggestive of gonococcal periarthritis–dermatitis syndrome. In this setting, the cervix would be the most likely site for a positive culture. Joint fluid aspiration could yield a positive culture, but the patient does not have joint effusions. Antinuclear antibody (ANA)

testing would be helpful if the patient's findings were more consistent with systemic lupus erythematosus (SLE) than gonorrhea. A patient with rheumatoid arthritis would be unlikely to have the skin findings, so rheumatoid factor is not a helpful test. Different skin and articular findings would be present in rheumatic fever, so streptococcal enzyme testing would be unlikely to yield a diagnosis.

Because gonorrhea is the most likely diagnosis, antibiotic treatment is required. Corticosteroids are contraindicated. Nonsteroidal anti-inflammatory agents (NSAIDs), local skin care, and splinting of joints may be useful ancillary measures but will not treat the primary problem of a bacterial infection.

6. The answer is D [VIII D]. This patient presents with characteristic features of scleroderma, a chronic illness in which unregulated immunologic processes (perhaps triggered by unknown environmental antigens) cause small vessel endothelial damage and widespread dermal and internal organ fibrosis. The small vessel endothelial damage leads to secondary vascular reactivity (Raynaud's phenomenon) and, possibly, ischemic tissue damage. The increased collagen synthesis by tissue fibroblasts, which leads to widespread fibrosis, is not unregulated; rather, it is caused by cytokine and growth factor secretion from lymphocytes, mast cells, and platelets. There is no evidence that scleroderma patients have tissue mucopolysaccharide infiltration or that there are tumors responsible for paraneoplastic dermal fibrosis.

7. The answers is D [VIII E 2 a]. Of the clinical manifestations listed, only renal disease is more likely to be found in diffuse systemic sclerosis than in the CREST syndrome. Also, pulmonary interstitial fibrosis typically worsens faster in the diffuse form. Both forms are characterized by esophageal motility dysfunction, distal skin thickening, and Raynaud's phenomenon. Telangiectasias also can occur in both forms of scleroderma, although they are more common and widespread in the CREST syndrome.

8. The answer is C [IX G 1]. Oral corticosteroids are the typical initial treatment for inflammatory myopathy. Nonsteroidal anti-inflammatory agents (NSAIDS), antimalarial drugs, bed rest, and aerobic exercise are not recognized treatments for polymyositis, although NSAIDs might help associated joint complaints and antimalarial drugs have been used for the skin features of dermatomyositis. Aerobic exercise is appropriate for patients with controlled disease but might be detrimental to those with active disease.

9. The answer is A [JV A 1 a (3)]. Enthesopathic inflammation (i.e., inflammatory lesions at ligamentous, cartilaginous, and tendinous attachments to bone) is a characteristic feature of all spondylarthropathies. Urethritis and oral ulcers are typical of Reiter's syndrome, and skin lesions are seen in Reiter's syndrome and psoriatic arthritis. Some patients with inflammatory bowel disease also have skin lesions (e.g., pyoderma gangrenosum), but the most typical feature other than rheumatic complaints is bowel inflammation.

10–12. The answers are: 10-D [XI E 2 a], **11-B** [XI F 2], **12-C** [XI G 3 b (2)]. This patient suffers from constitutional complaints (fatigue, malaise, 20-lb weight loss) and has clinical evidence of impaired functioning of multiple organs; these findings make vasculitis a distinct diagnostic possibility. Mononeuritis is an even more specific finding, suggesting a small to medium-sized vasculitis of vasa nervorum. The other clinical findings are compatible with vasculitic organ impairment as well and are typical of polyarteritis nodosa. Hypersensitivity vasculitis is unlikely, because patients with this disorder of the very small vessels almost always have distinct skin findings (e.g., palpable purpura) to support the diagnosis. Both rheumatoid arthritis and systemic lupus erythematosus (SLE) are systemic illnesses that can be complicated by a small to medium-sized vessel vasculitis, but the only findings supporting these diagnoses are the mild joint complaints. The absence of allergic history, eosinophilia, and chest x-ray infiltrate distinct from pulmonary edema makes Churg-Strauss syndrome unlikely.

Biopsy of involved tissue is the most direct way to make a diagnosis in polyarteritis nodosa. The foot numbness suggests that the sural nerve is involved. Without clinical abnormalities, biopsy of skin would be low yield. An alternative diagnostic tool would be three-vessel abdominal arteriography, which is positive in 80% of patients. Right arm arteriography would likely show nothing abnormal; the typical vessels imaged are larger than those involved in polyarteritis. Tests for rheumatoid factor and hepatitis B surface antigen (HBsAg), even if positive, are not specific for polyarteritis.

The most widely used treatments for polyarteritis nodosa include corticosteroids and immunosuppressive agents (e.g., cyclophosphamide). This patient's severe and progressive disease probably warrants the use of both types of agents. Five-year mortality rates have been dramatically improved for this disease since the advent of corticosteroids, and the addition of immunosuppressive treatment has likely improved survival further. Nonsteroidal anti-inflammatory drugs (NSAIDs), antibiotics, antimalarial agents, and cyclosporine are not accepted treatment for polyarteritis.

13–15. The answers are: 13-D [VII G 1; Table 10-8], **14-F** [X B], **15-I** [II B 4 d, 5]. This young woman has the sudden onset of a systemic febrile illness that includes findings suggestive of serositis (pleuritic chest pain), arthritis, and a facial skin rash (possibly a butterfly rash). New pretibial edema suggests the possibility of urinary protein loss from renal involvement (glomerulonephritis or nephrotic syndrome). Although laboratory data [including positive antinuclear antibodies (ANAs)] or radiographic support will be necessary to confirm possible organ abnormalities, systemic lupus erythematosus (SLE) is the most likely cause of these findings.

This man likely has primary Sjögren's syndrome. The dry eyes and dry mouth suggest lacrimal and salivary gland involvement in this disorder, and further ophthalmologic evaluation or labial salivary gland biopsy could confirm these suspicions. Arthralgias are a common feature of primary Sjögren's; the arthritis of rheumatoid arthritis should have more actual joint findings (tenderness, swelling, or limitation of motion) to be considered as a primary disease accompanied by a secondary form of Sjögren's. The purpuric lesions on the calves suggest the possibility of a small vessel vasculitis, a common skin feature of primary Sjögren's.

This patient's presentation is most consistent with a chronic degenerative arthritis and a superimposed acute inflammatory arthritis. The degenerative, bony changes involve unusual joints [wrist, metacarpophalangeals (MCPs)] and include an unusual feature (chondrocalcinosis on knee x-ray). These findings are most compatible with calcium pyrophosphate deposition (CPPD) disease causing atypical degenerative arthritis, and the superimposed acute knee inflammation (pseudogout) is likely caused by release of the CPPD crystals into the knee joint. Finding positively birefringent crystals under red-compensated, polarized light examination of synovial fluid would be diagnostic.

Chapter 11

Neurologic Disorders

Barney J. Stern

I.   **APPROACH TO THE PATIENT WITH A NEUROLOGIC COMPLAINT**

A. **Patient history.** The patient history is the cornerstone of the neurologic assessment.

1. **Key questions** to direct the patient interview might include:
   a. Did the symptoms have a gradual or sudden onset?
   b. Are the symptoms static, intermittent, or progressive?
   c. Has the problem remained limited in scope, or have new features been introduced over time?
   d. What concurrent problems does the patient have, and what medications or drugs are being used?
   e. Is there a family history of the disorder or predisposing conditions?
   f. What habits and toxin exposures might the patient have?

2. **Review of symptoms.** Depending on the clinical complaint, the patient should be asked if there is any history of:
   a. Headache or trauma to the head, neck, or spine
   b. Loss of consciousness, convulsive activity, mood alterations, confusion, or memory disturbances
   c. Impaired or double vision, facial numbness or weakness, impaired hearing or swallowing, or abnormal speech
   d. Arm or leg weakness or heaviness, slowness of movement, altered limb sensation, discomfort or tingling in the extremities
   e. Clumsiness, falling, or dizziness
   f. Bowel or bladder disturbances or sexual dysfunction

B. **Neurologic examination.** From the patient history, the physician can generate a series of diagnostic hypotheses that can be tested with a focused neurologic examination. Anatomic localization of the pathology within the nervous system is essential to this process (Figure 11-1).

1. **Mental status.** If the patient's mental status is abnormal, the history and those components of the physical examination that depend on patient cooperation must be approached within the proper context. For example, if the patient is confused, the sensory exam may be unreliable.
   a. The patient's level of arousal, orientation, short- and long-term memory, affect (i.e., mood), concentration and attention, fund of knowledge, insight, judgment, and constructional ability should be assessed.
   b. Linguistic abilities are evaluated by examining comprehension, repetition, fluency, naming, reading, and writing.
   c. The integrity of other cortical functions (e.g., graphesthesia, stereognosis, two-point discrimination, right–left disorientation) should be examined if parietal lobe dysfunction is suspected. The physician should search for extinction to double simultaneous visual and sensory stimulation, as evidence of neglect phenomena. (Patients with neglect may be unaware of their neurologic deficits.)

2. **Cranial nerves.** Examination of cranial nerves (CN) I–XII is necessary. (Table 11-1).
   a. In particular, visual acuity and fields should be checked, the optic nerve should be examined, and abnormalities of ocular motility including nystagmus and dysmetria should be documented (Table 11-2).
   b. Abnormalities of facial sensation (including the corneal reflex) and movement should be investigated as well.

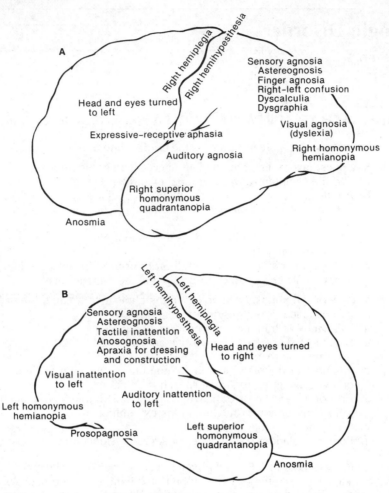

FIGURE 11-1. Summary of some of the outstanding neurologic signs and symptoms that occur with focal destructive lesions in the right or left cerebral hemisphere as detected upon neurologic examination. (*A*) Lateral view of the left cerebral hemisphere. (*B*) Lateral view of the right cerebral hemisphere. (Reprinted from NMS *Neuroanatomy*. Malvern, PA, Harwal Publishing, 1988, p 314.)

3. **Sensory system.** Regions of abnormal touch, pain (estimated by pinprick), temperature, vibration, and proprioception should be defined.
   a. Are the findings confined to one side of the body, the distribution of one or more dermatomes, or the territory of one or more peripheral nerves?
   b. Are the sensory changes found in a "stocking–glove" distribution?

4. **Motor system**
   a. The patient's **strength** should be defined as it pertains to individual muscles or groups of muscles. One conventional method of grading muscle strength for purposes of comparison and description is shown in Table 11-3.
   b. The presence of **atrophy, fasciculations, spasticity,** and **rigidity** should be noted.
   c. The patient's ability to perform **rapid alternating and other complex maneuvers** should be determined.
   d. The patient's **stance and gait** should be evaluated (Table 11-4).

5. **Coordination.** Finger-to-nose and heel-to-shin testing should be performed. The physician should look for **Romberg's sign** (i.e., the patient will sway or fall when standing with eyes closed and feet close together).

TABLE 11-1. Twelve Cranial Nerves

Number	Name	Summary of Function
I	Olfactory	Smells
II	Optic	Sees
III	Oculomotor	Moves eyeball and constricts pupil
IV	Trochlear	Moves eyeball
V	Trigeminal	Feels front half of head and chews
VI	Abducens	Moves eyeball
VII	Facial	Moves face; tears, tastes, and salivates
VIII	Vestibulocochlear	Equilibrates and hears
IX	Glossopharyngeal	Tastes, salivates, and swallows and monitors carotid body and sinus
X	Vagus	Tastes, swallows, lifts palate, and phonates; sensorimotor to thoracicoabdominal viscera
XI	Spinal accessory	Turns head and shrugs shoulders
XII	Hypoglossal	Moves tongue

Adapted from NMS *Neuroanatomy.* Malvern, Pa, Harwal Publishing, 1988, p 139.

TABLE 11-2. Innervation of the Eye by Its Six Nerves

Number and Name of Nerve	Innervation	Clinical Effects of Interruption of Nerve
Efferent		
CN III (oculomotor nerve)	Striated muscle: superior, medial, and inferior recti; inferior oblique	Diplopia, eye abducted and turned down
	Levator palpebrae	Ptosis (paralysis of volitional lid elevation)
	Smooth muscle: pupilloconstrictor	Pupil dilated and fixed to light
	Ciliary muscle	Loss of lens thickening
CN IV (trochlear nerve)	Striated muscle: superior oblique	Diplopia, most severe on looking down and in; eye extorted; head tilted to side opposite paralyzed eye
CN VI (abducens nerve)	Striated muscle: lateral rectuus	Diplopia, most severe on looking to side of paralysis; eye turned in (abducted)
Carotid sympathetic nerve	Smooth muscle: superior tarsal and pupillodilator	Horner's syndrome (ptosis, miosis, hemifacial anhidrosis, vasodilation)
Afferent		
CN II (optic nerve)	From retina	Blindness
CN V (trigeminal nerve)	Corneal/conjunctival afferents	Anesthesia of cornea with loss of corneal reflex

Adapted from NMS *Neuroanatomy.* Malvern, PA, Harwal Publishing, 1988, p 219.

TABLE 11-3. Medical Research Council of Great Britain Muscle Strength Grading Scale

Grade	Equivalent Patient Ability
5/5	Normal ability
4/5	Ability to overcome gravity and some resistance imposed by the examiner
3/5	Ability to overcome gravity only
2/5	Ability to move with gravity eliminated
1/5	Only a flicker of movement
0/5	Complete inability to move

6. **Muscle stretch reflexes.** The activity and symmetry of the brachioradialis (C5, C6), biceps (C5, C6), triceps (C7, C8), knee (L3, L4), and ankle (S1, S2) reflexes should be determined. The presence of the **Babinski response** should be assessed with plantar stimulation.

C. **Neurodiagnostic studies**

1. **Cerebrospinal fluid (CSF) evaluation**
   a. **Indications.** Study of the CSF can provide information about intracranial pressure (ICP) and infection, bleeding, malignancy, and sterile inflammation within the central nervous system (CNS).
   b. **Specific measurements and assays**
      (1) **Pressure.** The opening pressure should be determined. Pressure exceeding 180 mm H_2O is abnormal when the patient is relaxed and in a lateral decubitus position.
      (2) **Protein.** An elevated CSF protein level is a nonspecific indicator of inflammation or breakdown of the blood–brain barrier.
      (3) **Glucose. Hypoglycorrhachia** (i.e., CSF glucose less than 40 mg/dl or a simultaneous CSF–blood glucose ratio of < 0.6) suggests infection or sterile inflammation.

TABLE 11-4. Classification of Gait Disorders

Gait Disorder	Disequilibrium (Impaired Balance)	Gait Ignition Failure (Start/ Turn Hesitation) (Freezing)	Wide Base	Shortened Stride	Associated Findings
Cautious gait	Mild	Absent	Mild	Mild to moderate	. . .
Subcortical disequilibrium	Severe	Variable	Variable	Variable	Occasional parkinsonism; pyramidal signs
Frontal disequilibrium	Severe	Variable	Variable	Variable	Dementia, frontal release signs, and urinary incontinence; occasionally apraxia, parkinsonism, and pyramidal signs
Isolated gait ignition failure	None	Severe	Absent	Absent*	. . .
Frontal gait disorder	Moderate	Moderate to severe	Variable	Mild to moderate	Dementia, frontal release signs, and urinary incontinence; occasionally apraxia, parkinsonism, and pyramidal signs

Apraxia may be gauged by asking the patient to mime gestures with the arms or legs. Frontal release signs include gegenhalten hand and foot grasp reflexes, and rooting responses. In this table, "parkinsonism" refers to hypokinesia and difficulty executing rhythmic and repetitive alternating or sequential movements.
(Adaped with permission from Nutt JG, Marsden CD, Thompson PD: Human walking and higher-level gait disorders, particularly in the elderly. *Neurology* 43:272, 1993.)
* Steps would be of normal size and rhythm once walking was underway.

(a) Relatively common causes of hypoglycorrhachia include bacterial, fungal, or tuberculous infection, carcinomatous meningitis, and hypoglycemia.

(b) Less common causes include mumps, herpes simplex virus (HSV) or zoster infection, subarachnoid hemorrhage (SAH), sarcoidosis, syphilitic meningitis, and systemic lupus erythematosus (SLE).

(4) **White cell count.** A white cell count exceeding $5/\mu l$ of CSF is considered abnormal.

(a) **Excess neutrophils** suggest infection or, on occasion, sterile inflammation.

(b) **Excess mononuclear cells** suggest a viral infection, an indolent nonviral infectious process, or sterile inflammation.

(5) **Blood** may appear in the CSF as a result of the local trauma of a lumbar puncture (LP), or by CNS hemorrhage from multiple causes.

(a) A traumatic LP is suspected if gross blood exudes from the needle and then clears quickly, or if a large discrepancy exists between the number of red cells in the first drops of CSF obtained as compared to a later aliquot.

(b) A traumatic LP should not reveal a xanthochromic (yellow-tinged) CSF, because sufficient time would not have elapsed to cause breakdown of red cells.

(6) **Culture and Gram staining of CSF** are indicated to evaluate the possibility of infection. A CSF Venereal Disease Research Laboratories (VDRL) test is indicated if CNS syphilis is a diagnostic consideration.

(7) **Cytologic examination** is useful if malignancy is suspected.

(8) **Intrathecal immunoglobulin production** can be determined with the IgG index:

$$\frac{\text{CSF IgG/serum IgG}}{\text{CSF albumin/serum albumin}}$$

or through CSF electrophoresis, which reveals the presence of oligoclonal bands (discrete immunoglobulin aggregates). An elevated IgG index or oligoclonal bands are found in CNS inflammatory disorders, such as multiple sclerosis, and infections.

c. **Contraindications** to performing LP include:

(1) A **mass effect** sufficient to cause distortion of the lateral or third ventricles or a midline shift;

(2) A **posterior fossa mass;**

(3) A **coagulopathy** [e.g., a prothrombin time (PT) exceeding 3 seconds over control or a platelet count of less than 50,000 μl].

2. **Electroencephalography (EEG) and evoked potentials (EPs)**

a. **EEG** is indicated in the evaluation of **seizure disorders, encephalopathies, sleep disorders,** and **brain death.** Prolonged video EEG monitoring is the **gold standard** for evaluating seizure problems that are difficult to diagnose or treat.

b. **EPs** are repetitive afferent stimuli presented to the eye, ear, peripheral sensory nerves, or cerebral cortex that cause stereotypic wave forms that can be analyzed by computerized signal averaging methodology.

(1) **Visual, brain stem-auditory,** and **somatosensory EPs** can detect lesions, which are often clinically silent, in the anatomic pathways subserving these sensory systems.

(2) **Motor EPs** can be elicited by transcranial stimulation of the motor pathways. These studies provide information about the integrity of the motor system.

3. **Imaging studies**

a. **Computed tomography (CT) scanning** provides an image of the brain that allows definition of **hemorrhage, edema, atrophy, mass lesions,** and **ventricular size.**

(1) Intravenous contrast can be administered to define **regions where the blood–brain barrier is not intact.**

        (2) CT scanning can also visualize **the spinal cord** and **surrounding bony structures;** transverse images are especially well represented by CT scanning.

    b. Magnetic resonance imaging (MRI) provides excellent **anatomic depiction of the brain,** especially the posterior fossa, **and the spinal cord.** Disease of the cerebral white matter is particularly well defined. Intravenous contrast can detect sites of a disturbed blood–brain barrier.

    c. Single photon emission computed tomography (SPECT) provides an image-based estimate of **cerebral blood flow** following intravenous injection of a radioactive tracer.

    d. Noninvasive vascular studies

        (1) Duplex scanning provides an ultrasound image of the extracranial carotid and vertebral arteries together with a Doppler description of flow patterns.

        (2) Transcranial Doppler defines intracranial large artery flow patterns.

        (3) Magnetic resonance angiography uses magnetic resonance technology to image the vascular anatomy.

    e. Angiography. The vascular anatomy is best defined with cerebral angiography. This study is useful for identifying an aneurysmal source of SAH, evaluating occlusive cerebrovascular disease (especially if surgery is contemplated), defining vasculitis, and assessing arteriovenous malformations.

  4. Nerve conduction studies and electromyography (EMG)

    a. Nerve conduction studies can place peripheral nerve disease into sensory, motor, or sensorimotor categories; define primarily demyelinating or axonal dysfunction; and identify sites of conduction block. These distinctions help in making a diagnosis.

    b. EMG can differentiate problems affecting muscle into broad categories such as denervation and myopathy.

        (1) The **distribution of the observed changes** helps determine if the problem is myotomal (i.e., limited to a few nerve roots) or diffuse.

        (2) The **pattern of wave forms** provides information pertaining to ongoing muscular denervation and spontaneous reinnervation.

II.   LOSS OF CONSCIOUSNESS

  A. Syncope

    1. Definition. Syncope refers to a transient loss of consciousness that typically follows insufficient blood supply to the brain for more than a few seconds.

    2. Clinical signs. The patient is transiently unresponsive and muscle tone is diminished. A few generalized tonic spasms may occur, especially if the patient is prevented from lying down.

    3. Etiology. Cardiac and circulatory causes of syncope are discussed in Chapter 1 X. Most patients with syncope have a cardiac or circulatory basis for the event, although neurologic conditions need to be considered if the diagnosis remains elusive.

    a. Circulatory disturbances are particularly common.

        (1) Vasovagal syncope is commonly associated with emotional stress, fear, or pain, and is often seen in young people.

        (2) Postprandial syncope frequently affects the elderly, and often occurs following meals where alcohol was consumed.

        (3) Syncope can occur in diverse settings that have in common a **preceding Valsalva** or **straining maneuver** that decreases venous return and promotes parasympathetic tone.

    b. Cardiac output disturbances. Conditions that disturb cardiac output, other than arrhythmia or mechanical obstruction, should be considered.

(1) Vasodepressor (neurocardiogenic) syncope is caused by undue stimulation of afferent cardiac mechanoreceptors because of cardiac distention or strenuous contractions. This causes a decrease in sympathetic activity and an increase in parasympathetic activity that leads to vasodilatation, bradycardia, and subsequent hypotension.

(2) Carotid sinus hypersensitivity can lead to bradyarrhythmias and hypotension. Because carotid sinus hypersensitivity is present in many older men, it should be considered responsible for syncope only if other causes have been excluded.

    (a) Atropine may be used to treat **cardioinhibitory** carotid sinus hypersensitivity.

    (b) Epinephrine blocks the effects of **cardiodepressor** carotid sinus hypersensitivity.

    (c) Patients can exhibit both types of carotid sinus hypersensitivity.

c. Hypoglycemia causes a lack of nutrient supply to the brain and can lead to syncope. Hypoglycemia as a cause of syncope is particularly likely in insulin-dependent diabetics. Therapy involves the administration of glucose.

d. Neurologic disorders are relatively uncommon causes of syncope. Several conditions are important because they can lead to unresponsiveness and are therefore often considered during the evaluation of a patient with transient unresponsiveness.

(1) Seizures (see also IX A–B) are a cause of unresponsiveness that must be differentiated from syncope.

    (a) Rarely is a patient limp during a seizure.

    (b) Atonic seizures are rare in adults but do cause sudden collapse. Absence seizures, on the other hand, do not result in a fall.

    (c) Because some patients with syncope can exhibit involuntary movements, the possibility of a primary seizure is a consideration in these individuals. However, in most cases, the tonic or myoclonic activity tends to occur several seconds after consciousness is lost and merely reflects cerebral hypoperfusion, not a primary seizure disorder.

(2) Focal cerebral ischemia is rarely a cause of syncope.

    (a) Rarely, ischemia to the ascending **reticular activating system (RAS),** as found in the top-of-the-basilar syndrome, can cause transient unresponsiveness.

        (i) Cardiogenic emboli or extracranial or intracranial large artery occlusive disease may compromise perfusion.

        (ii) Sometimes small penetrating arteries arising from the rostral basilar artery can be responsible for transient unresponsiveness.

        (iii) Patients with vertebrobasilar occlusive disease may experience transient unresponsiveness as a result of focal ischemia. These patients typically have other symptoms and signs referable to focal ischemia [see VIII B 1 b].

    (b) Generally, unilateral carotid territory ischemia does not result in syncope.

(3) SAH can transiently increase ICP, compromising global cerebral perfusion. Clues to the diagnosis include persistent headache, meningismus, and papilledema.

(4) Basilar artery migraine (a unique type of migraine with aura) is a rare cause of unresponsiveness. A history of recurrent headache, recurrent episodes of unresponsiveness, and associated symptoms (e.g., visual distortion and dizziness) should lead the physician to consider this condition. In most instances, other causes of vertebrobasilar ischemia should be sought before assigning a diagnosis of basilar artery migraine.

(5) An **Arnold-Chiari malformation** (characterized by extension of the cerebellum into the spinal canal and brain stem distortion) can occasionally cause transient symptomatic hydrocephalus or compromise medullary function, leading to a brief loss of consciousness.

(6) Narcolepsy can cause episodes of sleep or cataplexy that can be mistaken for syncope.

(7) Glossopharyngeal neuralgia can cause bradycardia and vasodilation. Patients have paroxysms of pain in the pharynx or external auditory canal.

(8) A **colloid cyst of the third ventricle** can cause sudden obstructive hydrocephalus, leading to increased ICP and hypoperfusion.

e. Psychogenic unresponsiveness can be associated with anxiety, panic attacks, or hyperventilation, as well as somatoform (conversion) disorder.

4. Diagnosis. A history and physical examination can often provide clues to the proper diagnosis. If no clues are evident, it is generally appropriate to proceed with a cardiovascular evaluation as outlined in Chapter 1 X C.

   a. Neurologic testing frequently includes an EEG. Rarely is a CT scan diagnostic. In some patients, an MRI or imaging studies of the vascular system can be informative.

   b. Upright tilt testing, possibly with isoproterenol infusion, can provide evidence for a diagnosis of vasodepressor (neurocardiogenic) syncope, especially if the characteristic hemodynamic changes occur in less than 15 minutes without isoproterenol infusion.

5. Therapy depends on the underlying diagnosis. Neurocardiogenic syncope is treated with β-adrenergic blockers or disopyramide.

B. Coma

1. Definition. Coma is a state in which the patient is unresponsive to environmental stimuli and unable to communicate in any manner. Coma is associated with extensive damage to both cerebral hemispheres or to the ascending RAS in the diencephalon, mesencephalon, or pons.

2. Etiology. The many causes of coma can be broadly grouped as shown in Table 11-5.

TABLE 11-5. Causes of Coma

Category	Possible Etiologic Factors
Supratentorial (hemispheric) lesions	Epidural or subdural hematoma Intraparenchymal hemorrhage Large ischemic infarction Tumor Abscess Trauma
Infratentorial lesions	Pontine or cerebellar hematoma Basilar artery thrombosis Ischemic cerebellar infarction Tumor Abscess
Diffuse diseases, metabolic disorders, and toxins	Subarachnoid hemorrhage Meningitis Encephalitis Hydrocephalus Drugs (e.g., narcotics, alcohol, barbiturates, benzodiazepines) Hypo- or hyperglycemia Ischemic or hypoxic encephalopathy Hypercarbia Myxedema Hypothermia Hepatic or renal failure Thiamine deficiency
Psychogenic	

3. Approach to the patient. Complete and rapid assessment of the patient is critical for optimal care.

   a. Patient history. The physician should ascertain the following information:

   (1) The patient's **past medical status,** especially if the patient has a preexisting neurologic, cardiac, pulmonary, or renal condition

   (2) Prescription and **over-the-counter drugs** used by the patient

   (3) History of **drug abuse,** if applicable

   (4) Recent patient complaints

   (5) Details regarding the site where the patient was found (e.g., the presence of empty drug vials or evidence of a fall)

   b. The **physical examination** should be thorough. Extremes of blood pressure, pulse, or temperature, abnormal breathing patterns, evidence of head or neck trauma, and the presence of meningismus should be noted carefully. The patient's skin should be examined for signs of trauma or needle tracks. In addition, special attention should be directed to the patient's:

   (1) Pupils. Pupillary size and reactivity is dependent on sympathetic and parasympathetic innervation. Brain stem reflexes, such as the pupillary reaction to light, offer clues to the location of the lesion responsible for the coma.

   (a) Large, nonreactive pupils result from the disruption of the parasympathetic pupilloconstrictive impulses that arise from the mesencephalic Edinger-Westphal nucleus and travel as a component of the third cranial nerve to the eye.

   (b) Small, reactive pupils result from the disruption of the sympathetic pupillodilatory impulses that arise in the hypothalamus and course caudally through the periaqueductal gray matter and cervical spinal cord before travelling rostrally with the internal carotid artery toward the eye.

   (2) Ocular motility. Analysis of ocular motility allows the physician to assess damage to the brain stem and the cranial nerves that control eye movement.

   (a) The physician should first examine the resting position for spontaneous motion of the eyeballs. Although a comatose patient's eyes may move spontaneously, the eyes do not fixate or track in a purposeful manner.

   (b) If the eyes are immobile, movement can be elicited through the **vestibulo-ocular reflex** by moving the patient's head side to side (the **"doll's head"** or **oculocephalic maneuver**) or by elevating the patient's head 30° and irrigating the external auditory canal with ice water.

   (i) Conjugate deviation of the eyes bilaterally implies intact brain stem circuitry.

   (ii) Failure of an eye to abduct in response to these maneuvers implies dysfunction of pontine structures or sixth nerve compromise.

   (iii) Failure of an eye to adduct implies dysfunction of the medial longitudinal fasciculus or oculomotor nucleus or nerve.

   (iv) The presence of **conjugate nystagmus** contralateral to the side of ice water irrigation suggests psychogenic coma.

   (3) Motor functions. Quadriparesis, hemiparesis, or monoparesis may occur in comatose patients.

   (a) Quadriparesis and flaccidity suggest medullary compromise or a high cervical spinal cord insult.

   (b) Decorative posturing (i.e., leg extension with flexion of the arm, wrist, and fingers) can be unilateral or bilateral and suggests a hemispheral or diencephalic lesion.

   (c) Decerebrate posturing (i.e., leg and arm extension) also can be unilateral or bilateral and suggests midbrain or pontine compromise.

4. **Clinical features.** Once global brain stem dysfunction has developed, differentiation between supratentorial and infratentorial causes of coma cannot be made without diagnostic testing, unless a history and serial observations of the patient's clinical course can be documented.

   a. **Supratentorial causes of coma** are characterized by pathologic processes that result in **swelling of a cerebral hemisphere.**

      (1) This mass effect causes a midline shift of the affected hemisphere toward the contralateral side, compression of the ipsilateral third nerve as it courses near the medial temporal lobe (uncus), herniation of the medial temporal lobe below the tentorial notch (uncal herniation), distortion of the mesencephalon, and herniation of the cingulate gyrus under the midline falx (subfalcial herniation).

      (2) Typically, there is a progressive clinical deterioration characterized by increasing unresponsiveness, development of a third nerve palsy ipsilateral to the swollen hemisphere, and, ultimately, midbrain compromise (reflected by bilaterally nonreactive, dilated pupils).

   b. **Infratentorial causes of coma** can be suspected if ataxia, multiple asymmetric cranial nerve palsies, and unilateral or bilateral limb weakness or sensory loss develop prior to the development of more global, severe impairment of brain stem function (characterized by nonreactive pupils, absent ocular motility, and absent corneal and gag reflexes).

   c. **Diffuse, toxic, or metabolic causes of coma** can be suspected in a comatose patient if pupillary responses are intact, ocular motility is preserved, corneal reflexes can be elicited, a gag reflex is present, and limb movement in response to noxious local stimuli is observed. If pupillary responsiveness remains even when other brain stem and limb function is lost, a metabolic cause of coma should be considered.

   d. **Psychogenic coma** should be suspected if the patient has a history of psychiatric disease or if the findings on physical examination are nonphysiologic. Examples of nonphysiologic responses in a "comatose" patient include:

      (1) The presence of **nystagmus** when the patient's ears are irrigated with ice water

      (2) Adversive head and eye movements

      (3) Failure of the patient's arm, when held by the examiner over the patient's face, to fall upon the face when released by the examiner

      (4) Resistance to having the eyelids opened

5. **Therapy.** Ideally, care of the comatose patient is intertwined with the initial assessment of the patient and the development of etiologic hypotheses.

   a. **Initial therapy.** Maintaining an **adequate airway, optimal ventilation,** and **appropriate blood pressure** are priority concerns.

      (1) If there is a possibility of **cervical fracture, immobilization of the neck** is of great importance.

      (2) **Endotracheal intubation** is usually indicated to protect the airway.

      (3) **Blood samples** for a complete blood count (CBC), electrolytes, glucose, renal and liver function studies, coagulation profiles, blood gases, and toxicology should be obtained.

      (4) **Intravenous thiamine** (100 mg), one ampule of **50% glucose in water,** and **naloxone** (0.4 mg) are often administered. **Flumazenil** can be given if benzodiazepine or hepatic coma is suspected.

   b. **Additional therapy**

      (1) **Imaging.** If the patient's general medical condition permits, and if the cause of coma is not clearly cerebral anoxia following cardiopulmonary arrest or a drug overdose, most patients should have a brain **CT scan** to define the presence of an **intracranial mass, cerebral edema,** or **hydrocephalus.** Further management depends on the etiology of the coma.

      (2) **ICP evaluation and management**

         (a) **ICP evaluation.** Consideration of the patient's ICP is intimately tied to the evaluation of coma. The intracranial cavity has a finite volume and compliance.

      (i) Normally, modest volume additions to the intracranial contents, (e.g., from a small intraparenchymal hematoma), cause only a small rise in ICP.

      (ii) As the intracranial volume progressively increases, (e.g., from massive cerebral edema or a tumor), the intracranial compliance decreases and the ICP markedly increases.

      (iii) Because cerebral perfusion pressure is the result of the mean arterial pressure minus the ICP, an **excessive rise of the ICP** is associated with **impaired cerebral perfusion** and **progressive neurologic deterioration.**

    (b) **ICP management.** If a comatose patient is suspected of having a pathologic process associated with elevated ICP, emergency management of the patient should include steps to decrease, or at the very least, avoid increasing, the pressure. If possible, the cerebral perfusion pressure should be kept at greater than 60 mm Hg and the ICP should be maintained at less than 20 mm Hg. Optimal management of increased ICP often requires direct ICP monitoring as well as determination of hemodynamic parameters.

      (i) The patient can be hyperventilated with an Ambu bag prior to intubation. Intubation and endotracheal suctioning should be performed carefully in order to minimize elevation of ICP.

      (ii) Fever and agitation should be minimized.

      (iii) The patient's head should be elevated 30° and kept in midposition to optimize venous drainage.

      (iv) Osmotic therapy is used to dehydrate the brain and decrease the ICP. Patients are kept euvolemic and administered intravenous mannitol to achieve a hyperosmotic state.

C. **Vegetative state**

    1. Definitions

      a. The **vegetative state** is characterized by the patient's unawareness of self or external stimuli. Autonomic functions are relatively well maintained and a sleep–wake cycle exists.

        (1) The patient cannot interact with others in a meaningful fashion.

        (2) Patients can survive with medical and nursing support.

    2. A **persistent vegetative state** is defined as a vegetative state that persists for at least 1 month after the initial brain insult. If, with continued observation (usually 3 months for nontraumatic injury), there is no meaningful recovery, the likelihood of functional recovery can be judged to be nil and the patient can be said to be in a **permanent vegetative state.**

    3. Therapy. If a patient is in a persistent vegetative state, the family and physician should determine the level of treatment appropriate for the patient.

D. **Brain death**

    1. Definition. Death is recognized as occurring when there is irreversible cessation of all brain function. A brain insult sufficient to cause complete loss of cerebral function should be documented, if possible.

    2. Approach to the patient

      a. Physical examination. The patient is completely unresponsive to external visual, auditory, and tactile stimuli and is incapable of communication in any manner.

        (1) Pupillary responses are absent, and eye movements cannot be elicited by the vestibulo-ocular reflex or by irrigating the ears with cold water.

        (2) The corneal and gag reflexes are absent, and there is no facial or tongue movement.

        (3) The limbs are flaccid, and there is no movement, although primitive withdrawal movements in response to local painful stimuli, mediated at a spinal cord level, can occur.

b. Apnea test. Brain-dead patients have no respiratory function. An apnea test should be performed to ascertain that no respirations occur at a Pco_2 level of at least 60 mm Hg. The patient's oxygenation should be maintained as the Pco_2 is allowed to rise. The inability to develop respiration is consistent with medullary failure.

c. Exclusionary criteria. A diagnosis of brain death cannot be made in the setting of drug intoxication, hypothermia (defined as a core temperature of < 32 °C), severe hypotension (i.e., shock), or drug-induced paralysis.

d. Confirmatory tests are usually not necessary to diagnose brain death, but they can be used if doubt exists or if local statutes require them

(1) An **EEG** will not demonstrate any physiologic brain activity.

(2) Tests to assess cerebral blood flow fail to show cerebral perfusion.

e. A **period of observation** is necessary before a diagnosis of brain death can be made, unless there is gross evidence of a nonsurvivable insult to the brain.

(1) Two evaluations of the patient (at 6 hours and 12 hours) are usually sufficient to support a diagnosis of brain death.

(2) In the presence of anoxic brain damage, 24 hours of observation are appropriate before declaring brain death.

III. ALTERATION IN BEHAVIOR

A. Delirium

1. Definition. Delirium is a disorder of brain function affecting behavior and causing impaired attention and cognition, motor hyper- or hypoactivity, altered sleep–wake cycles, and altered states of arousal. It is often acute, reversible, and secondary to a medical or neurologic disorder.

2. Etiology. Generalized or focal causes of cerebral dysfunction are potential causes of delirium.

a. Generalized brain dysfunction can be caused by the following.

(1) Drugs, including anticholinergics, antiparkinsonians, analgesics, cimetidine, digoxin, benzodiazepines, antidepressants, and illicit substances, may produce delirium. Withdrawal from alcohol, barbiturates, and benzodiazepines is associated with delirium as well.

(2) Metabolic alterations, including hypoxia, hypercarbia, hyponatremia, uremia, hepatic failure, hyperglycemia, hypoglycemia, sepsis (septic encephalopathy), fever, dehydration, hypercalcemia, myxedema, hyperthyroidism, and thiamine and niacin deficiencies can cause delirium.

(3) Diffuse insults to the brain, such as meningitis, encephalitis, fat emboli, and disseminated intravascular coagulation (DIC), are associated with cognitive impairment.

(4) Nonconvulsive status epilepticus, including absence or complex partial seizures, may cause delirium. Postictal patients may also be delirious.

b. Focal cerebral disease. Differentiating a global cerebral disorder from a focal brain disease that may also cause altered behavior presents a clinical challenge. For example, focal brain disease can cause a subtle aphasia, which may be misinterpreted as delirium. Appropriate laboratory and neurodiagnostic tests should be performed based on the clinical presentation.

(1) Focal cerebral disease, typically due to stroke, involves the nondominant temporoparietal area, frontal lobes, head of the caudate nucleus, internal capsule, thalamus (the top-of-the-basilar syndrome), or occipital lobes, which may cause blindness. Patients suffering from a focal cerebral disease may be agitated and experience hallucinations.

(2) Mass lesions can also cause a confusional state, especially if they are located in the frontal lobes.

3. **Therapy** is aimed at identifying and treating, when possible, the causes of delirium. An offending agent may have to be withdrawn. Adequate nutrition should be maintained and the safety of the patient insured. If necessary, sedation with a low dose of haloperidol can be helpful.

B. Dementia

1. **Definition.** Dementia is a progressive mental disorder characterized by compromised abstract thinking ability, memory, and judgment. Unlike delirium, dementia is usually chronic and often results from primary degenerative brain disease or from a host of other conditions, such as multiple strokes.

2. **Etiology.** The causes of dementia are many. Identification of a treatable condition masquerading as a degenerative process is critical.
   a. Some **causes of dementia** include Alzheimer's disease, Parkinson's disease, multiple cerebral infarcts, Huntington's disease, Pick's disease, human immunodeficiency virus (HIV) infection, and Creutzfeldt-Jakob disease.
   b. **Potentially treatable conditions that can present as dementia** include depression (pseudodementia), normal pressure hydrocephalus (NPH), subdural hematoma, tumor, adverse drug effects, thyroid disease, vitamin B_{12} deficiency, thiamine deficiency, syphilis, heavy metal intoxication, and conditions causing hypersomnia (e.g., sleep apnea syndrome).

3. **Alzheimer's disease** is the **most common cause** of chronic dementia.
   a. **Definition.** Alzheimer's disease is a clinicopathologic entity characterized by progressive memory loss and other cognitive deficits. Onset commonly is late in life, although patients may be affected in middle age.
      (1) The disease usually arises spontaneously, but genetic factors have been identified. Familial cases have been mapped to chromosomes 1, 14, 19, and 21.
      (2) There is an association between the age of onset of Alzheimer's disease and the apolipoprotein E genotype. Patients with the APOE4/4 genotype are at the greatest risk for Alzheimer's disease at a given age.
   b. **Prevalence.** Alzheimer's disease is a burgeoning public health problem. It is estimated that 60%–80% of demented patients have Alzheimer's disease. The prevalence of Alzheimer's disease increases sharply with age, affecting 5%–15% of people over age 65 and about three times as many people age 85 and older (the fastest-growing segment of the population).
   c. **Pathology.** Although the cause and pathogenesis are unknown, Alzheimer's disease has a characteristic pathology consisting of **intracellular neurofibrillary tangles** and **extracellular neuritic plaques.**
      (1) The tangles are composed primarily of abnormally-phosphorylated, microtubule-associated tau proteins.
      (2) The plaques consist of β-amyloid protein, an abnormal fragment of amyloid precursor protein that is a transmembrane glycoprotein. The gene for amyloid precursor protein resides on chromosome 21 and may be involved in familial cases.
      (3) The pathologic processes associated with Alzheimer's disease disturb many neurotransmitters, particularly the cholinergic system.
   d. **Diagnosis**
      (1) The **clinical diagnosis** of **senile dementia of the Alzheimer's type (SDAT)** can be made if an otherwise alert patient exhibits progressive memory loss and other cognitive deficits, such as disorientation, language difficulties, inability to perform complex motor activities, inattention, visual misperception, poor problem-solving abilities, inappropriate social behavior, and, occasionally, hallucinations.
         (a) The **intellectual decline** should be present in two or more areas of cognition and be documented by clinical examinations such as the

TABLE 11-6. Mini-Mental State Examination

Maximum Score	Score	
		Orientation:
5	( )	What is the (year) (season) (date) (day) (month)?
5	( )	Where are we: (state) (county) (town) (hospital) (floor)?
		Registration:
3	( )	Name three objects: 1 second to say each. Then ask the patient all three after you have said them. Give 1 point for each correct answer. Then repeat them until he or she learns all three. Count trials and record. (No. of trials:)
		Attention and calculation:
5	( )	Serial 7's. 1 point for each correct. Stop after five answers. Alternatively spell "world" backwards.
		Recall:
3	( )	Ask for three objects repeated above. Give 1 point for each correct.
		Language:
9	( )	Name a pencil, and watch. (2 points)
		Repeat the following: "No ifs, ands, or buts." (1 point)
		Follow a three-stage command: "Take a paper in your right hand, fold it in half, and put it on the floor." (3 points)
		Read and obey the following: "Close your eyes." (1 point)
		Write a sentence. (1 point)
		Copy this design. (1 point)

Assess level of consciousness along a continuum.

Total score

Alert	Drowsy	Stupor	Coma

Reprinted with permission from Folstein M, Rovner B, Tune L, et al: The cognitively impaired patient. In *The Principles and Practice of Medicine,* 22nd ed. Edited by McGehee H, et al. East Norwalk, CT, Appleton & Lange, 1988, p 1136.

mini–mental state examination (Table 11-6) or the **Blessed dementia scale.**

- **(b) Formal neuropsychologic testing** can confirm the clinical impression and document progression of the disease. Tests that address recall (with or without cues) and delayed recall are especially sensitive for documenting early memory impairment.
- **(c)** Other systemic and neurologic diseases that could produce cognitive decline should be absent.

(2) Differential diagnosis. Patients with **pseudodementia (depression)** can exhibit many of the features of Alzheimer's disease. To complicate matters further, patients with Alzheimer's can present with depression.

- **(a)** A careful history and neuropsychological evaluation can often determine the proper diagnosis.
- **(b)** If doubt remains as to the role of depression in the clinical presentation, appropriate treatment for depression is warranted.

e. Therapy

(1) Medical therapy is useful in treating insomnia, agitation, and depression.

- **(a)** In general, drugs should initially be given at a low dose; the dose can be adjusted upwards slowly as clinically indicated.

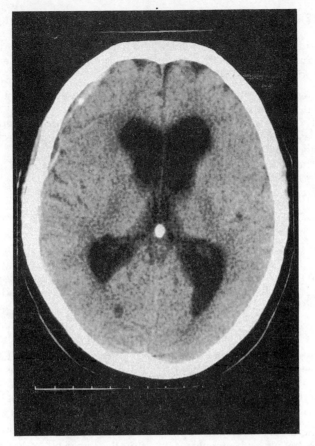

FIGURE 11-2. A nonenhanced computed tomography (CT) scan demonstrating hydrocephalus consistent with normal pressure hydrocephalus (NPH). Note the lack of cortical atrophy (sulcal effacement).

      (b) Medications with a short half-life and few anticholinergic side effects are best tolerated.

      (c) Cholinesterase inhibitors, such as tetrahydroaminoacridine, may improve memory function.

    (2) **Day care centers** (including day hospitals) and **respite care** are useful adjuncts to family supervision of the patient with Alzheimer's disease.

4. Normal pressure hydrocephalus (NPH)

  a. Definition. NPH is a condition characterized by cognitive impairment, urinary incontinence, and gait apraxia (i.e., impaired ambulation without evidence of primary motor, sensory, or cerebellar dysfunction).

  b. Etiology. In most patients, the cause of NPH is unknown. However, NPH can follow SAH or meningitis, sometimes even years later.

  c. Diagnosis. NPH should be suspected in a patient who presents with the clinical features noted in III B 4 a. The following tests may help to confirm the diagnosis.

    (1) Imaging studies

      (a) A CT scan reveals ventricular enlargement with relatively little cortical atrophy (Figure 11-2).

      (b) Cisternography involves injecting a radionuclide into the lumbar thecal sac and then taking serial determinations of the flow pattern of the radioactive bolus. In the presence of NPH, cisternography demonstrates persistent activity of the radionuclide in the lateral ventricles after 48 hours.

    (2) ICP monitoring for 24–48 hours can reveal transient pressure rises, if the diagnosis is in doubt.

    d. Therapy. Insertion of a **ventriculoperitoneal shunt** can improve the patient's condition, especially if performed within 6 months of the onset of the problem.

    5. Creutzfeldt-Jakob disease is a progressive, degenerative illness caused by **prions** (i.e., infectious proteinaceous particles).

      a. The gene for the prion protein is on **chromosome 20;** approximately 10% of cases are hereditary. Illness can develop because of **infection** or **somatic** and **germ cell mutations.**

      b. The **EEG** often demonstrates **periodic discharges** and an abnormal background rhythm.

      c. Death usually occurs within several months of the onset of the disease.

IV. HEADACHE.

is an extremely common patient complaint. Many patients are concerned that their headaches are due to a life-threatening condition, such as a brain tumor. Fortunately, this is rarely the case, but complaints of headache always deserve further evaluation.

A. Etiology

1. Non-neurologic causes of headache. Before assuming that cephalic discomfort is due to an intracranial disorder, the physician should consider the possibility of a non-neurologic cause. Disorders of the head and neck, such as sinus disease, glaucoma, dental infections, temporomandibular joint (TMJ) disease, ear pathology, muscular injury, or cervical spine problems can cause headache.

2. Intracranial stimulation of pain-sensitive structures can lead to headache. Problems that affect the meninges or distort the larger blood vessels cause pain.

B. Life-threatening causes of headache

1. An **intracranial mass** causes a headache that typically develops insidiously and progressively worsens.

    a. Clinical features. The **pain** is unlike any the patient has experienced and **may awaken the person** from sleep. Occasionally, the headache is worse early in the day. With time, **associated symptoms** (e.g., **nausea, vomiting,** and **exacerbation with lifting** and **straining**) can develop. Upon examination, the patient typically has evidence of **focal CNS disease.**

    b. Therapy is directed at the underlying lesion.

2. A **"sentinel" SAH** causes the apoplectic onset of headache in a previously healthy individual, or the sudden occurrence of headache that is of unique character in a chronic headache sufferer (see also VIII C 1).

    a. Clinical features. The possibility that a headache is a result of SAH is strengthened if the cephalic discomfort cannot be easily attributed to any of the usual causes of head pain. The patient may have no neurologic findings on examination, and meningismus may be absent.

    b. Diagnosis. Given the potential seriousness of the condition, the patient should have a **cranial CT scan.** If this is unrevealing, an **LP** will reveal the presence of subarachnoid bleeding.

C. Headache syndromes

1. Migraine

    a. Etiology. The cause of migraine is unknown, but several common precipitants have been observed.

      (1) Patients often have a **family history** of migraine.

(2) Headaches can be related to **stress, altered sleep patterns, menses, oral contraceptives, alcohol use, caffeine withdrawal, monosodium glutamate (MSG) intake,** and various **foodstuffs** (e.g., chocolate, nuts, aged cheeses, and meats containing nitrates).

(3) Migraine can develop **after seemingly minor head trauma;** recognition and treatment may prevent prolonged disability.

b. Pathophysiology. Hypotheses regarding pathophysiology center around the idea that a migraine attack is brought on by neurovascular disturbances.

(1) The classic **vasospasm–vasodilation theory** arose from clinical observations. Recent data suggest that oligemia occurs during a headache prodrome and persists into the headache phase. Hyperemia occurs subsequently and can persist after the headache subsides.

(2) Current theory maintains that **dysfunction** of the **trigeminovascular system,** resulting in the perivascular release of substance P, leads to migraine.

(3) Additional information implicates a slowly spreading area of **neuronal depolarization** (the cortical depression of Leao) as being involved in the pathogenesis of migraine.

c. Migraine syndromes

(1) Migraine without aura (common migraine) is an **intermittent** syndrome characterized by generalized or hemicranial **pulsatile** cephalic discomfort. Nausea, vomiting, photophobia, sonophobia, and anorexia may accompany the headache.

(2) Migraine with aura (classic migraine) presents with an aura, often a **vivid visual array** of colors in a geometric pattern involving one visual hemifield.

   (a) The **throbbing headache** is often **contralateral to the visual display,** and the patient may experience nausea, vomiting, photophobia, sonophobia, and anorexia.

   (b) Migraine with aura can also be associated with transient neurologic deficits such as visual field deficits and hemisensory loss.

   (c) On very rare occasions, stroke is a complication of migraine.

d. Therapy should first involve removal of inciting agents when possible.

(1) Abortive therapy for migraine

   (a) Ergotamine, available in oral, sublingual, and suppository forms, is a serotonin (5-HT$_1$)-receptor agonist that decreases substance P release at the trigeminovascular junction. Intravenous ergotamine [dihydroergotamine (D.H.E. 45)] has also proven to be efficacious; pretreatment with metoclopramide or prochlorperazine prevents nausea.

   (b) Aspirin, nonsteroidal anti-inflammatory drugs (NSAIDs), and isometheptene can abort a migraine. Analgesics may be administered for symptomatic relief as well.

   (c) Sumatriptan, a serotonin 5-HT$_1$–receptor agonist, is an effective agent for migraine treatment.

(2) Prophylactic measures include drug regimens and changes in patient behavior referable to headache precipitants.

   (a) Medical therapy. β-Blockers, tricyclic antidepressants, calcium channel blockers, NSAIDs, or valproic acid may be used to prevent migraines. Prophylactic medications, although of seemingly diverse types, may have in common a tendency to alter CNS serotonin activity.

     (i) The choice of medication is guided, in part, by the need to avoid or exploit a particular drug action (aside from the antiheadache effect) in a patient.

     (ii) Initially, a low dose should be administered, and the therapeutic benefits and undesirable side effects should be monitored as the dosage is increased. The dose can be increased until either a beneficial response is achieved or adverse side effects develop. A maximal dose is best maintained for several weeks before concluding that an agent is not effective.

(b) **Biofeedback therapy** may enable patients to lessen migraine events by helping them deal more effectively with stress.

2. A **muscle contraction,** or **tension headache,** is characterized by a band-like discomfort about the head.

a. **Clinical features.** This type of headache often develops during the course of the day and may be associated with emotional stress. Posterior cervical and occipital muscles are often tender and may be in spasm. The distinction between this type of headache and migraine without aura can be difficult.

b. **Therapy** entails reassurance, NSAIDs, muscle relaxants, moist heat, and, on occasion, antidepressant drugs and psychotherapy.

3. **Chronic daily headache**

a. **Etiology.** Patients with migraine or tension headache can develop chronic daily headaches, spontaneously or as a result of excessive use of analgesics or ergotamines.

b. **Therapy** consists of **withdrawal from excessive medications. Intravenous D.H.E.** 45 given for 2–3 days can help break the headache cycle. **Prophylactic migraine agents** can help prevent a headache recurrence.

4. **Cluster headache**

a. **Clinical features.** Cluster headaches are severe periorbital headaches, 30–90 minutes in duration, that occur once or several times daily over a period of several weeks or months. The unilateral pain may be accompanied by ipsilateral lacrimation, conjunctival injection, nasal congestion, and Horner's syndrome. The typical patient is a middle-aged man. Patients with cluster headaches often pace, as opposed to migraineurs, who seek quiet, dark places.

b. **Therapy**

(1) **Abortive and symptomatic treatment** includes the administration of 100% oxygen, ergotamines, analgesics, or sumatriptan.

(2) **Prophylactic therapy** incorporates lithium, calcium channel blockers, or corticosteroids.

5. **Temporal (giant cell) arteritis** (see also Chapter 10 XI E 6)

a. **Clinical features.** Patients over the age of 50 years who complain of a headache centered about one temple or located in the occipital area should be evaluated for giant cell arteritis. Associated symptoms include visual disturbances, jaw claudication, fever, arthralgias and myalgias, and weight loss. Polymyalgia rheumatica is also present in approximately 50% of patients who suffer from giant cell arteritis.

b. **Diagnosis.** The erythrocyte sedimentation rate is typically greater than 40 mm/hr. Biopsy of a temporal artery will confirm the diagnosis.

c. **Therapy. Corticosteroid treatment** can bring rapid relief.

6. **Benign intracranial hypertension (pseudotumor cerebri)** has no known cause but is associated with obesity, pregnancy, oral contraceptives, SLE, and a host of other conditions.

a. **Clinical features.** The development of a relatively constant, generalized headache in a patient with a clear sensorium, papilledema, and a normal neurologic examination is suggestive of benign intracranial hypertension. Visual obturations can occur, and visual loss is the most serious complication.

b. The **diagnosis** is suggested by a CT or MRI scan, which either will be normal or will demonstrate small ventricles. The diagnosis can be confirmed by finding an elevated CSF opening pressure and an otherwise normal CSF analysis.

c. **Therapy**

(1) Visual acuity and fields should be monitored.

(2) **Serial LPs** can relieve the syndrome.

(3) **Corticosteroids, acetazolamide, or furosemide** may be administered.

(4) Refractory disease has been managed with **lumboperitoneal shunting of CSF** or **optic nerve sheath fenestration.**

7. **Trigeminal neuralgia (tic douloureux)** is a syndrome that most often is idiopathic but has been associated with multiple sclerosis (MS), neoplasia, and vascular "loops" that impinge on the trigeminal nerve.
   a. **Clinical features.** Lightning-quick, severe facial pain, often associated with a trigger point, is suggestive of trigeminal neuralgia. The painful jabs are usually restricted to one or two divisions of the trigeminal nerve. There is no loss of facial sensation.
   b. **Therapy.** Therapeutic modalities include **carbamazepine, baclofen, and surgical intervention.**

8. **Indomethacin-responsive headaches** are characterized by severe, unilateral pain that may be relieved by treatment with indomethacin.
   a. **Chronic paroxysmal hemicrania** is characterized by painful, multiple attacks (up to 40 daily) that last from 2 minutes to 2 hours with nocturnal awakenings and associated autonomic features. Alcohol can precipitate the attacks.
   b. **Episodic paroxysmal hemicrania** is characterized by painful, multiple attacks (between 6 and 30 daily) that last up to 30 minutes and are associated with nocturnal awakenings and other autonomic features. Remissions lasting months to years can occur.

V. WEAKNESS.

Many disorders can cause weakness. In order to pinpoint the causative disorder, the physician must first determine which part of the nervous system is diseased.

A. **Anatomic and functional approach.** Weakness can result from dysfunction at various points in the CNS or peripheral nervous system. Localization of the site of the lesion depends on associated findings and the pattern of weakness.

1. **Upper motor neuron disorders.** Dysfunction of the descending corticospinal tracts (i.e., the cortical pyramidal cells and their axonal processes) results in a pattern of weakness such that the muscle flexor groups in the upper extremities tend to be stronger than the extensor muscles, whereas in the lower extremities, the extensor muscles remain stronger than the flexors.
   a. **Spasticity and hyperreflexia** are associated with upper motor neuron disorders, and often an extensor plantar response (Babinski's sign) may be elicited.
   b. Because of the relatively greater spatial dispersion of pyramidal cells and their axons rostral to the internal capsule, a large lesion in this area is necessary to cause widespread contralateral weakness; small lesions may produce somewhat restricted areas of weakness.
   c. Because of the relatively restricted spatial dispersion of the corticospinal tracts in the internal capsule and caudally, a small lesion targeting the corticospinal tracts can cause widespread contralateral weakness.

2. **Lower motor neuron disorders.** Dysfunction of the lower motor neurons, which, as part of a motor unit, innervate the skeletal muscles, causes a pattern of segmental e.g., as seen in poliomyelitis) or, in some cases, widespread weakness [e.g., as seen in amyotrophic lateral sclerosis (ALS)]. Muscle fasciculations, diminished muscle tone and bulk, and hyporeflexia often accompany lesions of the lower motor neurons.

3. **Nerve root and peripheral nerve disorders.** Pathologic processes involving the nerve roots or peripheral nerves (e.g., herniation of an intervertebral disk or carpal tunnel syndrome) cause selective patterns of weakness referent to the unique pattern of innervation of the impaired motor root or nerve.
   a. **Fasciculations** and **diminished muscle bulk** and **stretch reflexes** may occur.

b. More widespread weakness may be present, as in the **Guillain-Barré** syndrome.

4. Dysfunction of the neuromuscular junction, as in myasthenia gravis or botulism, results in either widespread or restricted weakness. Usually, reflexes are preserved and there is no decrease in muscle bulk. Fasciculations do not occur.

5. Muscle disease. Weakness attributable to muscle disease (such as polymyositis) typically presents with symmetric, proximal loss of strength. Muscle bulk may be decreased and muscle stretch reflexes depressed in proportion to the degree of weakness.

B. **Selected disorders characterized by weakness**

1. Facial weakness
  a. Upper motor neuron (central) facial weakness (e.g., as caused by a stroke) is characterized by preservation of forehead movement with accompanying lower facial weakness.
   (1) Any process affecting the facial upper motor neurons and descending fibers can cause the pattern of central facial weakness.
   (2) This pattern results from bilateral cortical innervation of forehead muscles and predominantly contralateral innervation of lower facial muscles.
   (3) **Therapy** depends on the underlying cause.
  b. Lower motor neuron (peripheral) facial weakness is characterized by weakness involving the forehead and lower face. A peripheral facial palsy may be accompanied by impaired tearing (decreased lacrimal gland function), hyperacusis (impaired stapedius muscle function), or impaired taste (chorda tympani dysfunction).
   (1) Etiology. Some cases are idiopathic (e.g., Bell's palsy). Others may be associated with Lyme disease, herpes zoster, trauma, otitis media, HIV infection, syphilis, sarcoidosis, diabetes, or neoplasia.
   (2) Therapy
     (a) Because the patient's ability to protect the cornea is impaired, the exposed eye should be frequently lubricated and gently taped closed during sleep.
     (b) Corticosteroid therapy is often used to treat an idiopathic peripheral facial palsy, barring any contraindications.

2. Amyotrophic lateral sclerosis (ALS) occurs in approximately 1 in 100,000 people. Half of the patients die within 3 years of the onset of the disease.
  a. Etiology. The cause of ALS is unknown.
   (1) The gene for familial ALS has been localized to **chromosome 21.**
   (2) An **excess of the excitatory amino acid glutamate** may play a role in the pathogenesis. There may be impaired synaptic reuptake of glutamate.
   (3) Antibodies to the ganglioside GM_1 and monoclonal paraproteinemia have been found in patients with ALS, raising the possibility of an immunopathogenesis.
  b. Diagnosis
   (1) Clinical features. The **hallmark of ALS is progressive weakness.**
     (a) Patients typically exhibit signs of **both upper and lower motor neuron dysfunction.** Rarely, patients have a preponderance of upper (primary lateral sclerosis) or lower (primary muscle atrophy) motor neuron features.
     (b) Loss of strength early in the course of the disease is usually focal and may only compromise speech, swallowing, or the use of one extremity.
   (2) Differential diagnosis. Other conditions may masquerade as ALS. Therefore, it is essential to evaluate the patient for the following conditions:
     (a) Cervical myelopathy or radiculopathy associated with cervical spondylosis
     (b) A mass lesion at the craniocervical junction

      (c) Thyrotoxicosis

      (d) Disorders of calcium metabolism

      (e) Multifocal motor neuropathy, a potentially treatable condition characterized by slowly progressive asymmetric weakness with multifocal demyelination and often associated with anti-GM_1 ganglioside antibodies

      (f) Diabetic amyotrophy

      (g) Postpolio syndrome

      (h) Lead intoxication

      (i) Hexosaminidase A deficiency

      (j) Spinocerebellar degeneration or multiple systems atrophy presenting with motor neuron dysfunction

      (k) Lower motor neuron dysfunction as a result of infection with polio or coxsackie virus

  c. Therapy is supportive; there is no cure. Particular attention should be paid to supporting a patient's breathing and swallowing functions.

    (1) Riluzole, a glutamate antagonist, minimally slows disease progression and prolongs life for a few months.

    (2) Patients with anti-ganglioside antibodies or paraproteinemias may be considered for **immunosuppressive therapy.**

    (3) Therapy with **nerve growth factors** is under investigation.

3. The **postpolio syndrome** occurs in patients 2–3 decades after an attack of poliomyelitis. Previously stable patients experience fatigue and further worsening of their lower motor neuron syndrome. Strengthening exercises may be beneficial.

VI. DISEQUILIBRIUM AND DIZZINESS

A. **Clumsiness** can be caused by cerebellar dysfunction or disorders of the motor or sensory system.

  1. Cerebellar dysfunction results in clumsiness. In addition to limb or truncal instability, as manifested by incoordination and impaired stance and gait, patients may exhibit hypotonia and ocular dysmetria.

    a. Acute cerebellar dysfunction (e.g., stroke, MS, neoplasia) typically presents with unilateral findings.

    b. Causes of relatively symmetric **subacute** or **chronic cerebellar dysfunction** include alcoholic cerebellar degeneration; drug intoxication (e.g., phenytoin); hypothyroidism; cerebellar or spinocerebellar degenerations; and paraneoplastic, immune-mediated degeneration.

  2. Motor or sensory disorders. A patient with strength in the 2/5–4/5 grade range (see Table 11-3) may appear clumsy, as may a patient with a sensory neuropathy, dorsal root ganglion disease, posterior column dysfunction, or parietal lobe disease (parietal ataxia).

B. **Dizziness**

  1. Approach to the patient

    a. History. Obtaining a thorough history will aid the physician in evaluating the patient. By paying special attention to associated symptoms, the physician may be able to identify pathology of the inner ear, eighth nerve, or CNS as the cause of the dizziness.

    b. The **physical examination** includes several screening techniques to search for evidence of structural disease.

      (1) Nystagmus is present in many patients who suffer from vertigo. The nystagmus can be observed spontaneously (when the patient gazes straight ahead, laterally, or vertically), or it may be elicited by using Fresnel lenses to block visual fixation, by having the patient shake his or her head during ophthalmoscopy, or by covering the contralateral eye during ophthalmoscopy (to decrease visual fixation).

(a) Horizontal or vertical nystagmus is characterized by a slow eye drift and a rapid shift in the opposite direction.

(b) Torsional nystagmus is characterized by a slow clockwise or counterclockwise rotation and a rapid movement in the opposite direction.

(c) The direction of nystagmus refers to the direction of the fast component of eye movement.

(2) Gaze mechanisms should be tested, including **saccadic speed** and **accuracy,** and the integrity of **smooth pursuits.** The presence of ocular dysmetria and the patient's visual acuity while shaking his or her head should be noted. Suppression of the vestibulo-ocular reflex (which may be tested by asking the patient to fixate on a target moving synchronously with the head) should be noted as well.

(3) The physician should check for the presence of **benign paroxysmal positional vertigo (BPPV)** by performing the Nylen-Bárány maneuver (i.e., by hyperextending the patient's neck and rotating the patient's head laterally as the patient is rapidly moved from a seated to a supine position.) Rotary nystagmus with a linear component that appears after a several-second latency period suggests BPPV.

(4) Vertigo that worsens when pressure is applied to the tragus may suggest a perilymphatic fistula.

2. Selected causes of dizziness

a. Labyrinthitis (vestibular neuronitis) is characterized by the acute onset of a spinning sensation (vertigo), exacerbated by movement, and associated with nausea and vomiting.

(1) The **etiology is often viral,** but labyrinthitis may also be caused by **trauma or inflammatory and vascular diseases.**

(2) Physical examination. Nystagmus is away from the affected ear (i.e., slow phase of eye movement is toward the side of the lesion). It is often of a mixed horizontal and torsional type.

b. Meniere's disease is characterized by episodic vertigo accompanied by nystagmus, tinnitus, fluctuating hearing loss, and aural discomfort.

c. BPPV occurs when the patient moves his or her head (e.g., by rolling over in bed, looking up, or standing up). This condition is usually idiopathic in nature but can be caused by trauma, viral or ischemic injury, or drug toxicity. A unique physical therapy technique that can be used to decrease symptoms of BPPV has been developed.

d. Drug-induced vestibulopathy can be caused by gentamicin, streptomycin, furosemide, and cisplatin.

e. Eighth cranial nerve disease can be associated with hearing loss. Causes include acoustic neuroma, metastatic disease, vasculitis, and basilar meningitis associated with infectious and inflammatory processes.

f. Lateral medullary syndrome (Wallenberg's syndrome) is due to occlusion of the vertebral or posterior inferior cerebellar artery.

(1) Patients often feel that the external world is "tilting" and complain of feeling propelled toward one side (usually the side of the lesion).

(2) Physical examination can reveal nystagmus (often horizontal–torsional and away from the lesion), ipsilateral ataxia, ipsilateral Horner's syndrome (characterized by ptosis, miosis, and anhidrosis), and ipsilateral facial sensory impairment with contralateral body sensory loss.

g. Cerebellar disease can be caused by stroke, tumor, infection, or degenerative and inflammatory disease. Paraneoplastic cerebellar degeneration is associated with anti-Yo antibodies (leading to Purkinje cell loss) and anti-Ri (antineuronal) antibodies. Physical examination reveals ataxia and postural instability and many types of nystagmus. Opsoclonus is associated with anti-Ri antibodies.

h. **Brain stem lesions** are typically associated with cranial nerve, motor, sensory, and cerebellar dysfunction.

i. **Other causes of dizziness** include postural hypotension, hyperventilation, hypoglycemia, hypothyroidism, epilepsy, migraine, psychiatric disorders (e.g., depression, anxiety, somatization disorders), and multisensory impairment (i.e., poor vision and positional sense).

3. **Therapy**
   a. Dizziness may be relieved by **treating the underlying disease.**
   b. If the underlying disease is unknown or otherwise untreatable, **acute symptomatic therapy** includes the use of meclizine, prochlorperazine, promethazine, topical scopolamine, and diazepam.
   c. **Vestibular and gait exercises** may help to habituate the vestibular pathways to the abnormal influences of the disease.
   d. **Chronic, poorly defined causes** of dizziness can be managed by withdrawing the patient from drugs that affect the vestibular system. This action may allow a better reevaluation of the patient. Teatment with a **low dose** of a **benzodiazepine** and **vestibular and gait exercises** may be effective.

VII. **PAIN SYNDROMES.** When a patient complains of pain, it is important to explore whether the pain is new-onset, long-standing, or intermittent, and whether it is static or progressive. The patient should be asked to identify exacerbating and alleviating factors as well as associated symptoms, such as weakness or numbness.

A. **Pain originating from the low back**

1. **Etiology**
   a. Diagnostic considerations include local muscular strain, traumatic conditions of the spine, degenerative and inflammatory arthritides, neoplastic and infectious processes, and nerve root irritation.
   b. Neurologic dysfunction commonly develops from impingement on nerve roots by disk material, bony overgrowth, or thickened ligaments.

2. **Disorders associated with low back pain**
   a. **Sciatica** denotes a syndrome of sharp pain radiating from the low back to the buttock, down the back of the thigh to the calf, and, at times, over the bottom or top of the foot. Sciatica is commonly associated with disk herniation but can result from other conditions that irritate nerve roots L4, L5, or S1.
      (1) **Clinical features.** Myotomal weakness and dermatomal numbness, along with appropriate muscle stretch reflex changes and pain that increases when the examiner raises the patient's extended leg, can occur.
      (2) **Diagnosis.** Persistent symptoms and neurologic deficits warrant in-depth investigation, which commonly includes the use of lumbosacral roentgenographs, lumbar MRI, and EMG. CT myelography may be indicated; conventional myelography is sometimes performed.
      (3) **Therapy.** Acute low back pain should be evaluated carefully. Therapy should be directed at the underlying disorder if possible.
         (a) Unless tumor or infection is the likely cause for sciatica, initial therapy should include **bed rest** and treatment with **NSAIDs.** If the patient shows signs of a **cauda equina syndrome** (i.e., a flaccid bladder, rectal dysfunction, and bilateral lower motor neuron leg weakness), **emergency surgery** is usually required.
         (b) **Long-term therapy.** As the acute syndrome remits, a regimen of **back-strengthening exercises** and **weight loss** (if applicable) can be

helpful. Surgery (e.g., **laminectomy**) may be necessary to relieve persistent symptoms.

   b. Lumbar stenosis is another common condition resulting in low back pain. Patients often have a congenitally small lumbar canal. Over time, bony and ligamentous overgrowth and disk protrusions may further encroach upon the neural and vascular contents of the canal and foramina.

   (1) Clinical features. Patients develop pain and, occasionally, **sensory loss** and **weakness** with **ambulation** and **prolonged standing** but are relatively comfortable at rest. The neurologic examination of the resting patient is often quite normal.

   (2) Therapy. It is necessary to differentiate pain caused by lumbar stenosis from that caused by vascular insufficiency. If symptoms are severe, **decompression surgery** is often pursued for treatment of lumbar stenosis.

B. **Pain originating from the neck**

   1. Etiology. Neck pain is often due to trauma (e.g., "whiplash"). Degenerative and inflammatory bone and disk disease can lead to nerve root irritation and is also a common source of neck pain. Local infection should be considered for acute symptoms; neoplasia may be the culprit when subacute symptoms exist.

   2. Disorders associated with neck pain

   a. Cervical radiculopathy. Pain can radiate in a dermatomal pattern with a parallel loss of sensation. Weakness may be in a myotomal distribution with a corresponding loss of muscle stretch reflexes.

   b. Arthritis. The cervical radiculopathy associated with cervical arthritis (spondylosis) can often be treated with a **soft cervical collar, NSAIDs, muscle relaxants,** and, occasionally, **surgery.**

C. **Selected pain syndromes**

   1. Herpes zoster

   a. Acute syndrome. "Shingles" is a painful condition caused by the activation of a latent herpes zoster infection, which affects the nerves that supply the skin. Although most common in the elderly, shingles can occur in immunosuppressed patients as well.

   (1) Clinical features. The rash, characterized by painful vesicles on an erythematous base, may be preceded by discomfort; the pain often abates when the skin lesions heal but may persist and lead to postherpetic neuralgia.

   (2) Therapy

   (a) Treatment with **corticosteroids** during the acute phase of shingles may lessen the risk of postherpetic neuralgia in nonimmunosuppressed patients over 60 years of age.

   (b) Treatment of **immunocompetent patients** with **famciclovir** decreases the duration of postherpetic neuralgia.

   (c) An **immunosuppressed patient** should be treated with **acyclovir** to hasten recovery.

   (d) Pain during the acute phase of the illness can be treated with **analgesics** and **tricyclic antidepressants.**

   b. Chronic syndrome

   (1) Once the vesicles have healed, residual discomfort can be managed with capsaicin ointment, vapo-coolant spray, or tricyclic antidepressants.

   (2) Therapy of postherpetic neuralgia includes the use of tricyclic antidepressants, carbamazepine, vapo-coolant spray, transcutaneous electrical nerve stimulation, and, occasionally, surgical intervention.

   2. Reflex sympathetic dystrophy (sympathetic maintained pain) is a chronic painful condition that can occur idiopathically or develop following trauma to a limb; at times the severity of the initial injury can be quite trivial.

   a. Clinical features. The affected limb is painful, with altered vasomotor tone and temperature. The skin may be thin.

    b. Diagnosis. In order to make a diagnosis, other local conditions that can cause pain must be eliminated. A differential nerve block via infiltration of paravertebral nerves with varying doses of local anesthesia will help the physician to differentiate between local somatic nerve hyperexcitability and the autonomic sympathetic dysfunction attributable to reflex sympathetic dystrophy. Intravenous phentolamine blockade can also provide evidence for reflex sympathetic dystrophy.

    c. Therapy includes **paravertebral sympathetic ganglion blocks** and **aggressive physical therapy.** Administration of tricyclic antidepressants or anticonvulsants is useful adjuvant therapy.

D. **Chronic pain syndromes.** Nonmalignant pain syndromes, when chronic, can be especially difficult to evaluate and manage.

    1. Care should be taken to assess the patient fully for remedial problems (e.g., lumbar stenosis).

    2. Use of **tricyclic antidepressants** and **supportive psychotherapy,** coupled with **attempts to improve the patient's functional status,** can be beneficial.

    3. An **interdisciplinary team approach** is best.

VIII. STROKE. is the most common neurologic disease causing serious morbidity and mortality.

A. **Introduction**

    1. Disease of the vascular system can disrupt blood supply to the CNS, leading to **neuronal dysfunction.** Some cerebrovascular diseases can be **asymptomatic.**

    2. **Optimal management** requires precise diagnosis for effective therapy. Stroke syndromes can be broadly classified into predominantly **ischemic** or **hemorrhagic processes.** In each category, asymptomatic lesions can predispose the patient to future disease.

        a. **General principles of management** of symptomatic patients include monitoring the patient for signs of clinical deterioration, ensuring adequate oxygenation, maintaining euvolemia, avoiding extremes of blood pressure without excessively lowering high blood pressure, treating infection and fever, and using normal saline (rather than glucose solutions) for intravenous hydration. Efforts should be made to prevent deep venous thrombosis and decubiti, avoid aspiration, maintain nutrition, and attend to bowel and bladder function.

        b. **Rehabilitation** of patients with persistent neurologic defects is important.

            (1) Multidisciplinary therapy involving physical, occupational, and speech therapy can be pursued on an inpatient or outpatient basis.

            (2) Depression occurs frequently in stroke patients and may be treated medically.

B. **Ischemic stroke**

    1. Introduction

        a. **Etiologies** include cardiogenic emboli, extracranial and intracranial large artery disease, small artery disease, and various systemic and hematologic disorders.

        b. **Clinical signs**

            (1) Impaired carotid circulation produces symptoms of contralateral weakness and sensory loss and aphasia or neglect syndromes and ipsilateral transient monocular blindness (amaurosis fugax). Typically, the weakness or numbness is greatest in the facial area, less pronounced in the arm, and still less pronounced in the leg.

(2) A diagnosis of vertebrobasilar disease is fairly certain if there is transient binocular blindness or other bilateral visual disturbances, diplopia, ataxia, quadriparesis, or vertigo associated with other neurologic symptoms.

c. Therapy. New therapies for acute ischemic stroke are under investigation, driven by the evidence that there may be a 3- to 4-hour "therapeutic window" during which intervention may lessen brain damage.

(1) Thrombolytic agents may be administered with a seemingly acceptable incidence of hemorrhagic infarction and intraparenchymal hematoma. A randomized, double-blind trial of intravenous recombinant **tissue plasminogen activator (t-PA)** administered no more than 3 hours after the onset of an acute ischemic stroke at a dose of 0.9 mg/kg (with 10% of the dose given as a bolus and the remainder infused over an hour) resulted in an improved clinical outcome at 3 months in patients treated with the active drug. t-PA–treated patients were more likely to sustain a symptomatic intracerebral hemorrhage during the first 36 hours; however, there was no significant difference in mortality between treated and untreated patients.

(a) This therapy appears to be beneficial for patients with small or large artery occlusive disease or cardioembolic stroke. Because there is such a narrow window of opportunity for the administration of t-PA, some patients destined to have a transient ischemic attack (TIA; see VIII B 2) will be inadvertently treated. However, this treatment is most suitable for ischemic stroke patients.

(b) Patients to be treated with t-PA must meet strict criteria to minimize the risk of hemorrhagic complications. In addition, no anticoagulants or antiplatelet agents should be administered for 24 hours following t-PA treatment, and blood pressure elevations should be treated. **Contraindications** for treatment include:

  (i) A rapidly improving neurologic deficit or minor symtoms
  (ii) A baseline CT scan showing evidence of intracranial hemorrhage
  (iii) A systolic blood pressure greater than 185 mm Hg or a diastolic blood pressure greater than 110 mm Hg
  (iv) A medication-induced or disease-related coagulopathy
  (v) A history of hemorrhagic stoke, recent surgery, or another invasive procedure

(2) A randomized, double-blind trial of **low-molecular-weight heparin** administered subcutaneously within 48 hours of acute ischemic stroke and continued for 10 days resulted in a significantly improved functional outcome after 6 months. Fifty-four percent of treated patients were independent at 6 months, as compared with thirty-six percent of the control patients.

(3) Other possible interventions to provide neuroprotection are based on altering the biochemical changes that follow cerebral ischemia. Options under investigation include the use of **calcium channel blockers, free radical scavengers,** and **excitatory amino acid antagonists.**

2. Transient ischemic attacks (TIAs) are short-lived neurologic deficits, often lasting minutes but at times up to 24 hours, attributable to ischemia in the carotid or vertebrobasilar arterial distributions. The distinction between a TIA and a stroke is arbitrary. Both warrant complete evaluation to determine the underlying pathophysiology and decrease the risk of subsequent ischemic events.

a. Etiologies. Although TIAs often result from atherosclerotic large vessel disease, other diagnostic possibilities deserve consideration, including cardiogenic emboli, other large artery disorders such as dissection and fibromuscular dysplasia, small artery disease, hematologic disorders, and migraine.

Other disease entities such as seizures, tumors, subdural hematomas, and multiple sclerosis sometimes masquerade as a TIA.

   b. **Diagnostic studies** should include a CBC, syphilis serology, a coagulation profile, and a CT scan or MRI. A transthoracic echocardiogram and 24-hour ambulatory ECG monitoring may be indicated.

      (1) A duplex examination of the extracranial carotid artery territory is often informative.

      (2) Transcranial Doppler studies and magnetic resonance angiography can provide insight into the intracranial arterial circulation.

      (3) Conventional interventional angiography is the definitive test to outline the vascular anatomy.

      (4) Patients with an unrevealing cardiac evaluation who are thought to have a cardiogenic embolus may benefit from a transesophageal echocardiogram.

      (5) If clinical suspicion exists, the possibility of CNS inflammation can be evaluated with a LP.

   c. **Therapy.** If atherosclerosis is suspected as the cause transient cerebral ischemia, control of risk factors for atherosclerosis is essential (see Chapter 1 III A 2). An evaluation for coronary artery disease is also appropriate.

      (1) Extracranial carotid artery disease. Carotid endarterectomy is superior to medical therapy in the prevention of ischemic stroke in patients experiencing a TIA ipsilateral to an angiographically demonstrated 70%–99% stenosis at the internal carotid artery origin.

         (a) Patients with less severe stenosis should be treated with aspirin. Ticlopidine is also effective in preventing stroke.

         (b) Anticoagulation therapy (heparin followed by warfarin) is occasionally used for patients sustaining a TIA secondary to internal carotid artery occlusion. Antiplatelet therapy can be used after several months.

      (2) Intracranial large artery disease. A TIA can result from large artery stenosis or occlusion. Some physicians prefer early anticoagulation therapy followed by antiplatelet therapy several months after the event. Others initiate treatment with an antiplatelet agent and reserve anticoagulation for patients with progressive symptoms.

      (3) Other causes of TIA. Therapy should be directed at the appropriate pathophysiologic process. For instance, anticoagulants are frequently used in patients with a source of cardiogenic emboli.

3. Cardiogenic embolic stroke

   a. **Etiology.** The most common cause of embolic stroke is nonvalvular atrial fibrillation.

      (1) Other conditions associated with cardiogenic emboli include recent myocardial infarction, an akinetic ventricular segment, dilated cardiomyopathy, a prosthetic heart valve, infective and nonbacterial thrombotic endocarditis, left heart myxoma, left atrial spontaneous contrast echo, and atrial septal aneurysm.

      (2) A patent foramen ovale or atrial septal defect predisposes the patient to paradoxical emboli, especially if there is a documented venous thrombosis.

      (3) Other cardiac conditions, such as mitral valve prolapse or a hypokinetic ventricular segment, are rarely associated with a cardiogenic embolus.

   b. **Diagnosis.** The diagnosis is most secure if there is an abrupt onset of neurologic dysfunction, an underlying cardiac condition known to predispose to emboli, strokes in multiple vascular territories, hemorrhagic arterial infarction, systemic emboli, an absence of concurrent conditions known to cause stroke, and angiography demonstrating (potentially transient) vessel occlusions in the absence of an intrinsic vasculopathy. Patients suffering from a cardiac embolism rarely present with all of these conditions.

   c. Therapy. An ischemic infarction caused by a cardiogenic embolus may develop into a hemorrhagic infarction, especially if reperfusion occurs or the infarction is large. Therefore, care must be taken to lessen the risk of parenchymal hemorrhage in the acutely ill patient while simultaneously taking measures to protect the patient from another embolic stroke.

     (1) If a patient has had a relatively small ischemic embolic infarction, a CT scan should be obtained. If no blood is present, a continuous infusion of heparin is administered. A PTT greater than twice the control value should be avoided to minimize the risk of hemorrhagic conversion of the ischemic infarction and clinical worsening.

     (2) If the patient has had a large ischemic embolic infarction, anticoagulation therapy should be withheld for 5–7 days. If the patient is recovering and a subsequent CT scan reveals no blood, heparin may be administered.

     (3) Subsequent treatment with oral anticoagulants depends on the underlying disease process and the patient's general condition.

4. Large artery disease

   a. Aortic arch atheromas or **thrombi,** as visualized by transesophageal echocardiography, can embolize to the cerebral circulation and cause stroke. Optimal management is yet to be defined but usually involves antiplatelet or anticoagulation therapy.

   b. Asymptomatic cervical bruit and carotid stenosis. The combination of an internal carotid artery bruit and atherosclerosis at the internal carotid artery origin is a marker for coronary artery disease as well as cerebrovascular disease. Approximately 2% of these patients will suffer an ischemic stroke each year. Patients with a hemodynamically significant or progressive stenosis are at increased risk for cerebral infarction.

     (1) Etiology. A midcervical bruit can be caused by a hyperdynamic circulation (as found in anemia, pregnancy, and thyrotoxicosis), an external carotid artery stenosis, and an internal carotid artery stenosis, or a venous hum.

     (2) Diagnosis. Noninvasive vascular testing (see I C 3 d) is helpful in determining if the bruit originates from atherosclerotic internal carotid artery disease and whether the lesion is hemodynamically significant. Angiography is employed if the patient is a surgical candidate.

     (3) Therapy

       (a) Control of risk factors for atherosclerosis (see Chapter 1 III A 2) is indicated. Aspirin is often prescribed, and a careful coronary artery evaluation is warranted.

       (b) Medical treatment. Patients with less than a 60% internal carotid artery stenosis should be managed medically.

       (c) Carotid endarterectomy

         (i) Patients with a 60%–99% stenosis who undergo **carotid endarterectomy** have less of a risk of ipsilateral stroke than patients managed medically if surgery can be achieved with less than a 3% risk of complications.

         (ii) Prophylactic carotid endarterectomy for asymptomatic internal carotid artery stenosis prior to major cardiac or vascular surgery is **usually inadvisable.**

   c. Ischemic infarction. An understanding of neuroanatomy is essential to localize the compromised area of the brain and to correlate this information with a likely site of vascular disease.

     (1) Etiologies

       (a) Large artery occlusive disease can cause ischemic infarction, either by being a source of artery-to-artery emboli or by causing hypoperfusion distal to a hemodynamically significant vascular stenosis. Large artery disease can involve the extracranial or intracranial portions of the cerebrovascular circulation.

(b) Vascular conditions other than atherosclerosis (e.g., **arterial dissection, arteritis, Takayasu's syndrome, fibromuscular dysplasia,** and **radiation-induced vasculopathy**) should be considered.

(2) **Diagnosis.** Diagnostic studies are pursued to define the vascular anatomy. Magnetic resonance angiography, carotid duplex, transcranial Doppler, and angiography can be used. The scope of testing is determined, in part, by the clinical condition of the patient and whether carotid endarterectomy or anticoagulation are therapeutic considerations. The more accurate the definition of the underlying cause of the infarction, the more precise the physician can be in defining prognosis and treatment.

(3) **Therapy**

(a) **Extracranial carotid artery disease.** If the patient has sustained a minor infarction with a functional recovery and has a 70%–99% atherosclerotic stenosis of the ipsilateral origin of the internal carotid artery, carotid endarterectomy is superior to medical therapy for prevention of subsequent stroke. If the stenosis is less than 70%, therapy with aspirin or ticlopidine (another antiplatelet agent) is appropriate.

(b) **Intracranial large artery disease**

(i) If the infarction is caused by a severe stenosis or occlusion of a large intracranial artery, and if the patient is stable, some physicians will treat the patient with anticoagulation agents (heparin, initially, followed by several months of warfarin therapy), before ultimately switching to antiplatelet therapy (i.e., aspirin or ticlopidine) if the patient is doing well.

(ii) Other physicians will first employ antiplatelet therapy and use anticoagulation agents only if the patient has new symptoms.

5. **Small artery disease.** The infarctions resulting from small artery disease typically are deep in the hemispheres or the pontomesencephalic region and are known as **lacunae.** The lesions are less than or equal to 15 mm in diameter.

a. **Etiology.** The underlying vascular lesion is usually hypertension-associated lipohyalinosis. A small atheromatous plaque blocking the ostium of an arteriole may, on occasion, be the cause of some occlusions, as may infectious or sterile inflammation, cardiogenic emboli, and large artery occlusive disease.

b. **Diagnosis**

(1) Ischemic events from small artery disease cause stereotypic syndromes such as pure motor or sensory stroke, sensorimotor stroke, clumsy hand-dysarthria syndrome, and ataxic hemiparesis.

(2) Patients should be screened for the possibility of cardiogenic emboli, large artery occlusive disease, and hematologic and inflammatory disorders (see VIII B) if the patient is not hypertensive or if the patient's history, examination, or routine diagnostic tests suggest a cause other than hypertension.

c. **Therapy** is directed at controlling hypertension. If another condition is defined as the cause of the infarction, appropriate intervention should be pursued. Aspirin or ticlopidine may be administered to decrease the likelihood of subsequent ischemic stroke.

6. **Hematologic and systemic conditions** can cause ischemic infarction.

a. Sickle cell disease, hyperviscosity associated with polycythemia and paraproteinemias, and hypercoagulability are conditions associated with ischemic stroke.

b. Hypercoagulability is associated with antiphospholipid antibodies (including anticardiolipins and the lupus anticoagulant syndrome), deficiency of proteins C and S, factor V mutation causing activated protein C resistance, antithrombin III deficiency, malignancy, nephrotic syndrome, and pregnancy, as well as several other conditions.

7. **The young ischemic stroke patient.** Patients younger than 45 years of age presenting with a stroke are often diagnostic challenges. The potential etiologies are vast and include, but are not limited to, the following conditions:
   a. Drug (especially cocaine) and alcohol abuse
   b. Hypercoagulable states
   c. Cardiogenic emboli
   d. Migraine
   e. Vasculitis and other rare arterial lesions
   f. CNS infection, including HIV-associated conditions
   g. Cancer
   h. Disorders of homocysteine metabolism
   i. Familial conditions (e.g., neurofibromatosis and von Hippel-Lindau disease)
   j. Pregnancy and the postpartum state

8. **The deteriorating ischemic stroke patient**
   a. **Pathophysiology**
      (1) An ischemic stroke patient's condition may deteriorate as a result of progressive occlusion of arteries from clot propagation or artery-to-artery emboli, or because of subsequent cardiogenic emboli. Deterioration can also result from excessive lowering of blood pressure or inadequate anticoagulation therapy.
      (2) Hemorrhagic infarction or a parenchymal hematoma can occur spontaneously or as a result of thrombolytic or anticoagulation therapy.
      (3) If the patient is being treated with heparin, the possibility of heparin-induced thrombosis (with associated thrombocytopenia) should be considered.
      (4) Cerebral edema can develop, causing shifting of brain structures and an increase in the ICP.
   b. **Approach to the patient.** Ideally, continuing efforts should be made to define the pathophysiology of the stroke.
      (1) The patient's blood pressure and degree of hydration should be checked.
      (2) A CT scan should be obtained to define mass effect and hemorrhagic complications.
      (3) As appropriate, a hematocrit, platelet count, and clotting profile should be obtained.
   c. **Therapy.** Patients should be confined to bed and extremes of blood pressure should be avoided.
      (1) Appropriate hydration should be maintained with normal saline, and increases in ICP should be treated as necessary.
      (2) If the patient is not already undergoing anticoagulation therapy, intravenous heparin is often administered. The efficacy of intravenous heparin is controversial.

C. **Hemorrhagic disorders**

1. **Subarachnoid hemorrhage (SAH)**
   a. **Etiology.** The most common causes of SAH are **trauma** and **ruptured berry aneurysms.**
      (1) Other causes include coagulopathies, mycotic aneurysm, arteriovenous malformation, vasculitis, and sympathomimetic drugs.
      (2) **Aneurysms** may be familial and are associated with polycystic kidney disease, coarctation of the aorta, fibromuscular dysplasia, moyamoya disease, polyarteritis nodosa, pseudoxanthoma elasticum, and Marfan and Ehlers-Danlos syndromes.
   b. **Diagnosis**
      (1) **Clinical signs.** Patients suffering from a ruptured berry aneurysm complain of an excruciating headache, but may not reveal many objective findings upon examination. Other patients can present with meningismus, altered states of arousal, and focal neurologic findings.

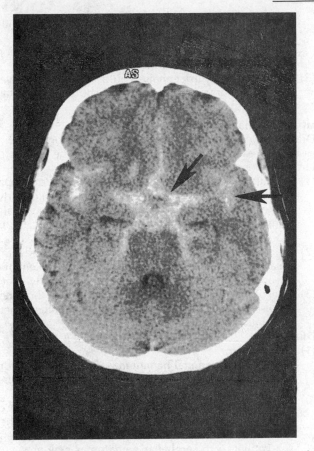

FIGURE 11-3. A nonenhanced computed tomography (CT) scan demonstrating a subarachnoid hemorrhage (SAH). Note the blood in the basal cisterns and the sylvian fissure.

      (2) Diagnostic studies. A **CT scan** will reveal the presence of subarachnoid blood in most patients (Figure 11-3). If the index of suspicion for an SAH is high, but a CT scan is unrevealing, an LP will provide the proper diagnosis. Conventional interventional angiography is necessary to localize the aneurysm.

   c. Therapy of aneurysmal SAH is aimed at **controlling** the **complications,** which include rebleeding, vasospasm leading to delayed ischemic stroke, hyponatremia, acute or chronic hydrocephalus, intraparenchymal and intraventricular hematoma, and cardiac arrhythmias. Unfortunately, the mortality rate from aneurysmal rupture approaches 50%, although recent studies suggest an improved outcome. Interventional neuroradiologic techniques are playing a larger role in the management of aneurysms.

      (1) Rebleeding most frequently occurs in the first 48 hours after aneurysmal rupture. **Early surgery** to isolate the aneurysm should be performed when possible to eliminate the threat of rebleeding.

      (2) Vasospasm. The course of vasospasm can be followed with transcranial Doppler studies.

         (a) The development of ischemic stroke from vasospasm is less likely when **nimodipine,** a calcium antagonist that may decrease small artery vasoconstriction or provide neuronal protection from ischemia, is administered.

         (b) Prophylaxis against symptomatic vasospasm also includes maintaining the patient in a euvolemic state and avoiding hypotension.

         (c) If the aneurysm has been surgically isolated from the circulatory system, symptomatic vasospasm may be treated with **hypervolemic therapy,** coupled with a moderate increase in blood pressure.

    (d) Refractory vasospasm may be amenable to angioplasty or selective intra-arterial papaverine infusion.

  (3) Symptomatic hydrocephalus can be treated with a ventricular drain, repeated LPs, or ventriculoperitoneal shunting, as dictated by clinical circumstances.

2. Intraparenchymal hematoma

  a. Diagnostic considerations. Chronic hypertension is often, but not invariably, associated with hemorrhage in the region of the putamen, thalamus, cerebellum, and pons.

    (1) An intraparenchymal hemorrhage that is not accompanied by a history of hypertension should prompt a search for an underlying cause of bleeding (e.g., coagulopathy, aneurysm, arteriovenous malformation, or tumor), particularly if the hemorrhage is not located in a region of the brain typically associated with hypertensive bleeding.

    (2) In the elderly patient, lobar hematomas, especially if multiple, may be indicative of amyloid angiopathy. The APOE4 allele may be a risk factor for amyloid angiopathy and amyloid angiopathy-related hemorrhage.

    (3) Coagulopathies (especially when induced by thrombolytic therapy) and the use of drugs such as cocaine and sympathomimetics are associated with intraparenchymal hematoma.

  b. Diagnosis

    (1) Clinical signs

      (a) A **large putaminal hematoma** causes impaired consciousness, contralateral hemiparesis and sensory loss, and gaze preference to the side of the hemorrhage.

      (b) Thalamic hemorrhage can lead to impaired consciousness, contralateral motor and sensory loss, diminished vertical gaze and small, poorly reactive pupils (i.e., Parinaud's syndrome).

      (c) Patients with **cerebellar hematomas** may present with impaired gait and stance and limb ataxia. If the hematoma is large, impaired consciousness, cranial nerve palsies (including eye movement abnormalities), and weakness can develop.

      (d) The classic signs of **pontine hematoma** include coma, pinpoint reactive pupils, impaired lateral ocular motility, and quadriplegia with decerebrate posturing. Small pontine hemorrhages cause more restricted pontine syndromes.

    (2) Diagnostic studies. A CT scan is central to diagnosis. A coagulation profile and drug toxicology screen should be performed. Angiography may be appropriate in normotensive patients and in those with hemorrhage at atypical sites.

  c. Therapy

    (1) Taking measures to lower the elevated ICP associated with parenchymal hematoma can improve outcome.

    (2) With cerebellar hematomas, surgical resection is a lifesaving measure. Surgical resection of hematomas at other sites is receiving increasing attention.

    (3) A coagulopathy should be treated appropriately.

3. An **arteriovenous malformation** may cause headaches, seizures, and intraparenchymal or, occasionally, subarachnoid hemorrhages. Therapeutic intervention can incorporate multiple modalities, including surgery, interventional radiology with embolization, and stereotactic radiosurgery.

IX.   **SEIZURES.** A seizure involves a **sudden abnormality of brain electrical activity.** Manifestations of seizure can include impairment or loss of consciousness and sensory, motor, or behavioral abnormalities. The term **epilepsy** describes a syndrome characterized by recurrent seizures.

A. **Classification.** Optimal management of the seizure patient depends on proper classification of the seizure type. Seizures can be categorized as being **generalized** or **partial.**

1. **Generalized seizures** are characterized by a sudden loss of consciousness.
   a. **Generalized convulsive seizures** consist of tonic, clonic, or tonic–clonic (grand mal) motor activity. Generalized onvulsions can result from a focal seizure disorder that has spread, involving the entire brain.
      (1) **Postictal obtundation** and **confusion** commonly last minutes, and occasionally, hours.
      (2) The EEG often shows generalized spikes or spikes and associated slow waves.
   b. **Generalized nonconvulsive (absence) seizures** are characterized by a brief, sudden loss of consciousness and minor motor activity such as blinking, sporadic myoclonic jerks, or automatisms. Typically, the EEG demonstrates generalized spikes and associated slow waves.

2. **Simple partial seizures** are not accompanied by an impairment of consciousness.
   a. There may be isolated clonic or tonic activity of a limb or transient altered sensory perceptions.
   b. The seizure activity may spread over one side of the body in a **jacksonian march** (e.g., the convulsive activity can start in the face, move to the ipsilateral arm and then to the leg, and may even evolve into a generalized seizure).
   c. The EEG may show a focal rhythmic discharge at the onset of a simple partial seizure, but occasionally, no ictal activity will be detected. Interictally, focal spikes with associated slow waves are frequently present.

3. **Complex partial seizures** are often characterized by an **aura** followed by **impaired awareness.** The EEG often reveals interictal spikes or spikes with associated slow waves in the temporal or frontotemporal areas and ictal focal rhythmic discharges.
   a. The **aura** may involve **hallucinations** (e.g., olfactory, visual, auditory, or gustatory) and complex **illusions** (e.g., of having experienced a new event or of never having experienced a commonplace event). However, patients frequently do not recall their aura.
   b. Nausea or vomiting, focal sensory perceptions, and focal tonic or clonic activity may accompany a complex seizure.
   c. Following the aura, there may be an episode of impaired consciousness, lasting seconds to several minutes, during which time automatisms may be observed. Return to baseline cognitive abilities can take several minutes.

4. **Status epilepticus** is defined as an episode of repeated or ongoing seizure activity with impaired arousal lasting at least 30 minutes. Status epilepticus can involve **convulsive** (generalized tonic–clonic activity) and **nonconvulsive** (absence or complex partial) seizures.
   a. Patients experiencing convulsive seizures are at risk for hypoxia, aspiration, acidosis, hypotension, hyperthermia, myoglobinuria, hypoglycemia, and multiple physical injuries.
   b. A patient experiencing a nonconvulsive seizure can appear to be delirious. A fluctuating sensorium and subtle automatisms or myoclonic jerks are clues to the diagnosis, and the EEG is confirmatory.

B. **Etiology.** Table 11-7 outlines some of the many causes of seizures.

C. **Diagnosis**

1. **Patient history** and **physical examination** can aid in the determination of whether or not a seizure, or some other transient event, was responsible for the patient's symptoms.

TABLE 11-7. Selected Causes of Seizures

Idiopathic	Infection
Genetic predisposition	Meningitis, abscess, and encephalitis
Mesial temporal sclerosis	Degenerative diseases
Metabolic abnormalities	Alzheimer's disease
Hyponatremia	Trauma
Hypo- or hyperglycemia	Eclampsia
Hypocalcemia	Drugs
Hypomagnesemia	Theophylline
Uremia	Lidocaine
Vascular disease and stroke	Cocaine
Infarction, especially cortical	Drug and substance withdrawal
Vascular malformation	Anticonvulsant medications
Vasculitis	Benzodiazepines
Inflammatory causes	Alcohol
Systemic lupus erythematosus (SLE)	Psychogenic causes
Neoplasia	
Metastatic and primary brain tumors	

    a. A **family history** of **epilepsy** or a **history** of **febrile convulsions** is relevant information.

    b. An **accurate description of the event by an observer** is helpful in defining the problem.

    c. **Urinary incontinence, back pain** (from a vertebral compression fracture), **myalgias,** and **oral lacerations** are clues to the proper diagnosis.

    d. Seizures can be provoked by **fever, fatigue, stress,** and **menses.**

  2. Differential diagnosis. Other conditions that may produce a sudden loss of consciousness are discussed in II A. Psychogenic seizures should be considered if the patient exhibits nonstereotypic events, has an unexpected resistance to antiepileptic drugs, or has a psychiatric disorder.

  3. Diagnostic studies

    a. The **EEG** is central to the evaluation of the seizure patient. The best technique for fully characterizing a seizure disorder is continuous video EEG monitoring of the patient, but this is not usually employed as an initial diagnostic test.

    b. An **MRI** scan is the most useful modality for detecting lesions that may cause seizures.

    c. **SPECT** and **positron emission tomography (PET)** can provide additional information to help localize a seizure focus.

    d. **Laboratory studies** are indicated to evaluate potential metabolic or toxic causes.

 D. **Therapy**

  1. Therapy for a seizure

    a. General principles. If a seizure is the suspected diagnosis, decisions about therapy depend on the underlying cause.

      (1) Correction of hyponatremia, hypoglycemia, or drug intoxication may be all that is necessary.

      (2) Patients with a neurologic condition known to be associated with recurrent seizures often require medication.

      (3) Anticonvulsant therapy is often not initiated in patients with a single, unprovoked convulsion, a normal neurologic examination, and a normal brain imaging study and EEG unless they experience a second seizure.

    b. Medical therapy

      (1) General principles. An attempt is usually made to prevent subsequent seizures using a **single agent,** in order to limit toxic effects. The drug should be administered in **progressive doses** until seizure control has been achieved or until drug toxicity occurs. Only if monotherapy fails should a second drug be added to the patient's regimen. If control is then obtained, the first agent might be carefully withdrawn.

(2) **Specific agents.** The choice of medication should be based on the seizure type, bearing in mind possible contraindications and side effects.

(a) Typically, generalized convulsive, simple partial, and complex partial seizures are treated with carbamazepine, phenytoin, valproic acid, phenobarbital, or primidone.

(b) Valproic acid or ethosuximide is used for generalized nonconvulsive spells (absence seizures).

(c) Valproic acid is particularly effective for controlling myoclonic epilepsy of Janz (a disorder characterized by myoclonic seizures).

(d) **Lamotrigine** and **gabapentin** are adjunctive medications for the treatment of patients with refractory partial seizures.

c. **Surgical therapy.** Patients refractory to medical control of seizures may be candidates for surgery to control the epilepsy. **Temporal lobe resection, ablation** of a **cortical seizure focus,** and **corpus callosum sectioning** are able to reduce seizure frequency in some patients who meet specific criteria.

2. **Control of status epilepticus.** Generalized convulsive status epilepticus can be a life-threatening condition; therefore, management of convulsive status epilepticus requires making certain that the patient's airway is unobstructed and maintaining adequate oxygenation, blood pressure, and hydration. Definition of the underlying problem is essential.

a. **Glucose** and **thiamine** should be administered after blood samples for glucose, electrolytes, renal function, anticonvulsant drug levels, and toxicology have been obtained.

b. Often, **intravenous diazepam** or **lorazepam** is given to stop the convulsions. Lorazepam carries less of a risk of respiratory depression or arrest and remains effective longer.

c. Administration of a benzodiazepine is followed by administration of either **phenytoin** or **phenobarbital,** or both, if one fails to arrest the seizure.

d. If convulsions continue after loading doses of phenytoin and phenobarbital have been administered, intravenous **midazolam** or **pentobarbital** can be given in a carefully supervised setting, with continuous EEG monitoring, until the seizure discharges are eliminated from the EEG.

e. Diminished cardiac output, bradycardia, and hypotension often limit the dose of intravenous anticonvulsants.

(1) **Fluid resuscitation** and **vasopressors** may be used.

(2) The new prodrug, **phosphenytoin,** may cause less adverse cardiac effects than phenytoin.

3. **Psychosocial issues** are important to attend to when managing epilepsy.

a. Patients may be depressed, have behavioral disturbances, and often require vocational support services. Frequently, community support services are available to the patient.

b. Reviews of the patient's driving status and work and play environment are necessary.

c. Family and friends need to be counseled as to how to manage a convulsion.

X. MOVEMENT DISORDERS

A. Parkinson's disease

1. **Pathology.** Parkinson's disease is characterized by a degeneration of cells in the substantia nigra, which causes a deficiency of dopamine (a neurotransmitter) in the CNS, leading to a series of changes in motor control pathways. The mecha-

nism behind the degeneration of these cells is unknown, although hypotheses center about free radical damage and impaired mitochondrial oxidative function.

2. **Diagnosis**
   a. **Clinical symptoms and signs**
      (1) Parkinson's disease patients often complain of "slowing up;" they have trouble dressing, arising from a seated position, climbing or descending stairs, writing, and turning over in bed.
      (2) On examination, **rigidity** and **akinesia** or **bradykinesia** are present and a **resting tremor** and **postural instability** are often evident. Signs are often asymmetrical early in the disease.
      (3) Cognitive impairment develops in over 50% of patients over time.
   b. **Differential diagnosis.** The diagnosis is a clinical determination, although, at times, testing to exclude other entities presenting as parkinsonism is indicated.
      (1) Sometimes **serial observations** are necessary to determine if the parkinsonian state is the harbinger of another neurologic illness; this is of special concern in patients who do not have the **characteristic "pill-rolling"** or **resting tremor** of **Parkinson's disease** or fail to respond to levodopa therapy.
      (2) Conditions that may produce parkinsonian symptoms similar to those found in patients suffering from Parkinson's disease include NPH, multiple strokes, hypothyroidism, drug effects [e.g., neuroleptics (dopamine-blocking agents), metoclopramide, diltiazem, and reserpine], Wilson's disease, anoxic encephalopathy, and intoxication [e.g., by carbon monoxide, manganese, or n-methyl-4-phenyl-1,2,3,6-tetrahydropyridine (MPTP)].
      (3) Rare neurologic disorders that may have parkinsonian features are summarized in Table 11-8.

3. **Therapy.** Parkinson's disease is a progressive disease. Therefore, management protocols vary depending on the patient's symptoms and the extent of functional impairment.
   a. **Early therapy.** Several medications are available to treat Parkinson's disease.
      (1) **Deprenyl,** a monoamine oxidase (MAO) type B inhibitor, may slow the

TABLE 11-8. Key Features of Selected Conditions Causing Parkinsonism

Disorder	Distinguishing Clinical Characteristics
Progressive supranuclear palsy	Impaired vertical gaze; early axial rigidity with postural instability
Multiple systems atrophy (Shy-Drager syndrome)	Autonomic insufficiency; cerebellar dysfunction; upper and lower motor neuron dysfunction
Diffuse Lewy body disease	Dementia early in illness
Cortical-basal ganglionic degeneration	Asymmetric findings on examination of sensory loss and apraxia; unilateral rigidity; unilateral stimulus-sensitive myoclonus
Huntington's disease	Parkinsonian features prominent in young patients; family history, choreoathetosis
Olivopontocerebellar atrophy*	Cerebellar dysfunction; autonomic dysfunction
Basal ganglia calcification	Calcification visible on computed tomography (CT) scan
Neuroacanthocytosis	Acanthocytes in wet peripheral blood smear

*May be the same as multiple systems atrophy.

clinical progression of Parkinson's disease and delay the need for other medications.

    (2) Carbidopa/levodopa combinations are the mainstay of treatment for Parkinson's disease. This treatment should begin when the disease impairs the patient's functional status.

        (a) Levodopa is converted to dopamine by the presynaptic neuron and therefore increases the amount of neurotransmitter available to the postsynaptic dopamine receptor.

        (b) Carbidopa blocks systemic conversion of levodopa to dopamine, thereby decreasing the undesirable systemic effects of levodopa.

    (3) Anticholinergics, which improve the cholinergic–dopaminergic balance in the basal ganglia, are particularly helpful in treating tremor.

    (4) Amantadine, which increases the availability of dopamine to the postsynaptic neuron, can be effective early in the course of the disease or as an adjunctive therapy later in the disease course to help "smooth out" motor function. It may lose its effectiveness after approximately 6 months of use.

  b. Advanced therapy. In the later stages of the disease, therapy is directed at optimizing the patient's functional status and avoiding adverse effects of medication.

    (1) Dopamine agonists. If the therapeutic response to carbidopa/levodopa therapy is inadequate, or if the patient cannot tolerate the medication, **pergolide** or **bromocriptine** may be administered.

        (a) These drugs are **direct postsynaptic dopamine-receptor agonists.**

        (b) A combination of carbidopa/levodopa and pergolide or bromocriptine seems to be particularly effective and is often well-tolerated. Dopamine agonists help decrease motor fluctuations when used in conjunction with carbidopa/levodopa.

        (c) Occasionally, dopamine agonists are used early in the course of Parkinson's disease as monotherapy.

    (2) Management of Parkinson's disease becomes increasingly difficult as the disease progresses. **"Wearing off"** effects, dyskinesias, and wide, random swings in the patient's mobility (**"on–off" phenomena**) develop. A sustained-release form of carbidopa/levodopa (alone or in combination with pergolide or bromocriptine) can be used.

  c. Ancillary therapy

    (1) Other therapeutic maneuvers include the **strategic reduction of medication** if the patient is experiencing dyskinesia and **judicious use** of **psychotropic agents** to treat the various untoward behavioral consequences of Parkinson's disease (e.g., insomnia, hallucinations, and agitation).

    (2) Dietary manipulations that **redistribute** or **limit protein** intake during the day may improve levodopa's efficacy.

    (3) Physical therapy and an **exercise program** help optimize mobility.

    (4) Pallidotomy offers a new therapeutic option for refractory Parkinson's disease patients.

    (5) The role of surgical implants of dopamine-containing cells for the treatment of Parkinson's disease remains experimental.

B. **Hyperkinetic disorders**

  1. Tremor

    a. Benign essential tremor is characterized by a posture-related 5–9 Hz oscillation of the hands and forearms that impairs performance of fine motor tasks.

      (1) This type of tremor is often **familial** and may be accompanied by **titubation (head tremor).**

      (2) Consumption of alcohol may temporarily suppress the tremor; stress, caffeine, or sleep deprivation may exacerbate the condition.

      (3) β**-adrenergic blocking agents** and **primidone** are effective treatments.

b. An **action (kinetic) tremor** is evident when the patient moves his or her arms; there may be a relatively mild accompanying postural and intention component. **Clonazepam** treatment can be useful.

2. **Chorea** describes **rapid, "dance-like" distal limb** and **facial movements.** Causes include hyperthyroidism, drugs (e.g., birth control pills, levodopa), Sydenham's chorea, pregnancy, SLE, antiphospholipid syndrome, stroke, porphyria, Wilson's disease, Lyme disease, Huntington's disease, and neuroacanthocytosis.

3. **Athetosis** describes a **moderately rapid, principally distal, somewhat rotary "snake-like" movement in the distal extremities.** Causes include Wilson's disease, Huntington's disease, anoxic encephalopathy, trauma, birth control pills, and several rare hereditary disorders.

4. **Dystonia** describes **slow, writhing, sustained** and **involuntary contractions of the proximal limb, trunk,** and **neck musculature.** The gene for autosomal dominant, idiopathic, generalized torsion dystonia is on chromosome 9. Dystonia is associated with Wilson's disease, Parkinson's disease, Huntington's disease, trauma, neuronal storage disorders, encephalitis, drugs (e.g., neuroleptics and levodopa), and other rare hereditary conditions.
    a. Some patients with idiopathic dystonia are particularly responsive to carbidopa/levodopa therapy; other patients may respond to high doses of trihexyphenidyl.
    b. Focal dystonias, such as writer's cramp, blepharospasm, spastic dysphonia, and torticollis, can occur; treatment with local botulinum toxin infiltration can be beneficial.
    c. Some patients may exhibit chorea and athetosis with dystonia.

5. **Hemiballismus** describes **wild, flinging, prinicipally proximal movements** of the **arms** or **legs.** It is often caused by an infarct in the subthalamic nucleus. Haloperidol can decrease the involuntary movements.

6. **Blepharospasm** can occur in isolation or as part of a more widespread disorder such as Parkinson's disease, stroke, or Meige's syndrome (this is a syndrome distinct from that associated with ovarian cancer.) Blepharospasm can be of such severity as to cause functional blindness.
    a. Many drugs have been tried in an attempt to control the problem with modest effect.
    b. Infiltration of botulinum toxin about the eyes can provide relief by decreasing neuromuscular transmissions.

7. **Neuroleptic-associated movement disorders** represent a spectrum of disorders related to the acute or chronic administration of neuroleptic medications (although for selected conditions, other drugs are implicated as well).
    a. **Acute dystonia** typically occurs shortly after the first few doses of a neuroleptic agent.
        (1) **Clinical signs** include uncontrollable face, neck, tongue, and eye muscle (oculogyric crisis) spasms.
        (2) **Therapy** consists of the administration of anticholinergics or diphenhydramine.
    b. **Parkinsonism** can develop with neuroleptic use. Therapy consists of decreasing the dose of the neuroleptic, changing to another neuroleptic agent, administering an anticholinergic agent, or using amantadine, a carbidopa/levodopa preparation, or clozapine.
    c. **Tardive dyskinesia** describes an almost constant writhing movement of the tongue and otomandibular area, which may be accompanied by blepharospasm, respiratory grunts, choreoathetosis, and truncal hyperactivity. Ill-fitting dentures or an edentulous state can cause mouthing movements that are mistaken for tardive dyskinesia.

      (1) Tardive dyskinesia is usually an adverse side effect of neuroleptic agents; occasionally other drugs such as amphetamines, antihistamines, and carbamazepine are causally implicated.

      (2) If medication is implicated as the cause of the problem, the offending agent should be discontinued if possible. Clonazepam, propranolol, clonidine, reserpine, and other drugs have been used to treat tardive dyskinesia with variable success. Clozapine use is another option.

   d. Other neuroleptic-associated movement disorders include tardive dystonia, akathisia (motor restlessness), and the rabbit syndrome (rhythmic lip movements).

   e. Neuroleptic malignant syndrome (NMS) is an idiosyncratic reaction to neuroleptics. It can also occur in Parkinson's disease patients following the abrupt discontinuation of antiparkinsonian medications. Dopamine receptor blockade is thought to be the cause of NMS.

      (1) Clinical signs include altered mentation, high fever, rigidity, autonomic instability, high creatine kinase (CK) levels, and myoglobinuria.

      (2) Therapy for this potentially lethal condition includes hydration, cooling blankets, antipyretics, dantrolene, and levodopa/carbidopa preparations or bromocriptine, although the use of antiparkinsonian drugs is controversial.

8. Meige's syndrome (orofacial dystonia) is an idiopathic condition that has features of dystonia and tardive dyskinesia, particularly blepharospasm.

   a. This diagnosis cannot be made if the patient has recently taken neuroleptic agents or other drugs implicated as a cause of tardive dyskinesia.

   b. No single medication is consistently effective in treating this condition; clonazepam is a reasonable first-line agent. Botulinum toxin infiltration can be used to treat the blepharospasm.

9. Hemifacial spasm describes lightning-quick spasms of muscles innervated by the facial nerve.

   a. The condition is most often caused by irritation of the facial nerve by a vascular "loop."

   b. Rarely, it occurs following facial nerve paralysis or is associated with tumors, multiple sclerosis, or other irritative processes.

   c. Botulinum toxin infiltration, clonazepam, and **carbamazepine** have been used to treat **hemifacial spasm;** microsurgical decompression may be successful.

10. Tics are brief involuntary movements, sounds, or sensations that occur within the context of normal neurologic function.

   a. Types of tics

      (1) Simple motor tics are isolated movements such as an eyeblink, shoulder shrug, or facial grimace. **Complex motor tics** include touching, smelling, and jumping.

      (2) Simple phonic tics include throat clearing, sniffling, and grunting. **Complex phonic tics** include the repetition of words and coprolalia.

      (3) Sensory tics often accompany motor and phonic tics and are characterized by focal sensations of pressure, tickle, warmth, or cold.

   b. Tourette's syndrome

      (1) Tourette's syndrome has the following **characteristics:**

         (a) Multiple motor and one or more phonic tics (that has been present at some time over the course of the illness)

         (b) Tics that occur many times a day, nearly every day, for more than 1 year

         (c) Tics that change over time in their anatomic location, number, frequency, complexity, type, and severity

         (d) Onset of illness before age 21

         (e) The absence of other conditions that can cause similar, but isolated, symptoms (e.g., neuroleptic drug effects, seizures, chorea)

(2) Etiology. Tourette's syndrome is thought to be inherited in an autosomal dominant pattern with incomplete and sex-specific penetrance (males are affected more commonly than females) and variable expression. Striatal dopamine receptor supersensitivity and an abnormality in the endogenous opioid system may be responsible for some of the clinical manifestations.

(3) Associated behavioral disturbances include **obsessive–compulsive disorder** and **attention deficit hyperactivity disorder.**

(4) Therapy consists of education and counseling of the patient, family, and other appropriate parties. Clonidine, pimozide, or haloperidol can be used to manage disabling tics. Behavioral disturbances should respond to appropriate psychoactive medications.

XI. DEMYELINATING DISEASES

A. **Multiple sclerosis (MS)** is characterized by multiple foci of CNS demyelination. Patients either experience clinical remissions (often followed by relapses) or chronic, progressive symptoms.

1. **Pathophysiology.** Although the cause of MS remains unknown, a predominant theory contends that MS is an immunologic disorder associated with CNS immunoglobulin production and alteration of T lymphocytes. The **pathologic hallmark** of MS is inflammation associated with areas of **demyelination scattered about CNS white matter.**

2. **Diagnosis**
   a. **Clinical signs**
      (1) The diagnosis is most secure if neurologic problems occur over an extended length of time and involve several white matter pathways.
      (2) Several patterns emerge that are suggestive of MS, including **optic neuritis** and **internuclear ophthalmoplegia** or either of these conditions in association with corticospinal tract or cerebellar signs. Long-term follow-up reveals that 74% of women and 34% of men presenting with isolated optic neuritis ultimately develop MS.
      (3) Neurologic signs that can be localized to a single discrete area in the CNS, such as the brain stem or craniocervical junction, should make the diagnosis suspect.
   b. **Differential diagnosis.** There is no specific diagnostic marker for MS; the physician needs to exclude other conditions that can masquerade as MS. Among these disorders are somatization disorder, SLE, brain stem or spinal vascular malformation, Sjögren's syndrome, Lyme disease, HIV infection, vitamin B_{12} deficiency, brain stem neoplasm, vasculitis, sarcoidosis, and adrenomyeloleukodystrophy.
   c. **Diagnostic studies**
      (1) MRI is an excellent technique for visualizing white matter lesions. Although its diagnostic specificity is poor, the contrast agent **gadolinium-DTPA** indicates areas of breakdown of the blood–brain barrier. Serial MRI studies reveal white matter lesions that may come and go without clinical manifestations.
      (2) Examination of the **CSF** can reveal a sterile inflammation with a mild protein elevation, modest, predominantly mononuclear pleocytosis, an elevated IgG index, oligoclonal bands, and increased myelin basic protein. Only occasionally are all of these abnormalities present in a single patient.
      (3) Visual, brain stem–auditory, and **somatosensory EPs** and **central motor conduction studies** can demonstrate clinically silent disruption of white matter tracts.

3. **Therapy.** There is no cure for MS.

    a. **Corticosteroid therapy** may hasten maximal recovery from an acute exacerbation. If optic neuritis is treated, high doses of intravenous corticosteroids are preferable to lower, oral doses.

    b. **Interferon-β** (IFN-β) therapy decreases the frequency of relapses, especially moderate and severe attacks. As judged by serial MRI studies, disease activity is lessened with IFN-β treatment.

    c. **Copolymer** also decreases the frequency of relapses, especially for patients with mild disease.

    d. Otherwise, therapy is directed at **symptoms.**

        (1) **Amantadine** and **pemoline** can improve **fatigue.**

        (2) **Isoniazid** and **carbamazepine** may help **cerebellar tremor.**

        (3) **Baclofen** and **diazepam** improve **spasticity.**

        (4) **Urologic dysfunction** can be helped by a **variety of agents,** depending on the specific problem.

B. **Central pontine myelinolysis**

1. **Etiology.** Demyelination of the basis pontis and other myelinated areas has been associated with the **excessively rapid correction** of **severe hyponatremia.** Central pontine myelinolysis has been seen in alcoholics, malnourished patients, and in association with diuretic use in women.

2. **Diagnosis.** Patients develop **impaired arousal, quadriparesis,** and **pseudobulbar signs. MRI** or **CT scan** will confirm the diagnosis.

3. **Therapy.** Optimal therapy is controversial. Hyponatremia should be corrected **slowly,** and hypernatremia should be avoided.

XII. MYELOPATHY AND OTHER SPINAL CORD DISORDERS

A. **Etiology.** Selected causes of myelopathy are listed in Table 11-9.

B. **Clinical signs.** Disease affecting the spinal cord can present with principally "**long tract signs**" or a combination of long tract signs and **local radicular features.**

TABLE 11-9. Selected Causes of Myelopathy

Vertebral column disorders	Multiple sclerosis
Trauma	Vascular disease
Cervical stenosis	Infarction
Disk protrusion	Vascular malformation
Odontoid subluxation	Metabolic diseases
Rheumatoid arthritis	Vitamin B_{12} deficiency (subacute combined degeneration)
Down syndrome	
Neoplasia	Vitamin E deficiency
Epidural spinal cord compression	Adrenomyeloneuropathy
Intradural extramedullary mass	Radiation effects
Intramedullary mass	Syringomyelia
Infection	Spinocerebellar degeneration
Spinal epidural abscess	
Human immunodeficiency virus (HIV)	
Human T-cell lymphotropic virus type I (HTLV-I)	

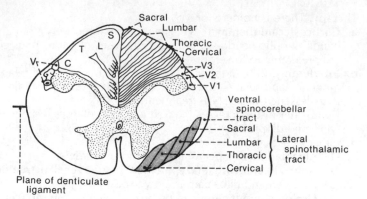

FIGURE 11-4. Cross section of the spinal cord at C1. It shows the lamination of ascending sensory axons by the level of entry in the dorsal columns (discriminative modalities) and ventrolateral columns (pain and temperature). *V1, V2,* and *V3* refer to the first, second, and third sensory divisions of CN V, the trigeminal nerve. (Reprinted from NMS *Neuroanatomy.* Malvern, PA, Harwal Publishing, 1988, p 115.)

1. **Long tract motor signs** result from the disruption of descending corticospinal fibers, which causes **weakness, spasticity, and hyperreflexia.**

2. **Impaired sensation** results from disordered function of ascending spinothalamic and dorsal column pathways (Figure 11-4).

3. **Bowel, bladder, and erectile function may be compromised.**

4. **Local radicular symptoms and signs include radiating pain, weakness,** and **sensory loss** referable to one or several myotomes and dermatomes. These findings help define the rostral–caudal extent of a lesion (Figure 11-5).

5. The **Brown-Séquard syndrome** is caused by a lesion compromising the right or left hemispinal cord at a discrete level. There is caudal ipsilateral upper motor neuron weakness and loss of proprioception and vibratory sensibility as well as contralateral loss of pain and temperature sensation.

C. Selected conditions

1. **Syringomyelia**
   a. **Definition.** Syringomyelia is a condition of unknown cause resulting in **cavitation of the spinal cord.** Syringomyelia can occur in isolation or in association with the **Arnold-Chiari malformation** (i.e., descent of the cerebellar tonsils into the cervical spinal canal).
   b. **Diagnosis**
      (1) **Signs of lower motor neuron dysfunction** develop on a segmental basis and are accompanied by **upper motor neuron signs** caudal to the cavity.
      (2) **Dermatomal loss of pain and temperature sensibility** results from local disruption of the spinothalamic tract by the cavity (syrinx). Impaired ascending dorsal column sensibility occasionally occurs caudal to the cavity.
      (3) **MRI** of the spine is the **optimal diagnostic test** (Figure 11-6).
   c. **Therapy. Surgery** is occasionally indicated to decompress the fluid-filled spinal cord cavity and to biopsy the wall to evaluate the possibility of a cavitary neoplasm. **Otherwise, treatment is supportive.**

2. **Transverse myelitis.** Inflammation of the spinal cord can cause an acute myelopathy.
   a. **Etiology.** Although many cases of segmental transverse inflammation are idiopathic, MS, SLE, and various infectious agents may cause transverse myelitis.
   b. **Diagnosis.** The patient may experience localized back or radicular pain, fol-

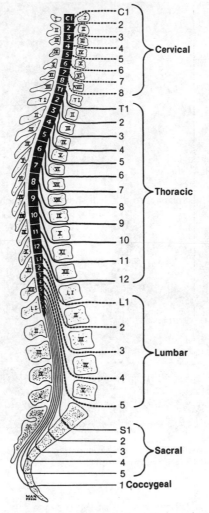

FIGURE 11-5. Topographic relationship among nerve roots, spinal cord segments, and the bodies and spinous processes of the vertebrae, which are indicated by *Roman numerals.* (Adapted with permission from Haymaker W, Woodhall B: *Peripheral Nerve Injuries,* 2nd ed. Philadelphia, WB Saunders, 1953, p 32.)

lowed by prickling or burning sensations and progressive weakness in the legs. Bowel and bladder disturbances are usually present.

   c. Corticosteroid therapy is often advocated but is of unproven value.

3. Anterior spinal artery occlusion

   a. Etiology. Blockage of a radicular artery to the spinal cord can cause an ischemic infarction.

      (1) In many cases, it is the **artery of Adamkiewicz,** a branch of the aorta supplying the anterior two-thirds of the lumbar spinal cord, that is compromised.

      (2) Thrombosis can be caused by aortic dissection, local atherosclerosis, vasculitis, and hyperviscosity.

   b. Diagnosis. The patient presents with flaccid, hyporeflexic paraplegia, impaired lower extremity pain and temperature sensation, and compromised bladder and bowel function. However, position and vibration senses are usually preserved.

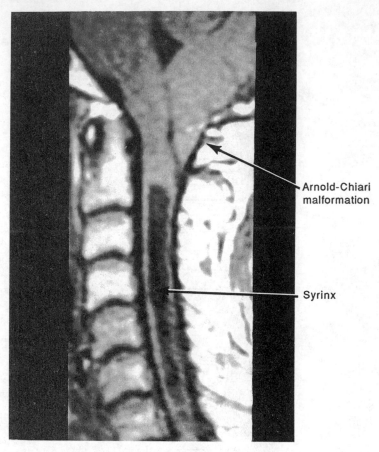

FIGURE 11-6. Nonenhanced T_1-weighted magnetic resonance imaging (MRI) scan demonstrating syringo-myelia and an associated Arnold-Chiari malformation.

       c. Therapy calls for treatment of the disease responsible for the spinal cord infarction.

XIII. NEUROPATHY

  A. **Classification.** Neuropathies may be classified by:

    1. Course (acute, subacute, or chronic)

    2. The type of symptoms and signs (sensory, motor, autonomic, or any combination of the three)

    3. The presence of pain (hyperesthesia or dysesthesia)

    4. Distribution (generalized, focal, or multifocal)

    5. NCV/EMG features (disruption of the axon, myelin sheath, or both)

  B. **Etiology.** Selected causes of neuropathy are listed in Tables 11-10A and 11-10B.

  C. **General principles of therapy.** Control of the underlying disease process is critical.

    1. If impaired sensation renders the patient prone to injury, protective measures should be taken.

TABLE 11-10A. Selected Types and Causes of Neuropathy

Neuropathy	Causes		
	Acute	**Subacute or Chronic**	
Sensory neuropathy		Diabetes mellitus	Toxins
		Uremia	Vitamin B_6 intoxication
		Alcohol abuse	Sjögren's syndrome*
		Deficiencies	Paraneoplastic (anti-Hu antibody)*
		Vitamins B_1, B_6, B_{12}, niacin	Paraproteinemia**
		HIV	Cryoglobulinemia
		Hereditary neuropathies	Amyloidosis
		Drugs	Leprosy
		Vinca alkaloids	Anti-sulfatide antibodies
		Cisplatin	
		Phenytoin	
		2', 3'-dideoxycytidine	
Motor neuropathy	Guillain-Barré syndrome	CIDP	
	Diabetes mellitus (proximal ischemic neuropathy)	Lead intoxication	
		Multifocal motor neuropathy	
	Critical illness polyneuropathy	Antibodies to GM_1 and asialo-GM_1 gangliosides	
	Porphyria	Charcot-Marie-Tooth disease	
Sensorimotor neuropathy		Diabetes mellitus	CIDP
		Uremia	Charcot-Marie-Tooth disease
		Critical illness polyneuropathy	Other hereditary neuropathies
		Vasculitis	Metachromatic leukodystrophy
		Hypothyroidism	
		Lyme disease	Refsum disease
		Paraproteinemia**	Adrenomyeloneuropathy
		Cryoglobulinemia	Lipoprotein deficiencies
		Paraneoplastic	
		Drugs	
		Toxins	
Autonomic neuropathy	Gullain-Barré syndrome	Diabetes mellitus	
	Porphyria	Amyloidosis	
		Familial dysautonomia	

HIV = human immunodeficiency virus; CIDP = chronic inflammatory demyelinating polyneuropathy.
* Also, sensory neuronopathy.
** Including myelin-associated glycoprotein (MAG) antibody and monoclonal gammopathy.

2. Weakness (e.g., wrist or foot drops) calls for appropriate splinting and physical therapy.

3. Autonomic insufficiency is difficult to manage; orthostatic hypotension can be treated with agents that expand blood volume (e.g., fludrocortisone) and increase vascular tone (e.g., ephedrine and yohimbine).

4. Tricyclic antidepressants, carbamazepine, phenytoin, and capsaicin can help patients suffering from pain.

TABLE 11-10B. Selected Types and Causes of Neuropathy Classified by Other Features

Neuropathy	Causes
Dysesthetic neuropathy	Diabetes mellitus Alcohol abuse HIV 2'3'-dideoxycytidine
Axonal neuropathy	Diabetes mellitus Uremia Drugs and toxins Critical illness polyneuropathy Vasculitis Paraproteinemia Cryoglobulinemia Vitamin B_{12} deficiency Hereditary neuropathies
Demyelinating neuropathy	Guillain-Barré syndrome CIDP Paraproteinemia* Hereditary neuropathies
Multifocal (mononeuritis multiplex) neuropathy	Diabetes mellitus Vasculitis Lyme disease Leprosy Sarcoidosis Hereditary liability to pressure palsy Malignant infiltrates

HIV = human immunodeficiency virus; CIDP = chronic inflammatory demyelinating polyneuropathy.
* Including myelin-associated glycoprotein (MAG) antibody and monoclonal gammopathy.

D. **Selected syndromes**

1. **Compression neuropathies.** Nerves can be damaged by repeated wear against firm surfaces, typically bone or fibrous tissue. Motor and sensory loss develop, referent to the affected nerve. A nerve conduction velocity examination will reveal a "conduction block" at the site of injury because of focal demyelination. If the compression is severe, evidence of axonal injury may appear (e.g., muscle wasting, denervation on the EMG).
   a. Common sites of compression leading to focal nerve dysfunction include the **median nerve** at the wrist (carpal tunnel), the **ulnar nerve** at the elbow, the **peroneal nerve** at the fibula head, and the **tibial nerve** at the ankle (tarsal tunnel).
   b. The **carpal tunnel syndrome** can result from repetitive wrist movements, trauma, carpal tunnel stenosis, arthritides (rheumatoid arthritis and crystal-induced synovitis), diabetes mellitus, myxedema, pregnancy, birth control pills, acromegaly, and infiltrative processes, such as amyloidosis.
   c. **Therapy. Treatment of underlying conditions** is important. Splinting often alleviates the condition, especially if aggravating maneuvers can be eliminated. **Surgical decompression** of the nerve is necessary at times.

2. **Guillain-Barré syndrome**
   a. **Definition and etiology.** Guillain-Barré syndrome is a predominantly demyelinating motor polyneuropathy that usually occurs in an otherwise healthy individual. The illness can follow a nonspecific viral syndrome or be associated with HIV infection, *Campylobacter jejuni* infection, hepatitis, infectious mononucleosis, *Mycoplasma pneumoniae* infection, vaccination, surgery, lymphoma, or SLE.

b. Diagnosis
  (1) Clinical signs
    (a) Classically, the disease presents with **foot** and **leg weakness** that ascends to involve other regions of the body; weakness can, however, begin in the arms or face. Progression of the disease should not extend beyond 4 weeks.
    (b) Generalized paralysis can develop gradually or relatively acutely, impeding respiratory function.
    (c) Relatively minor sensory signs and symptoms occur; however, the patient may complain of painful extremities.
    (d) The **autonomic nervous system** is often involved. Involvement of the autonomic nervous system can lead to early mortality as a result of **cardiac arrhythmias** and **wide swings in blood pressure.**
  (2) Diagnostic studies
    (a) Examination of the CSF demonstrates an elevated protein and less than 50 mononuclear cells/μl (albuminocytologic dissociation).
    (b) The motor nerve conduction velocity can be slowed.
    (c) An abnormally small compound muscle action potential amplitude obtained with distal stimulation of a peripheral nerve (a measure of the integrity of the most distal parts of the axonal portion of the nerve) is associated with a poor prognosis.
c. Therapy
  (1) Plasmapheresis can shorten the length of time that the patient is dependent on a respirator and unable to ambulate. Criteria to initiate plasmapheresis include the inability of a patient to walk or rapid progression of the disease.
  (2) Intravenous immunoglobulin treatment is also efficacious. Therapy with intravenous immunoglobulin carries lower morbidity rates than plasmapheresis, but may be less successful in maintaining a beneficial clinical response. Some physicians combine plasmapheresis and intravenous immunoglobulin treatment.

3. Diabetic neuropathy (see also Chapter 9 IV A 7 e). Diabetes mellitus causes several neuropathic syndromes. The nerve injury may be secondary to chronic hypoxia (related to microvascular disease) that leads to axonal damage.
  a. Types
    (1) A predominantly sensory, distal, symmetric, small fiber polyneuropathy can be dysesthetic and involve pain and temperature modalities more than vibration and position senses.
    (2) A predominantly sensory, distal, symmetric, large fiber polyneuropathy may occur, affecting vibration and position modalities.
    (3) A sensorimotor neuropathy can develop.
    (4) An autonomic neuropathy or a mononeuropathy or mononeuritis multiplex can occur.
    (5) Proximal diabetic neuropathy represents injury to large nerves that causes weakness and pain; it commonly involves the lumbosacral plexus.
  b. Therapy. Aldose reductase inhibitors may be effective therapy for diabetic neuropathy. As a group, patients with better blood glucose control have a less severe polyneuropathy, though in individual patients, symptoms usually do not respond to tighter blood glucose control.

XIV. DISORDERS OF THE NEUROMUSCULAR JUNCTION

A. **Myasthenia gravis**

  1. Etiology. Antibodies directed against the acetylcholine receptor on the muscle surface cause an increased rate of receptor destruction and lead to weakness.

   2. **Diagnosis**
      a. **Clinical signs.** Patients are often young women or older men. Complaints of double vision, difficulty swallowing and speaking, and limb weakness and fatigue are common. A thymoma is present in 10%–25% of patients.
      b. **Diagnostic studies**
         (1) Administration of **intravenous edrophonium** (a cholinesterase inhibitor) usually produces a transient improvement in strength in patients suffering from myasthenia gravis. Patients with respiratory compromise or excessive oral secretions should not be given edrophonium because they may be unable to compensate for the increase in secretions that occurs following administration of this agent.
         (2) **Repetitive nerve stimulation studies** can demonstrate a decremental response of the motor unit action potential voltage.
         (3) **Acetylcholine receptor antibodies** can be detected in the blood of 80%–90% of patients.
         (4) A **thoracic CT** or **MR scan** will reveal the presence of a thymoma.
   3. **Therapy**
      a. The mainstay of therapy is **administration** of a **cholinesterase inhibitor** (e.g., pyridostigmine).
      b. **Thymectomy** can often lead to improvement; the presence of a thymoma is a definite indication for surgery.
      c. **Corticosteroids, immunosuppressive agents, intravenous immunoglobulin,** or **plasmapheresis** are effective in patients with refractory disease.

B. **Eaton-Lambert myasthenic syndrome**

   1. **Pathophysiology.** This syndrome results when antibodies directed against the calcium channels on the presynaptic membrane of the neuromuscular junction interfere with the calcium-mediated release of acetylcholine vesicles in response to nerve stimulation. This syndrome is often associated with an underlying malignancy, especially small-cell carcinoma of the lung.
   2. **Diagnosis**
      a. **Clinical signs.** Patients complain of weakness and fatigue, have diminished muscle stretch reflexes, and may have impaired autonomic function, leading to a dry mouth and poor visual accommodation.
      b. **Diagnostic studies.** Repetitive nerve stimulation studies show an incremental response of the motor action potential voltage.
   3. **Therapy.** Guanidine, diaminopyridine, plasmapheresis, or immunosuppressive therapy may be helpful.

XV. DISORDERS OF MUSCLE

A. **Muscular dystrophies**

   1. **Types of muscular dystrophies**
      a. **Duchenne muscular dystrophy (DMD)** is an X-linked recessive disorder that is caused by a defect in the dystrophin gene, which codes for a muscle membrane protein that is not detectable in patients with DMD.
         (1) Although distal muscles are eventually affected as well, patients experience initial progressive proximal muscular weakness.
         (2) **Prednisone treatment** slows progression of weakness.
         (3) **Death** usually occurs in the third decade of life, often as a result of pneumonia.
      b. **Becker's muscular dystrophy (BMD)** is an X-linked recessive disorder of muscle that is caused by a defect in the dystrophin gene, which codes for a muscle protein that is altered or present in reduced quantity in BMD. Patients have a **more benign course than those with DMD, with a 50%** survival rate beyond age 50.

c. **Myotonic muscular dystrophy** is an autosomal dominant disorder localized to chromosome 19. Patients with myotonic dystrophy have an increased number of CTG trinucleotide repeats in a gene that may code for a protein kinase. The severity of the disease can increase in successive generations, and the CTG repeats increase proportionately (a phenomenon known as "anticipation.")

(1) **Clinical signs** include a characteristic muscle myotonia (i.e., persistent muscle activity in response to contraction or percussion), distal weakness, cataracts, frontal balding, impaired intellect, hypersomnia, testicular atrophy, cardiomyopathy, mitral valve prolapse, and cardiac conduction defects.

(2) **Death** occurs in the fifth or sixth decade and typically is attributable to respiratory compromise or cardiac arrhythmia.

d. **Facioscapulohumeral muscular dystrophy** is an autosomal dominant disorder characterized by progressive weakness about the face, neck, upper torso, and proximal arms. The responsible gene is located on chromosome 4.

e. **Limb-girdle muscular dystrophy** is an autosomal recessive disorder characterized by progressive loss of motor strength of the trunk and proximal limbs.

(1) This disorder may actually represent a group of conditions with different genotypic origins. One candidate gene is located on chromosome 15.

(2) Some patients actually have a disorder of dystrophin. A mutation in the adhalin gene, which produces adhalin (a component of the muscle membrane dystrophin–glycoprotein complex), can also cause the phenotypic appearance of limb-girdle muscular dystrophy.

2. **Diagnosis.** Patients typically have an **elevated serum CK level. EMG** demonstrates a "myopathic" pattern (i.e., brief, small amplitude muscle potentials). A **muscle biopsy** is often informative. **Genetic studies** are increasingly pursued.

B. **Acquired myopathy**

1. **Etiology.** Muscle disease can be caused by inflammatory, toxic or metabolic processes (Table 11-11).

2. **Diagnosis**

a. **Clinical signs.** A patient history and examination may provide clues to the diagnosis.

TABLE 11-11. Selected Causes of Acquired Myopathy

Polymyositis
  Idiopathic
  Associated with other connective tissue diseases, infectious agents (including HIV), and drugs
Dermatomyositis
  Associated with malignancy
Inclusion body myositis
  Associated with connective tissue diseases
Electrolyte disorders
  Hypokalemia
  Hyperkalemia
  Hypercalcemia
  Hypomagnesemia
  Hypophosphatemia
	Endocrine disorders
	  Hypothyroidism
	  Hyperthyroidism
	  Cushing's disease and iatrogenic corticosteroid administration
	  Addison's disease
	  Acromegaly
	Alcohol abuse
	Drugs (e.g., lovastatin, ε-aminocaproic acid, procainamide, zidovudine, phencyclidine, L-tryptophan)

HIV = human immunodeficiency virus.

        (1) Weakness is usually proximal and symmetric; disease onset can be acute, subacute, or chronic.

        (2) Swallowing and breathing can be compromised, and myoglobinuria may result from rapid muscle destruction, leading to renal insufficiency.

     b. Diagnostic studies. The serum CK level may be elevated. The EMG will reveal a "myopathic" pattern. A muscle biopsy is often informative.

   3. Selected syndromes

     a. Corticosteroid myopathy is usually caused by chronic corticosteroid therapy and is associated with proximal muscle weakness and wasting. The serum CK level is normal, and the EMG is usually unremarkable.

     b. Polymyositis. The infiltration of lymphocytes associated with polymyositis destroys muscle fiber (see Chapter 10 IX D).

     c. Inclusion body myositis is an inflammatory myopathy characterized by a resistance to corticosteroid therapy and by distal and proximal weakness that may be asymmetric.

        (1) Diagnosis. Muscle biopsy demonstrates inflammation and inclusion bodies (including "rimmed vacuoles") that contain amyloid. Cytotoxic T (Tc) cells are active against a muscle antigen.

        (2) There is **no accepted therapy.**

     d. Polymyalgia rheumatica (PMR) is not a myopathy but can masquerade as one.

        (1) Clinical signs

           (a) Patients often appear weak, but the major symptom is **painful (tender, aching,** and **stiff) muscles.**

           (b) Activities such as ascending stairs may be difficult to perform and upon formal strength testing, the patient may appear slightly weak, presumably because the pain prevents maximal effort. It has been found that if the pain can be relieved, strength is preserved.

           (c) Temporal (giant cell) arteritis is present in 15%–20% of patients.

        (2) Diagnostic studies. The erythrocyte sedimentation rate usually is significantly elevated but may be normal. The serum CK level is normal, and the EMG is unremarkable. Muscle histology is normal; biopsy is usually not performed.

        (3) NSAID or corticosteroid therapy should bring about a rapid resolution of symptoms.

C. **Nondystrophic myotonias (channelopathies)** are characterized by prolonged muscle relaxation after voluntary contraction or mechanical stimulation.

   1. Table 11-12 summarizes the **clinical features** of the nondystrophic myotonias.

   2. Therapy includes the use of quinine, procainamide, and phenytoin.

D. **Metabolic myopathies** include disorders of carbohydrate and lipid metabolism.

E. **Myoglobinuria** can be caused by crush injuries, vascular occlusions, infection, toxins, drugs, metabolic myopathies, hyperthermia, and severe inflammation.

   1. Diagnosis is aided by documenting an elevated serum CK level and urinary myoglobin. The latter can be suspected upon the finding of dark (brownish) urine and a positive dipstick for blood along with a paradoxical absence of red blood cells in the urine.

   2. Therapy should be directed at the underlying cause. Patients must be kept vigorously hydrated to prevent kidney damage.

XVI. INFECTION

A. **Meningitis, encephalitis, and neurologic complaints associated with HIV infection** are discussed in Chapter 8.

TABLE 11-12. Clinical Features of the Nondystrophic Myotonias

Feature	Sodium Channel Diseases		Chloride Channel Diseases Myotonia Congenita	
	Hyperkalemic Periodic Paralysis	Paramyotonia Congenita	Thompsen's	Becker's
Periodic paralysis	Yes	Yes	No	Yes
Potassium-induced weakness	Yes	In some families	No	No
Cold-induced weakness	No	Yes	No	No
Paradoxical myotonia	Occasional	Yes	No	No
Progressive weakness	Variable	Variable	No	Rare
Systemic involvement	No	No	No	No
Genetic transmission/ chromosome locus	AD/17	AD/17	AD/7	AR/7

Adapted with permission from Ptacek LJ, Johnson KJ, Griggs RC: Genetics and physiology of the myotonic muscle disorders. *N Engl J Med* 328(7):483, 1993.
AD = autosomal dominant; AR = Autosomal recessive.

B. **Brain abscess**

1. **Etiology.** An abscess can occur following neurosurgery or penetrating head trauma, in association with otitis media or poor oral hygiene, in patients with a bacteremia, and in individuals with a pulmonary arteriovenous malformation or cardiac right-to-left shunt.

2. **Diagnosis**
   a. **Clinical signs.** A brain abscess can present with headache, seizures, an altered sensorium, and focal neurologic symptoms and signs.
   b. **Diagnostic studies. CT** or **MR scanning** can easily detect a brain abscess, though differentiation from a neoplastic lesion can be difficult.

3. **Therapy.** Empiric therapy should be directed against aerobic and microaerophilic gram-positive streptococci and anaerobes, including Bacteroides fragilis.
   a. **Antibiotic therapy** often includes penicillin, chloramphenicol, metronidazole, and cefotaxime or trimethoprim–sulfamethoxazole. The clinical setting can help define the most likely pathogen.
   b. Therapy is monitored by serial brain imaging techniques.
   c. Often, **surgical excision** of the abscess **can be avoided. Stereotactic biopsy and drainage of an abscess** occasionally is required.

C. A **spinal epidural abscess** is usually caused by hematogenous seeding of an infective organism and is characterized by local pain and tenderness, fever, and neurologic signs and symptoms appropriate to the site of the infection.

1. **Diagnosis** can be aided by **spinal MRI** or **CT scans** and **myelography.**

2. **Surgical drainage** is indicated along with **antibiotic therapy.**

D. **Neurosyphilis**

1. **Stages and clinical signs**
   a. **Asymptomatic disease.** CSF abnormalities may be the only sign of infection.
   b. **Acute syphilitic meningitis** usually develops within 2 years of primary infec-

tion. Headache, meningismus, hydrocephalus, and cranial nerve palsies can occur.

    c. Cerebrovascular (meningovascular) syphilis presents months to years after primary infection with ischemic strokes (often associated with headache) and behavioral abnormalities.

    d. General paresis develops 1–2 decades after primary infection and is characterized by a progressive dementia.

    e. Tabes dorsalis also presents 10–20 years after primary infection with lightning pains, paresthesias, bladder dysfunction, gait instability, Argyll Robertson pupils (i.e., impaired pupillary light reaction with preserved pupillary constriction to accommodation, perhaps is a result of a midbrain tegmental lesion), areflexia (especially at the ankles), and loss of position and vibration sensibility.

2. Diagnostic studies. Patients with HIV infection should be particularly suspect for having neurosyphilis.

    a. Almost all patients with neurosyphilis have a **reactive serum fluorescent treponemal antibody (FTA-ABS) test.** A patient with a nonreactive CSF FTA-ABS test does not have neurosyphilis.

    b. The **CSF VDRL** test is often reactive in neurosyphilis, but a nonreactive CSF VDRL test is found in 25% of patients with neurologic disease years removed from the primary infection.

    c. Other CSF findings include a predominantly mononuclear pleocytosis and an elevated protein and IgG index.

3. Therapy. Penicillin is the treatment of choice for neurosyphilis. Patients with concurrent HIV infection develop neurosyphilis earlier and may be more resistant to therapy than immunocompetent patients.

XVII. PRIMARY CNS TUMORS, though relatively uncommon malignancies, seem to be of increasing incidence.

A. Astrocytic neoplasms

1. Astrocytomas are neoplasms with slight hypercellularity and pleomorphism. **Anaplastic astrocytomas** are characterized as having moderate cellularity and pleomorphism and some vascular proliferation.

    a. Clinical signs. Astrocytomas and anaplastic astrocytomas typically present with focal hemispheric neurologic dysfunction, convulsions, or headache.

    b. Prognosis is inversely related to the patient's age and the presence of tumor necrosis. Other predictors of outcome include the patient's functional status and the amount of residual tumor after initial surgery.

    c. Therapy. Anaplastic astrocytomas can be treated with **surgery** and **radiotherapy; chemotherapy** may be helpful. The survival rate after 2 years is 38%–50%.

2. Glioblastoma multiforme has moderate to marked hypercellularity, pleomorphism, and necrosis; vascular proliferation may be present.

    a. Clinical signs are similar to those of less aggressive tumors. CT or MRI scans typically reveal an enhancing, irregular mass (Figure 11-7).

    b. Glioblastoma multiforme has a **poor prognosis** with a survival rate of 10% after 24 months.

    c. Therapy includes **corticosteroid therapy** (for edema reduction), **surgical debulking, radiotherapy,** and **chemotherapy.**

B. Oligodendrogliomas are infiltrating tumors that commonly present with headache and convulsions; focal neurologic deficits can develop.

1. Prognosis. The overall median length of survival is 53 months.

2. Therapy. Anaplastic oligodendrogliomas seem to be responsive to **radiotherapy** and **chemotherapy. Surgery** is the mainstay of treatment.

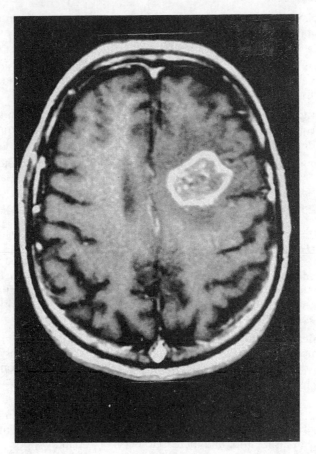

FIGURE 11-7. An enhanced T$_1$-weighted magnetic resonance imaging (MRI) scan demonstrating a glioblastoma multiforme.

C. **Meningiomas** are tumors that arise from the meninges and slowly enlarge, causing a mass effect that displaces normal structures. Angioblastic meningiomas are locally invasive.

1. **Clinical signs.** Headache, seizures, and focal neurologic signs can occur.

2. **Therapy is surgical resection; radiotherapy** can be used for invasive tumors.

3. **Prognosis.** If the entire tumor can be surgically resected, the majority of patients do well. If the entire tumor cannot be removed, the patient will experience recurrence of symptoms.

D. **Schwannomas** of the eighth cranial nerve (acoustic neuroma) typically arise from the vestibular component of the nerve. They can enlarge and displace structures about the cerebellopontine angle.

1. **Clinical signs.** Patients develop dizziness, hearing loss, and tinnitus. A diminished corneal reflex may be a sign of trigeminal nerve compromise by an enlarging mass.

2. **Diagnostic studies.** Diagnosis is best made with an enhanced MRI.

3. **Therapy. Surgical resection** is the preferred treatment.

4. **Prognosis.** Small tumors can be surgically cured. If residual tumor remains, recurrent symptoms can develop, usually years later.

E. **Primary CNS lymphoma** is increasing in incidence, especially in immunocompromised patients. Occasionally, primary CNS lymphoma presents as meningeal lymphomatosis.

1. **Imaging studies** reveal one or more intensely enhancing lesions, typically in a periventricular distribution. The diagnosis can be established with stereotactic biopsy.

2. **Therapy.** Although initial treatment with corticosteroids can lead to a rapid decrease in the size of the mass, ultimate survival depends on radiation therapy and chemotherapy.

3. **Prognosis.** The development of multimodality treatment protocols has extended patient survival for years, especially in immunocompetent patients.

XVIII. HEREDITARY DISORDERS

A. **Wilson's disease (hepatolenticular degeneration)** is an autosomal recessive disease localized to chromosome 13. It is associated with the accumulation of copper in the brain, liver, and other tissues because of a deficiency of the copper-binding protein ceruloplasmin.

1. **Clinical signs** include hepatic disease, a Kayser-Fleischer ring in Descemet's membrane of the cornea, behavioral problems (including psychosis), movement disorders (e.g., incoordination, tremor, masked facies, dystonia, and athetosis), and hemolytic anemia.

2. **Diagnostic studies**
   a. Diagnosis is made by finding a low serum ceruloplasmin level, excessive 24-hour urine copper excretion, a Kayser-Fleischer ring upon examination with a slit lamp, and increased levels of hepatic copper.
   b. MRI can reveal atrophy of the caudate and putamen with increased signal intensity on T_2-weighted images.

3. **Therapy** consists of **copper chelation.**

B. **Neurofibromatosis**

1. **Neurofibromatosis type 1 (NF 1, von Recklinghausen's disease)** is an autosomal dominant disorder. The responsible gene is located on chromosome 17.
   a. A patient meeting two or more of the following criteria can be diagnosed as suffering from NF 1.
      (1) **Neurofibromas** (two or more, or one plexiform neurofibroma)
      (2) **Café-au-lait macules** (six or more measuring 1.5 cm in their greatest dimension)
      (3) **Freckling** in the **axillary or inguinal areas**
      (4) **Optic glioma**
      (5) Two or more **iris hamartomas (Lisch nodules)**
      (6) **Sphenoid dysplasia** or **thinning of the cortex of the long bones**
      (7) An **immediate relative** with NF 1
   b. **Complications** of NF 1 include astrocytic tumors, optic glioma, neurofibrosarcoma, compressive peripheral neuropathies, compressive myelopathy, pheochromocytoma, and scoliosis.
   c. **Therapy** is directed at the complications of the disease.

2. **Neurofibromatosis type 2 (NF 2)** is an autosomal dominant disorder localized to chromosome 22 and characterized by bilateral acoustic neurofibromas.

C. **von Hippel-Lindau disease** is an autosomal dominant disorder localized to chromosome 3 and characterized by **cerebellar** and **retinal hemangioblastomas.**

1. Hemangioblastomas may also be found throughout the CNS. The kidneys, pancreas, and liver can harbor hemangiomas. Pheochromocytomas may develop.

2. Polycythemia is associated with cerebellar hemangioblastoma.

D. **Osler-Weber-Rendu disease (hereditary hemorrhagic telangiectasia)** is an autosomal dominant disorder characterized by telangiectatic skin lesions, CNS vascular malformations, and pulmonary arteriovenous fistulae. A brain abscess may occur, as may ischemic stroke, secondary to a paradoxical embolus via a pulmonary arteriovenous fistula.

E. **Tuberous sclerosis** is an autosomal dominant disorder localized to chromosome 9.

1. **Criteria for diagnosis** include multiple facial angiofibromas, ungual fibromas, retinal hamartoma, cortical tubers, subependymal glial nodules (often calcified), and multiple renal angiomyolipomas.

2. **Some associated features** are hypomelanotic macules, a shagreen patch, multicystic kidneys, seizures, and mental retardation. Benign giant cell astrocytomas can develop, often near the foramen of Monro.

F. **Down syndrome (trisomy 21)** is characterized by mental retardation, epicanthal folds, Brushfield spots on the iris, a transverse palmar crease, and cardiac malformations. By age 50, most patients develop Alzheimer's disease. Myelopathy may develop because of atlantoaxial dislocation.

G. **Huntington's disease** is an autosomal dominant disorder. The responsible gene, which is localized to chromosome 4, has an excess of trinucleotide repeats and codes the protein huntingtin. Patients develop a progressive cognitive decline and choreoathetosis between 30 and 50 years of age. Depression frequently occurs. Atrophy of the caudate nucleus is characteristic.

H. **Cerebellar atrophies** are associated with multisystem degenerative processes within two broad, heterogeneous sets of conditions: the spinocerebellar atrophies and the olivopontocerebellar atrophies.

1. **Etiology.** These diseases can be transmitted as autosomal dominant or recessive disorders, or they may be sporadic. Autosomal dominant cerebellar ataxia has been mapped to chromosome 6 and is characterized by an excess number of trinucleotide repeats. Molecular genetics will allow further genotypic classification of these disorders. Cerebellar atrophies have been associated phenotypically with deficiencies of glutamate dehydrogenase, pyruvate dehydrogenase complex, hexosaminidase, and vitamin E and elevated very long–chain fatty acids.

2. **Clinical signs.** Spinocerebellar and olivopontocerebellar atrophies can be characterized by the development of various combinations of slowly progressive ataxia, parkinsonism, cognitive impairment, and myelopathy.

I. **Peroxisome disorders.** The peroxisome is a cellular organelle that is involved with fatty acid oxidation.

1. **Adrenoleukodystrophy** is an X-linked disorder characterized by progressive intellectual decline, spasticity, and visual loss. **Adrenomyeloneuropathy,** also an X-linked disorder, is characterized by a progressive myelopathy and neuropathy.
   a. White matter changes are visible on CT and MRI scans in adrenoleukodystrophy.
   b. Both conditions result in excessive levels of very long–chain fatty acids in the blood, perhaps as a result of defective β-oxidation.

2. **Refsum disease** is an autosomal recessive disorder characterized by a sensorimotor neuropathy, retinal pigmentation, ataxia, anosmia, hearing loss, skin lesions, and elevated CSF protein.
   a. There is an excess of phytanic acid in the blood because of a defect in IgA-oxidation of this fatty acid.

b. Dietary control of phytanic acid intake and plasmapheresis can help control the neurologic problems.

J. **Mitochondrial disorders.** Mitochondrial DNA codes for components of the mitochondrial respiratory chain and oxidative phosphorylation enzymatic complexes. Disorders of mitochondrial DNA are transmitted by nonmendelian, maternal inheritance. The mitochondrial encephalopathies and myopathies have ragged red fibers in muscle. The ragged red fibers represent abundant abnormal mitochondria that are demonstrated using a modified Gomori trichrome stain. Patients often have elevated blood lactic acid levels.

1. **Kearns-Sayre syndrome** is characterized by progressive external ophthalmoplegia, pigmentary retinopathy, complete heart block, CSF protein levels greater than 100 mg/dl, ataxia, and myopathy. Deletions in the mitochondrial DNA are found.

2. **Myoclonic epilepsy with ragged red fibers (MERRF)** presents with myoclonus, epilepsy, and ataxia. There is a point mutation in the mitochondrial genome.

3. **Mitochondrial encephalomyopathy with lactic acidosis and stroke-like events (MELAS)** is characterized by intermittent vomiting and headaches, recurrent ischemic strokes, and seizures. Sensorineural hearing loss and short stature can be present. Point mutations are present in the mitochondrial DNA.

4. **Leber's hereditary optic neuropathy** presents with subacute bilateral central vision loss with retinal microangiopathy. It is caused by point mutations in the mitochondrial genome.

XIX. TOXIC AND METABOLIC DISORDERS

A. **Vitamin B_{12} deficiency.** Combined systems degeneration results from a deficiency of vitamin B_{12}.

1. **Pathophysiology.** Deprivation of vitamin B_{12} leads to demyelination and axonal degeneration, affecting the peripheral nerves, the spinal cord (where the posterior and lateral columns are demyelinated) and the cerebrum.

2. **Diagnosis**
   a. **Clinical signs.** Neurologic manifestations include cognitive impairment, diminished position and vibratory sensation, upper motor neuron signs with abnormal gait, and sensory peripheral neuropathy.
   b. **Diagnostic studies.** Patients typically have anemia, macrocytosis, and a low vitamin B_{12} level. Neurologic disease, however, can occur without anemia or macrocytosis. If the diagnosis remains suspect in a patient with a normal or marginally decreased serum vitamin B_{12} level, the finding of elevated serum methylmalonic acid and total homocysteine can confirm the presence of vitamin B_{12} deficiency.

3. **Therapy** is administration of **cobalamin.**

B. **Acute intermittent porphyria**

1. **Pathophysiology.** This autosomal dominant disorder is caused by a defect in the activity of uroporphyrinogen I synthetase, which leads to increased activity of δ-aminolevulinic acid synthetase and elevated levels of δ-aminolevulinic acid.

2. **Diagnosis.** Acute intermittent porphyria causes delirium, seizures, and autonomic, sensory, and motor neuropathies; a Guillain-Barré–like illness can develop. During an acute attack, the **Watson-Schwartz test** will reveal elevated levels of urinary porphobilinogen.

3. **Therapy. Hematin administration** can decrease clinical manifestations. Precipitants such as barbiturates, phenytoin, starvation, and infection should be avoided in susceptible individuals.

C. **Complications of alcohol abuse.** Alcohol may affect the nervous system by itself (i.e., alcohol intoxication, addiction, or withdrawal) or in tandem with a nutritional deficiency.

1. **Complications from intoxication, addiction, and withdrawal**
   a. **Acute alcohol intoxication** causes delirium and incoordination.
      (1) Severe intoxication can lead to metabolic coma with respiratory depression.
      (2) Alcoholic **"blackouts"** are characterized by the inability to form new memories in spite of preservation of consciousness.
   b. **Alcohol withdrawal** causes early symptoms of tremulousness and hallucinosis. Delirium tremens is seen during late withdrawal from alcohol. Benzodiazepines may be used to treat alcohol withdrawal symptoms.
   c. **Alcohol-related seizures ("rum fits")** are brief, generalized tonic–clonic convulsions that frequently occur in clusters.
      (1) Classically, alcohol-related seizures were thought to occur primarily in the 48 hours following withdrawal from chronic alcohol intake. However, alcohol-related seizures may also be caused by chronic alcohol intoxication and represent a toxic effect of alcohol on the brain, not a withdrawal phenomenon.
      (2) Typically, the patient is alert shortly after the seizure. Patients do not have seizure discharges on an interictal EEG.
      (3) **Therapy** should be directed at the underlying alcohol abuse. Anticonvulsant medications are not indicated for typical alcohol-related seizures.
   d. Alcohol abuse is associated with **cerebral atrophy** and **cognitive impairments** and may **predispose a patient to stroke.**
   e. Alcoholic patients may develop a **myopathy** that is acute or chronic and predominantly affects the proximal muscles. **Rhabdomyolysis** can complicate the acute disorder.

2. **Complications related to nutritional deficiencies**
   a. **Wernicke's encephalopathy** is seen in the malnourished alcoholic patient who has a **thiamine deficiency.** Other conditions (e.g., hyperemesis, renal dialysis, malnutrition) are associated with thiamine deficiency and can lead to Wernicke's encephalopathy, even in patients who do not abuse alcohol.
      (1) **Clinical signs.** Patients typically are delirious, have nystagmus and sixth cranial nerve palsies, and ataxia. Disorders of consciousness and hypothermia can occur.
      (2) **Therapy.** Thiamine administration can resolve the acute illness.
   b. **Korsakoff psychosis** is a chronic encephalopathy that is seen in alcoholic patients with a thiamine deficiency.
      (1) **Clinical signs** include retrograde and anterograde memory deficits, apathy, and impaired problem solving abilities.
      (2) **Therapy.** The patient may not improve with abstinence from alcohol or thiamine administration.
   c. **Sensory neuropathy** is caused by alcohol and often leads to dysesthesia. Although this axonal (though some authors suggest demyelinative) neuropathy is probably related to concurrent malnutrition, alcohol itself may be toxic to nerves.
   d. **Cerebellar degeneration** may occur in alcoholics.
      (1) The anterior and superior vermis are particularly affected.
      (2) **Clinical signs.** Patients have difficulty with gait and stance; nystagmus and arm ataxia are not prominent.

D. **Drug abuse**

1. Use of **cocaine** or **"crack"** can result in seizures, ischemic stroke, subarachnoid and intraparenchymal hemorrhage, and rhabdomyolysis. Hemorrhagic strokes may be associated with an underlying vascular lesion; angiography is usually indicated to search for an aneurysm or arteriovenous malformation.

2. Use of **heroin** can cause a metabolic coma; miosis is a characteristic finding in heroin users. Heroin has been associated with rhabdomyolysis, chronic myopathy, transverse myelitis, and peripheral neuropathies.

3. Ingestion of **phencyclidine (PCP)** can cause a wide range of neurologic disturbances ranging from acute psychosis to coma. Nystagmus, miosis, ataxia, myoclonus, dystonic posturing, generalized rigidity, dyskinesias, and seizures can occur.

XX. SLEEP DISORDERS

A. **Narcolepsy** is characterized by hypersomnia with short latency periods for the onset of daytime sleep and the early development of rapid eye movement (REM) sleep. Patients awaken refreshed from sleep attacks.

1. **Etiology.** Narcolepsy is probably an autosomal dominant disorder with variable penetrance; it has been mapped to chromosome 6. The vast majority of patients have antigens for HLA-DR2 or HLA-DQw1.

2. **Clinical signs** include **cataplexy** (i.e., transient episodes of diminished muscle tone), **sleep paralysis,** and **vivid dreams** at the beginning and end of sleep.

3. **Therapy.** Methylphenidate or pemoline can diminish the hypersomnia, and protriptyline or imipramine can decrease cataplexy.

B. **Sleep apnea,** or hypoventilation during sleep, can be attributable to obstructive causes (e.g., obesity, a small oropharynx) or to nonobstructive (CNS) causes. Sleep apnea is commonly "mixed" and represents both CNS and obstructive problems.

1. **Clinical signs.** Patients have daytime hypersomnia and can develop nocturnal hypoxia, pulmonary hypertension, and cardiac arrhythmias.

2. **Therapy.** Treatment options include weight loss, continuous positive airway pressure (CPAP), uvulopalatopharyngoplasty (UPPP), and tracheostomy.

C. **Periodic movements in sleep** involve flexor contractions in the legs. Patients can also experience sleep myoclonus and dystonia and restless legs syndrome while awake.

1. **Clinical signs.** The patient is momentarily aroused, and therefore nocturnal sleep quality is poor, leading to daytime hypersomnia.

2. **Therapy.** Treatment options include carbidopa/levodopa combinations, opiates, and clonazepam.

XXI. TRAUMA

A. **Brain injury**

1. A **concussion** is a momentary disruption of brain function following head injury that results in a brief loss of consciousness.
   a. **Clinical signs.** After awakening, patients complain of impaired memory, poor concentration, blurred vision, tinnitus, dizziness, and nausea.
   b. Symptoms can persist for days or weeks as the **postconcussion syndrome.**
   c. **Post-traumatic migraine** can develop but may be alleviated using antimigraine agents.

2. **Severe head trauma** can cause brain contusion, epidural and subdural hematoma, penetrating brain injuries, SAH, and CSF leaks.

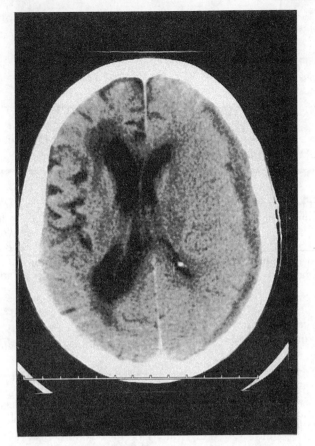

FIGURE 11-8. A nonenhanced computed tomography (CT) scan showing a chronic subdural hematoma. Note the mass effect on the lateral ventricle and the absence of sulci.

        a. Clinical signs. Progressive mental status changes leading to coma and focal neurologic signs can develop.

        b. Diagnostic studies. Emergent CT scanning can help delineate the extent of the problem.

        c. Therapy. Control of ICP and neurosurgical evaluation are indicated as appropriate.

    3. A **subdural hematoma** can result from acute head trauma and present with an altered sensorium and focal neurologic findings (e.g., hemiparesis). A subdural hematoma is also associated with minor trauma and can present with subtle subacute or chronic behavioral changes and mild focal deficits. At times, no history of trauma is elicited; this is especially true in elderly patients.

        a. Diagnostic studies. A CT scan is very helpful in documenting the presence of a subdural hematoma (Figure 11-8).

        b. Therapy. Neurosurgical intervention is usually indicated for an acute subdural hematoma; a chronic subdural hematoma may not require surgery.

B. **Spinal cord injury** can result in an acute paraparesis or quadriparesis. A central cord syndrome can follow a hyperextension injury to the cervical spinal cord and is characterized by lower motor neuron dysfunction affecting the cervical myotomes, mild sensory loss in the arms, and a myelopathy.

    1. Diagnostic studies. Because the vertebral column may not be stable, the patient should be immobilized while a radiographic assessment is made.

    2. Therapy. High-dose methylprednisolone therapy given within 8 hours of injury can improve outcome.

STUDY QUESTIONS

DIRECTIONS: Each of the numbered items or incomplete statements in this section is followed by answers or by completions of the statement. Select the ONE lettered answer or completion that is BEST in each case.

1. A 70-year-old retired professor complains of weakness and fatigue. Any physical activity is an effort, and he cannot find a comfortable position at rest. He has lost 5 pounds over the past month. Physical examination is normal. The most likely diagnosis is

(A) depression
(B) hypokalemia
(C) temporal (giant cel) arteritis
(D) polymyalgia rheumatica (PMR)
(E) polymyositis

2. A 29-year-old woman suddenly develops a left hemiparesis. The patient experienced a deep venous thrombosis in her right leg 3 years ago. The most likely cause of this patient's deficit is

(A) nonvalvular atrial fibrillation
(B) lupus anticoagulant
(C) mitral valve prolapse
(D) multiple sclerosis (MS)
(E) astrocytoma

3. An assembly-line worker complains of awakening at night with right-hand discomfort that resolves after several minutes. After 3 weeks of continuing symptoms, he seeks medical advice. Examination discloses mild weakness of thumb abduction and diminished pain sensibility on the palmar aspect of the thumb and index finger. The most likely diagnosis is

(A) carpal tunnel syndrome
(B) cervical radiculopathy
(C) reflex sympathetic dystrophy
(D) tendonitis
(E) left middle cerebral artery ischemic attacks

4. A 32-year-old woman complains that she has had difficulty walking for the past week. Examination reveals leg weakness, to a lesser extent, arm weakness, and areflexia. The patient is unable to walk across the room. The best treatment would be administration of

(A) corticosteroids
(B) penicillin
(C) phenytoin
(D) levodopa
(E) intravenous immunoglobulin

5. A 73-year-old woman presents with a 6-month history of deteriorating gait and low-back discomfort, exacerbated by walking. Examination is unremarkable except for hypoactive muscle stretch reflexes in the legs. X-rays of the lumbosacral area show the expected degenerative changes associated with a woman of her age. The most likely diagnosis is

(A) acute lumbar disk herniation
(B) lumbar stenosis
(C) myopathy
(D) normal pressure hydrocephalus (NPH)
(E) cervical stenosis

6. A 45-year-old right-handed man complains that he has had difficulty holding and using a writing instrument for the past year. He notes the development of right-hand and forearm spasms only when writing. Physical examination is unremarkable. The most likely diagnosis is

(A) Parkinson's disease
(B) focal dystonia
(C) carpal tunnel syndrome
(D) cervical radiculopathy
(E) benign essential tremor

7. A previously healthy, 68-year-old woman develops auditory hallucinations. She cannot provide many details but believes her mother is speaking to her. She has difficulty cooperating during the interview and physical examination, which is unremarkable. The most likely diagnosis is

(A) complex partial seizures
(B) Alzheimer's disease
(C) adverse medication effect
(D) hyperthyroidism
(E) peduncular hallucinosis

8. A 24-year-old construction worker with a 2-year history of low-back pain complains of an acute onset of bilateral leg weakness and incontinence. The best management tactic would be

(A) administration of nonsteroidal anti-inflammatory drugs (NSAIDs)
(B) emergency surgery
(C) strict bed rest
(D) lumbar traction
(E) back exercises

9. A 32-year-old man presents with repetitive generalized motor convulsions that continue for 35 minutes until 10 mg of diazepam are administered intravenously. The next course of action should be to administer

(A) phenytoin intravenously
(B) carbamazepine orally
(C) pentobarbital intravenously
(D) ethosuximide orally

10. A 78-year-old woman complains of experiencing headaches and progressive confusion for the past month. She has a left hemianopia and cannot dress herself. A computed tomography (CT) scan demonstrates a large, irregularly enhancing mass in the right parietal lobe. There is no obvious systemic disease. The most likely diagnosis is

(A) brain abscess
(B) glioblastoma multiforme
(C) meningioma
(D) metastasis
(E) central nervous system (CNS) lymphoma

11. A 63-year-old woman develops intermittent dizziness. Examination discloses a diminished right corneal reflex and mild hearing loss in the right ear. The most likely diagnosis is

(A) cerebellopontine angle tumor
(B) benign paroxysmal positional vertigo (BPPV)
(C) lateral medullary syndrome
(D) Meniere's disease

12. A previously vigorous 80-year-old woman collapses when getting out of bed. Examination of her legs reveals bilateral weakness, loss of pain and temperature sensation, and areflexia. Her bladder is distended. The remainder of the examination is unremarkable. The most likely diagnosis is

(A) Guillain-Barré syndrome
(B) anterior cerebral artery occlusion
(C) cauda equina syndrome
(D) anterior spinal artery occlusion
(E) thoracic spinal cord compression

13. A 70-year-old man reports that over the past 2 months, he has had progressive difficulty walking. Examination demonstrates distal (greater than proximal) weakness in the arms and legs and the absence of muscle stretch reflexes. Motor nerve conduction velocities are slowed. The most likely diagnosis is

(A) Guillain-Barré syndrome
(B) lead poisoning
(C) chronic inflammatory demyelinating polyneuropathy (CIDP)
(D) amyotrophic lateral sclerosis (ALS)
(E) polymyositis

14. A 56-year-old man presents with a 2-year history of impotence and not feeling "right." Examination reveals masked facies, bradykinesia, rigidity, mild ataxia, and postural hypotension. The diagnosis is

(A) Parkinson's disease
(B) combined systems degeneration
(C) multiple systems atrophy
(D) spinocerebellar degeneration
(E) vitamin E deficiency

A patient with a subarachnoid hemorrhage (SAH) caused by a right anterior communicating artery aneurysm undergoes successful surgery 2 days after the hemorrhage. Three days later, right arm weakness develops. The most likely diagnosis is

(A) hydrocephalus
(B) meningitis
(C) repeat hemorrhage
(D) vasospasm

16. A 17-year-old high school varsity diver develops a headache, dizziness, left-sided arm and leg clumsiness, and loss of pain and temperature sensation in the left facial and right body areas following a practice session. The most likely diagnosis is

(A) benign paroxysmal positional vertigo (BPPV)
(B) multiple sclerosis (MS)
(C) vertebral artery dissection
(D) astrocytoma
(E) labyrinthitis

DIRECTIONS: Each set of matching questions in this section consists of a list of four to twenty-six lettered options (some of which may be in figures) followed by several numbered items. For each numbered item, select the ONE lettered option that is most closely associated with it. To avoid spending too much time on matching sets with large numbers of options, it is generally advisable to begin each set by reading the list of options. Then, for each item in the set, try to generate the correct answer and locate it in the option list, rather than evaluating each option individually. Each lettered option may be selected once, more than once, or not at all.

Items 17–19

(A) Baclofen
(B) Amitriptyline
(C) Indomethacin
(D) Corticosteroids

Select the most effective therapy for each headache.

17. Migraine

18. Temporal (giant cell) arteritis

19. Paroxysmal hemicrania

ANSWERS AND EXPLANATIONS

1. The answer is D [IV C 4 a–b; XV B 3 d (1)–(2)]. Polymyalgia rheumatica (PMR) is characterized by muscle discomfort, and patients often present with vague complaints, as in this case. By definition, the neuromuscular examination is normal. Temporal (giant cell) arteritis can occur with PMR, but this patient has no complaint of headache or symptoms referable to vision. Depression can cause fatigue and diminished activity but discomfort is less frequently a complaint. A normal erythrocyte sedimentation rate, which is elevated in the presence of PMR, would support a diagnosis of depression. Hypokalemia can cause muscle weakness but discomfort is not a typical feature. Polymyositis can cause muscle discomfort, but there should be accompanying weakness. The serum creatine kinase (CK) level is often elevated.

2. The answer is B [VIII B 4 b]. The lupus anticoagulant (an antiphospholipid antibody) is associated with peripheral venous thrombosis and ischemic (arterial) stroke. In patients with a history of deep venous thrombosis, the possibility of a paradoxical embolus causing a stroke (via a right-to-left cardiac shunt) should also be considered. Nonvalvular atrial fibrillation is a common cause of stroke in the elderly but there is no reason to suspect a rhythm disturbance in this patient. Mitral valve prolapse has been associated with cardiogenic emboli and stroke, but other causes of stroke should always be searched for since mitral valve prolapse is a relatively common entity. Multiple sclerosis (MS) and an astrocytoma can cause neurologic deficits in young patients; however, these conditions are not associated with deep venous thrombosis unless the patient is immobilized. These diagnoses should be considered in the evaluation of patients with hemiparesis, but the patient's history can often serve as a clue to guide diagnostic thinking.

3. The answer is A [XIII D 1 a–b]. People such as assembly-line workers or typists are particularly prone to carpal tunnel syndrome because their daily activities require repetitive wrist movements, which may, in time, compress the median nerve, causing neuropathy.

Awakening at night with hand discomfort is a common complaint, and the findings upon examination support the diagnosis. A cervical radiculopathy can cause some of the findings on examination of this patient. However, the history is more suggestive of carpal tunnel syndrome. Patients with a cervical radiculopathy often have a concurrent carpal tunnel syndrome and vice versa. The history and examination are not supportive of a diagnosis of tendonitis or reflex sympathetic dystrophy. Transient ischemic attacks (TIAs) rarely cause discomfort and are not associated with neurologic deficits after 24 hours have elapsed.

4. The answer is E [XIII D 2 b (1), c (2)]. The patient probably has Guillain-Barré syndrome. Administration of intravenous immunoglobulin has been found to hasten clinical improvement in these patients. Plasmapheresis is the preferred therapy. Corticosteroids ae not indicated for the treatment of Guillain-Barré syndrome but can be used to treat chronic inflammatory demyelinating polyneuropathy (CIDP). This illness can present with chronic progressive weakness, and, occasionally, subacute weakness, and it needs to be distinguished from the Guillain-Barré syndrome. Clues to a diagnosis of CIDP include early, marked slowing of nerve conduction velocities and disease progression beyond 4 weeks. Penicillin is used to treat Lyme disease, which can present with multiple radiculopathies and thereby cause difficulty ambulating. Examination of cerebral spinal fluid (CSF) typically reveals a pleocytosis. The patient has no stigmata of Parkinson's disease other than difficulty ambulating; therefore, levodopa therapy is inappropriate. Phenytoin is used, on occasion, to treat painful polyneuropathies. There is no need for such treatment in this patient, because she has not complained of pain.

5. The answer is B [III B 4 a; VII A 2 b; XV B 2 a]. Lumbar stenosis is caused by degenerative changes in the lumbosacral spine, often in association with a congenitally small lumbosacral intraspinal space. The history is often that of vague low-back discomfort associated with subtle findings upon examination referable to impingement on motor and sensory roots. Diagnosis can be made by the characteristic finding of an "hourglass" appearance on magnetic resonance (MR) scans. An acute disk herniation is characterized by low-back discomfort and pain extending in a radicular fashion down one or both legs. Examination is often consistent with impingement on a single sensory or motor root. A myopathy can cause an impaired gait, low-back discomfort because of weakness, and hypoactive muscle stretch reflexes, typically at the knees. However, this condition is much less common than lumbar stenosis and therefore is not the most likely diagnosis. Normal pressure hydrocephalus (NPH) causes an apractic gait (i.e., difficulty in walking in spite of an intact motor, sensory, and cerebellar examination), cognitive impairment, and urinary incontinence. The clinical picture is not consistent with this diagnosis. Cervical stenosis can cause a myelopathy and resultant gait problem. The patient did not exhibit signs of a myelopathy, and therefore this diagnosis is unlikely.

6. The answer is B [X A 2 a (1)–(2), B 1 a, 4 b; XIII D 1 a–b]. Writer's cramp is a focal dystonia of unknown cause. Patients develop symptoms of cramps or spasms with altered hand and arm posture when attempting the specific task of writing. Examination of the patient is otherwise normal. Micrographia is a symptom of Parkinson's disease but is usually accompanied by signs of rigidity and bradykinesia, and often tremor, upon examination. Carpal tunnel syndrome is caused by pressure on the median nerve as it enter the hand via the carpal tunnel. Median nerve dysfunction leads to hand weakness and loss of sensibility, which can affect writing. A cervical radiculopathy can lead to hand numbness and weakness and hyporeflexia. The exact distribution of findings depends on the nerve roots involved. A benign essential tremor is characterized by a distal upper extremity tremor during a task. There is no accompanying rigidity or bradykinesia. Handwriting in particular may suffer. However, carpal tunnel syndrome, cervical radiculopathy, and benign essential tremor are all unlikely because the patient's examination reveals no signs or symptoms other than difficulty with writing.

7. The answer is B [III B 3 d; IX A 3 a]. Alzheimer's disease is a cause of new-onset auditory hallucinations in the elderly. Typically, evidence of cognitive impairment is present, although on occasion, watchful waiting is nec-

essary before other manifestations of Alzheimer's disease become apparent. Low doses of haloperidol can be quite helpful in treating auditory hallucinations associated with Alzheimer's disease. Complex partial seizures can cause auditory hallucinations, but usually the patient reports simple sounds rather than words or complex sound patterns. Many medications can cause hallucinations, but this woman was "previously healthy;" therefore, it is unlikely that she was receiving medical therapy. Hyperthyroidism, especially apathetic hyperthyroidism, is a cause of delirium in the elderly. It is not particularly associated with auditory hallucinations. Peduncular hallucinations are primarily visual hallucinations due to rostral mesencephalic ischemia. This phenomenon is part of the "top-of-the-basilar" syndrome, which involves an ischemic insult to the territory of the rostral basilar artery.

8. The answer is B [VII A 2 a (2) (a)]. The patient probably has an acute disk herniation causing a cauda equina syndrome, an indication for emergency surgery. Surgery should be considered as an elective intervention for those patients with sciatica, disabling neurologic deficits, and disk herniation (as demonstrated by appropriate imaging techniques) who fail to respond to 6 weeks of conservative management. Nonsteroidal anti-inflammatory drugs (NSAIDs) can be helpful in the treatment of acute, and possibly chronic, low-back pain; however, they are not indicated as primary therapy for patients with acute, severe neurologic disability. Strict bed rest is very helpful for the treatment of acute back pain, but this therapy is not appropriate for this patient. The intradisk pressure is lowest in the supine position. Bed rest for 2–7 days is usually suggested; prolonged bed rest results in deconditioning. Lumbar traction is probably not effective for the treatment of low-back pain. Patients typically cannot exercise during the first few days of acute back pain. However, as the acute pain subsides, an exercise program may help prevent future problems.

9. The answer is A [IX D 1 b (2) (a)–(b), 2 c]. Administration of intravenous diazepam should be followed by the administration of phenytoin or phenobarbital in order to control status epilepticus because diazepam's duration of actin is measured only in minutes. Therefore, unless there is a contraindication, the patient should receive a loading dose of phenytoin intravenously. Carbamazepine is an effective anticonvulsant, but it cannot be given intravenously or intramuscularly. Therefore, a therapeutic level cannot be rapidly achieved given a drug half-life of 8–12 hours. Intravenous pentobarbital can be used to control repetitive seizures. However, since the patient is not currently convulsing, induction of barbiturate coma is not indicated. Ethosuximide is indicated for the treatment of absence seizures. Therefore, this is not an appropriate therapy for generalized motor convulsions.

10. The answer is B [XVI B 1, 2; XVII A 2, C, E 1]. A large, irregularly enhancing central nervous system (CNS) mass in an elderly patient without systemic cancer is highly suggestive of a glioblastoma multiforme. However, a biopsy is necessary before a definitive diagnosis can be made. The patient has no predisposing condition for a brain abscess, such as poor dentition or intravenous drug abuse. A meningioma can occur in the parietal area and distort the brain; however, a "convexity" meningioma is typically a homogeneously enhancing lesion. In the absence of systemic cancer, a brain metastasis is an unlikely cause of the patient's problem. However, without a biopsy the diagnosis of metastatic disease cannot be excluded. CNS lymphoma typically presents as a homogeneously enhancing mass lesion. Patients suffering from the human immunodeficiency virus (HIV) and other immunocompromised patients are prone to CNS lymphoma; in other populations, CNS lymphoma is rare.

11. The answer is A [VI B 2 b–c, e–f; XVII D 1–3]. A cerebellopontine angle tumor, such as a schwannoma, can cause intermittent dizziness. The tumor can arise from the eighth cranial nerve, thereby also affecting hearing, and can press on the trigeminal nerve, causing impairment of the corneal reflex. Benign paroxysmal positional vertigo (BPPV) causes intermittent brief dizziness that is dependent on postural changes. Nystagmus is characteristic, but there are no other neurologic deficits. A lateral medullary syndrome usually causes constant dizziness that is exacerbated with movement. Although the corneal reflex can be depressed, hearing is normal. Meniere's disease causes intermittent dizziness and hearing loss, but the corneal reflex is not diminished.

12. The answer is D [VII A 2 a (2) (a); XII C 3 b; XIII D 2 b (1)]. Thrombosis of the caudal anterior spinal artery leads to a flaccid paraplegia, loss of pain and temperature sensation,

and bowel and bladder dysfunction. The blood supply to the caudal spinal cord arises from the aorta via lumbar radicular arteries. The perfusion territory of the anterior spinal artery involves the anterior horn cells and the pain and temperature pathways. The Guillain-Barré syndrome rarely develops suddenly. Loss of temperature and pain sensation can occur but rarely without a concurrent loss of position and vibration sense. Sensory loss is usually less severe than motor loss. Generalized areflexia is common. An anterior cerebral artery thrombosis, especially when bilateral, can cause leg weakness, but there is no sensory loss. Upper motor neuron signs are present in the leg.

A cauda equina syndrome can cause a flaccid paraplegia, but all sensory modalities may be compromised because sensory nerve roots, which carry sensory fibers of all types, are involved in the disease process.

Thoracic spinal cord compression is often associated with back pain and produces upper motor neuron dysfunction in the legs. In the acute condition, the bladder may be distended but with time, its capacity is typically reduced.

13. The answer is C [V B 2 b (1); XII D 2 b (2); Table 11-10 A & B]. Chronic inflammatory demyelinating polyneuropathy (CIDP) is characterized by progressive weakness that occurs over an extended time (e.g., 4 weeks or more), absent muscle stretch reflexes, and slowed motor nerve conduction velocities. The Guillain-Barré syndrome should not cause progressive worsening of strength beyond 4 weeks. Typically, only some motor nerves demonstrate slowing, usually in a segmental, rather than a generalized, fashion. Lead poisoning can cause a motor neuropathy in children but only rarely in adults. Amyotrophic lateral sclerosis (ALS) causes progressive weakness, but motor nerve conduction velocities are unremarkable and muscle stretch reflexes are often hyperactive. Polymyositis causes progressive proximal (greater than distal) weakness and is not associated with impaired motor nerve conduction velocities are unremarkable and muscle stretch reflexes are often hyperactive. Polymyositis causes progressive proximal (greater than distal) weakness and is not associated with impaired motor nerve conduction velocities.

14. The answer is C [V B 2 b (2) (j); X A 2 a (2); XIX A 2 a; Table 11-8]. The signs and symptoms are most consistent with multiple systems atrophy (Shy-Drager syndrome). The early appearance of autonomic dysfunction (impotence and postural hypotension) and ataxia are against the diagnosis of Parkinson's disease. Combined systems degeneration is due to vitamin B_{12} deficiency. Parkinsonian features are not a feature of the disease. Spinocerebellar degeneration is characterized by cerebellar dysfunction and an accompanying upper motor neuron syndrome. Extrapyramidal and autonomic dysfunction are not prominent features. Vitamin E deficiency can masquerade as spinocerebellar degeneration.

15. The answer is D [VIII C 1 c (2)]. Vasospasm can develop several days after an aneurysmal subarachnoid hemorrhage (SAH). Patients present with progressive weakness and alterations in behavior. Early in the course, a computed tomography (CT) scan may not reveal an ischemic infarction. Hydrocephalus can occur immediately following an SAH or weeks to months later. Symptoms are typically nonfocal and, if the hydrocephalus develops acutely, it is often accompanied by a depressed level of consciousness. Bacterial meningitis can develop after a craniotomy. Typically, there is fever and impaired arousal. Focal signs can develop but are rarely the presenting feature. Although a repeat hemorrhage can occur following clipping of an aneurysm if the aneurysm is not completely isolated from the circulation, it is unusual for this to happen and present with a focal deficit, as opposed to depressed consciousness.

16. The answer is C [VI B 2 f; VIII B 2 c (1) (b), 6 d]. The patient has manifestations of a lateral medullary syndrome. In a young patient, who has subjected himself to strenuous neck movements, the most likely etiology is vertebral artery dissection.

Benign paroxysmal positional vertigo (BPPV) causes sudden episodes of dizziness, typically with changes in position. However, there are no associated neurologic symptoms or signs other than nystagmus. Multiple sclerosis (MS) can cause dizziness and clumsiness. However, the constellation of findings in this patient, which are referable to a single site within the brain and are of sudden onset, make the diagnosis of MS less likely. An astrocytoma can cause dizziness and unsteadiness. Often there is a headache. The onset is typically insidious, and the symptoms progressive. Labyrinthitis causes severe vertigo. Patients find it difficult to move about and prefer to remain still. Gait instability can occur because of the profound dizziness, but there are no cerebellar deficits. There are no neurologic signs other than nystagmus.

17–19. The answers are: 17-B [IV C 1 d (2) (a)], **18-D** [IV C 4 c], **19** [IV C 7]. Migraine headaches respond well to treatment with tricyclic antidepressants, such as amitriptyline. Temporal (giant cell) arteritis responds to corticosteroids. Paroxysmal hemicrania is responsive to indomethacin treatment. In fact, a positive response to treatment with indomethacin can serve to confirm a diagnosis of paroxysmal hemicrania.

Comprehensive
Examination

DIRECTIONS: Each of the numbered items or incomplete statements in this section is followed by answers or by completions of the statement. Select the ONE lettered answer or completion that is BEST in each case.

1. If present, which one of the following features distinguishes upper tract (kidney) from lower tract (bladder) infection in women?

(A) Fever >38.5°C
(B) Colony count >10^5/ml
(C) White blood cells in urinalysis
(D) Burning on urination

2. The most potent stimulus for the development of pulmonary hypertension in chronic obstructive pulmonary disease (COPD) is

(A) obliteration of the pulmonary vascular bed
(B) alveolar membrane damage
(C) left ventricular failure
(D) hypoxia
(E) acidosis

3. Chvostek's sign is a contraction of the facial muscles and upper lip when the examiner taps the facial nerve in front of the ear. A positive sign suggests which one of the following conditions?

(A) Hypercalcemia
(B) Hypocalcemia
(C) Hyperkalemia
(D) Acidosis
(E) Hypophosphatemia

4. A 50-year-old woman complains of redness, swelling, and stiffness in the distal interphalangeal (DIP) joints of her hands, but has no other joint complaints. The most likely diagnosis is

(A) erosive osteoarthritis
(B) rheumatoid arthritis
(C) systemic lupus erythematosus (SLE)
(D) ankylosing spondylitis
(E) scleroderma

5. A patient with chronic renal failure due to long-standing, severe hypertension is seen because of chest pain. The patient has received hemodialysis twice weekly for the last 2 years and has recently experienced episodes of hypotension at the beginning of treatment. The chest pain is located over the trapezius muscle. It is moderately reduced by assuming the upright position and exacerbated by deep breathing. The most likely cause of this patient's chest pain is

(A) pericarditis
(B) coronary artery disease
(C) diffuse esophageal spasm
(D) pulmonary embolism
(E) costochondritis

6. A 45-year-old man who has been in excellent health, except for mild obstructive lung disease as a result of smoking one pack of cigarettes per day (up until 3 years ago), is evaluated by his internist for numbness and tingling in his fingers with painful paresthesias. The internist refers the patient to a neurologist, who does laboratory studies to rule out vitamin B_{12} deficiency and diabetes. The patient has a normal hematologic profile and chemistry panel. His neurologic exam is only notable for sensory neuropathy in the hands accompanied by mild proprioception and vibratory loss. His physical examination otherwise is unremarkable. The patient has a normal chest x-ray. A computed axial tomography (CAT) scan of the chest and abdomen reveals a 3.5 × 4 cm anterior mediastinal mass. Mediastinotomy is performed and tissue is obtained. An extensive metastatic workup reveals no other evidence of disease outside of the mediastinum. The most appropriate therapy for this patient would be

(A) etoposide (VP-16-213), cisplatin, and concurrent radiation therapy to the chest
(B) VP-16-213, cisplatin, and bleomycin
(C) cyclophosphamide, doxorubicin, vincristine, and prednisone
(D) cyclophosphamide, doxorubicin, vincristine, and prednisone, followed by radiation to the chest if there is any residual abnormality in the anterior mediastinum.

7. A 30-year-old intravenous drug addict develops right-sided weakness and headache over a period of 2 days. Examination reveals an afebrile, poorly nourished individual with a mild right hemiparesis. The most likely diagnosis is

(A) bacterial endocarditis
(B) human immunodeficiency virus (HIV) meningitis
(C) brain abscess
(D) cryptococcal meningitis
(E) foreign body embolus

8. A previously normal 65-year-old black man presents with benign prostatic hypertrophy. A urinary infection is treated with sulfamethoxazole-trimethoprim. One week later, routine laboratory tests reveal new normocytic anemia with hemoglobin 8.9 g/dl. The most likely diagnosis is

(A) glucose-6-phosphate dehydrogenase (G6PD) hemolysis
(B) occult blood loss from cecal carcinoma
(C) occult blood loss from renal carcinoma
(D) sickle cell trait
(E) favism

9. A 45-year-old man with cirrhosis has had generalized abdominal pain for 24 hours without nausea or vomiting. His temperature is 38.3°C, and he has a distended abdomen with a clear fluid wave. There is diffuse tenderness on abdominal palpation. Paracentesis shows a clear fluid with 816 leukocytes/μl (85% polymorphonuclear cells, 15% lymphocytes). Gram stain shows no bacteria. The most likely diagnosis is

(A) peptic ulcer disease
(B) primary peritonitis
(C) pancreatitis
(D) cholecystitis
(E) liver abscess

10. A 17-year-old boy arrives at the clinic complaining of swelling of his face and legs for the last several weeks. He has been in good health until the onset of this problem and has not seen a physician for the last 3 years, except for school examinations. He denies any medication use and any other medical problems. On physical examination, the young man does not appear to be in any acute distress. His blood pressure is 110/80 mm Hg, his pulse is 60 bpm, his respiratory rate is 15, and his temperature is 98.6°F. The only abnormalities relate to the marked peripheral edema, which is visible up to mid-thigh, and some facial puffiness. On laboratory examination, blood urea nitrogen (BUN) is 10 mg/dl and creatinine is 1.1 mg/dl. The rest of the laboratory studies are normal. Urinalysis reveals 4 + protein and is negative for blood and glucose. Microscopic examination reveals several hyaline casts but no other cellular elements. The urine protein is 16.4 g/24 hr. Which disease best explains this clinical disorder?

(A) Minimal change nephropathy
(B) Membranous glomerulonephritis
(C) Henoch Schönlein purpura
(D) Acquired immune deficiency syndrome (AIDS) nephropathy
(E) Systemic vasculitis

11. A 24-year-old woman complains of generalized weakness. Which of the following physical findings would be most suggestive of polymyositis as the cause of her weakness?

(A) Difficulty combing hair
(B) Difficulty unscrewing a lid from a jar
(C) Prominent tenderness in the weak muscles
(D) Difficulty with heel-toe walking
(E) Involvement of facial and skeletal muscles

12. A 65-year-old man reads in the newspaper that prostate-specific antigen is a good screening test for cancer and asks his internist to have this drawn. The test reveals mildly elevated prostate-specific antigen levels of 10.4 ng/ml. Digital rectal examination reveals a normal-sized prostate, but ultrasound reveals a small hypoechoic area measuring 5×7 mm in the right lobe. The next appropriate step would be to

(A) perform a bone scan
(B) repeat assays for prostate-specific antigen in 3 months to check for further elevation
(C) perform a transrectal biopsy of the abnormal area revealed by ultrasound
(D) begin leuprolide depot therapy
(E) perform a computerized axial tomography (CAT) scan of the retroperitoneum, pelvis, and prostate

13. Pulmonary crackles are frequently heard in patients with which one of the following conditions?

(A) Pneumothorax
(B) Pulmonary fibrosis
(C) Pleural effusion
(D) Lung cancer
(E) Cor pulmonale

14. Although most cases of acute viral hepatitis resolve spontaneously, complications may occur. Which of the following statements best describes the complications of hepatitis B infection?

(A) The chronic carrier state is associated with an increased risk of hepatoma
(B) Chronic persistent hepatitis usually leads to progressive deterioration of liver function and must be treated aggressively
(C) Chronic active hepatitis can be diagnosed within 2–4 weeks of the acute infection with hepatitis B virus
(D) Chronic active hepatitis is characterized on liver biopsy by a periportal lymphocytic infiltrate without fibrosis or extraportal extension
(E) Fulminant hepatitis is characterized by rapidly rising transaminase levels in an enlarging liver

15. An 80-year-old woman with a history of congestive heart failure develops angina pectoris. Her medications are adjusted to include furosemide, digoxin, nitroglycerin, and potassium supplements. Shortly thereafter, she develops intermittent frontal throbbing headaches. What should the physician do first?

(A) Perform a temporal artery biopsy
(B) Begin propranolol
(C) Begin sublingual ergotamine
(D) Obtain a brain computed tomography (CT) scan
(E) Discontinue nitroglycerin

16. A 55-year-old man who has smoked 30 cigarettes daily since he was 25 is seen because of hemoptysis. He reports no symptoms except for a cough that produces 5–10 ml of sputum each morning. Results found on physical examination and x-ray are normal. The most likely cause of this man's hemoptysis is

(A) bronchogenic carcinoma
(B) pulmonary tuberculosis
(C) bronchiectasis
(D) α_1-antitrypsin deficiency
(E) chronic bronchitis

17. Which one of the following statements is true regarding renovascular hypertension?

(A) Renovascular hypertension is associated with an increased renin release
(B) This condition does not respond to treatment with captopril
(C) It is frequently seen in young men as a complication of fibromuscular disease
(D) Renovascular hypertension is easy to control

18. A 45-year-old asymptomatic woman has a random serum glucose level of 165 mg/dl on routine examination. Which of the following studies should be used next to evaluate this finding?

(A) Urine glucose
(B) Glucose tolerance test
(C) Fasting serum glucose
(D) 2-hour postprandial serum glucose
(E) Hemoglobin A_{1C} measurement

19. A 65-year-old patient presents with right knee pain, warmth, and swelling. Which one of the following findings would be most useful for making a diagnosis of pseudogout in this patient?

(A) Enlarged proximal interphalangeal (PIP) and distal interphalangeal (DIP) joints
(B) Elevated serum uric acid level
(C) Negatively birefringent crystals in the knee fluid
(D) Meniscal calcium on a radiograph of the involved knee
(E) Inflammatory fluid on aspirate

20. A 25-year-old woman visits her family physician, complaining of nasal blockage and rhinorrhea. She is not pregnant and has not been taking medication recently, except for nasal decongestant spray, which she uses occasionally to relieve her symptoms. She says a recent spell of humid weather has made the symptoms more severe. Nasal speculum examination, skin tests, and cytologic nasal smear reveal no evidence of infection or of anatomic or immunologic abnormality. The most likely diagnosis is

(A) nasal decongestant spray abuse
(B) allergic rhinitis
(C) eosinophilic nonallergic rhinitis
(D) vasomotor rhinitis

21. An 18-year-old man develops a persistent headache and fever and, after 5 days, has a focal seizure. A computed tomography (CT) scan of the head shows a ring-enhancing lesion in the right frontal lobe and an air-fluid level in the right frontal sinus. Neurosurgical aspiration of the lesion would be most likely to show

(A) small mononuclear cells suggestive of Burkitt's lymphoma
(B) *Toxoplasma gondii* cysts and tachyzoites (trophozoites)
(C) *Escherichia coli* and *Bacteroides fragilis*
(D) α-hemolytic streptococcus and mixed anaerobes
(E) budding yeast organisms with hyphal elements

22. A 20-year-old Asian woman presents with a new left lower extremity deep venous thrombosis. She has a history of mild thrombocytopenia and two miscarriages; she was treated for syphilis 2 years ago due to a positive rapid plasma reagin (RPR) test, even though antitreponemal antibody testing was negative. Her collective medical history most likely represents

(A) phospholipid antibody syndrome
(B) systemic lupus erythematosus (SLE)
(C) Ro antibody syndrome
(D) Takayasu's arteritis
(E) mixed connective tissue disease

23. A 60-year-old gardener presents with a change in personality. The family states that several weeks ago he complained of a painful wrist and 1 week ago he had transient facial asymmetry. A particularly pertinent issue to address is

(A) toxin exposure
(B) sexual habits
(C) tick bite
(D) mosquito bite

24. A 40-year-old woman in good general health has sudden chest pain, fever, and shortness of breath. She is a heavy smoker and takes no medicines, except oral contraceptives. Tachypnea and a temperature of 38°C are found on physical examination. Chest auscultation, percussion, and x-ray findings are normal. The most likely diagnosis is

(A) tracheobronchitis
(B) atypical pneumonia
(C) pulmonary embolus
(D) bacterial pneumonia
(E) lung cancer

25. A 70-year-old man has had intravesical chemotherapy for recurrent transitional cell carcinoma of the bladder. All of his previous lesions have been noninvasive, but his last cystoscopy showed a large ulcerating lesion that appeared to have muscle invasion. The patient refuses cystectomy and undergoes a course of radiation therapy accompanied by cisplatin chemotherapy. Unfortunately, 1 year later, the patient develops multiple pulmonary nodules. The appropriate chemotherapy regimen would be

(A) MVAC [methotrexate, vinblastine, doxorubicin (Adriamycin), and cisplatin]
(B) carboplatin
(C) cyclophosphamide, doxorubicin, and 5-fluorouracil (5-FU)
(D) etoposide (VP-16-213) and cisplatin

26. Which one of the following features is most suggestive of systemic lupus erythematosus (SLE) rather than rheumatoid arthritis?

(A) An active urinary sediment (red cells, white cells, cellular casts, no bacteria)
(B) Inflammatory arthritis of the metacarpophalangeal (MCP) and proximal interphalangeal (PIP) joints
(C) Pleural effusion on chest x-ray
(D) Anemia
(E) Abnormal liver function tests

27. A patient with lung carcinoma develops nausea, vomiting, and lethargy, and is found to have a serum calcium level of 13.4 mg/dl. Which of the following agents should be the first treatment step?

(A) Intravenous etidronate
(B) Intravenous mithramycin
(C) Intravenous glucocorticoids
(D) Intravenous saline and furosemide
(E) Subcutaneous calcitonin

Questions 28–30

A 27-year-old woman enters the emergency ward complaining of dyspnea and pleuritic chest pain. She also complains that over the past 4 days her right calf and thigh have become swollen and tender. Deep venous thrombosis, which may have led to pulmonary embolism, is suspected on the basis of the clinical presentation.

28. Which one of the following pieces of information in the patient history best supports this diagnosis?

(A) History of smoking cigarettes
(B) History of diabetes mellitus in the patient's family
(C) History of lower extremity injury
(D) History of hypertension

29. The first test the physician should order to establish the diagnosis is

(A) cardiac catheterization
(B) contrast venography
(C) impedance plethysmography
(D) lung ventilation and perfusion scans

30. The definitive diagnosis of pulmonary embolism is best made by

(A) arterial blood gas analysis
(B) chest x-ray
(C) electrocardiography (ECG)
(D) nuclear scanning of the lung
(E) pulmonary arteriography

31. A 42-year-old man with a history of seizure disorder experiences a grand mal seizure. His laboratory tests, taken shortly afterward, reveal the following: serum sodium = 140 mEq/L, serum potassium = 4.1 mEq/L, serum chloride = 97 mEq/L, plasma bicarbonate concentration $[HCO_3^-]$ = 16 mEq/L, arterial pH = 7.15, and P_{CO_2} = 46 mm Hg. The acid-base disturbance is best characterized as

(A) respiratory acidosis
(B) metabolic acidosis
(C) metabolic acidosis plus respiratory acidosis
(D) metabolic acidosis plus respiratory alkalosis

32. A 56-year-old woman has an elevated serum calcium level of 12.2 mg/dl. She has no history of any illness or treatment associated with hypercalcemia. Which one of the following studies would be most helpful in making a diagnosis of primary hyperparathyroidism?

(A) Serum ionized calcium
(B) Serum phosphate
(C) Serum parathyroid hormone (PTH)
(D) Computerized tomography (CT) of the neck
(E) 24-Hour urine calcium excretion

33. In a 23-year-old woman with a history of easy bruising and menorrhagia, coagulation laboratory studies reveal a normal prothrombin time (PT), a prolonged partial thromboplastin time (PTT), a normal platelet count, and a prolonged template bleeding time. The most likely diagnosis is

(A) hemophilia A
(B) factor IX deficiency
(C) factor VII deficiency
(D) aspirin ingestion
(E) von Willebrand's disease (vWD)

34. A 23-year-old woman complains of generalized weakness and easy fatigability of 8 months duration. She has no other symptoms. Her blood pressure is 126/86 mm Hg; otherwise, the physical examination is unremarkable. Laboratory studies reveal the following: serum sodium = 142 mEq/L, serum potassium = 2.2 mEq/L, serum chloride = 86 mEq/L, and plasma bicarbonate concentration $[HCO_3^-]$ = 44 mEq/L. The most likely cause of the hypokalemic alkalosis in this patient is

(A) primary aldosteronism
(B) Cushing's syndrome
(C) chronic diarrhea
(D) surreptitious vomiting
(E) licorice abuse

35. A 27-year-old hospital employee has induration at the site of a purified protein derivative (PPD) test done as a part of routine screening. Which of the following features would argue against chemoprophylaxis with isoniazid?

(A) Induration of 4-mm diameter
(B) Negative PPD skin test 1 year earlier
(C) Positive PPD skin test 1 year earlier
(D) Recent extensive exposure to a neighbor with active tuberculosis

36. A 66-year-old woman presents with a painless deterioration in walking. Examination reveals a mildly spastic gait, poor position and vibration sense at the toes, 3+ muscle stretch reflexes at the knees, and absent ankle reflexes. The most likely diagnosis is

(A) multiple sclerosis (MS)
(B) vitamin B_{12} deficiency
(C) normal pressure hydrocephalus (NPH)
(D) human T-cell lymphotropic virus type I (HTLV-I) infection

37. Which one of the following statements best describes patients with obstructive sleep apnea?

(A) They have different clinical presentations than patients with other forms of sleep apnea
(B) They respond well to respiratory stimulants
(C) They respond well to nasal continual positive airway pressure (CPAP)
(D) They are not likely to fall asleep during the day
(E) They are not likely to develop cor pulmonale

Question 38–39

A 30-year-old man develops pain and swelling in the right testicle. His physician orders an ultrasound, which reveals a testicular mass measuring 2 × 2.5 cm. Inguinal exploration and orchiectomy are performed. The pathology reveals a pure seminoma. A computed axial tomography (CAT) scan of the chest, abdomen, and pelvis reveals two 3-cm retroperitoneal nodes that are enlarged. Blood counts, chemistries, and tumor markers are all within normal limits.

38. The oncologist and radiation therapist agree that the best therapeutic approach would be

(A) radiation therapy to a total dose of 2500–3000 cGy to the ipsilateral iliac, retroperitoneal nodes, and mediastinum
(B) radiation therapy to a total dose of 2500–3000 cGy to the ipsilateral iliac and retroperitoneal nodes
(C) radiation therapy to a total dose of 3500–4000 cGy to the ipsilateral iliac and retroperitoneal nodes and mediastinum
(D) radiation therapy to a total dose of 3500–4000 cGy to the ipsilateral iliac and retroperitoneal nodes

39. The same patient is followed with monthly chest x-rays and computed axial tomography (CAT) scans of his chest every 8–12 weeks. One year after completion of his radiation therapy, the patient's CAT scan reveals a 4-cm mediastinal mass. The oncologist recommends

(A) mediastinal radiation
(B) therapy with etoposide (VP-16-213), cisplatin, and bleomycin
(C) mediastinoscopy
(D) needle biopsy of the mass, guided by CAT

40. Which one of the following juvenile rheumatoid arthritis patients is at greatest risk for developing chronic, erosive, disabling arthritis?

(A) A patient with oligoarthritis with axial spine involvement
(B) A patient with oligoarthritis without axial spine involvement
(C) A patient with systemic-onset juvenile rheumatoid arthritis
(D) A patient with polyarticular arthritis who is seropositive for rheumatoid factor
(E) A patient with polyarticular arthritis who is seronegative for rheumatoid factor

41. A 42-year-old woman has recently experienced fatigue, sleepiness, dry skin, constipation, and a 10-pound weight gain. Her thyroid is firm and twice the normal size. Which one of the following laboratory tests is most likely to confirm the suspected diagnosis of hypothyroidism?

(A) Serum thyroxine (T_4)
(B) Serum triiodothyronine (T_3)
(C) T_3 resin uptake
(D) Serum thyroid-stimulating hormone (TSH) measurement
(E) Antithyroid antibodies

42. A 71-year-old man presents with acute onset of gout. This problem has been recurrent for several years and has usually manifested itself as an acute monoarticular arthritis involving the first metatarsal proximal intertarsal joint. The patient also has a long history of chronic renal insufficiency, with serum creatinine values of 4–6 mg/dl over the past 5 years. In addition, he has long-standing hypertension, which has been treated with a variety of agents, including diuretics and α-adrenergic blocking agents. On physical examination, his blood pressure is 170/105 mm Hg, his pulse is 72 bpm, his respiratory rate is 15, and his temperature is 98.6°F. Physical examination further reveals moderate cardiomegaly with third heart sound (S_3) and fourth heart sound (S_4) gallops and a swollen, tender right first metatarsal joint. Laboratory studies reveal the following: blood urea nitrogen (BUN) = 63 mg/dl, creatinine = 5.1 mg/dl, serum sodium = 136 mEq/L, serum potassium = 5.9 mEq/L, serum chloride = 100 mEq/L, CO_2 = 19 mEq/L, and uric acid = 9.3 mg/dl. The most likely cause of this patient's condition is

(A) chronic lead nephropathy
(B) primary overproduction of uric acid
(C) chronic interstitial nephritis related to analgesic abuse
(D) hypertensive nephropathy
(E) renovascular disease

43. A 28-year-old woman with a history of migraine develops a constant pressure-like headache associated with photophobia and a temperature of 102.4°F. A lumbar puncture (LP) demonstrates a cerebral spinal fluid (CSF) protein level of 62 mg/dl, a glucose level of 76 mg/dl, and 26 mononuclear cells/μl. Two days later, the patient is afebrile and has a headache only upon arising. The most likely diagnosis for this patient now is

(A) migraine
(B) septic meningitis
(C) aseptic meningitis
(D) muscle contraction headache
(E) post-LP headache

44. A 26-year-old woman is diagnosed with hypothalamic amenorrhea. Which of the following treatments would be most likely to restore normal ovulation and menstruation?

(A) Gonadotropin-releasing hormone (GnRH) injected every 24 hours
(B) GnRH injected every 4 hours
(C) GnRH injected every 90–120 minutes
(D) A long-acting GnRH analog injected every 24 hours
(E) A long-acting GnRH analog injected every 12 hours

45. A 17-year-old girl has a diffuse, red skin rash, a fever of 39.4°C, and mild, watery diarrhea. She had a sore throat recently, for which sulfamethoxazole was administered. She began her menses 3 days ago. Physical examination shows diffuse erythematous changes of the skin with early desquamation. The mouth and conjunctivae are red. Which one of the following infections explains the process?

(A) *Salmonella* bacteremia
(B) Toxic shock syndrome (TSS)
(C) Tuberculosis
(D) Epstein-Barr virus mononucleosis

46. A 24-year-old woman complains that her hands turn white and then blue in the cold. Which one of the following features is most suggestive of scleroderma as a cause of Raynaud's phenomenon in this patient?

(A) Distal skin thickening extending proximally to the metacarpophalangeal (MCP) joints
(B) Anticentromere antibody in serum
(C) Antinuclear antibody (ANA) in serum
(D) Distal capillary changes on evaluation of the nailbed
(E) Esophageal spasm on manometry

47. A 73-year-old man attends a family dinner celebration and has a grand evening. As he leaves the restaurant he collapses. The most likely diagnosis is

(A) seizure
(B) cardiac arrhythmia
(C) carotid sinus hypersensitivity
(D) colloid cyst of the third ventricle
(E) postprandial syncope

48. A 36-year-old woman is evaluated for sore throat and cervical adenopathy. She has a temperature of 37°C, a pulse of 90 bpm, and a blood pressure of 110/70. The right anterior cervical node measures 2.5 × 3 cm. No supraclavicular, axillary, epitrochlear, or inguinal adenopathy is palpable. The patient's abdominal exam is unremarkable. Over the next 6 months, the patient is reevaluated for recurrent upper respiratory tract infections. During this time period, she has some regression of her cervical node, but it seems to wax and wane in size in response to antibiotics. Because of her persistent adenopathy, the patient is referred to a surgeon and a node biopsy is formed. Which one of the following would describe the histopathology corresponding to this patient's diagnosis?

(A) Follicular small cleaved cell lymphoma
(B) Diffuse large cell lymphoma
(C) Immunoblastic lymphoma
(D) Burkitt's lymphoma
(E) Normal lymph node

49. In human immunodeficiency virus (HIV) infection, diffuse lymphadenopathy in a person who is clinically well is usually a sign of

(A) lymphoma
(B) Kaposi's sarcoma
(C) tuberculosis
(D) no specific infection or tumor

50. Which physiologic change occurs during a normal pregnancy?

(A) Hyperuricemia
(B) Proteinuria
(C) Hypertension
(D) A 40% increase in the glomerular filtration rate (GFR)
(E) Metabolic alkalosis

51. A 35-year-old man with polyuria has a dehydration test. After fluid restriction, his maximum urine osmolality is 550 mOsm/kg and his plasma osmolality is 295 mOsm/kg. One hour after a subcutaneous injection of 5 U of aqueous vasopressin, his urine osmolality is 860 mOsm/kg. Which one of the following diagnoses is likely?

(A) No disease
(B) Diabetes insipidus
(C) Partial diabetes insipidus
(D) Nephrogenic diabetes insipidus
(E) Diabetes mellitus

52. What percentage of patients with cystic fibrosis live to be 18 years of age or older?

(A) <10
(B) 10–20
(C) 20–30
(D) 30–40
(E) >40

53. A previously healthy 17-year-old girl has a total white blood cell count (WBC) of 500 cells/μl (9% neutrophils, 91% lymphocytes) and a fever of 39.1°C. Piperacillin and amikacin therapy is initiated. This therapy is

(A) inappropriate because no antifungal therapy is included
(B) appropriate because infection progresses quickly if untreated
(C) inappropriate because no cultures are available to corroborate bacterial infection
(D) appropriate because *Staphylococcus aureus* is the pathogen likely to be found
(E) inappropriate because *Pseudomonas aeruginosa* is not likely to be inhibited

54. The use of diuretics in the treatment of hypertension may be associated with side effects. These include which one of the following?

(A) Hypoglycemia
(B) Bronchospasm
(C) Prerenal azotemia
(D) Hemolytic anemia

55. A 42-year-old woman with menorrhagia from uterine fibroid tumors presents with anemia characterized by a hemoglobin level of 8.0 g/dl. The mean corpuscular volume (MCV) is 70 μm^3, and the blood smear reveals a uniform collection of both hypochromic and microcytic cells. The most likely diagnosis is

(A) pernicious anemia
(B) sickle cell anemia
(C) iron deficiency anemia
(D) sideroblastic anemia
(E) glucose-6-phosphate dehydrogenase (G6PD) deficiency

56. A 50-year-old patient with Down syndrome develops changes in personality, impaired memory, and difficulty with speech. The most likely diagnosis is

(A) hypothyroidism
(B) multiple strokes
(C) hydrocephalus
(D) senile dementia of the Alzheimer type (SDAT)
(E) dementia associated with prions

57. The most common nonalcoholic cause of acute pancreatitis in the United States is

(A) thiazides
(B) hypercalcemia
(C) hyperlipidemia
(D) gallstones
(E) pancreas divisum

58. Eosinophilia is most likely to be found in which of the following settings?

(A) Pneumococcal pneumonia
(B) Diarrhea caused by *Giardia lamblia*
(C) Schistosomiasis
(D) Measles
(E) Corticosteroid therapy

59. Osteoarthritis is a more likely diagnosis than rheumatoid arthritis in which one of the following patients?

(A) A patient with an inflammatory synovial effusion
(B) A patient with radiographic evidence of joint damage
(C) A patient with arthritis who has lost weight and experiences prominent fatigue
(D) A patient with arthritis who experiences only transient morning stiffness daily
(E) A patient with arthritis who has a firm nodule just distal to the olecranon process of the ulna

60. A 62-year-old man has sudden onset of sharp right-sided chest pain. He has a long history of smoking and has used bronchodilators for 6 years. Six months earlier, he had a stroke, which resulted in dense left hemiplegia. He has a slight increase in cough with some reddish-yellow sputum, a temperature of 38.1°C, and diffuse rhonchi and wheezing without a noticeable increase in shortness of breath. The following test results were obtained:

Mycoplasma pneumoniae antibody: negative
Chest x-ray: patchy consolidation in right lower lobe
Noninvasive studies of leg veins: no evidence of clot
Sputum Gram stain: many polymorphonuclear cells, rare squamous cells, many short gram-negative rods, rare gram-positive cocci in chains, rare gram-negative cocci; culture results pending
Ventilation–perfusion scan: small, nonsegmental matched defects; larger defect in perfusion of right lower lobe. Which of the following drugs would be most reasonable?

(A) Heparin
(B) Tetracycline
(C) Erythromycin
(D) Ceftriaxone
(E) Warfarin

61. While camping in late August, a 56-year-old man with a previous history of ischemic heart disease experiences sharp pain in the right forearm. Local erythema develops quickly, followed by diffuse urticaria and mild hoarseness. Within 20 minutes, the patient is brought to an emergency facility and found to be hypotensive, lethargic, and in moderate respiratory distress. Consultation with the patient's cardiologist reveals ongoing treatment with propranolol and an antihyperlipidemic agent. In light of this information, which one of the following constitutes an appropriate follow-up treatment measure?

(A) Intravenous pressors and hydrocortisone
(B) Nebulized β_2-adrenergic agonists
(C) Nebulized epinephrine
(D) Intravenous aminophylline

Questions 62–63

A 45-year-old white man enters the emergency room complaining of squeezing chest pain and nausea. The pain began approximately 1 hour prior to his arrival in the emergency room. On physical examination, the blood pressure is 110/70 and the pulse is 72 and irregular. The patient is diaphoretic. Auscultation of the lungs reveals bibasilar rales. Cardiac examination is unremarkable. An electrocardiogram (ECG) reveals S-T segment elevation in leads V_1 through V_4, with S-T segment depression in leads 2, 3, and aVF.

62. The most likely diagnosis is

(A) inferior myocardial infarction
(B) anterior myocardial infarction
(C) pulmonary embolism
(D) peptic ulcer disease
(E) pericarditis

63. The most appropriate initial therapy for this patient would be

(A) close observation on a general ward
(B) administration of streptokinase (provided there are no contraindications)
(C) administration of atropine
(D) intramuscular administration of morphine sulfate to relieve the patient's pain and anxiety

64. A 44-year-old man calls the physician's office on Labor Day and complains of "the worst headache of his life." He is awake and oriented but does not want to leave the comfort, quiet, and darkness of his bedroom. The patient comes to the hospital and refuses to have a computed tomography (CT) scan. A difficult lumbar puncture (LP) yields a lightly blood-tinged sample with a red blood cell count of 300,000/μl, a white blood cell count of 55,000/μl (90% polymorphonuclear cells), a protein level of 88 mg/dl, and a glucose level of 20 mg/dl. Gram stain is negative. The most appropriate therapy is

(A) ϵ-aminocaproic acid
(B) intravenous ceftriaxone
(C) heparin
(D) erythromycin

65. A 50-year-old man is admitted to the hospital with a temperature of 102°F and a tensely swollen right knee with markedly decreased range of motion. A 50-ml sample of purulent fluid is removed from the patient's knee, which has a white cell count of 60,000/μl (95% neutrophils) but contains no crystals or organisms. The most likely diagnosis is

(A) bacterial infection
(B) calcium pyrophosphate arthropathy
(C) rheumatoid arthritis
(D) gout
(E) Reiter's (reactive) arthritis

Questions 66–67

A 44-year-old white woman enters the emergency ward complaining of acute shortness of breath on exertion. The patient states that she has a history of both heart disease and emphysema. She was in her usual state of health until 3:00 A.M. when she was awakened by the sudden onset of severe dyspnea. There was no chest pain associated with her dyspnea; however, she did note a cough productive of pinkish sputum. On physical examination, she is dyspneic and in obvious distress. Her blood pressure is 200/110. Her pulse is 110 and regular. Her temperature is 100°F, and her respiratory rate is 36. Her neck veins are not distended. Examination of the thorax reveals pulmonary rales up to the level of the scapulae and bilateral wheezes. The cardiac examination reveals a summation gallop and no murmurs. There is no evidence of peripheral edema. An electrocardiogram (ECG) shows normal sinus rhythm and nonspecific S-T segment changes. A chest x-ray demonstrates an enlarged heart and fluffy bilateral alveolar densities. Arterial blood gases drawn on room air reveal a P_{O_2} of 59, a P_{CO_2} of 25, and a pH of 7.45.

66. Her most likely diagnosis is

(A) emphysema exacerbated by pneumonia
(B) pulmonary embolism
(C) adult respiratory distress syndrome (ARDS)
(D) acute cardiogenic pulmonary edema
(E) hypertensive crisis

67. The most appropriate initial therapy for this patient is administration of

(A) oxygen
(B) quinidine sulfate
(C) digoxin
(D) penicillin

DIRECTIONS: Each set of matching questions in this section consists of a list of four to twenty-six lettered options (some of which may be in figures) followed by several numbered items. For each numbered item, select the ONE lettered option that is most closely associated with it. To avoid spending too much time on matching sets with large numbers of options, it is generally advisable to begin each set by reading the list of options. Then, for each item in the set, try to generate the correct answer and locate it in the option list, rather than evaluating each option individually. Each lettered option may be selected once, more than once, or not at all.

Items 68–72

(A) Painful feet
(B) Acute delirium
(C) Progressive hemiparesis
(D) Acute hemiparesis
(E) Progressive leg weakness

Select the appropriate symptom for each problem that can occur in a human immunodeficiency virus (HIV) seropositive patient.

68. Nonbacterial thrombotic endocarditis

69. Chronic inflammatory demyelinating polyneuropathy (CIDP)

70. Chronic sensory polyneuropathy

71. Central nervous system (CNS) lymphoma

72. Cryptococcal meningitis

Items 73–76

(A) Cushing's disease due to pituitary adrenocorticotropic hormone (ACTH) excess
(B) Cushing's syndrome due to an adrenal tumor
(C) Ectopic ACTH syndrome
(D) Adrenal insufficiency
(E) No adrenal disease

A patient is suspected of having Cushing's disease. For diagnostic purposes, dexamethasone is given in a low dose (2 mg daily) for 2 days and a high dose (8 mg daily) for 2 days. For each change in urinary 17-hydroxycorticoids and urinary free cortisol levels, select the diagnosis it indicates.

73. They fall distinctly with low-dose dexamethasone and high-dose dexamethasone

74. They do not change with low-dose dexamethasone but fall distinctly with high-dose dexamethasone

75. They do not fall with either low-dose or high-dose dexamethasone; the plasma ACTH level is elevated

76. They do not fall with either low-dose or high-dose dexamethasone; the plasma ACTH level is low

Items 77–81

(A) Nitroblue tetrazolium (NBT) test
(B) Serum calcium level
(C) Platelet number and morphology
(D) Surface iC3b receptor activity
(E) Lymphocyte count

Match each of the immunodeficiency disorders listed below with the relevant assay.

77. Wiskott-Aldrich syndrome

78. Severe combined immunodeficiency (SCID)

79. Chronic granulomatous disease

80. DiGeorge syndrome

81. Leukocyte adhesion deficiency

Items 82–88

(A) Respiratory alkalosis
(B) Respiratory acidosis
(C) Metabolic alkalosis
(D) Metabolic acidosis

Match each clinical condition with the simple acid-base disturbance associated with it.

82. Myasthenia gravis

83. Cardiogenic shock

84. Early gram-negative septicemia

85. Heroin overdose

86. Normal pregnancy

87. Diuretic abuse

88. Diabetic coma

Items 89–93

(A) Inhibits sympathetic outflow from the central nervous system (CNS)
(B) Reduces smooth muscle tone, producing vasodilation
(C) Blunts the renin-angiotensin mechanism for the reabsorption of sodium and water
(D) Directly dilates arteries and arterioles
(E) Antagonizes norepinephrine's stimulation of α-adrenergic receptors

Match each antihypertensive agent with its mechanism of action.

89. Metoprolol

90. Nifedipine

91. Prazosin

92. Methyldopa

93. Minoxidil

Items 94–98

(A) Ulcerative colitis
(B) Laxative abuse
(C) Pseudomembranous colitis
(D) Viral gastroenteritis
(E) *Campylobacter* infection
(F) Collagenous colitis

For each patient with diarrhea described below, select the most likely cause of the diarrhea.

94. A healthy 20-year-old man has an acute diarrheal disease characterized by bloody stool, crampy abdominal pain, and low-grade fever. His symptoms resolve spontaneously in 5 days and do no recur.

95. A healthy 20-year-old man has an acute onset of bloody diarrhea, crampy abdominal pain, and fever. His symptoms persist for several weeks, after which he consults a physician who notes bleeding, friable mucosa on proctosigmoidoscopy.

96. A 30-year-old woman develops severe, watery diarrhea, 2 weeks after undergoing antibiotic therapy for pelvic inflammatory disease (PID). Proctosigmoidoscopy shows plaque-like lesions covering the mucosa.

97. A 30-year-old woman complains of chronic watery diarrhea. Stool examination shows an osmolarity of 300 mEq/dl, a sodium (Na^+) concentration of 30 mEq/dl, and a potassium (K^+) concentration of 45 mEq/dl. Shortly after she is hospitalized for evaluation and begun on a 48-hour fast, her diarrhea disappears.

98. A 56-year-old woman complains of intermittent nonbloody watery diarrhea over the past several years. All stool, radiographic, and endoscopic evaluations are normal, but the sedimentation rate is elevated slightly and biopsy of the colon shows a prominent eosinophilic band in the subepithelial layer.

Items 99–103

(A) Folic acid deficiency
(B) Vitamin B_{12} deficiency
(C) Deficiency of either folic acid or vitamin B_{12}
(D) No vitamin deficiency

For each condition described below, select the vitamin status with which it is most closely associated.

99. Pancytopenia with macrocytic anemia and megaloblastic marrow

100. Gastric carcinoma

101. An abnormal Schilling test

102. Neuropathy of the spinal cord

103. Alcoholism

Items 104–107

(A) Hormone therapy
(B) Radical prostatectomy or radiotherapy
(C) Observation
(D) Radical radiotherapy
(E) Radical radiotherapy with boost doses to the prostate gland

Match each of the following stages of prostatic carcinoma with its appropriate therapy.

104. Stage A_2

105. Stage B

106. Stage C

107. Stage D

Items 108–112

| | O_2 | | | | |
	PO$_2$ (mm Hg)	Saturation (%)	Pco$_2$ (mm Hg)	[HCO$_3^-$] (mEq/L)	pH
(A)	120	99	20	19	7.60
(B)	104	99	24	12	7.25
(C)	81	95	51	45	7.58
(D)	62	92	34	23	7.46
(E)	38	65	65	26.2	7.22

For each of the following clinical conditions, select the patient with the appropriate data.

108. Fulminant status asthmaticus

109. Long-standing pyloric obstruction

110. Hysterical hyperventilation

111. Diabetic ketoacidosis

112. Emphysematous chronic obstructive pulmonary disease (COPD)

Items 113–115

(A) IgG anti-insulin-receptor antibodies
(B) IgE anti-insulin antibodies
(C) IgG anti-insulin antibodies in circulating immune complexes
(D) T-cell cytotoxicity
(E) IgG anti-insulin antibodies

For each of the clinical scenarios described below, select the pathogenic mechanism with which it is likely to be associated.

113. After the initiation of insulin therapy, local erythema, swelling, and pruritus develop at multiple injection sites. Despite antihistamine therapy, subsequent injections of insulin lead to generalized urticaria and angioedema.

114. A gradually increasing insulin requirement is noted in a patient with a past history of frequent local reaction and intermittent insulin therapy.

115. A 60-year-old diabetic woman requires increasing amounts of insulin. Arthralgias then develop, along with pigmented lesions of the axilla and groin.

Items 116–120

(A) Polycythemia vera
(B) Anemia of chronic disease
(C) Renal failure
(D) Aplastic anemia
(E) Secondary polycythemia of hepatoma

For each abnormality of erythropoietin described, match the correlating clinical condition.

116. High plasma erythropoietin titers; poor response to exogenous erythropoietin

117. Low to absent plasma erythropoietin

118. Diminished erythropoietin secretion; good response to exogenous erythropoietin

119. Near normal to slightly elevated plasma erythropoietin; variable response to exogenous erythropoietin

120. Extremely elevated plasma erythropoietin levels

Items 121–124

(A) Small-cell lung cancer
(B) Testicular cancer
(C) Breast cancer
(D) Pancreatic cancer

Match each of the following syndromes with the appropriate tumor.

121. Eaton-Lambert syndrome

122. Syndrome of inappropriate antidiuretic hormone (SIADH)

123. Gynecomastia

124. Trousseau's syndrome [chronic disseminated intravascular coagulation (DIC) associated with malignancy]

Items 125–127

(A) X-ray of sacroiliac joints
(B) Joint fluid Gram stain and culture
(C) Serum rheumatoid factor determination
(D) Antibody titer to *Borrelia burgdorferi*
(E) Erythrocyte sedimentation rate
(F) X-ray of lumbar spine
(G) Paired blood cultures
(H) Abdominal arteriogram

For each of the following case descriptions, select the most appropriate test to be used to arrive at a diagnosis.

125. A 28-year-old man complains of a 3-month history of morning low back pain, lasting 2 hours each day. He has also noticed a "sausage-like" swelling of his left second toe for 2 months, and has had pain in the bottoms of both heels when he walks. He reports that he had "pink eye" 1 year ago, around the time of an episode of bloody diarrhea that was treated by his family doctor with an antibiotic.

126. A 24-year-old woman has experienced extreme fatigue and polyarticular joint pain for 6 months. She has taken aspirin irregularly over that time with some relief, but she still complains of prolonged morning stiffness as well as bilateral pain and swelling in her wrists and metacarpophalangeal (MCP) and proximal interphalangeal (PIP) joints. She has no history of fever or other complaints. The only remarkable findings upon physical examination are swelling of the joints and mild limitation of motion of the involved joints due to pain.

127. A 60-year-old man, who had a red, target-shaped rash on his leg during the summer, experiences fatigue, radicular left arm pain and numbness, and difficulty using his left hand for gripping in September. Two months later, he notices pain and swelling of the left wrist and right knee.

Items 128–132

(A) Chronic lymphocytic leukemia (CLL)
(B) Chronic myelogenous leukemia (CML)
(C) Both CLL and CML
(D) Neither CLL nor CML

For each clinical situation, select the disease state with which it is most closely associated.

128. Elevated leukocyte alkaline phosphatase (LAP) level

129. Elevated lymphocyte count

130. Slow, steady disease progression

131. Termination in acute leukemia

132. Splenomegaly

Items 133–138

(A) Pernicious anemia
(B) Dye and printing chemicals
(C) Asbestos
(D) Ulcerative colitis
(E) Epstein-Barr virus

Match each of the following tumors with the associated risk factor.

133. Burkitt's lymphoma

134. Bladder carcinoma

135. Gastric carcinoma

136. Colorectal carcinoma

137. Lung carcinoma

138. Nasopharyngeal cancer

ANSWERS AND EXPLANATIONS

1. The answer is A [Chapter 8 V F 3]. Fever is a variable feature in pyelonephritis and prostatitis but is never found with simple cystitis. Irritative voiding symptoms do not distinguish between upper and lower tract infections. White blood cell casts are formed in renal tubules and represent upper tract disease, but white blood cells are present in both upper and lower tract infections. Quantitative urine cultures do not distinguish between upper and lower tract infections.

2. The answer is D [Chapter 2 VII C 1]. Pulmonary hypertension in patients with chronic obstructive pulmonary disease (COPD) is due primarily to the vasoconstrictive effect of hypoxia. This response may be increased by acidosis, which also has a direct, although less dramatic, vasoconstrictive effect on the pulmonary vasculature. Pulmonary vasoconstriction puts a strain on the right ventricle, leading to its eventual failure (cor pulmonale). Left ventricular failure occurs independently of right ventricular failure and usually is caused by atherosclerotic coronary artery disease. In patients with emphysema, a loss of the pulmonary capillary bed also may contribute to pulmonary hypertension.

3. The answer is B [Chapter 9 III B 3 a (1) (b)]. Chvostek's sign suggests hypocalcemia. A decrease in ionized calcium leads to increased neuromuscular irritability. In addition to Chvostek's sign, patients may have numbness and tingling of the extremities, twitching and cramps of the muscles, and muscular fatigue and weakness. Severe hypocalcemia, if untreated, can cause laryngeal spasm and seizures.

4. The answer is A [Chapter 10 I E 1]. Erosive osteoarthritis typically involves the distal interphalangeal (DIP) joints in middle-aged women. It is unlikely that such prominent distal joint symptoms would occur in a patient with rheumatoid arthritis or systemic lupus erythematosus (SLE) without more generalized joint complaints. There is no evidence to suggest ankylosing spondylitis or scleroderma.

5. The answer is A [Chapter 6 Part I: III E 2]. The chest pain experienced by this patient is typical of pericarditis and inflammation of the pericardium, which are common complications in chronic renal failure patients on hemodialysis. These patients also may have inflammation in various serosal linings, including the peritoneum, the pleura, and various joint spaces; the mechanism of this complication is unknown. Although coronary artery disease is common in dialysis patients, the characteristics of the pain in this individual suggest that this disease is not the diagnosis. Esophageal disease also is common in dialysis patients and should be specifically excluded as a possible cause. In addition, musculoskeletal pain due to various causes is typically seen in dialysis patients and may be due to the abnormalities of calcium and phosphorus metabolism, which lead to calcific deposits in various components of the musculoskeletal system.

6. The answer is A [Chapter 4 VII D 2–3, G 2 a (1) (a); Table 4-27]. Small-cell lung cancer often presents with paraneoplastic syndromes, including a variety that affect the central nervous system (CNS), the most common of which is Eaton-Lambert myasthenia. Other neuropathies, including sensory neuropathies, have been reported. Small-cell lung cancer can be cured if disease is limited to the chest. The most effective therapy for small-cell lung carcinoma (SCLC) limited to the chest is etoposide (VP-16-213) and cisplatin with concurrent radiation therapy.

7. The answer is C [Chapter 11 XVI B 1–2]. Intravenous drug addicts are prone to develop a bacteremia, which can in turn cause a brain abscess and progressive neurologic dysfunction. Patients with a brain abscess are typically afebrile unless there is an accompanying endocarditis or other endovascular source of infection. Intravenous drug addicts are predisposed to develop bacterial endocarditis and neurologic deficits can occur apoplectically because of a septic embolus to the brain. However, patients are typically febrile. Human immunodeficiency virus (HIV) meningitis causes headache and evidence of meningeal irritation, but focal neurologic deficits do not occur. Cryptococcal meningitis typically presents with altered behavior and headache. The patient is afebrile. However, stroke-like events are rare. Intravenous drug abuse can lead to a foreign body embolus and apoplectic neurologic problems. An embolus can reach the brain via a right-to-left cardiac shunt or pulmonary arteriovenous malformation if the injection is venous. The embolus may enter the cerebral circulation directly if the injection is intracarotid.

8. The answer is A [Chapter 3 1 C 2 b (2) (c) (i)]. Glucose-6-phosphate dehydrogenase (G6PD) deficiency is common in blacks, with a gene incidence of 10%. The gene is sex-linked, so hemolytic disease manifests mainly in males. The deficiency in blacks is relatively mild, and only older red blood cells are critically enzyme-deficient and liable for oxidant-induced hemolysis. Thus, hemolytic episodes are relatively mild (rarely is hemoglobin less than 7.5 g/dl), well tolerated, and quickly reversible. This is very different from the Mediterranean variant, favism, in which the enzyme deficit is so severe that all red blood cells are liable for hemolysis and fatalities can result. Sulfa antibiotics are a classic precipitant. Occult blood loss causes chronic iron loss, and the resulting anemia would be expected to be microcytic. Sickle cell trait is asymptomatic hematologically, and an anemia would not be expected.

9. The answer is B [Chapter 8 V E 1 a]. The most likely diagnosis is primary peritonitis. Although it may be difficult to distinguish primary (spontaneous) peritonitis from rupture of a hollow viscus and peritoneal soiling, the presence of fever and the elevated white blood cell count (WBC) in the ascitic fluid suggest some kind of peritoneal infection. Liver abscess tends to be a subacute illness without prominent peritoneal findings. Abdominal pain in cholecystitis is in the right upper quadrant, and there is usually nausea and vomiting. Pancreatitis is characterized by severe localized (midepigastric) pain, which radiates quickly to the back. Nausea and vomiting generally are not associated with acute pancreatitis.

10. The answer is A [Chapter 6 Part I: X B]. The most likely cause of this syndrome is minimal change nephropathy. This entity is the most common cause of nephrotic syndrome in children and adolescents. The disease has an excellent prognosis. Patients typically respond quite well to steroid therapy; although recurrent treatments are frequently necessary, complete remission eventually occurs in most patients. Renal biopsy is the only way to definitively diagnose minimal change nephropathy. Typically, no serologic abnormalities are associated with minimal change disease. Poststreptococcal glomerulonephritis and Henoch Schönlein purpura are associated with a nephritic picture [i.e., with an active urinary sediment (red blood cells and casts) and heavy proteinuria]. Acquired immune deficiency syndrome (AIDS) nephropathy may present with a bland urinalysis and findings similar to those in minimal change nephropathy; however, associated renal insufficiency is much more common. The absence of systemic manifestations of human immunodeficiency virus (HIV) infection also makes this diagnosis highly unlikely in this patient. Finally, vasculitis rarely produces proteinuria as the sole renal manifestation. More frequently, vasculitis produces renal insufficiency, a glomerulonephritic picture, or both, along with systemic manifestations.

11. The answer is A [Chapter 10 IX E 1 d (1) (a)]. Difficulty combing hair and arising from a sitting position are cardinal symptoms of the proximal muscle weakness typical of polymyositis. Unscrewing a lid and heel-toe walking involve distal muscle strength, which would be more likely affected by a neuropathic problem. Facial muscle involvement is not typical of polymyositis but is common in myasthenia gravis, in which involvement of eyelid and extraocular muscles is common. Tenderness in a muscle is a nonspecific finding that is not usually present in typical polymyositis; also, the avoidance of contracting a painful muscle could simulate weakness.

12. The answer is C [Chapter 4 IX C 4 a (5), b (1)]. Prostate-specific antigen is a test that can be used to screen for prostate cancer. However, prostate-specific antigen levels can also be mildly elevated in benign prostatic hypertrophy. A transrectal ultrasound can identify small lesions not palpable on rectal examination. If the patient has an elevation in prostate-specific antigen and an ultrasound has confirmed an abnormal area, this area can be biopsied transrectally under ultrasound guidance. Patients with prostate cancer generally undergo a metastatic workup, which includes a bone scan; chest x-ray; computed axial tomography (CAT) scan of the retroperitoneum and pelvis; or magnetic resonance imaging (MRI) of the retroperitoneum and pelvis with special attention to the prostate, accompanied by laboratory studies. Metastatic prostate cancer can be treated with leuprolide, a luteinizing hormone releasing hormone (LH-RH) agonist that suppresses testicular testosterone production. Leuprolide therapy is equivalent to orchiectomy or estrogen therapy in the treatment of metastatic prostate cancer.

13. The answer is B [Chapter 2 XII D 2]. Crackles are produced by fluid in alveoli or by fibrotic airways. Therefore, they can be heard in patients with pulmonary fibrosis or congestive heart failure.

14. The answer is A [Chapter 5 IX A 1 f (1)–(4)]. The chronic carrier state for hepatitis B virus is associated with an increased risk of hepatoma and is found in 0.2% of the population of the United States. Chronic active hepatitis cannot be diagnosed until at least 6 months following the acute infection with hepatitis B. In chronic active hepatitis, the inflammation and fibrosis extend past the portal area and, thus, correlate with profuse deterioration of liver function, which may result in cirrhosis or liver failure. Fulminant hepatitis occurs in approximately 1%–2% of cases of hepatitis B, C, and non-A, non-B, non-C hepatitis. This rare complication usually is associated with falling transaminase levels as liver tissue is destroyed and the liver decreases in size.

15. The answer is E [Chapter 11 IV C 1 a (2), d (1) (a), 4 a–b]. Nitroglycerin can cause throbbing "vascular" headaches; therefore, the simplest management option is discontinuation of the nitroglycerin preparation and use of an alternate cardiac medication if possible. Temporal arteritis should always be considered as a possible cause of headache in patients over 50 years of age. An elevated erythrocyte sedimentation rate; jaw claudication; arthralgias and myalgias; and a tender, indurated temporal artery make the diagnosis more likely. Propranolol is an effective anti-migraine medication. However, before anti-migraine medication is prescribed, potential precipitants of migraine should be eliminated. Ergotamine is an effective abortive therapy for migraine. However, because it is a vasoconstrictor, it should not be used in patients with angina pectoris. A brain computed tomography (CT) scan should be considered in the evaluation of an elderly patient with the new onset of headache. In this case, if the headache can be eliminated simply by stopping the nitroglycerin, a CT scan is unnecessary.

16. The answer is E [Chapter 2 II A 1 a, E 2 a (2); IV A 4 c]. By definition (i.e., cough and sputum production), this patient has chronic bronchitis. Normal results on chest x-ray do not absolutely rule out carcinoma, but make it unlikely. The same is true for tuberculosis and bronchiectasis. A smoker in this age-group would require bronchoscopy if the hemoptysis did not subside soon or if the clinical situation changed. Alpha$_1$-antitrypsin deficiency is a genetic factor that predisposes to emphysema. Unlike chronic bronchitis, emphysema is associated with little or no cough and expectoration.

17. The answer is A [Chapter 6 Part I: XIV C, Part III: II B 1]. Renovascular hypertension is associated with an increased renin release. Diminished renal blood flow stimulates the kidney to release increasing amounts of renin, which activate the renin-angiotensin-aldosterone axis, leading to hypertension. Because captopril prevents the conversion of angiotensin I to angiotensin II (a vasoconstrictor, this drug would be expected to be particularly effective in this disease. Young women, much more frequently than young men, develop fibromuscular obstruction of the renal arteries, leading to renovascular hypertension. Renovascular hypertension is notoriously difficult to control; this difficulty often raises the suspicion that it is present.

18. The answer is D [Chapter 9 IV A 5 a–d, 8 d (3) (c) (i)–(ii)]. The two-hour postprandial glucose level is a more sensitive test for early diabetes than the fasting glucose level, because in mild, early cases of diabetes, the glucose level often rises excessively after a meal and is slow to fall, but may return to normal levels before the next meal. Measurement of hemoglobin A$_{1C}$ and, occasionally, urine glucose, may be useful in evaluating the glycemic control in patients with diabetes, but they are not sufficiently reliable or standardized enough to be very useful in the diagnosis of diabetes. The glucose tolerance test is the most precise test for the diagnosis of diabetes, but it is seldom needed.

19. The answer is D [Chapter 10 II B 5 b]. The finding of meniscal calcium on a radiograph of the involved knee is a diagnostic feature of calcium pyrophosphate dihydrate (CPPD) disease, and is therefore suggestive that the knee inflammation is caused by pseudogout. The finding of positively birefringent crystals on red-compensated polarized light examination of synovial fluid is specific for a diagnosis of pseudogout. Serum urate elevation is associated with gout, not CPPD. Enlargement of proximal interphalangeal (PIP) and distal interphalangeal (DIP) joints suggests only osteoarthritis and not a specific cause. Likewise, there are many causes of an inflammatory effusion other than CPPD.

20. The answer is D [Chapter 7 III E 2 a–h]. The woman's symptoms are likely caused by vasomotor rhinitis, which is a syndrome characterized by nasal blockage and rhinorrhea without evidence of immunologic or infectious nasal disease. Symptoms of vasomotor rhinitis often worsen after affected patients endure emotional stress, change in body or environmental temperature, change in body position, or humid weather. Vasomotor rhinitis does not respond well to medication. Although nasal blockage and rhinorrhea are symptoms of eosinophilic nonallergic rhinitis, this disorder is characterized by pronounced nasal eosinophilia, an immunologic abnormality that would have shown up on the nasal smear. Nasal polyps are another symptom of eosinophilic nonallergic rhinitis. Allergic rhinitis, which is an IgE-mediated sensitivity disorder, would be characterized by a pale, boggy nasal mucosa, nasal eosinophilia, and positive skin tests. Decongestant spray abuse is not indicated in the patient's history. The woman's history also rules out pregnancy and deviated septum, both of which are possible causes of rhinorrhea and nasal blockage.

21. The answer is D [Chapter 8 V A 3 a, b]. Neurosurgical aspiration of the lesion would most likely show α-hemolytic streptococcus and mixed anaerobes. Brain abscess may well occur in teenagers. Usually, frontal lobe disease is associated with sinusitis and reflects oral flora. *Escherichia coli* and *Bacteroides fragilis* are more commonly found in brain abscesses of otic origin. Primary brain lymphoma and toxoplasmosis are rarely seen in immunocompetent people. In people with severe acidosis, *Zygomycetes* can cause brain abscess, but these fungi have no yeast phase.

22. The answer is A [Chapter 10 VII G 3 b]. This patient has several subtle manifestations of phospholipid antibody syndrome, which, taken together, make it a likely diagnosis. A positive rapid plasma reagin test (RPR) with negative treponemal test results probably reflect antibodies cross-reacting to the cardiolipin or phospholipid components of treponemal antigens. Thrombocytopenia is commonly seen in this entity, probably due to platelet–endothelial cell interactions and clotting induced by the antibodies. Miscarriages can be caused by clotting of small placental vessels. Deep venous thromboses or even major arterial clotting can be caused by the consequent hypercoagulability. No other evidence is presented for systemic lupus erythematosus (SLE), although phospholipid antibodies can be detected in approximately one-third of the patients. Takayasu's arteritis classically occurs in young Asian women, but no evidence is given for the large vessel arterial ischemia characteristic of this entity. Finally, no features of the Ro antibody syndrome or mixed connective tissue disease are described.

23. The answer is C [Chapter 8 V A 2 a; VII F 3 b, c]. Lyme disease is transmitted by a tick bite. Neurologic complications include cranial neuropathy, radiculopathy, and encephalopathy. The patient's outdoor activities put him at risk for exposure to Lyme disease if he lives in an endemic area and the suggestion of wrist arthritis is consistent with the systemic manifestations of Lyme disease. Toxin exposures can cause confusion but should not cause an arthritis or facial weakness. High-risk sexual behavior can predispose to human immunodeficiency virus (HIV) infection, which can cause a facial nerve palsy and encephalopathy. However, given this patient's history and presentation, Lyme disease is more likely. A mosquito bite can transmit viral encephalitis. However, there is no history of fever and the wrist arthritis and facial weakness are against a diagnosis of early viral encephalitis.

24. The answer is C [Chapter 8 V C 3, 4]. The most likely diagnosis is a pulmonary embolus. Acute onset rules out atypical pneumonia and makes lung cancer very unlikely. Without evidence of productive cough, tracheobronchitis—also a subacute illness—is unlikely. Bacterial pneumonia is very unlikely in conjunction with a normal chest x-ray. Smoking and oral contraceptive use both predispose to deep venous thrombosis and pulmonary embolus.

25. The answer is A [Chapter 4 IX B 7 b]. Following chemotherapy with MVAC [methotrexate, vinblastine, doxorubicin (Adriamycin), and cisplatin], 87% of patients with metastatic bladder cancer will achieve a partial or complete response. Complete responses have been observed in approximately 30% of patients. In many cases the responses are long-lasting, but there is no curative therapy at the present time for metastatic bladder cancer.

26. The answer is A [Chapter 10 III G; VII G 1; Table 10-8]. An active urinary sediment suggests glomerulonephritis, a feature common in patients with systemic lupus erythematosus (SLE) but not in those with rheumatoid arthritis. Arthritis of the metacarpophalangeal (MCP) and proximal interphalangeal (PIP) joints, pleural effusions, and anemia could be seen in either disease. Abnormal liver function can be an atypical feature of SLE but would more commonly be due to drug-related hepatic dysfunction [e.g., due to non-steroidal anti-inflammatory drugs (NSAIDs)] in either disease.

27. The answer is D [Chapter 9 III A 6 a, b, d, 7 c (1), (3), (4)]. Hypercalcemia caused by diseases other than hyperparathyroidism may be treated with intravenous saline and furosemide. Fluid replacement with intravenous saline, followed by forced diuresis with saline and intravenous furosemide, is a rapid and safe way to lower serum calcium and should be tried first. Etidronate, mithramycin, or calcitonin may be added if additional lowering of the calcium level is needed. Glucocorticoids are effective in treating hypercalcemia caused by vitamin D excess, sarcoidosis, and some hematologic malignancies, but do not lower calcium levels in most cases of hypercalcemia associated with solid tumors.

28–30. The answers are: 28-C [Chapter 1 VIII A 2 d, 3 a], **29–C** [Chapter 1 VIII A 4 a–b], **30-E** [Chapter 2 VIII E 6 a–c, 7–8 a]. Lower extremity injury may lead to blood clot formation and the development of thrombophlebitis. Other factors that contribute to the development of deep venous thrombosis include the use of estrogen-containing compounds (e.g., oral contraceptives) and lower limb immobilization (e.g., during surgery or prolonged bed rest), which leads to venous stasis. Hypertension, diabetes mellitus, and intravenous drug abuse have no association with deep venous thrombosis. The dyspnea and pleuritic pain in this patient suggest that the suspected deep venous thrombosis has led to pulmonary embolism—the most common cause of which is the migration of a thrombus from the veins in the lower extremities or pelvis to the pulmonary artery.

Lower extremity plethysmography is a noninvasive test that is useful for establishing a diagnosis of deep venous thrombosis. Contrast venography provides a definitive diagnosis in almost every case; however, this invasive test actually can cause thrombophlebitis in a minority of cases. Cardiac catheterization and lung scanning would not be of any use in diagnosing deep venous thrombosis.

The most sensitive and specific test for pulmonary embolism is pulmonary arteriography. Nuclear scanning of the lung is another useful technique, but is not as specific as arteriography. Although a normal scan virtually rules out pulmonary embolism, scanning results often fall into the intermediate probability range, making a definitive diagnosis impossible. In most cases of pulmonary embolism, the electrocardiogram (ECG) is normal. Acute right axis deviation noted on the ECG may lead to the erroneous diagnosis of anterior myocardial infarction. Hypoxia, hypocapnia, and respiratory alkalosis are classic findings on arterial blood gas analysis but are not specific for pulmonary embolism. The chest x-ray may be normal, especially if infarction has not occurred.

31. The answer is C [Chapter 6 Part II: IV B–D]. The patient has significant acidemia (low arterial pH), which is associated with a low serum HCO_3^- concentration; thus, metabolic acidosis must be present. This condition is due to lactate accumulation, which is due to seizure activity. Another clue is the elevated anion gap. In addition, the patient also has respiratory acidosis, as evidenced by the elevated P_{CO_2}. Hyperventilation often accompanies grand mal seizure.

32. The answer is C [Chapter 9 III A 5 b]. An elevated level of serum parathyroid hormone (PTH), in the absence of renal failure or other cause of secondary hyperparathyroidism, is strong evidence for primary hyperparathyroidism. In hypercalcemia of other causes, such as cancer, sarcoidosis, or excessive vitamin D intake, the PTH level is suppressed by the hypercalcemia and is low (or normal).

33. The answer is E [Chapter 3 V D 1 b]. von Willebrand's disease (vWD) is a genetic defect with variable transmissions that results in the deficiency or derangement of the large antigenic portion of factor VIII (VIII^{ag}). This molecule is associated with both the intrinsic coagulation pathway and platelet–vessel wall interaction. Thus, in vWD, there is prolongation of both the partial thromboplastin time (PTT) [indicative of defects in the intrinsic coagulation cascade] and bleeding time (indicative of a defect in the platelet–VIII^{ag}–vessel wall interaction). The hemophilias, either factor VIII or factor IX varieties, affect males due to sex linkage of the genes. Isolated prolongations of PTT are characteristic. Other coagulation tests, including bleeding time, are normal. Factor VII is in the extrinsic arm of the coagulation cascade, and deficiency of this factor prolongs prothrombin time (PT) only. Aspirin, as well as many other nonsteroidal anti-inflammatory drugs (NSAIDs), inhibits platelet prostaglandin synthesis, which results in defective platelet function and prolongation of bleeding time. Other coagulation tests are normal.

34. The answer is D [Chapter 6 Part II: III B 2 a (1)]. Although hypokalemia can occur in each of these conditions, the patient's hypokalemic alkalosis is most likely the result of surreptitious vomiting. Chronic diarrhea is characterized by acidosis rather than alkalosis. Although the remaining conditions are typically associated with alkalosis, surreptitious vomiting is the only condition associated with absence of hypertension due to extracellular volume contraction. The other conditions typically are associated with expansion of extracellular volume and hypertension, due to increased mineralocorticoid activity.

35. The answer is A [Chapter 8 VII C 3]. Induration of 4-mm diameter at the site of a purified protein derivative (PPD) test would argue against chemoprophylaxis with isoniazid. All adults younger than 35 years with positive PPD test results should have isoniazid chemoprophylaxis unless they cannot tolerate isoniazid, have already received a full course, or are known to have been exposed to isoniazid-resistant tuberculosis. Usually, induration of at least 10 mm is required to call a test positive. Lesser degrees of induration may represent cross-reactions to other mycobacteria or fading skin test reactivity, and PPD testing may be repeated in a couple of weeks.

36. The answer is B [Chapter 11 III B 4 a; XI A; XIX A 2 a]. Vitamin B$_{12}$ deficiency causes combined systems degeneration. Patients can present with a gait disturbance characterized by spasticity and diminished vibratory and position sense. A mild neuropathy may be present, causing depressed ankle reflexes. Because this is a treatable cause of abnormal gait, identification of vitamin B$_{12}$ deficiency is important. Multiple sclerosis (MS) does not typically present in this age group. Absent ankle reflexes are not a common feature of MS; rather, hyperactive reflexes are consistent with the upper motor neuron findings commonly found.

Normal pressure hydrocephalus (NPH) is a cause of deteriorating gait. However, cognitive decline is often present and patients can have urinary incontinence. Impaired vibration and position sense and absent ankle reflexes are not typical of NPH. Human T-cell lymphotropic virus type I (HTLV-I) infection is a cause of myelopathy and should be suspected in patients who have had blood transfusions, abuse intravenous drugs, or have resided in endemic areas. It is not evident from the patient history that this patient has any risk factors for this infection.

37. The answer is C [Chapter 2 XV B–E]. Patients with obstructive apnea respond very well to nasal continual positive airway pressure (CPAP), which acts to splint the obstructed posterior pharynx. Patients with sleep apnea, whether central, obstructive, or mixed, are indistinguishable clinically; sleep studies are necessary to determine which type of apnea is present. Although some patients with obstructive apnea may respond to respiratory stimulants, others require more drastic measures. Patients with all forms of sleep apnea are sleepy during the day and, for reasons unknown, all are at risk for developing cor pulmonale.

38–39. The answers are: 38-B [Chapter 4 X G 2], **39-D** [Chapter 4 VII E 2–4]. Testicular cancer is the most common cancer in young adult males. The most common varieties are seminomas and nonseminomatous germ cell tumors, both of which are curable even in advanced stages. Seminomas are exquisitely sensitive to radiation therapy; therefore, patients with stage II disease (i.e., disease limited to the testicle and nodes above the diaphragm) may be treated with low doses of radiation. Because of bone marrow toxicity from mediastinal radiation therapy, prophylactic radiation to the mediastinum is no longer indicated.

Patients with a history of seminoma should be evaluated for recurrent disease. If disease recurs outside of the radiation field, the patient should undergo diagnostic procedures to confirm the diagnosis, followed by combination chemotherapy with etoposide (VP-16-213), cisplatin, and bleomycin. The diagnosis may be made by needle biopsy under computed axial tomography (CAT) guidance. If this does not provide the diagnosis, a mediastinotomy or mediastinoscopy may be required. Mediastinal radiation alone would not be sufficient to eliminate the recurrent disease.

40. The answer is D [Chapter 10 V E 2 c (1), H 2 a]. The subset of juvenile rheumatoid arthritis patients most likely to develop chronic, erosive, and severe arthritis is the polyarticular group that is seropositive for rheumatoid factor. This form of the disease is also most similar to adult rheumatoid arthritis and most likely to require a second-line agent (e.g., gold).

41. The answer is D [Chapter 9 II A 5]. Serum thyroid-stimulating hormone (TSH) measurement is most likely to confirm a suspected diagnosis of hypothyroidism. In a mild case of primary hypothyroidism, TSH usually rises to abnormal levels before serum thyroxine (T_4) or serum triiodothyronine (T_3) have fallen below the normal range. The T_3 resin uptake is not a highly accurate test of thyroid function, but is used mainly to exclude abnormalities in thyroid-hormone-binding proteins. A high titer of antithyroid antibodies would indicate the presence of chronic thyroiditis, the most common cause of hypothyroidism, but would not indicate whether or not hypothyroidism is present.

42. The answer is A [Chapter 6 Part I: XII B 2 b]. Chronic lead nephropathy is the most likely cause of this patient's condition. Lead nephropathy is associated with an impairment in uric acid excretion and typically is associated with the clinical syndrome of gout. While gout and chronic renal failure from other etiologies could coexist, the current evidence suggests that lead toxicity is responsible for the bulk of cases in which both diseases are concurrent. Analgesic abuse should not be associated with an increased incidence of gout, although the renal findings could be similar. Hypertensive nephropathy also may explain the findings, although it would not explain the occurrence of gout in this patient. Renovascular hypertension could be present

in this patient but is typically associated with more severe hypertension when renal failure occurs. Furthermore, renovascular hypertension is not usually associated with gout. However, imaging of the renal vascular tree would be necessary in order to completely exclude this diagnosis.

43. The answer is E [Chapter 8 V A 1 a (1) (a)–(b); Chapter 11 IV C 2]. The patient most likely had a self-limited aseptic meningitis and developed a postural, post-lumbar puncture (LP) headache upon arising. Associated symptoms can include nausea, blurred vision, tinnitus, and vomiting. Diminished cerebral spinal fluid (CSF) pressure may be the cause of an LP-associated headache. Treatment options include bed rest, analgesics, and a lumbar epidural blood patch which may, in part, plug a dural tear. Although the patient has a history of migraine, it is unusual for vascular headaches to occur only when standing. Septic meningitis is a rare complication of an LP. However, since the patient is afebrile and only has a headache when upright, this diagnosis is unlikely. Likewise, it is unlikely that the headache is due to persistent aseptic meningitis. Patients can develop tender, tight cervical muscles following aseptic meningitis. This can be confused with persistent meningismus. However, it is more likely that this patient is suffering from a headache as a result of complications from the LP.

44. The answer is C [Chapter 9 VI B 1]. Normal hypothalamic secretion of gonadotropin-releasing hormone (GnRH) consists of pulsatile release every 90–120 minutes. If GnRh is injected by infusion pump in a way that mimics the normal pattern, luteinizing hormone (LH) and follicle-stimulating hormone (FSH) are secreted normally and cyclic ovarian function may follow. Continuous, rather than pulsatile, blood levels of GnRH, which are produced by injection of long-acting analogs, have the opposite effect and suppress LH and FSH production.

45. The answer is B [Chapter 8 VII D 1 a, 2 b]. *Salmonella* bacteremia, toxic shock syndrome (TSS), tuberculosis, and Epstein-Barr mononucleosis can be accompanied by fever, but a diffuse desquamative rash should suggest TSS, severe drug reaction (e.g., Stevens-Johnson syndrome), Kawasaki disease, or scarlet fever. The skin rash associated with *Salmonella* is very subtle and evanescent (Rose spots). Tuberculosis is not characterized by diffuse skin and mucous membrane involvement or watery diarrhea.

46. The answer is A [Chapter 10 VIII F 1]. Skin thickening is a defining characteristic of scleroderma; if it is limited to distal areas it may be a manifestation of the CREST variant of scleroderma (i.e., scleroderma that involves the coexistence of subcutaneous calcinosis, Raynaud's phenomenon, esophageal motility dysfunction, sclerodactyly, and telangiectasia). Patients with Raynaud's phenomenon who are seropositive for antinuclear antibody (ANA) or anticentromere antibody or who exhibit digital capillary changes are at higher risk for developing scleroderma than a patient with Raynaud's phenomenon who does not have these features. Distal esophageal dysmotility, spasm, or stricture are possible features of scleroderma but are nonspecific.

47. The answer is E [Chapter 11 II A 3 a (2), b (2), d (1) (8)]. Postprandial syncope is a common cause of fainting in the elderly. Alcohol intake can also lead to syncope and often is a contributing factor. Postprandial syncope may occur when blood is shunted to the mesenteric bed, resulting in relative cerebral hypoperfusion. The patient shows no signs of convulsive activity; therefore, a seizure is unlikely. A cardiac arrhythmia and carotid sinus hypersensitivity can cause syncope and should always be considered in the elderly patient. However, the setting in which this patient fainted makes postprandial syncope a more likely cause. A colloid cyst of the third ventricle is a rare cause of sudden unconsciousness. The small cyst acts like a ball valve and obstructs flow through the foramen of Monro, causing acute hydrocephalus.

48. The answer is A [Chapter 4 XV C 2, D 2]. Follicular small cleaved cell lymphoma, previously called nodular poorly differentiated lymphocytic lymphoma, is one of the most common varieties of the indolent non-Hodgkin's lymphomas. These patients often present with Stage III or IV disease. Even without treatment, patients may have waxing and waning of adenopathy, but over time, the disease will progress and the patient will require chemotherapy. A small percentage of patients will develop a more aggressive lymphoma, usually of the large cell or immunoblastic varieties.

49. The answer is D [Chapter 8 VIII G 1 b]. Diffuse lymphadenopathy in a human immu-

nodeficiency virus (HIV)-infected person who is clinically well is usually a sign that there is no specific infection or tumor involved. Although all of the answers can be true, people with multiple enlarged lymph nodes, tuberculosis, or malignancy tend to be ill. Most often they will also experience weight loss and fevers. Lymphoma is more likely to present with organ involvement in HIV-infected patients than in other patients. Kaposi's sarcoma may have lymphatic involvement, but generally this is found only in late-stage disease with extensive cutaneous and mucosal lesions. Moderate lymphadenopathy is a common finding in mid-stage HIV infection. Its exact etiology is unknown, but the disappearance of long-standing lymphadenopathy may precede clinical deterioration.

50. The answer is D [Chapter 6 Part I: XV A 1, 2]. The glomerular filtration rate (GFR) increases by approximately 40% in pregnancy. In fact, a fall in serum uric acid level typically occurs, as does a rise in uric acid clearance. Proteinuria normally is not seen in pregnancy, and the finding of increased urinary protein excretion suggests the presence of underlying renal disease or preeclampsia. The blood pressure typically falls in pregnancy; therefore, any degree of elevation represents important hypertension. Finally, respiratory alkalosis, not metabolic alkalosis, typically occurs, and this condition leads to a fall in serum bicarbonate level.

51. The answer is C [Chapter 9 I B 1 c; Table 9-2]. The patient probably has partial diabetes insipidus. The definite response by the patient to the injection of antidiuretic hormone (ADH) indicates that he did not produce maximally effective levels of ADH after fluid restriction and, therefore, he has either partial or complete diabetes insipidus. The ability to achieve normal or near-normal urine concentration, however, indicates that the ADH deficit is only partial. The response to ADH rules out nephrogenic diabetes insipidus. Diabetes mellitus, another cause of polyuria, is diagnosed by blood and urine glucose levels rather than studies of renal water handling.

52. The answer is E [Chapter 2 IV B 2 b]. More than 40% of patients with cystic fibrosis will live to be 18 years of age or older. Until the 1960s, cystic fibrosis was purely a pediatric disease. At that time, the median age of cystic fibrosis patients shifted to the teens. This was primarily due to the availability of antibiotics that are more specific to the pathogenic bacteria and due to the better understanding of the need for nutritional supplementation and exogenous pancreatic replacement. In 1991, the median age of patients with cystic fibrosis was over 29 years.

53. The answer is B [Chapter 8 II A 3 b; IV H]. While recommendations about treatment regimens for patients with profound neutropenia always change, the general principle is that infection with enteric gram-negative rods and *Pseudomonas aeruginosa* is likely and will quickly lead to a poor clinical outcome if left untreated. Piperacillin and amikacin may be good initial choices, depending on the antibiotic susceptibility of gram-negative rods in the community and the hospital. Antifungal therapy may be needed in a few days if there is no response to these antibiotics. Staphylococcal infections, common in patients with indwelling vascular catheters, are less likely to lead to cataclysmic deterioration.

54. The answer is C [Chapter 6 Part III: IV C 2 a (2)]. The use of diuretics in the treatment of hypertension may be associated with several side effects, including prerenal azotemia. Hypokalemia, hyperglycemia, hyperlipidemia, hyperuricemia, and hypercalcemia are also side effects of diuretic therapy. Bronchospasm is a side effect of β-blockade, and hemolytic anemia is a side effect of methyldopa, a centrally acting adrenergic antagonist. Both β-blockers and centrally acting adrenergic antagonists are alternative therapies for hypertension.

55. The answer is C [Chapter 3 I A 1]. The setting and history of this case are appropriate for a diagnosis of iron deficiency anemia. The excessive menses represent a source of iron loss. The hypochromia and microcytosis revealed by the blood smear establish that there is no deficiency of vitamin B_{12}; therefore, pernicious anemia is unlikely. The blood smear also excludes sickle cell anemia. Although blood smear reveals a microcytic cell population in cases of sideroblastic anemia, it also shows a normal or slightly macrocytic population existing with the microcytic component. Glucose-6-phosphate dehydrogenase (G6PD) deficiency is unlikely because it presents as hemolysis, for which there is no evidence in this case.

56. The answer is D [Chapter 11 XVIII F]. Patients with Down syndrome are at high risk of developing senile dementia of the Alzheimer type (SDAT) at approximately age 50. The pathology found is that of senile plaques and neurofibrillary tangles. Certainly hypothyroidism and hydrocephalus might occur in patients with Down syndrome, but the onset of dementia at are 50 is highly typical of developing Alzheimer's disease. Likewise, multiple strokes can lead to dementia, but stroke is not a usual cause of dementia in a 50-year-old Down syndrome patient. Creutzfeldt-Jakob disease is associated with prions and causes dementia.

57. The answer is D [Chapter 5 VII A 1]. Like alcoholic pancreatitis, gallstone pancreatitis accounts for approximately 30%–40% of all cases of acute pancreatitis in the United States. Thiazide therapy, hypercalcemia, and pancreas divisum are less common causes of acute pancreatitis. Hyperlipidemia is an associated finding in 15% of cases, but it also may be causative.

58. The answer is C [Chapter 8 VII B 1, 2]. Of the choices, eosinophilia is most likely to be found in schistosomiasis. Eosinophilia is a characteristic finding in infections due to multicellular, tissue-invasive parasites, such as *Schistosoma, Trichinella, Ascaris,* and *Strongyloides* species. Pinworm infestation is a purely luminal process, which does not elicit eosinophilia. Protozoal infections, such as giardiasis and amebiasis, rarely are associated with eosinophilia; the same is true of bacterial and viral infections, such as measles. Corticosteroids may be administered to individuals with underlying eosinophilia due to asthma or allergy to reduce the eosinophilia.

59. The answer is D [Chapter 10 I F 1 b]. Patients with joint conditions that are noninflammatory (e.g., osteoarthritis) typically exhibit morning stiffness of less than 1 hour's duration, whereas patients with inflammatory disorders (e.g., rheumatoid arthritis) have stiffness persisting longer than 1 hour. Patients with either rheumatoid arthritis or osteoarthritis have radiographic evidence of joint damage. A patient with rheumatoid arthritis is much more likely to have inflammatory synovial effusions, constitutional complaints (e.g., weight loss, malaise), and rheumatoid nodules.

60. The answer is D [Chapter 8 V C 4 c]. Although the studies do not completely exclude the possibility of a pulmonary embolus, bacterial pneumonia is likely. According to the Gram stain results, *Haemophilus influenzae* is the most likely causative organism, although pneumococcus is still possible. Ceftri-axone is effective against both. Bacterial resistance to tetracycline and erythromycin make these suboptimal choices.

61. The answer is A [Chapter 7 V G 2 a–f]. A hypersensitivity reaction to an insect sting is likely to be the cause of the patient's symptoms. Immediately following such a sting, most individuals experience local discomfort. The progressive occurrence of diffuse pruritus or urticaria, however, indicates a systemic hypersensitivity reaction, culminating in respiratory and cardiovascular embarrassment. Recent or concurrent use of β-antagonists such as propranolol reduces the efficacy of β-adrenergic agonists and predicts a more severe and protracted course of the anaphylactic reaction. In patients who have been taking β-blockers, measures not dependent upon β-adrenergic receptor stimulation are preferred; thus pressor agents and intravenous hydrocortisone are preferred over intravenous aminophylline, nebulized epinephrine, and nebulized β_2-adrenergic agonists.

62–63. The answers are: 62-B [Chapter 1 III A 5 b (1), (2) (a)–(b)], **63-B** [Chapter 1 III A 5 b (4) (a) (i)–(ii), (5) (a)–(b)]. The patient is experiencing anterior myocardial infarction. The S-T segment elevation in the anterior precordial leads indicates a current of myocardial injury. The S-T segment depression in the inferior leads is probably a reciprocal change reflecting the S-T segment elevation in the opposite (anterior) wall. Although pericarditis can mimic the clinical presentation of myocardial infarction, the electrocardiogram (ECG) in pericarditis demonstrates diffuse S-T segment elevation without S-T segment depression.

The most appropriate initial therapy for this patient would be the administration of streptokinase. Thrombolysis with streptokinase may allow for reperfusion of the myocardium, thus reducing infarct size and the chance of patient mortality. Reperfusion therapy is most effective within the first 4 hours after the beginning of the infarction. All patients with myocardial infarction or suspected myocardial infarction should be monitored in an intensive care unit, not a general ward. The patient's heart rate and blood pressure are adequate. Administration of atropine would increase the heart rate, causing further increases in myocardial oxygen consumption and possibly worsening the myocardial infarction. Pain relief is an important therapy in myocardial infarction, but intramuscular injections should be avoided when treating this condition. By relieving pain, one relieves anxiety, which decreases oxygen consumption and may also decrease the incidence of arrhythmias.

64. The answer is B [Chapter 8 V A 1 a]. All information is not in, but the weight of the evidence suggests that this patient has bacterial meningitis. The presence of blood can confuse the interpretation of lumbar puncture (LP) results. The number of white blood cells is more than expected for simple blood contamination. There is no role for oral or intravenous erythromycin in the treatment of meningitis. Heparin would be contraindicated until the diagnosis of subarachnoid bleed can be totally ruled out. Although there may be a role for a clot stabilizer in documented subarachnoid bleeds, the most urgent matter in this case is to treat for possible bacterial meningitis.

65. The answer is A [Chapter 10 VI D, E]. Bacterial infection is the most likely diagnosis in any patient who presents with a fever and an inflammatory monoarthritis, unless crystals are seen under polarized light examination of the synovial fluid. The absence of crystals in this patient's joint fluid eliminates gout and pseudogout as diagnoses. A joint fluid white cell count exceeding $50,000/\mu l$ also makes the diagnosis of septic arthritis more likely.

66–67. The answers are: 66-D [Chapter 1 I D 1 e, 2 a–g], **67-A** [Chapter 1 I F 3 a]. The patient is suffering from acute cardiogenic pulmonary edema. The rapid onset of the symptoms, in addition to the pinkish sputum, the gallop rhythm, and the bilateral infiltrates on the chest x-ray, strongly suggest this diagnosis, particularly in a patient with antecedent heart disease. Although one could not rule out the possibility that a bilateral pneumonitis could be exacerbating the patient's emphysema, the acute onset and the absence of purulent sputum militate against this diagnosis.

Because the patient is dyspneic, hypoxic, and hypocarbic, administration of oxygen should be the first course of action. Although one must be cautious of administering oxygen to emphysemic patients, the fact that this patient is hypocarbic suggests that she will not retain CO_2 when a prudent amount of oxygen is administered. Since there is no evidence of an acute myocardial infarction, her occasional extrasystoles do not require therapy with quinidine at this time. Although digoxin may be of some benefit in the long-range therapy of congestive heart failure, it has little immediate effect because it takes many hours to provide the patient with an adequate loading dose.

68–72. The answers are: 68-D [Chapter 11 VIII B 2 c (1) (a)–(b)], **69-E** [Chapter 11 XIII D 2], **70-A** [Table 11–10], **71-C** [Chapter 11 XVII E], **72-B** [Chapter 8 VII G 1 c (1)]. Acute ischemic stroke can occur in patients with acquired immune deficiency syndrome (AIDS), leading to acute hemiparesis. Stroke can be due to nonbacterial thrombotic endocarditis and an associated embolus, human immunodeficiency virus (HIV)-associated vasculitis, meningovascular syphilis, and the vasculopathy associated with cryptococcal and tuberculous meningitis, lymphoma, and herpes zoster.

Progressive leg weakness can be due to chronic inflammatory demyelinating polyneuropathy (CIDP) or an acute Guillain-Barré-type demyelinating polyneuropathy, a chronic sensorimotor polyneuropathy, myelopathy, and myopathy.

A predominantly small fiber sensory polyneuropathy with diminished pain and temperature sensibility and pedal discomfort is a common finding in patients with AIDS and AIDS-related complex (ARC).

Central nervous system (CNS) lymphoma can cause a progressive hemiparesis. The tumor often originates deep in the brain, close to the corticospinal tracts. Imaging studies will reveal at least one intensely-enhanced mass.

Cryptococcal meningitis can cause an acute deterioration in cognition. Delirium in a patient with AIDS can be caused by many conditions including HIV encephalopathy and CNS toxoplasmosis. A cerebral spinal fluid (CSF) evaluation, computed tomography (CT), and magnetic resonance imaging (MRI) can be very helpful in distinguishing among the possibilities.

73–76. The answers are: 73-E, 74-A, 75-C, 76-B [Chapter 9 V B 3 b (2), c, d (2); Table 9–13]. Although basal cortisol levels may be increased by physical or emotional stress, even low doses of dexamethasone usually result in normal suppression in such cases.

The pituitary secretion of adrenocorticotropic hormone (ACTH) in Cushing's disease can be suppressed by dexamethasone or other glucocorticoids. Larger-than-normal doses of dexamethasone, however, are necessary for suppression.

The production of ACTH by oat cell carcinoma of the lung and other tumors is not suppressed by dexamethasone. Therefore, even high doses do not lower cortisol levels. The increased blood ACTH levels are helpful in distinguishing ectopic ACTH syndrome from adrenal tumors, in which ACTH (of pituitary origin) is suppressed.

Cortisol production by adrenal adenomas and carcinomas is autonomous; it is not under the control of pituitary ACTH. ACTH levels are, in fact, suppressed by the increased circulating cortisol. Therefore, even high doses of dexamethasone will not lower cortisol levels by suppressing pituitary excretion of ACTH.

77–81. The answers are: 77-C [Table 7–9], **78-E** [Table 7–8], **79-A** [Table 7–5], **80-B** [Table 7–7], **81-D** [Table 7–5]. Wiskott-Aldrich syndrome is characterized clinically by susceptibility to infection during the first year of life, eczema, and purpura. The immunologic response deficiency is accompanied by a reduction in both the number and size of platelets.

Profound lymphopenia ($<1500/\mu l$) is a cardinal feature of the severe combined immunodeficiency (SCID) disorders. This heterogeneous group of disorders usually presents in infancy with frequent bouts of otitis media, pneumonia, cutaneous infections, diarrhea, and sepsis. Opportunistic infections frequently lead to death before the age of two years.

The nitroblue tetrazolium (NBT) test is a simple screening procedure for chronic granulomatous disease; failure to reduce the nitroblue tetrazolium dye during phagocytosis constitutes a positive result. This disorder is characterized by an absence of the usual respiratory burst due to abnormal function of the reduced form of nicotinamide-adenine nucleotide phosphate (NADPH).

DiGeorge syndrome (thymic hypoplasia) results from dysmorphogenesis of the third and fourth pharyngeal pouches, leading to aplasia or hypoplasia of the thymus and parathyroid glands. Neonatal tetany secondary to hypoparathyroid-induced hypocalcemia may be the first clinical manifestation; thus, assessing the serum calcium level is appropriate. Mandibular hypoplasia; hypertelorism; low-set, notched ears; and conotruncal heart lesions are common. The magnitude of the immune deficiency is variable, and patients with congenital heart defects have the least favorable prognosis.

Delayed umbilical cord separation followed by persistent omphalitis suggests leukocyte adhesion deficiency. The diagnosis is confirmed using a monoclonal antibody technique to detect a marked reduction in iC3b receptors on phagocytes. Affected children typically develop recurrent deep soft-tissue or superficial cold abscesses.

82–88. The answers are: 82-B [Chapter 6 Part II: IV B 2 b c], **83-D** [Chapter 6 Part II: IV D 2 a (1), (2)] **84-A** [Chapter 6 Part II: IV C 2 f], **85-B** [Chapter 6 Part II: IV B 2 d], **86-A** [Chapter 6 Part II: IV C 2 h], **87-C** [Chapter 6 Part II: IV E 2 c], **88-D** [Chapter 6 Part II: IV D 2 a (1), (2)]. Diseases (e.g., myasthenia gravis and other myopathies) that lead to thoracic wall dysfunction and hypoventilation lead to carbon dioxide retention and respiratory acidosis.

Conditions of tissue hypoperfusion, including severe decreases in cardiac output, lead to anaerobic glycolysis, increased lactate production, and decreased hepatic lactate metabolism. The result is lactic acidosis, a metabolic acidosis that is characterized by an increased anion gap.

Tachypnea and hyperpnea are early clinical signs of endotoxemia. The resulting decrease in Pco_2 leads to a pure respiratory alkalosis. As septicemia proceeds to septic shock, lactic acidosis may supervene.

Drugs that depress the central ventilatory center (e.g., heroin) will induce hypoventilation, carbon dioxide retention, and respiratory acidosis.

During normal pregnancy, progesterone stimulates the ventilatory center, producing a mild respiratory alkalosis.

The chloruresis and volume depletion induced by diuretic use lead to augmented proximal reabsorption of sodium bicarbonate, causing metabolic alkalosis.

Diabetic ketoacidosis is a metabolic acidosis associated with a wide anion gap. It occurs secondary to ketone body formation in the insulin-deficient state.

89–93. The answers are: 89-C [Chapter 6 Part III: IV C 2 b], **90-B** [Chapter 6 Part III: IV C 2 f], **91-E** [Chapter 6 Part III: IV C 2 e], **92-A** [Chapter 6 Part III: IV C 2 c], **93-D** [Chapter 6 Part III: IV C 2 g]. Metoprolol is a β-adrenergic blocking agent. It is theorized that this class of drugs reduces hypertension by reducing cardiac output and blunting the renin-angiotensin mechanism for the reabsorption of water. Nifedipine is a calcium channel antagonist that modulates calcium release in smooth muscle, reducing smooth muscle tone and producing vasodilation. Alpha-adrenergic blocking agents, such as prazosin, reduce blood pressure by antagonizing norepinephrine's stimulation of α-adrenergic receptors.

Methyldopa, a centrally acting adrenergic antagonist, inhibits sympathetic outflow from the central nervous system (CNS) by stimulating central α-adrenoreceptors, which reduces peripheral resistance and blood pressure. Minoxidil, a vasodilator, directly dilates arteries and arterioles.

94–98. The answers are: 94-E [Chapter 5 IV D 4 f], **95-A** [Chapter 5 V D 2], **96-C** [Chapter 5 V I], **97-B** [Chapter 5 IV D 3 d], **98-F** [Chapter 5 V H]. *Campylobacter* infection is the most common cause of bacterial diarrhea. The diarrhea can be severe and bloody, and proctosigmoidoscopy during the acute phase can show ulcerated, friable mucosa. The disease is self-limited, however, and complete healing of the mucosa takes place.

Ulcerative colitis may present as an acute diarrheal illness that fails to resolve. Proctosigmoidoscopy shows diffuse friability, bleeding, and ulceration of the mucosa. Biopsy of the involved mucosa characteristically shows abscesses in the crypts of Lieberkühn.

Pseudomembranous colitis may arise as a complication of therapy with broad-spectrum antibiotics (e.g., clindamycin). Clindamycin suppresses most anaerobic bacteria of the colon but actually causes an overgrowth of the anaerobe *Clostridium difficile,* which produces an enterotoxin that is responsible for the development of pseudomembranous colitis. The characteristic lesion is a white plaque (pseudomembrane), which is seen in the sigmoid of 75%–90% of patients. The diagnosis can be established by measuring the toxin of *C. difficile* in the stool of patients in whom disease is confined to the right side of the colon.

Laxative abuse is an important cause of both secretory and osmotic diarrhea. Secretory diarrhea, which is diagnosed on the basis of the absence of an osmotic gap on stool electrolyte studies, may be caused by such laxatives as castor oil, bisacodyl, and phenolphthalein. Osmotic diarrhea, which is diagnosed on the basis of the presence of an osmotic gap, may be caused by such laxatives as milk of magnesia, lactulose, sorbitol, and magnesium-containing antacids. Because the only other causes of osmotic diarrhea are disaccharidase deficiency and maldigestion, the presence of an osmotic gap on stool electrolyte studies always should raise the suspicion of laxative abuse.

Collagenous colitis has been reported in middle-aged women who may have associated polyarthritis or thyroid disease.

Detectable abnormalities may comprise only an elevated sedimentation rate (in about half of the patients) and a thickened colonic subepithelial collagen band (15–100 μ in diameter). Stool frequency is characteristic of a secretory diarrhea and may be due to incomplete absorption through the thickened band of collagen in the colonic submucosa.

99–103. The answers are: 99-C [Chapter 3 I B 3 a], **100-B** [Chapter 3 I B 3 a (1)], **101-B** [Chapter 3 I B 3 c (3)], **102-B** [Chapter 3 I B 3 c (2)], **103-A** [Chapter 3 I B 3 a (2)]. Both folic acid and vitamin B_{12} deficiencies cause detective DNA synthesis and, thus, impaired cell maturation. Deficient DNA synthesis is the main characteristic of classic megaloblastic marrow (i.e., marrow cells with immature nuclei but mature cytoplasm) and macrocytic anemia. Because all marrow cell lines are affected, there is pancytopenia.

Vitamin B_{12} deficiency can result from absence of the gastric intrinsic factor needed to bind the vitamin and, thus, aid its absorption into the terminal ileum. This form of vitamin B_{12} deficiency, termed pernicious anemia, is associated with gastric atrophy, achlorhydria, and gastric carcinoma. The inability to absorb vitamin B_{12} into the ileum, which is corrected by administration of intrinsic factor, is identified by an abnormal Schilling test.

Due to the role of vitamin B_{12} in myelin metabolism, deficiency causes neuropathy in the lateral and posterior columns of the spinal cord. Folic acid deficiency causes blood findings that are similar to those caused by vitamin B_{12} deficiency; however, folic acid deficiency is not associated with neuropathy. Usually, folic acid deficiency results from dietary deficiency due to poor intake (e.g., in the case of alcoholism).

104–107. The answers are: 104-D [Chapter 4 IX C 5 a, 6 a], **105-D** [Chapter 4 IX C 5 b], **106-E** [Chapter 4 IX C 5 c], **107-A** [Chapter 4 IX C 5 d, 6 b]. Stage A_1 prostatic tumors are low morbidity lesions that usually are found in a routine examination for benign obstructive disease. Close follow-up may be adequate for Stage A_1 tumors, which are well differentiated. Stage A_2 tumors are confined to the prostate gland and can be cured with radical radiotherapy (7000 cGy) or surgery.

Stage B tumors are the true, classic prostate nodules that are found on rectal examination. These tumors are confined to the gland and, therefore, theoretically can be cured with radical prostatectomy or radiotherapy.

Stage C tumors are cancers that are associated with metastasis to local structures (e.g., the seminal vesicles) but not to distant sites. These tumors cannot be treated surgically. However, radical radiotherapy with boost doses to the prostate gland has proved to be curative.

Stage D tumors are cancers that have distant metastases, and, therefore, local measures do not suffice as therapy. Stage D prostatic carcinoma requires systemic treatment, such as hormone therapy or chemotherapy.

108–112. The answers are: 108-E [Chapter 2 III E 3], **109-C** [Chapter 6 Part II: IV B, E], **110-A** [Chapter 6 Part II: IV C 1–2 a], **111-B** [Chapter 6 Part II: IV D 2 a (1), 4 b], **112-D** [Chapter 2 II E 2 a (1) (a)]. Patient E has status asthmaticus with respiratory failure. The patient has retained carbon dioxide from severe airway obstruction (as indicated by an arterial P_{CO_2} above the normal level of 40 mm Hg). The combination of abnormally high P_{CO_2} and abnormally low P_{O_2} (i.e., below the normal level of 80–100 mm Hg) in this patient indicates the presence of respiratory failure.

The blood gas data for patient C exemplify hydrochloric acid loss from pyloric-outlet obstruction. The high arterial pH (i.e., above the normal value of 7.40), increased arterial P_{CO_2}, and increased bicarbonate level (i.e., above the normal level of 24 mmol/L) indicate the presence of metabolic alkalosis with a compensatory respiratory acidosis.

A patient with hysterical hyperventilation has no obvious pulmonary disease and, therefore, should have no alveolar-arterial P_{O_2} gradient. This is the case with patient A. The excessive elimination of carbon dioxide by this patient results in pure respiratory alkalosis, which is characterized by below-normal arterial P_{CO_2} and bicarbonate levels and increased arterial pH.

Patient B does not have lung disease but, rather, shows a primary metabolic acidosis with a compensatory respiratory alkalosis. This condition is defined by a decrease in both arterial pH and arterial bicarbonate concentration and a lower than predicted arterial P_{CO_2} value (as determined using Winter's formula). This condition is seen in patients with diabetic ketoacidosis.

Patient D shows signs of the emphysematous type of chronic obstructive pulmonary disease (COPD). (The other classic type of COPD)—bronchitic COPD—is dominated by signs and symptoms of chronic bronchitis.) Pulmonary function testing in patients with emphysematous COPD reveals only mild hypoxia and hypocapnia, which are demonstrated in this patient by slight decreases in oxygen saturation and arterial Pco_2. In contrast, patients with bronchitic COPD demonstrate severe hypoxia and hypocapnia on pulmonary function testing.

113–115. The answers are: 113-B [Chapter 7 VII D 3 a (1)], **114-E** [Chapter 7 VII D 3 b (2)], **115-A** [Chapter 7 VII D 3 b (2)]. IgE-mediated hypersensitivity is implicated in local reactions at the site of insulin injections. Such reactions often subside in a few weeks. Improper injection techniques may also be responsible for local reactions to insulin.

High titers of circulating IgG antibodies to insulin may be associated with a rising insulin requirement (i.e., up to 200 U/day). An uncommon cause of insulin resistance, this phenomenon develops most frequently during the first year of therapy in patients with histories of local allergic reactions, intermittent insulin therapy, and administration of impure insulin preparations. Spontaneous remission is observed within 6 months in over half of affected patients.

Elderly diabetic women are at risk of developing type B insulin resistance syndrome, a disorder characterized by an increasing insulin requirement, acanthosis nigricans, and lupus-like symptoms. Associated laboratory findings include IgG anti-insulin-receptor antibodies, elevated sedimentation rate, and antinuclear antibodies (ANAs). Spontaneous improvement is rare, and immunosuppressive therapy may be required.

116–120. The answers are: 116-D [Chapter 3 I C 1 a], **117-A** [Chapter 3 II C 2 b (2) (a)], **118-C** [Chapter 3 I C 1 c], **119-B** [Chapter 3 I A 2 a–b], **120-E** [Chapter 3 II C 2 b (1)]. Aplastic anemia patients have deficient stem cells and thus cannot respond to their own endogenously elevated erythropoietin or to exogenously administered erythropoietin.

Polycythemia vera is a neoplastic disease characterized by marrow synthesis of blood cells independent of erythropoietin and, therefore, lowered renal erythropoietin synthesis.

Renal failure patients lose renal erythropoietin synthetic ability along with renal function. Their erythropoiesis is intrinsically normal and responds well to exogenous erythropoietin.

In the anemia of chronic disease, adaptive mechanisms result in marrow less responsive to either endogenous or exogenous erythropoietin.

Secondary erythrocytosis syndromes associated with specific malignancies develop due to normal marrow responding to very high levels of tumor-synthesized erythropoietin analogues.

121–124. The answers are: 121-A [Chapter 4 Table 4-27], **122-A** [Chapter 4 VII D 3 b], **123-B** [Chapter 4 X E 4], **124-D** [Chapter 4 XVI B 2 a]. Patients with small-cell lung cancer can present with Eaton-Lambert syndrome. These patients often have muscle weakness that improves with exercise. Skeletal muscles and the muscles of respiration may be affected.

Other neurologic paraneoplastic syndromes are also associated with small-cell lung cancer. Many patients with small-cell lung cancer will have hyponatremia due to the syndrome of inappropriate antidiuretic hormone (SIADH). This improves with therapy.

Patients with nonseminomatous germ cell tumors and seminoma of the anaplastic variety can have elevations in human chorionic gonadotropin (β-hCG). These tumors are associated with gynecomastia, which resolves as the tumor responds to therapy.

Trousseau's syndrome is chronic disseminated intravascular coagulation (DIC) associated with increased incidence of deep venous thrombosis in patients with malignancy. This occurs in patients with adenocarcinomas of the pancreas, stomach, and prostate, and occasionally with other tumor cell types of adenocarcinomatous histology.

125–127. The answers are: 125-A [Chapter 10 IV B 1 d (2), e (4), 2 d, e (4) (b)], **126-C** [Chapter 10 III F] **127-D** [Chapter 8 VII F]. Radiographic evidence of sacroiliac and spinal involvement should be sought to confirm this patient's diagnosis. This patient's morning low back pain associated with prolonged stiffness sounds like the inflammatory symptoms associated with spondylarthropathies. The "sausage toes" and heel pain are probably manifestations of the enthesopathic features of Reiter's syndrome, a diagnosis made more likely by the association with conjunctivitis. The onset after an episode of bloody diarrhea suggests that an infectious gastroenteritis triggered the reactive musculoskeletal findings.

This patient has had 6 months of a polyarticular inflammatory arthritis (prolonged morning stiffness and joint swelling suggest an inflammatory process), and the symmetrical involvement of wrists and the metacarpophalangeal (MCP) and proximal interphalangeal

(PIP) joints is typical of rheumatoid arthritis. Certainly other diagnoses [e.g., systemic lupus erythematosus (SLE), sarcoidosis, psoriatic arthritis] must be considered, but the chronicity and character of the joint complaints are more typical of rheumatoid arthritis. Seropositivity for rheumatoid factor would help confirm the diagnosis; the erythrocyte sedimentation rate is likely to be elevated but nonspecific.

High levels of immunoglobulin M (IgM) antibody and increasing levels of IgG antibody to one or more *B. burgdorferi* antigens corroborate clinical suspicions of Lyme disease. The combination of a painful radiculitis and an oligoarthritis should support the likelihood of Lyme disease in an endemic area, even if no skin features are present and no tick bite was noted. Onset of these later features after the summer months is another piece of helpful evidence, since most cases start with a tick bite in the spring or summer.

128–132. The answers are: 128-D, 129-A, 130-A, 131-B, 132-C [Chapter 3 III A 2 b (1), B 3 a (3)]. Chronic lymphocytic leukemia (CLL) is a steadily progressive disease characterized by an accumulation of mature lymphocytes in the tissues and peripheral blood. Clinical manifestations of CLL vary with the extent of disease progression, which is broken down into stages (0 through 4). Examples include splenomegaly (a stage-2 CLL presentation) and anemia (a stage-3 CLL presentation). In time, CLL causes marrow failure and death.

Chronic myelogenous leukemia (CML) is characterized by excessive granulocytes and granulocyte precursors in the blood and tissues. These cells lack the normal leukocyte alkaline phosphatase (LAP) level. Splenomegaly is a common finding with CML. This disease, which often terminates in acute leukemia, is characterized by an accelerated progression.

133–138. The answers are: 133-E [Chapter 4 XV B 2 a], **134-B** [Chapter 4 IX B 2 a], **135-A** [Chapter 5 II B 1 b (1)], **136-D** [Chapter 5 V G 3 b (3) (a)], **137-C** [Chapter 4 VII B 2], **138-E** [Chapter 4 XI B 6]. Studies have shown

clustering of cases of non-Hodgkin's lymphomas, which suggests that infectious agents may play a causative role. In particular, Epstein-Barr virus has been implicated in the development of Burkitt's lymphoma, a disease commonly found in Africa.

Bladder carcinoma has been linked to tobacco as well as to certain chemical and biologic carcinogens. For example, there is a well-documented association between occupational exposure to dye and printing chemicals and the development of bladder tumors.

Several relationships have been noted in the etiology of gastric carcinoma. Up to 10% of patients with achlorhydria, atrophic gastritis, and pernicious anemia develop gastric cancer. An increased concentration of nitrosamine compounds in gastric juice has been suggested as an underlying factor in these relationships.

Colorectal carcinoma is a common malignancy in the United States, for which several precancerous lesions are known. Chronic ulcerative colitis of long duration has a documented and statistically significant association with the incidence of colorectal cancer.

In the United States, lung cancer is the primary cause of cancer-related deaths in men and is second only to breast cancer as the leading cause of cancer deaths in women. Cigarette smoking largely is implicated as a cause of lung cancer, but other etiologic factors have been noted, such as exposure to industrial carcinogens. One of these, asbestos, classically has been linked to the more rare mesothelioma; however, asbestos exposure also has a clear and strong association with lung cancer.

Head and neck tumors are highly unusual in the Mormon population, which abstains from both alcohol and tobacco. This fact exemplifies the statistically-based claims that the use of tobacco and alcohol is associated with an increased risk of head and neck cancers. Another noted risk factor is the Epstein-Barr virus, which has been linked to the unusual nasopharyngeal carcinoma that is unique to Asians.

CASE STUDIES IN CLINICAL DECISION MAKING

Case 1: Coma in a Diabetic Patient

A 20-year-old college student is rushed to the emergency room by ambulance after being found comatose by her roommate in her dormitory room. She is known to have insulin-dependent diabetes mellitus (type I diabetes) that has been well controlled by diet and insulin.

QUESTIONS

1. *What are your immediate concerns about this patient?*

2. *What are possible mechanisms of coma in a diabetic patient?*

3. *What is at the top of your differential diagnosis?*

DISCUSSION

The causes of coma that are directly related to diabetes are diabetic ketoacidosis, hypoglycemia, and hyperosmolar nonketotic coma. The latter occurs mainly in elderly patients with noninsulin-dependent (type II) diabetes, so the first diagnostic impressions when this patient arrives in the emergency room are diabetic ketoacidosis and hypoglycemia.

Diabetic ketoacidosis occurs when there is a severe deficiency of insulin, which causes an inability to utilize glucose and leads to hyperglycemia, ketosis, and acidosis. Hypoglycemia in a diabetic patient is usually the result of an imbalance between the factors that lower the blood glucose level, namely administered insulin, oral hypoglycemic agents, and exercise, and the factors that raise the blood glucose level, namely food ingestion and hepatic output of glucose. Diabetic ketoacidosis and hypoglycemia should be ruled out before serious consideration is given to other causes of coma such as drug overdose, seizures, stroke, or meningitis.

When the patient first arrives in the emergency room, an adequate airway should be assured, vital signs should be measured to assess circulatory status, intravenous access should be established, and blood should be drawn for chemistries, arterial blood gas measurements, and a fingerstick glucose determination. Then additional information should be obtained from the patient's friend.

The roommate recalls that the patient has been complaining of an "upset stomach" for 2 days, with some nausea, anorexia, mild diarrhea, and increasing abdominal pain. She seemed a bit groggy that morning, and did not go to classes. She did not take her morning insulin dose because she was unable to eat breakfast. The roommate returned from class at 3:00 P.M. and found the patient lying in bed, breathing deeply, and unresponsive to her questions.

QUESTIONS

1. *What risk factors does this patient have for the development of diabetic ketoacidosis?*

2. *What is the significance of each of the patient's complaints?*

693

DISCUSSION

The apparently gradual onset over a period of hours, the preceding illness, and the omission of an insulin dose strongly suggest diabetic ketoacidosis rather than hypoglycemia as the most likely diagnosis. Illness such as upper respiratory infection or gastroenteritis may increase the need for insulin because of stress-related increases in catecholamines, cortisol, and glucagon; omitting insulin doses because of the illness makes matters worse. The gastrointestinal symptoms at the onset of illness suggest that gastroenteritis was the precipitating event, although the increasing abdominal pain could have been caused also by the developing ketoacidosis.

Why does abdominal pain sometimes occur in diabetic ketoacidosis? Gastric distention may be a factor, and it is known that ketosis from other causes, such as starvation, may lead to gastrointestinal symptoms such as anorexia, nausea, and vomiting. But the precise cause of abdominal pain in diabetic ketoacidosis is not known. The grogginess that the patient experienced earlier in the day suggests that the process leading to mental obtundation had already started. A gradual onset over several hours is typical of the symptoms of diabetic ketoacidosis, while the mental changes of hypoglycemia commonly have a relatively sudden onset, usually preceded by adrenergic symptoms such as sweating, tremor, and palpitations.

On examination the patient is unresponsive, with dry skin and mucous membranes and rapid, deep respirations. Her blood pressure is 100/60 mm Hg supine, falling to 80/50 mm Hg when the head of the bed is raised. The neck veins are collapsed when the patient is lying supine. Her pulse rate is 110 bpm, her respiratory rate is 24/min, and her temperature is 98.6°F. She winces when moderate pressure is applied to her abdomen. The deep tendon reflexes are hypoactive.

QUESTIONS

1. Do these physical findings aid in differentiating between diabetic ketoacidosis and hypoglycemia?

2. What is the significance of the patient's respiratory pattern?

DISCUSSION

These physical findings are highly suggestive of diabetic ketoacidosis. Insufficient insulin action makes glucose unavailable to the tissues, and the liver responds by producing ketones as an alternative fuel. The rising blood levels of glucose and ketones cause an osmotic diuresis, producing dehydration and intravascular volume depletion, with orthostatic hypotension. The osmotic diuresis leads to urinary losses of potassium and other electrolytes; hypokalemia causes muscle weakness and decreased reflexes. Abdominal pain and tenderness, perhaps caused by the ketosis, may be severe. The rapid, deep respirations, called Kussmaul's respirations, are caused by stimulation of the respiratory center by acidosis. This leads to respiratory alkalosis, which partially offsets the metabolic acidosis.

Blood glucose by fingerstick, determined soon after the patient's arrival in the emergency room, is found to be greater than 400 mg/dl. Urine dipstick testing is strongly positive for glucose and ketones. Treatment is started with an intravenous infusion of normal saline solution at a rate of 1000 ml/hr.

QUESTIONS

1. What is the rationale behind ordering these laboratory tests?

2. What initial steps should be taken at this point to manage this patient's condition?

DISCUSSION

The elevated blood and urine glucose levels and urine ketone levels confirm the diagnosis of diabetic ketoacidosis. The first priority in treatment is fluid replacement, which can be started while the initial laboratory results are awaited. An infusion of normal saline (1 L/hr for the first 2 hours) should be given if intravascular volume depletion is severe, as indicated in this patient by the orthostatic hypotension and decreased central venous pressure (decreased neck vein filling). Once the diagnosis of diabetic ketoacidosis is confirmed, insulin therapy should be started.

Intravenous infusion of regular insulin is started at a rate of 5 U/hr. Initial laboratory results include the following serum findings: glucose level of 520 mg/dl, sodium level of 132 mEq/L, potassium level of 3.3 mEq/L, and normal phosphate, calcium, and chloride levels. Blood urea nitrogen (BUN) and creatinine are slightly elevated, as is serum amylase. The white blood cell count is 14,500/μl. Arterial blood gas analysis reveals a pH of 7.20, bicarbonate of 8 mEq/L, and a pattern consistent with high anion gap metabolic acidosis.

QUESTIONS

1. *How do these laboratory values affect your differential diagnosis?*

2. *What is the significance of the elevated amylase?*

3. *What is the significance of the leukocytosis?*

4. *What processes are included in your differential diagnosis for high anion gap acidosis?*

DISCUSSION

These laboratory findings are typical of moderately severe diabetic ketoacidosis. The metabolic acidosis is caused by the hepatic production of ketone bodies, which must be buffered by bicarbonate. Sodium tends to be low because of the osmotic effect of hyperglycemia, which increases extracellular water, thus diluting serum sodium. Potassium, although initially high due to movement out of cells, falls to low levels as urinary losses occur. Although serum phosphate may be normal initially, large urinary losses often lead to depletion of total body phosphate, which should be replaced. The BUN and creatinine tend to be slightly increased because of the effect of volume depletion on renal function.

Serum amylase often is increased, but this usually is attributed to transient leakage from the salivary glands as well as the pancreas and does not usually indicate pancreatitis.

Leukocytosis is common in diabetic ketoacidosis; if infection is not present, the increased white cell count may be attributed to dehydration and increased glucocorticoid activity, which occurs in response to stress and may cause leukocytosis.

The high anion gap is caused by the presence of an unmeasured anion, in this case ketone bodies. Other important causes of high anion gap acidosis include renal failure, alcoholic ketoacidosis, lactic acidosis, and toxic substances such as salicylates, ethylene glycol, and methanol.

After 6 hours of treatment, the patient is awake, breathing comfortably at a rate of 18 respirations per minute, and able to respond to questions. The serum glucose level is 210 mg/dl, the arterial blood pH is 7.34, and the serum bicarbonate level is 14 mEq/L. Urine ketones are now only weakly positive.

QUESTIONS

1. *What other types of acute care might this patient require?*

2. *What are some of the potential complications of diabetic ketoacidosis?*

DISCUSSION

Because insulin therapy is still needed to treat the resolving ketosis and acidosis, glucose should now be added to the intravenous fluids to prevent hypoglycemia. Potassium and phosphate should be replaced as indicated by blood values.

In spite of careful treatment, patients with diabetic ketoacidosis have a mortality rate of 5%–10%. Death may be caused by overwhelming infection, by irreversible shock, or by arterial thrombosis causing myocardial infarction or stroke. Cerebral edema occasionally occurs in young patients who appear to be responding well to treatment, and may cause death. A more rapid fall in glucose levels in blood than in the cerebrospinal fluid (CSF) causes fluid to enter the relatively hyperosmolar CSF compartment, leading to increased intracranial pressure (ICP) and cerebral edema.

Case 2: Syncope

A 64-year-old man is walking around a shopping mall with his wife when he suddenly loses consciousness and falls to the ground. An ambulance brings him to the emergency room. Upon arrival at the hospital, the man is awake and alert and complaining only of pain in his right elbow, which he apparently injured when he fell. He is placed on a cardiac monitor and blood is drawn for laboratory work, which includes a complete blood count (CBC) and electrolyte, glucose, calcium, and cardiac enzyme studies.

QUESTIONS

1. What is the definition of syncope?

2. What are some of the causes of a sudden loss of consciousness?

DISCUSSION

Syncope is a sudden, temporary loss of consciousness caused by a lack of cerebral perfusion. The causes of sudden loss of consciousness can be divided into three major categories—cardiovascular, neurologic, and metabolic.

Cardiovascular syncope occurs when the cardiovascular system fails to maintain adequate blood pressure for cerebral perfusion. Inadequate stroke volume, inadequate heart rate, or inadequate total peripheral resistance all could be pathophysiologic causes of cardiovascular syncope. Impairment in stroke volume severe enough to cause syncope may be seen in ischemia and myocardial infarction, dehydration or hemorrhage, or as a result of tachyarrhythmias, which impair ventricular filling. Mitral, aortic, or idiopathic hypertrophic subaortic stenosis, atrial myxoma, and pulmonary embolism may also cause syncope by obstructing cardiac inflow or outflow. Severe bradycardia (i.e., a heart rate less than 40 bpm), such as occurs in heart block and sick sinus syndrome, may cause syncope. In some circumstances, cardiac output is adequate but total peripheral resistance is reduced, leading to a fall in blood pressure. Autonomic dysfunction or the use of vasodilators may reduce total peripheral resistance to the extent that syncope results. A common manifestation of syncope induced by reduced total peripheral resistance is the "vasovagal faint," which approximately 50% of the population experiences at some point during the course of a lifetime.

Head trauma, stroke, or cerebrovascular disease may all cause loss of consciousness. Sudden increases in intracranial pressure (ICP) can compromise cerebral perfusion and cause a loss of consciousness, even in the setting of normal systemic blood pressure. A classic example would be a colloid cyst of the third ventricle that acts as a ball valve and causes sudden obstructive hydrocephalus. Only rarely do disorders of the cerebrovascular system compromise perfusion to such an extent as to cause syncope. Therefore, syncope should not be viewed as a usual manifestation of a transient ischemic attack (TIA). Rarely, patients with compromise of distal basilar artery circulation (the "top-of-the-basilar" syndrome) experience a sudden loss of consciousness because of impaired perfusion of the ascending reticular activating system (RAS).

Another condition that is commonly considered in the differential diagnosis of syncope is seizure. However, seizures in the adult rarely cause a loss of consciousness that is not associated with repetitive motor activity. It should be noted that some patients with syncope attributable to cardiac or circulatory failure will have some generalized involuntary motor activity resulting from impaired cerebral perfusion, but this motor activity does not represent a primary convulsive event.

Finally, impaired delivery of essential nutrients to the brain (e.g., as a result of hypoglycemia or hypoxia) can cause a sudden loss of consciousness. Usually, however, metabolic disturbances worsen gradually and cause obtundation prior to loss of consciousness; therefore, the true definition of syncope is not usually met.

Additional history reveals that the fall was not preceded by an aura and that the patient remained continent during the episode. He awoke spontaneously and was not confused upon awakening. The patient has had several previous episodes of light-headedness during exertion but says he never lost consciousness during those episodes. The patient does not recall anything unusual about the day prior to his syncopal episode, except that he experienced mild angina that was immediately relieved by a single sublingual nitroglycerin tablet.

QUESTIONS

1. *What is significant about the onset and recovery of this syncopal episode?*
2. *Based on the above limited history, what process do you most suspect as a cause of this patient's syncope?*

DISCUSSION

The abrupt onset of loss of consciousness is characteristic of a cardiac cause. There were no warning symptoms to suggest the aura of a seizure, no discrete neurologic symptoms characteristic of a TIA, and no diaphoresis, nausea, and wooziness, such as would be associated with a vasovagal or hypoglycemic episode. The fact that the patient remained continent during the event supports a cardiac or vasovagal cause, although this information is probably not very helpful in decision making. The continence of a patient during a seizure is more likely related to whether or not the patient's bladder is full at the time of the event. The lack of confusion upon awakening argues against a seizure episode, although patients with atonic seizures can very rapidly regain normal cognition. Patients with a complex partial seizure do have a period of confusion often lasting several minutes. An important question to ask the patient's wife is whether or not the patient had any involuntary motor activity while unconscious. If he remained "limp," this would argue strongly against the event being a seizure.

The patient's history of several prior episodes of light-headedness suggests an underlying abnormality of the cardiovascular system. In particular, this history in an older patient should direct attention to the heart. This impression is reinforced by the fact that the patient apparently has a history of angina and has been taking nitroglycerin.

In summary, a cardiac cause of syncope is highly likely in this patient, due to the abrupt onset of the loss of consciousness and the history of angina. Because coronary disease should be particularly suspect in someone of this patient's age, the possibility of an arrhythmia would be particularly important to consider.

Past medical history for this patient is significant because of sporadic bouts of angina, for which the patient takes nitroglycerin. The angina has not recently increased in frequency or intensity. An exercise stress test was performed 3 years ago and was negative. The patient has had a heart murmur for many years but has been told that it is not

significant. He takes no regular medications. His father died of a heart attack at age 60, and his mother had a mild stroke at 70 but she did not die until 10 years later.

QUESTION

1. What is the significance of the patient's angina, stress test, family history, and heart murmur?

DISCUSSION

The patient's angina suggests the possibility of coronary artery disease. Although the patient had a negative exercise stress test 3 years ago, this does not preclude the possibility of progression of atherosclerotic disease. It is entirely possible that mild coronary disease that was present then has now progressed to the point that it is causing symptoms. However, one must ask why the patient had a stress test. If he had it because of his chest pain, and his chest pain was not caused by ischemia 3 years ago (as suggested by the negative stress test), then his pain quite possibly may not be ischemic now.

The significance of the family history is hard to judge. Although a "heart attack" at age 60 in the patient's father does suggest premature coronary disease, many patients who are labeled as heart attack victims have not truly suffered a myocardial infarction. The patient's mother's stroke at age 70 might represent atherosclerotic disease (at a relatively advanced age) or a hemorrhagic event. Certainly, the patient's history raises the possibility that atherosclerosis of the coronary or cerebral arterial circulation is causing the patient's symptoms. Although stroke or TIA due to large artery occlusive disease rarely is a cause of syncope, some patients with bilateral severe internal carotid artery stenosis can have syncopal events. The physician should also bear in mind the possibility of a "top-of-the-basilar" syndrome. The significance of the murmur is unclear from the history alone, but its existence suggests that underlying structural cardiac disease could be contributing to the patient's symptoms.

Although it is very likely that this patient has suffered syncope from a cardiovascular cause, the additional information does not help sway our clinical judgement one way or the other. It adds some "soft" features suggestive of coronary artery or valvular heart disease, which might in turn be responsible for a cardiac arrhythmia leading to syncope. However, this additional history is also entirely consistent with the absence of significant heart disease.

Physical examination reveals a well-developed, well-nourished white man in no acute distress. His vital signs include a pulse of 88 bpm, respirations of 14/min, blood pressure of 108/74 mm Hg, and a temperature of 98.9°F. The patient's skin is warm and dry, his pupils are equal and reactive to light and accommodation, and his lungs are clear. Cardiac examination reveals a normal first heart sound (S_1), a soft second heart sound (S_2), and a fourth heart sound (S_4). He has a harsh, late-peaking systolic ejection murmur that is loudest in the aortic area and radiates to both carotids. His carotids demonstrate delayed upstroke and low volume. There are no carotid bruits and no jugular venous distention. Examination of his abdomen and extremities reveals no abnormalities, with the exception of a bruise on his right elbow. Neurologic examination is completely within normal limits.

QUESTIONS

1. Which of these signs and symptoms are significant?

2. How does this physical examination influence your differential diagnosis?

3. What studies would you like to obtain?

DISCUSSION

The patient's appearance does not suggest a systemic illness. Obtaining supine and upright blood pressure and pulse determinations is important in light of the patient's relatively low blood pressure. The patient does have a slightly high pulse, which suggests dehydration. That his skin is dry also raises the possibility of dehydration, as well as autonomic failure with resultant postural hypotension. His preserved pupillary accommodation attests to preservation of parasympathetic nervous function but leaves open the possibility of sympathetic nervous system failure. The harsh, late peaking, systolic ejection murmur, the delayed and reduced carotid upstrokes, and the soft S_2 are highly suggestive of aortic stenosis, an important cause of syncope. The lack of carotid bruits must be considered within the context of a patient with a loud precordial murmur that is already radiating into the neck; critical carotid stenoses can be missed because of masking sounds (as in this patient). Patients with preocclusive stenosis at the internal carotid artery origin may not have enough forceful perfusion to generate an audible bruit.

The information from the examination directs attention to the heart. Of particular concern is the possibility of structural heart disease as a cause of impaired aortic area outflow. Given the patient's history, consideration also should be given to the possibility of associated coronary artery disease and, less likely, carotid artery disease.

Usually the next studies that are ordered in patients suspected of having cardiac disease are the electrocardiogram (ECG) and the chest x-ray. However, in this case neither is likely to be very informative. The ECG may show evidence of left ventricular hypertrophy, but some patients with severe aortic stenosis fail to demonstrate this finding. Thus, a negative ECG should not dissuade one from the diagnosis. Typically, the chest x-ray in aortic stenosis shows a normal size heart, sometimes with a boot-shaped configuration indicative of concentric left ventricular hypertrophy. Again, this finding is not specific.

The most important study to be ordered at this time is an echocardiogram with Doppler evaluation of the aortic valve. The echocardiogram will demonstrate the concentric left ventricular hypertrophy typical of aortic stenosis. Further, it will demonstrate severe restriction of the aortic valve leaflets. Both of these findings are consistent with the diagnosis but do not help quantify the disease's severity. However, Doppler evaluation of the aortic valve can precisely quantify the transvalvular aortic gradient. In most cases the echo Doppler study is adequate to confirm the diagnosis and to arrive at a decision regarding surgery. However, because this patient is in the coronary disease age-group and because of the history of angina, cardiac catheterization to confirm the aortic valve gradient and to define the coronary anatomy with coronary arteriograms should also be performed.

An ECG shows left ventricular hypertrophy but no evidence of past or present ischemia. A chest x-ray is within normal limits and an x-ray of the right elbow is also normal. Laboratory values are noncontributory. The patient is sent for an electroencephalogram (EEG) and for an echocardiogram with Doppler examination. The echocardiogram reveals a calcified aortic value and left ventricular hypertrophy, both consistent with calcific aortic stenosis. The aortic valve gradient is 70 mm Hg. The patient is admitted to the hospital for a cardiac catheterization and probable aortic valve replacement, because only 50% of patients with aortic stenosis who have syncope achieve a 3-year survival if left untreated.

QUESTIONS

1. What are some of the causes of aortic stenosis?

2. What is the pathophysiology underlying the physical signs and symptoms that characterize aortic stenosis?

DISCUSSION

Causes of aortic stenosis include congenital, rheumatic, and calcific conditions. In this patient's age-group, calcific aortic stenosis is of particular concern. There is no evidence of subaortic stenosis, such as asymmetric septal hypertrophy.

In aortic stenosis, the heart muscles force blood through a stenotic valve, which results in pressure overload on the left ventricle and subsequent concentric left ventricular hypertrophy. The clinical triad of angina, syncope, and heart failure are typical of aortic stenosis. The angina is the result of impaired blood flow limiting oxygen to the enlarged myocardium. The syncope can be caused by a decrease in the heart's ability to increase cardiac output across the stenotic valve. Syncope can also occur because of arrhythmias resulting from calcification within the cardiac conduction system. The patient's low systemic blood pressure is a consequence of his impaired cardiac output. The diminished S_2 is the result of impaired valve motion from the aortic disease. The S_4 is a result of decreased left ventricular compliance.

This patient illustrates that, with an appropriate history and physical examination, clues to the cause of a patient's syncope can be defined. Further evaluation can then be tailored to the patient. However, in many patients, a cause for syncope is not readily evident. In these situations, a review of the patient's history may be informative. For instance, did the syncope occur following a meal or during straining at defecation? In the patient with recurrent syncope, a Holter monitor to examine for arrhythmias, a stress test to try and induce the arrhythmia responsible for the syncope, autonomic testing to examine the integrity of postural reflexes, and an echocardiogram to search for underlying cardiac pathology are warranted. If arrhythmias are the suspected cause, electrophysiologic stimulation may provoke the causative arrhythmia. If occlusive cerebrovascular disease is suspected, a carotid duplex examination, magnetic resonance angiography, transcranial Doppler studies, or interventional angiography should be considered. If a neurologic etiology is suspected, an EEG to look for seizure activity and magnetic resonance imaging (MRI) to look for structural brain abnormalities are warranted.

Case 3: Dyspnea

A 58-year-old man calls an ambulance complaining that he "cannot get enough air" and that he is "suffocating." Upon arrival, the paramedics find that the man is alert and oriented but that he cannot speak more than one or two words at a time because of shortness of breath. On the way to the emergency room, the paramedics insert an intravenous line and administer oxygen at a rate of 15 L/min via mask.

QUESTIONS

1. What are your immediate concerns about this patient?

2. How would you define dyspnea?

3. What are some of the mechanisms that produce dyspnea?

DISCUSSION

From his complaints and physical appearance, this patient appears to be suffering from symptoms of dyspnea. Dyspnea has many causes, most of which are cardiac or pulmonary in origin. The overriding concern in a dyspneic patient is to rule out the possibility of serious cardiac or pulmonary causes of the symptoms. Evaluation of this man should begin with a check of vital signs, including blood pressure, pulse and respiratory rates, and temperature, to begin to narrow the list of potential major cardiac or pulmonary causes of dyspnea. Conditions that are associated with symptoms of dyspnea include pulmonary vascular disease [e.g., pulmonary embolism, pulmonary hypertension secondary to chronic obstructive pulmonary disease (COPD)], interstitial lung disease, asthma, COPD, neuromuscular disease, chest wall disease, and congestive heart failure (including that caused by the various types of heart disease including valvular disease, hypertension, cardiomyopathy, and pulmonary edema). Although chest pain would be a more common presenting symptom of myocardial infarction than would dyspnea, myocardial infarction should be considered and ruled out with cardiac enzyme studies and an electrocardiogram (ECG).

Another concern in this case (i.e., a new patient without a known cause of dyspnea) is the administration of oxygen at a high flow rate (i.e., 15 L/min), which may be the wrong approach if this man has obstructive pulmonary disease with carbon dioxide retention. Delivery of inspired oxygen at a high concentration can worsen carbon dioxide retention.

Dyspnea is defined as any uncomfortable awareness of breathing; it involves both the perception of an abnormal sensation and a reaction to that perception.

Upon arrival at the emergency room, the man is still short of breath and breathing at a rate of 28 respirations/min. His other vital signs show a pulse of 110 bpm, a blood pressure of 150/85 mm Hg, and a temperature of 100.5°F. Initial history reveals that 6 days ago, the patient developed an upper respiratory infection with rhinorrhea and a cough productive of thick yellow sputum. He has been short of breath for the past few days, but his symptoms worsened in the past several hours. He notes that he is more short of breath with minimal exertion and often begins to cough as a result of any effort. He denies chest pain or tightness.

The patient's past medical history is significant because of two previous hospital admissions for similar episodes. He also has a history of hypertension, for which he is supposed to take a mild diuretic once a day; however, he ran out of the drug and has not yet refilled his prescription. He uses an inhaler as needed but denies other medications or drug allergies. The patient says that he has smoked two packs of cigarettes per day for 30 years and that he drinks three to four beers per night. He is not married and recently lost his job in construction because he tires too easily.

QUESTIONS

1. *How do these descriptions of the patient's symptoms help you in thinking about your differential diagnosis?*

2. *How can you differentiate between cardiac and pulmonary causes of dyspnea?*

DISCUSSION

The subsequent history is more suggestive of a chronic process (e.g., chronic lung disease with congestive heart failure or upper respiratory infection exacerbation) than an acute process (e.g., acute myocardial infarction, pulmonary embolism). The differential diagnosis at this point includes obstructive pulmonary disease, asthma, congestive heart failure, infection, and a tumor (a possibility in a patient with COPD and a history of cigarette smoking). The physician should also keep in mind the possibility of work-related exposures, such as asbestos, asthma-sensitizers, and other occupational pulmonary toxins. Although the chronicity of symptoms points more toward a chronic than an acute process, the possibility of an acute myocardial infarction should still be ruled out. Recurrent pulmonary embolism still is a possibility at this point, and ventilation–perfusion scanning with lower extremity Doppler studies may be indicated.

Physical examination shows a well-developed, slightly overweight, white man in moderate respiratory distress with vital signs as noted above. His skin is moist without cyanosis, his neck shows mildly dilated jugular veins, his lungs reveal a prolonged expiratory phase with expiratory wheezes in all lung fields and poor respiratory effort, and examination of his heart reveals a prominent third heart sound (S_3) but no murmurs. Examination of his abdomen is unremarkable, revealing a slightly enlarged liver, and his extremities show 2+ peripheral edema.

QUESTIONS

1. *What do these physical signs suggest?*

2. *What disease process would be at the top of your differential diagnosis now?*

3. *What laboratory tests or studies would you like to obtain?*

DISCUSSION

The expiratory wheezing and increased respiratory effort noted on physical examination of this patient suggest the presence of obstructive lung disease. Additionally, there is an S_3 gallop and peripheral edema. The S_3 and dilated jugular veins suggest left-sided heart failure, and the enlarged liver and peripheral edema suggest right-sided heart failure. The wheezes may be associated with either obstructive lung disease or congestive heart failure. At this point, it is essential to differentiate cardiac from pulmonary causes of this man's distress in order to plan an effective treatment. A chest x-ray along with an ECG, cardiac enzyme studies, and a complete blood count (CBC) with differential would help to determine whether the patient has either or both underlying conditions.

The emergency room physician calls for the patient's old records, orders some laboratory tests (including arterial blood gas studies on oxygen, a CBC, a serum electrolyte panel, a cardiac enzyme analysis, a sputum culture, a stat ECG, and a portable x-ray). The ECG suggests some right axis deviation and sinus tachycardia but no ischemic changes. The results of the arterial blood gas studies are returned promptly and show a pH of 7.44, a PaO_2 of 81 mm Hg, a $PaCO_2$ of 50 mm Hg, and an O_2 saturation of 95% on 3 L FIO_2 by nasal cannula.

QUESTION

1. What sort of pattern do the arterial blood gas findings suggest?

DISCUSSION

The arterial blood gas findings represent adequate oxygenation (normal PaO_2 = 80 mm Hg or above) with mild hypercarbia (normal $PaCO_2$ = 40 mm Hg) and a normal pH. The normal pH suggests a chronic process.

The patient's chest x-ray suggests a mild prominence of the pulmonary vascular markings. Otherwise, there are no radiographic changes.

QUESTION

1. Which diagnoses are less likely because of these x-ray results?

DISCUSSION

The radiographic findings make the possibility of post-obstructive pneumonitis, tumor, or pneumonia much less likely and are more compatible with a COPD exacerbation with some mild congestive heart failure. There is no mass to suggest a tumor and no infiltrates to suggest pneumonia.

Because the patient continues to have respiratory distress and is very uncomfortable without the oxygen, he is admitted to the hospital. His old records reveal that his previous admissions were for exacerbations of bronchitis. He is started on oxygen and diuretics and a broad-spectrum antibiotic.

QUESTIONS

1. What are your goals for therapy for this patient?

2. How can you prevent similar episodes from happening again?

DISCUSSION

The goals for this patient are to control the exacerbation of his bronchitis with antibiotics and bronchodilators and to return him to baseline respiratory status. Peak flow measurements should be obtained before and after bronchodilators are administered, and the possibility of using corticosteroids along with the routine bronchodilator therapeutic regimen should be entertained. The possibility of underlying heart disease also should be addressed. An echocardiogram would be indicated at this time to determine if there is any cardiac functional abnormality. The most likely diagnosis here is chronic bronchitis exacerbated by an upper respiratory infection without pneumonia, with an underlying possibility of mild congestive heart failure. Future prophylaxis should include immunization against influenza as well as a pneumococcal vaccine. In addition, the possibility of entering a pulmonary rehabilitation program should be discussed with the patient.

Case 4: Gastrointestinal Bleeding

A 54-year-old white man presents to his general practitioner's office complaining of fatigue. He says that he tires easily and often feels light-headed and short of breath after climbing a single flight of steps or taking a short walk. He says that he is having difficulty at work because he is "just not himself."

QUESTIONS

1. *What are some possible causes of generalized fatigue and weakness?*

2. *What other questions would you like to ask this patient?*

DISCUSSION

Fatigue and weakness are common complaints that can be psychogenic or physical in origin. It is important to differentiate between these broad etiologic categories. Psychogenic causes consist of anxiety states and depression. Physical causes include infectious disease, metabolic disorders, blood dyscrasias, renal disease, liver disease, chronic pulmonary disease, chronic cardiovascular disease, neoplastic diseases, and neuromuscular disease. Specific examples of physical causes of fatigue include tuberculosis, diabetes mellitus, hypothyroidism, hyperparathyroidism, Addison's disease, anemia, lymphoma, leukemia, acute and chronic renal failure, acute and chronic hepatitis, cirrhosis, and common neoplastic diseases such as carcinoma of the lung, breast, colon, pancreas, prostate, ovary, or endometrium.

To narrow the diagnostic possibilities for this patient's fatigue and weakness, additional history should be obtained. The patient should be questioned about whether he has experienced weight loss, fever, chills, chest pain, paroxysmal nocturnal dyspnea, orthopnea, pedal edema, abdominal pain, changes in bowel habits, melena, hematochezia, polyuria, polydipsia, polyphagia, intolerance to heat or cold, or insomnia. A positive answer to these questions often, although not always, would indicate a physical or organic cause of fatigue and weakness.

Further history reveals that the patient's symptoms started about 2 months ago and have steadily worsened. He claims he was in excellent health until this time; in fact, he has not had a routine physical examination in approximately 2 years because he has felt healthy. The patient takes no medications, except for the occasional use of acetaminophen or laxatives. He is an executive in a publishing company who smokes approximately half a pack of cigarettes per day and drinks a martini or two at lunch. He has no significant family history, except that an estranged older brother died after an

abdominal operation for an unknown cause. The patient denies chest pain or palpitations but has occasional shortness of breath and dyspnea on exertion, as described above. He has had no loss of appetite and even jokes that he can eat even on days when he is a bit "irregular." When asked about his constipation, he notes that he sometimes has difficulty passing his stool, but the stool is of normal consistency. He also reports that his stools have seemed a bit darker lately, but he thought it might be due to laxatives he took for constipation; he has not noticed any bright red blood in the stool and denies hematemesis, nausea, vomiting, or diarrhea.

QUESTION

1. Which of these signs and symptoms concern you?

DISCUSSION

This patient's history raises several points of concern. His symptoms began 2 months ago, meaning they are chronic complaints, and they have steadily worsened—an ominous sign. Acute complaints could be attributed to an acute viral or self-limited illness. That the patient was in excellent health until 2 months ago also indicates a change from a preexisting pattern. For example, a history of chronic abdominal pain and a change in bowel habits, if acutely present over 2–3 days or a week, could be compatible with an acute viral enteritis. Symptoms that have been present for a long time (2–3 years or more) suggest a chronic nonprogressive illness such as irritable bowel syndrome. However, in a patient who was previously symptom-free and in excellent health, a 2-month history of symptoms that have steadily worsened would suggest a new and potentially serious change that could be compatible with inflammatory bowel disease, infectious states (e.g., giardiasis), or even malignant disease involving the gastrointestinal tract, particularly the colon.

The absence of medications would eliminate the possibility that a side effect of a drug (e.g., an antihypertensive agent) is responsible for the fatigue and shortness of breath. Smoking is clearly associated with numerous malignancies, including bronchogenic and pancreatic carcinoma, in addition to its known cardiovascular and pulmonary effects. The family history of an abdominal operation for an unknown cause raises the specter of possible colonic carcinoma, which has a two- to threefold increased incidence in first-degree relatives. Dyspnea on exertion could signify a cardiovascular cause but could also be associated with an anemic state. The patient's "abnormally dark stools" might be indicative of melena, which would suggest that the upper gastrointestinal tract (above the ligament of Treitz) is the source of bleeding; dark red or mahogany-colored stools could indicate blood emanating from the right colon.

Physical examination reveals a well-developed, overweight white man with a somewhat-rapid respiratory rate (i.e., 20 respirations/min). Other vital signs show a pulse of 94 bpm, a blood pressure of 110/60 mm Hg, and a normal temperature. The patient's skin is pale, as are his mucous membranes. His lungs are clear upon auscultation and his heart rhythm is regular, with a normal first and second heart sound (S_1 and S_2) and no third or fourth heart sound (S_3 or S_4). His abdomen is soft, without tenderness or obvious masses. His extremities show no cyanosis or edema; he has prolonged capillary refill. His rectal examination shows no palpable masses, but a dark, heme-positive stool is noted.

QUESTIONS

1. Based on this physical examination, what do you suspect is the cause of this man's fatigue?

2. What are some of the causes of melena?

3. What sorts of disorders produce hematochezia?

4. How would you proceed in working up the heme-positive stool?

DISCUSSION

Physical examination reveals an individual whose skin and mucous membranes are pale and who has heme-positive stool. These signs suggest that the patient has gastrointestinal bleeding and is most likely anemic, possibly the reason he is feeling fatigued.

Melena is the passage of dark, tarry stools due to the presence of blood altered by intestinal juices. Melena is most commonly caused by upper gastrointestinal bleeding, e.g., duodenal ulcer disease, gastric ulcer disease, hemorrhagic gastritis, erosive esophagitis, esophageal varices or Mallory-Weiss tears, or arteriovenous malformation of the stomach. In the setting of an individual who is not acutely ill, peptic ulcer disease would be the most common cause of melena; esophageal varices or a Mallory-Weiss tear of the distal esophagus would be unlikely.

Hematochezia is the passage of blood from the rectum, which varies in color from dark red or mahogany (from bleeding in the right colon) to bright red (as a result of bleeding from a more distal colonic source or the anal ring itself). Hematochezia may be caused by colonic diverticulosis and angiodysplasia, hemorrhoids, fissures, colon polyps, colon carcinoma, ulcerative colitis, infectious dysentery (especially *Shigella, Campylobacter,* and amebic colitis), and ischemic colitis. Hematochezia, unlike melena, is often a sign of neoplastic lesions of the gastrointestinal tract; therefore, the patient should be evaluated for these disorders. Occasionally, an upper gastrointestinal source (e.g., brisk bleeding from a peptic ulcer) could lead to the passage of bright red blood from the rectum. Generally, this occurrence is seen in a patient who is otherwise hemodynamically unstable and would be identified by the finding of blood upon the passage of a nasogastric tube into the stomach.

The initial workup for heme-positive stool depends on the patient's history and physical examination. If the history and examination are suggestive of an upper gastrointestinal source, initial workup with a double-contrast upper gastrointestinal examination or an upper endoscopy is indicated. However, in most cases of occult gastrointestinal bleeding, a lower gastrointestinal evaluation would be indicated. Colonoscopy or flexible sigmoidoscopy combined with an air contrast barium enema would be the appropriate initial tools for evaluation of a patient with occult gastrointestinal bleeding. If this workup is unrevealing, an upper gastrointestinal source should be pursued, including evaluation of the small bowel. If no upper gastrointestinal source is identified, small bowel enteroclysis or small bowel enteroscopy would be indicated.

A nasogastric tube is inserted but does not reveal any evidence of blood. The physician has an anoscope in his office, but anoscopy does not reveal any obvious lesions. In-office hemoglobin and hematocrit tests reveal values of 9.4 g/dl and 36%, respectively. The physician decides to refer the patient immediately to a gastroenterologist for further workup of his gastrointestinal bleeding.

QUESTIONS

1. Why does the physician first look for evidence of upper gastrointestinal bleeding?

2. What are the most common causes of lower gastrointestinal bleeding in this age-group?

DISCUSSION

The patient's history suggested a dark stool but, on the basis of the history, the physician could not determine whether the stool was black. Therefore, an upper gastrointestinal source was sought by the passage of a nasogastric tube. In approximately 75%–80% of cases, an upper gastrointestinal bleeding source can be identified by blood in the nasogastric tube. Occasionally, bleeding from a duodenal ulcer will be so slight it will cause a gastric aspirate to be negative for blood.

In this age-group, the two most common causes of lower gastrointestinal bleeding are diverticulosis and angiodysplasia. The differential diagnosis would also include those conditions known to cause hematochezia, as discussed earlier. Also to be considered would be a bleeding diathesis caused by a primary hematologic source such as leukemia, thrombocytopenia, hemophilia, or disseminated intravascular coagulation (DIC).

The gastroenterologist sees the patient immediately, and some laboratory tests are performed. A complete blood count (CBC) reveals a white cell count of 7.2/μl, a platelet count of 525,000/μl, and hemoglobin and hematocrit consistent with the previous values. Red cell indices show a mean corpuscular volume (MCV) of 70 μm^3 and a mean corpuscular hemoglobin (MCH) of 25 pg. Serum iron and transferrin are decreased. Prothrombin time (PT) and partial thromboplastin (PTT) are normal, as are electrolyte, blood urea nitrogen (BUN), and creatinine levels.

QUESTIONS

1. What type of anemia do these values suggest?

2. Which of the previously mentioned differential diagnoses can be ruled out by the laboratory values?

3. What conditions are the highest on your differential?

4. What are your immediate management plans?

DISCUSSION

The laboratory findings suggest a microcytic, hypochromic anemia. The MCV of 70 μm^3 and the MCH of 25 pg are compatible with this diagnosis. An elevated platelet count is often seen in patients with chronic blood loss. The differential diagnosis of this type of anemia includes iron deficiency, due to poor intake or lack of absorption, or chronic blood loss. The usual source of chronic occult blood loss is from the gastrointestinal tract. Iron chelation therapy for lead intoxication may also cause this type of anemia. Congenital anemia, such as thalassemia, is also associated with hypochromic, microcytic anemia. Iron deficiency states are characterized by a low serum iron, a high total iron binding capacity, and a low ferritin level.

The normal PT and PTT make a bleeding diathesis and a primary hematologic problem unlikely. Anemia of chronic renal insufficiency would be ruled out by the normal BUN and creatinine levels.

The most likely causes of this patient's problem are those involving chronic gastrointestinal blood loss (i.e., colonic polyp, colonic neoplasm, or angiodysplasia). Of particular concern is colonic neoplasm, in light of the patient's recent history of a change in bowel habits (constipation). Immediate management goals would include fluid replacement, correcting hypovolemia if present, monitoring serial hemoglobin and hematocrit values to be certain the patient does not have ongoing bleeding, arresting any active hemorrhage, and preventing recurrent hemorrhage.

The gastroenterologist arranges for a colonoscopy. During the colonoscopy, several polyps are noted in the descending portion of the colon. The polyps are 1–2 cm in size, and most are pedunculated. These lesions are removed by snare cautery and sent to pathology for evaluation.

QUESTIONS

1. What other procedures could have been employed to investigate this problem?

2. Why was colonoscopy useful in this case?

3. What would have prevented colonoscopy from being a useful diagnostic tool?

DISCUSSION

If bleeding were active and profuse, a technetium-labeled red blood cell scan, angiography, or both could locate a bleeding source, especially if the blood loss exceeded 2 ml/min. Otherwise, a high-quality air contrast barium enema and flexible sigmoidoscopy would have been an acceptable means of evaluating the colon. Colonoscopy is particularly useful, because it can be both diagnostic and therapeutic if a colonic polyp is discovered.

In this patient, colonoscopy was useful because there was no active bleeding to limit total examination of the colonic mucosa. However, if the bowel lumen had been coated with blood, a small polyp or arteriovenous malformation could have been missed. Also, if hemodynamic instability makes the patient a poor candidate for adequate sedation, a thorough evaluation of the colon may not be possible.

Pathology reveals villous adenomatous polyps with no foci of carcinoma. The patient is reassured, treated with iron supplements, and told to return in 1 year for a follow-up colonoscopy. If unremarkable, a repeat colonoscopy at 3 years would be indicated.

QUESTIONS

1. What factors about polyps increase the risk of adenocarcinoma?

2. What would the treatment have been if foci of malignant cells had been found?

DISCUSSION

Adenomatous and villous adenomatous polyps are considered precursors for adenocarcinoma. The risk of adenocarcinoma in patients with colonic polyps increases in proportion to the amount of villous tissue present in the polyp. Polyps that are sessile or greater than 2 cm in diameter also carry an increased risk for developing into carcinoma.

Management of a malignant focus in a colonic polyp depends on the type of polyp. If a polyp is pedunculated on a long stalk and the carcinomatous cells have not invaded the stalk, the patient could be cured by simple colonoscopic polypectomy. However, if the carcinomatous cells have invaded the stalk, or if the polyp is sessile and the carcinomatous cells reach the margins of resection, the patient would require a segmental colonic resection. In either case, follow-up colonoscopy is indicated on a periodic basis in patients who have large or multiple colonic polyps, or if a malignancy is identified in any such lesions.

Case 5: Acute Low Back Pain

A 35-year-old man presents to the emergency room with a 2-day history of severe low back pain. The pain is worse when he sits up and better when he lies flat on his back. He claims to be well, although he recently experienced polyarthralgias, chills, and sweating. He reports that he was hospitalized for some form of hepatitis 2 years ago; he says it resolved uneventfully and he does not know what caused it. He denies alcohol or drug abuse.

QUESTIONS

1. What are your immediate concerns about this patient's low back pain?

2. What additional information do you want to know about the pain?

3. What are some of the mechanisms of low back pain?

DISCUSSION

The history of chills and sweats makes one consider an infectious process more seriously than other possible causes of this patient's sudden low back pain. The pain is described as severe, making it more worrisome. The fact that the pain is worse when sitting upright and better with recumbency is not particularly helpful in suggesting a specific, potentially serious cause of this patient's back complaint; most discogenic and mechanical low back pain presents in this manner.

Ninety percent of low back pain is caused by self-limited biomechanical or strain problems, but it is important to look for features that make an acute medical condition more likely. There is important information still to be obtained about the nature of this patient's back pain.

Pain that is insidious in onset, associated with prolonged morning stiffness, relieved by exercise, and worsened by rest suggests underlying inflammatory back pain, typically the sacroiliitis of the spondylarthropathies. In contrast, mechanical low back pain often is sudden in onset, worsened by exercise, and improved by rest. Pain that is ripping or tearing and perhaps associated with abdominal complaints is typical of an expanding abdominal aortic aneurysm. Pain associated with bladder or bowel incontinence and saddle anesthesia suggests a mid-line lumbar disk herniation with cauda equina compression; pain associated with leg sensory or motor complaints suggests lateral disk herniation and spinal nerve compression. Back pain associated with gastrointestinal or genitourinary complaints suggests a need to investigate an intra-abdominal source as the cause. Constitutional complaints such as fever and chills make an infection more likely. Pain increasing with recumbency (the opposite of this patient's complaint) suggests a possible tumor; mid-line pain suggests either a tumor, an infection, or a compression fracture.

On initial examination, the patient is writhing in discomfort and asking for intramuscular narcotics. His temperature is 100.8°F, and prominent "needle tracks" are observed on his hands and legs. Diffuse tenderness and guarding are noted on the abdominal exam, marked tenderness is noted over the entire low back paraspinal region, and prominent percussion tenderness is noted over the costovertebral angle and over several lumbar and sacral vertebrae. The patient cooperates poorly with strength testing, but deep tendon reflexes and sensation are intact and anal wink and perianal sensations are normal. The patient complains of hamstring tenderness when either leg is raised in a straightened, extended position.

QUESTIONS

1. How do the findings on physical examination help you in thinking about your differential diagnosis?

2. What conditions might cause referred back pain? Which should be ruled out?

3. What information should you seek from laboratory tests and procedures at this time?

DISCUSSION

Several findings on physical examination make self-limited musculoskeletal pain retreat far down the differential diagnosis list. For one thing, we know that the patient is likely abusing intravenous drugs, even though he denied this in the history. Narcotic drug-seeking behavior makes the physical examination more difficult to interpret, because exaggerated responses to physical examination maneuvers are common in drug-abusing patients. We also know that the patient has a fever and prominent findings on abdominal and back palpation as well as on spinal and costovertebral angle percussion. Intravenous drug abuse and fever make an infectious process (e.g., epidural abscess, paraspinal or perirectal collection, septic sacroiliitis) much more likely. No specific evidence for an aortic aneurysm exists on abdominal exam, and there is no neurologic evidence for cauda equina compression or discogenic nerve compression. No evidence has been presented for a potential referred source of pain, such as a penetrating duodenal ulcer (gastrointestinal source) or a renal infection or stone (genitourinary source), and there is no evidence of a spondylarthropathy.

A complete blood count (CBC) might help with evaluation of an infectious process, particularly if leukocytosis is present. Amylase would be increased with pancreatitis and bowel emergencies (e.g., small bowel obstruction). The erythrocyte sedimentation rate is nonspecific but if significantly elevated might also suggest an infection, particularly osteomyelitis. Urinalysis is important for discovering a potential genitourinary infection. Three sets of paired blood cultures should be obtained, because bacterial endocarditis can present with musculoskeletal complaints, and any bacterial process in the low back might be associated with bacteremia. Plain x-rays of the low back and sacroiliac joints quite likely might be normal, although patients with diskitis can have intervertebral narrowing and vertebral end-plate destruction; those with sacroiliitis can have sacroiliac joint erosions and sclerosis. A lumbar computed tomography (CT) scan would be of great help in evaluating bony detail for bone tumor or infection, and magnetic resonance imaging (MRI) would be best for evaluating soft tissue or intraspinal collections.

The test results come back as follows: hemoglobin is 11.3 g/dl, the white blood cell count is 15,000/μl, and the platelet count is 500,000/μl. The Westergren erythrocyte sedimentation rate is 100 mm/hr. Chemistries reveal only an elevated alkaline phosphatase; amylase is normal. Urinalysis is negative. Chest x-ray, lumbar spine x-ray, and pelvic x-rays are unrevealing. MRI of the lumbar spine is scheduled for the following day.

One day later, the patient has required high doses of intramuscular narcotic for pain control but still complains of severe low back pain. He says that he is having difficulty walking to the bathroom due to leg weakness. His maximum temperature is 102°F. Physical examination reveals continuing poor cooperation with strength testing, but the patient appears to be severely weak (3/5 on muscle strength testing) in all lower extremity muscle groups. He also has decreased sensation to pinprick from the toes to the navel and prominent increased deep tendon reflexes in the lower extremities with four beats of clonus bilaterally.

QUESTIONS

1. What are the remaining most likely diagnoses at this point?

2. What additional diagnostic tests are appropriate to confirm a diagnosis?

3. What therapeutic approach is most appropriate now?

DISCUSSION

The neurologic findings (leg weakness, abdominal sensory level, increased reflexes, and clonus) suggest spinal cord compression with features of an upper motor neuron lesion. Adding the history of intravenous drug abuse, fever, low back pain, and progressive neurologic deficit, the differential diagnosis narrows markedly. The patient's sensory level to about T12 suggests that the cord compression is occurring at this level, probably from an epidural abscess. Still possible are transverse myelitis or an ischemic myelopathy at T12 cord level or a mid-line herniated thoracic disk, but these diagnoses are less likely to explain the fever or to be associated with intravenous drug abuse.

The best procedure for confirming a diagnosis would be an MRI scan. This test will best discriminate between an intrinsic cord lesion (e.g., transverse myelitis) and an extrinsic compression (e.g., due to an abscess or herniated disk). The test should be done emergently, because early surgical intervention is critical to preservation of lower extremity function.

The emergency MRI scan reveals an epidural abscess at T12 and surgical débridement is carried out immediately. *Staphylococcus aureus* **grows from one set of the blood cultures and the abscess.**

QUESTION

1. What remaining treatment modalities should be used now?

DISCUSSION

The patient should be treated for 4–6 weeks with antibiotics effective against *S. aureus,* initially intravenously. He should be carefully watched for features of bacterial endocarditis, despite the fact that only one blood culture was positive. Furthermore, the patient should receive intensive physical therapy once the acute pain subsides so that he can recover lower extremity strength and the ability to walk.

Case 6: Breast Lump

A 41-year-old white woman goes to her physician after discovering a lump in her left breast while doing a breast self-examination in the shower. She had thought in the past that she might have felt something in the same location, but now feels that the lump has gotten larger.

QUESTION

1. What additional historical information would you like to have from this patient?

DISCUSSION

Eighty percent of patients with breast lumps will find the lump while performing a breast self-examination. As part of this patient's history, the physician should ask the patient about her risk factors for breast cancer. One should also ask how long the patient has been aware of the lump, what its original size was, when it increased in size, and by how much. It might also be helpful to know whether the mass changed in size in conjunction with the patient's menstrual period, because benign disease can regress following the menstrual cycle. If the mass is not clinically suspicious, it might be appropriate to reevaluate the patient following her next menstrual cycle when the flow ends—if the mass persists, intervention is necessary. Did the patient experience any discharge from the nipples? If so, was it bloody or clear? The presence of breast edema, discoloration, or pain is important to ascertain. Finally, the patient should be asked whether she has had any mammograms in the past.

Further history from the patient reveals that she first discovered the lump in the upper, outer quadrant of her left breast about 4 months ago, but she did not seek medical attention because she has always had large, "lumpy" breasts. The patient's menstrual period does not seem to have any effect on the presence of the lump. She has not experienced nipple discharge, breast edema or discoloration, or pain.

The patient has no previous medical or surgical history and takes no medications. She has one cousin who died from breast cancer, but none of her other female relatives have had any cancer. Both of her parents are alive; her father has hypertension and coronary artery disease. The patient first began to menstruate at age 12 and has had regular periods lasting 4 days on a 30-day cycle. She has not experienced any symptoms of menopause. She has one daughter who is 7 years old. She uses a diaphragm for birth control. The patient had a baseline mammogram at age 35, but has not had one since and she has not seen a gynecologist for over 1 year.

QUESTIONS

1. What risk factors does this patient have for developing breast cancer?

2. What diseases might be included in your differential diagnosis at this point?

DISCUSSION

Although most breast cancers are found in the upper, outer quadrant, location should not change the physician's approach to excluding malignancy. Similarly, a patient's lack of risk factors for breast cancer should not dissuade the physician from performing the necessary procedures to rule out malignancy. The most important risk factors for breast cancer are family history (especially if the patient has a first-degree relative who developed premenopausal breast cancer), a history of fibrocystic disease, a history of previous breast biopsies, early onset of menarche, late onset of menopause, a first pregnancy after the age of 30 and, possibly, the use of high-dose estrogens by a postmenopausal patient.

A young, premenopausal woman with a breast lump could have a benign mass, such as a fibroadenoma or a cyst. Breast lumps are benign in 80% of cases, but malignancy must be ruled out. If the lump is indeed malignant, the patient has a higher chance of lymph node metastasis and micrometastatic disease as the tumor increases in size.

Physical examination reveals a well-developed, thin, white woman who is slightly anxious, but in no acute distress. The examination is normal, except for the presence of a 2-cm mass in the upper, outer quadrant of the left breast. The mass appears firm and somewhat mobile. There is no obvious asymmetry between breasts, skin dimpling, or redness. No axillary nodes can be palpated, and there are no masses in the right breast.

QUESTION

1. What would you do next to evaluate this patient?

DISCUSSION

All patients with a definable mass should have a mammogram; because this patient has not had a mammogram in 6 years, having one now would probably be especially worthwhile. Twenty percent of the time, a breast lump will be seen on mammogram alone. However, mammograms are often difficult to interpret in premenopausal patients or postmenopausal patients taking estrogen, because estrogen causes dense, white, glandular tissue that may obscure white tumor masses of similar density. When a woman goes through menopause, the mammogram shows a gray background, because the breast consists of mostly fibrofatty tissue. Thus, gray serves as an ideal background for identification of new breast abnormalities, which appear whiter in contrast to the normal breast tissue. A negative mammogram does not necessarily imply that a patient's mass is not cancerous.

In addition to having a mammogram, this patient should be referred to a surgeon for needle aspiration to evaluate for the presence of fluid. If the mass disappears with aspiration of the fluid, then this is a benign cyst (assuming the cytology is negative). Less than 1% of patients in whom the mass totally disappears will have malignant cells seen on cyst aspiration. If the mass is solid, the contents of the needle should be placed on a slide and submitted for cytology. Even if the cytology is benign, a malignant lesion still cannot be ruled out. If the mass persists after the patient's next menstrual period, an excisional biopsy should be performed to rule out cancer.

If an aspiration is not done, ultrasound can determine if the mass is solid or cystic. If the lesion is cystic, the cyst seen on ultrasound examination should be the same size as the palpable mass. If there are no internal echoes within the cyst, then a solid lesion cannot be ruled out and carcinoma is still a possibility.

Attempted fine needle aspiration does not produce any fluid. A mammogram is done and the report shows a well-defined 2.2-cm density in the left upper, outer quadrant. There are no other densities or calcifications noted.

The suspicious mammogram, coupled with the enlarging, palpable mass and the failure to aspirate fluid, lead the physician to recommend that the patient undergo a biopsy of the lesion. The patient is referred to a surgeon and a biopsy with needle localization is performed. The pathology report reveals an infiltrating adenocarcinoma.

QUESTIONS

1. *How would you stage this patient's cancer?*

2. *What would be your preferred mode of treatment?*

3. *What is the patient's prognosis?*

DISCUSSION

This patient would be classified as having stage II disease, because the tumor measures between 2 and 5 cm in diameter and there are no fixed nodes or distant metastases. Most patients with stage I or II breast cancer can be offered the option of lumpectomy, axillary dissection, and radiation therapy to the breast (and node-bearing areas, if the nodes are positive). This procedure's cure rates are equivalent to those for a modified radical mastectomy, if the patient meets certain criteria. Because this particular patient does not have multicentric disease in the breast, more than one breast primary, subareolar primaries, or a tumor greater than 5 cm in diameter, she is an optimal candidate for radiation therapy. The presence of collagen vascular disease must also be taken into consideration, because these patients tolerate radiation poorly.

Before the decision is made to perform a lumpectomy and axillary dissection, the patient should be seen by a radiation therapist. If the radiation therapist feels that the patient is not an optimal candidate, then a modified radical mastectomy is warranted. If the patient chooses to have a modified radical mastectomy, she has the option of undergoing breast reconstruction surgery at the time of the mastectomy or at some future time.

Adjuvant hormonal therapy, chemotherapy, and radiation therapy (i.e., radiation therapy for purposes other than breast conservation) also may play a role in treating patients with breast cancer.

Prognosis varies widely in breast cancer patients. Approximately 50% of patients with operable breast cancer will develop recurrent disease unless they receive adjuvant chemotherapy or hormone therapy. Prognostic factors include the patient's axillary node status, the histopathology of the tumor, the patient's hormone receptor status, the S-phase fraction and DNA index, and oncogene expression.

Case 7: HIV Infection

A 37-year-old man, who was diagnosed with HIV-1 infection 4 years ago, has experienced good overall health for 3 years despite a falling CD4 count. Fourteen months ago he developed headaches and mild confusion at a time when his CD4 count was 94 cells/mm^3. Imaging studies and spinal fluid analysis confirmed the diagnosis of cryptococcal meningitis, and the patient responded well to antifungal therapy.

QUESTIONS

1. *What is the value of the CD4 count in monitoring patients who are infected with HIV-1?*

2. *What are the major neurologic problems encountered in people with HIV-1 infection?*

DISCUSSION

It is very common for patients infected by HIV-1 to experience a long period of clinical latency. There is active viral replication during all phases of the disease, but symptoms usually do not become apparent until there has been a substantial reduction in host immune function. The stage of HIV disease can be inferred from evaluation of clinical parameters (such as weight loss, decreasing functional capacity, and development of one or more specific problems) and laboratory tests (such as the enumeration of CD4 cells or quantitation of viral RNA). The CD4 count can be performed in many hospital and reference laboratories. When levels of circulating CD4 cells drop below certain thresholds, various interventions such as infection prophylaxis or antiretroviral therapy should be offered to the patient. [For example, when the CD4 count drops below 200 cells/mm^3, prophylaxis for *Pneumocystis carinii* pneumonia (PCP) should be initiated.]

Several neurologic infections can complicate HIV-1 infection. The two most common are cryptococcal meningitis and toxoplasmic encephalitis. Both of these infections occur relatively late in the course of HIV-1 infection at a time when there are clinical or laboratory clues of strikingly diminished cellular immunity. Cryptococcal infection commonly presents as a chronic meningitis characterized by headache and diffuse, often mild, neurologic symptoms. Toxoplasmosis more often presents with focal neurologic findings or seizures. Dementia secondary to HIV-1 infection is also common late in the course of the disease. Less common neurologic complications include progressive multifocal leukoencephalopathy, central nervous system (CNS) lymphoma, neurosyphilis, *Listeria* meningitis, herpes simplex encephalitis, and cytomegalovirus (CMV) encephalitis.

The patient was able to go back to work as a financial planner, and he seemed to be tolerating his medicines. His regimen consisted of trimethoprim– sulfamethoxazole 3 days a week, isoniazid daily, zidovudine, lamivudine, and fluconazole. During this office visit, the patient says he is less peppy than usual following a bout of a gastrointestinal illness consisting of watery diarrhea and crampy abdominal pain. He thinks he may have had some fevers over the past 2 weeks, but he has not taken his temperature.

QUESTIONS

1. *What is the purpose of each of the medications the patient is currently taking?*

2. *What is the differential diagnosis of watery diarrhea in a person with advanced HIV infection?*

3. *What diagnostic tests can be done to determine the cause of watery diarrhea?*

4. *Of what significance is fever in a person with advanced HIV infection?*

DISCUSSION

This patient is receiving a number of medications that are common to patients with HIV infection. Trimethoprim–sulfamethoxazole is used to prevent *P. carinii* infection, but it is also partly effective in preventing symptomatic toxoplasmosis and in reducing the number of bacterial infections. Zidovudine and lamivudine are two of the growing list of antiretroviral drugs available for direct suppression of HIV. The fluconazole is to prevent a recurrence of the patient's previously documented cryptococcal meningitis. Because the rate of symptomatic recurrence of cryptococcal meningitis is high, fluconazole should be given for the duration of the patient's life. The isoniazid is used to prevent tuberculosis in a patient who has already been infected [i.e., one who tested positive using the purified protein derivative (PPD) test]. There is no accepted indication for monotherapy in patients with active tuberculosis.

Watery diarrhea is a common complication of HIV infection. Many cases are self-limited and no specific etiology is determined. However a wide variety of pathogens have been associated with this syndrome. The most common and perhaps the hardest to treat is *Cryptosporidium parvum*. Other protozoans that can cause diarrhea of this nature are

Giardia lamblia, microsporidia, and *Isospora belli.* Common bacterial agents of watery diarrhea include *Escherichia coli, Salmonella,* and *Campylobacter.* Diarrhea secondary to the toxin produced by *Clostridium difficile* should always be considered when a patient is undergoing or has recently completed a course of antibacterial therapy.

Diagnostic tests for watery diarrhea should be ordered when the diarrhea is persistent or extremely symptomatic. Usually, stool specimens are sent for microscopic assessment of protozoa (some laboratories call this test the ova and parasites test). The laboratory should be notified that cryptosporidia and other unusual protozoa are being sought. Stool cultures should also be sent. If the patient is currently undergoing or has just completed a course of antibacterial therapy, toxin tests for *C. difficile* should be ordered as well. If these noninvasive tests do not yield a result, further evaluation could entail endoscopic studies of the lower gastrointestinal tract or aspiration of the upper intestinal contents. A definitive diagnosis can be elusive if the first few stool tests are negative.

Fever is a very nonspecific problem in patients with advanced HIV infection. The development of new fever should prompt a careful history and physical evaluation. In addition to the large spectrum of infections that can produce a fever, there are a number of noninfectious processes, such as malignancies and drug reactions, that should be considered. If the patient history, physical examination, chest radiographs, and routine laboratory tests do not suggest an organ-specific abnormality, disseminated infections such as *Mycobacterium avium-intracellulare,* histoplasmosis, CMV, and HIV itself should be considered as causes of the fever.

On examination, the patient looks alert but pale. His temperature is 38°C, but otherwise, his vital signs are normal. The patient has lost 6 pounds since his last visit, 6 weeks earlier. Otherwise, there are no focal abnormalities. Laboratory testing shows a hemoglobin of 9.0 g/dl and a white blood cell count of 3400 cells/mm^3 with a normal differential. The mean corpuscular volume (MCV) is 99 μm^3 and the serum vitamin B$_{12}$ level is at the lower limit of normal. The patient's CD4 count is 32 cells/mm^3. Chemistries show mild elevation of aspartate aminotransferase (AST) and alanine aminotransferase (ALT).

QUESTIONS

  1. What is the differential diagnosis of the macrocytic anemia?

  2. What is the significance of the weight loss?

DISCUSSION

Macrocytic anemia is fairly common in patients with advanced HIV infection. Although nutritional deficiencies should be considered as potential causes of macrocytic anemia, the disorder is far more commonly associated with drug therapy—zidovudine or the antimetabolites of trimethoprim–sulfamethoxazole can cause macrocytic anemia. In many cases, the anemia is mild and only bears watching, but sometimes patients are given leucovorin (folinic acid) to combat the folate depletion brought on by zidovudine or trimethoprim–sulfamethoxazole. The serum levels of vitamin B$_{12}$ can be depressed in AIDS patients, but there is rarely a response to injections of vitamin B$_{12}$.

Weight loss is a sign of active disease associated with HIV infection. In many patients, there is no obvious malabsorption, infection, or malignancy to account for weight loss, so efforts are directed at increasing the lean body weight. Nutritional supplements and hormonal manipulations are the most common interventions. Many infections are associated with weight loss, but in the absence of malabsorption or organ dysfunction, disseminated infections should be considered first.

Blood cultures for mycobacteria are reported as positive 2 weeks later. The patient's fever has persisted and he has lost 3 more pounds. He still has no localizing complaints. Repeat complete blood count and chemistry tests show no change.

QUESTION

1. What is the most likely explanation for the positive blood cultures?

DISCUSSION

Most likely, the positive blood cultures represent infection with *M. avium-intracellulare,* rather than *Mycobacterium tuberculosis.* Disseminated tuberculosis without any organ involvement is rare. It is even rarer to find positive blood cultures for *M. tuberculosis* at all (except in patients with overwhelming, possibly terminal, tuberculosis). And it would be even more unusual (although not impossible) for cultures to be positive when the patient is on prophylactic isoniazid therapy. *M. avium-intracellulare* is a commonly seen late complication of HIV infection and would most likely account for the weight loss seen in this patient. Patients infected by *M. avium-intracellulare* have infiltration of many organs (with very little tissue reaction) and often have high titers of mycobacteria in the blood and bone marrow. Many of these patients experience a partial or complete reversal of weight loss when the infection is brought under control.

The patient is started on therapy with three oral agents, ofloxacin, clarithromycin, and rifabutin. There is gradual reduction in fevers, and he is able to return to work full time. His weight stabilizes and he is comfortable except for intermittent nausea from the large number of pills that he takes daily.

QUESTION

1. What is the patient's prognosis?

DISCUSSION

M. avium-intracellulare infection may be controlled but is essentially never cured in people with AIDS. Although *M. avium-intracellulare* infection is rarely considered to be the cause of death in people with AIDS, mycobacteremia is a predictor of earlier mortality and increased morbidity. Treatment of mycobacteremia seems to benefit those people who can tolerate the therapy and who are not moribund at its inception.

Case 8: Newly Discovered Renal Failure

A 62-year-old man visits his physician for a routine physical examination. He mentions that he has to get out of bed more frequently than he used to (two to three times each night) to urinate, that he has difficulty initiating and maintaining a urinary stream, and he has experienced mild shortness of breath upon walking two to three flights of stairs. He also says that his regular biweekly workouts at the gym have been much more difficult for him lately. Physical examination reveals moderate pallor, a blood pressure of 150/105 mm Hg, a pulse of 80 bpm, and a respiratory rate of 18 respirations per minute. There is trace pedal edema. Examination of the chest and heart reveals no abnormalities. Examination of the abdomen reveals slight fullness in the lower abdomen but neither tenderness nor pain are elicited. Laboratory work is obtained, including a complete blood count, electrolyte, glucose, calcium, and renal studies. The results of these studies are as follows: blood urea nitrogen (BUN), 88 mg/dl; creatinine, 6.4 mg/dl; sodium, 137 mEq/L; potassium, 5.9 mEq/L; chloride, 112 mEq/L; bicarbonate, 16 mEq/L; hemoglobin, 8.7 g/dl.

QUESTIONS

1. *What is the first determination you should make with respect to this patient?*

2. *What additional information might help you make this determination?*

3. *What is the most likely cause of this patient's renal insufficiency? Does the patient's altered electrolyte and acid-base metabolism support this diagnosis?*

DISCUSSION

The determination of onset of renal failure is crucial in order to determine the proper therapeutic approach. Acute renal failure implies the potential for reversibility and therefore every effort must be made to identify any ongoing injurious agents that adversely affect the kidney. In addition, acute support via some form of dialytic therapy may be required to sustain the patient until renal recovery can occur. On the other hand, the presence of chronic renal failure suggests that the patient has sustained irreversible injury. The patient must then be treated in a way to prevent further loss of kidney function; chronic renal replacement therapy, either through dialytic support or through transplantation, may be necessary.

The determination of chronicity of renal failure can be difficult. In patients with acute renal failure, a clear precipitating event (e.g., exposure to nephrotoxic agents such as gentamicin, sepsis, shock) can usually be identified. The determination of the onset of chronic disease is more problematic. The time of initiation of subtle symptoms consistent with renal failure (e.g., pruritus) may be helpful in determining the onset of the disease. Renal ultrasound provides information about kidney size, which typically is reduced in chronic renal failure and normal in acute renal failure. Exceptions include diabetic nephropathy and amyloidosis, which may be associated with normal or enlarged kidneys, and polycystic kidney disease, which may be associated with extremely large kidneys despite coexistent renal failure. Chronic renal failure is typically associated with secondary hyperparathyroidism; subperiosteal resorption is typically seen radiographically. In addition, generalized bone demineralization, loss of bone mass at the acromial-clavicular joint, or mottling of the skull may be important findings. Anemia is typically seen in chronic renal failure because erythropoietin levels are reduced as kidney mass is reduced. However, anemia may develop rather rapidly and occasionally. Severe anemia is seen in patients with acute renal failure as well as those with chronic renal failure and likely explains the dyspnea in this patient.

This patient most likely has acute renal insufficiency as a result of chronic obstructive uropathy. This conclusion stems from the history of difficulty voiding, the presence of bladder fullness on physical examination, and the findings of renal failure, hyperkalemia, and metabolic acidosis. Other common causes of acute renal failure in the ambulatory setting include toxic nephropathy from medication use and acute glomerulonephritis. In men, the most common cause of chronic obstructive nephropathy is prostatic hypertrophy, but bladder cancer or prostatic cancer are possible as well. The patient demonstrates hyperchloremic hypobicarbonatemia with associated hyperkalemia. This constellation of findings is common in patients with chronic renal insufficiency, particularly in association with obstructive uropathy. The hypobicarbonatemia suggests metabolic acidosis but could also be caused by chronic respiratory alkalosis. The presence of renal insufficiency makes metabolic acidosis the most likely cause of the hypobicarbonatemia in this patient. The high chloride level reflects the fact that electrical neutrality must be maintained by body fluids and as bicarbonate levels fall, preferential chloride reabsorption with sodium occurs in the renal tubules. Because the kidney is unable to generate new bicarbonate in order to restore the levels reduced by ingestion of dietary precursors of various mineral acids, bicarbonate levels fall. A reduced bicarbonate level is typical of all forms of renal failure. The increase in serum potassium is an important indication of obstructive uropathy. Potassium is secreted in the distal nephron but requires adequate amounts of aldosterone as well as a normally responsive distal tubule potassium transport system for normal excretion. Chronic obstructive uropathy is associated with impairment of potassium excretion, occasionally secondary to reduced aldosterone levels but more typically due to a direct tubular abnormality. Correction of the underlying obstructive process leads to a normalization of potassium excretion and a return of serum potassium levels to the normal range.

Renal ultrasound is performed and confirms the diagnosis of obstructive uropathy. A Foley catheter is put in place.

QUESTION

1. What clinical problem should be anticipated following relief of obstruction?

DISCUSSION

It is typical for patients with obstructive uropathy to undergo, upon relief of obstruction, a striking diuresis. The source of the diuresis is a combination of excretion of previously retained solutes and fluids as well as a mild residual tubular defect in sodium and water conservation. This massive diuresis typically remits once the patient's BUN and creatinine have leveled off. Dialysis, either by hemodialysis or peritoneal dialysis, may be necessary in patients with renal insufficiency secondary to obstructive uropathy, but attempts should always be made to correct the obstructive uropathy prior to initiating hemodialysis. The decision to perform dialysis must be made on an individual basis and defies simple categorization. Hemodialysis is indicated in patients with pericarditis. Congestive heart failure may also be an indication for dialytic therapy in order to achieve fluid removal. Institution of dialysis should not be made on the basis of the absolute BUN level alone, although most clinicians feel that the BUN should be maintained below 150 mg/dl.

Index

Note: Page numbers in *italics* denote figures; those followed by (t) denote tables; those followed by Q denote questions; and those followed by E denote explanations.